Handbook of
Child
Psychopathology
THIRD EDITION

Handbook of
Child
Psychopathology

THIRD EDITION

Edited by

Thomas H. Ollendick

Virginia Polytechnic Institute
and State University
Blacksburg, Virginia

and

Michel Hersen

School of Professional Psychology
Pacific University
Forest Grove, Oregon

Plenum Press • New York and London

Library of Congress Cataloging-in-Publication Data

Handbook of child psychopathology / edited by Thomas H. Ollendick and
Michel Hersen. -- 3rd ed.
    p.   cm.
  Includes bibliographical references and index.
  ISBN 0-306-45321-5
  1. Child psychopathology--Handbooks, manuals, etc. I. Ollendick,
Thomas H. II. Hersen, Michel.
  RJ499.3.H36 1998
  618.92'89--dc21   97-40923
                                              CIP

ISBN 0-306-45321-5

© 1998, 1989, 1983 Plenum Press, New York
A Division of Plenum Publishing Corporation
233 Spring Street, New York, N.Y. 10013

http://www.plenum.com

10 9 8 7 6 5 4 3 2 1

Printed in the United States of America

Contributors

THOMAS M. ACHENBACH, Department of Psychiatry, University of Vermont, Burlington, Vermont 05401-3456

LISA ARMISTEAD, Department of Psychology, Georgia State University, Atlanta, Georgia 30302-5010

SANDRA T. AZAR, Frances L. Hiatt School of Psychology, Clark University, Worcester, Massachusetts 01610

BRET G. BENTZ, Department of Psychology, Louisiana State University, Baton Rouge, Louisiana 70803

JOSEPH BIEDERMAN, Joint Program in Pediatric Psychopharmacology, Massachusetts General Hospital and McLean Hospital, Boston, Massachusetts 02114; and Harvard Medical School, Cambridge, Massachusetts 02138

SUSAN J. BRETON, Frances L. Hiatt School of Psychology, Clark University, Worcester, Massachusetts 01610

SUSAN B. CAMPBELL, Department of Psychology, University of Pittsburgh, Pittsburgh, Pennsylvania 15260

MARJORIE H. CHARLOP-CHRISTY, Department of Psychology, Claremont McKenna College, Claremont, California 91711

THOMAS L. CREER, Department of Psychology, Ohio University, Athens, Ohio 45701

JAN L. CULBERTSON, Child Study Center, Department of Pediatrics, University of Oklahoma Health Sciences Center, Oklahoma City, Oklahoma 73117

LYNNDA M. DAHLQUIST, Department of Psychology, University of Maryland Baltimore County, Baltimore, Maryland 21228

CYNTHIA R. ELLIS, Medical College of Virginia, Virginia Commonwealth University, Richmond, Virginia 23298-0489

MARILYN T. ERICKSON, Psychology Department, Virginia Commonwealth University, Richmond, Virginia 23284-2018

MONICA H. FERRARO, Frances L. Hiatt School of Psychology, Clark University, Worcester, Massachusetts 01610

REX FOREHAND, Psychology Department, University of Georgia, Athens, Georgia 30602

95187

JEAN FRAZIER, Pediatric Psychopharmacology Unit, Department of Psychiatry, Massachusetts General Hospital, Boston, Massachusetts 02114; and Harvard Medical School, Cambridge, Massachusetts 02138

PAUL J. FRICK, Department of Psychology, University of Alabama, Tuscaloosa, Alabama 35487

ALICE G. FRIEDMAN, Department of Psychology, Binghamton University, Binghamton, New York 13905

GOLDA S. GINSBURG, Division of Applied Psychology and Quantitative Methods, University of Baltimore, Baltimore, Maryland 21201

TRACY R. G. GLADSTONE, Judge Baker Children's Center, Boston, Massachusetts 02115

ALAN M. GROSS, Department of Psychology, University of Mississippi, University, Mississippi 38677

BARBARA HENKER, Department of Psychology, University of California, Los Angeles, Los Angeles, California 90095

MARTIN HERBERT, Department of Psychology, University of Exeter, Exeter EX4 4QG, England

SUZANNE BENNETT JOHNSON, Center for Pediatric Psychology and Family Studies, University of Florida Health Science Center, Gainesville, Florida 32610-0165

NADINE J. KASLOW, Department of Psychiatry and Behavioral Sciences, Emory University School of Medicine, Atlanta, Georgia 30335

BETH KOTCHICK, Psychology Department, University of Georgia, Athens, Georgia 30602

ELISE E. LABBÉ, Department of Psychology, University of South Alabama, Mobile, Alabama 36688

SUSAN A. LATHAM, Department of Psychology, Binghamton University, Binghamton, New York 13905

BRIAN P. MARX, Department of Psychology, Oklahoma State University, Stillwater, Oklahoma 74047

NORMAN A. MILGRAM, Department of Psychology, Tel Aviv University, Ramat Aviv 69978, Israel

DIANE MORIN, Centre de Consultation Psychologique et Éducationnelle, Montréal, Quebec H3C 3P8, Canada

STEVEN J. ONDERSMA, College of Medicine, University of Oklahoma Health Sciences Center, Oklahoma City, Oklahoma 73190

DONALD P. OSWALD, Medical College of Virginia, Virginia Commonwealth University, Richmond, Virginia 23298-0489

JODIE Y. RABALAIS, Department of Psychology, Louisiana State University, Baton Rouge, Louisiana 70803

JOHANNES ROJAHN, Nisonger Center for Developmental Disabilities and Department of Psychology, Ohio State University, Columbus, Ohio 43210

SANDRA W. RUSS, Psychology Department, Case Western Reserve University, Cleveland, Ohio 44106-7123

FLOYD R. SALLEE, Department of Psychiatry and Behavioral Science, Medical University of South Carolina, Charleston, South Carolina 29425-0742

LAURA SCHREIBMAN, Department of Psychology, University of California, San Diego, La Jolla, California 92093-0109

JENNIFER A. J. SCHWARTZ, Department of Psychiatry and Behavioral Sciences, Emory University School of Medicine, Atlanta, Georgia 30335

WENDY K. SILVERMAN, Child and Family Psychosocial Research Center, Department of Psychology, Florida International University, Miami, Florida 33199

NIRBHAY N. SINGH, Medical College of Virginia, Virginia Commonwealth University, Richmond, Virginia 23298-0489

THOMAS J. SPENCER, Pediatric Psychopharmacology Unit, Department of Psychiatry, Massachusetts General Hospital, Boston, Massachusetts 02114; and Harvard Medical School, Cambridge, Massachusetts 02138

EVE G. SPRATT, Department of Psychiatry and Behavioral Science, Medical University of South Carolina, Charleston, South Carolina 29425-0742

RIC STEELE, Psychology Department, University of Georgia, Athens, Georgia 30602

MARC J. TASSÉ, Départment de psychologie, Université du Quebéc à Montréal, Montréal, Quebéc H3C 3P8, Canada

C. EUGENE WALKER, College of Medicine, University of Oklahoma Health Sciences Center, Oklahoma City, Oklahoma 73190

CAROL K. WHALEN, Department of Psychology and Social Behavior, University of California, Irvine, Irvine, California 92697

TIMOTHY E. WILENS, Pediatric Psychopharmacology Unit, Department of Psychiatry, Massachusetts General Hospital, Boston, Massachusetts 02114; and Harvard Medical School, Cambridge, Massachusetts 02138

DONALD A. WILLIAMSON, Department of Psychology, Louisiana State University, Baton Rouge, Louisiana 70803

RICHARD A. WINETT, Center for Research in Health Behavior, Virginia Polytechnic Institute and State University, Blacksburg, Virginia 24061

Preface

In our first edition of the *Handbook* in 1983, we noted that child psychopathology should no longer be viewed as a downward extension of adult psychopathology. Rather, we suggested that children should be viewed as children, not as miniature adults, and that a merger of the disciplines of clinical child psychology and developmental psychology must occur for this evolution to be fully realized. In the second edition of the *Handbook* in 1989, we asserted that the synthesis of these two fields of inquiry was underway, at least on a conceptual level. At that time, however, we also acknowledged that much remained to be accomplished, not only in the conceptual arena but also on the front line of clinical practice with children, adolescents, and their families. That is, although important conceptual advances were being made, there was little evidence of this movement in the day-to-day practice of clinical child psychology. Children were still being viewed as miniature adults in clinical practice, as evidenced by downward extensions of adult assessment and treatment protocols from adults for, or to, children. Perhaps not unlike the proverbial parenting dictum, children were being "seen" but not "heard."

Fortunately, much has occurred in the 15 years since that first edition of this work. Of critical importance, the field of developmental psychopathology has emerged and, although its influence has not yet been fully assimilated into our clinical armamentarium, its presence is being felt. Concern with development and developmental variations throughout and across the life span characterizes this approach. Basically, developmental psychopathology studies the origins and course(s) of maladaptive behavior, whatever the causes, whatever the age of onset, whatever the transformations in behavioral expression, and however complex the developmental pattern may prove to be. It strives to integrate these two disciplines in an intimate and oftentimes complex manner.

Careful attention to issues of development and other contextual issues relevant to children, adolescents, and their families guided us in our efforts to solicit contributors for this third edition. All the contributors are active researchers and clinicians in the field of child psychopathology, and all are keenly aware of the interface between clinical child psychology and developmental psychology. In addition, all the contributors are conceptually and empirically minded; as a result, the chapters are databased and theory-driven and include the most up-to-date knowledge available. However, as research-based knowledge is more evident in some areas of child psychopathology than others, the chapters necessarily vary in length and scope.

Like the second edition, this edition is organized into four parts: "Basic Issues," "Specific Childhood Psychopathologies," "Psychological Aspects of Physical Conditions," and "Prevention and Treatment." In the first part, developmental, etiological, diagnostic, and taxonomic issues are considered in detail. Furthermore, clinical formulation of psychopathology is addressed. The purpose of this part is to provide the background and a framework for the specific psychopathologies that follow. In the second part, a wide variety of psychopathologies are examined. Each chapter is organized around a set of specific issues, including definition, taxonomy or diagnosis, etiology, assessment, and treatment. Furthermore, each chapter includes a case study in which the process of clinical formulation is illustrated. Although not exhaustive, this section samples a wide array of child behavior problems. As in the second edition, we include a set of chapters on the psychological aspects of a host of physical conditions in the third part, including pediatric headaches, childhood asthma, juvenile diabetes, childhood cancer, and pediatric AIDS. We also offer chapters on child abuse and neglect and on children under stress. Each of the chapters in this section reflects the tremendous impact of the field of behavioral medicine and its welcome sibling, pediatric psychology, on the practice of clinical child psychology. Finally, in the fourth part, psychodynamic, behavioral, and psychopharmacological treatments are carefully reviewed and evaluated. Special attention is afforded the empirical support of use of these various modalities of treatment. New and exciting preventive strategies, couched within a proactive-developmental-ecological perspective, are highlighted in the final chapter of this edition. All in all, like the first and second editions of this book, the third edition is intended to be a sourcebook detailing the current status of, and highlighting future directions for, research and practice in the broad fields of child psychopathology and clinical child psychology.

In a comprehensive project such as this, many persons are to be acknowledged. Among the foremost is our distinguished list of contributors. Quite obviously, without them, up-to-date and scholarly treatment of topics could hardly have been possible. We would also like to acknowledge Ms. Mariclaire Cloutier, Mr. Eliot Werner, and the various professionals at Plenum Publishing Corporation, whose support over the years has been untiring and invaluable. In addition, we would also like to give special thanks to the many children and adolescents who have, perhaps unknowingly and unwittingly, served as the impetus for this third edition. As students of child psychopathology, we are grateful for what they have taught us. Although we have learned much from them over the past 15 years, we have much more to learn in the years ahead. We look forward to this continued process.

Finally, we would like to thank our own children, Laurie and Katie (THO) and Jonathan and Nathaniel (MH). When we completed the first edition of this book in 1983, they were children; in 1989, at the time of second edition, they were adolescents. Now, they are young adults. They, too, have taught us much—especially about development and developmental variations that have occurred across their own development—and ours. To them, we dedicate this effort.

Thomas H. Ollendick
Michel Hersen

Contents

PART III. PSYCHOLOGICAL ASPECTS OF PHYSICAL CONDITIONS

Basic Issues

I

Developmental Perspectives

SUSAN B. CAMPBELL

INTRODUCTION

Although it is obvious to any student of child development that behavior, whether "normal" or "abnormal," must be examined within a developmental context, it is only in the last decade that child psychiatry and clinical child psychology have begun to incorporate a developmental perspective. Both theory and nomenclature were originally adapted from work with adults, and the important changes in behavior and cognitive capacity that occur as a function of physical maturation and psychological development were largely overlooked. Instead, attempts were made to extend adult models downward, and theories of adult psychopathology were unsuccessfully adapted to childhood problems.

More recently, there has been an upsurge of interest in clinical problems among developmental psychologists as well as an effort to apply concepts and findings from normal development to the understanding of developmental processes in populations of infants and children at risk (e.g., Cicchetti & Richters, 1993; Greenberg, Speltz, & DeKlyen, 1993; Rutter & Garmezy, 1983; Sroufe & Rutter, 1984). The hallmark of this work is a transactional and ecological view that assumes the coherence and predictability of development and adaptation, despite change and transformation (e.g., Sroufe, 1979), and emphasizes the importance of family and social environmental factors in understanding the nature and direction of that change (e.g., Belsky, 1984; Coie & Jacobs, 1993; Reid, 1993).

Although conceptualizations of adult problems may provide some insights into childhood disorders and vice versa, it is now generally recognized that both research and practice in the child psychopathology field are complicated by a host of factors that influence problem definition, course, and outcome, as well as treatment decisions. Among these are the child's chronological age, level of cognitive and social development, family background, and a variety of other social and cultural factors. Indeed, it is virtually meaningless to consider child behavior in isolation from social context and developmental stage.

At the most basic level, problem definition depends on the age of the child. Behaviors considered symptomatic of disturbance at one age may be considered typical at another. Thus, bedwetting, inability to read, stranger anxiety, or sep-

SUSAN B. CAMPBELL • Department of Psychology, University of Pittsburgh, Pittsburgh, Pennsylvania 15260.

Handbook of Child Psychopathology, 3rd edition, edited by Ollendick & Hersen. Plenum Press, New York, 1998.

aration distress are not considered problems among 1- and 2-year-olds, but are worthy of concern in 12-year-olds. Refusal to go to sleep before midnight might be a cause of concern to parents of infants, but not to those of adolescents. Other potentially problematic behaviors appear to change with age. For example, a frequent concern of parents is defiant behavior, which is more common among toddlers and adolescents than among 8-year-olds. However, its manifestations obviously vary as a function of age.

The cognitive-developmental level of the child similarly influences how a particular behavior is perceived, interpreted, and labeled by adults. For example, aggressive behavior is a common referral complaint among school-age and adolescent males seen in child mental health facilities. However, interpretations of aggressive behavior vary with the age of the child, and aggressive behavior in 2- and 3-year-old males rarely leads to referral. Parents may describe their youngster as "rough" and note that he does not "mean" to hurt the other child. Inherent in this is a distinction between the child's behavior and intentions as well as some notion of perspective-taking. The toddler, who has not yet reached the stage of cognitive development that permits him to take the viewpoint of others into account, does not connect his behavior (i.e., hitting) with its effect on another person (i.e., inflicting pain). Further, aggressive encounters between 2- and 3-year-olds are frequently struggles over a toy (Shantz, 1987), reflecting the egocentrism of this stage of cognitive and social development. Both think of "me" and do not consider the fact that the other wants the toy just as much as they do. Thus, the egocentrism and lack of perspective-taking typical of toddlerhood lead adults to construe particular negative behaviors as less problematic in young children than these same behaviors would be viewed in older children.

Similarly, the prognostic implications of behaviors at different ages vary considerably, although much empirical work remains to be done in this area. Parents of toddlers frequently complain of noncompliance, tantrums, and aggression toward peers, but they are more likely than parents of older children to perceive these behaviors as transient developmental phenomena, reflecting a stage of normal development. At less extreme levels, these behaviors do appear to be age-appropriate and typical manifestations of the struggle for autonomy and development of a sense of self (Campbell, 1990). Data on the long-term consequences of these behaviors in young children, however, suggest that, at the extremes, these behaviors may persist and become indicators of more serious problems (e.g., Campbell, 1994; Campbell & Ewing, 1990; Richman, Stevenson, & Graham, 1982). However, clinicians generally do not interpret such behavior as likely to predict later antisocial behavior or interpersonal problems in toddlers and preschoolers, whereas disobedience toward adults and aggression toward peers in school-age youngsters are often seen as more likely to predict serious problems. Indeed, a growing body of research links aggression and noncompliance in school-age youngsters, especially boys, with antisocial behavior in adolescence and young adulthood (e.g., Loeber et al., 1993; Moffitt, 1990; Robins, 1966). Thus, clinicians would be more likely to be concerned about the potentially negative prognosis of such behaviors in a school-age as opposed to a preschool child.

Age of onset and chronicity of symptoms are also relevant to the conceptualization of problem behavior in children and to probable prognosis. Thus, overactive and defiant behavior in a 10-year-old boy that is described as having been present since infancy or toddlerhood is more likely to be seen as a serious problem with a relatively poor prognosis than the same behaviors occurring in a 10-year-old boy in response to parental divorce. Whereas early onset and chronicity would contribute to a diagnosis of a bona fide syndrome, late onset of an acute disorder in response to a specific stressor could most likely be viewed as a reactive disorder that is time-limited and has a good prognosis. Thus, the same overt behaviors in children of the same age and sex may elicit different diagnostic formulations and treatment recommendations depending partly on the developmental factors of age of onset and chronicity.

Treatment recommendations are likewise influenced by the child's age and cognitive-developmental level. In terms of more traditional dynamic therapy, play therapy is most often used with children in preschool and the primary grades who are less likely to be clearly aware of their problems or to have the verbal sophistication to discuss them directly in a therapeutic situation. However, some clinicians find play an ideal vehicle for communicating with and gaining insight into the problems of young children (e.g., Axline, 1969). On the other hand, older children with average intelligence and good verbal skills are more likely to be seen in verbal psychotherapy.

From the perspective of more empirically validated treatments, young children's problems are most frequently dealt with by working with parents to modify parenting style and disciplinary practices (e.g., Webster-Stratton, 1990). Although behavioral approaches are used with children of all ages, usually with parent or teacher as the behavior change agent, the nature and frequency of rewards will be likely to vary with age: More immediate rewards are more likely to be effective with younger children, whereas older children are more likely to have the cognitive capacity to bridge the delay required by the use of tokens. Self-monitoring and self-reinforcement approaches or the use of peers as behavior modifiers (e.g., Colletti & Harris, 1977) are more common with older children.

Cognitive-developmental factors also play a role in treatment outcome. For example, cognitive-behavioral approaches that attempt to teach the child more efficient problem-solving strategies appear to work better with school-age youngsters (see Kendall, Lerner, & Craighead, 1984) who have attained a certain level of cognitive development and can think about the short-term consequences of their behavior than with younger children (Cohen, Sullivan, Minde, Novak, & Helwig, 1981) who are less likely to engage in consequential thinking.

Similarly, cognitive-developmental level is seen as influencing diagnostic labels. It has been suggested that the "here and now" orientation of children up to age 8 or 9 and a tendency not to reason about the future preclude the development of true affective disorders as defined in adults. Because a feeling of hopelessness and pessimism about the future is often conceptualized as central to a diagnosis of depression (e.g., Beck, 1972), a certain degree of cognitive development would appear to be a necessary prerequisite to a sense of future time. Thus, although it is clear that young children can experience periods of tearfulness and dysphoric mood, the debate continues as to whether or not a true syndrome of depression can be identified in prepubertal children (Angold & Costello, 1993; Puig-Antich, 1986; Quay & La Greca, 1986; Rutter, 1986).

Taken together, then, these examples illustrate the important role that cognitive, social, and affective development play in determining who is perceived as a problem, how the problem is conceptualized and labeled, what treatment recommendations are made, and what the likely outcome of the problem is.

PROBLEM BEHAVIOR AND ADULT EXPECTATIONS: WHOSE PROBLEM IS IT?

Whereas most adults who reach mental health facilities initiate contact themselves and have at least some notion that they have a problem, children almost uniformly are seen because a parent, teacher, or physician has expressed concern; they may or may not be aware of the problem themselves. Indeed, they may not have a problem at all. The first task of the clinician working with children and families is to determine whether or not a problem actually exists. Intolerance, ignorance, and misconceptions on the part of adults often lead to referral. All too often, when there is a problem, the problem may reside more in the family system or in the way parents are managing their child's behavior, though this is often a difficult concept to convey to parents. Further, parents' perceptions of child behavior are often influenced by their own emotional state.

For example, Shepherd, Oppenheim, and Mitchell (1971), in a large epidemiological study of childhood psychopathology, compared a group of clinic attenders with matched controls who were rated as having problems of equivalent severity but whose parents had never sought treatment. The main factors that differentiated clinic attenders from nonattenders were maternal perceptions of the problem as serious versus transient, maternal feelings of competence, family disruption, and maternal depression. Sandberg, Wieselberg, and Shaffer (1980) noted an association between ratings of behavior problems and maternal psychiatric distress. Similarly, Richman et al. (1982), in a study of behavior problems in 3-year-olds, found that high ratings of behavior problems were associated with maternal depression, marital dysfunction, and high stress, suggesting that maternal tolerance also plays a large role in defining behavior problems in young children. Similar findings linking family distress to children's problems have been obtained in more recent studies (e.g., Koot, 1993; Newth & Corbett, 1993).

The well-documented association between marital problems and childhood behavior disorders (e.g., Emery, 1982; Hetherington & Martin, 1986) also suggests the importance of the family climate in the perception and definition of childhood problems. Not only is marital distress associated with higher rates of behavior problems, but Jouriles and colleagues (Jouriles et al., 1991) found that parental disagreements over childrearing predicted behavior problems in 3-year-old boys over and above global marital adjustment. This suggests that family stress in general, as well as specific issues around the parenting role may lead to the identification of the child as a problem and to referral.

In a study of referral patterns among general

practitioners in London, Gath (1968) reported that in at least two-thirds of the cases referred to a child psychiatry clinic, parental attitudes had been the key factor leading to referral. Other evidence indicates that family stress influences both perceptions of child behavior and the emotional tone of mother–child interaction (Campbell, Pierce, March, & Ewing, 1991; Conger, McCarty, Yang, Lahey, & Kropp, 1984; Dumas & Wahler, 1985). In general, more family stress and social isolation are associated with more negative, less appropriate parenting. Taken together, then, these findings suggest that parental conceptualizations of the nature of the problem and their own psychological state influence their tolerance for and ability to handle child behavior and, thus, may have considerable impact on referral patterns.

In our own work with parent-identified hard-to-manage toddlers and preschoolers, we were consistently impressed with the variations we saw in parental tolerance (Campbell, 1990). Although a few parents rationalized as "just being a boy" a range of destructive, aggressive, and inappropriate behaviors, other parents seemed unable to accept even the mildest temper outburst or expression of defiance in 2- or 3-year-olds and called the project to seek help "before things get out of hand." Some parents in our project defined "normal" and age-appropriate attempts to be independent as "problem" behavior and engaged in a negative and escalating cycle of coercive control (Patterson, DeBaryshe, & Ramsey, 1989). Clearly, parental tolerance and its influence on parenting style and child management skills play an important role in the definition of childhood problems as well as in their development and maintenance.

This issue is further complicated by the fact that not everyone in the child's environment will perceive the same behaviors, interpret a behavior as a problem, or perceive a problem the same way. Thus, parent and teacher ratings of behavior problems often show only modest agreement (see Achenbach, McConaughy, & Howell, 1987, for a review), and disagreement between parents and physicians has also been reported (Jenkins, Bax, & Hart, 1980). Finally, even within families, parents do not always agree on the existence or severity of problem behavior (e.g., Ferguson, Partyka, & Lester, 1974). This is not totally surprising as children behave in different ways in different situations and with different individuals (e.g., Lytton, 1979; Lytton & Zwirner, 1975). Taken together, adult variations in tolerance and expectations, their differential effects on child behavior, and the situational specificity of behavior also contribute to difficulties assessing when and whether a problem exists.

EPIDEMIOLOGICAL STUDIES OF CHILDHOOD BEHAVIOR PROBLEMS: PREVALENCE RATES AS A FUNCTION OF AGE AND SEX

Although definitions of "normal" or "abnormal" behavior are impossible to arrive at, and it is clear that age, sex, cultural, and other factors determine what is and is not considered appropriate, some attempts have been made to provide normative data on the frequencies of specific behaviors in representative samples of children of a particular age. Thus, a number of large-scale survey studies of representative groups of children have been carried out to determine the rates of specific problem behaviors in the general population. The bulk of these studies have been conducted in great Britain (e.g., Richman et al., 1982; Rutter, Tizard, & Whitmore, 1970; Shepherd et al., 1971) and the United States (e.g., Lapouse & Monk, 1958; MacFarlane, Honzik, & Allen, 1954; Werry & Quay, 1971). This work has been critically reviewed by Links (1983).

Studies of very young children have been rare. However, in one study (Jenkins et al., 1980), parental concerns were examined. The sample consisted of about 97% ($N = 418$) of the 6-week-old to 4½-year-old children in a geographic catchment area of North London.

Problems in infancy were relatively rare, and the focus, not surprisingly, was on sleeping problems, on feeding difficulties and colic, and on crying. Between ages 1 and 2, problems began to increase somewhat, but feeding and sleeping problems continued to predominate. Bowel and bladder problems emerged at age 2 and problems peaked at age 3 when the major complaint became difficulties with management and discipline. Parents expressed concerns about specific behaviors, but few saw their children as demonstrating significant or severe problems, an observation with which the examining general practitioner usually agreed. These cross-sectional findings generally confirm results of the Berkeley Growth Study (MacFarlane et al., 1954), which followed a representative sample of children from 21 months to 14 years.

The majority of large-scale studies of children's behavior have been concerned with children of preschool and school age. Despite differences in methodology, age of child, sample characteristics, locale, and sources of data, major findings have been remarkably consistent. When frequencies of specific behaviors considered to be of psychiatric significance are studied in large populations of children, it is evident that symptomatic behaviors are very common among nonreferred children of preschool age (e.g., Crowther, Bond, & Rolf, 1981; Kohn, 1977; MacFarlane et al., 1954; Newth & Corbett, 1993; Stallard, 1993) and school age (e.g., Rutter et al., 1970; Werry & Quay, 1971). Further, boys are perceived as having more problems than girls, especially behaviors associated with conduct disorders and hyperactivity (McGee, Silva, & Williams, 1984; Offord, Boyle, Fleming, Blum, & Rae-Grant, 1989; Rutter et al., 1970; Werry & Quay, 1971), although sex differences in behaviors are found less consistently with younger children (Crowther et al., 1981; Hughes, Pinkerton, & Plewis, 1979; Kohn, 1977; MacFarlane et al., 1954; Richman et al., 1982; Stallard, 1993). Age changes in specific behaviors are also apparent, with a general tendency for problems such as fears and worries, nightmares, enuresis, and tantrums to decrease with age in preschool

(Coleman, Wolkind, & Ashley, 1977; MacFarlane et al., 1954) and school-age samples (Lapouse & Monk, 1958; Werry & Quay, 1971).

Prevalence estimates for certain behaviors are extremely high and underline the importance of considering the frequency, intensity, and chronicity of clusters of symptoms within a developmental and social context when defining psychiatric disorders (Richman et al., 1982; Rutter et al., 1970). Isolated behaviors in and of themselves do not determine whether or not a disorder exists. Furthermore, rare behaviors do not indicate disturbance any more than frequent behaviors indicate normality. However, it is important to note that many behaviors considered of psychiatric significance are extremely common in nonclinical samples.

For example, among the defining symptoms of attention-deficit/hyperactivity disorder (ADHD) are restlessness, distractibility, and short attention span (American Psychiatric Association, 1994). According to Werry and Quay's (1971) data, teachers described 49.7% of kindergarten through grade 2 boys in a Midwestern college town as restless, 43.5% were described as having a short attention span, and 48.2% were rated as distractible. Similarly, a large proportion of mothers in Buffalo, New York, rated their 6- to 12-year-olds as overactive (49%) and restless (30%) (Lapouse & Monk, 1958). ADHD or hyperactivity is rarely diagnosed in Great Britain (Rutter et al., 1970), and the prevalence rates of associated behaviors are somewhat lower. However, Shepherd et al. (1971) still found that 20% of the mothers of boys between 5 and 14 years old, sampled in the Buckinghamshire survey, described their sons as restless. Rutter et al. (1970) found that parents rated 34.8% of the general population of 10- and 11-year-old boys on the Isle of Wight as restless and 25.2% as having poor concentration. Comparable figures for teacher ratings were 15.7 and 35.3%, respectively. Across all four studies, fewer girls were rated as showing these behaviors and younger children showed them more often than older children.

What are the implications of these data? First,

if the epidemiological cutoff of 10% is utilized (e.g., Shepherd et al., 1971) and it is agreed that rarity means abnormality, we would be forced to conclude that, assuming that these ratings by teachers and parents are valid reflections of the behavior in question, these behaviors are essentially normal. That is, restlessness and attentional problems are so common in young boys as to be virtually meaningless in terms of diagnostic significance. Indeed, even calling these behaviors problematic might be misleading. An alternative interpretation might be that an epidemic of hyperactivity has spread from North America to Great Britain. Furthermore, the data on cross-sectional age differences might suggest that overactive behavior and attentional problems are outgrown as children get older. However, all of these conclusions would be wrong.

Data on isolated behaviors cannot really answer questions about the presence of an actual psychological disorder or its course. Diagnostic formulations require information on patterns of symptoms that covary and on their change over time within subjects showing the disorder. In fact, hyperactivity is one of the most common diagnoses given to school-age boys seen in child mental health facilities in North America (Barkley, 1990). Furthermore, some studies suggest that these problems are also common in preschool samples (Behar, 1977; Coleman et al., 1977; Kohn, 1977; Richman et al., 1982) and that they may have prognostic significance for later school functioning (Campbell, 1994; Campbell & Ewing, 1990; Coleman et al., 1977; Kohn, 1977; Richman et al., 1982). Follow-up studies of hyperactive school-age youngsters indicate that problems in social and academic functioning persist, although the specific behavioral manifestations of the disorder change somewhat with age (Barkley, Fischer, Edelbrock, & Smallish, 1990; Gittelman, Mannuzza, Shenker, & Bonagura, 1985; Weiss & Hechtman, 1993). Thus, the clinical findings parallel the epidemiological findings in that the problems are common, are more often found in boys, and show some changes with age. However, were we to conclude from the epidemiological studies that the problems were merely transient developmental disturbances or behaviors that were so common as to be clinically meaningless, we would be wrong. The frequency of occurrence of the specific behavior in the population as a whole, as well as its variation in the population as a function of age and sex, may highlight the need to be cautious in diagnosing disorder. However, it tells us little about the prevalence, developmental course, or likely outcome of a syndrome that includes the specific behavior in question.

Thus, it is important to distinguish between isolated behaviors that may be characteristic of both "normal" and disturbed children and clusters of symptoms that tend to covary and to interfere with adaptive functioning and the mastery of developmental tasks, which therefore are considered indicative of psychiatric disorder (Rutter et al., 1970). Several epidemiological studies have examined prevalence rates of disorder over and above examining the frequencies of specific symptomatic behaviors. Gersten, Langner, Eisenberg, Simcha-Fagan, and McCarthy (1976) noted that 12% of their subjects residing in midtown Manhattan had significant behavior problems, and Bower (1969) reported problems in 10% of Los Angeles schoolchildren. Rutter et al. (1970) screened all 10- and 11-year-olds on the Isle of Wight (England) in 1965 ($N = 3316$) and, on the basis of empirically derived cutoff scores on parent and teacher behavior rating scales, selected 13% for intensive psychiatric assessment. On the basis of this assessment, 5.4% of the total population were diagnosed as having a psychiatric disorder. Problems were more common in boys. However, sex differences were also apparent in the type of problem. Not surprisingly, conduct disorders were more frequent among boys and neurotic problems were more common in girls. Finally, interpersonal problems and concentration difficulties were the most common symptoms found across all diagnostic groups.

Two more recent epidemiological studies conducted in Ontario, Canada, and Dunedin, New Zealand, provide a similar picture. In the Ontario Child Health Study, 18% of 4- to 16-year-olds showed evidence of a psychiatric disorder (Offord, Boyle, Fleming, Blum, & Rae Grant, 1989). In the Dunedin study, rates of disorder were found to vary widely based on whether both parent and teacher had to agree, on how disorder was defined, and on whether stability of problems was considered. However, regardless of these factors, boys were seen as having more antisocial problems than girls who were seen as more anxious and depressed (e.g., McGee, Feehan, Williams, & Partridge, 1990; McGee, Silva, & Williams, 1984). In addition, girls show an increase in depression and anxiety in early adolescence, surpassing boys in overall frequency of problem behavior (Offord et al., 1989; Rutter et al., 1970). Here again, the findings of prevalence of disorder parallel findings examining frequencies of specific behaviors. Developmental issues also become important in interpreting findings from epidemiological studies.

Richman et al. (1982) reported a prevalence rate of 7% "moderate to severe" problems and 15% "mild" problems among a representative sample of 3-year-olds in London, roughly similar to the rates reported by Rutter et al. Richman and her colleagues did not find sex differences in rates of disorder, but family problems were associated with childhood disturbances. These findings were confirmed by Hughes et al. (1979) in London and by Minde and Minde (1977) in a smaller nonrepresentative sample of 3- to 4-year-olds in Toronto. Four more recent studies of the prevalence of problems in young children confirm overall rates of about 10–12% in 2- to 4-year-olds (Cornely & Bromet, 1986; Koot, 1993; Newth & Corbett, 1993; Stallard, 1993). Furthermore, behavior problems in toddlers and preschoolers appear to be associated with a high incidence of delayed language development (Baker, Cantwell, & Mattison, 1980; Richman et al., 1982).

Finally, there is general consensus from a large number of studies that problems in toddlers, preschoolers, and school-age youngsters fall into two primary categories of disorder: internalizing or inner-directed clusters of behavior such as neurotic, withdrawn, depressed, and somatic problems and externalizing or outer-directed clusters of behavior such as conduct problems, hyperactivity, and aggressive and antisocial disorders (e.g., Achenbach & Edelbrock, 1983; Achenbach, Howell, Quay, & Conners, 1991; Behar, 1977; Kohn, 1977; Quay, 1986); and like specific symptoms, age changes and sex differences are found when clusters of behavior are examined (e.g., Achenbach et al., 1991).

In summary, symptomatic behaviors are common across the age range from early to later childhood, although estimates of actual disorder seem relatively low. Furthermore, family functioning and parental tolerance as well as the age of the child influence whether or not a child will actually be referred for an evaluation and whether or not a problem will be diagnosed. These factors also will determine, in part, whether a problem is perceived by the clinician as potentially serious or as a transient developmental problem typical of a particular stage of development. It is to these that we now turn.

COMMON DEVELOPMENTAL PROBLEMS

As already noted, problem definition and the prognostic implications of specific behaviors vary with age. It is also clear, however, that certain problem behaviors are characteristic of a particular developmental stage and appear to be transient. Common developmental problems may reflect the exaggeration of age-appropriate behaviors or difficult transitions from one stage of development to the next. Although the turbulence of adolescence and the defiance of toddlerhood are the most frequently cited examples of common developmental problems, problems are common at all ages; they may be particularly intense at one age (e.g., toddlerhood) and more subtle at another (e.g., early

school-age or "latency"). However, common developmental problems are often a source of serious concern to parents (e.g., Mesibov, Schroeder, & Wesson, 1977). Further, the assumption is often made by both parents and professionals that improper handling of a difficult developmental phase may lead to later problems and, conversely, that if early problems are handled sensitively and appropriately, the development of difficulties at a later stage may be prevented (e.g., Sroufe, 1979; Thomas, Chess, & Birch, 1968).

Among young children, common developmental difficulties rarely reach the mental health practitioner; rather, the family physician or pediatrician is frequently consulted about the behavioral and developmental concerns of parents of infants and toddlers. Often, such difficulties reflect misunderstandings on the part of parents about the normal course of development and the particular tasks of a developmental stage; further, these common developmental problems are often exacerbated by parental mismanagement, family stress, or their combined impact. Thus, it is important to bear in mind that these childhood problems can best be conceptualized within a model that examines the reciprocal influences of parents on children and children on parents (Bell & Harper, 1977; Sameroff & Chandler, 1975). Several typical problems characteristic of different stages from infancy through school age will be discussed with particular emphasis on their developmental aspects, both typical and potentially problematic.

Infancy

The "Difficult" Infant

Infants are rarely referred to mental health professionals except in severe cases of gross disorder or developmental delay, although parental concerns often do reach the pediatrician (Carey, 1972). Much clinical, theoretical, and research attention has focused on very early individual differences in infants or infant "temperament," especially those behavioral characteristics that may be potential precursors of childhood difficulties (e.g., Bates & Bayles, 1988). Individual differences in the frequency and duration of crying, infant cuddliness and consolability, activity level, alertness, and self-quieting (e.g., Brazelton, 1973; Korner, 1971; Vaughn, Taraldson, Crichton, & Egeland, 1980) can have profound effects on parental behavior and the quality of the developing parent–infant relationship (e.g., Korner, 1971; Osofsky, 1976) as well as on parental mood and self-esteem (Cutrona & Troutman, 1986; Hopkins, Campbell, & Marcus, 1987). It seems obvious that an active, alert, and easily consoled infant will elicit different behaviors from caretakers and have different requirements for caretaking than an active but irritable infant who cries frequently and is not easily calmed.

The possibility that early infant temperamental characteristics could influence the quality of early parenting as well as later infant development and family relationships was initially articulated by Thomas et al. (1968) in a classic prospective study of early infant temperament and the development of behavior disorders in young children. These authors noted the importance of "goodness of fit" between an infant's behavioral style and parental tolerance, sensitivity, and methods of childrearing. These notions of mutual regulation of parent–child interaction and individual differences in the specifics of interaction patterns have been spelled out within a more sophisticated theoretical framework in Sameroff and Chandler's (1975) transactional model of development and have been operationalized by several investigators of infant development (Brazelton, Koslowski, & Main, 1974; Stern, 1974). More recently, Campos, Mumme, Kermoian, and Campos (1994) have discussed the regulation of negative affect as a prime indicator of difficult temperament in infancy that may have implications for the quality of parent–child interaction.

Thomas and his associates suggested that infants who were irritable, slow to adapt to changes in routine, intense in reaction, and irregular in biological functioning were more difficult to care for and more likely to develop later behavior problems. However, intensive clinical follow-up of a sample of families in New York City indicated that difficult infants who were handled sensitively, whose parents effectively modulated their intensity and permitted them time to warm up to new stimuli, were more likely to weather this often difficult developmental period with no ill effects. On the other hand, parents who were rough, intolerant, or who forced their difficult infants to adapt to changes in routine quickly and often were more likely to suffer the consequences later on, as their difficult infants grew into negative and defiant toddlers with early peer problems. On the other hand, easy infants—that is, infants who were positive in mood, reasonably regular in patterns of sleeping and eating, and adaptable to change—adjusted to a wider range of parental management styles and were less likely to develop later problems, although they were not immune from them. This early study, although methodologically flawed, has become a classic in the field and has generated a number of more sophisticated research studies into the relationship between early infant temperament and later behavior.

It is clear from the longitudinal work of Thomas et al. (1968) that not all difficult infants become behavior-problem toddlers. However, retrospective data from several studies support the contention that children who are described as active and aggressive in toddlerhood and early preschool (e.g., Campbell, Szumowski, Ewing, Gluck, & Breaux, 1982) are more likely to be described by parents as irritable and difficult-to-sooth infants who had irregular and unpredictable patterns of eating and sleeping. Similarly, difficult temperament is associated with later aggression in boys (Olweus, 1980). Although the problems of collecting such data retrospectively are obvious, findings are at least suggestive of a relationship between difficult infant temperament and later behavior problems.

It is likely that a cycle of negative interactions

develops early in some proportion of difficult infants and their mothers and that it escalates, partly as a function of ongoing environmental events. For example, Cutrona and Troutman (1986) reported that infant irritability affected maternal mood directly and also indirectly through the impact of infant irritability on maternal feelings of competence and self-efficacy. Crockenberg's (1981) data indicated that the development of an insecure attachment in some mother–infant pairs was mediated by the impact of limited social support and lack of help with child care on mothers who were already stressed by the demands of caring for an infant who was irritable and difficult to console. These findings illustrate the complex relationships among child characteristics, parental behavior, and environmental factors, all of which contribute to an understanding of developmental outcome.

Continued work in this area is required, especially research that systematically assesses the relationships among infant temperamental characteristics, early parent–child relations, and later behavior problems. It does seem safe to conclude, however, that some infants are easier to care for than others; further, difficulties during this period may indeed be a precursor of later problems, although it also appears that parental behavior can influence whether or not difficult infant behavior will develop into later behavior problems or will merely reflect a difficult phase of development that is eventually outgrown. Research evaluating the specific aspects of both infant and parental behavior and their changes over time is beginning to address these questions.

Prospective studies confirm that infant difficultness is associated with a range of problems in adaptation over the course of the first few years of life. Effects on the mother and the mother–infant relationship have been reported. Two studies indicate an association between infant difficultness and maternal depression in the immediate postpartum period (Cutrona & Troutman, 1986; Hopkins et al., 1987), as well as feelings of inadequacy as a parent (Cutrona &

Troutman, 1986). Crockenberg (1981) reported that infant difficultness was associated with lowered maternal responsiveness in early infancy and that the combination of infant irritability and limited social support predicted an insecure infant–mother attachment at 1 year. Other studies likewise have found a relationship between infant difficultness and lowered maternal responsiveness during the first year of life (Bates, Freeland, & Lounsbury, 1979; Campbell, 1979). In a large-scale longitudinal study of difficult infants, Bates and his colleagues reported that infant difficultness predicted negative and conflicted mother–child encounters at 2 years (Lee & Bates, 1985) and maternal reports of persistent problems with aggression and noncompliance at 3 and 5 years (Bates, Maslin, & Frankel, 1985). Sanson and colleagues (Sanson, Oberklaid, Pedlow, & Prior, 1991) in a large-scale prospective study of infants in Australia also found that early ratings of difficult temperament predicted ratings of behavior problems during the preschool years. Taken together, these findings and others (e.g., Maccoby, Snow, & Jacklin, 1984) suggest that infant difficultness can have a profound impact on maternal mood and behavior as well as on the developing mother–infant relationship.

Problems in Attachment

It has long been assumed by clinicians and theorists of child psychopathology that the early mother–infant relationship is a primary determinant of later development and subsequent mental health (e.g., Bowlby, 1969; A. Freud, 1965; Mahler, 1968; Winnicott, 1957). Whereas early theorists hypothesized a unidirectional and causal relationship between early maternal behavior and an infant's psychological development, recent theoretical advances underscore the complex and mutually regulated interaction that develops between mother and infant (Tronick, 1989). The major reconceptualization in this area falls under the rubric of attachment theory (Ainsworth, 1969; Bowlby, 1969), which combines ethological, cognitive, and social constructs and stresses the biological advantage of developing a secure attachment between the infant and primary caregiver. Research on qualitative aspects of the mother–infant relationship confirms some, but not all, of the ideas put forth by attachment theorists.

Over the course of the first year of life, infants develop a specific and enduring relationship with primary caretakers (usually parents) that has been termed *attachment* (Ainsworth, 1969; Bowlby, 1969). Attachment is a reciprocal relationship that develops gradually through stages during the first year and is mediated by the quality, timing, and pacing of adult–child encounters (Ainsworth, Blehar, Waters, & Wall, 1978). Initially, the infant directs social responses (crying, smiling, sucking, clinging) indiscriminantly to any responsive adult. However, as cognitive capacities develop, the infant begins to respond differentially to familiar and unfamiliar figures, usually by the end of the third month. By 6 or 7 months, the infant actively seeks to maintain contact with attachment figures, is active in initiating contact, protests at separation, and is beginning to show wariness of strangers. As the attachment relationship consolidates, the primary attachment figure serves as a secure base from which the infant explores the environment and is the main source of comfort in times of distress, fear, or illness. Although the establishment of attachment is a universal feature of infant social-emotional development (except in cases of early infantile autism where failure to form an attachment is a significant feature of the disorder), variations in maternal and infant behavior can influence the quality of the attachment relationship that develops.

Individual differences in patterns of attachment have been explored in depth by Ainsworth and her colleagues (e.g., Ainsworth et al., 1978; Ainsworth & Wittig, 1969; Stayton, Hogan, & Ainsworth, 1971), as well as by others (e.g., Belsky, Taylor, & Rovine, 1984; Isabella & Belsky, 1991; Main & Solomon, 1986; Vaughn, Egeland, Sroufe, & Waters, 1979). Findings from these studies indicate that early maternal behavior influences later infant–mother attachment.

Mothers who are sensitive to their infant's cues and responsive across a range of situations including feeding, responsiveness to crying, early face-to-face play, and the provision of opportunities to explore, foster the development of a secure attachment relationship.

Mothers who respond to their infants abruptly, who are unresponsive, or who pace their behavior to their own needs and schedules foster the development of an anxious or ambivalent attachment characterized by excessive anger, clinging, and/or avoidance behavior on the part of the infant. Mothers whose behavior with their infants is grossly distorted, because they are either abusive or severely mentally ill, are more likely to have infants whose behavior is disorganized and disturbed during separation and reunion situations. These disorganized infants are unable to use their mothers to help them relieve distress (e.g., Carlson, Cicchetti, Barnett, & Braunwald, 1989; DeMulder & Radke-Yarrow, 1991; Lyons-Ruth, Repacholi, McLeod, & Silva, 1991; Radke-Yarrow, Cummings, Kuczynski, & Chapman, 1985). In general, insecure infants seem unable to rely on their mothers for support or comfort in stressful situations, given their prior experiences with maternal rejection and/or unresponsiveness.

Quality of attachment at 1 year appears to build on earlier mother–infant interaction patterns and has also been found to relate to later problem-solving ability (Frankel & Bates, 1990; Matas, Arend, & Sroufe, 1978), competence with peers (Waters, Wippman, & Sroufe, 1979), and willingness to comply with maternal requests (Londerville & Main, 1981). Securely attached infants appear to develop in more optimal directions both cognitively and socially, although findings are more equivocal and less robust in the less extreme ranges of insecurity and maternal rejection (Lamb, 1987), suggesting the potential importance of alternative caregivers as well as the resilience of some insecure infants (e.g., Cicchetti, Rogosch, Lynch, & Holt, 1993).

Research using a prospective design suggests that maternal behavior interacts with infant characteristics and life circumstances to influence the pattern of attachment. Neonatal difficulties, as measured by the Brazelton Neonatal Behavioral Assessment Scale, were associated with anxious attachments at 1 year among a sample of families at risk because of poverty and other stressful life events (Vaughn et al., 1979; Waters, Vaughn, & Egeland, 1980). Furthermore, severe environmental disruption predicted changes in the quality of the attachment relationship. Securely attached infants became insecure as their environments became less stable and their mothers were less available to meet their needs (Vaughn et al., 1979). Similarly, the Crockenberg (1981) study, cited earlier, indicated that the combination of infant irritability and limited social support contributed to the development of an insecure attachment.

Studies are also beginning to assess the impact of more extreme forms of deviance in caretaking on the developing mother–infant relationship. One study found that abused and neglected infants were much more likely than comparison infants to evidence anxious insecure attachments or disorganized attachments at 12 and 18 months (Carlson et al., 1989; Schneider-Rosen, Braunwald, Carlson, & Cicchetti, 1985). Furthermore, longitudinal data indicated that, over time, a higher proportion of maltreated infants showed avoidant and/or resistant behavior, most likely a result of continued family instability, which exacerbated conflict between mother and toddler at a time when young children grapple with the balance between needs for sensitive support and closeness with strivings for autonomy.

The impact of maternal psychopathology on infant–mother attachment has been examined by Radke-Yarrow and her colleagues (DeMulder & Radke-Yarrow, 1991; Radke-Yarrow et al., 1985) in the context of an in-depth longitudinal study of the offspring of depressed parents. Attachment theory predicts that the social withdrawal and unavailability of women with major psychiatric disorders should translate into insensitive and unresponsive caregiving that is ultimately associated with insecure attachment

patterns. Radke-Yarrow and colleagues' data partly confirm these theoretical predictions in that both the nature and the severity of maternal disorder were associated with insecure attachment. Infants of mothers with bipolar disorder were more likely to demonstrate an insecure, disorganized attachment. Further, chronicity of disorder in severely ill women was associated with an extremely impaired mother–infant relationship, with infant behavior becoming especially disorganized during brief separation and reunion episodes. However, toddlers of mothers with major depression were not more likely to be insecurely attached than toddlers of comparison women (DeMulder & Radke-Yarrow, 1991). Other studies of attachment patterns in the infants of depressed women have also been equivocal (Campbell & Cohn, 1997), suggesting that a multiplicity of risk factors may be associated both with insecure attachment and with the development of problems. Additional longitudinal studies are needed that focus on the impact of family context and parenting factors and that index both short-term disruptions and more chronic aberrations in caregiving.

Attachment theory also predicts that insecure attachment in infancy will have long-term implications for the quality of a child's functioning, mediated by the effect of maternal rejection, unavailability, and insensitivity on the child's developing sense of self-esteem, feelings of self-efficacy, and ability to relate to others (Bretherton, 1985; Sroufe & Fleeson, 1986). Thus, from this theoretical perspective, insecure attachment should be associated with the onset of behavior problems in young children. The few studies to examine this question have yielded conflicting results.

Sroufe (1983) reported that insecure children from the high-risk sample described earlier (Vaughn et al., 1979) evidenced a variety of adaptational and interpersonal difficulties in preschool. For example, insecure children were more dependent on teachers, less compliant, less socially engaged with peers, more likely to lash out negatively to initiations from others, and less empathic with peers. Lewis, Feiring,

McGuffog, and Jaskir (1984) followed up a sample of white middle-class infants at age 6 and examined the association between attachment security at 1 year and later maternal reports of social competence and behavior problems on the Child Behavior Checklist. Overall, insecurely attached boys, but not girls, were seen as having significantly more behavior problems, especially those of an internalizing nature. Further, the combination of an insecure attachment in infancy and ongoing environmental stress predicted problem behavior at school entry. However, those insecure males who resided in a more stable family environment were less likely to develop problems; in addition, a secure attachment appeared to buffer boys living in stressful circumstances from developing problems.

These data are consistent with predictions from attachment theory, but they were not supported by Bates and Bayles (1988), who also followed a middle-class sample from infancy to age 5 and found no relationship between attachment security and maternal reports of problem behavior. Lyons-Ruth (1992), however, did link insecurity, especially disorganized attachment patterns, to later behavior problems in a high-risk sample. In addition, Speltz, Greenberg, and DeKlyen (1990) reported that preschool boys with diagnosed disruptive behavior problems were much more likely to be insecure than demographically similar nonreferred control boys, also suggesting an association between insecurity and problem behavior.

These findings are provocative and underline the importance of continued research on these questions. In particular, we require research that examines the impact of a variety of psychological and social variables on the development of attachment; more research on the relationship between early attachment and later psychological adjustment and maladjustment is sorely needed. Many clinicians working with infants and families tend to assume that early problems in attachment will inevitably lead to later interpersonal problems. Although it seems logical that disordered attachment is a risk factor increasing the probability of later problems, findings from the studies cited above also indicate that some children growing up in less than advantageous circumstances develop normally and are reasonably invulnerable to influences that would be deleterious to others (Garmezy, 1987; Lewis et al., 1984; Schneider-Rosen et al., 1985; Werner, 1993). Thus, research must continue to probe those factors that potentiate problem behavior and those that protect children at risk. Delineating the mechanisms by which early attachment relationships interact with other risk or protective factors to lead to either good or poor developmental outcomes clearly requires additional theoretical and empirical work (Cicchetti et al., 1993).

Toddlerhood and Preschool Age

Defiance or Independence?

The achievement of independence is among the major developmental tasks of toddlerhood. Children must make the shift from being dependent infants to being mobile, verbal children who explore the world and begin to interact outside the nuclear family. This is a stage of rapid cognitive development as youngsters begin to develop a sense of themselves as individuals, to learn that their behavior has effects on others, to spend time experimenting on the inanimate world, and to test their own limits. Although parents expect children to develop independence at this stage in areas such as feeding, toileting, and even dressing, independence in other areas can lead to parent–child conflict. Often the child's headlong move toward independence and environmental mastery leads to a period of intense struggle with parents over limits and control (Brazelton, 1974; Campbell, 1990).

Although children at this age are rarely brought to mental health clinics, pediatricians must deal with questions about behavior management on a daily basis. This is an extremely difficult time for parents who are often afraid to set limits or are unable to accept the defiance that is typical of this stage. Amazingly little research has been done on behavior problems in this age group, although the few survey studies cited earlier (Jenkins et al., 1980; Koot, 1993; MacFarlane et al., 1954; Richman et al., 1982) indicate that noncompliance or management problems are the prominent parental concern. Jenkins et al. reported that whereas only 5% of parents of infants expressed excessive concern about behavior, 23% of parents of 3-year-olds were unsure about how to discipline their toddler. MacFarlane et al. (1954) found that negativism peaked at age 3 for boys and was associated with hyperactivity and tantrum behavior. This is confirmed by our own data on behavior-problem toddlers in which disciplinary problems and concerns about when and how to set limits are the major concerns expressed by parents of $2\frac{1}{2}$- to $3\frac{1}{2}$-year-olds (Campbell, 1990; Campbell et al., 1982).

Several research studies on compliance in this age group are enlightening. It is well known from the behavioral literature (e.g., Forehand & Scarboro, 1975) that excessive and/or ambiguous parental commands are associated with increased noncompliance in children. In an elegant study of parent–child interaction in toddlers, Lytton and Zwirner (1975) carried out extensive home observations of a large sample of 2- and 3-year-old boys. Sequential analyses indicated that these youngsters were more likely to comply after a parental suggestion than after a command or prohibition. Further, less conflict-laden situations were associated with more compliant behavior. Finally, physical control and negative interaction were associated with more noncompliance, which in turn led to a negative and controlling response from the parent and the cycle escalated. Lytton (1979) also reported that when physical control was paired with a command or prohibition, compliance was even less likely to occur. This escalating and negative cycle of conflict in preschoolers has been described in detail by Patterson (1976).

Minton, Kagan, and Levine (1971) observed 90 firstborn children at home when the child was 27 months of age. They reported that children were on the whole obedient and suggested that the notion of the "terrible twos" was a myth, at least for this sample. They did, however, note social class differences in parenting style and sex differences in child behavior. Mothers from lower educational levels tended to use more prohibitions and more physical punishment; boys tended to be more disobedient than girls especially in response to maternal prohibitions. College-educated mothers, on the other hand, tended to use more reasoning and to explain prohibitions. These findings are consistent with a number of earlier studies that found social class differences in childrearing and differential effects of authoritarian versus democratic childrearing practices on child behavior (see Maccoby & Martin, 1983). In addition, studies suggest that compliance is facilitated when the ongoing relationship between mother and toddler is warm and supportive (Londerville & Main, 1981).

It is obvious that parental behavior can maintain noncompliant behavior at a high rate, but it is also likely that some degree of "defiant" or "independent" behavior is both age-appropriate and necessary for the child's normal development as an individual. Toddlers must learn to separate from parents, to be aware of and to express their own needs, and to learn about their capacities. Crockenberg and Litman (1990) distinguish between noncompliance that reflects self-assertion, in the service of independence striving and self-definition, and noncompliance indicative of angry defiance. This is a subtle distinction, and often behavior considered to be "independent" by tolerant and knowledgeable parents is considered "defiant" or "noncompliant" by less tolerant or aware parents. In toddlerhood, noncompliance may also reflect a lack of understanding of adult expectations (Kaler & Kopp, 1990). As with many problems of childhood, the problem may be in the eye of the beholder.

In our own work with toddlers and their families, we have been impressed with the variations in parental tolerance, their impressions of their child's intent, and the management strategies they employ (Campbell, 1990). Parents who complain that their toddler "never listens" or that no form of discipline ever "works" are often those with inconsistent management approaches who shout and threaten but tend not to follow through to effectively enforce limits. Or they use a good deal of physical punishment, which exacerbates the cycle of conflict. Their children are irritable and the battles between them constant. They are often amazed at the cooperation that a quiet, yet direct and firm approach achieves. Such parents often perceive any attempt at independence as a test of their authority as a parent—something they attempt to squelch almost automatically. At the other extreme, we see parents who are at their wit's end, unable to set appropriate limits on their toddlers' defiance, parents who are being tyrannized by their 2-year-olds. Parental knowledge of normal developmental tasks, paired with training in the use of subtle and proactive controls (Holden, 1983) and the enforcement of firm limits when appropriate (Kuczynski, Radke-Yarrow, Kochanska, & Girnius-Brown, 1987; Zahn-Waxler, Radke-Yarrow, & King, 1979), would appear necessary to interrupt the development of such a negative cycle of parent–child interaction. Data from two longitudinal studies suggest that a negative and conflicted parent–child relationship in early childhood is predictive of continued problems at school entry and beyond (Campbell, 1990; Campbell & Ewing, 1990; Richman et al., 1982).

In conclusion, the striving for independence typical of toddlerhood is often perceived by parents as defiance. Further, it appears that attempts by parents at overcontrol can lead to an escalation of noncompliant behavior. Although clinical lore predicts that in most instances excessive defiance in toddlerhood is a stage-specific developmental phenomenon, it also appears that especially insensitive handling of this stage may increase the likelihood that problems will develop and perhaps even persist. This issue is addressed in more detail in Campbell (1995).

Aggressive Behavior

Aggressive behavior toward peers is a common complaint of parents and teachers of preschoolers, and when descriptions of the behavior of young children are factor-analyzed, an aggressive factor invariably emerges (Achenbach, Edelbrock, & Howell, 1987; Behar, 1977; Kohn & Rosman, 1972). Coleman et al. (1977) noted that 53% of their sample were described as having difficulty with peers at age 3. Crowther et al. (1981) found that approximately 25% of 4- and 5-year-old boys in their sample of day-care attenders were seen as moderately to highly aggressive with peers according to caregivers' reports; the comparable figure for girls was about 10%. Observations of nonclinical samples in preschools confirm that aggressive encounters are reasonably common occurrences (Blurton-Jones, 1972; Laursen & Hartup, 1989; Smith & Green, 1975).

Some studies of peer interaction among toddlers and preschoolers indicate not only that aggressive behavior is fairly common, but also that it tends to be successful. Both Patterson, Littman, and Brickner (1967) and Smith and Green (1975) reported that the majority of aggressive acts among preschoolers resulted in the aggressor getting his or her way, a conclusion questioned more recently by Shantz (1987). However, when outcomes are inequitable, the interaction is likely to be discontinued (Laursen & Hartup, 1989). Studies also indicate that aggressive interchanges are more common between boys than between girls or mixed-sex dyads (Pedersen & Bell, 1970; Smith & Green, 1975) and that the majority are property conflicts over the use of a toy (Blurton-Jones, 1972; Houseman, 1973; Smith & Green, 1975).

Smith and Green (1975) noted that 73% of the aggressive incidents they observed in 15 different preschool classrooms were property conflicts. Houseman (1973) reported that 67% of the conflicts she witnessed during 63 hours of observation in preschools were related to the possession or use of materials or space. Conflicts averaged 13.6 per hour per child and lasted a mean of 12.4 seconds. Further, frequency of conflict varied with activity setting. For example, fights were more likely to develop when children were playing with blocks than when they were engaged in an art activity. There is evidence that this form of instrumental or object-oriented aggression declines with age (Hartup, 1974).

Feshbach and Feshbach (1972) suggested that aggressive behavior is a response readily available in the repertoire of young children and a direct way of reaching a goal such as obtaining a toy. With development, children learn alternate, more adaptive means such as sharing and negotiating. However, Feshbach and Feshbach pointed out that it is often difficult to distinguish between an instrumental aggressive act that is determined solely by self-interest (obtaining a toy) and hostile or person-oriented aggression where the intent is to hurt the other child. Intent may be a factor that differentiates "normal" aggressive behavior from aggressive behavior that is more problematic.

However, descriptive studies of preschool aggression have usually failed to take into account the nature of the relationships among the children involved. Recent work indicates that this is important. For example, one study found that the resolution of disputes in preschoolers is partly a function of the closeness of the relationship between preschool peers. Hartup, Laursen, Stewart, and Eastenson (1988) compared naturally occurring conflicts between friends and acquaintances in their preschool classrooms. Although conflicts between acquaintances and between friends did not differ in frequency or duration, they did differ in intensity, with conflicts between friends resolved before they escalated in intensity. Friends were more likely to disengage or negotiate and the outcome of the dispute was more likely to be equal than was the case with acquaintances. Finally, friends were more likely to continue to play together after the dispute than nonfriends. This underlines the importance of relationship quality, even to young children.

Both peer popularity and the ability to engage in a dyadic relationship with a friend are probably also related to the frequency and nature of aggression, with more aggressive children at a clear disadvantage. This has been well documented in school-age children (see Coie & Cillessen, 1993, for a brief review), but has received less attention in preschool children. However, studies do indicate that children who are consistently aggressive in preschool are less popular with peers; conversely, prosocial behavior is associated with greater peer popularity (Hartup, 1983). In addition, observational studies suggest that aggressive behavior elicits negative behavior from peers, especially when boys are the aggressors (Fagot, 1984), whereas positive interaction elicits more compliance and prosocial behavior (Hartup, 1983).

Several studies also found relationships among high-intensity behaviors. That is, preschool children who tend to be active and boisterous also tend to be more aggressive, to initiate peer interaction, and to attempt to dominate peers (Battle & Lacey, 1972; Billman & McDevitt, 1980; Buss, Block, & Block, 1980). Thus, youngsters who engage in behavior at a high rate and are more involved with peers are also more likely to become aggressive than more quiet, passive children. Moreover, there is evidence that these patterns persist through the preschool period (Fagot, 1984) and into the early school years (Battle & Lacey, 1972; Buss et al., 1980; Halverson & Waldrop, 1976; Kohn, 1977).

More recent research has begun to examine the links between family and peer relationships, on the assumption that the nature of childrearing strategies and relationships among family members are an important arena in which children learn social skills and social understanding (e.g., Dunn, 1988; Hartup, 1989). Data do suggest that more positive, inductive, and child-centered parenting styles are associated with more prosocial behavior in the peer group. It is also logical to argue that parenting styles should influence children's behavior in the peer group, especially aggressive behavior and social competence (Hartup, 1989; Maccoby & Martin, 1983). Thus, youngsters raised in homes in which punitive, power-assertive discipline is favored over the use of reasoning and induction, would be expected to be more aggressive with peers. In a recent study, Hart, DeWolf, Wozniak, and Burts (1992) found that preschool children with more power-assertive parents were more aggressive and disruptive when observed on the playground, whereas children whose mothers used inductive reasoning and explained the consequences of behavior were more likely to show prosocial behavior with peers.

Thus, there is evidence that aggressive exchanges between young children are common, particularly between boys, and that aggressive behavior influences peer acceptance even in preschool. Short-term longitudinal studies suggest that early aggressive behavior may develop into less adaptive, competent forms of social behavior. However, the meaning or long-term implications of aggressive behavior in young children, especially young children who have not been identified as behavior problems, are unclear. It seems unlikely that lack of sharing and struggles over toys in preschool will have long-term negative implications for later social development and peer relations. In most instances, such conflicts will facilitate the development of socially appropriate behaviors by teaching children alternative prosocial strategies such as negotiating and turn-taking (Shantz, 1987). However, it is likely that peer problems in preschool, when paired with other behavioral problems that are mismanaged by parents or that occur in the context of a disturbed or discordant family situation, will persist and have a poor prognosis (Campbell, Ewing, Breaux, & Szumowski, 1986; Richman et al., 1982).

Studies that directly examine aggressive behavior in groups of clinically identified preschoolers have been rare. Schleifer et al. (1975) observed parent-identified hyperactive preschoolers in a research nursery and found that they were more aggressive with peers than nonhyperactive controls. Moreover, follow-up of these same youngsters into elementary school indicated that problems persisted (Campbell, Endman, & Bernfeld, 1977).

We have been engaged in a comprehensive assessment and follow-up study of parent-identified hard-to-manage toddlers and preschoolers. Aggression towards peers was a prominent concern of mothers who reported behavior problems with their children (Campbell, 1994; Campbell et al., 1982). In two cohorts of hard-to-manage preschool children, the problem group was rated as significantly more aggressive by both parents and teachers (Campbell, 1994; Campbell & Cluss, 1982). Observations of peer interaction in preschool confirmed that children identified as problems were significantly more likely than control children to engage in aggressive encounters with peers (Campbell & Cluss, 1982; Campbell, Pierce, March, Ewing, & Szumowski, 1994). Although most of these interchanges were struggles over a toy, consistent with the observations of Smith and Green (1975), several children were observed to approach other children and lash out physically by pushing, hitting, kicking, or biting. At times, these outbursts appeared to be unprovoked; at other times, they appeared to be overreactions to approaches from others. Whereas conflicts and resolutions over sharing toys may be an important facet in normal social development that facilitates more positive peer relations as sharing and perspective-taking develop, the angry, aggressive, and apparently unprovoked attacks we witnessed from several of our subjects may indeed be early precursors of more severe social problems. The more aggressive children in our sample continued to have difficulties at age 9 (Campbell & Ewing, 1990), including continued oppositional behavior, peer problems, and general difficulties in social adjustment at home and school.

Social Withdrawal

Although studies of social withdrawal are relatively rare, factors that include shy, withdrawn, and solitary behaviors usually emerge from factor-analytic studies of behavioral descriptions of young children (Achenbach, Edelbrock, & Howell, 1987; Behar, 1977; Kohn & Rosman,

1972). However, adults complain much less about excessively shy and withdrawn behavior than they do about aggression and management difficulties. For example, in the Crowther et al. (1981) study, caregivers rated fewer than 10% of 3- to 5-year-olds as highly bashful, avoidant of peer contact, or fearful of everyday situations or people. It may be that behaviors that are less attention-getting and annoying are rated as less severe problems or noted less often because they are less salient. However, Kohn and Parnes (1974) provided some data suggesting that teacher ratings of social withdrawal are valid reflections of amount of peer interaction. Preschoolers who were rated high on the apathetic-withdrawn dimension of Kohn's Social Competence Scale were also observed to interact less with peers, to be more solitary, and to cope less effectively with aggression from peers.

In a detailed analysis of the peer interactions of "normal" and "disturbed" preschoolers, Leach (1972) found that 3-year-olds who had difficulty separating from their mothers were less competent with peers. They initiated less interaction with peers, were less responsive to initiations from peers, and tended to withdraw or give in to aggressive interactions, for example, when a peer grabbed a toy. Over time, these children continued to interact less and to be less integrated into the peer group. Although newcomers into nursery school often show some initial social withdrawal and other adjustment problems (Hughes et al., 1979), they become integrated into the group relatively rapidly and over time are indistinguishable from peers (Feldbaum, Christenson, & O'Neal, 1980; McGrew, 1972). However, this was not the case with the youngsters in Leach's sample.

Early research on social withdrawal emphasized amount of interaction on the assumption that quantity of peer contact is a reflection of social competence. However, Gottman (1977a,b) questioned this assumption. He reported (1977a) that children selected because of a limited amount of peer interaction were not necessarily less popular with peers as assessed by sociometric measures of peer acceptance, and he

argued that peer rejection may be more important to examine than quantitative measures of peer interaction in the identification of high-risk children. Observational and sociometric data obtained on a large sample of preschool children in Head Start programs suggested that one group of poorly accepted children was frequently "tuned out" when alone. Rather than showing just low rates of social interaction, these youngsters were higher on observations of shy, anxious, and fearful behavior. Gottman argued that these were the true social isolates, as their incompetent social behavior was also associated with limited popularity with peers.

More recently, Rubin and his colleagues (Rubin, Hymel, Mills, & Rose-Krasnor, 1991; Rubin & Mills, 1988) have argued that the significance of social isolation, as reflected in shy, withdrawn, and socially incompetent behavior, has been underemphasized as one pathway to peer rejection and persistent social problems. In a prospective longitudinal study from kindergarten to Grade 5, Rubin et al. (1991) selected an extreme group of socially isolated children based on observations of play behavior. Children who spent more than the average amount of time as onlookers, unoccupied, or in solitary (usually less mature) play made up this group. There was evidence for a moderate degree of stability in this form of self-imposed social isolation, and these children were less assertive, took less social initiative, and their requests were more likely to be ignored by peers in elementary school than those of less socially isolated children. Although Rubin et al. (1991) argued that this form of social incompetence should lead to loneliness and depression, it is not entirely clear that these children are really at risk for clinically significant problems or that their social isolation continues indefinitely. Indeed, these youngsters were not rejected by peers or seen as significantly different from peers by teachers.

Several other studies also suggest that socially isolated behaviors show some temporal stability. Buss et al. (1980) found that teacher ratings of 3-year-olds as shy and reserved, withdrawn, and solitary were negatively correlated with objective and independent measures of activity level at age 3 and that these relationships persisted at ages 4 and 7. Kohn (1977) reported that children rated as apathetic-withdrawn in day care were less engaged with peers and continued to be perceived as socially withdrawn by their classroom teachers in Grade 3. They were also functioning less well academically than their more socially competent peers. However, other studies indicate that social withdrawal tends to be a transient phenomenon in preschoolers (Fagot, 1984; Fischer, Rolf, Hasazi, & Cummings, 1984).

This issue, therefore, is far from resolved. Further research on the empirical description of preschool children who are quiet and withdrawn and either ignored or overtly rejected by peers is obviously a priority if the socially incompetent preschool child is to be better understood. Although there is accumulating evidence that shy and quiet children are less at risk than their aggressive and disruptive peers (Asher, 1983; Parker & Asher, 1987), it is also true that this group is more difficult to define, and studies have been rare. For example, no studies could be found that followed severely anxious preschoolers with separation anxiety over time.

Taken together, these studies suggest that children who are perceived by their preschool teachers as socially withdrawn may continue to have problems, although these youngsters seem to be less likely to come to the attention of mental health professionals than their more active and aggressive counterparts. In addition, the relationship between social withdrawal and other signs of internalizing problems in preschoolers, such as excessive fearfulness, separation anxiety, and dysphoric mood, needs to be better understood before the long-term implications of these behaviors can be determined.

School Age

School Problems

Problems related to school functioning are among the most common reasons for referral to child mental health facilities. School problems tend to be relatively pervasive and to encompass learning and achievement problems, attentional and conduct problems, and impaired relationships with teachers and peers. They can run the gamut from delayed reading achievement and distractibility, which are reasonably common complaints of both parents and teachers (Rutter et al., 1970; Shepherd et al., 1971), to truancy and disruptive, aggressive behavior, which appear to vary with age, family dysfunction, and social conditions (Patterson et al., 1989; Robins, 1966).

There is wide agreement that achievement and behavior problems in school tend to covary, that they are associated with family disturbance, and that they are more common in boys (e.g., McGee et al., 1984; Moffitt, 1990; Offord et al., 1989; Rutter et al., 1970; Shepherd et al., 1971). For example, in the study by Shepherd et al., teachers rated approximately one-third of the boys and one-fourth of the girls in a sample of over 6000 youngsters as "below average" in school attainment. Poor achievers were also more likely to be rated as showing disruptive, uncooperative, and restless behavior in the classroom. However, when stricter, more specific, and more objective criteria of poor achievement are employed, rates go down. Rutter et al. (1970) classified children as showing specific reading retardation only if they were 28 months behind in reading and of average intelligence. The prevalence rate given these criteria was only 3.7% of 10- to 11-year-olds on the Isle of Wight. Reading disorders were associated with other cognitive deficits including poor spelling and arithmetic achievement and language dysfunction. Furthermore, poor readers came from larger families and were more likely to have conduct disorders in school.

Several large screening studies of school maladjustment in the United States indicate that when combined assessments are made utilizing teacher ratings and school achievement indices, roughly 30% of primary-school children are classified as "at risk" (Cowen et al., 1975; Glidewell & Swallow, 1969). For example, Cowen and his colleagues conducted a massive screening, intervention, and follow-up study of children identified by teacher ratings as "at risk" in the primary grades. Children identified as potentially maladjusted differed from classroom controls on measures of school achievement and peer popularity. Furthermore, within the high-risk group, family variables were related to patterns of disturbance. Children from families low in pressure to succeed in school were rated as less socially competent and more likely to have learning problems than other referred children (Gesten, Scher, & Cowen, 1978). Family crises were also associated with referral patterns. Children whose parents had recently separated or divorced were more likely to be referred to the mental health project for conduct disturbances than children not in family crisis (Felner, Stolberg, & Cowen, 1975). Overall, referral to the school-based program was associated with more stressful life events and family disruption as well as more chronic illness in the child (Cowen, Weissberg, & Guare, 1984). In particular, separation/divorce, remarriage, family illness, and financial hardship were more frequent in the families of poorly functioning children than in controls. Other studies have found a link between parental divorce (Guidubaldi & Perry, 1984) and other family stresses (Richman et al., 1982) and children's academic functioning.

Similarly, Bower (1969) screened over 5000 children in Grades 4 through 6 in California. Roughly 10% of the population were rated by teachers as showing some degree of maladjustment in school, and roughly 5% were referred for help. Referred children differed from classmates on a number of measures that closely parallel the findings of other studies (Cowen et al., 1975; Love & Kaswan, 1974). Referred children were behind their classmates in reading and arithmetic, scored lower on a measure of intelligence, had poorer self-esteem, and were more likely to be perceived negatively by peers.

Taken together, then, a number of studies indicate that problems in school are a source of concern to parents and teachers and that relatively large numbers of children do not function optimally in the school environment. Furthermore, children identified by school personnel as showing poor adjustment perform less well than peers on measures of achievement, are less competent socially, and are more likely to have behavior problems in school. Finally, these deficits are associated with varying types and degrees of family disturbances, as well as with poor peer relationships (e.g., Patterson et al., 1989).

Peer Problems

It is obvious from the preceding section that school, family, and peer problems tend to occur together, and there is increasing interest in the important role peer interaction plays in both normal (Hartup, 1983) and deviant development (Campbell, 1990; Coie & Cillessen, 1993; Parker & Asher, 1987). It is widely accepted among child development theorists that many aspects of socialization are facilitated by give-and-take within the peer group (Hartup, 1983). Furthermore, there is a converging body of evidence linking success with peers to psychological adjustment and academic achievement across a wide age span (e.g., Ladd, 1990). Children who are both socially and academically competent tend to be more popular with peers (Asher, 1983; Hartup, 1983), whereas unpopular children or children who are not socially competent are more likely to experience adjustment difficulties and to achieve less academically (Coie & Cillessen, 1993; Hartup, 1983).

A number of studies also indicate that children with externalizing symptoms such as hyperactivity, aggressivity, and disruptive behavior in school are perceived more negatively by peers (Klein & Young, 1979; Pelham & Bender, 1982). For example, Klein and Young (1979) reported that hyperactive boys were perceived more negatively by their classmates and were observed to engage in more negative interactions than active but normal classroom controls. Pelham and Bender (1982) found that hyperactive children were rejected by peers after only brief interactions in newly formed play groups.

Parents and teachers also are likely to rate referred children as having more problems with peers than controls (Campbell & Paulauskas, 1979; Cowen et al., 1984; Klein & Young, 1979; Love & Kaswan, 1974). For instance, Love and Kaswan (1974) found that children referred to a school-based mental health program were more likely to receive a high rating from teachers on a series of items reflecting "negative social impact," while they were perceived as lower in "social assets" than controls. Independent observations by "blind" observers indicated that referred children disrupted peer play on the playground more often than controls. Other studies of referral patterns to school-based mental health programs indicate that referred youngsters are perceived by teachers as having problems getting along with other children, because they are either too aggressive and domineering or too timid and unassertive (Bower, 1969; Cowen et al., 1975; Gesten et al., 1978).

Whereas it is thus relatively clear that poor peer relations are a concomitant of problem behavior in referred groups, it is also true that behaviors that may be construed as symptomatic of peer difficulties are relatively common in the general population. For example, teachers in the Werry and Quay (1971) study rated roughly 30% of the boys in the sample as aggressive and uncooperative in group situations. Ratings of shyness were also common; 33% of boys and 41% of girls were perceived as shy. Approximately 13% of children in the Isle of Wight study (Rutter et al., 1970) were rated by teachers as "not liked" by peers and 15% were rated as solitary. Furthermore, children who were rated high on number of problems were also more likely to be perceived as "not liked" by both parents and teachers.

Attempts have been made to define differences between popular and unpopular children in behavioral terms so as to better understand why some children are not liked by peers. Distinctions have been made between subgroups of unpopular children, that is, those who are rejected, those who are neglected or ignored, as well as children of high social impact termed *controversial* (Coie & Cillessen, 1993; Coie & Kupersmidt, 1983). These subgroups, selected on the basis of positive and negative peer nominations, have been compared with popular and average children (Coie & Kupersmidt, 1983; Dodge, 1983). Findings indicate that many rejected children tend to engage in inappropriate, disruptive, and aggressive behaviors, whereas neglected children appear shy and withdrawn, as well as somewhat inappropriate in their play (Coie & Kupersmit, 1983; Dodge, 1983). Controversial children, on the other hand, engage in high rates of both prosocial and negative, disruptive behaviors that appear to elicit both admiration and annoyance from peers. In one recent study, Bierman, Smoot, and Aumiller (1993) differentiated between aggressive-rejected and nonaggressive-rejected 6- to 12-year-old boys, using peer nominations and extensive observations in the natural environment. They found that nonaggressive-rejected boys were shy and socially awkward and were inept at reading social cues, but they were not social isolates.

Prospective studies of group formation indicate that the aggressive and provocative behaviors characteristic of many rejected children lead to rejection by peers, rather than vice versa; negative reputation does not, by itself, elicit inappropriate behavior (Dodge, 1983). Other studies reveal that children who are rejected because of aggressive and disruptive behavior in one group behave similarly in a new group and that negative social status is quite stable. Children who are rejected consistently not only tend to show aggression, they tend to show limited prosocial behavior or concern for others (Coie & Cillessen, 1993), and they tend to bully peers and violate social norms (Coie, Dodge, Terry, & Wright, 1991). However, children who are neglected in one setting may not be so in another, highlighting some situational factors in shy and withdrawn behavior (Asher, 1983).

Dodge (1986) proposed a theory of social information processing that posits that encoding, cue interpretation, and response evaluations all influence the utilization of social information, which, in turn, should influence social behavior. He demonstrated that processing biases in aggressive children (Dodge & Frame, 1982) tend to increase the likelihood of aggressive responses to the behavior of others in ambiguous situations involving threats to self-esteem or provocations. Aggressive boys are more likely to attribute aggressive intentions to others in ambiguous circumstances and then to retaliate aggressively. Dodge, Pettit, McClaskey, and Brown (1986) also have demonstrated relationships among social information processing, social behavior, and peers' evaluations of social competence, indicating that cognitive processing biases clearly do influence actual behavior with peers. In addition, parenting factors have been implicated in the development of aggressive behavior and negative attributional biases (Weiss, Dodge, Bates, & Pettit, 1992). Harsh, punitive discipline predicted later aggression with peers, and was mediated, in part, by hostile attributional biases. The implications of these findings for prevention and intervention appear obvious (Coie & Jacobs, 1993; Reid, 1993); they are being applied in the multisite, multimodal prevention program called FAST Track (Conduct Problems Prevention Research Group, 1992) in which parenting styles, social information processing, and peer relations in high-risk children, identified as noncompliant and aggressive, are among the targets of intervention.

Studies have also examined the social behavior of clinically defined groups. As noted above, children with externalizing symptoms are more negative and disruptive when observed with peers in the classroom (Abikoff, Gittelman, & Klein, 1980; Klein & Young, 1979) and in relatively unstructured play groups (Pelham & Bender, 1982). Pelham and Bender observed 5- to 9-year-old hyperactive children with normal peers during both free play and cooperative, structured activities over five sessions. Hyperactive (ADD) children were more talkative, disruptive, aggressive, and noncompliant and engaged in more teasing and name calling than controls. Furthermore, disruptive and annoying behavior was more pronounced during free

play. Although these behaviors appear to reflect presenting complaints that may lead to peer rejection (Dodge, 1983; Pelham & Bender, 1982), there is also evidence to suggest that children with behavior problems, like the aggressive boys studied by Dodge, process social information in ways that increase their tendency to behave inappropriately.

Learning-disabled and hyperactive youngsters have been found to communicate with peers less efficiently than controls in several studies (e.g., Bryan, 1977; Whalen & Henker, 1985). In referential communication tasks and tasks requiring group decision-making, hyperactive children are less responsive to communications from others, more likely to ignore peers or behave inappropriately, and less likely to provide partners with task-relevant information (see Whalen & Henker, 1985, for a review). Milich and Dodge (1984) extended work on social information processing biases to clinical populations. Hyperactive-aggressive boys were more likely to attribute hostile intent to peers, to report that they would retaliate with aggression in ambiguous situations, and to make rapid decisions about the behavior of others in the absence of complete information. These data may be interpreted to suggest that the impulsivity and inattention characteristic of hyperactive children interfere with social information processing and also contribute to their well-documented problems with peers. These issues are addressed more fully by Whalen and Henker (this volume).

In summary, it appears that social competence with peers is reflected in peer popularity and that more skilled children also are better adjusted. Continued research on the specific behaviors that contribute to more versus less competent peer relations is an important goal. However, this area has seen remarkable progress in the last few years, with clear evidence linking harsh and dysfunctional family processes, children's hostile and negative attributional biases, and low social competence (Conduct Problems Prevention Research Group, 1992; Weiss et al., 1992). Prevention and treatment programs that include social behavior and social cognitive processes as foci of intervention along with parenting styles offer one hopeful avenue for changes in developmental processes that have seemed relatively resistant to less comprehensive, more piecemeal approaches.

LONGITUDINAL PERSPECTIVES: THE NATURAL COURSE OF CHILDHOOD PROBLEMS

A thorough understanding of the developmental features of childhood behavior problems hinges on knowledge of the developmental course of the more common symptoms and disorders. Although studies on the developmental course of behavior problems can only give clues to etiology, they provide important information on who is at risk for continued disorder, who is likely to improve without treatment, and who is likely to develop a disorder at a later date. In addition, correlates of positive and negative outcome help define populations that are vulnerable to the onset or persistence of disorder. Although cross-sectional studies suggest that changes in symptoms occur as a function of age (e.g., Lapouse & Monk, 1958; Werry & Quay, 1971), only follow-up studies that examine the same children over time can provide accurate information on changes in problem behaviors and the relative prognostic importance of particular clusters of symptoms. Gersten et al. (1976) found that several behaviors that appeared to decrease with age when examined cross-sectionally, failed to show similar changes when data were analyzed longitudinally so as to assess stability and change over time in the same subjects; this highlights the problems of making longitudinal inferences from cross-sectional findings.

From both a research and a clinical perspective, then, it is essential that we learn more about the meaning and prognostic significance of potentially problematic behaviors. For example, which difficult infants are truly at risk to develop later problems and which problems specifically? What aspects, if any, of preschool aggression or social withdrawal are early precursors of later problems? What family processes and childrearing strategies are likely to exacerbate or ameliorate early problems? Only prospective studies will provide clear answers to such questions. Related issues of primary prevention and early intervention are beyond the scope of this chapter.

Early longitudinal studies of nonclinical populations (MacFarlane et al., 1954) suggested that the majority of symptoms experienced by young children were transient developmental phenomena. Such findings led Robins (1979) to conclude that patterns of symptoms appearing before age 6 were of little predictive significance. However, a review of several recent follow-up studies of young children suggests that this conclusion was incorrect.

In an early study, Westman, Rice, and Bermann (1967) reported that ratings of poor adjustment in preschool were associated with use of mental health services during elementary and high school. Family problems and poor peer relationships were predictive of later problems, whereas "immaturity" was not. Two additional follow-up studies of nonclinical samples of preschoolers suggested that patterns of angry-defiant behavior and apathetic-withdrawn behavior persisted into the early elementary school grades and that aggressive and hyperactive behaviors were also associated with poorer cognitive functioning in the primary grades (Halverson & Waldrop, 1976; Kohn, 1977). On the other hand, symptoms such as enuresis and fears declined with increasing age, whereas others such as discipline problems and poor peer relationships did not (Coleman et al., 1977; Richman et al., 1982).

Hughes et al. (1979) followed a sample of preschoolers for 18 months after school entry. Thirteen percent were assessed by teachers as showing serious adjustment problems initially. Many of these problems were transient reactions that appeared to abate as the child adapted to school, although as many as 56% of those children having initial difficulties continued to have specific problems. Similarly, Chazan and Jackson (1974) reported that 43% of 5-year-olds who were identified as having problems continued to experience problems when followed at age 7. Fischer et al. (1984) reported that externalizing, but not internalizing, problems persisted in approximately 30% of children identified as having difficulties 7 years earlier in preschool.

Several large-scale studies are consistent with the view that early externalizing problems persist and become clinically significant in a relatively large proportion of children. Moreover, ongoing and concurrent family stresses and severity of initial symptoms appear to predict outcome. Richman et al. (1982) followed up a sample of 96 behavior-problem preschoolers, identified at age 3 in an epidemiological study conducted in London. Each problem child was matched with a control child from a larger, representative sample. At 1-year follow-up, mothers continued to rate 63% of the problem group as showing at least mild problems; ratings of problem behavior were confirmed by clinician judgments. Continued follow-up to age 8 indicated at least mild problems in 62% of the problem group, with 43% scoring above a cutoff indicative of high risk for behavioral and emotional disorder. Teacher ratings confirmed parental reports. Boys with more severe initial problems, characterized as overactive and difficult to manage, were most likely to have continuing problems. At age 8, problem children were described as more inattentive, fidgety, difficult to control, and as less competent with peers than controls. Family problems including maternal depression, marital distress, and a poor mother–child relationship were associated with concurrent problems at each time period. Furthermore, persistent and severe family problems were associated with the onset of difficulties in children who had not had earlier problems. However, problems in girls and internalizing problems were more likely to be transient.

Two other recent studies provide findings convergent with those of Richman and her colleagues. In our own work, we have followed a sample of parent-identified hard-to-manage 3-year-olds and controls. Half of the problem group continued to evidence clinically significant difficulties at school entry (Campbell et al., 1986). Maternal ratings of hyperactivity, aggression, and peer problems were confirmed by observational measures in the classroom and by teacher ratings. Social class, severity of initial symptoms, and a negative mother–child interaction predicted persistent problems at age 9, and concurrent family stress also was associated with parental reports of problem behavior (Campbell & Ewing, 1990). Persistent problems through age 9 were also predictive of problems in early adolescence (Ewing & Campbell, 1995). We have now replicated these findings in a second cohort of hard-to-manage preschool boys with externalizing symptoms. More extreme early problems were likely to persist and persistent problems were associated with family stress and maternal depression (Campbell, 1994).

Data from the Dunedin study of child health and development (e.g., McGee et al., 1984, 1990; Moffitt, 1990) also suggest that problems identified at preschool age and in the early elementary school grades may persist; consistent with the findings of both Richman and Campbell, family adversity was associated with a poorer outcome in middle childhood and adolescence. In addition, more severe and continuing problems were associated with cognitive difficulties in the Dunedin sample (Moffitt, 1990). This work is reviewed more thoroughly in Campbell (1995). Numerous studies also indicate that problems identified in early elementary school are likely to persist into adolescence (e.g., Barkley et al., 1990; Gersten et al., 1976; Rutter et al., 1970; Weiss & Hechtman, 1993) and young adulthood (Robins, 1966; Weiss & Hechtman, 1993). Indeed, work by Eron and Huesmann (1990) suggested that aggressive and antisocial behavior in childhood is stable across generations and is implicated in arrest records, marital distress, and inept parenting (see also Patterson et al., 1989).

Thus, accumulating evidence suggests that a small proportion of children with early problems continue to show later difficulties, often at a clinically significant level of symptomatology. Moreover, developmental models of child psychopathology (e.g., Campbell, 1990; Cicchetti & Richters, 1993; Greenberg et al., 1993; Patterson et al., 1989; Reid, 1993) implicate early problems involving management and self-control in the onset of later more pervasive and serious externalizing disorders. Both research and theoretical models also underscore the importance of parenting style, family dysfunction, parent–child conflict, and maternal mental health problems as likely precursors and/or correlates of child maladjustment and suggest directions for early intervention efforts (e.g., Conduct Problems Prevention Research Group, 1992; Greenberg et al., 1993; Reid, 1993).

On the other hand, internalizing disorders including neurotic, withdrawn, anxious, and psychosomatic complaints appear less persistent. Rates of adult disturbance did not differentiate Robins's (1996) neurotic child guidance cases from controls. Similarly, Gersten et al. (1976) found less stability among internalizing behaviors such as social isolation and anxiety than among more aggressive behaviors. Other studies of clinical groups report findings consistent with these, indicating that neurotic symptoms in childhood are less likely than externalizing symptoms to be associated with serious adult disorders (e.g., Hafner, Quast, & Shea, 1975). However, very little research has focused on internalizing disorders in young children or examined the developmental coarse of anxiety, social isolation, and severe separation anxiety.

Continued research into early precursors of behavior disturbances and their family and environmental correlates, as well as on predictors of good and poor outcome, is a priority if we are to progress beyond the level of description and classification of childhood problems to an understanding of developmental processes and developmental course. Although this review has emphasized the persistence of externalizing problems, it is also the case that between 50 and 70% of children with early signs of attentional, conduct, and peer problems improve over time, underlining the importance of identifying both risk and protective factors (Garmezy, 1987; Werner, 1993). Finally, successful amelioration of potential problems requires the design and initiation of appropriately targeted prevention and early intervention programs that must select at-risk populations likely to develop significant and persistent disorders, and focus on processes thought to initiate and/or maintain early problems (e.g., Conduct Problems Prevention Research Group, 1992). Data on precursors, correlates, and outcome of disorders in children are an essential first step in this endeavor.

SUMMARY

This chapter examined childhood behavior problems from a developmental perspective. Several ways in which developmental factors may influence problem definitions, diagnostic formulations, treatment recommendations, and predictions about outcome were briefly explored. It was noted that patterns of childhood referral and parental help-seeking about childhood problems are largely a function of the expectations adults have about child behavior rather than a result of clearly deviant behavior. Furthermore, the psychological state of parents influences parental tolerance and plays a role in determining which children are referred and treated.

Epidemiological studies of specific problem behaviors and prevalence rates of actual disorder as a function of age and sex were reviewed next. Although it is clear that symptomatic behaviors are common in the general population, estimates of actual disorder, based on clusters of symptoms that interfere with functioning, are relatively low. Furthermore, rates of both symptoms and disorders appear to vary with the age and sex of the sample.

Several common developmental problems were examined in the next section, with emphasis on their appearance at a particular stage of development. They were conceptualized as exaggerations of age-appropriate behaviors, reflections of difficult transitions from one developmental stage to the next, or as age-related but maladaptive reactions to environmental, particularly family, stress. Examples include attachment problems in infancy, defiance and aggression among toddlers and preschoolers, and peer difficulties among older children. Research on these behaviors was critically examined, integrating studies on both "normal" and clinical populations when possible. An attempt also was made to draw inferences about the potential long-term developmental impact of such behaviors. In general, it appears that common developmental problems may be a warning signal; the skill with which they are handled at a particular stage of development will partly determine whether such problems are indeed transient or are precursors of more severe and persistent difficulties.

Finally, follow-up studies were examined. They generally suggest that problems among preschoolers are not transient as was once assumed, especially when associated with family dysfunction or parental psychopathology. When behavior disorders in school-age samples include primarily externalizing symptoms, they appear to have a poorer prognosis than disorders characterized primarily by internalizing symptoms. However, research and conceptual models need to focus on mechanisms rather than description before clear guidelines for prevention or intervention can be established.

REFERENCES

Abikoff, H., Gittelman, R., & Klein, D. F. (1980). Classroom observation code for hyperactive children: A replication of validity. *Journal of Consulting and Clinical Psychology, 48,* 555–565.

Achenbach, T. M., & Edelbrock, C. (1983). *Manual for the Child Behavior Checklist and the Revised Child Behavior Profile.* Burlington, VT: Queen City Printers.

Achenbach, T. M., Edelbrock, C., & Howell, C. T. (1987).

Empirically based assessment of the behavioral/emotional problems of 2- and 3-year-old children. *Journal of Abnormal Child Psychology, 15,* 629–650.

Achenbach, T. M., Howell, C. T., Quay, C. T., & Conners, C. K. (1991). National survey of problems and competencies among four-to-sixteen-year olds: Parents' reports from normative and clinical samples. *Monographs of the Society for Research in Child Development, 56*(Serial No. 225).

Achenbach, T. M., McConaughy, S. H., & Howell, C. T. (1987). Child/adolescent behavioral and emotional problems: Implications of cross-informant correlations for situational specificity. *Psychological Bulletin, 101,* 213–232.

Ainsworth, M. D. S. (1969). Object relations, dependency, and attachment: A theoretical review of the infant–mother relationship. *Child Development, 40,* 969–1025.

Ainsworth, M. D. S., Blehar, M., Waters, E., & Wall, S. (1978). *Patterns of attachment.* Hillsdale, NJ: Erlbaum.

Ainsworth, M. D. S., & Wittig, B. A. (1969). Attachment and exploratory behavior of one-year-olds in a strange situation. In B. M. Foss (Ed.), *Determinants of infant behavior* (Vol. IV, pp. 113–136). London: Methuen.

American Psychiatric Association. (1994). *Diagnostic and statistical manual of mental disorders* (4th ed. rev.). Washington, DC: Author.

Angold, A., & Costello, E. J. (1993). Depressive comorbidity in children and adolescents: Empirical, theoretical, and methodological issues. *American Journal of Psychiatry, 150,* 1779–1791.

Asher, S. (1983). Social competence and peer status: Recent advances and future directions. *Child Development, 54,* 1427–1434.

Axline, V. M. (1969). *Play therapy* (rev. ed.). New York: Ballantine Books.

Baker, L., Cantwell, D. P., & Mattison, R. E. (1980). Behavior problems in children with pure speech disorders and in children with combined speech and language disorders. *Journal of Abnormal Child Psychology, 8,* 245–256.

Barkley, R. A. (1990). *Hyperactive children: A handbook for diagnosis and treatment.* New York: Guilford Press.

Barkley, R. A., Fischer, M., Edelbrock, C., & Smallish, L. (1990). The adolescent outcome of hyperactive children diagnosed by research criteria: I. An 8-year prospective follow-up study. *Journal of the American Academy of Child and Adolescent Psychiatry, 29,* 546–557.

Bates, J. E., & Bayles, K. (1988). The role of attachment in the development of behavior problems. In J. Belsky & T. Nezworski (Eds.), *Clinical implications of attachment* (pp. 253–299). Hillsdale, NJ: Erlbaum.

Bates, J. E., Freeland, C. A. B., & Lounsbury, M. L. (1979). Measurement of infant difficultness. *Child Development, 50,* 794–803.

Bates, J. E., Maslin, C. A., & Frankel, K. A. (1985). Attachment security, mother–child interaction, and temperament as predictors of behavior problem ratings at age three years. In I. Bretherton & E. Waters (Eds.), Growing points of attachment theory and research. *Monographs of the Society for Research in Child Development, 50*(Serial No. 209). 167–193.

Battle, E. S., & Lacey, B. (1972). A context for hyperactivity in children over time. *Child Development, 43,* 757–773.

Beck, A. T. (1972). *Depression: Causes and treatment.* Philadelphia: University of Pennsylvania Press.

Behar, L. (1977). The Preschool Behavior Questionnaire. *Journal of Abnormal Child Psychology, 5,* 265–276.

Bell, R. Q., & Harper, L. V. (1977). *Child effects on adults.* Hillsdale, NJ: Erlbaum.

Belsky, J. (1984). Determinants of parenting: A process model. *Child Development, 55,* 83–96.

Belsky, J., Taylor, D. G., & Rovine, M. (1984). The Pennsylvania Infant and Family Development Project, III: The origins of individual differences in infant–mother attachment: Maternal and infant contributions. *Child Development, 55,* 718–728.

Bierman, K. L., Smoot, D. L., & Aumiller, K. (1993). Characteristics of aggressive-rejected, aggressive (nonrejected), and rejected (nonaggressive) boys. *Child Development, 64,* 139–151.

Billman, J., & McDevitt, S. C. (1980). Convergence of parent and observer ratings of temperament with observations of peer interaction in nursery school. *Child Development, 51,* 395–400.

Blurton-Jones, N. (1972). Categories of child–child interaction. In N. Blurton-Jones (Ed.), *Ethological studies in child behavior* (pp. 97–128). London: Cambridge University Press.

Bower, E. M. (1969). *Early identification of emotionally handicapped children in school* (2nd ed.). Springfield, IL: Charles C. Thomas.

Bowlby, J. (1969). *Attachment and loss: Vol 1. Attachment.* New York: Basic Books.

Brazelton, T. B. (1973). *The Neonatal Behavioral Assessment Scale.* Clinics in Developmental Medicine, No. 50. Philadelphia: Lippincott.

Brazelton, T. B. (1974). *Toddlers and parents.* New York: Delta.

Brazelton, T. B., Koslowski, B., & Main, M. (1974). The origins of reciprocity: The early mother–infant interaction. In M. Lewis & L. Rosenblum (Eds.), *The effect of the infant on its caregiver* (pp. 49–76). New York: Wiley.

Bretherton, I. (1985). Attachment theory: Retrospect and prospect. In I. Bretherton & E. Waters (Eds.), Growing points of attachment theory and research. *Monographs of the Society for Research in Child Development, 50*(Serial No. 209), 3–35.

Bryan, T. H. (1977). Learning disabled children's comprehension on non-verbal communication. *Journal of Learning Disabilities, 10,* 36–41.

Buss, D. M., Block, J. H., & Block, J. (1980). Preschool activity level: Personality correlates and developmental implications. *Child Development, 51,* 401–408.

Campbell, S. B. (1979). Patterns of mother–infant interaction and maternal ratings of temperament. *Child Psychiatry and Human Development, 10,* 67–76.

Campbell, S. B. (1990). *Behavior problems in preschool children: Clinical and developmental issues.* New York: Guilford Press.

Campbell, S. B. (1994). Hard-to-manage preschool boys: Externalizing behavior, social competence, and family context at two-year follow-up. *Journal of Abnormal Child Psychology, 22,* 147–166.

Campbell, S. B. (1995). Behavior problems in preschool children: A review of recent research. *Journal of Child Psychology and Psychiatry, 36,* 113–149.

Campbell, S. B., & Cluss, P. (1982). Peer relations of young children with behavior problems. In K. H. Rubin & H. S. Ross (Eds.), *Peer relationships and social skills in childhood* (pp. 323–351). Berlin: Springer-Verlag.

Campbell, S. B., & Cohn, J. F. (1997). The timing and chronicity of postpartum depression: Implications for infant development. In L. Murray & P. Cooper (Eds.), *Postpartum depression and child development* (pp. 165–197). New York: Guilford Press.

Campbell, S. B., Endman, M., & Bernfeld, G. (1977). A three-year follow-up of hyperactive preschoolers into elementary school. *Journal of Child Psychology and Psychiatry, 18,* 239–250.

Campbell, S. B., & Ewing, L. J. (1990). Hard-to-manage preschoolers: Adjustment at age nine and predictors of continuing symptoms. *Journal of Child Psychology and Psychiatry, 31,* 871–889.

Campbell, S. B., Ewing, L. J., Breaux, A. M., & Szumowski, E. K. (1986). Parent-referred problem three-year-olds: Follow-up at school entry. *Journal of Child Psychology and Psychiatry, 27,* 473–488.

Campbell, S. B., & Paulauskas, S. L. (1979). Peer relations in hyperactive children. *Journal of Child Psychology and Psychiatry, 20,* 233–246.

Campbell, S. B., Pierce, E., March, C., & Ewing, L. J. (1991). Noncompliant behavior, overactivity, and family stress as predictors of negative maternal control in preschool children. *Development and Psychopathology, 3,* 175–190.

Campbell, S. B., Pierce, E., March, C., Ewing, L. J., & Szumowski, E. K. (1994). Hard-to-manage preschool boys: Symptomatic behavior across contexts and time. *Child Development, 65,* 836–851.

Campbell, S. B., Schleifer, M., & Weiss, G. (1978). Continuities in maternal reports and child behaviors over time in hyperactive and comparison groups. *Journal of Abnormal Child Psychology, 6,* 33–45.

Campbell, S. B., Szumowski, E. K., Ewing, L. J., Gluck, D. S., & Breaux, A. M. (1982). A multidimensional assessment of parent-identified behavior problem toddlers. *Journal of Abnormal Child Psychology, 10,* 569–592.

Campos, J., Mumme, D. L., Kermoian, R., & Campos, R. G. (1994). A functionalist perspective on the nature of emotion. In N. A. Fox (Ed.), The development of emotion regulation. *Monographs of the Society for Research in Child Development, 59*(2–3), 284–303.

Carey, W. B. (1972). Measurement of infant temperament in pediatric practice. In J. C. Westman (Ed.), *Individual differences in children* (pp. 293–308). New York: Wiley.

Carlson, V., Cicchetti, D., Barnett, D., & Braunwald, K. (1989). Disorganized/disoriented attachment relationships in maltreated infants. *Developmental Psychology, 25*, 525–531.

Chazan, M., & Jackson, S. (1974). Behaviour problems in the infant school: Changes over two years. *Journal of Child Psychology and Psychiatry, 15*, 33–46.

Cicchetti, D., & Richters, J. E. (1993). Developmental considerations in the investigation of conduct disorder. *Development and Psychopathology, 5*, 331–344.

Cicchetti, D., Rogosch, F. A., Lynch, M., & Holt, K. D. (1993). Resilience in maltreated children: Processes leading to adaptive outcome. *Development and Psychopathology, 5*, 629–647.

Cohen, N. J., Sullivan, J., Minde, K., Novak, C., & Helwig, C. (1981). Evaluation of the relative effectiveness of methylphenidate and cognitive behavior modification in the treatment of kindergarten-aged hyperactive children. *Journal of Abnormal Child Psychology, 9*, 43–54.

Coie, J. D., & Cillessen, A. H. (1993). Peer rejection: Origins and effects on children's development. *Current Directions in Psychological Science, 2*, 89–92.

Coie, J., Dodge, K. A., Terry, R., & Wright, V. (1991). The role of aggression in peer relations: An analysis of aggression episodes in boys' play groups. *Child Development, 62*, 812–826.

Coie, J. D., & Jacobs, M. R. (1993). The role of social context in the prevention of conduct disorder. *Development and Psychopathology, 5*, 263–275.

Coie, J. D., & Kupersmidt, J. B. (1983). A behavioral analysis of emerging social status in boys' groups. *Child Development, 54*, 1400–1416.

Coleman, J., Wolkind, S., & Ashley, L. (1977). Symptoms of behaviour disturbance and adjustment to school. *Journal of Child Psychology and Psychiatry, 18*, 201–210.

Colletti, G., & Harris, S. L. (1977). Behavior modification in the home: Siblings as behavior modifiers, parents as observers. *Journal of Abnormal Child Psychology, 5*, 21–30.

Conduct Problems Prevention Research Group. (1992). A developmental and clinical model for the prevention of conduct disorder: The FAST Track Program. *Development and Psychopathology, 4*, 509–527.

Conger, R. D., McCarty, J. A., Yang, R. K., Lahey, B. B., & Kropp, J. P. (1984). Perception of child, child-rearing values, and emotional distress as mediating links between environmental stressors and observed maternal behavior. *Child Development, 55*, 2234–2247.

Cornely, P., & Bromet, E. J. (1986). Prevalence of behavior problems in three-year-old children living near Three Mile Island: A comparative analysis. *Journal of Child Psychology and Psychiatry, 27*, 489–498.

Cowen, E. L., Trost, M. A., Izzo, L. D., Lorion, R. P., Dorr, D., & Isaacson, R. V. (1975). *New ways in school mental health. Early detection and prevention of school maladaptation.* New York: Human Sciences Press.

Cowen, E. L., Weissberg, R. P., & Guare, J. (1984). Differentiating attributes of children referred to a school mental health clinic. *Journal of Abnormal Child Psychology, 12*, 397–410.

Crockenberg, S. B. (1981). Infant irritability, mother responsiveness, and social support influences on the security of mother–infant attachment. *Child Development, 52*, 857–865.

Crockenberg, S., & Litman, C. (1990). Autonomy as competence in 2-year-olds: Maternal correlates of child defiance, compliance and self-assertion. *Developmental Psychology, 26*, 961–971.

Crowther, J. K., Bond, L. A., & Rolf, J. E. (1981). The incidence, prevalence and severity of behavior disorders among preschool-age children in day care. *Journal of Abnormal Child Psychology, 9*, 23–42.

Cutrona, C. E., & Troutman, B. R. (1986). Social support, infant temperament, and parenting self-efficacy: A mediational model of postpartum depression. *Child Development, 57*, 1507–1518.

DeMulder, E. K., & Radke-Yarrow, M. (1991). Attachment with affectively ill and well mothers: Concurrent behavioral correlates. *Development and Psychopathology, 3*, 227–242.

Dodge, K. A. (1983). Behavioral antecedents of peer social status. *Child Development, 54*, 1386–1399.

Dodge, K. A. (1986). A social information processing model of social competence in children. In M. Perlmutter (Ed.), *Minnesota Symposium on Child Psychology* (Vol. 18, pp. 77–125). Hillsdale, NJ: Erlbaum.

Dodge, K. A., & Frame, C. L. (1982). Social cognitive biases and deficits in aggressive boys. *Child Development, 53*, 620–635.

Dodge, K. A., Pettit, G. S., McClaskey, C. L., & Brown, M. M. (1986). Social competence in children. *Monographs of the Society for Research in Child Development, 51*(Serial No. 213).

Dumas, J., & Wahler, R. G. (1985). Indiscriminate mothering as a contextual factor in aggressive-oppositional child behavior: "Damned if you do and damned if you don't." *Journal of Abnormal Child Psychology, 13*, 1–18.

Dunn, J. (1988). *The growth of social understanding.* Cambridge, MA: Harvard University Press.

Emery, R. E. (1982). Interparental conflict and the children of discord and divorce. *Psychological Bulletin, 92*, 310–330.

Eron, L. D., & Huesmann, L. R. (1990). The stability of aggressive behavior - even into the third generation. In M. Lewis & S. Miller (Eds.), *Handbook of developmental psychopathology* (pp. 147–156). New York: Plenum Press.

Ewing, L. J., & Campbell, S. B. (1995, April). *Hard-to-manage preschoolers: Social competence, externalizing behavior, and social competence at early adolescence.* Poster presented at the Society for Research in Child Development, Indianapolis, IN.

Fagot, B. (1984). The consequents of problem behavior in toddler children. *Journal of Abnormal Child Psychology, 1,* 248–256.

Feldbaum, C. L., Christenson, T. E., & O'Neal, E. C. (1980). An observational study of the assimilation of the newcomer to the preschool. *Child Development, 51,* 497–507.

Felner, R. D., Stolberg, A., & Cowen, E. L. (1975). Crisis events and school mental health referral patterns of young children. *Journal of Consulting and Clinical Psychology, 43,* 305–310.

Ferguson, L. R., Partyka, L. B., & Lester, B. M. (1974). Patterns of parent perception differentiating clinic from non-clinic children. *Journal of Abnormal Child Psychology, 2,* 169–182.

Feshbach, N., & Feshbach, S. (1972). Children's aggression. In W. W. Hartup (Ed.), *The young child: Reviews of research* (Vol. 2, pp. 284–302). Washington, DC: National Association for the Education of Young Children.

Fischer, M., Rolf, J. E., Hasazi, H. E., & Cummings, L. (1984). Follow-up of a preschool epidemiological sample: Cross-age continuities and predictions of later adjustment with internalizing and externalizing dimensions of behavior. *Child Development, 55,* 137–150.

Forehand, R., & Scarboro, M. E. (1975). An analysis of children's oppositional behavior. *Journal of Abnormal Child Psychology, 3,* 27–32.

Frankel, K. A., & Bates, J. E. (1990). Mother–toddler problem solving: Antecedents in attachment, home behavior, and temperament. *Child Development, 60,* 810–819.

Freud, A. (1965). *Normality and pathology in childhood.* New York: International Universities Press.

Garmezy, N. (1987). Stress, competence, and development: The search for stress-resistant children. *American Journal of Orthopsychiatry, 57,* 159–174.

Gath, D. (1968). Child guidance and the general practitioner. A study of factors influencing referrals made by general practitioners to a child psychiatric department. *Journal of Child Psychology and Psychiatry, 9,* 213–227.

Gersten, J. C., Langner, T. S., Eisenberg, J. G., Simcha-Fagan, O., & McCarthy, E. D. (1976). Stability and change in types of behavioral disturbances of children and adolescents. *Journal of Abnormal Child Psychology, 4,* 111–128.

Gesten, E. L., Scher, K., & Cowen, E. L. (1978). Judged school problems and competencies of referred children with varying family background characteristics. *Journal of Abnormal Child Psychology, 6,* 247–256.

Gittelman, R., Mannuzza, S., Shenker, R., & Bonagura, N. (1985). Hyperactive boys almost grown up: I. Psychiatric status. *Archives of General Psychiatry, 42,* 937–947.

Glidewell, J. C., & Swallow, C. S. (1969). *The prevalence of maladjustment in elementary school: A report prepared for the*

Joint Commission on the Mental Health of Children. Chicago: University of Chicago Press.

Gottman, J. (1977a). The effects of a modeling film on social isolation in preschool children: A methodological investigation. *Journal of Abnormal Child Psychology, 5,* 69–78.

Gottman, J. (1977b). Toward a definition of social isolation in children. *Child Development, 48,* 513–517.

Greenberg, M. T., Speltz, M. L., & DeKlyen, M. (1993). The role of attachment in the early development of disruptive behavior problems. *Development and Psychopathology, 5,* 191–213.

Guidubaldi, J., & Perry, J. D. (1984). Divorce, socioeconomic status, and children's cognitive-social competence at school entry. *American Journal of Orthopsychiatry, 54,* 459–468.

Hafner, A. J., Quast, W., & Shea, M. J. (1975). The adult adjustment of one thousand psychiatric and pediatric patients: Initial findings from a twenty-five-year follow-up. In R. D. Wirt, G. Winokur, & M. Roff (Eds.), *Life history research in psychopathology* (Vol. 4, pp. 167–186). Minneapolis: University of Minnesota Press.

Halverson, C. F., & Waldrop, M. (1976). Relations between preschool activity and aspects of intellectual and social behavior at age 7 ½. *Developmental Psychology, 12,* 107–112.

Hart, C. H., DeWolf, D. M., Wozniak, P., & Burts, D. C. (1992). Maternal and paternal disciplinary styles: Relations with preschoolers' playground behavioral orientation and peer status. *Child Development, 63,* 879–892.

Hartup, W. W. (1974). Aggression in childhood: Developmental perspectives. *American Psychologist, 29,* 336–341.

Hartup, W. W. (1983). Peer relations. In E. M. Hetherington (Ed.), *Socialization, personality, and social development* (Vol. IV, pp. 103–196). In P. Mussen (Series Ed.), *Handbook of child psychology* (4th ed.). New York: Wiley.

Hartup, W. W. (1989). Social relationships and their developmental significance. *American Psychologist, 44,* 120–126.

Hartup, W. W., Laursen, B., Stewart, M. I., & Eastenson, A. (1988). Conflict and the friendship relations of young children. *Child Development, 59,* 1590–1600.

Hetherington, E. M., & Martin, B. (1986). Family factors and psychopathology in children. In H. C. Quay & J. S. Werry (Eds.), *Psychopathological disorders of childhood* (3rd ed., pp. 332–390). New York: Wiley.

Holden, G. W. (1983). Avoiding conflict: Mothers as tacticians in the supermarket. *Child Development, 54,* 233–240.

Hopkins, J., Campbell, S. B., & Marcus, M. (1987). The role of infant-related stressors in postpartum depression. *Journal of Abnormal Psychology, 96,* 237–241.

Houseman, J. A. (1973, August). *Interpersonal conflicts among nursery school children in free play settings.* Paper presented at the American Psychological Association, Montreal, Canada.

Hughes, M., Pinkerton, G., & Plewis, I. (1979). Children's difficulties in starting infant school. *Journal of Child Psychology and Psychiatry, 20,* 187–196.

Isabella, R. A., & Belsky, J. (1991). Interactional synchrony and the origins of infant–mother attachment: A replication study. *Child Development, 62,* 373–384.

Jenkins, S., Bax, M., & Hart, H. (1980). Behaviour problems in pre-school children. *Journal of Child Psychology and Psychiatry, 21,* 5–18.

Jouriles, E. N., Murphy, C. M., Farris, A. M., Smith, D. A., Richters, J. E., & Waters, E. (1991). Marital adjustment, parental disagreements about child rearing, and behavior problems in boys: Increasing the specificity of the marital assessment. *Child Development, 62,* 1424–1433.

Kaler, S. R., & Kopp, C. B. (1990). Compliance and comprehension in very young toddlers. *Child Development, 61,* 1997–2003.

Kendall, P. C., Lerner, R. M., & Craighead, W. E. (1984). Human development and intervention in childhood psychopathology. *Child Development, 55,* 71–82.

Klein, A. R., & Young, R. D. (1979). Hyperactive boys in their classroom: Assessment of teacher and peer perceptions, interactions, and classroom behaviors. *Journal of Abnormal Child Psychology, 7,* 425–442.

Kohn, M. (1977). *Social competence, symptoms, and underachievement in childhood: A longitudinal perspective.* Washington, DC: Winston.

Kohn, M., & Parnes, B. (1974). Social interaction in the classroom—A comparison of apathetic-withdrawn and angry-defiant children. *Journal of Genetic Psychology, 125,* 165–175.

Kohn, M., & Rosman, B. L. (1972). Social Competence Scale and Symptom Checklist for the preschool child: Factor dimensions, their cross-instrument generality, and longitudinal persistence. *Developmental Psychology, 6,* 430–444.

Koot, H. M. (1993). *Problem behavior in Dutch preschoolers.* Unpublished doctoral dissertation, Erasmus University, Rotterdam.

Korner, A. F. (1971). Individual differences at birth: Implications for early experience and later development. *American Journal of Orthopsychiatry, 41,* 608–619.

Kuczynski, L., Radke-Yarrow, M., Kochanska, G., & Girnius-Brown, O. (1987). A developmental interpretation of young children's noncompliance. *Developmental Psychology, 23,* 799–806.

Ladd, G. W. (1990). Having friends, keeping friends, making friends, and being liked by peers in the classroom: Predictors of children's early school adjustment. *Child Development, 61,* 1081–1100.

Lamb, M. (1987). Predictive implications of individual differences in attachment. *Journal of Consulting and Clinical Psychology, 55,* 817–824.

Lapouse, R., & Monk, M. A. (1958). An epidemiologic study of behavior characteristics in children. *American Journal of Public Health, 48,* 1134–1140.

Laursen, B., & Hartup, W. W. (1989). The dynamics of preschool children's conflicts. *Merrill-Palmer Quarterly, 35,* 281–297.

Leach, G. M. (1972). A comparison of the social behaviour of some normal and problem children. In N. Blurton-Jones (Ed.), *Ethological studies in child behaviour* (pp. 244–284). London: Cambridge University Press.

Lee, C. L., & Bates, J. E. (1985). Mother–child interaction at age two years and perceived difficult temperament. *Child Development, 56,* 1314–1325.

Lewis, M., Feiring, C., McGuffog, C., & Jaskir, J. (1984). Predicting psychopathology in six-year-olds from early social relations. *Child Development, 55,* 123–136.

Links, P. S. (1983). Community surveys of the prevalence of childhood psychiatric disorders: A review. *Child Development, 54,* 531–548.

Loeber, R. Wung, P., Keenan, K., Giroux, B., Stouthamer-Loeber, M., van Kammen, W. B., & Maughan, B. (1993). Developmental pathways in disruptive child behavior. *Development and Psychopathology, 5,* 103–133.

Londerville, S., & Main, M. (1981). Security of attachment, compliance, and maternal training methods in the second year of life. *Developmental Psychology, 17,* 289–299.

Love, L. R., & Kaswan, J. W. (1974). *Troubled Children: Their families, schools, and treatments.* New York: Wiley.

Lyons-Ruth, K. (1992). Maternal depressive symptoms, disorganized infant–mother attachment relationships and hostile-aggressive behavior in the preschool classroom: A prospective longitudinal view from infancy to age five. In D. Cicchetti & S. Toth (Eds.), *Developmental perspectives on depression. Rochester Symposium on Developmental Psychopathology* (Vol. 4, pp. 131–172). Rochester: University of Rochester Press.

Lyons-Ruth, K. B., Repacholi, B., McLeod, S., & Silva, E. (1991). Disorganized attachment behavior in infancy: Short-term stability, maternal and infant correlates, and risk-related subtypes. *Development and Psychopathology, 3,* 377–396.

Lytton, H. (1979). Disciplinary encounters between young boys and their mothers and fathers. Is there a contingency system? *Developmental Psychology, 15,* 256–268.

Lytton, H., & Zwirner, W. (1975). Compliance and its controlling stimuli observed in a natural setting. *Developmental Psychology, 11,* 769–779.

Maccoby, E. E., & Martin, J. A. (1983). Socialization in the context of the family: Parent–child interaction. In E. M. Hetherington (Ed.), *Socialization, personality, and social development* (Vol. IV, pp. 1–102). In P. Mussen (Series Ed.), *Handbook of child psychology* (4th ed.). New York: Wiley.

Maccoby, E. E., Snow, M. E., & Jacklin, C. N. (1984). Children's dispositions and mother–child interaction at 12 and 18 months: A short-term longitudinal study. *Developmental Psychology, 20,* 459–472.

MacFarlane, J. W., Honzik, M. P., & Allen, L. (1954). *A devel-*

opmental study of the behavior problems of normal children between twenty-one months and fourteen years. Berkeley: University of California Press.

Mahler, M. (1968). *On human symbiosis and the vicissitudes of individuation.* New York: International Universities Press.

Main, M., & Solomon, J. (1986). Discovery of an insecure disorganized/disoriented attachment pattern: Procedures, findings and implications for the classification of behavior. In M. Yogman & T. B. Brazelton (Eds.), *Affective development in infancy* (pp. 95–124). Norwood, NJ: Ablex.

Matas, I., Arend, R. A., & Sroufe, L. A. (1978). Continuity of adaptation in the second year: The relationship between quality of attachment and later competence. *Child Development, 49,* 547–556.

McGee, R., Feehan, M., Williams, S., & Partridge, F. (1990). DSM-III disorders in a large sample of adolescents. *Journal of the American Academy of Child and Adolescent Psychiatry, 29,* 611–619.

McGee, R., Silva, P. A., & Williams, S. (1984). Perinatal, neurological, environmental, and developmental characteristics of children with stable behaviour problems. *Journal of Child Psychology and Psychiatry, 25,* 573–586.

McGrew, W. C. (1972). Aspects of social development in nursery school children with emphasis on introduction to the group. In N. Blurton-Jones (Ed.), *Ethological studies in child behaviour* (pp. 129–156). London: Cambridge University Press.

Mesibov, G. B., Schroeder, C. S., & Wesson, L. (1977). Parental concerns about their children. *Journal of Pediatric Psychology, 2,* 13–17.

Milich, R., & Dodge, K. A. (1984). Social information processing in child psychiatric populations. *Journal of Abnormal Child Psychology, 12,* 471–490.

Minde, K. K., & Minde, R. (1977). Behavioral screening of preschool children: A new approach to mental health. In P. J. Graham (Ed.), *Epidemiological approaches in child psychiatry* (pp. 121–143). New York: Academic Press.

Minton, C., Kagan, J., & Levine, J. A. (1971). Maternal control and obedience in the two-year-old. *Child Development, 42,* 1873–1894.

Moffitt, T. E. (1990). Juvenile delinquency and attention deficit disorder: Boys' developmental trajectories from age 3 to age 15. *Child Development, 61,* 893–910.

Newth, S. J., & Corbett, J. (1993). Behaviour and emotional problems in three-year-old children of Asian parentage. *Journal of Child Psychology and Psychiatry, 34,* 333–352.

Offord, D. R., Boyle, M. H., Fleming, J., Blum, H. M., & Rae Grant, N. (1989). Ontario Child Health Study: Summary of selected results. *Canadian Journal of Psychiatry, 34,* 483–491.

Olweus, D. (1980). Familial and temperamental determinants of aggressive behavior: A causal analysis. *Developmental Psychology, 16,* 644–660.

Osofsky, J. (1976). Neonatal characteristics and mother–infant interaction in two observational situations. *Child Development, 47,* 1138–1147.

Parker, J. G., & Asher, S. R. (1987). Peer relations and later personal adjustment: Are low accepted children at risk? *Psychological Bulletin, 102,* 357–389.

Patterson, G. R. (1976). The aggressive child: Victim and architect of a coercive system. In E. J. Mash, L. A. Hamerlynck, & L. C. Handy (Eds.), *Behavior modification and families* (pp. 267–316). New York: Brunner/Mazel.

Patterson, G. R., DeBaryshe, B. D., & Ramsey, E. (1989). A developmental perspective on antisocial behavior. *American Psychologist, 44,* 329–335.

Patterson, G. R., Littman, R. A., & Brickner, W. (1967). Assertive behavior in children: A step toward a theory of aggression. *Monographs of the Society for Research in Child Development, 32,* Whole No. 5 (Serial No. 113).

Pedersen, F. A., & Bell, R. Q. (1970). Sex differences in preschool children without histories of complications of pregnancy and delivery. *Developmental Psychology, 3,* 10–15.

Pelham, W., & Bender, M. E. (1982). Peer relations in hyperactive children: Description and treatment. In K. Gadow & I. Bialer (Eds.), *Advances in learning and behavioral disabilities* (Vol. 1, pp. 365–436). Greenwich, CT: JAI Press.

Puig-Antich, J. (1986). Psychobiological markers: The effects of age and puberty. In M. Rutter, C. E. Izard, & P. B. Read (Eds.), *Depression in young people: Developmental and clinical perspectives* (pp. 341–381). New York: Guilford Press.

Quay, H. C. (1986). Classification. In H. C. Quay & J. S. Werry (Eds.), *Psychopathological disorders of childhood* (pp. 1–34). New York: Wiley.

Quay, H. C., & La Greca, A. (1986). Disorders of anxiety, withdrawal, and dysphoria. In H. C. Quay & J. S. Werry (Eds.), *Psychopathological disorders of childhood* (pp. 73–110). New York: Wiley.

Radke-Yarrow, M., Cummings, E. M., Kuczynski, L., & Chapman, M. (1985). Patterns of attachment in two- and three-year-olds in normal families and families with parental depression. *Child Development, 56,* 884–893.

Reid, J. (1993). Prevention of conduct disorder before and after school entry: Relating interventions to developmental findings. *Development and Psychopathology, 5,* 243–262.

Richman, N., Stevenson, J., & Graham, P. (1982). *Preschool to school: A behavioural study.* New York: Academic Press.

Robins, L. N. (1966). *Deviant children grown up.* Baltimore: Williams & Wilkins.

Robins, L. N. (1979). Follow-up studies. In H. C. Quay & J. S. Werry (Eds.), *Psychopathological disorders of childhood* (2nd ed., pp. 415–450). New York: Wiley.

Rubin, K. H., Hymel, S., Mills, R., & Rose-Krasnor, L. (1991). Conceptualizing different developmental pathways to social isolation in children. In D. Cicchetti & S. Toth

(Eds.), *Internalizing and externalizing expressions of dysfunction: Vol. 2. Rochester Symposium on Developmental Psychopathology.* Hillsdale, NJ: Erlbaum.

Rubin, K. H., & Mills, R. (1988). The many faces of social withdrawal in childhood. *Journal of Consulting and Clinical Psychology, 56,* 916–924.

Rutter, M. (1986). The developmental psychopathology of depression: Issues and perspectives. In M. Rutter, C. E. Izard, & P. B. Read (Eds.), *Depression in young people: Developmental and clinical perspectives* (pp. 3–30). New York: Guilford Press.

Rutter, M., & Garmezy, N. (1983). Developmental psychopathology. In E. M. Hetherington (Ed.), *Socialization, personality, and social development.* (Vol. IV, pp. 775–912). In P. Mussen (Series Ed.), *Handbook of child psychology.* New York: Wiley.

Rutter, M., Tizard, J., & Whitmore, K. (1970). *Education, health, and behaviour.* London: Longman.

Sameroff, A. J., & Chandler, M. J. (1975). Reproductive risk and the continuum of caretaking casualty. In F. D. Horowitz (Eds.), *Review of child development research.* (Vol. 4, pp. 187–241). Chicago: University of Chicago Press.

Sandberg, S. T., Wieselberg, M., & Shaffer, D. (1980). Hyperkinetic and conduct problem children: Some epidemiological considerations. *Journal of Child Psychology and Psychiatry, 21,* 293–312.

Sanson, A., Oberklaid, F., Pedlow, R., & Prior, M. (1991). Risk indicators: Assessment of infancy predictors of preschool behavioural maladjustment. *Journal of Child Psychology and Psychiatry, 32,* 609–626.

Schleifer, M., Weiss, G., Cohen, N. J., Elman, M., Cvejic, H., & Kruger, E. (1975). Hyperactivity in preschoolers and the effect of methylphenidate. *American Journal of Orthopsychiatry, 45,* 38–50.

Schneider-Rosen, K., Braunwald, K. G., Carlson, V., & Cicchetti, D. (1985). Current perspectives in attachment theory: Illustrations from the study of maltreated infants. In I. Bretherton & E. Waters (Eds.), Growing points of attachment theory and research. *Monographs of the Society for Research in Child Development, 50*(Serial No. 209), 194–210.

Shantz, C. (1987). Conflicts between children. *Child Development, 58,* 283–305.

Shepherd, M., Oppenheim, B., & Mitchell, S. (1971). *Childhood behavior and mental health.* New York: Grune & Stratton.

Smith, P. K., & Green, M. (1975). Aggressive behavior in English nurseries and play groups: Sex differences and responses of adults. *Child Development, 46,* 211–214.

Speltz, M. L., Greenberg, M. T., & DeKlyen, M. (1990). Attachment in preschoolers with disruptive behavior: A comparison of clinic-referred and non-problem children. *Development and Psychopathology, 2,* 31–46.

Sroufe, L. A. (1979). The coherence of individual development. *American Psychologist, 34,* 834–841.

Sroufe, L. A. (1983). Infant–caregiver attachment and patterns of adaptation in preschool: The roots of maladaptation and competence. In M. Perlmutter (Ed.), *Minnesota Symposium on Child Psychology* (Vol. 16, pp. 41–79). Hillsdale, NJ: Erlbaum.

Sroufe, L. A., & Fleeson, J. (1986). Attachment and the construction of relationships. In W. Hartup & Z. Rubin (Eds.), *The nature and development of relationships* (pp. 51–71). Hillsdale, NJ: Erlbaum.

Sroufe, L. A., & Rutter, M. (1984). The domain of developmental psychopathology. *Child Development, 55,* 17–29.

Stallard, P. (1993). The behaviour of 3-year-old children: Prevalence and parental perception of problem behaviour: A research note. *Journal of Child Psychology and Psychiatry, 34,* 413–421.

Stayton, D., Hogan, R., & Ainsworth, M. D. S. (1971). Infant obedience and maternal behavior: The origins of socialization reconsidered. *Child Development, 42,* 1057–1069.

Stern, D. (1974). Mother and infant at play: The dyadic interactions involving facial, vocal, and gaze behaviors. In M. Lewis & L. Rosenblum (Eds.), *The effects of the infant on its caregiver* (pp. 187–214). New York: Wiley.

Thomas, A., Chess, S., & Birch, H. G. (1968). *Temperament and behavior disorders in children.* New York: New York University Press.

Tronick, E. Z. (1989). Emotions and emotional communication in infants. *American Psychologist, 44,* 112–119.

Vaughn, B., Egeland, B., Sroufe, L. A., & Waters, E. (1979). Individual differences in infant–mother attachment at 12 and 18 months: Stability and change in families under stress. *Child Development, 50,* 971–975.

Vaughn, B. E., Taraldson, B., Crichton, L., & Egeland, B. (1980). Relationships between neonatal behavioral organization and infant behavior during the first year of life. *Infant Behavior and Development, 3,* 47–66.

Waters, E., Vaughn, B. E., & Egeland, B. R. (1980). Individual differences in infant mother attachment relationships at age one: Antecedents in neonatal behavior in an urban, economically disadvantaged sample. *Child Development, 51,* 208–216.

Waters, E., Wippman, J., & Sroufe, L. A. (1979). Attachment, positive affect, and competence in the peer group: Two studies in construct validation. *Child Development, 50,* 821–829.

Webster-Stratton, C. (1990). Long-term follow-up of families with young conduct problem children: From preschool to grade school. *Journal of Clinical Child Psychology, 19,* 144–149.

Weiss, B., Dodge, K. A., Bates, J. E., & Pettit, G. S. (1992). Some consequences of early harsh discipline: Child aggression and a maladaptive social information processing style. *Child Development, 63,* 1321–1335.

Weiss, G., & Hectman, L. T. (1993). *Hyperactive children grown up* (2nd ed.). New York: Guilford Press.

Werner, E. E. (1993). Risk, resilience, and recovery: Perspectives from the Kauai Longitudinal Study. *Development and Psychopathology, 5,* 503–515.

Werry, J. S., & Quay, H. C. (1971). The prevalence of behavior symptoms of younger elementary school children. *American Journal of Orthopsychiatry, 41,* 136–143.

Westman, J. C., Rice, D. L., & Bermann, E. (1967). Nursery school behavior and later school adjustment. *American Journal of Orthopsychiatry, 37,* 725–731.

Whalen, C., & Henker, B. (1985). The social worlds of hyperactive (ADDH) children. *Clinical Psychology Review, 5,* 447–478.

Winnicott, D. W. (1957). *Mother and child: A primer of first relationships.* New York: Basic Books.

Zahn-Waxler, C., Radke-Yarrow, M., & King, R. A. (1979). Childrearing and children's responses to victims of distress. *Child Development, 50,* 319–330.

2

Etiological Factors

MARILYN T. ERICKSON

INTRODUCTION

This chapter examines the genetic, prenatal, perinatal, demographic, and postnatal factors that have been empirically associated with children's behavior disorders. The review of postnatal factors includes social/psychological conditions such as family stressors, parent psychological characteristics, child psychological characteristics, and parent–child interactions.

Up to the last few decades, clinicians tended to conceptualize etiology in relatively simplistic ways that may be characterized as one-to-one relationships. That is, specific behavior problems were viewed as having single causes. For example, depending on the time period, the cause of juvenile delinquency was attributed to heredity *or* society *or* poor parenting. In addition, different eras seemed to have "popular" etiologies. Prior to World War II, heredity was viewed as the primary etiological factor for many behavior problems. After World War II, strong acceptance of psychodynamic theory supported a be-

lief that behavior/emotional problems were caused primarily by parents (i.e., mothers). As learning theory and behavior therapy began to gain advocates in the 1970s, so did the belief that behavior problems were primarily manifestations of learned behavior, often reflecting inappropriately placed reinforcement. In parallel, other investigators were discovering biological hazards that increased the probability of developmental and behavior problems in children and adolescents.

In many instances, the labeling of risk factors is arbitrary; most risk factors are confounded with or related to other risk factors. In general, environmental factors interact with genetic factors such that behavioral effects can only rarely be attributed to one type of factor *or* another. Furthermore, experiencing one risk factor increases the probability of experiencing additional risk factors, and therefore the impact of a given risk factor likely depends on other risk factors to which the child has been exposed.

A contemporary approach necessitates a multifaceted view of etiological factors and examines the additive and interactive effects of multiple factors on risk for developing behavior disorders. As therapists have moved toward more eclectic orientations, so have they also become more accepting of the possibility that the

MARILYN T. ERICKSON • Psychology Department, Virginia Commonwealth University, Richmond, Virginia 23284-2018.

Handbook of Child Psychopathology, 3rd edition, edited by Ollendick & Hersen. Plenum Press, New York, 1998.

same behavior may have several causes or various combinations of causes.

GENETIC RISK FACTORS

Clinical child psychology's interest in genetic influences on behavior has been low until relatively recently. However, the identification of chromosomal abnormalities as the basis for particular syndromes associated with developmental disabilities has stimulated increased attention to hereditary influences on a wide range of child and adolescent behavior disorders. Moreover, twin studies in which statistical analyses estimate the amount of variance in behavior related to genetic factors, shared environment, and unshared environment are beginning to examine the relative contributions of heredity and environment to a variety of psychological disorders.

Great progress has been made in our knowledge about chromosomes; methods for laboratory staining of the chromosomes (called *banding techniques*) and other chromosome-mapping methods have permitted parts of the chromosomes and their locations on the chromosomes to be identified clearly. Applications based on the mapping of chromosomes include the possibility of prenatal identification of individuals who will not manifest serious hereditary disorders until later in life. In 1989, molecular biologists embarked on a 15-year project to identify the exact sequence of all 3 billion nucleotide pairs that together encode all inherited human traits.

Chromosomal Abnormalities

The clinical syndrome first found to be associated with an abnormal number of chromosomes was Down syndrome or "mongolism." Lejeune, Gautier, and Turpin (1959) discovered that chromosome 21 was represented in triplicate (trisomy) instead of duplicate, thus increasing the chromosome count in each cell to 47 instead of 46. Trisomies of other autosomal chromosomes have subsequently been described in the research literature. Many of the possible chromosomal abnormalities have been found only in spontaneously aborted fetuses, suggesting that most abnormalities in the number of chromosomes are incompatible with life. Chromosomal defects can be identified in about 2.5% of newborn infants (Willis & Walker, 1989). Many chromosomal errors are not inherited; rather they are caused by environmental factors.

In an early large-scale survey of newborn infants, 11 out of 4400 were found to have abnormalities in the number of sex chromosomes (Leonard, Landy, Ruddle, & Lubs, 1974). Prospective studies of children diagnosed at birth as having sex chromosome abnormalities have found higher than expected rates of developmental, learning, and behavior problems (e.g., Robinson, Bender, Borelli, Puck, & Salenblatt, 1983).

A large number of inherited metabolic disorders have been discovered, and some of them are associated with behavior disorders. These conditions are almost always autosomal recessive or sex-linked and the result of one defective gene. The abnormalities are detected by means of urine and blood tests that evaluate amino acid levels. A number of the metabolic disorders can be treated by restricting or providing particular foods, chemicals, or drugs.

Psychological Studies of Genetic Factors

The area of behavior genetics encompasses a variety of approaches for determining the hereditary basis of behavior. Animal studies, which utilize selective breeding techniques, have yielded the most direct measures of the influence of heredity. Studies with humans, being necessarily correlational in design, have measured the contribution of heredity indirectly as a function of the genetic relationships among the persons examined.

Pedigree Analysis

One of the earliest techniques for evaluating the hereditary contributions to behavior involved the initial identification of an individual (proband) who had the behavior (or trait) and the tracing of the incidence of this trait in the proband's ancestors, siblings, and children. Galton (1869) used this method in his study of the families of eminent men. Family aggregation of emotional and behavior problems has also been used in a community population survey (Szatmari, Boyle, & Offord, 1993). Pedigree studies have a number of methodological shortcomings, not the least of which is the confounding of hereditary and environmental influences. Galton's eminent men, for example, whose abilities he believed were the result of hereditary factors, were raised in intellectually stimulating environments. In addition, reliable descriptions of family members beyond a few generations are seldom possible. The chances of locating hereditary abnormalities are more likely, however, when families with more than one defective individual are studied. Out of an institutionalized population of 3000 people, Wright, Tarjan, and Eyer (1959) found 61 families with more than one resident, and 9 of these families had identifiable hereditary disorders.

Twin Studies

The results of several dozen twin studies have suggested that heredity is the primary factor in determining the differences among people with respect to intellectual functioning, accounting for between 50 and 70% of the variance (Plomin, 1989). Such findings have often been misunderstood to mean that intelligence is fixed or predetermined, when, in fact, they only describe the contribution of heredity under the environmental conditions experienced by that particular group of subjects. There is nothing inherent in the attribution of heritability that precludes a specially designed environment from increasing intellectual abilities. Theoretically, if all people lived under environmental conditions that permitted them to realize their potential, then all remaining individual differences would be attributable to heredity. Scarr-Salapatek (1971) found that heritability of intelligence was considerably higher for children in the upper socioeconomic groups than for children from lower socioeconomic environments.

Studies of behavior genetics indicate that identical twins have a higher concordance rate for a variety of behaviors during infancy than do same-sex fraternal twins. More recent research has utilized structural equation modeling to examine heritability of behavior problems in large samples of twins. For example, Silberg et al. (1994) found significant heritability for maternal ratings of both internalizing and externalizing behavior problems in 8- to 16-year-old twins as well as significant contributions of shared and unshared environments. Plomin (1994) argued that because genetic influence on developmental psychopathology has only rarely accounted for more than half of the variance, genetic research provides the best evidence for the importance of environmental influences.

One objection to the twin method has been the assumption that the environments of identical and fraternal twins are the same. In a sense, this argument is not compelling, as (1) the natural environment of twins reared together is likely to be extremely similar and (2) any differences in the environments of twins reared together have a higher probability of being related to behaviors resulting from genetic factors than of being related to random environmental variations. That is, environmental differences are as likely to be dependent on the idiosyncratic behaviors of each twin as on differences in the environment per se.

Generalizations to the population from the data of twin studies have also been criticized on the basis that twins differ from the population. They tend to weigh less at birth, to have older mothers, and to show small but consistently higher levels of both internalizing and externalizing behavior problems (Gau, Silberg, Erickson, & Hewitt, 1992).

In twin studies, all concordance is attributed to heredity, and discordance is considered to reflect the influences of environment. It is possible that not all concordance reflects the direct influence of the genetic constitution. For example, a particular complication during pregnancy could affect identical twins similarly and fraternal twins differentially, because fraternal twins are more likely to be at different embryological stages at the time of the complication. In such instances, the prenatal factors may be of primary importance in terms of prevention. Some of the discordance found in identical twins may also be related to prenatal and perinatal events that affect only one of the twins (e.g., lack of oxygen during a difficult delivery). As heredity and environment are confounding beginning with conception, and perhaps prior to conception (Erickson, 1967), the relationship between heritability figures and psychopathology should be carefully interpreted.

PRENATAL RISK FACTORS

A number of prenatal factors have been implicated in the etiology of behavior disorders, but much of our information comes from correlational research. Although some experimental research has been conducted with animals, generalizations of the findings to humans must be made with extreme caution. For ethical reasons, experimental designs cannot be utilized with humans in most instances.

A primary source of correlational information has been the determination of those prenatal factors that have been associated with increased infant mortality rates. The factors that cause death in some infants are also likely to cause other infants brain damage that may be manifested later in learning and behavior problems.

Much of the available information in this area has been derived from retrospective studies. Children with particular developmental or behavior problems are first identified; then, their prenatal histories are examined for evidence of detrimental conditions. There are a number of possible weaknesses in this approach, especially the reliance on poorly documented medical and hospital records. The errors involved in the poor recordkeeping are often those of omission, which reduces the chances of identifying a significant factor. When retrospective studies are carefully designed, however, they do add substantially to our statistical understanding of the role of prenatal factors in the etiology of developmental and behavior problems. It should be emphasized that such knowledge does not permit the specification of etiology in the individual case. When a prenatal event known to be detrimental on a statistical basis has occurred, its causal role cannot be established because very few complications of pregnancy, labor, and delivery affect all children in the same way. Although certain pregnancy complications may increase the mortality rate of the infants who experience them, most of the infants survive, and most of the survivors show little or no adverse effects. It is generally recognized that the child is most vulnerable during the first trimester (3 months) of gestation.

Prospective, longitudinal studies have also contributed to our understanding of prenatal etiological factors, but they are relatively rare because of their expense and the great lengths of time involved. One substantial study, the Collaborative Perinatal Project (Hellmuth, 1967), involved 14 institutions of higher learning and 20,000 children whose mothers were studied during pregnancy. The children received physical and psychological examinations at regular intervals from infancy through 8 years of age. This project has provided significant information regarding the impact of prenatal events on developmental disabilities.

Nutrition

The mother's nutritional status has long been recognized as one of the most important determinants of infant status. The condition of the child at birth depends not only on the mother's nutrition during pregnancy but also on the mother's entire nutritional history. If the mother was poorly nourished during her own development, her physical condition during pregnancy will be less than optimal, and the probability of adverse conditions for the child in utero will be increased. Even optimal nutrition during pregnancy will not counteract the deficiencies of a physically malfunctioning mother.

After genetic factors, nutritional history most strongly determines differences in height, weight, physical development, and morbidity rates. In the United States, the adolescent girl is likely to be the most poorly nourished member of the family. This problem is at least partly the result of the culture's emphasis on slimness and the preponderance of easily available but relatively nonnutritious foods. Unfortunately, poor dietary habits developed in adolescence may continue into adulthood. Because approximately 25% of mothers having their first child are less than 20 years old, adolescent nutrition becomes an important factor. Loss of body fat from dieting or exercise can cause fertility problems; fat tissue exerts a regulatory effect on the reproductive ability of women (Frisch, 1988).

Experimental studies with lower animals have shown that nutritional deficiencies are capable of producing serious disturbances in the growth and development of the embryo and fetus. Experimental research involving the deprivation of particular nutritional substances prior to conception and during pregnancy has demonstrated an increased rate of fetal death and congenital abnormalities (absence of eyes, small eyes, harelip, cleft palate, underdevelopment of lungs and kidneys). The timing of the nutritional deficiency during pregnancy is also important in determining whether or not a specific congenital defect will result. Genetic factors are also involved; studies have shown that different strains of the same species respond differently to the same nutritional deficiency.

One of the earliest experimental studies with humans to demonstrate the substantive effect of maternal diet on the health of the infant was that of Ebbs, Tisdall, and Scott (1942). These investigators studied a group of women all of whom were originally poorly nourished. Nearly half of the original group was given a diet that increased their intake of protein, calcium, iron, and calories to a desirable level. Women on the supplemental diet and their infants did better on all criteria than did women who remained on their usual diet. Poor diet was significantly associated with poor prenatal status, prolonged labor and convalescence, and a three- to fourfold greater incidence in illness of the infants during the first 6 months of life. Nearly 12% of poor-diet infants were lost through miscarriage, stillbirth, or later death, whereas all of the supplemented-diet infants survived.

Similarly, studies of women living under wartime conditions with very strict rationing of food have shown that about half of them stopped menstruating and the other half experienced irregular menstrual periods. For the women who did conceive, the rate of premature births, stillbirths, and congenital malformations of the infants was increased considerably (Smith, 1947). Children who were malnourished in utero have also been found to have poorer verbal comprehension and expressive language skills (Walther & Ramaekers, 1982).

Maternal nutrition has also been found to influence the intelligence of children. Harrell, Woodyard, and Gates (1955) conducted a study that examined the influence of vitamin supplementation of pregnant and lactating women's diet on the intelligence of their children. The study involved over 2000 women whose diets had been judged as poor. Four kinds of vitamin supplements and a placebo were administered in such a way that no participant knew the contents of the tablets. When tested at 4 years of age, children of mothers who were given supplements surpassed the placebo group by an average of 5.2 Stanford–Binet IQ points. The average for the B-complex groups exceeded that of the placebo group by 8.1 points. High caloric supplementation from birth to 2 years has also been found to predict higher levels of social involvement, both happy and angry affect, and moderate activity level at school age, whereas low supplementation was associated with passivity, dependency, and anxious behavior (Barrett, Radke-Yarrow, & Klein, 1982).

Maternal Age

Difficulties during pregnancy and birth, as well as the frequency of developmental abnormalities, have been shown to be highly correlated with age of mother. Available evidence indicates ages 23 to 28 years as being optimal for pregnancy in the United States, as this age span is associated with the highest survival rates for mother and child and lowest spontaneous abortion, miscarriage, stillbirth, prematurity, and malformation rates.

The higher incidence of problems at younger ages has been attributed in part to the immaturity of the reproductive system; the pelvic organs are not fully developed until at least 10 years after the beginning of menstruation. It has been estimated that over one-third of females between 15 and 20 years of age in the United States have at least one unwanted pregnancy. Whereas some have chosen abortion or adoption, many teenagers are choosing to give birth and keep their infants. Many of these young mothers also endanger their own psychological welfare by curtailing their education and thereby create for themselves and their children lives of poverty. Prematurity and child abuse are significant risk factors associated with teenage parenting.

After the age of 28 years, a gradual increase in the rate of problems associated with pregnancy begins, and this rate accelerates after the age of 35, when the reproductive system begins to lose efficiency. Higher rates of mental retardation and other behavior disorders have been found to be related with increased age of the mother.

Viral and Bacterial Infections of the Mother

At one time it was believed that a mother's diseases could not affect the fetus. As the number of investigations has increased, however, evidence has accumulated that both viruses and bacteria can be transmitted from mother to child. A number of these infections are capable of seriously affecting the development of the fetus. We have also learned that when the mother is immunized during pregnancy the fetus itself will receive maternal antibodies and will be immune for several months after birth.

The idea that viruses could affect the embryo or fetus was resisted strongly at one time. This position was understandable given that most of the common viral diseases, such as mumps, measles, and chickenpox, usually occurred during childhood, providing the future mother immunity that lasted through childbearing years. Because relatively few pregnant women developed these diseases, data were sparse. Rubella (German measles), however, is likely to occur in young adulthood. Being a relatively mild communicable disease, rubella can be very damaging to the fetus during the first trimester of pregnancy. Prenatal exposure to rubella virus greatly increases the risk of pathological eye conditions, deafness, dental defects, cleft palate, cardiac defects, mental retardation, and microcephaly. Several prospective studies have indicated that the risk of a major defect is 50% if the mother is infected with rubella in the first month of pregnancy, 25% in the second month, 17% in the third, 11% in the fourth, 6% in the fifth, and essentially no risk in subsequent months.

A number of other formerly common childhood diseases, such as measles and mumps, can lead to spontaneous abortions and possibly congenital defects. The *live* vaccines for communicable diseases may harm the fetus and should not be given to pregnant women. Prevention of these problems would be largely accomplished if all parents were careful about having their children immunized early in life and maintaining recommended immunization schedules.

Our most recent concern about viruses involves pediatric AIDS or human immunodeficiency virus (HIV) infection (Task Force on Pediatric AIDS, 1989). At present, child cases of

AIDS constitute less than 2% of the total reported AIDS cases in the United States. About 19% of reported child AIDS cases are the result of transfusions of HIV-contaminated blood, but this proportion is expected to decrease with improved screening of the blood supply. The majority of cases involve transmission from the mother to child either prenatally or during delivery. The mother's infection can usually be traced to her own or her sexual partner's use of intravenous drugs. Prenatal and perinatal infection increases the risk for the development of HIV symptoms. In addition to frequent illnesses, these children are also likely to show failure to thrive and delayed development.

As a group, bacterial infections of the pregnant woman have not been associated with congenital deformities of the child, but many of these infections are transmitted to the child from the mother. Toxoplasmosis is a protozoan disease that is essentially symptomless in the adult but has serious consequences for the child in utero. Congenital toxoplasmosis is related to hydrocephalus (large head associated with an excessive amount of fluid in the cranium), serious damage to the eyes, convulsions, and calcification (hardening) of small areas of the brain. Hydrocephalus occurs in about 80% of the cases. Mental retardation is almost always present, varying from mild to profound. Because toxoplasmosis is a relatively common disease, women are given a skin test early in pregnancy, and those with negative reactions are reexamined at intervals during pregnancy. Prevention programs include avoiding cats (which may transmit the disease through their stools) and eating only well-cooked meat.

Maternal Dysfunction

This section considers those physical conditions of the mother, other than infections, that bear on the subsequent status of the child.

Obesity has been associated with an increased mortality rate for both mother and child. Obese women also have higher risk for a variety of other physical problems. Because of these relationships, physicians have exerted considerable pressure on pregnant women to gain only moderate amounts of weight. More recently, there have been concerns that physicians have been too stringent in their standards for weight gain, and that some mothers and infants have thereby been subjected to possible nutritional deficiencies. Obstetricians are currently advising the average pregnant woman that a weight gain of 25 pounds is optimal.

The *toxemias* (presence of toxic substances in the blood) of pregnancy, preeclampsia and eclampsia, whose causes are currently unknown, affect about 5% of pregnant women. The symptoms of preeclampsia include excessive weight gain because of fluid retention in the tissues, a rise in blood pressure, and the detection of albumin in the urine. Eclampsia includes the foregoing symptoms plus maternal convulsions. Toxemia is the principal cause of maternal death, although the majority of cases can now be prevented. There is evidence that the brain of a toxemic woman's fetus can be affected adversely.

Pregnant women who have high blood pressure, or *hypertension,* also have higher rates of fetal and maternal mortality, especially when the mother was hypertensive in her nonpregnant condition. Hypertension often alters the development of the placenta such that oxygen deficiency occurs, which results in a slower growth rate of the fetus.

Sickle-cell anemia is a genetically determined blood disorder primarily affecting African Americans. This condition, when present in pregnant women, increases the rate of abortions, stillbirths, and abnormalities; there is also a tendency for children to have low birth weight. Those who survive are either carriers of the trait or manifest the condition themselves.

Diabetes is characterized by deficiency in the supply of insulin, which controls the metabolism of carbohydrates. The principal symptoms are excessive urination, sugar in the urine, high blood sugar, excessive thirst and hunger, weakness, and loss of weight. Diabetes during pregnancy may create significant risks for both mother and child. Probably because of the hyperactivity of its pancreas, the fetus grows at a greater than usual rate, reaching the weight of an average newborn several weeks before the end of gestation. If permitted to go to full term, the newborn may be injured during the birth process. Early diagnosis and treatment have greatly improved the originally poor prognosis (Sells, Robinson, Brown, & Knopp, 1994). Dietary treatment and early delivery of the child can save the lives of virtually all infants of diabetic mothers. Special precautions after birth must be maintained, however. Even though quite large, the newborn of the diabetic mother is very much like a premature infant and must be handled as such in the hospital after delivery.

Medications and Addictive Substances

The thalidomide tragedy during the 1960s increased our awareness of the effects of medication on the developing fetus. Thalidomide was prescribed as a mild tranquilizer in Europe, primarily in Germany. When taken early in pregnancy, it caused the absence or shortening of the infant's limbs. Thousands of physically handicapped children were born before thalidomide was identified as the cause and taken off the market.

Medication and drugs are being manufactured and consumed in great quantities. Many of the foods we eat contain additives and preservatives. Although there are laws that govern the testing of drugs and other substances consumed by humans, much of the research has not been adequate. It is true that medications that are to be administered to adults must be tested on adults, but these drugs may not have been tested for their effects on the unborn child. There is ample evidence that the adult's reaction to a particular drug does not adequately predict its effect on the fetus. Drugs taken by a pregnant woman may affect the fetus, but this effect depends on the particular drug, the period of pregnancy, the amount taken, and the genetic constitutions of mother and child.

Moreover, adverse effects may not become apparent for a number of years after the pregnant woman has been given the medication. For example, in the early 1970s, it was discovered that the synthetic estrogen DES, used for threatened miscarriage during the 1950s and 1960s, increased the rate of vaginal cancer beginning in early adulthood of the female offspring. This group of women may also have a higher risk of spontaneous abortions and lowered fertility rates, which are probably the result of uterine structural abnormalities.

A number of case studies in the medical literature link the ingestion of particular medications to fetal abnormalities. Because many medications have not been evaluated with respect to their risk of causing developmental abnormalities, physicians are being extremely cautious in prescribing medication to pregnant women and are advising them against taking any drugs, even over-the-counter preparations, without consultation. Evidence is beginning to accumulate that a variety of substances ingested by the male may affect his reproductive system as well and thus may contribute to birth defects in the child.

Drugs given during labor and delivery may present hazards to the fetus. Most anesthetics, analgesics, and sedatives produce depressed physiological functioning of the mother and, as a result, may alter the oxygen supply to the fetus. Premature infants are especially vulnerable to adverse effects of anesthetics. For these reasons, obstetric drugs are used judiciously (Finster, Petersen, & Morishima, 1983).

A woman who is addicted to narcotics during pregnancy will produce a child who is physiologically a drug addict. The baby appears normal at birth but within a day or two begins to show marked agitation, sleeplessness, tremors, convulsions, breathing difficulties, and feeding problems. The severity of the symptoms is directly related to the drug dosage taken by the mother. If the mother is deprived of drugs during pregnancy, the fetus manifests withdrawal symptoms by excessive kicking. It is current practice not to have the mother go through withdrawal therapy during pregnancy because of the risk of harming the baby in utero. Narcotics-addicted pregnant women have a high rate of complications; their infants have perinatal medical problems, impaired interactive and state control behavior during early infancy, and cognitive and psychomotor deficits. The mother who is a drug addict can also transmit narcotics to her infant through breast milk.

With the increasing number of persons using illicit drugs has come an increase in the number of women who use illicit drugs during pregnancy. Recent surveys indicate that up to 18% of newborn infants have been exposed to substance abuse prenatally. A high proportion of these infants have been exposed to cocaine. The results of research on prenatal cocaine exposure have been equivocal; a recent study suggests that earlier negative effects may have been related primarily to low socioeconomic status rather than cocaine per se (Hurt et al., 1995).

Jones, Smith, Ulleland, and Streissguth (1973) described a pattern of physical defects and behavioral problems found in children of chronic alcoholic mothers. This pattern, "fetal alcohol syndrome," includes physical growth deficiency, abnormal development of the heart, defects of the joints, and facial abnormalities, especially the eyes. The children of chronically alcoholic women have a high death rate during infancy, and close to half of the survivors may be retarded, even if they are raised in good foster homes. Behavioral and cognitive problems are also common (Steinhausen, Williams, & Spohr, 1994). Heavy drinking (four or five drinks per day) or binge drinking (multiple drinks during a 1- to 3-day period in the first trimester of pregnancy) is associated with fetal alcohol syndrome, low birth weight, and infants with physical problems and/or developmental delays (Willis & Walker, 1989).

Women who smoke give birth to children who weigh less than the children of nonsmoking women. Furthermore, prematurity rates rise in direct relation to the number of cigarettes smoked per day (Cardozo, Gibb, Studd, & Cooper, 1982). Cigarette smoking in pregnant wom-en is related to decreases in placental blood flow, fetal activity, and fetal breathing movements. Experimental studies with animals have also shown that offspring of rats and rabbits exposed to tobacco smoke during pregnancy weigh less at birth than offspring of control subjects.

Psychological Factors

Pregnant women's attitudes and feelings have been found to be related to later incidence of complications of pregnancy, labor, and delivery in prospective studies. Davids, DeVault, and Talmadge (1961) noted that anxiety was higher for a group of women who later gave birth to children with developmental problems than for a control group. Erickson (1965), in a study of pregnant middle-class patients, found that multigravidas (women having their second or subsequent children) who later experienced one or more perinatal complications expressed more fears for self and baby, irritability, and depression than did multigravidas who were to have no complications. In the context of sociopolitical violence in Chile, women living in neighborhoods with high rates of violence had increased risk of pregnancy complications (Zapata, 1992).

Animal studies have suggested that prenatal stress may produce important effects. Herrenkohl (1979) found that female rats whose mothers were under stress during pregnancy subsequently experienced more spontaneous abortions, longer pregnancies, and fewer live-born young than did female rats whose mothers were subjected to stress; the offspring weighed less and were less likely to survive the neonatal period. It was hypothesized that prenatal stress influences the balance of hormones in the fetus and thereby produces reproductive dysfunction in adulthood. Further, an experimental study with squirrel monkeys demonstrated impairment of neuromotor development when mothers were socially stressed repeatedly during pregnancy; a short period of stress during the middle of gestation did not result in adverse effects, however (Schneider & Coe, 1993).

PERINATAL RISK FACTORS

The dividing line between prenatal and perinatal factors in the etiology of childhood disorders is difficult to establish as the child's condition at birth is, quite obviously, a product of both genetic and prenatal influences. The perinatal factors to be discussed in this section will thus be a combination of those variables that seem to be relevant during labor and delivery and other variables that begin to be relevant earlier in pregnancy but that manifest themselves primarily during and immediately after the birth process. Mothers' self-report of perinatal complications has been associated with poorer school achievement in children with learning problems (Gray, Davis, McCoy, & Dean, 1992).

Anoxia

Oxygen lack is most likely to occur immediately before, during, and immediately after the child is born. It is estimated that difficulty in the initiation and maintenance of respiration occurs in 5 to 10% of newborns. Anoxia can occur if the placenta detaches too soon (placenta previa), if the umbilical cord becomes knotted, or if the cord gets wrapped tightly around the baby's neck. Even though anoxia has received considerable research attention, its effects are not clearly understood. The primary reason for our inability to interpret the findings is the confounding of anoxia with other factors. Indeed, the possibility exists that other physical problems prevent the infant from withstanding the effects of anoxia. Correlational studies with human subjects have found that anoxia at birth is associated with mild impairments of intelligence, neurological status, and personality functioning.

Windle's (1958) classic experimental studies with monkeys involved depriving full-term infant monkeys of oxygen for specific periods of time after they had been delivered by Cesarean

section. He found that anoxia at birth resulted in impaired motor functioning; longer periods of oxygen deprivation were associated with more profound motor problems.

In humans, anoxia is correlated both with very rapid labors (less than 1 or 2 hours) and with very long labors (more than 24 hours). Although the fetus and newborn are quite resistant to the adverse effects of oxygen deprivation, the brain is the first organ to be affected when minimum oxygen needs are not met. The brain requires more oxygen and has a more active metabolism than any other organ of the body. Within the central nervous system, the different parts vary in their vulnerability to oxygen deprivation, with the higher levels, such as the cortex and cerebellum, being least resistant, and the spinal cord and sympathetic ganglia being most resistant to anoxia.

Prematurity and Postmaturity

An infant is considered to be premature when its birth weight is $5\frac{1}{2}$ lb (2500 g) or less. The premature infant whose gestational age is less than full term has a decreased risk for later problems relative to the infant who is born underweight at term, a condition suggesting chronic problems in utero. Prematurity occurs more often under conditions of poor nutrition and inadequate medical care and is correlated with many pregnancy complications; low socioeconomic status may exacerbate the negative effects of low birth weight (Liaw & Brooks-Gunn, 1994).

Without the technology of modern medicine many more premature infants would succumb. Most infants weighing over 3 lb at birth can now be expected to survive; infants weighing between 500 and 999 g (about 1.1 to 2.2 lb) have survival rates ranging between 13 and 65%.

In one recent study, Hack et al. (1994) matched a surviving group of children with birth weights under 750 g with a group weighing between 750 and 1499 g at birth and a group born at term. At school age, the rates of mental retardation (IQ < 70) in the three groups were

21, 8, and 2%, and the rates of cerebral palsy were 9, 6, and 0%, respectively; the children with the lowest birth weight had poorer psychomotor and social skills, poorer academic achievement, and more behavior and attention problems.

Current research suggests that environmental factors beginning at birth contribute significantly to the premature infant's future cognitive and behavioral status (Cohen, 1995). Thompson et al. (1994) identified maternal stress as one such environmental "marker." Lee and Barratt (1993) maintained that environmental influences eventually overshadowed the biological influences in their longitudinal study of 5- to 8-year-old low-birth-weight children.

Birth Injury

Several situations may cause a difficult delivery and thus increase risk to the child. Sometimes the infant is in a position other than head first; such deliveries are much more difficult, and the risk of anoxia or injury is increased. If aware of the abnormal position of the baby early enough, the physician may try to change the baby's position manually. If the physician is concerned about the baby's status, forceps may be used to deliver the head more quickly. Mid and high forceps are used with caution because of damage they might cause to the head. The use of low forceps ranges widely; some hospitals report physicians using them for a majority of deliveries, whereas others report their use only infrequently.

DEMOGRAPHIC RISK FACTORS

Demographic risk factors are usually simply descriptive variables that are assumed not to have a causal role in and of themselves; that is, other (often unknown) risk factors are responsible for the findings associated with demographic risk factors. Socioeconomic status (SES) would usually be included in this section, but our understanding of the risk factors associated with SES prompted its placement in the following section on postnatal risk factors.

Gender

The human male is more biologically vulnerable than the female, beginning at conception and continuing through old age. Between 130 and 150 males are conceived for every 100 females, but only 105 boys are born for every 100 girls. Reproductive wastage in the form of abortions and miscarriages affects more males than females. Because such a large percentage of spontaneously aborted fetuses show chromosomal abnormalities, and because a large number of chromosomal abnormalities involve the sex chromosome, it is possible to hypothesize that the male is more vulnerable on a genetic basis as well. This explanation is more plausible when it is remembered that males express recessive genes on the sex chromosomes because there is no opportunity for a counteracting gene on the other sex chromosome. The male dies more often during the neonatal period and through childhood until the sex ratio of live persons approaches 100 males to 100 females during adolescence.

Proctor, Vosler, and Murty (1992) examined the demographic characteristics of children referred to an outpatient child guidance clinic and found that boys, minorities, and low SES children were more likely to receive a serious psychiatric diagnosis. Many studies have reported that boys have more behavior problems than do girls. During childhood, boys also show more aggression (Maccoby & Jacklin, 1980). Research on sex-steroid hormones with adolescents indicates that the *variability* of a person's hormone levels may be more predictive of behavior than *absolute amounts* of circulating hormones. For example, Inoff-Germain, Arnold, Nottelman, and Susman (1988) found that both boys and girls whose circulating levels of testosterone varied widely from day to day were more likely to show anger.

Adoption

Being adopted is a risk factor for behavior problems during childhood and adolescence (Goldberg & Wolkind, 1992). The basis for this risk appears to include prenatal factors, such as young age, substance abuse, and chronic psychological stress of the mother, and perinatal factors, such as prematurity and other complications of labor and delivery. If the infant is not placed in a stable home environment within the first few months of life, then attachment processes may not be optimal.

Age

The number and types of behavior problems reported for children vary with age. Many children with developmental and cognitive problems are not diagnosed until after they have started school. The peaks for referrals to clinics occur within a few years after school entry and again within a few years after onset of adolescence. A significant number of problems are recognizable during preschool years, but there has been a tendency for physicians to delay referral of the preschool child hoping that the child will "grow out of it." Some abnormal conditions, especially those associated with congenital abnormalities, can be recognized at birth, whereas others can be diagnosed only later.

Just as the normal behaviors of children change as a function of age or developmental status, so do abnormal behaviors change. Indeed, genetic factors could be expected to influence behaviors differently at different ages; in addition, pre- and perinatal factors may affect behaviors at some ages and not others. Although behavior patterns have traditionally been viewed as relatively unstable during childhood, recent research suggests substantial stability for general types of behavior problems, such as externalizing behavior disorders, but that specific characteristics may vary with age (Campbell, 1990; Cohen, Cohen, & Brook, 1993).

POSTNATAL RISK FACTORS

The range of postnatal risk factors is extremely wide in that it includes both physical and psychological factors that increase risk of abnormal behavior, interactive effects of physical and psychological factors, and interactive effects with the previously described risk factors (i.e., genetic, prenatal, and demographic). Contemporary research has only begun to examine the combined or interactive effects of risk factors.

Neglect

Neglect refers to parents' withholding or not providing adequate resources for their child's physical well-being. Child neglect may include inadequate food, shelter, clothing, or caring. In some instances, parents do not provide these necessities for the child because of poverty and/or ignorance, whereas in other instances, parents choose to deprive their children of these basic necessities.

Obviously, neglect occurs on a continuum. Extreme neglect inevitably leads to the child's death, and intermediate levels may be associated with chronic malnutrition and illnesses that increase the risk for other developmental and behavioral problems.

Malnutrition

It has been estimated that 40 to 60% of children worldwide are mildly or moderately undernourished; the exact incidence of undernourishment in the United States continues to be debated (Lozoff, 1989). Nutrition is an important factor in determining physical and behavioral status throughout postnatal life. Severe nutritional deficiencies during infancy and later preschool years have been associated with detrimental alterations in brain development, which in turn retard physical growth and behavioral development (Stoch, Smythe, Moodie, & Bradshaw, 1982; Winick, 1979).

Galler (1984) reported a study conducted in Barbados comparing a group of children severely undernourished only in the first year of life with similar children who had no history of undernourishment. The undernourished children eventually caught up in physical growth, but they continued to show deficits in cognitive and behavioral functioning. The undernourished children had IQ scores that were 12 points lower, and 60% of them displayed symptoms associated with attentional problems. Moreover, these symptoms persisted throughout the school years.

Undernourished children tend to come from the most disadvantaged families—characterized by low incomes, poor housing and medical care, and mothers with low intelligence. Children who are undernourished become less active and demand even less from environments that are already poorly equipped to give them attention and stimulation. Grantham-McGregor, Schofield, and Powell (1987) found that their psychosocial stimulation program in the home was able to remediate the psychological deficits of severely malnourished children. Children from low-income families who participate in school breakfast programs have been shown to score higher on achievement tests in the elementary school grades; participating children also have lower rates of school absence and tardiness (Meyers, Sampson, Weitzman, Rogers, & Kayne, 1989).

Accidents

Minor injuries to the head are quite common in infancy and childhood, but little is known about the effects of these everyday occurrences. Physically, the skull does not offer as much protection to the brain during the first 6 months of life as it does later in the child's life. Accidents, especially those involving automobiles, and physical abuse are responsible for many cases of brain damage. Laws requiring use of seat belts and compliance with this requirement contribute significantly to reductions in head injury cases. However, about 1 million children each year sustain closed head injuries, and a large number of these children will have physical, cognitive, and/or behavior problems as a result (Telzrow, 1987). Both the families, in particular, and society, in general, pay enormous costs, economically and psychologically, in their attempts to rehabilitate children with traumatic brain injury.

Abuse

Child abuse is receiving considerable professional and public attention because of resulting physical injuries, including brain damage, and assorted psychological sequelae. In earlier times, children were considered property of their parents and parents wanted healthy children who could contribute to the family's economic welfare. In modern times, children do not usually contribute significantly to a family's income; therefore, the economic consequence of child abuse and neglect may be felt more by society than by the individual family. Belsky (1993) proposed a developmental-ecological analysis of child maltreatment that includes community, cultural, and evolutionary contexts. All states have laws that require professionals to report suspected and known instances of child neglect and abuse to local social service authorities, who investigate the case to determine whether court action, therapy, or other services are needed by the family.

Reports of child abuse have doubled over the last decade, and a large body of research has focused on both short- and long-term psychological consequences of child maltreatment (Cicchetti, 1994). This research suggests that early maltreatment is associated with poor social relationships, poor self-perceptions, and depression. As adults, people who have been abused appear to have a higher risk for aggressive and violent acts as well as self-injurious and suicidal behavior. A history of physical abuse has also been associated with adult psychological problems such as anxiety and depression (Malinosky-Rummell & Hansen, 1993).

A review of 45 studies by Kendall-Tackett, Williams, and Finkelhor (1993) demonstrated that sexually abused children had more psychological symptoms than nonabused children, with abuse accounting for between 15 and 45% of the variance; the most frequently occurring symptoms were fears, posttraumatic stress disorder, behavior problems, sexualized behaviors, and poor self-esteem. However, no specific behavioral syndrome was found for children who had been sexually abused. Degree of symptomatology was affected by penetration, duration and frequency of abuse, force, relationship of perpetrator to the child, and maternal support. Another review of the long-term correlates of child sexual abuse revealed that child sexual abuse survivors reported higher rates of substance abuse, binge eating, somatization, and suicidal behavior (Polusny & Follette, 1995).

Environmental Hazards

What children ingest and breath may be harmful to their development. For example, lead is capable of producing severe inflammation of the brain with resulting hemorrhage and lesions. Of children hospitalized with lead poisoning, more than one-fourth die, and an equal number sustain permanent brain damage. Several studies have demonstrated that less-than-toxic levels of lead may also be detrimental. Results show a continuous inverse relationship between intelligence and relatively low levels of lead in the body (Fergusson, Horwood, & Lynskey, 1993); higher levels of cognitive functioning appear to be affected before any signs of motor impairment are seen (Thatcher, Lester, McAlaster, Horst, & Ignatius, 1983). Classroom behavior, particularly the ability to attend, to inhibit distracting stimuli, and to follow directions, seems to be sensitive to lead's effects (Fergusson, Fergusson, Horwood, & Kinzett, 1988; Needleman & Bellinger, 1984).

Poisoning is more likely to occur when parents are neglectful or do not anticipate the development of children's locomotion skills. Young children are prone to ingest substances that resemble food or drinks and may be especially attracted to colorful containers. Childproof caps and other devices no doubt prevent some poisonings. Food additives have been hypothesized to have a role in children's behavior problems, such as hyperactivity; however, the research data indicate that only a small number of children may be significantly affected by additives such as food dyes (Weiss, 1984).

Disease and Illness

Several diseases are known to cause brain damage in children. *Meningitis* involves an inflammation of the meninges, the covering of the brain. It is usually a bacterial infection and can be treated with antibiotics, thereby offering the possibility of preventing adverse effects, if the disease is diagnosed early enough. The acute illness, if untreated, lasts for 2 weeks or more followed by gradual recovery. In almost all cases, complete recovery is never achieved. Intellectual functioning may be grossly impaired, and behavioral changes can be profound.

Encephalitis is usually a viral infection that involves inflammation of the brain itself. There is often no medical treatment available, and risk of serious consequences is always present. Encephalitis is known to occur as a complication following common childhood diseases, especially measles but also chickenpox, scarlet fever, and whooping cough. Immunization programs for measles significantly reduce the likelihood of encephalitis. In the case of epidemic encephalitis, or sleeping sickness, about one-third of the patients die; of the two-thirds who recover, half become physically or mentally disabled.

Infections in young children are sometimes accompanied by high fevers. Parents are usually advised by their physicians to use procedures such as cool baths and medications to reduce high fevers because of the possibility of damage to the brain. Middle ear infections are among the most common infections during the first 3 years of life; chronic ear infections may cause partial or temporary deafness that is associated with later language problems (Secord, Erickson, & Bush, 1988).

Children who suffer from chronic physical illness, especially during the preschool years, may be at risk for later developmental and psychological problems because their pain and medical interventions may prevent them from learning what their agemates are learning and from having age-appropriate life experiences.

Social Factors

Societies vary in their definitions of behavior disorders; a behavior that is condoned and reinforced in one culture may be disapproved of or punished in another. The well-adjusted person, then, may be conceptualized as one whose behaviors are compatible with the prevailing norms of the dominant culture in the society. Almost all countries have a variety of subcultures within them (e.g., tribes, religious sects), but the United States is unique in its collection of people whose ancestors come from all over the earth. Children may perhaps be expected to encounter greater problems when they are subjected to cultural demands that differ markedly from those of their subculture.

As each succeeding wave of immigrants arrived, they were assigned to the lowest rung of the social ladder. Many individuals were eventually able to better their situation; in most cases, their success was correlated with their adoption of the dominant cultural standards. Being white, Anglo-Saxon, and Protestant has been a significant advantage throughout our history.

Success in our society is also correlated with (and defined by) certain behaviors. For adults, those behaviors include being achievement oriented, intelligent, and nonemotional, and having a job that is dependent on mental, rather than manual, activity. Children who are raised by parents possessing these characteristics have a higher probability of acquiring these characteristics than do children whose parents are poor, undereducated, blue-collar workers.

Family Life Events

Family life events are changes or stressors that affect the family unit. Some life events affect one or both parents directly and the child indirectly, other events affect the child directly, and still others effect directly all members of the family unit. There is a growing body of research suggesting that short-term (up to 1 year) accumulations of stressors have small but significant negative effects on children's behavior (Johnson & Bradlyn, 1988). The effects of life span-accumulated life events on children's behavior have not yet been studied adequately, although we are beginning to understand the effects of particular life events over the course of development. The adverse effects of life events may be decreased when social support systems are available and, in contrast, may be increased when such systems are deficient or unavailable.

Changes in children's environments, particularly changes related to the people in those environments, have long been associated with later psychological problems. Such changes may vary from death or long-term hospitalization of the mother to inconsistent attention to the child by the mother; in the former instance, the mother is lost to the child, and in the latter, the child experiences relatively smaller losses on a continuous but unpredictable basis. Potentially traumatic life changes for children also include such experiences as marital separation and divorce, parental conflict/violence, parental substance abuse, and sexual or physical abuse. A recent study has indicated that negative life events experienced by the parents increase adolescent depression by undermining both the emotional health of the parents and their disciplinary practices (Ge, Conger, Lorenz, & Simmons, 1994).

Socioeconomic Status

Low SES has been associated with a higher prevalence of behavior disorders. Low SES, however, is also related to other etiological factors. For example, low-SES mothers are apt to have had poor nutrition during their own development; during pregnancy, they have a higher incidence of almost all complications, including nutritional deficiencies. Their children are more likely to be born prematurely and to experience problems during the perinatal period. A special issue of the *Journal of Clinical Child Psychology* (Routh, 1994) reviewed the impact of short- and long-term poverty and described a number of correlated factors such as prenatal methadone exposure, low birth weight, racial and ethnic minority status, and neighborhood disadvantage.

Family Composition

Increased mobility has created change in the composition of families in recent years. A few generations ago, the average person was raised in a small town where most of the individual's relatives also resided. The person was trained to do a job that would in some way benefit the community, usually married a person from the community, and spent the rest of his or her life there. In these small towns everyone knew everyone else, and parents were soon informed when their children's behavior did not measure up to the expectations of the community. In a sense, the whole community participated in childrearing. Many of the old neighborhoods in more populated areas also demonstrated community rearing of children. But now, the transient quality of contemporary living precludes such participation. On the other hand, mobility has created certain advantages that facilitate the development of individuality.

Older models of being parents seem, at least retrospectively, to have been correlated with fewer behavior problems in children. The extended (inclusion of other relatives) family, now relatively uncommon in our society, appears to have been a situation in which children were

likely to receive more individual attention from adults, and parents were less likely to be overwhelmed by childrearing responsibilities. That is, all adults in the family shared in the childrearing activities. Multiple "parents" are fairly common in so-called primitive societies; in some groups, children call their paternal uncles "father," and their relationships with the uncles are no different than their relationships with their biological fathers.

Clinicians have supported the belief that the family should be composed of a mother, a father, and their children. Deviations from that pattern have been felt to be detrimental to all members of the family, especially the children. In comparison with two-parent families, single parents are more socially isolated, work longer hours, receive less emotional and parental support, have less stable social networks, and experience more stressful life events (Weintraub & Wolf, 1983). Kallam, Ensminger, and Turner (1977) reported that a higher risk for problem behavior in children is associated with mother-only and mother/stepfather family structures; in their poor, urban, black sample, mother/grandmother family structures were nearly as effective as mother/father structures.

The emphasis on having both a mother and a father in the home has been related to the appropriate gender role development of the children. That is, children were assumed to need strong and continuous models of both genders in order to become adequate men and women. And yet, a study comparing children reared in lesbian and single-parent households found no differences between the groups in terms of their gender identity, gender role behavior, sexual orientation, or other psychological characteristics (Golombok, Spencer, & Rutter, 1983). Similarly, over 90% of adult sons of gay men have been found to be heterosexual (Bailey, Bobrow, Wolfe, & Mikach, 1995).

Adolescent Parenthood

It is well known that many adolescents in our society are sexually active, but we have not been able to agree on how to decrease the sexual activity or how to prevent pregnancies that occur as a result. Many sexually active teenagers do not use reliable birth control methods and do not have an accurate understanding of reproduction.

Having a child during adolescence not only increases the child's physical risk, but increases long-term psychological risks to the child. Children born to teenage mothers show poorer social and intellectual competence than do children born to older mothers (Roosa, Fitzgerald, & Carlson, 1982). Current attention on the mental health problems of adolescent mothers suggests that depression and/or drug abuse may be important factors in determining which mothers and their children will have poor outcomes (Zuckerman, Amaro, & Beardslee, 1987). The responsibility of rearing a child may force the single mother to curtail her education and thereafter be confined to an existence at or near the poverty level. Moreover, few adolescents are prepared for the demands of parenthood; their inadequate parenting skills may have a negative impact on the developing child (Sugar, 1984) and increase their risk for becoming abusive parents.

Separation and Divorce

Half of all children born during the 1980s were likely to experience their parents' divorce; the majority of these children will also experience the remarriage of their parents (Hetherington, Stanley-Hagan, & Anderson, 1989). Most children initially experience their parents' divorce as stressful. The long-term effects of parental divorce are related to the child's age, gender, and temperament, the qualities of the home environment, and the social and economic support systems available to the family.

When a marital relationship is terminated, it has been customary for the mother to assume custody of the children, with the father providing all or some of the financial support. Whether or not she has worked prior to separation, the probability is high that the mother will have to be employed in addition to having the major responsibility of childrearing. Although the father

is required to contribute to the support of the family, total amount of available income may still be considerably less than what the family had to live on before the separation. Mother's working may mean that preschool children will have inadequate caregivers and that older children will be unsupervised after school. When mother arrives home from work, she may be confronted with all of the household duties. The single parent and children may be faced with considerable change in their circumstances, and this change is likely to be the key factor in determining child behavior. Recent research suggests that marital conflict is predictive of children's behavior disorders; parental conflict is more likely to occur during the separation and divorce process and often continues long after divorce.

In a 3-year longitudinal study, Katz and Gottman (1993) found that husbands' angry and withdrawn pattern predicted teachers' ratings of children's internalizing behavior problems, whereas a mutually hostile pattern predicted teachers' ratings of children's subsequent externalizing behavior problems. Interparental verbal and physical conflict placed 3- to 6-year-olds from low-income families at high risk for both conduct and emotional problems, the latter of which were worse when the mothers and children resided in a shelter; the authors hypothesized that shelter placement deprived the children of coping mechanisms available in their natural environment, leaving them less protected from stress (Fantuzzo et al., 1991).

In a study of 7- to 17-year-old children of divorce, age at the time of divorce was not related to level of adjustment, but different patterns of emotional and behavior problems were associated with different ages (Kalter & Rembar, 1981). In addition, girls generally demonstrate better adjustment to divorce than do boys (Guidubaldi, Perry, & Cleminshaw, 1984).

Parent Factors

It is generally acknowledged that parental psychological characteristics have considerable potential for influencing their children's behavior. Many of the behaviors learned by children, particularly those learned early in life, are learned from parents.

Parents' psychological health may have a large impact on their everyday behavior toward the child. It has been assumed that mental illness and certain personality characteristics may lead the parent to behave in ways that deprive the child of needed interpersonal relationships and/or that create anxiety in the child.

In examining the relationship between parent psychological status and child behavior disorders, two subject selection procedures have been utilized by investigators. One procedure involves examining children of parents who have been clinically diagnosed as abnormal. In general, children of parents with psychological problems have a higher risk for psychological problems than do children of parents without diagnosed psychological problems. However, the children's problems may not be the same as the parents' problems. Such relationships have been found for most types of parental psychopathology. For example, Orvaschel, Walsh-Allis, and Ye (1988) found that 41% of children of parents with recurrent depression met criteria for at least one psychological disorder compared with 15% of control children. High-risk children also had significantly greater rates of affective and attentional disorders. A review of 34 studies indicated that the children of depressed parents were at greater risk for both internalizing and externalizing behavior problems (Forehand, McCombs, & Brody, 1987).

The second procedure for examining the relationship between parent and child psychological status is to assess the parents of children who have been clinically diagnosed as abnormal. Huschka (1941), using clinical records of children with behavior disorders, found that 42% of the mothers had neurotic symptoms, depression, suicidal impulses, or paranoid tendencies; he concluded that mother's psychological status greatly affected children at all stages of development. A number of studies using objective personality tests for assessing the adjustment of parents of children with behavior problems have also been conducted. Wolking, Quast, and Lawton (1966) administered the Minnesota Multiphasic Personality Inventory (MMPI) to parents of six diagnostic groupings of children. They found elevations of several MMPI clinical scales for all groups of parents with behavior-problem children in comparison with control parents, but no relationship between parental profile types and specific child disorders could be determined.

These correlational studies have typically been interpreted as reflecting that parental characteristics cause children's behavior problems and rarely the possibility that behavior problems in children adversely affect the parents (Erickson, 1968) or that some other variable could be responsible for both the parent and child findings.

Parental alcohol and substance abuse has been implicated as another risk factor for child psychopathology, including an increased rate of alcohol and substance abuse in children (Phares & Compas, 1992). A review of studies on children of alcoholic parents revealed a higher incidence of psychological symptoms in the children; however, the authors (West & Prinz, 1987) cautioned that "neither all nor a major portion of the population of children from alcoholic homes are inevitably doomed to childhood psychological disorder" (p. 204). A large-scale study of adults who experienced childhood exposure to parental problem drinking found an increased incidence of psychological symptoms and marital instability but no increased risk for problems in occupational functioning (Greenfield, Swartz, Landerman, & George, 1993).

Much has been written that blames parents for children's psychological problems and infers parental psychopathology as the reason for poor parenting. In many instances, however, parents may behave inappropriately toward their children through modeling of important adults in their own childhood and out of ignorance of long-term consequences. For example, most adults living today were probably hit or spanked by their parents during childhood, and some of them are simply following the example modeled by their parents. In addition, many parents today do not believe that there is potential harm to physical punishment. They are impressed with the quick results that such interventions often produce. Furthermore, the line between physical punishment and child abuse is sometimes not easy to draw. Parents may begin by spanking a child for *specific* serious infractions, then they spank to reduce *any* unwanted behavior, and finally may hit the child whenever the child reminds them of something unpleasant (e.g., the child is perceived as requiring too much work). Improved education for parenting and psychological support of parents would likely reduce at least some ineffective and damaging parental practices.

Child Factors

Just as parents vary in their personal characteristics, so do children, even from birth. For a long period, individual differences among infants and young children did not receive very much attention from clinicians because it was assumed that behavioral variability in children was caused by variations in parenting. Beginning in the 1960s, a longitudinal study of infants by Chess and Thomas (Thomas & Chess, 1977; Thomas, Chess, & Birch, 1968) began to demonstrate the implications of infants' behavioral characteristics.

Thomas and Chess (1977) identified three constellations of temperament: easy, slow-to-warm-up, or difficult. Easy children were high in rhythmicity and adaptability and not extreme in any other dimension. Slow-to-warm-up children showed slower adaptability with mildly intense and negative responsivity, but adapted positively over time. Difficult children were irregular in their biological functioning, resisted changes in their environment, and cried a lot. Thomas and Chess hypothesized that particular temperament styles would be associated with later psychopathology; their research stimulated a change in professionals' perceptions of infants.

Infants began to be perceived as having their own style or temperament virtually from birth.

In an ongoing longitudinal study, Kagan and his colleagues have reported a relationship between social inhibition in the second and third years of life and numbers of fears several years later; similarly, the laboratory index of inhibition in the second year of life had a .52 correlation with an aggregate index of behavioral inhibition at $5\frac{1}{2}$ years. Although early dispositions of children tended to be preserved through $7\frac{1}{2}$ years of age, environmental events appeared to modify these characteristics (Kagan, Reznick, & Snidman, 1990).

There has been evidence that infant temperament is somewhat stable during the preschool years, but that stability may gradually erode over time (Garrison & Earls, 1987, p. 48). Moderate heritability has been found for the temperamental traits of sociability, emotionality, and activity (Plomin & Rowe, 1977). Although it would be interesting to consider temperament as primarily a hereditary characteristic, we must consider that prenatal and postnatal factors could affect temperament as well as other behaviors.

Parent–Child Interaction

The influences of all of the aforementioned risk factors notwithstanding, parent–child interaction has captured the attention of theorists and clinicians alike. Freud's theory placed the origin of adult neuroses in pathological parent–child interactions during infancy and the preschool years. Behaviorists, on the other hand, being less interested in the *origin* of behavior disorders, focused on parents as *maintainers* of children's behavior problems. Both theoretical orientations have made significant contributions to our understanding of behavior problems. Possibly Freud's greatest contribution was his drawing attention to the great influence of experience during infancy and the preschool period and the potentially detrimental effects of extremely harsh parenting behaviors. The behaviorists' contribution has been their strong focus on empirical research and the ways that parental behavior affects the behavior of children and adolescents.

Parent–child interaction begins in earnest at birth with a complex series of exchanges in which behaviors of each affect behaviors of the other. It seems obvious that the infant who is "good" and whose behavior is what the parents expect is likely to get better responses from parents, but real-life practice is much more complex. For example, the young infant's cry is the only signal that the infant has to indicate need (hunger, pain, boredom); the infant who doesn't cry is more likely to be neglected. Therefore, being "good" should not mean absence of crying. Unfortunately, many parents often don't know what behavior to expect from infants and children.

From the child's point of view, the cumulative daily interactions and meeting of needs are what determines his or her perception of people and self. Perhaps the most critical factor during the preschool period is child care.

Child Care

At one time, orphanages for young children were much more common than they are today. The primary reason for their demise was the increasing awareness that children who were placed into institutional settings at an early age had high rates of mortality and behavior problems. Goldfarb (1944), Spitz (1945), and Bowlby (1952) described the conditions in which many of the orphans lived. The basic needs of the children were quite adequate; that is, they were fed, kept clean, and protected against contagious diseases. In spite of these efforts, between 30 and 75% of the children were dying within 2 years of being placed in the institutions and were found to be extremely susceptible to disease and other illnesses. Each child was typically placed in a crib whose sides were draped in sheets, thus effectively preventing the infants from seeing other children and the rest of the room. Unless the children could stand up in the crib, they were confined to a world almost totally lacking in visual stimulation. Social contact between caretakers and infants was extremely brief, and the children were usually not held, even for feeding.

Observers interpreted the high mortality, poor development, and emotional apathy (depression) as reflecting the children's having been separated from their mothers. Bowlby (1952) proposed that normal mental health requires a continuous relationship with a mother or mother substitute during infancy. Casler (1961) and Yarrow (1964), however, suggested that the devastating effects of institutions on infants and young children may not have been caused by separation from the mother per se but by the deprivation of the stimulation that the mother provided and mediated.

Research evidence has demonstrated that group care for infants and young children can be designed to be as effective, and sometimes better than that given by some mothers. A review by Belsky and Steinberg (1978) concluded that high-quality day care does not adversely affect IQ scores, is not disruptive to the emotional bond between mother and child, and increases both positive and negative peer interactions. More recent research suggests that 1-year-olds in day care may be more likely to avoid their mothers after brief separations and to be more aggressive with their peers a few years later; Clarke-Stewart (1989) recommended that future research focus on factors that may moderate or mediate the effects of infant day care.

Baydar and Brooks-Gunn (1991) found that timing of mother's employment in the first year of life affected children's cognitive and behavioral functioning 3 years later. Mothers who began (or resumed) work in the fourth quarter had higher functioning children; beginning work during the second quarter appeared to be more detrimental than beginning in the first quarter. More negative effects were found for children whose mothers worked 10–19 hours a week compared with mothers who worked fewer than 10 or more than 20 hours. The authors suggested that stability of child care may have been the important determinant of these interesting findings. In a larger study, Bates et al. (1994) found a small but statistically significant relationship between extent of child care and subsequent adjustment problems during kindergarten.

Related to child care and the larger context of parent–child interactions is the concept of attachment. Bowlby's original concern about children in orphanages led to a quest by himself and others, most notably Mary Ainsworth, to understand the nature of attachment and its implications for psychological health. The caretaker–child attachment process occurs primarily in the first 1 to 2 years of life. The infant who becomes securely attached has a lower risk for later psychological problems compared with infants who are insecurely attached. It would appear that any life event that interrupts the caretaker–infant relationship might affect future attachment. Interestingly, modern life has greatly increased the probability of physical separation of mothers and infants as compared with earlier times when mothers had to breast-feed their children. Research has only begun to identify the family life experiences that affect attachment. For example, Shaw and Vondra (1993) found that cumulative family adversity, such as parental criminality, maternal depression, and overcrowding in the home, differentiated secure from insecure 12-month-olds.

It is extremely important that infants and children receive the care and stimulation that will optimize their physical and psychological development. Although it has not yet given exact specifications, research has at least provided some information about the most salient variables. In general, infants and children need adults to care for their physical needs (food, water, shelter, protection from harm, temperature control, cleanliness) and to give them experiences (visual, language, and tactile stimulation) that will facilitate their learning about people and the environment. Included in this care from adults should be the message that adults care about them and that they should care for others.

The child's need for care continues until adulthood (and sometimes later), but the type of parental caring behaviors vary as the child matures. The parents' principal goal is attending to the *socialization* of the child, that is, ensuring that the child's behavior "fits" with the general expectations of society. Methods by which parents approach this goal appear to affect the development of behavior disorders during childhood and adolescence. Considerable research has shown that children and adolescents whose parents are authoritative (both accepting and strict) are better adjusted than those whose parents are neglectful (neither accepting nor strict), authoritarian (overly strict), or indulgent (overly accepting). A meta-analysis of 172 studies published from 1952 to 1987 revealed significant differences in how parents socialize boys and girls (Lytton & Romney, 1991). Parents tended to encourage sex-typed activities and used more physical punishment with boys.

Finally, a recent study with adolescents examined differences in adjustment that were associated with parenting styles over a 1-year period and found them to be either maintained or increased. Adolescents from authoritative homes showed increases in self-reliance and academic self-concept and a decrease in behavior problems, whereas adolescents from neglectful homes showed a sharp increase in behavior problems (Steinberg, Lamborn, Darling, Mounts, & Dornbusch, 1994).

SUMMARY

Cumulative research findings indicate that a biopsychological theoretical orientation will probably optimize our understanding of the etiology of children's behavior disorders. Although accounting for only a small percentage of empirical studies, behavior genetic twin research has shown that heredity plays a significant role in both externalizing and internalizing behavior problems; this research also indicates that environmental factors usually contribute larger proportions of the variance, however.

Physical factors during the prenatal, perinatal, and postnatal periods, such as maternal substance abuse and prematurity, increase children's risk for later developmental and behavior problems. Many of these physical risk factors can be reduced through medical and psychological prevention and early intervention programs. Psychological risk factors, particularly stressful family life events, also increase the risk for psychopathology, especially when they occur in conjunction with hereditary and other physical risk factors.

Age of the child seems to play a complex role in determining the child's vulnerability to behavior disorders. That is, physical and psychological trauma may have quite different outcomes depending on the child's age at the time of the event.

Although our understanding of etiological factors is more "balanced" on the biological–psychological continuum than it has ever been, we continue to be ignorant about the relative importance of the risk factors described. Research that includes measures of all of the known risk factors on the same subjects will be necessary for our knowledge to progress. That research should also utilize both categorical and continuous measures of children's behavior disorders to help in evaluating the utility of both approaches.

Acknowledgments

I wish to express my appreciation to Teresa Southall Parr and Cassandra Stanton for their careful reading and comments on the manuscript.

REFERENCES

Bailey, J. M., Bobrow, D., Wolfe, M., & Mikach, S. (1995). Sexual orientation of adult sons of gay fathers. *Developmental Psychology, 31,* 124–129.

Barrett, D. E., Radke-Yarrow, M., & Klein, R. E. (1982). Chronic malnutrition and child behavior: Effects of early calorie supplementation on social and emotional functioning at school age. *Developmental Psychology, 18,* 541–556.

Bates, J. E., Marvinney, D., Kelly, T., Dodge, K. A., Bennett, D. S., & Pettit, G. S. (1994). Child care history and kindergarten adjustment. *Developmental Psychology, 30,* 690–700.

Baydar, N., & Brooks-Gunn, J. (1991). Effects of maternal employment and child-care arrangements on preschoolers' cognitive and behavioral outcomes. *Developmental Psychology, 27,* 932–945.

Belsky, J. (1993). Etiology of child maltreatment: A developmental-ecological analysis. *Psychological Bulletin, 114,* 413–434.

Belsky, J., & Steinberg, L. D. (1978). The effects of day care: A critical review. *Child Development, 49,* 929–949.

Bowlby, J. (1952). *Maternal care and mental health.* Geneva: World Health Organization.

Campbell, S. B. (1990). *Behavior problems in preschoolers: Clinical and developmental issues.* New York: Guilford Press.

Cardozo, L. D., Gibb, D. M. F., Studd, J. W. W., & Cooper, D. J. (1982). Social and obstetric features associated with smoking in pregnancy. *British Journal of Obstetrics and Gynaecology, 89,* 622–627.

Casler, L. (1961). Maternal deprivation: A critical review of the literature. *Monographs of the Society for Research in Child Development, 26,* No. 2.

Cicchetti, D. (Ed.). (1994). Special issue: Advances and challenges in the study of the sequelae of child maltreatment. *Development and Psychopathology, 6,* 1–247.

Clarke-Stewart, K. A. (1989). Infant day care: Maligned or malignant? *American Psychologist, 44,* 266–273.

Cohen, P., Cohen, J., & Brook, J. S. (1993). An epidemiological study of disorders in late childhood and adolescence: II. Persistence of disorders. *Journal of Child Psychology and Psychiatry and Allied Disciplines, 34,* 869–877.

Cohen, S. (1995). Biosocial factors in early infancy as predictors of competence in adolescents who were born prematurely. *Developmental and Behavioral Pediatrics, 16,* 36–41.

Davids, A., DeVault, S., & Talmadge, M. (1961). Anxiety, pregnancy, and childbirth abnormalities. *Journal of Consulting Psychology, 25,* 74–77.

Ebbs, J. H., Tisdall, F. F., & Scott, W. A. (1942). The influence of prenatal diet on the mother and child. *The Milbank Memorial Fund Quarterly, 20,* 35–36.

Erickson, M. T. (1965). Relationship between psychological attitudes during pregnancy and complications of pregnancy, labor, and delivery. *Proceedings of the American Psychological Association, 1,* 213–214.

Erickson, M. T. (1967). Prenatal and preconception environmental influences. *Science, 157,* 1210.

Erickson, M. T. (1968). MMPI comparisons between parents of young emotionally disturbed and organically retarded children. *Journal of Consulting and Clinical Psychology, 32,* 701–706.

Fantuzzo, J. N., DePaola, L. M., Lambert, L., Martino, J., Anderson, G., & Sutton, S. (1991). Effects of interparental violence on the psychological adjustment and competencies of young children. *Journal of Consulting and Clinical Psychology, 59,* 258–265.

Fergusson, D. H., Fergusson, J. E., Horwood, L. J., & Kinzett, N. G. (1988). A longitudinal study of dentine lead levels, intelligence, school performance and behavior. Part III. Dentine lead levels and attention/activity. *Journal of Child Psychology and Psychiatry, 29,* 811–824.

Fergusson, D. M., Horwood, L. J., & Lynskey, M. T. (1993). Early dentine lead levels and subsequent cognitive and behavioral development. *Journal of Child Psychology and Psychiatry and Allied Disciplines, 34,* 215–227.

Finster, M., Petersen, H., & Morishima, H. O. (1983). Principles of fetal exposure to drugs used in obstetric anesthesia. In B. Krauer, F. Krauer, F. E. Hythen, & E. Del-Pozo (Eds.), *Drugs and pregnancy.* New York: Academic Press.

Forehand, R. L., McCombs, A., & Brody, G. H. (1987). The relationship between parental depressive mood state and child functioning. *Advances in Behavior Research and Therapy, 9,* 1–20.

Frisch, R. E. (1988). Fatness and fertility. *Scientific American, 258,* 88–96.

Galler, J. R. (Ed.). (1984). *Human nutrition: A comprehensive treatise: Nutrition and behavior* (Vol. 5). New York: Plenum.

Galton, F. (1869). *Hereditary genius.* London: Macmillan.

Garrison, W. T., & Earls, F. J. (1987). *Temperament and child psychopathology.* Newbury Park, CA: Sage.

Gau, J. S., Silberg, J. L., Erickson, M. T., & Hewitt, J. K. (1992). Childhood behavior problems: A comparison of twin and non-twin samples. *Acta Genetica Medicae, 41,* 53–63.

Ge, X., Conger, R. D., Lorenz, F. O., & Simons, R. L. (1994). Parents' stressful life events and adolescent depressed mood. *Journal of Health and Social Behavior, 35,* 28–44.

Goldberg, D., & Wolkind, S. (1992). Patterns of psychiatric disorder in adopted girls. *Journal of Child Psychology and Psychiatry, 33,* 935–950.

Goldfarb, W. (1944). The effects of early institutional care on adolescent personality: Rorschach data. *American Journal of Orthopsychiatry, 14,* 441–447.

Golombok, S., Spencer, A., & Rutter, M. (1983). Children in lesbian and single-parent households: A psychosexual and psychiatric appraisal. *Journal of Child Psychology and Psychiatry and Allied Disciplines, 24,* 551–572.

Grantham-McGregor, S., Schofield, W., & Powell, C. (1987). Development of severely malnourished children who received psychosocial stimulation: Six-year follow-up. *Pediatrics, 79,* 247–254.

Gray, J. W., Davis, B., McCoy, K., & Dean, R. S. (1992). Mothers' self-reports of perinatal information as predictors of school achievement. *Journal of School Psychology, 30,* 233–243.

Greenfield, S. F., Swartz, M. S., Landerman, L. R., & George, L. K. (1993). Long-term psychosocial effects of childhood exposure to parental problem drinking. *American Journal of Psychiatry, 150,* 608–613.

Guidubaldi, J., Perry, J. D., & Cleminshaw, H. K. (1984). The legacy of parental divorce. In B. B. Lahey & A. E. Kazdin (Eds.), *Advances in clinical child psychology* (Vol. 7, pp. 109–151). New York: Plenum Press.

Hack, M., Taylor, H. G., Klein, N., Eiben, R., Schatschneider, C., & Mercuri-Minich, K. (1994). School-age outcomes in children with birth weights under 750 g. *New England Journal of Medicine, 331,* 753–759.

Harrell, R. F., Woodyard, E., & Gates, A. I. (1955). *The effects of mothers' diets on the intelligence of offspring.* New York: Teachers College.

Hellmuth, J. (Ed.). (1967). *Exceptional infant* (Vol. 1). New York: Brunner/Mazel.

Herrenkohl, L. R. (1979). Prenatal stress reduces fertility and fecundity in female offspring. *Science, 206,* 1097–1099.

Hetherington, E. M., Stanley-Hagan, M., & Anderson, E. R. (1989). Marital transitions: A child's perspective. *American Psychologist, 44,* 303–312.

Hurt, H., Brodsky, N. L., Betancourt, L., Braitman, L. E., Melmud, E., & Giannetta, J. (1995). Cocaine-exposed children: Follow-up through 30 months. *Developmental and Behavioral Pediatrics, 16,* 29–35.

Huschka, M. (1941). Psychopathological disorders in the mother. *Journal of Nervous and Mental Disease, 94,* 76–83.

Inoff-Germain, G., Arnold, G. S., Nottelmann, E. D., & Susman, E. J. (1988). Relations between hormone levels and observational measures of aggressive behavior of young adolescents in family interactions. *Developmental Psychology, 24,* 129–139.

Johnson, J. H., & Bradlyn, A. S. (1988). Life events and adjustment in childhood and adolescence. In L. H. Cohen (Ed.), *Life events and psychological functioning* (pp. 64–95). Newbury Park, CA: Sage.

Jones, K. L., Smith, D. W., Ulleland, C. N., & Streissguth, A. P. (1973). Pattern of malformation in offspring of chronic alcoholic mothers. *Lancet, 1,* 1267–1271.

Kallam, S. G., Ensminger, M. E., & Turner, R. J. (1977). Family structure and the mental health of children. *Archives of General Psychiatry, 34,* 1012–1022.

Kagan, J., Reznick, J. S., & Snidman, K. (1990). The temperamental qualities of inhibition and lack of inhibition. In M. Lewis & S. M. Miller (Eds.), *Handbook of developmental psychopathology* (pp. 219–226). New York: Plenum Press.

Kalter, N., & Rembar, J. (1981). The significance of a child's age at the time of parental divorce. *American Journal of Orthopsychiatry, 51,* 85–100.

Katz, L. F., & Gottman, J. M. (1993). Patterns of marital conflict predict children's internalizing and externalizing behaviors. *Developmental Psychology, 29,* 940–950.

Kendall-Tackett, K. A., Williams, L. M., & Finkelhor, D.

(1993). Impact of sexual abuse on children: A review and synthesis of recent empirical studies. *Psychological Bulletin, 113,* 164–180.

Lee, H., & Barratt, M. S. (1993). Cognitive development of preterm low birth weight children at 5 to 8 years old. *Journal of Developmental and Behavioral Pediatrics, 14,* 242–249.

Lejeune, J., Gautier, M., & Turpin, R. (1959). Le mongolisme: Premier example d'aberration autosomique humaine. *Annales de Genetique, 1,* 41.

Leonard, M. F., Landy, G., Ruddle, F. H., & Lubs, H. A. (1974). Early development of children with abnormalities of the sex chromosomes: A prospective study. *Pediatrics, 54,* 208–212.

Liaw, F., & Brooks-Gunn, J. (1994). Cumulative familiar risks and low-birthweight in children's cognitive and behavioral development. *Journal of Clinical Child Psychology, 23,* 360–372.

Lozoff, B. (1989). Nutrition and behavior. *American Psychologist, 44,* 231–236.

Lytton, H., & Romeny, D. M. (1991). Parents' differential socialization of boys and girls: A meta-analysis. *Psychological Bulletin, 109,* 267–296.

Maccoby, E. E., & Jacklin, C. O. (1980). Sex differences in aggression: A rejoinder and reprise. *Child Development, 51,* 964–980.

Malinosky-Rummell, R., & Hansen, D. J. (1993). Long-term consequences of childhood physical abuse. *Psychological Bulletin, 114,* 68–79.

Meyers, A. F., Sampson, A. E., Weitzman, M., Rogers, B. L., & Kayne, H. (1989). School breakfast program and school performance. *American Journal of Diseases of Children, 143,* 1234–1239.

Needleman, H. L., & Bellinger, D. (1984). The developmental consequences of childhood exposure to lead. In B. B. Lahey & A. E. Kazdin (Eds.), *Advances in clinical child psychology* (Vol. 7, pp. 195–220). New York: Plenum.

Orvaschel, H., Walsh-Allis, G., & Ye, W. (1988). Psychopathology in children of parents with recurrent depression. *Journal of Abnormal Child Psychology, 16,* 17–28.

Phares, V., & Compas, B. E. (1992). The role of fathers in child and adolescent psychopathology. *Psychological Bulletin, 111,* 387–412.

Plomin, R. (1989). Environment and genes: Determinants of behavior. *American Psychologist, 44,* 105–111.

Plomin, R. (1994). Genetic research and identification of environmental influences. *Journal of Child Psychology and Psychiatry and Allied Disciplines, 35,* 817–834.

Plomin, R., & Rowe, D. C. (1977). A twin study of temperament in young children. *Journal of Psychology, 97,* 107–113.

Polusny, M. A., & Follette, V. M. (1995). Long-term correlates of child sexual abuse: Theory and review of the empirical literature. *Applied and Preventive Psychology, 4,* 143–166.

Proctor, E. K., Vosler, N. R., & Murty, S. (1992). Child demographics and DSM diagnosis: A multi-axis study. *Child Psychiatry and Human Development, 22,* 165–183.

Robinson, A., Bender, B., Borelli, J., Puck, M., & Salenblatt, J. (1983). Sex chromosomal anomalies: Prospective studies in children. *Behavior Genetics, 13,* 321–329.

Roosa, M. W., Fitzgerald, H. E., & Carlson, N. A. (1982). Teenage parenting and child development: A literature review. *Infant Mental Health Journal, 3,* 4–18.

Routh, D. K. (1994). Impact of poverty on children, youth, and families: Introduction to the special issue. *Journal of Clinical Child Psychology, 23,* 346–348.

Scarr-Salapatek, S. (1971). Race, social class, and I.Q. *Science, 14,* 1285–1295.

Schneider, M. L., & Coe, C. L. (1993). Repeated social stress during pregnancy impairs neuromotor development of the primate infant. *Journal of Developmental and Behavioral Pediatrics, 14,* 81–87.

Secord, G. J., Erickson, M. T., & Bush, J. P. (1988). Neuropsychological sequelae of otitis media in children and adolescents with learning disabilities. *Journal of Pediatric Psychology, 13,* 531–542.

Sells, C. J., Robinson, N. M., Brown, Z., & Knopp, R. H. (1994). Long-term developmental follow-up of infants of diabetic mothers. *Journal of Pediatrics, 125,* 59–77.

Shaw, D. S., & Vondra, I. (1993). Chronic family adversity and infant attachment security. *Journal of Child Psychology and Psychiatry and Allied Disciplines, 34,* 1205–1215.

Silberg, J. L., Erickson, M. T., Meyers, J. M., Eaves, L. J., Rutter, M. L., & Hewitt, J. K. (1994). The application of structural equation modeling to maternal ratings of twins' behavioral and emotional problems. *Journal of Consulting and Clinical Psychology, 62,* 510–521.

Smith, C. A. (1947). Effects of maternal undernutrition upon the newborn infant in Holland (1944–45). *Journal of Pediatrics, 30,* 229–243.

Spitz, R. A. (1945). Hospitalism: An inquiry into the genesis of psychiatric conditions in early childhood. *Psychoanalytic Study of the Child, 1,* 53–64.

Steinberg, L., Lamborn, S. D., Darling, N., Mounts, N. S., & Dornbusch, S. M. (1994). Over-time changes in adjustment and competence among adolescents from authoritative, authoritarian, indulgent, and neglectful families. *Child Development, 65,* 754–770.

Steinhausen, H.-C., Williams, J., & Spohr, H.-L. (1994). Correlates of psychopathology and intelligence in children with fetal alcohol syndrome. *Journal of Child Psychology and Psychiatry and Allied Disciplines, 35,* 323–331.

Stoch, M. B., Smythe, P., Moodie, A. D., & Bradshaw, D. (1982). Psychosocial outcome and CT findings after gross undernourishment during infancy: A 20-year developmental study. *Developmental Medicine and Child Neurology, 24,* 419–436.

Sugar, M. (1984). Infants of adolescent mothers: Research perspective. In M. Sugar (Ed.), *Adolescent parenthood* (pp. 101–108). New York: Spectrum.

Szatmari, P., Boyle, M. H., & Offord, D. R. (1993). Family aggregation of emotional and behavioral problems in childhood in the general population. *American Journal of Psychiatry, 150,* 1398–1403.

Task Force on Pediatric AIDS, American Psychological Association. (1989). Pediatric AIDS and human immunodeficiency virus infection. *American Psychologist, 44,* 258–264.

Telzrow, C. F. (1987). Management of academic and educational problems in head injury. *Journal of Learning Disabilities, 20,* 536–545.

Thatcher, R. W., Lester, M. L., McAlaster, R., Horst, R., & Ignatius, S. W. (1983). Intelligence and lead toxins in rural children. *Journal of Learning Disabilities, 16,* 355–359.

Thomas, A., & Chess, S. (1977). *Temperament and development.* New York: Brunner/Mazel.

Thomas, A., Chess, S., & Birch, H. G. (1968). *Temperament and behavior disorders in children.* New York: New York University Press.

Thompson, R. J., Goldstein, R. F., Oehler, J. M., Gustafson, K. E., Catlett, A. T., & Brazy, J. E. (1994). Developmental outcome of very low birth weight infants as a function of biological risk and psychosocial risk. *Journal of Developmental and Behavioral Pediatrics, 15,* 232–238.

Walther, F. J., & Ramaekers, L. H. J. (1982). Language development at the age of 3 years of infants malnourished in utero. *Neuropediatrics, 13,* 77–81.

Weintraub, M., & Wolf, B. M. (1983). Effects of stress and social supports on mother–child interactions in single and two-parent families. *Child Development, 54,* 1297–1311.

Weiss, B. (1984). Food additive safety evaluation: In B. B. Lahey & A. E. Kazdin (Eds.), *Advances in clinical child psychology* (Vol. 7, pp. 221–251). New York: Plenum.

West, M. O., & Prinz, R. J. (1987). Parental alcoholism and childhood psychopathology. *Psychological Bulletin, 102,* 204–218.

Willis, D. J., & Walker, C. E. (1989). Etiology. In T. H. Ollendick & M. Hersen (Eds.), *Handbook of child psychopathology* (2nd ed., pp. 29–51). New York: Plenum Press.

Windle, W. F. (Ed.). (1958). *Neurological and psychological deficits of asphyxia neonatorium.* Springfield, IL: Thomas.

Winick, M. (Ed.). (1979). *Human nutrition: A comprehensive treatise. Volume 1: Pre- and postnatal development.* New York: Plenum.

Wolking, W. D., Quast, W., & Lawton, J. J. (1966). MMPI profiles of parents of behaviorally disturbed children and parents from the general population. *Journal of Clinical Psychology, 22,* 39–48.

Wright, S. W., Tarjan, G., & Eyer, L. (1959). Investigations of families with two or more mentally defective siblings: Clinical observations. *American Journal of Diseases of Children, 97,* 445–456.

Yarrow, L. J. (1964). Separation from parents during early childhood. In M. L. Hoffman & L. W. Hoffman (Eds.), *Review of child development research* (Vol. 1, pp. 89–136). New York: Russell Sage Foundation.

Zapata, B. C. (1992). The influence of social and political violence on the risk of pregnancy complications. *American Journal of Public Health, 82,* 685–690.

Zuckerman, B. S., Amaro, H., & Beardslee, W. (1987). Mental health of adolescent mothers: The implications of depression and drug use. *Developmental and Behavioral Pediatrics, 8,* 111–116.

3

Diagnosis, Assessment, Taxonomy, and Case Formulations

THOMAS M. ACHENBACH

INTRODUCTION

Diagnostic terminology is widely used by mental health professionals. In the United States, diagnostic concepts have become dominated by the *Diagnostic and Statistical Manual* (DSM) published by the American Psychiatric Association (1980, 1987, 1994). Because reimbursement has become increasingly dependent on DSM diagnoses, mental health professionals are understandably concerned about such diagnoses.

To third-party payers, it may seem logical to model reimbursements for psychopathology on diagnosis-based reimbursement for physical disorders. It may also seem logical to model reimbursement for child psychopathology on diagnosis-based reimbursement for adult psychopathology. (For brevity, I will use the term *child* to include *adolescents*.) However, those who work with children know that children's behavioral/emotional problems and needs seldom fit

neatly into the diagnostic categories favored by third-party payers. Instead, children's problems often vary from one context to another. Consequently, interventions involve working with parents, teachers, and others, rather than merely applying a reimbursable treatment to the child. In addition, because troubled children may qualify for multiple diagnoses, they may receive the best-reimbursed diagnoses, rather than diagnoses that best reflect their problems and needs.

Efforts by third-party payers to control fee-for-service costs have greatly augmented interest in diagnoses for children's behavioral/emotional problems. However, mismatches between reimbursable diagnoses and children's actual problems argue for broader approaches to diagnosis. Moreover, the growing displacement of traditional fee-for-service models by capitated managed care is changing the incentive structure for service providers. Whereas fee-for-service providers are reinforced for using maximally reimbursable diagnoses and procedures, capitated managed care providers are reinforced for keeping clients healthy and satisfied at the lowest possible cost. In managed care systems, accurate assessment that facilitates more effective

THOMAS M. ACHENBACH • Department of Psychiatry, University of Vermont, Burlington, Vermont 05401-3456.

Handbook of Child Psychopathology, 3rd edition, edited by Ollendick & Hersen. Plenum Press, New York, 1998.

prevention and early intervention therefore becomes more valuable than the reimbursability of particular diagnoses and procedures.

To elucidate diagnostic concepts, I will first distinguish among the multiple meanings of diagnosis. Alternative terms are then provided to reduce confusion among the different components of diagnosis. Thereafter, problems and solutions specific to child psychopathology are presented, followed by illustrative applications.

DIAGNOSTIC CONCEPTS

Mental health workers devote a great deal of time to diagnostic issues during their clinical training. Yet, there is little agreement about the proper nature and role of diagnosis with respect to child psychopathology. Psychodynamically oriented workers, for example, think of diagnosis in terms of underlying personality structures and forces inferred from clinical interviews and projective tests. Behaviorally oriented workers, by contrast, may limit diagnosis to documentation of specific behaviors and their supporting contingencies. Family therapists are apt to diagnose children's problems as symptoms of disturbed family systems, whereas physicians look for symptoms from which to infer underlying illness. And psychometricians may think in terms of traits measured in terms of standardized tests.

Even among workers who share similar theoretical orientations, disagreements often arise about specific cases. Case conferences may be enlivened, for example, by disputes about whether a child manifesting conduct problems is actually suffering from an underlying depression. Yet, diagnostic conclusions about whether the child has a conduct disorder or is depressed seldom dictate specific treatments of proven efficacy for the child's problems. Instead, interventions may be dictated more by reimbursability or by the predilections of the practitioner than by well-validated relations between diagnosis and specific interventions.

If diagnosis does not usually lead to more effective help for children, it should not be surprising that many practitioners disparage diagnosis. Yet, to improve our understanding of children's problems and our ability to help, we need better ways of determining what the problems are in the first place and how differences between problems should affect the choice of intervention.

To *diagnose* literally means "to distinguish" or "to know apart" (from Greek *dia,* "apart," and *gignoskein,* "to know"). Confusion arises, however, because the term *diagnosis* is used in the three different ways discussed next.

Diagnosis in the Narrow Sense: Formal Diagnosis

In its narrowest meaning, *diagnosis* is "the medical term for classification," according to a leading psychiatric diagnostician (Guze, 1978, p. 53). In this narrow sense, to diagnose means to assign cases to the categories of a system for classifying diseases. Such systems are called *nosologies.* Examples include the DSM and the *International Classification of Diseases* (ICD; World Health Organization, 1992). A diagnosis in the sense of classification is called a *formal diagnosis.* For example, if we decide that 11-year-old Jason meets criteria for a DSM diagnosis of attention-deficit/hyperactivity disorder (ADHD), we are making a formal diagnosis.

Diagnosis in the Broad Sense: Diagnostic Formulation

Beside being the medical term for classification, *diagnosis* is used in a broader sense to mean "a statement or conclusion concerning the nature or cause of some phenomenon" (Woolf, 1977, p. 313). When used in this sense, diagnosis refers to a *diagnostic formulation;* that is, the formulation of conclusions about a problem.

Even though Jason's formal diagnosis is ADHD, we need to provide a comprehensive diagnostic formulation on which to base an intervention strategy. This formulation should be based on information about Jason's developmental history, family, physical condition, school situation, strengths, and vulnerabilities, as well as whatever is captured by the formal diagnosis of ADHD.

Diagnosis as an Activity: Diagnostic Process

Jason's formal diagnosis of ADHD and the diagnostic formulation of his case are both products of data that have been obtained about him. The activity of gathering the data is also known as diagnosis, or, more specifically, *diagnostic process*. Neither the diagnostic classification nor the diagnostic formulation can be any better than the data on which they are based. Yet, the criteria for making the formal diagnosis of ADHD do not specify what data should be obtained, by what means, or from whom. Although the DSM does stated that "reports from multiple informants . . . are helpful" (American Psychiatric Association, 1994, p. 83), it does not say how such reports are to be obtained. Nor does it say how to resolve discrepancies among reports in order to make yes-or-no judgments of such criteria as "often talks excessively" and "often has difficulty awaiting turn" (p. 84). The procedures for obtaining data, the sources of the data, the ways in which practitioners combine data, and the inferences drawn from the data all affect formal diagnoses and diagnostic formulations.

Distinguishing among the Meanings of Diagnosis

To distinguish more clearly among the multiple meanings of diagnosis, the following sections deal with processes, objectives, and products that are often merged within the terminology of diagnosis but each of which nonetheless deserves explicit attention in its own right. The following terms are substituted for the various meanings of diagnosis: As a substitute for *diagnostic process, assessment* refers to gathering data

about cases so as to identify their distinguishing features; as a substitute for *formal diagnosis, taxonomy* refers to grouping cases according to their distinguishing features; and as a substitute for *diagnostic formulation, case formulation* refers to a comprehensive summary of the case. Reflecting the author's view that we need to expand knowledge about child psychopathology, the emphasis will be on advancing the empirical basis for assessment, taxonomy, and case formulation.

ASSESSMENT

The DSM Approach to Assessment

In the DSM and ICD approach to child psychopathology, diagnostic categories and criteria for defining each category are chosen by committees. After the categories and criteria have been chosen, assessment procedures are designed to determine which children meet criteria for the diagnostic categories.

Since the introduction of explicit diagnostic criteria by DSM-III (American Psychiatric Association, 1980), structured interviews have become popular for assessing child psychopathology. Examples include the *Diagnostic Interview Schedule for Children* (DISC; Costello, Edelbrock, Dulcan, Kalas, & Klaric, 1984; Shaffer, 1992) and the *Diagnostic Interview for Children and Adolescents* (DICA; Herjanic & Reich, 1982; Reich & Welner, 1992). These interviews consist of questions designed to yield yes-or-no answers about whether a child meets each criterion specified for each diagnostic category. The criteria include current behavioral characteristics, a minimum period over which the behaviors are required to be present, an age by which the symptoms had to have occurred, and other criteria specific to the diagnosis.

For example, in using a structured diagnostic interview to determine whether 11-year-old Jason qualifies for a DSM-IV diagnosis of ADHD, we must obtain yes-or-no judgments of criteria such as the following: Does Jason often talk excessively? Have at least six symptoms of inattention or hyperactivity-impulsivity persisted for at least 6 months to a degree that is maladaptive and inconsistent with developmental level? Were some symptoms that caused impairment present before age 7? Is some impairment from symptoms present in two or more settings (e.g., school and home)? Is there clear evidence of clinically significant impairment in social, academic, or occupational functioning? Do the symptoms occur exclusively during the course of certain other disorders or are they better accounted for by another disorder? (paraphrased from DSM-IV, American Psychiatric Association, 1994, pp. 84–85).

According to the DSM model, "yes" judgments of all of the criterial features required for the diagnosis mean that Jason has ADHD. On the other hand, if any of the required criteria are not affirmed, Jason does not qualify for the ADHD diagnosis.

Empirically Based Assessment

The empirically based approach to assessment follows a different strategy from the DSM approach. The general strategy of the DSM approach is to "work from the top down" by starting with definitional criteria for diagnostic categories and then determining which children meet the criteria. The empirically based approach, by contrast, "works from the bottom up" by starting with large pools of items for reporting behavioral and emotional problems that are considered to be important in their own right. These items are then scored for large clinical and normative samples to determine how well they discriminate between children who are considered to need professional help versus children considered to be relatively normal.

Derivation by Syndromes from Assessment Data

In addition to testing the discriminative power of candidate items, the empirically based approach uses data obtained with these items to derive syndromes of problems that are found to co-occur in clinical samples. Specifically, multivariate methods, such as factor analysis and principal components analysis, are used to identify sets of problems that tend to co-occur. These sets of co-occurring problems are viewed as syndromes in the generic sense of "a set of concurrent things" (Gove, 1971, p. 2320). In deriving syndromes, we do not make any assumptions about why particular problems co-occur. The syndromes may result from genetic factors, nongenetic physical abnormalities, environmental factors, or any combination of these. Rather than defining assessment criteria on the basis of assumptions about what disorders exist, the empirically based approach uses assessment data to identify patterns of problems as a basis for a taxonomy of disorders.

The Relevance of Normative Data

Just as empirically based assessment does not make a priori assumptions about what disorders exist, it also does not assume that particular problems or syndromes have precisely the same meaning for both sexes, all ages, and all sources of data. For example, a problem such as "often talks excessively" might have different clinical significance for boys versus girls, younger versus older children, and reports by parents, teachers, and the children themselves. To make valid judgments about particular problems and syndromes, it is necessary to know their distributions for each sex at different ages and according to different sources of data. The empirically based approach therefore employs data from normative samples, as assessed via different sources, to provide a frame of reference for judging problems reported for individual children.

For example, in the empirically based assessment of 11-year-old Jason, we would evaluate problems reported by his parents, his teacher, and Jason himself in relation to problems reported for reference samples of boys of the same age by their parents, teachers, and the boys themselves. This is done by comparing Jason's score on empirically based syndromes with the scores of normative samples of nonreferred boys who have been randomly selected to be representative of boys who are relatively normal. By using standard scores (such as *T* scores) or percentiles, we can determine whether Jason's score on each syndrome is relatively low, medium, or high, as compared with the scores of his nonreferred peers. We may find, for example, that even though Jason's mother reports problems such as "often talks excessively," his score on the syndrome that includes this problem corresponds to the 50th percentile of scores obtained by his nonreferred peers, as scored by their parents. In fact, in a national sample of nonreferred 11-year-old boys, their parents reported that over 40% talked excessively (Achenbach, 1991a). Consequently, if Jason's mother reported that he talked excessively and also reported other problems of the syndrome that collectively summed only to a score at the 50th percentile of the normative sample, we would not judge Jason to be deviant.

Even if Jason's mother's reports do not indicate deviance from norms for his peers, his teacher's reports might yield a different picture. For example, if the problems scored by Jason's teacher summed to a score that was above the 98th percentile for his nonreferred peers, this would indicate considerable deviance from the level of problems reported for most other boys by their teachers.

It would not be unusual for data from parents and teachers to yield different pictures of a child's problems. In fact, meta-analyses of numerous studies have yielded a mean correlation of only .27 between parent and teacher reports of children's problems (Achenbach, McConaughy, & Howell, 1987). Although this correlation was statistically significant, its modest size reflects considerable variation between the problems reported by children's parents and their teachers. To take account of the variations between different sources of data, empirically based assessment employs a multiaxial approach, as presented in the next section.

Multiaxial Assessment

The DSM defines multiaxial assessment in terms of the following five axes: Axis I—clinical disorders and other conditions that may be a focus of clinical attention; Axis II—personality disorders and mental retardation; Axis III—general medical conditions; Axis IV—psychosocial and environmental problems (a statement of problems such as "victim of child neglect"); Axis V—global assessment of functioning, as rated from 1 for extremely poor functioning to 100 for superior functioning (American Psychiatric Association, 1994). Axes I–III thus comprise different types of diagnostic categories, whereas Axis IV comprises the diagnostician's summary of problems thought to be diagnostically relevant and Axis V comprises a rating based on the diagnostician's global judgment. For all five axes, the diagnostician's judgment determines what assessment data are obtained, how the data are combined, and what diagnostic conclusions are specified.

The empirically based approach employs a different concept of multiaxial assessment. Instead of comprising different kinds of diagnostic conclusions, multiaxial empirically based assessment comprises data obtained from different sources. The sources that are relevant to comprehensive assessment of most children are grouped according to the following five axes: Axis I—parent reports; Axis II—teacher reports; Axis III—tests of cognitive functioning and achievement; Axis IV—physical assessment; and Axis V—direct assessment of the child, which may include observations, interviews, and self-ratings. Table 1 summarizes the components of empirically based multiaxial assessment. Additional sources of data, such as observations of family interactions, may also be relevant in many cases.

Instruments Designed for Multiaxial Empirically Based Assessment

Table 1 lists several instruments that are designed to obtain standardized ratings of chil-

Table 1. Examples of Multiaxial Assessment

Age range	Axis I Parent reports	Axis II Teacher reports	Axis III Cognitive assessment	Axis IV Physical assessment	Axis V Direct assessment of child
0–2	Child Development Inventory (Ireton, 1992) Developmental history Parent interview		Developmental tests, e.g., Bayley Infant Scales (1993)	Height, weight Medical exam Neurological exam	Observations during developmental testing
2–5	Child Behavior Checklist (CBCL) Developmental history Parent interview	Caregiver-Teacher Report Form (C-TRF) School records Teacher interview	Intelligence tests, e.g., McCarthy (1972) Scales of Children's Ability Perceptual-motor tests Speech and language tests	Height, weight Medical exam Neurological exam	Observations during play interview Direct Observation Form (DOF)
6–11	CBCL Developmental history Parent interview	TRF School records Teacher interview	Intelligence tests, e.g., WISC-III (Wechsler, 1991) Achievement tests Perceptual-motor tests Speech and language tests	Height, weight Medical exam Neurological exam	DOF Semistructured Clinical Interview for Children and Adolescents (SCICA)
12–18	CBCL Developmental history Parent interview	TRF School records Teacher interview	Intelligence tests, e.g., WISC-III Achievement tests Speech and language tests	Height, weight Medical exam Neurological exam	Youth Self-Report (YSR) SCICA Self-concept measures Personality tests

Note: CBCL, C-TRF, TRF, DOF, SCICA, and YSR are discussed and referenced in the following sections.

dren's functioning in a coordinated fashion from different informants, as described in the following sections. In later sections, we will consider how taxonomic constructs are derived from them and how data from multiple sources can be coordinated as a basis for case formulations.

The Child Behavior Checklist (CBCL)

The CBCL is designed to obtain parents' ratings of their children's functioning in a standardized fashion. In recognition of developmental differences in problems and competencies, there are separate versions of the CBCL for

ages 2–3 (CBCL/2–3; Achenbach, 1992) and ages 4–18 (CBCL/4–18; Achenbach, 1991a). Both instruments have lists of items that describe behavioral/emotional problems which can be reported by most parents with a minimum of inference. Parents score each item as 0 = not true of their child; 1 = somewhat or sometimes true; and 2 = very true or often true. To take account of the rapid changes among 2- and 3-year-olds, parents are asked to base their ratings on the previous 2 months, whereas parents of 4- to 18-year-olds are asked to use a 6-month rating period.

To tap social and academic competencies, the CBCL/4–18 requests parents to list the child's favorite sports and nonsports activities, organizations the child belongs to, and jobs and chores. Parents are also required to rate the amount and quality of the child's participation in the activities that they have listed and to rate the child's relationships with significant other people. In addition, parents are requested to rate the child's school performance in each academic subject and to provide information on other aspects of functioning in school. The competence items are scored on scales entitled *Activities, Social,* and *School* that provide percentiles and *T* scores based on a national sample of children who had not been referred for mental health services in the preceding 12 months. The problem items are scored on syndromes that will be described in the section on empirically based taxonomy.

The Teacher's Report Form (TRF)

The TRF is designed to obtain teachers' ratings of many of the same behavioral/emotional problems that the parents rate on the CBCL, plus other problems specific to the school setting. There is a version for ages 2–5 [Caregiver-Teacher Report Form (C-TRF/2–5); Achenbach, 1997a] that can be completed by day-care providers as well as preschool and kindergarten teachers. The version for ages 5–18 (TRF/5–18; Achenbach, 1991b) is designed for teachers who see children in more structured academic settings. It includes items that are scored on scales for academic performance and adaptive functioning. Norms for the TRF/5–18 are based on subjects from the same national sample as the CBCL/4–18.

The Youth Self-Report (YSR)

For ages 11–18, the YSR (Achenbach, 1991c) obtains self-ratings of problems and competencies similar to those on the CBCL/4–18. In place of CBCL problem items that are inappropriate for adolescents, the YSR provides 16 socially desirable items that most adolescents endorse. Norms for the YSR are based on subjects from the same national sample as the CBCL/4–18 and TRF/5–18.

The Direct Observation Form (DOF)

The DOF is designed to combine the advantages of customized descriptions of children's behavior with quantitative ratings, norms, and comparisons with the behavior of other children in the same environment (Achenbach, 1991a). It does this by having observers write narrative descriptions of the children's behavior during 10-minute observation periods. The narrative is written in a space provided on the DOF, adjoining the problem items that are to be rated. At the end of each minute within the 10-minute period, the observer scores the child as being on task or not on task. At the end of the 10-minute period, the on-task scores are summed to yield an on-task score ranging from 0 to 10. In addition, the observer rates each problem item on scales ranging from 0 for not observed, to 3 for a definite occurrence with severe intensity or greater than 3 minutes' duration. The problem items are then scored in terms of empirically based syndromes derived from the DOF.

To take account of variations in children's behavior, it is recommended that a child be observed for three to six 10-minute periods on different occasions, such as the mornings and afternoons of different days. In addition, to compare a child with other children in the same setting, it is recommended that two control subjects of the same sex as the target subject be observed on the same occasions. For example, if a girl is observed on four occasions in her second-grade classroom, a control girl who sits far away from the target subject should be observed for 10 minutes on each occasion just before the target subject is observed. A second control girl who sits far away from the target subject in a different direction should be observed for 10 minutes just after the target subject. A computer program is available that averages the target subject's scores over all observations and separately averages both control subjects' scores.

The program can then be used to print profiles that display the mean of the target subject's scores versus the mean of the control subjects' scores on each scale and item. Norms are also displayed to enable users to determine whether scores of the target subject and control subjects deviate from those of a normative reference group, as well as from each other.

The Semistructured Clinical Interview for Children and Adolescents (SCICA)

The SCICA is designed to provide a format for clinical interviews that is flexible and encourages behavioral and verbal self-expression by subjects (McConaughy & Achenbach, 1994). The SCICA also provides standardized quantitative scoring and a basis for comparing problems observed in the interview with those observed elsewhere, problems observed in interviews on different occasions, and problems observed for different children.

The SCICA includes a semistructured protocol of questions and assessment activities, such as a Kinetic Family Drawing, reading and arithmetic achievement tests, and gross and fine motor tasks. The sequence of the interview can be altered if necessary in response to the child's behavior. For example, the interviewer starts by asking about the child's favorite activities, and then asks about school. However, if the child begins to spontaneously discuss family relationships, the interviewer is free to skip ahead to the portion of the protocol dealing with the family and then to return to school-related questions later.

The interviewer takes notes to document the child's comments and behavior. After the interview, the interviewer rates 120 observational items and 114 self-report items according to criteria like those of the DOF. The item scores are then summed in terms of empirically based syndromes. Additional self-report items are scored for ages 13–18 on the basis of the subject's answers to direct questions about somatic complaints, substance use, and trouble with the law.

TAXONOMY

The term *taxonomy* may be unfamiliar and seem overly technical as a substitute for *formal diagnosis*. However, it emphasizes the goal of grouping cases according to important features of the cases themselves. Identifying important features and constructing groupings based on them are viewed as scientific activities. Because we do not know in advance which features and which ways of grouping cases will be most useful, it is necessary to test taxonomic procedures in order to determine how well they achieve particular goals.

The DSM Approach to Taxonomy

The main basis for the DSM diagnostic categories of childhood disorders has been decisions by the architects of DSM about which categories to include and how to define each category. Clinical experience, inferences from the existing literature, and the influence of various stakeholders may all have contributed to the categories that were ultimately selected for each edition of the DSM.

Starting with DSM-III (American Psychiatric Association, 1980), each diagnostic category has been defined according to explicit rules that specify the criterial features that must be present for a child to qualify for the category. Many of the diagnostic categories for childhood disorders have changed from DSM-III, to DSM-III-R, and again to DSM-IV (American Psychiatric Association, 1980, 1987, 1994). In addition, categories that retained the same name from one edition to another underwent important changes in criteria. As a result, children who received a particular diagnosis, such as conduct disorder (CD), according to one edition, often failed to qualify for that diagnosis in the next edition and vice versa (Lahey et al., 1990).

In preparation for DSM-IV, field trials were conducted to evaluated candidate criteria for some childhood disorders (e.g., Frick et al.,

1994; Lahey et al., 1994). However, the diagnostic categories were not derived from findings on the co-occurrence of the various candidate criteria. Instead, the candidate criteria were evaluated largely on the basis of how they performed in relation to diagnostic entities that were already assumed to exist, such as CD and ADHD. In other words, the process did not include construction of a taxonomy of problems or disorders.

Empirically Based Taxonomy

A major reason for developing empirically based taxonomy was to advance knowledge of child psychopathology by providing explicit data-based foci for research, communication, training, and treatment. The paucity of official diagnostic categories for child psychopathology prompted early efforts to identify syndromes of problems via multivariate analyses (e.g., Achenbach, 1966; Miller, 1967; Quay, 1964). Although official nosologies have since added many diagnostic categories for child psychopathology, the new categories have not been derived from taxonomic research to identify the actual patterns of co-occurring problems nor to test different approaches to taxonomy. There is thus a continuing need to advance the empirical basis for taxonomy, both by identifying patterns of co-occurring problems and by testing the value of these patterns in relation to other variables.

Steps in Constructing Empirically Based Taxonomies

The empirically based approach was previously described as "working from the bottom up." That is, it starts with large pools of items that are tested for their ability to discriminate between subjects who are considered to be relatively normal versus deviant and are analyzed to detect syndromes of co-occurring problems, typically via factor analysis or principal components analysis.

Any single analysis of any single sample may yield syndromes that do not replicate in other analyses. To develop a taxonomy of problem patterns, we therefore need to identify those elements that replicate in multiple analyses and samples. Those elements that are found to replicate in multiple analyses and samples can be used to define taxonomic constructs that then provide conceptual foci for research, theory, training, and services. Because each construct may be measured using more than one assessment procedure, the constructs can be thought of in statistical terms as *latent variables*. That is, they are inferred variables that may not be exhaustively measured by any single assessment procedure. Instead, they can be estimated from multiple procedures that tap them in different ways. The steps taken to develop an empirically based taxonomy of syndromes scored from parent, teacher, and self-ratings (Achenbach, 1993) will be used to illustrate one strategy, although other strategies are also possible.

The CBCL/4–18, TRF/5–18, and YSR were first tested and revised through a series of pilot editions that were completed by the appropriate respondents in diverse settings. The resulting version of the CBCL/4–18 was then completed by parents of 4455 children seen in 52 mental health settings, the TRF/5–18 was completed by teachers of 2815 children seen in 58 mental health and special education settings, and the YSR was completed by 1272 youths seen in 26 mental health settings. The 0–1–2 scores on each problem item were then analyzed as follows, with all analyses being done separately for each sex within particular age ranges:

1. Correlations among Problem Items. Separately for each instrument, correlations were computed between each item and every other item.

2. Derivation of Syndromes from Each Instrument. a. To identify syndromes that might be detected by any of the instruments, the correlations among all items (except very rare ones) on a particular instrument were subjected to principal components analysis with varimax rotations of various numbers of the resulting components.

b. To identify syndromes that could potentially be detected by all three instruments, the 89 problem items that have counterparts on all three were subjected to principal components/varimax analyses.

3. Selection of Robust Syndromes in Each Sex/Age Group. All of the varimax rotations from 2a and 2b were compared to select one for each sex/age group that had the best representations of syndromes that emerged from multiple rotations.

4. Identification of Syndromes that Were Similar across Multiple Sex/Age Groups on Each Instrument. The syndromes that were derived from a particular instrument via steps 2a, 2b, and 3 were compared across all of the sex/age groups for a particular instrument to identify syndromes that were similar for multiple groups.

5. Derivation of Core Syndromes from Each Instrument. For each syndrome that was found for multiple sex/age groups on a particular instrument, a *core syndrome* was formed that consisted of the problem items that were common to the versions of the syndrome for a majority of the sex/age groups.

6. Derivation of Cross-Informant Syndrome Constructs. For each core syndrome having counterparts in at least two of the three instruments, a *cross-informant syndrome construct* was formed, which comprised the problem items that were present in the core syndromes for at least two of the instruments. (Note that a *core syndrome* comprises items that were common to multiple versions of a syndrome on a *particular instrument*. A *cross-informant construct,* by contrast, comprises items that were common to core syndromes derived from *at least two of the three instruments.*)

The eight constructs that were thus derived provide the basis for a taxonomy of syndromes that can be scored for both sexes, different ages, and parent, teacher, and self-reports. The eight cross-informant syndrome constructs are designated as: Aggressive Behavior, Anxious/Depressed, Attention Problems, Delinquent Behavior, Social Problems, Somatic Complaints, Thought Problems, and Withdrawn. A few additional syndromes were specific to particular sex/age groups scored on a single instrument, but we will focus on the eight that qualified as cross-informant constructs.

To operationalize the constructs in terms of practical assessment procedures, syndrome scales were constructed for each instrument. Each syndrome scale consists of the instrument-specific versions of the items that define the construct. Some of the scales on particular instruments include additional items that were included in the core syndrome for that instrument. For example, the following items that are scored only on the TRF are included in the TRF scale for scoring the Attention Problems syndrome: fidgets, difficulty following directions, has difficulty learning, apathetic or unmotivated, and messy work.

To enable users to view a child's scores on each syndrome scale in relation to the scores of normative samples of nonreferred peers, the syndromes are displayed in a profile format. The profile provides T scores and percentiles that enable users to compare a child's syndrome scores with those of a national normative sample of nonreferred peers, as rated by the same type of informant as rated the target child. Figure 1 summarizes the steps involved in developing the taxonomy of cross-informant syndrome constructs and the scales for scoring them on the CBCL/4–18, TRF/5–18, and YSR. Figure 2 illustrates a computer-scored profile scored for 12-year-old Kelly from the CBCL completed by her mother.

Correlates of Empirically Based Syndromes

How useful are the taxonomic constructs? This can be judged in several ways. If the constructs directly reflect patterns of co-occurring

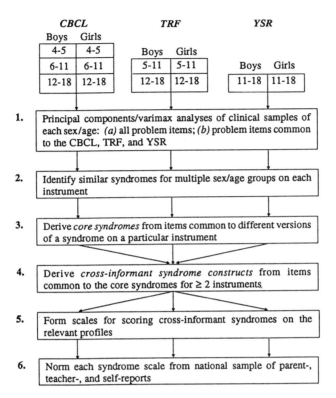

Figure 1. Development of cross-infant syndrome constructs and scales for scoring them on the CBCL/4–18, TRF/5–18, and YSR. (From Achenbach, 1993.)

characteristics, they can help us conceptualize and communicate about children's problems more effectively than if we had to focus on each child's characteristics one by one. The constructs may also have heuristic value in that they can suggest hypotheses about differences between patterns of problems that may not be evident when focusing on each problem in isolation.

Aggressive versus Delinquent Syndromes. As an example, numerous empirically based efforts to identify patterns of conduct problems have yielded separate syndromes comprising overtly aggressive behavior, such as physically attacking people, versus covertly delinquent behavior, such as lying, stealing, and truancy (e.g., Quay, 1993). Even though both kinds of conduct problems are combined in the DSM-IV criteria for

CD, the empirically based syndromes suggest that overtly aggressive versus covertly delinquent behaviors may be sufficiently distinct to serve as markers for other important differences among children.

Many differences have in fact been found between the correlates of the Aggressive versus Delinquent syndromes. For example, several studies have yielded stronger biochemical correlates and higher heritabilities for the Aggressive than the Delinquent syndrome (e.g., Edelbrock, Rende, Plomin, & Thompson, 1995; Hanna, Yuwiler, & Coates, 1995; Stoff, Pollock, Vitiello, Behar, & Bridger, 1987; Van den Oord, Boomsma, & Verhulst, 1994). Furthermore, children manifesting the Aggressive syndrome have been found to differ from those manifesting the Delinquent syndrome with respect to moral reasoning, empathy, stimulus seeking, psycho-

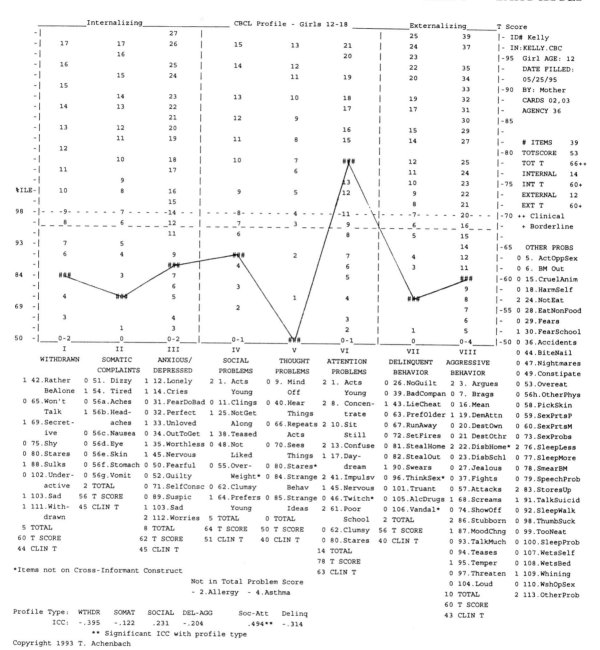

Figure 2. Profile scored for 12-year-old Kelly from the CBCL completed by her mother.

physiological responses, adaptation to institutional settings, and postrelease outcomes (Henn, Bardwell, & Jenkins, 1980; Quay, 1993). Significantly greater developmental stability has also been found for the Aggressive than for the Delinquent syndrome (Stanger, Achenbach, & Verhulst, 1997). The different correlates of the Aggressive versus Delinquent syndromes thus suggest that their underlying determinants differ enough to warrant a taxonomic distinction that DSM-IV does not make.

Associations between DSM Diagnoses and Empirically Based Syndromes. Some findings on the correlates of empirically based syndromes argue for taxonomic differences from the DSM's categories. However, numerous studies have also shown significant associations between syndrome scores and DSM diagnoses (e.g., Edelbrock & Costello, 1988; Edelbrock, Costello, & Kessler, 1984; Gould, Bird, & Jaramillo, 1993; Weinstein, Noam, Grimes, Stone, & Schwab-Stone, 1990). Other studies have tested relations between various cut points on the empirically based syndromes and specific operational definitions of DSM diagnoses. For example, a cut point on scores for the Attention Problems syndrome was

identified that yielded 96% accuracy in classifying children who were diagnosed as ADHD by the Kiddie Schedule for Affective Disorders and Schizophrenia (K-SADS) (Chen, Faraone, Biederman, & Tsuang, 1994).

Because DSM-IV has not yet generated much published research on relations between the syndromes and DSM diagnoses, most of the published studies used DSM-III or DSM-III-R criteria. However, based on the DSM-III and III-R findings, plus the descriptive features of DSM-IV diagnostic categories, relations between the two systems can be outlined as in Table 2.

Table 2 shows that many of the common DSM diagnoses for children's behavioral/emotional problems have counterparts among the empirically based syndromes. Still, this does not mean that there are one-to-one relations between the DSM's diagnostic categories and the empirically based syndromes. The empirically based assessment instruments are designed to measure relatively common behavioral/emotional problems occurring within a particular window of time, as scored by different informants who see children under a variety of conditions. These instruments are not designed to assess extremely rare behaviors, such as those characteristic of autism, nor to make judgments about age of onset,

Table 2. Approximate Descriptive Relations between DSM-IV Diagnoses and Empirically Derived Syndromes

DSM-IV	CBCL/TRF/YSR	DOF	SCICA
Attention-Deficit/Hyperactivity Disorder	Attention Problems	Hyperactive	Attention Problems
Avoidant Disorder	Withdrawn	Withdrawn-Inattentive	Withdrawn
Conduct Disorder	Aggressive Behavior Deliquent Behavior	Aggressive	Aggressive Behavior
Dysthymic Disorder	Anxious/Depressed	Depressed	Anxious/Depressed
Generalized Anxiety Disorder	Anxious/Depressed	Nervous-Obsessive	Anxious
Major Depressive Disorder	Anxious/Depressed	Depressed	Anxious/Depressed
Oppositional Defiant Disorder	Aggressive Behavior	Aggressive	Aggressive Behavior
Schizotypal Personality Disorder	Thought Problems	—	Strange
Somatization Disorder	Somatic Complaints	—	—
Gender Identity Disorder	Self-Destructive/Identity Problems (YSR boys only) Sex problems (CBCL ages 4–11 only)	—	—

persistence, or impairment, which are included in DSM criteria for many disorders.

The DSM has numerous diagnoses that lack counterparts among the empirically based syndromes. Conversely, some empirically based syndromes lack clear counterparts among the DSM categories. An example is the cross-informant Social Problems syndrome, which includes acts too young for age, too dependent, doesn't get along with other kids, gets teased a lot, not liked by other kids, clumsy, and prefers being with younger kids. Despite its absence from DSM, this syndrome has been found to have high heritability (Edelbrock et al., 1995) and to be developmentally quite stable (McConaughy, Stanger, & Achenbach, 1992).

The Social Problems syndrome has also yielded exceptionally good cross-informant agreement between mothers, fathers, teachers, and youths. In an Australian sample (Sawyer, 1990; see Achenbach, 1991c), the mean correlation of .62 among parent, teacher, and self-ratings for 362 11- to 16-year-olds was higher than for any other syndrome. Furthermore, the Social Problems syndrome has shown very good discrimination between referred and non-referred children rated by parents and teachers (Achenbach, 1991a,b). The Social Problems syndrome thus appears to represent an important pattern of behavioral/emotional problems.

Predictive Correlates in Childhood and Adolescence. Between birth and maturity, humans undergo massive changes in physique, cognitive functioning, social status, competencies, and behavioral/emotional problems. The kinds of problems and disorders found among infants are apt to differ greatly from those found among preschoolers, school-age children, adolescents, and young adults. To distinguish between problems that are relatively transitory versus those that have long-term sequelae, we need longitudinal research on the developmental course of problems and their correlates. Because the prevalence, pathognomicity, and pat-

terning of problems may change with development, we also need assessment and taxonomic procedures that are sensitive to these changes.

Even for disorders that persist over long developmental periods, it is unlikely that the same criteria will identify them with equal accuracy in both sexes at every age. Some types of problems occurring at older ages may be later manifestations of disorders that could potentially be detected at younger ages. For example, adolescent truancy and substance abuse may be continuations of earlier patterns that do not include these specific behaviors.

To take account of age differences in problems and in the prediction of relations between them, several longitudinal studies have applied empirically based assessment and taxonomic procedures. Starting at the youngest ages for which standardized empirically based assessment of behavioral/emotional problems has been standardized, longitudinal analyses have shown that some syndromes assessed at age 2 yielded substantial predictive correlations with scores on corresponding syndromes as much as 7 years later (Achenbach, 1992). The highest 7-year correlation was .55 for Aggressive Behavior, even though the instruments and many of the specific problems differed at ages 2 and 9. The predictive correlation was much lower for the Somatic syndrome ($r = .11$). The findings thus indicate that the problem pattern reflected in the Aggressive Behavior syndrome is considerably more stable from the toddler to the elementary school years than is the pattern reflected in the Somatic syndrome. As evidence that these findings were not just artifacts of parental perceptions, the predictive correlations from parents' ratings at age 2 to teachers' ratings at age 9 showed similar patterns.

Predictive correlations have also been tested over later ages. For general population samples of U.S. and Dutch children originally assessed at ages 4–12 and reassessed 6 years later, the Aggressive Behavior syndrome showed the highest correlation ($r = .52$ in the U.S. sample; $r = .55$ in the Dutch sample; Achenbach, Howell, Mc-Conaughy, & Stanger, 1995a; Verhulst & van der Ende, 1992). Like findings for ages 2–9, the Somatic syndrome showed a relatively low correlation (U.S. $r = .24$; Dutch $r = .29$). Similar findings were also obtained in a long-term follow-up of a U.S. clinical sample (Stanger, MacDonald, McConaughy, & Achenbach, 1996).

In addition to testing the prediction of later syndrome scores from earlier syndrome scores, the longitudinal studies have also tested prediction of various signs of disturbance from earlier syndrome scores. The signs of disturbance are outcomes that are of concern whether or not they are associated with particular syndromes or diagnoses. U.S. and Dutch studies have both found that signs of disturbance such as suicidal behavior, trouble with the law, referral for mental health services, school behavior problems, and academic problems could be significantly predicted over periods of 6 years from combinations of syndrome scores, family variables, and stressful experiences (Achenbach, Howell, McConaughy, & Stanger, 1995b; Verhulst, Koot, & van der Ende, 1994). The Attention Problems and Delinquent Behavior syndromes were especially good predictors of signs of disturbance.

Predictive Correlates in Adulthood. Although the empirically based paradigm was originally developed to cope with the lack of nosological differentiation for childhood disorders, it is being increasingly applied to the early adult years. One reason for extending the empirically based paradigm to adults is that subjects in several longitudinal studies of psychopathology are reaching their adult years (Achenbach, Howell, McConaughy, & Stanger, 1995c; Ferdinand, Verhulst, & Wiznitzer, 1995; Reinherz, 1995). There has been a paucity of empirically based measures geared to the young adult years that could provide continuity of assessment from the preadult years. Instead, assessment of adults has typically focused on disorders assumed to characterize ages 18 and older, whereas assessment of preadults has focused on disorders assumed

to characterize ages below 18. For example, structured psychiatric interviews are designed either for adults (e.g., Kessler et al., 1994) or for preadults (e.g., Shaffer, 1992). Consequently, criteria for child/adolescent disorders are not included in the adult interviews and vice versa. This makes it difficult to identify specific continuities and discontinuities between preadult and adult problems.

To facilitate identification of continuities and discontinuities between preadult and adult years, upward extensions of the CBCL/4–18 and YSR have been developed. Designed for ages 18–30, the Young Adult Behavior Checklist (YABCL) is completed by parents, while the Young Adult Self-Report (YASR) is completed by the subjects themselves. The YABCL and YASR have many counterparts of CBCL/4–18 and YSR items, but with wording appropriate for young adults. These instruments also have additional items that tap problems and issues related to the various developmental paths followed by young adults. For example, subjects who are pursuing higher education are asked to respond to items concerning their educational situation; subjects who have jobs are asked to respond to job-related items; and subjects who are married or have similar conjugal relationships are asked to respond to items pertinent to these relationships.

Principal components/varimax analyses of the YABCL and YASR have yielded eight cross-informant syndromes designated as Aggressive Behavior, Anxious/Depressed, Attention Problems, Delinquent Behavior, Intrusive, Somatic Complaints, Thought Problems, and Withdrawn (Achenbach, 1997b). Strong predictive correlations were found between syndromes assessed in adolescence and the adult syndromes bearing the same names assessed 3 years later.

The Intrusive syndrome, which does not have a clear preadult counterpart, includes problems such as bragging, demanding attention, showing off (the highest loading item), talking too much, teasing, and being unusually loud. It was strongly predicted by the preadult Aggressive

Behavior syndrome. Because the adult Aggressive Behavior syndrome was also strongly predicted by the preadult Aggressive Behavior syndrome, this suggests that some aggressive adolescents remain overtly aggressive into adulthood, whereas others become less overtly aggressive but manifest the socially obnoxious behavior of the Intrusive syndrome.

Strongly predicted by the preadult Attention Problems syndrome, the adult Attention Problems Syndrome shares the following items with the preadult version: acts too young for age, can't concentrate, daydreams, impulsive, and poor school (or job) performance. However, the adult version syndrome lacks the item can't sit still that is on the preadult syndrome and it includes fails to finish things, irresponsible (the highest loading item), and trouble making decisions. Thus, although overactivity is not part of the adult pattern, the attention problems of the preadult syndrome are present and are joined by problems that reflect inadequacy in coping with adult responsibilities.

In addition to young adult syndromes as outcome variables, young adult signs of disturbance have also been predicted from a combination of scores on preadult syndromes, family variables, and stressful experiences. The signs of disturbance include suicidal behavior, trouble with the law, referral for mental health services, fired from a job, dropping out of school without a high school diploma, substance abuse, and unwed pregnancy (Achenbach, Howell, McConaughy, & Stanger, submitted).

CASE FORMULATION

The preceding sections distinguished between "diagnostic process" and "formal diagnosis" in terms of "assessment" and "taxonomy." We turn now to "diagnostic formulation," which can be more neutrally designated as "case formulation." This refers to the stage of the clinical process where the practitioner integrates all that is known about the case into a comprehensive picture that provides a basis for decisions. Clinical experience and creativity are especially important at this stage, because the practitioner must judiciously weigh various kinds of evidence. The empirically based assessment procedures described earlier facilitate direct comparisons of data from different sources.

When all of the evidence points to a single type of problem, such as attention problems, the case formulation is relatively easy. However, even in these rare cases, the practitioner must still take account of multiple sources of data in order to rule out additional problems in the child, family, and school that may be camouflaged by an exclusive focus on attention problems. The practitioner also needs a clear picture of the child's competencies and of family and school variables so as to judge how to maximize the efficacy of particular interventions, such as stimulant medication and behavior modification for attention problems.

In the many cases where the data do not uniformly point to a single type of problem, the practitioner must weigh the evidence to make judgments such as the following:

1.   Is there consistent multisource evidence for a complex pattern of problems, such as high scores on the Attention Problems and Delinquent Behavior syndromes, or high scores on the Aggressive Behavior and Anxious/Depressed syndromes?

2.   Is there evidence that the child's behavior differs markedly between contexts, as seen by different informants? For example, do ratings from both parents yield high scores on the Aggressive Behavior syndrome, whereas ratings by several teachers yield high scores on the Withdrawn syndrome? If so, this would suggest that the child's problem patterns are significantly affected by the situational context and that different interventions may be needed at home and school.

3.   Is there evidence that reports by a partic-

ular informant are very discrepant from everything else that is known about the child? For example, suppose that ratings by 12-year-old Kelly's mother and father, ratings by several teachers, and Kelly's self-ratings all yield high scores only on the Attention Problems syndrome, but her math teacher's ratings instead yield a high score for the Aggressive Behavior syndrome. It would be important to determine whether Kelly is in fact more aggressive in math class than elsewhere. Is there something about the math class or teacher that evokes aggressive behavior, or is the difference less in Kelly's behavior than in her math teacher's perception of it? Large differences in reports by different teachers would argue for having a classroom observer rate samples of Kelly's behavior in the classes whose teachers had provided discrepant reports. By using data from the DOF, the practitioner can determine whether Kelly in fact displays more aggressive behavior and fewer attention problems in math class than elsewhere. The narrative description recorded on the DOF would also provide information about the teacher's behavior, the behavior of students interacting with Kelly, and other contextual factors that might be affecting Kelly.

Discrepancies between particular combinations of informants may provide valuable information for case formulations and interventions. For example, if the profile of syndromes scored from a mother's CBCL ratings differs from the profile scored from the father's CBCL ratings, this would provide a basis for interviewing the parents about their different perceptions of their child. If the parents are reasonably sophisticated, the practitioner can even show them the profiles scored from their respective CBCLs and ask why they think there are discrepancies. It may be found, for example, that their child displays certain behavior only in the presence of one parent, who may play a role in evoking the behavior. Or it may be found that one parent has too little contact with the child to observe the problems reported by the other parent. Another possibility is that the parents differ in their thresholds for noticing or reporting certain kinds of behavior. Support for any of these explanations could provide a basis for designing interventions to modify the parents' behavior or judgments.

Aids to Cross-Informant Comparisons

Cross-Informant Computer Program

To help the practitioner make explicit comparisons among data from different informants, a cross-informant computer program is available (Arnold & Jacobowitz, 1993). This program enables the user to enter CBCL, TRF, and YSR data from any combination of up to five respondents. The program will print separate item scores, scale scores, and profiles from each informant. In addition, the program displays the item and scale scores from all informants side by side so that the user can identify specific areas of agreement and disagreement among informants. The scale scores are in T score units that are based on national normative samples, as scored by each type of informant. For example, the T scores for the Attention Problems syndrome scored for 12-year-old Kelly from her mother's and father's CBCLs are based on a national normative sample of adolescent girls rated by their parents. Similarly, the T score for the Attention Problems syndrome scored from Kelly's YSR is based on a national normative sample of adolescent girls' YSRs. And the T score for the Attention Problems syndrome scored from Kelly's teachers' TRFs are based on TRFs for a national normative sample of adolescent girls.

Because the syndrome scores are all displayed in terms of T scores, the user can see at a glance the degree of deviance on each syndrome that is indicated by each informant's ratings, as compared with the relevant national norms. The program also prints a cross beside each scale score that is in the borderline clinical range and two crosses beside each scale score that is in the clinical range. Figure 3 illustrates a cross-informant printout for 12-year-old Kelly. As discussed

T Scores for 8 Syndrome Scales Common to CBCL, YSR and TRF

Scale	Mo.CBCL.1	Fa.CBCL.2	Slf.YSR.3	Tch.TRF.4	Tch.TRF.5
1. Withdrawn	60	63	63	58	54
2. Somatic Complaints	56	56	56	50	57
3. Anxious/Depressed	62	64	66	61	58
4. Social Problems	64	66	68+	66	66
5. Thought Problems	50	50	55	50	50
6. Attention Problems	78++	78++	72++	76++	65
7. Delinquent Behavior	56	56	54	55	66
8. Aggressive Behavior	60	63	66	62	74++

+Borderline Clinical Range
++Clinical Range

	Mo.CBCL.1	Fa.CBCL.2	Slf.YSR.3	Tch.TRF.4	Tch.TRF.5
Internalizing	60+	60+	62	56	56
Externalizing	60+	60+	60+	58	70++
Total Problems	66++	71++	69++	70++	71++

- -

Q Correlations Between 8 Scale Scores from Different Informants

For Reference Samples

For this Subject		25th %ile	Mean	75th %ile	Agreement between
Mo.CBCL.1 x Fa.CBCL.2 =	.65	.35	.58	.89	Mother and Father is average.
Mo.CBCL.1 x Slf.YSR.3 =	.51	-.11	.26	.60	Mother and Youth is average.
Mo.CBCL.1 x Tch.TRF.4 =	.55	-.14	.23	.60	Mother and Teacher is average.
Mo.CBCL.1 x Tch.TRF.5 =	-.19	-.14	.23	.60	Mother and Teacher is below average.
Fa.CBCL.2 x Slf.YSR.3 =	.30	-.11	.26	.60	Father and Youth is average.
Fa.CBCL.2 x Tch.TRF.4 =	.50	-.14	.23	.60	Father and Teacher is average.
Fa.CBCL.2 x Tch.TRF.5 =	-.18	-.14	.23	.60	Father and Teacher is below average.
Slf.YSR.3 x Tch.TRF.4 =	.25	-.15	.17	.50	Youth and Teacher is average.
Slf.YSR.3 x Tch.TRF.5 =	-.20	-.15	.17	.50	Youth and Teacher is below average.
Tch.TRF.4 x Tch.TRF.5 =	.35				There is no reference sample for this combination

- -

Intraclass Correlations (ICCs) with Cross-Informant Profile Types from Different Informants

Cross-Informant Profile Types

ICC from	WITHDR	SOMAT	SOCIAL	DEL-AGG	SOC-ATT	DEL
Mo.CBCL.1	-.395	-.122	.231	-.204	.494**	-.314
Fa.CBCL.2	.012	-.268	.174	-.528	.464**	-.290
Slf.YSR.3	.209	-.435	.420	-.542		
Tch.TRF.4	.105	.152	.312	.088		
Tch.TRF.5	.051	.249	.230	.394		

** Significant ICC with profile type

Figure 3. Cross-informant printout of scale scores and *Q* correlations for 12-year-old Kelly.

earlier, Kelly's CBCLs, YSR, and some TRFs indicated deviance on the Attention Problems syndrome (two crosses in Figure 3), whereas her math teacher's TRF (Tch.TRF.5) indicated deviance on the Aggressive Behavior syndrome.

As Figure 3 shows, the printout displays not only the scores obtained from each informant, but also correlations between the scores from each pair of informants. These correlations (called *Q* correlations) indicate the degree to which the scores from two informants agree with each other. To help the user evaluate the level of agreement between particular informants, the printout also displays *Q* correlations between similar pairs of informants from large reference samples. For example, Figure 3 shows that, in the reference sample, the 25th percentile correlation between pairs of parents is .35, the mean correlation is .58, and the 75th percentile correlation is .89. The correlation of .65 between Kelly's parents is considered to be average for pairs of parents, because it is in the middle 50%, between the 25th and 75th percentiles. The printout states for each combination of informants whether the agreement is average, below average, or above average, as compared with the reference sample.

For informants whose agreement is below average, the practitioner can explore the reasons, as illustrated earlier. For example, in Kelly's case, the correlations between all pairs of informants were average, except for the below average correlation with the math teacher whose TRF yielded a deviant score for Aggressive Behavior but not Attention Problems. This below average correlation and disagreement about the kind of behavior that was deviant would prompt the practitioner to investigate the reasons for the discrepancy, as discussed earlier. The side-by-side display of item and scale scores enables the user to pinpoint specific discrepancies among informants. If the reason can be determined, such as the math teacher's unusual perception of Kelly's behavior or classroom factors that evoke actual aggressive behavior, this would be included in the case formulation.

Taxonomic Decision Tree

The cross-informant program discussed in the preceding section enables users to make item-by-item and scale-by-scale comparisons among the specific scores from different informants. Another approach to comparing data from multiple sources is to consider the syndromes that are deviant on various combinations of instruments. Figure 4 illustrates a taxonomic decision tree that maps a sequence of binary decisions based on syndrome scores from multiple sources.

In Figure 4, the potential sources of data displayed at the top are the CBCL, TRF, YSR, SCICA, and DOF. Not all of these instruments are necessary for the decision-making strategy depicted by the taxonomic decision tree. Other instruments can also be substituted if they have enough scales in common to permit binary decisions about deviance versus nondeviance in each of several areas. Because multiple instruments may have some but not all scales in common, a user may choose to apply the decision tree to just those scales that are common to several instruments.

Applying the decision tree to Kelly's CBCLs from both parents, her YSR, and TRFs, we start with Box 1, at the initial screening level near the top of the tree in Figure 4. As shown in Box 1, we first ask, "Are any scales in the clinical range?" As we saw in Figure 3, the Attention Problems scale was in the clinical range on all forms, except the math teacher's TRF, which yielded a T score in the clinical range on the Aggressive Behavior syndrome but a lower score on the Attention Problems syndrome. The answer to the initial screening question in Box 1 is thus "yes," some scales are in the clinical range.

We then move to Box 3, where we ask, "Is deviance confined to a single syndrome in all sources?" Here the answer is "no," because the math teacher's TRF yielded a deviant score on the Aggressive Behavior syndrome, in contrast to the Attention Problems syndrome that was deviant in the other informants' ratings.

Moving down to Box 5, we ask, "Are the same syndromes deviant in all sources?" Again the answer is "no," because the math teacher's ratings yielded deviance in a different area than did the other informants' ratings. We therefore move to Box 7, where we ask, "Does the child's behavior actually differ much among contexts?" To answer this question, we need additional data, which might include the SCICA, DOF, and/or an interview with the math teacher.

As part of a comprehensive evaluation, the practitioner interviewed Kelly, using the SCICA. The SCICA yielded relatively high scores on the Attention Problems scale, based on Kelly's behavior in the interview, but also on the Aggres-

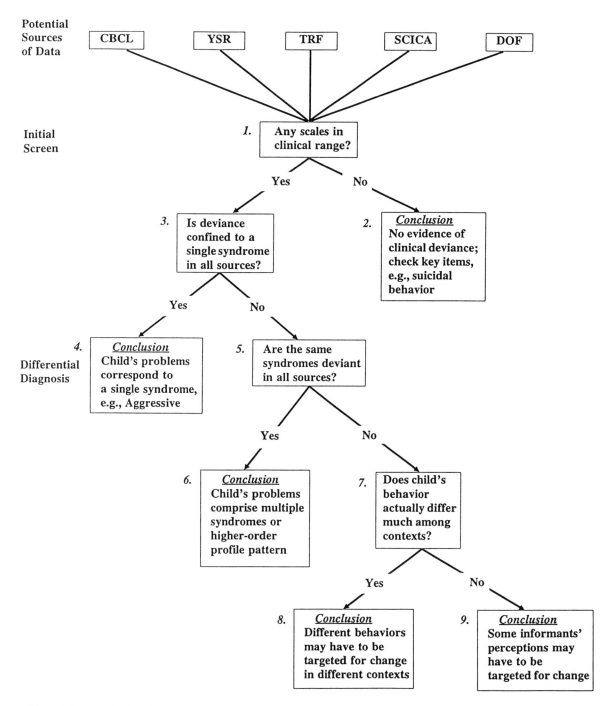

Figure 4. Taxonomic decision tree for guiding decisions about syndrome scores obtained from multiple sources. (From Achenbach, 1993.)

sive Behavior scale, based on her comments about aggressive behavior in math class. In addition, the DOF yielded a relatively high score for aggressive behavior from observations in math class. In a phone interview, the math teacher described several specific episodes of aggressive and defiant behavior like those to which Kelly had alluded during the SCICA.

It thus appeared that Kelly was quite aggressive in math class but not in the contexts observed by other informants, who noticed mostly her attention problems. Our answer to the question raised in Box 7 of the decision tree is thus "yes," Kelly's behavior does differ among contexts. Moving to Box 8, our conclusion is that different behaviors may have to be targeted for change in different contexts, i.e., attention problems in most contexts, but also aggressive behavior in math class.

Other Types of Data

As part of our case formulation, we would take account of other types of data, including developmental history, family and school contexts, medical data, and cognitive and achievement tests. The developmental history reported by Kelly's mother indicated normal physical development but rather high levels of activity and distractibility since the preschool period. Kelly's school performance had been in the average range until she reached middle school, where it began to decline. She was now failing math and was barely passing her other sixth-grade subjects.

It was learned from the developmental history that Kelly was an only child who had been quite close to both parents until 2 years earlier, when her parents began to argue about a possible move to a different area of the country. This evidently placed pressure on Kelly to side with either her mother or her father. The question of a move was still unresolved when Kelly was seen for assessment because of her declining school performance, failure to do schoolwork, apparent inability to handle the middle

school environment, and aggressive behavior in math class.

A recent medical examination had revealed normal pubertal development, with no physical abnormalities. Cognitive testing yielded a WISC-III verbal IQ of 96, performance IQ of 110, and full-scale IQ of 103. Kelly's lowest subtest score was on Coding, where her scale score of 6 reflected moderate difficulty in remaining on task. Her Peabody Individual Achievement Test scores were about one standard deviation below her cognitive scores, but not low enough to quality for special education.

Deviance primarily in the area of attention problems and secondarily in aggressive behavior may seem unusual for a 12-year-old girl. However, longitudinal research that has tested the predictive power of empirically based syndromes separately for each sex shows that girls who obtain high scores on the Attention Problems syndrome later tend to manifest elevated rates of academic problems, school behavior problems, and aggression (Achenbach et al., 1995a,b). Furthermore, the same longitudinal research shows that, although attention problems have high long-term stability among girls, stressful experiences can further exacerbate them.

Applying the research findings to Kelly's case formulation, it appears likely that Kelly has long had more problems with attention than most other girls her age, but not enough to meet DSM criteria for ADHD, which are based mainly on the more conspicuous problems of attention, overactivity, and impulsivity manifested by boys. The stress of conflicts between her parents just as Kelly was making a difficult transition from her self-contained elementary school class to the complexities of a departmentalized middle school, plus having to deal with the biological and social challenges of puberty, would account for a decline in school functioning for a girl who may already have had problems with attention. The aggressive behavior that reached the clinical range only in math class could be provoked by the greater demands of math for learning specific new concepts and skills than in other classes. Kelly's attentional problems and avoidance of schoolwork could create a gap between what was expected and what she accomplished that was especially salient in math, causing distress to which she reacted with anger and defiance. The longitudinal research indicating that early attention problems predict later aggressive behavior among girls suggests that this behavior may become serious in adolescence, unless effective interventions are applied.

Based on the case formulation, it seems clear that interventions should focus on the following issues: (1) alleviation of interparental issues that place Kelly in conflict about siding with her mother versus father, e.g., through couples or conjoint family therapy; (2) efforts to help Kelly with her attention problems, e.g., through a trial of stimulant medication; (3) counseling to help Kelly adapt to the stresses of the middle school, e.g., in small groups run by school counselors for students who are having similar problems; (4) a behavioral contract system for reinforcing completion of schoolwork and more acceptable behavior in math class, coupled with one-to-one tutoring in math as long as needed for her to catch up to her class.

To evaluate the effectiveness of the interventions and make changes as needed, Kelly should be reassessed in 3 months by repeating the empirically based rating forms. Because these include teachers' ratings of academic performance and several kinds of adaptive behavior in school, they can indicate whether Kelly is learning more effectively, as well as whether her behavior problems have diminished. The empirically based rating forms can be readministered in the following school year to determine whether further interventions are needed. Annual group achievement tests can be used to determine whether Kelly's academic skills are at the level expected from her cognitive abilities.

Although the empirically based assessment, taxonomic, and case formulation process may seem elaborate and costly, it is not. Most of the initial data and all of the follow-up data from parents, teachers, and Kelly herself could be obtained at little cost from standardized forms that

were scored by clerical workers on their desktop computers. The more expensive individually administered tests and interviews would have been included in any comprehensive evaluation. The direct observations from which the DOF were scored could be done by a paraprofessional, such as a teacher's aide. The multiaxial data can also be used to determine whether Kelly meets criteria for any DSM diagnoses. Her deviance on the Attention Problems syndrome according to multiple informants indicates that ADHD is the diagnosis she would most likely receive. The particular combination of procedures may vary from case to case, but the typical sequence would proceed from empirically based assessment, taxonomy, and case formulation, to intervention, outcome assessment, and follow-up assessment.

SUMMARY

Diagnostic terminology is widely used by mental health professionals. However, the multiple meanings of diagnosis can sow confusion. To distinguish among three meanings of diagnosis, the term *assessment* can be substituted for *diagnostic process,* i.e., gathering data about a case; *taxonomy* can be substituted for *formal diagnosis,* i.e., grouping cases according to their distinguishing features; and *case formulation* can be substituted for *diagnostic formulation,* i.e., a comprehensive summary of a case.

The DSM approach starts with definitional criteria for diagnostic categories and then determines which children meet the criteria. The empirically based approach, by contrast, starts with assessment data on large samples of children and then identifies syndromes of co-occuring problems as a basis for taxonomy. The empirically based approach also employs distributions of scores obtained from normative and clinical samples, separately for each sex in different age ranges, as seen by different informants. Rather than applying the same fixed cut points to all sources of data on children of both sexes and all ages, the empirically based approach provides standard scores and percentiles with which to compare individual children to normative samples of peers. In addition to this quantitative basis for judging the degree of deviance manifested by a child, the empirically based approach provides cut points that discriminate significantly between children referred for mental health services and demographically matched nonreferred peers. Empirically based syndromes have numerous significant correlates, such as DSM diagnoses, biochemical and genetic variables, and differences in long-term outcomes in childhood, adolescence, and adulthood.

To provide comprehensive evaluations, the empirically based approach employs data from multiple sources, including parents, teachers, interviews, self-reports, direct observations, tests, and medical procedures. Because agreement between different sources is often modest, no single source can substitute for all of the others. Instead, data from different sources must be compared as part of the case formulation. Inconsistencies among the findings from different sources may reveal important information both about situational influences on a child's behavior and about differences in the ways informants perceive the child. Such information can be valuable in planning interventions to change the behavior of both the child and various interaction partners, if need be.

A cross-informant computer program and taxonomic decision tree can aid users in drawing conclusions from complex multisource data. As capitated managed care changes the incentive structure for service providers, detailed multiaxial assessment, taxonomy, and case formulations are likely to become more cost-effective than categorical diagnoses of child and adolescent psychopathology.

REFERENCES

Achenbach, T. M. (1966). The classification of children's psychiatric symptoms: A factor-analytic study. *Psychological Monographs, 80.*

Achenbach, T. M. (1991a). *Manual for the Child Behavior Checklist/4–18 and 1991 Profile.* Burlington: University of Vermont Department of Psychiatry.

Achenbach, T. M. (1991b). *Manual for the Teacher's Report Form and 1991 Profile.* Burlington: University of Vermont Department of Psychiatry.

Achenbach, T. M. (1991c). *Manual for the Youth Self-Report and 1991 Profile.* Burlington: University of Vermont Department of Psychiatry.

Achenbach, T. M. (1992). *Manual for the Child Behavior Checklist/2–3 and 1992 Profile.* Burlington: University of Vermont Department of Psychiatry.

Achenbach, T. M. (1993). *Empirically based taxonomy: How to use syndromes and profile types derived from the CBCL/4–18, TRF, and YSR.* Burlington: University of Vermont Department of Psychiatry.

Achenbach, T. M. (1997a). *Guide for the Caregiver-Teacher Report Form for Ages 2–5.* Burlington: University of Vermont Department of Psychiatry.

Achenbach, T. M. (1997b). *Manual for the Young Adult Self-Report and Young Adult Behavior Checklist.* Burlington: University of Vermont Department of Psychiatry.

Achenbach, T. M., Howell, C. T., McConaughy, S. H., & Stanger, C. (1995a). Six-year predictors of problems in a national sample of children and youth: I. Cross-informant syndromes. *Journal of the American Academy of Child and Adolescent Psychiatry, 34,* 336–347.

Achenbach, T. M., Howell, C. T., McConaughy, S. H., & Stanger, C. (1995b). Six-year predictors of problems in a national sample of children and youth: II. Signs of disturbance. *Journal of the American Academy of Child and Adolescent Psychiatry, 34,* 488–498.

Achenbach, T. M., Howell, C. T., McConaughy, S. H., & Stanger, C. (1995c). Six-year predictors of problems in a national sample: III. Transitions to young adult syndromes. *Journal of the American Academy of Child and Adolescent Psychiatry, 34,* 658–669.

Achenbach, T. M., Howell, C. T., McConaughy, S. H., & Stanger, C. Six-year predictors of problems in a national sample: IV. Young adult signs of disturbance. (submitted).

Achenbach, T. M., McConaughy, S. H., & Howell, C. T. (1987). Child/adolescent behavioral and emotional problems: Implications of cross-informant correlations for situational specificity. *Psychological Bulletin, 101,* 213–232.

American Psychiatric Association. (1980, 1987, 1994). *Diagnostic and statistical manual of mental disorders* (3rd ed., 3rd rev. ed., 4th ed.). Washington, DC: Author.

Arnold, J., & Jacobowitz, D. (1993). *The Cross-Informant Program for the CBCL/4–18, YSR, and TRF.* Burlington: University of Vermont Department of Psychiatry.

Bayley, N. (1993). *Bayley Scales of Infant Development* (2nd ed.). New York: Psychological Corporation.

Chen, W. J., Faraone, S. V., Biederman, J., & Tsuang, M. T. (1994). Diagnostic accuracy of the Child Behavior

Checklist scales for attention-deficit hyperactivity disorder: A receiver-operating characteristic analysis. *Journal of Consulting and Clinical Psychology, 62*, 1017–1025.

Costello, A. J., Edelbrock, C., Dulcan, M. K., Kalas, R., & Klaric, S. H. (1984). *Report on the Diagnostic Interview Schedule for Children (DISC)*. Pittsburgh, PA: University of Pittsburgh Department of Psychiatry.

Edelbrock, C., & Costello, A. J. (1988). Convergence between statistically derived behavior problem syndromes and child psychiatric diagnoses. *Journal of Abnormal Child Psychology, 16*, 219–231.

Edelbrock, C., Costello, A. J., & Kessler, M. D. (1984). Empirical corroboration of attention deficit disorder. *Journal of the American Academy of Child Psychiatry, 23*, 285–290.

Edelbrock, C., Rende, R., Plomin, R., & Thompson, L. A. (1995). A twin study of competence and problem behavior in childhood and early adolescence. *Journal of Child Psychology and Psychiatry, 36*, 775–785.

Ferdinand, R. F., Verhulst, F. C., & Wiznitzer, M. (1995). Continuity and change of self-reported problem behaviors from adolescence into young adulthood. *Journal of the American Academy of Child and Adolescent Psychiatry, 34*, 680–690.

Frick, P. J., Lahey, B. B., Applegate, B., Kerdyck, L., Ollendick, T., Hynd, G. W., Garfinkel, B., Greenhill, L., Biederman, J., Barkley, R. A., McBurnett, K., Newcorn, J., & Waldman, I. (1994). DSM-IV field trials for the disruptive behavior disorders: Symptom utility estimates. *Journal of the American Academy of Child and Adolescent Psychiatry, 33*, 529–539.

Gould, M. S., Bird, H., & Jaramillo, B. S. (1993). Correspondence between statistically derived behavior problem syndromes and child psychiatric diagnoses in a community sample. *Journal of Abnormal Child Psychology, 21*, 287–313.

Gove, P. (Ed.). (1971). *Webster's third new international dictionary of the English language*. Springfield, MA: Merriam.

Guze, S. (1978). Validating criteria for psychiatric diagnosis: The Washington University approach. In M. S. Akiskal & W. L. Webb (Eds.), *Psychiatric diagnosis: Exploration of biological predictors* (pp. 49–59). New York: Spectrum.

Hanna, G. L., Yuwiler, A., & Coates, J. K. (1995). Whole blood serotonin and disruptive behaviors in juvenile obsessive-compulsive disorder. *Journal of the American Academy of Child and Adolescent Psychiatry, 34*, 28–35.

Henn, F. A., Bardwell, R., & Jenkins, R. L. (1980). Juvenile delinquents revisited. Adult criminal activity. *Archives of General Psychiatry, 37*, 1160–1163.

Herjanic, B., & Reich, W. (1982). Development of a structured psychiatric interview for children: Agreement between child and parent on individual symptoms. *Journal of Abnormal Child Psychology, 10*, 307–324.

Ireton, H. (1992). *Child Development Inventory*. Minneapolis: Behavior Science Systems.

Kessler, R. C., McGonagle, K. A., Zhao, S., Nelson, C. B., Hughes, M., Eshleman, S., Wittchen, H. U., & Kendler,

K. S. (1994). Lifetime and 12-month prevalence of DSM-III-R psychiatric disorders among persons in the United States. *Archives of General Psychiatry, 51*, 8–19.

Lahey, B. B., Applegate, B., McBurnett, K., Biederman, J., Greenhill, L., Hynd, G. W., Barkley, R. A., Newcorn, J., Jensen, P., Richters, J., Garfinkel, B., Kerdyk, L., Frick, P. J., Ollendick, T., Perez, D., Hart, E. L., Waldman, I., & Shaffer, D. (1994). DSM-IV field trials for Attention Deficit Hyperactivity Disorder in children and adolescents. *American Journal of Psychiatry, 151*, 1673–1685.

Lahey, B. B., Loeber, R., Stouthamer-Loeber, M., Christ, M. A. G., Green, S., Russo, M. F., Frick, P. J., & Dulcan, M. (1990). Comparison of DSM-III and DSM-III-R diagnoses for prepubertal children: Changes in prevalence and validity. *Journal of the American Academy of Child and Adolescent Psychiatry, 29*, 620–626.

McCarthy, D. (1972). *McCarthy Scales of Children's Abilities*. New York: Psychological Corporation.

McConaughy, S. H., & Achenbach, T. M. (1994). *Manual for the Semistructured Clinical Interview for Children and Adolescents*. Burlington: University of Vermont Department of Psychiatry.

McConaughy, S. H., Stanger, C., & Achenbach, T. M. (1992). Three-year course of behavioral/emotional problems in a national sample of 4- to 16-year-olds: I. Agreement among informants. *Journal of the American Academy of Child and Adolescent Psychiatry, 31*, 932–940.

Miller, L. C. (1967). Louisville Behavior Checklist for males, 6–12 years of age. *Psychological Reports, 21*, 885–896.

Quay, H. C. (1964). Personality dimensions in delinquent males as inferred from the factor analysis of behavior ratings. *Journal of Research in Crime and Delinquency, 1*, 33–37.

Quay, H. C. (1993). The psychobiology of undersocialized aggressive conduct disorder: a theoretical perspective. *Development and Psychopathology, 5*, 165–180.

Reich, W., & Welner, Z. (1992). *DICA-R-C. DSM-III-R version. Revised version of DICA for children ages 6–12*. St. Louis, MO: Washington University Department of Psychiatry.

Reinherz, H. Z. (1995). *Entering adulthood: A longitudinal community study*. Boston: Simmons College of Social Work.

Sawyer, M. G. (1990). *Childhood behavior problems: Discrepancies between reports from children, parents, and teachers*. Unpublished doctoral dissertation. University of Adelaide, Australia.

Shaffer, D. (1992). *Diagnostic Interview Schedule for Children, Version 2.3*. New York: Columbia University Division of Child Psychiatry.

Stanger, C., Achenbach, T. M., & Verhulst, F. C. (1997). Accelerated longitudinal comparisons of aggressive versus delinquent syndromes. *Development and Psychopathology, 9*, 43–58.

Stanger, C., MacDonald, V., McConaughy, S. H., & Achenbach, T. M. (1996). Predictors of cross-informant syndromes among children and youth referred for mental health services. *Journal of Abnormal Child Psychology, 24*, 597–614.

Stoff, D. M., Pollack, L., Vitiello, B., Behar, D., & Bridger, W. H. (1987). Reduction of ^{3}H-imipramine binding sites on platelets of conduct disordered children. *Neuropsychopharmacology, 1,* 55–62.

Van den Oord, E. J. C. G., Boomsma, D. I., & Verhulst, F. C. (1994). A study of problem behaviors in 10- to 15-year-old biologically related and unrelated international adoptees. *Behavior Genetics, 24,* 193–205.

Verhulst, F. C., Koot, H. M., & van der Ende, J. (1994). Differential predictive value of parents' and teachers' reports of children's problem behaviors: A longitudinal study. *Journal of Abnormal Child Psychology, 22,* 531–546.

Verhulst, F. C., & van der Ende, J. (1992). Six-year developmental course of internalizing and externalizing problem behaviors. *Journal of the American Academy of Child and Adolescent Psychiatry, 31,* 924–931.

Wechsler, D. C. (1991). *Wechsler Intelligence Scale for Children* (3rd ed.). San Antonio, TX: Psychological Corporation.

Weinstein, S. R., Noam, G. G., Grimes, K., Stone, K., & Schwab-Stone, M. (1990). Convergence of DSM-III diagnoses and self-reported symptoms in child and adolescent inpatients. *Journal of the American Academy of Child and Adolescent Psychiatry, 29,* 627–634.

Woolf, H. B. (Ed.). (1977). *Webster's new collegiate dictionary.* Springfield, MA: Merriam.

World Health Organization. (1992). *Mental disorders: Glossary and guide to their classification in accordance with the Tenth Revision of the International Classification of Diseases.* Geneva: Author.

II

Specific Childhood Psychopathologies

4

Mental Retardation

NIRBHAY N. SINGH, DONALD P. OSWALD, AND CYNTHIA R. ELLIS

INTRODUCTION

Mental retardation is a social construct devised to categorize individuals with a variety of symptoms, etiologies, and outcomes. Most definitions of mental retardation include deficits in learning and social adaptation, and the disorder is typically viewed within a life-span developmental context, ecology, and culture of the individual. Given that notions of mental retardation are not universal, our understanding of the disorder is predicated on the prevailing beliefs, attitudes, and values of our particular culture. Thus, what we mean by the term *mental retardation* varies between and even within cultures (Singh, 1995a). How we define the term and view individuals with the disorder are important considerations because policies, resource allocation, prevention, treatment, and care practices follow directly from our assumptions of the capabilities of individuals with mental retardation.

NIRBHAY N. SINGH, DONALD P. OSWALD, AND CYNTHIA R. ELLIS • Medical College of Virginia, Virginia Commonwealth University, Richmond, Virginia 23298-0489.

Handbook of Child Psychopathology, 3rd edition, edited by Ollendick & Hersen. Plenum Press, New York, 1998.

PHENOMENOLOGY

Mental retardation has been defined and characterized in a number of different ways since it was first distinguished from mental illness in the Middle Ages. At that time, individuals with mental retardation were thought to be possessed by the devil and were frequently banished from society. Indeed, it was not until the 1600s and 1700s that a more humanistic attitude was adopted toward individuals with mental retardation. Furthermore, it was not until the twentieth century that a more objective view began to be accepted, with the first classification of individuals as mentally retarded based on intelligence test scores in 1916.

It is now well recognized that mental retardation is not a specific disease and there is no single cause, mechanism, course, or prognosis. Rather, it is a behavioral syndrome representing subaverage levels of individual functioning. Individuals with mental retardation are not a homogeneous group; they represent a wide spectrum of abilities, clinical presentations, and behaviors. Although it was once thought that individuals with mental retardation were without the capacity for emotion and basic sensory acuities, even to the point that they were thought to lack the ability to discriminate hot from cold, it is now accepted that they experience the full range of emotions and, thus, may manifest the same behavior and psychiatric problems seen in the general population. Indeed, we now know that the prevalence of psychopathology and problem behaviors is up to five times higher in individuals with mental retardation than in the general population (Rutter, Tizard, & Whitmore, 1970).

DIAGNOSIS

Over the years, a number of different systems have been used to diagnose individuals with mental retardation and classify them within that diagnostic category. These have evolved from a basis solely on scores obtained on standardized tests of general intelligence to current definitions that consider cognitive abilities, adaptive behavior, and age of onset. The most widely accepted definition is the one offered by the American Association on Mental Retardation (AAMR; Luckasson et al., 1992):

> *Mental retardation* refers to substantial limitations in present functioning. It is characterized by significantly subaverage intellectual functioning, existing concurrently with related limitations in two or more of the following applicable adaptive skill areas: communication, self-care, home living, social skills, community use, self-direction, health and safety, functional academics, leisure, and work. Mental retardation manifests before age 18. (p. 1)

This definition refers to a state of impaired cognitive and adaptive functioning within the community rather than an inherent trait of the individual. The essential features of this definition have also been incorporated into the diagnostic criteria for mental retardation in the fourth edition of the *Diagnostic and Statistical Manual of Mental Disorders* (DSM-IV; American Psychiatric Association, 1994). In both diagnostic schemes, *significantly subaverage intellectual functioning* is defined as an IQ of approximately two standard deviations below the mean (about 70 to 75 or below), based on a standardized, individually administered general intelligence test. Concurrent deficits in present adaptive functioning refers to a functional impairment in two or more of the adaptive skill areas necessary to meet everyday life demands and achieve "standards of personal independence expected of someone in their particular age group, sociocultural background, and community setting" (American Psychiatric Association, 1994, p. 40). Manifests before age 18 refers to manifestation of the above during the developmental period. Despite the similarities in criteria used to diagnose mental retardation, there are substantial differences in the assignment of levels of severity or disability between the AAMR and DSM-IV diagnostic systems. Rather than subdividing individuals with mental retardation into degrees of severity based on their level of intellectual functioning (see Table 1) as in the DSM-IV, the AAMR diagnostic scheme subclassifies these individuals into four levels based on the intensities and patterns of supports they require (i.e., intermittent, limited, extensive, and pervasive).

Mental retardation should be diagnosed whenever the diagnostic criteria are met, regardless of the presence or absence of other disorders. The diagnosis, however, can be difficult to make with certainty in the presence of a number of organic and environmental factors, such as a severe sensory impairment, a severe emotional or behavioral disorder, being reared in an impoverished environment, or the interference with cognitive and neurological functioning reported with some drugs (Aman, Hammer, & Rojahn, 1993). The differential diagnosis of mental retardation includes Learning Disorders, Communication Disorders, Pervasive Development Disorders, and dementia. In the Learning and Communication Disorders, there will be a delay in specific areas of development, such as mathematics or expressive language, without a generalized impairment in cognitive and adaptive functioning. Pervasive Developmental Disorder is usually characterized by qualitative impairments in the development of communi-

Table 1. Classification of Mental Retardation by Severity

IQ level[a]	DSM-IV diagnostic classification	Educational classification	Old terminology	Approximate % of population with MR
50–55 to approx. 70	Mild Mental Retardation	Educable	Feebleminded moron	85%
35–40 to 50–55	Moderate Mental Retardation	Trainable	Feebleminded imbecile	10%
20–25 to 35–40	Severe Mental Retardation	Severely/Profoundly Handicapped	Feebleminded imbecile	3–4%
Below 20–25	Profound Mental Retardation	Severely/Profoundly Handicapped	Feebleminded idiot	1–2%

[a]Based on scores obtained on one or more standardized individually administered general intelligence tests.

cation skills (verbal and nonverbal) and reciprocal social interaction or the presence of stereotyped behavior, interests, and activities relative to the individual's developmental level or mental age. Individuals with mental retardation can have a comorbid diagnosis of a Learning Disorder, Communication Disorder, or Pervasive Developmental Disorder provided the specific deficit is out of proportion to the severity of the mental retardation. Dementia is a significant decline in cognitive functioning and memory following a period of previously higher functioning. Mental retardation with onset following a period of documented normal development may qualify for an additional diagnosis of dementia.

Mental retardation may be suspected prenatally (through amniocentesis) or in a young infant (with congenital anomalies or an abnormal newborn screen) if a condition associated with mental retardation is diagnosed (e.g., Down syndrome). Alternatively, the first indication of mental retardation may be the presence of developmental delay in a child previously thought to have normal cognitive abilities, the presentation of which typically depends on the severity of the condition. For example, severe and profound mental retardation often presents as motor delay in the first months of life whereas moderate mental retardation may present in a toddler with normal motor development as delayed language development. Furthermore, mild mental retardation may not be

evident until a child enters school and demonstrates poor educational and social development relative to his or her peers. Mental retardation may also arise suddenly as a result of a postnatal event or illness, such as head trauma. Mild mental retardation differs significantly from the more severe forms of the disorder in terms of its presentation, prevalence, etiology, associated features, management, and prognosis. Indeed, some school-age children with mild mental retardation who receive appropriate training are able to develop adequate adaptive skills such that they no longer meet the criteria for deficits in adaptive functioning as an adult and, thus, "graduate" from the diagnosis of mental retardation. The course of mental retardation, however, is highly individual and is influenced by a number of medical, psychological, environmental, and cultural factors.

ETIOLOGY

Although there may be a single, identifiable biological (e.g., a genetic syndrome) or environmental factor (e.g., childhood lead poisoning) associated with a specific case of mental retardation, the majority of cases are presumed to be multifactorial in origin, even if one factor is determined to be of primary importance. Further, in 30 to 40% of cases, no predisposing or risk factors can be identified despite a comprehensive evaluation. However, the more severe the mental retardation, the greater is the likelihood that a responsible etiological agent can be identified.

There are a large number of conditions and disorders associated with mental retardation and they can be classified according to the phase of development during which they exert their impact: (1) prenatal (e.g., hereditary disorders and early alterations of embryonic development), (2) perinatal (e.g., later pregnancy and neonatal problems), (3) postnatal (e.g., acquired childhood diseases or accidents, environmental influences, and other mental disorders), and (4) unknown. Although a comprehensive review is beyond the scope of this chapter, a list of the more common conditions associated with mental retardation is presented in Table 2.

EPIDEMIOLOGY

Although the prevalence of mental retardation is generally reported to be about 3%, a number of studies have reported different prevalence rates depending on the definition used, method of assessment, and population studied. For example, prevalence varies with the age group studied, with peak prevalence being about age 10 to 14 years, and a decrease in prevalence after adolescence. In addition, prevalence varies with the severity of mental retardation. Within the population of individuals with mental retardation, its prevalence decreases with increasing severity such that the majority of these individuals have mild mental retardation. The male-to-female ratio for mental retardation is about 1.6:1 (McLaren & Bryson, 1987) but,

Table 2. Etiological Factors Associated with Mental Retardation

Predisposing factor	Approximate % of population with MR	Examples of specific disorders or conditions
Hereditary disorders (based on parental genotype, may have variable expression)	5%	Inborn errors of metabolism (e.g., Tays–Sachs disease, Hurler's syndrome, phenylketonuria, galactosemia), other single-gene abnormalities (e.g., neurofibromatosis, tuberous sclerosis), chromosomal aberrations (e.g., translocation Down syndrome, fragile X syndrome)
Early alterations of embryonic development	30%	Chromosomal abnormalities (e.g., Down syndrome related to trisomy 21), prenatal exposure ot toxins (e.g., maternal alcohol consumption or substance abuse, intrauterine infections)
Later pregnancy and perinatal problems	10%	Fetal malnutrition, placental insufficiency, prematurity, hypoxia, trauma, low birth weight, intracranial hemorrhage, respiratory disorders, sepsis, hyperbilirubinemia
Acquired childhood diseases/accidents	5%	Infections (e.g., meningitis, encephalitis, slow virus infections), demyelinating or degenerative disorders (e.g., leukodystrophies), malnutrition, head trauma (e.g., car or household accidents, child abuse), poisoning (e.g., lead, mercury), environmental deprivation (psychsocial disadvantage, neglect, or deprivation)
Environmental influences and other mental disorders	15–20%	Deprivation, child abuse, severe mental disorders
Unknown	30–40%	

again, the results vary depending on study characteristics. The critical factor to note is that, in most of these studies, mental retardation has been defined solely in terms of IQ, with a two standard deviation cutoff, without a consideration of adaptive behavior. Current prevalence estimates are around 1% when both IQ and adaptive behavior are included in the definition of mental retardation (Baroff, 1986).

Among individuals with mental retardation, there is a high prevalence of associated disorders. Epilepsy is the most common single associated disorder and it tends to increase with greater severity of mental retardation (Pond, 1979). Other associated disorders include cerebral palsy, motor impairments, and psychiatric/ behavior problems (McLaren & Bryson, 1987). The prevalence of blindness and deafness is also much higher in individuals with mental retardation than in the general population (Baroff, 1986).

ASSESSMENT

Traditionally, the assessment of mental retardation has consisted of a measure of intellectual ability and a measure of adaptive functioning. Indeed, these two areas continue to comprise the bulk of assessment activities in individuals with mental retardation. In recent years, however, two additional areas have emerged and produced a burgeoning literature in mental retardation: assessment of psychopathology and quality of life. Although our review is limited to recent developments and the general state of the art in only these four assessment domains, we recognize the fact that a multimodal assessment is necessary to fully evaluate the strengths of an individual before interventions can be planned. Multimodal assessments may include the evaluation of motor, physiological, emotional, and cognitive behavior, among other domains. These assessments may include a number of strategies, including interviewing, checklists and rating scales, self-reports, self-monitoring,

direct observation, peer-referenced assessment, physiological and neuropsychological assessments, intellectual and achievement testing, and projective techniques (Ollendick & Hersen, 1993).

Intellectual Assessment

The need to assess individuals' intelligence has spawned an entire industry that has experienced considerable growth in recent years. The development, standardization, and marketing of intelligence tests is a major undertaking that entails a wide range of conceptual, technical, social, and political issues. Thus, the appearance of new, or newly revised, intelligence tests is a relatively rare event and the number of intellectual assessment instruments available to assist in the diagnosis of mental retardation is relatively small. Further, because the assessment of intelligence in the moderate-to-profound range of impairment is not the principal use of the instruments, there are a number of issues that limit their usefulness. Among these is the perennial problem of insufficient floor, particularly on the low end of the age ranges covered. Insufficient floor refers to a shortage of tasks that are accessible to individuals with significant cognitive impairment, and tests that are so characterized cannot discriminate levels of ability at the lower end of the continuum. Several of the most commonly used instruments for intellectual assessment in individuals with mental retardation are discussed below.

The Wechsler intelligence tests remain the most widely used set of IQ assessment devices in the United States. Relatively recent revisions of the children's scales have kept the Wechsler scales current and close to the state of the art in intellectual assessment. The adult scale is aging but continues to have wide use and acceptance.

The Wechsler Preschool and Primary Scale of Intelligence-Revised (WPPSI-R; Wechsler, 1989) is designed for the individual assessment of intelligence in children aged 3 years through 7 years 3 months and yields the traditional Full

Scale IQ, Verbal IQ, and Performance IQ. In addition, scaled scores are produced for each of 12 subtests, with 2 subtests (Animal Pegs and Sentences) that are optional and can be substituted for other Performance IQ and Verbal IQ subtests, respectively, in the computation of IQ scores. The table for deriving Full Scale IQ scores on the WPPSI-R does not extend below an IQ of 41 while the lower limits of the tables for Verbal IQ and Performance IQ are 46 and 45, respectively. For children whose performance falls below the lower limits of the tables, a "test age" may be determined to "gain a coarse understanding of the child's absolute level of performance" (Wechsler, 1989, p. 10). The manual contains cautions about the interpretation of test age scores though these are perhaps understated. The term *test age* is unquestionably preferable to *mental age* but the concept is still problematic.

The Wechsler Intelligence Scale for Children-Third Edition (WISC-III; Wechsler, 1991) is the latest version of Wechsler's individually administered intelligence test for children aged 6 years through 16 years 11 months. Thirteen subtests are included in the scale and all global scale scores can be derived without the administration of the 13th subtest (Mazes). The WISC-III yields scaled scores for each subtest, IQ scores (Full Scale, Verbal, and Performance), and scores for four scales (Verbal Comprehension, Perceptual Organization, Freedom from Distractibility, and Processing Speed) derived from a factor analysis of subtest scores. These factor scores are provided on the same distribution as IQ scores (mean = 100; SD = 15) and offer an alternate way of interpreting the subtest profile. WISC-III Full Scale IQs extend down to 40 while Verbal IQs and Performance IQs extend down to 46. Like the WPPSI-R, the child must obtain raw scores greater than zero on three verbal subtests and three performance subtests in order to derive the Full Scale IQ, Verbal IQ, and Performance IQ.

The problem of insufficient floor in the assessment of children with mental retardation is less critical with the WISC-III, in part because the age range overlaps with the WPPSI-R on the lower end. Thus, for children between the ages of 6 years and 7 years 3 months who are suspected of having limited intellectual ability, the WPPSI-R offers an alternative with a substantially lower floor. The WISC-III manual discusses the derivation of a child's "test age," but, unfortunately, without the modest cautionary remarks found in the WPPSI-R. Clinicians who use test age in the interpretation or explanation of intelligence test results should be aware that, despite the intuitive appeal of the notion of "test age," they are on decidedly thin conceptual and statistical ice in doing so.

The Wechsler Adult Intelligence Scale-Revised (WAIS-R; Wechsler, 1981) is an individually administered intelligence scale for adults aged 16 through 74 years. The scale includes 11 subtests, with scaled scores from the first 6 subtests summed to derive a Verbal IQ and scores from the last 5 summed to derive a Performance IQ. Scaled scores from all 11 subtests are summed to derive a Full Scale IQ. The lower limits for IQ score tables are different for each age group but range from 46 to 54 for Verbal IQ, from 47 to 61 for Performance IQ, and from 45 to 51 for Full Scale IQ. Thus, the WAIS-R's capacity to assess mental retardation is restricted in the upper and lower extremes of the age distribution. The WAIS-R differs from the children's scales in that no guidance is provided in the manual for dealing with subtest raw scores of zero but common sense suggests that an IQ is highly suspect unless it is derived from a profile with at least three Verbal IQ and three Performance IQ subtests whose raw scores are greater than zero.

The limited floor at the lower extreme of the age distribution can be circumvented by using the WISC-III for 16-year-olds suspected of intellectual limitation. However, the floor limitations are even more severe at the upper end of the age distribution (i.e., above age 54 years) and there are no alternatives in the Wechsler scales for this age group. This presents a problem when tracking the intellectual functioning of individuals with mental retardation across the life span.

The Stanford–Binet, Fourth Edition (SB:FE;

Thorndike, Hagen, & Sattler, 1986) is an individually administered intelligence test for individuals aged 2 years through 23 years 11 months. The test includes 15 subtests but no age group is administered more than 13. The SB:FE yields a Composite Standard Age Score roughly equivalent to a Full Scale IQ although the mean of 100 and standard deviation of 16 slightly lower the cutoff point for intellectual functioning in the range for mental retardation; two standard deviations below the mean is a score of 68 on the SB:FE rather than the score of 70 that is typical for other intelligence tests. In addition, the SB:FE yields four Area Standard Age Scores (Verbal Reasoning, Abstract/Visual Reasoning, Quantitative Reasoning, and Short-Term Memory) also with a mean of 100 and standard deviation of 16.

The SB:FE has a serious floor problem at the lower end of the age range. The lowest Composite Standard Age Score that a child of 2 years 0 months can receive is 95. The instrument cannot classify a child's intellectual functioning as falling in the range of mental retardation until age 3 years 3 months and intellectual functioning at the moderate mental retardation level cannot be identified until age 4 (Sattler, 1992). This limited floor is one of the chief complaints of this test.

The AAMR definition (Luckasson et al., 1992) stresses the need to consider "cultural and linguistic diversity as well as differences in communication and behavioral factors" when administering assessment instruments and interpreting the results. Although few would argue with the intent of such a qualifying statement, the practical impact of attempting to comply remains to be seen. One can easily imagine some clinicians throwing up their hands in despair over such a mandate, at a loss over just how to go about considering each of those factors and how to incorporate those considerations into a diagnosis. On the other hand, a more pernicious hypothetical scenario might involve the deliberate manipulation of a diagnostic decision that is retrospectively attributed to these considerations. Issues of diversity in the assessment of mental retarda-

tion continue to plague practitioners in the 1990s; those issues are, if anything, more clearly drawn and troubling than at any time in the history of this field. The AAMR definition does little to assist in addressing these issues and introduces an additional set of problems that have not begun to be satisfactorily addressed (MacMillan, Gresham, & Siperstein, 1995).

Adaptive Behavior

The alternatives available for the assessment of adaptive behavior are even fewer than those for intellectual assessment. The measurement of the construct of adaptive behavior is still at a relatively primitive stage although the most recent generation of instruments represents a significant advance in the field. To the extent that clinicians seek to follow it, the AAMR definition of mental retardation (Luckasson et al., 1992) introduces further complexity in the assessment of adaptive behavior. The requirement to document limitations in 2 of the 10 specified adaptive skill areas presupposes a sophistication in adaptive skill assessment that this field currently does not possess (MacMillan et al., 1995). Luckasson et al. also set forth a high standard with regard to the selection of adaptive skill assessment instruments including "technically adequate . . . designed for the particular population, the functional purpose, and the specific adaptive skills intended . . . [and] normed within community environments on individuals who are of the same age grouping as the individual being evaluated" (pp. 41–42). Such virtues are difficult to document in even the most respected instruments in use today. Several commonly used adaptive behavior assessment devices are discussed below.

The Vineland Adaptive Behavior Scales (VABS; Sparrow, Balla, & Cicchetti, 1984) is a revision of Doll's (1953) original Vineland Social Maturity Scale that was intended to assess personal and social sufficiency in individuals from birth through adulthood. There are three versions of the VABS: (1) Interview Edition, Survey

Form; (2) Interview Edition, Expanded Form; and (3) Classroom Edition. Each of the versions assesses adaptive behavior in four domains: Communication, Daily Living Skills, Socialization, and Motor Skills, with each of these domains including several subdomains constituting conceptually meaningful divisions of skills within the domain.

The Interview Edition of the VABS are administered as semistructured interviews with a caretaker who reports on the subject's abilities in a wide variety of adaptive skills. The Expanded Form is more comprehensive than the Survey Form, offering a more detailed picture of the individual's skill profile for the purpose of educational and habilitation planning. The Classroom Edition is a questionnaire completed by the subject's teacher. The VABS yields Standard Scores for each of the domains and a total adaptive behavior score is derived from the sum of the domain standard scores for the Adaptive Behavior Composite. Additional domain and composite scores may be derived, including confidence intervals, percentiles, stanines, and age equivalents. At the subdomain level, scores are limited to "Adaptive Level" (high, moderately high, adequate, moderately low, and low) and age equivalent.

The AAMD Adaptive Behavior Scale (ABS; Nihira, Foster, Shellhaas, & Leland, 1974) is a revision of the original 1969 version. The ABS includes 10 adaptive behavior domains and 14 domains related to personality and behavior disorders. Scoring the ABS yields a percentile rank for each of the domains. Percentiles are based on a sample of approximately 4000 individuals living in facilities for individuals with mental retardation in the United States and are available for 11 age groups. A common criticism of the ABS is the varying range of skills assessed in the domains; some subtests include many kinds of skills across a wide range of difficulty while others are relatively narrow in scope. Although the ABS offers some information about a variety of adaptive behavior domains, using the derived percentile rank scores as the sole documentation of limitations in at least 2 of the 10 AAMR

definition of adaptive skills areas is probably an inappropriate use of the instrument.

The AAMR Adaptive Behavior Scale—School: Second Edition (ABS-S:2; Lambert, Nihira, & Leland, 1993) is a revision of the earlier version of this scale designed to assess school-age children's personal and community independence as well as personal and social performance and adjustment. Norms are available for individuals aged 3 through 21 years. The instrument is completed by someone who has personal knowledge of the individual or who has interviewed a person who has a good knowledge of the target individual. The first part of the ABS-S:2 focuses on personal independence in nine behavior domains, and the second part focuses on social behaviors and consists of seven domains. The ABS-S:2 yields percentiles, standard scores, and age equivalents for each of these domains. In addition, similar scores can be calculated for each of five subscales empirically derived by factor analysis of the entire scale.

The Inventory for Client and Agency Planning (ICAP; Bruininks, Hill, Weatherman, & Woodcock, 1986) contains an adaptive behavior assessment section consisting of 77 adaptive behavior items drawn from a more extensive instrument, the Scales of Independent Behavior (SIB; Bruininks, Woodcock, Weatherman, & Hill, 1984). These instruments assess adaptive behavior in four domains: Social/Communication Skills, Personal Living Skills, Community Living Skills, and Motor Skills. The ICAP has been used widely in community settings for individuals with mental retardation and the adaptive behavior portion has been found to be related to measures of community adjustment and integration as defined by economic independence, independence in daytime activities and living arrangements, and independence from community support services (McGrew, Bruininks, & Thurlow, 1992).

Psychopathology

The assessment of psychopathology in individuals with mental retardation has received increasing attention in recent years, yielding a handful of problem behavior and diagnostic checklists. As illustrative examples, we review a problem behavior checklist, a screening instrument for psychiatric disorders, and a diagnostic instrument for psychopathology. A recent comprehensive review of instruments for assessing behavior problems and psychopathology in this population is available elsewhere (Aman, 1991).

The Aberrant Behavior Checklists (ABC) are rating scales for assessing inappropriate and maladaptive behavior of persons with mental retardation. They were designed to monitor treatment effects and may be used with children and adults. Two versions of the ABC are available; the original version was designed for individuals with mental retardation in residential settings (ABC-Residential; Aman & Singh, 1986) and the more recent community version (ABC-Community; Aman & Singh, 1994) was designed to provide a parallel measure for individuals with mental retardation in community settings.

The ABC consists of 58 items that are rated by someone who has regular contact with the individual and knows him or her well. The five subscales of the ABC have been empirically derived through factor analysis. The ABC-Residential includes normative data in the form of mean subscale scores (and standard deviations) for two large samples of persons with mental retardation in institutional settings. Mean scores are reported by gender and age. The ABC-Community provides an extended range of normative information, translating raw scores into selected percentiles, ranging from the 50th to the 98th. Normative data for each subscale are offered in several formats by age, gender, and level of retardation. The ABC has high internal consistency and item–total correlations and good test–retest and interrater reliabilities. A wide range of validity studies including factor replications, criterion group validity, and congruent validity have provided broad and robust support for the scales (Aman, 1991).

The Reiss Screen for Maladaptive Behavior (Reiss, 1988) is intended to identify individuals with mental retardation who are likely to have a significant mental health problem. The instrument was designed for individuals 12 years and older with all levels of mental retardation. It is an informant-report instrument and requires ratings from two or more persons familiar with the subject. The Reiss Screen consists of 38 items, 26 of which are included in one or more of the scales' seven empirically derived subscales. Of the remaining 12 items, 4 are included in an Autism subscale, 6 are scored individually as special symptoms that describe serious behavior problems, and 2 are experimental items. A 26-item Total Score may also be derived. Cutoff scores (indicating a need for further assessment) are provided for each of the subscales, the total scale, and the special symptoms.

Psychometric data on the Reiss Screen indicate generally adequate item interrater reliability and subscale internal consistency. Validity studies have been supportive of the instrument as a screen for the presence of some mental disorder although few data are available regarding the scale's power to screen for *specific* diagnoses (Aman, 1991).

The Psychopathology Instrument for Mentally Retarded Adults (PIMRA; Matson, 1988) was designed to diagnose psychopathological conditions, to help plan mental health treatment, and to assess treatment in individuals with mental retardation. The PIMRA is intended to be used with adolescents and adults with mild to profound retardation. Two versions are available: a self-report version for individuals with mild (and, in some cases, moderate) mental retardation and an informant version.

The PIMRA consists of 56 items divided into eight subscales. Each subscale includes seven items and endorsement of four of the seven items on a subscale constitutes evidence for the diagnosis. Items included in the PIMRA were based on major diagnostic categories in the DSM-III (American Psychiatric Association, 1980) and were grouped into subscales. Empirical studies of the reliability and internal consistency of the subscales have been mixed; the validity of subscales is largely uninvestigated although there is some support for the Affective Disorder subscale (Aman, 1991) and the Schizophrenia subscale (Swiezy, Matson, Kirkpatrick-Sanchez, & Williams, 1995).

Quality of Life

The notion of including measures of quality of life in the assessment of individuals with mental retardation has gained increasing acceptance in recent years. Quality of life is an emerging construct for which increasingly refined conceptual models are beginning to appear (e.g., Felce & Perry, 1995). Hughes, Hwang, Kim, Eisenman, and Killian (1995) identified 15 dimensions of quality of life in their review of the literature, some of which included 10 or more specific components, but they reported that the field appeared to be converging on a multidimensional and interactional concept that relates to personal competence and successful community adjustment.

The quality of life construct appears to be far too broad for a single comprehensive instrument to cover. The psychometric properties of many available instruments and indicators are largely unknown and there are no assessment devices with enough history and research to be called standards in the field. However, practitioners and researchers interested in quality of life may be assured that they do not need to begin from scratch; Hughes et al. (1995) offer a compilation of sources that will help the dedicated reader to avoid mistakes and pitfalls and to build on the considerable efforts of others. Meaningful, psychometrically sound measurement of quality of life is perhaps the next frontier in the assessment of persons with mental retardation.

An indirect method of assessing the quality of life has recently been suggested that entails evaluating the nature of their care and living environments of individuals with mental retardation (Singh, 1995b). The suggestion is that there is a consensus among professionals, parents, advocates, and the consumers themselves regarding the nature and quality of services that ought to be provided in different domains (e.g., psychological, educational, psychiatric, medical, nursing, and dental services; living environments; civil rights) regardless of where individuals with mental retardation live. In this view, the question of institution versus community placement does not arise because the central issue is not residential location but the nature of services provided. Indeed, "living in the community is not inherently better if the services we provide to individuals with mental retardation in the community are not of the same quality as those we provide for ourselves. . . . We have the choice of providing a quality life-style in the community to individuals with mental retardation or making the community a larger institution for them." (Singh, 1995b, p. 144).

TREATMENT

Although our society has not yet developed a system of care that provides all individuals with mental retardation appropriate treatment and services to ensure that their quality of life is comparable to that of the mainstream of society (Singh, 1995b), there has been a significant evolution in our philosophy regarding the treatment, care, and rights of individuals with mental retardation. From early Greek and Roman civilizations (also termed the "era of extermination") through the Middle Ages, there was little time, resources, or tolerance for individuals with any handicapping conditions and they were frequently removed and isolated from the community. By the early 1800s, society in general had adopted a more humanitarian attitude toward handicapped individuals but these individuals, including those with mental retardation, were still grouped together with criminals and denied most privileges and rights. Indeed, it was not until 1837 that the first public residential institution for individuals with mental retardation was established in Europe and 1848 before the first such facility was opened in Massachusetts. Although the interest was initially in providing for education and treatment to individuals with mental retardation, there was a gradual transition of these schools to custodial institutions. The schools were viewed as failures when they were unable to teach the skills of self-independence necessary to live in mainstream society and, thus, their emphasis was changed to teach skills suitable for life "inside" the institution. At the same time, the movement for segregation and eugenics strengthened in this country, leading to the "era of institutionalization." Since the 1950s, however, there has been an increase in public concern for individuals with mental retardation, including efforts to depopulate institutions and integrate residential programs into the community and to improve the health, educational, and social services for persons with mental retardation. This trend was significantly influenced by the active interest and role of President Kennedy as well as Congressional action advocating for individuals with mental retardation and the recognition of their civil rights by the courts.

Since the 1950s, there have been a number of legislative and court decisions having a direct impact on improving the quality of the lives of individuals with mental retardation, particularly in areas related to their rights to education, appropriate treatment, and community living (Singh, Guernsey, & Ellis, 1992). For example, in 1954, *Brown v. Board of Education* established that separate education did not represent equal opportunity. Although this case specifically dealt with racial segregation, it was applicable to students with mental retardation as well and led the way for other legislative action and litigation on their behalf. The passage of PL 94-142 (the Education for All Handicapped Children Act) in 1975 guaranteed public education and services to all children, including (1) free, appropriate education and related services (e.g., speech pathology, psychological services, and medical evaluations), (2) procedures to test and evaluate children that are nondiscriminatory in terms of race and culture, (3) written Individualized Educational Plans (IEPs), and (4) educa-

tion in the least restrictive environment. This was followed in 1986 by PL 99-457, which extended entitlement of educational and related services to children 3 to 5 years of age and provided incentives for the provision of services to children under 3 years of age. There have also been landmark decisions establishing the rights of individuals with mental retardation to such things as appropriate treatment in the least restrictive environment (e.g., *Wyatt v. Stickney* in 1972 and *Youngberg v. Romeo* in 1982) and Congressional action enacting the Civil Rights of Institutionalized Persons Act (1981) granting legal power to the Justice Department to protect the rights of institutionalized individuals with mental retardation (see Singh et al., 1992).

This evolution in the philosophy of care and treatment for individuals with mental retardation has had a significant influence on our current perspective on services for this population today. There is now an emphasis on deinstitutionalization and placement of all individuals with mental retardation in the community (Singh, 1995b). In addition, it is recognized that the education and training of all children and adults with mental retardation should include an interdisciplinary assessment (including parents), due process, placement in the least restrictive environment (mainstreaming or inclusion), and the development of written IEPs and FSPs (Family Service Plans). Probably most important, however, is the realization that the definition of education needs to be broadened to include the teaching of skills that enhance the individual's quality of life, whether they be academic, social, or self-care skills. Furthermore, it has been recognized that this population has special medical and psychiatric needs and it is important that they be provided adequate and appropriate medical/psychiatric diagnoses and treatment. The protective and advocacy measures enacted by the Congress and judicial system are dedicated to ensuring that all individuals are provided with the quality of life they are entitled to, whether or not they have mental retardation.

Given the broad range of needs, individuals

with mental retardation require a diversity of services, including treatment for behavioral excesses, skills training for behavioral deficits, and psychiatric services for emotional disorders. In addition, they need the same array of services (e.g., medical, dental) that is provided for the general population. In the following sections, we briefly discuss some conceptual issues in behavioral intervention that can be used to enhance the quality of life of individuals with mental retardation. There are numerous books and thousands of research papers that describe in great detail behavioral strategies that can be used to reduce problem behaviors and remediate behavioral deficits in this population. Thus, there is little necessity for us to repeat this information here and the interested reader should consult these sources for descriptions of various behavioral procedures typically found useful with individuals with mental retardation (e.g., Carr et al., 1994; Repp & Singh, 1990; Singh, 1996; Van Houten & Axelrod, 1993). In addition, we present an overview of the various psychotropic drugs that have been used to control behavior problems and treat psychiatric problems in this population.

Behavioral Interventions

Behavioral approaches are based on the notion that we can reduce problem behaviors and remediate skills deficits through learning-based procedures. To achieve the best results, behavior reduction programs are often paired with skills acquisition programs in an effort to produce meaningful changes in the lives of these individuals.

Behavioral Excesses

Typically, in the absence of organic causes, behavioral excesses are thought to result from faulty or incomplete learning and, therefore, most amenable to behavioral treatment. The assessment, analysis, and treatment of behavior problems is a multistage process that includes

(1) a structural analysis of the problem behavior; (2) descriptive analysis of the target and collateral behaviors; (3) hypothesis formation; (4) experimental analysis under analog or natural conditions; (5) development, implementation, and evaluation of the treatment; and (6) maintenance and generalization of treatment effects (Axelrod, 1987; Mace, Lalli, & Shea, 1992). A structural analysis includes an assessment of the impact of the physical and biological environments on the individual's problem behaviors. This type of analysis requires a collaboration between the behavioral psychologist and a physician specializing in the unique problems of individuals with developmental disabilities. If the analysis indicates that the behavioral excess (e.g., self-injury) is maintained by the individual's physical environment (e.g., staff, workplace demands), one aspect of the treatment will focus on the manipulation of the environment; if it is maintained by the individual's biological environment (e.g., otitis media), the treatment will focus on medical management. Undertaking a structural analysis before a formal functional analysis is advised because it may save a substantial amount of time, lead to easily implemented environmental or medical interventions, and can make a dramatic change in the individual's quality of life without the labor-intensive manipulation of the individual's response contingencies.

A descriptive analysis requires structured or unstructured observations in the natural setting, interviews with staff who know the individual and the conditions under which the target behavior occurs, and data collection on antecedents, target behaviors, and consequences using a partial interval recording procedure. Analysis of the data thus obtained provides the basis for deriving tentative hypotheses about the functional relationships between various motivational variables and the occurrence of a target behavior. These hypotheses can be informally tested in the natural environment of the individual to determine the primary motivation for the behavior in each setting in which it occurs. An informal assessment strategy is useful because it allows the behavior to be assessed in the actual environment in which it occurs and in which it will be treated. Thus, all of the naturally occurring antecedents and consequences are in play during the assessment and treatment. Further, it obviates the need for deliberately escalating the problem behavior in an effort to determine its motivation. In the few cases where such a strategy proves unsuccessful, the presumed motivation for the behavior can be tested under analog conditions (Iwata, Vollmer, & Zarcone, 1990).

Regardless of whether an informal or formal functional analysis is used, once the function of the target behavior is identified, this information can be used to design an appropriate intervention. There are many ways in which the behavioral excess can be controlled and positive behaviors of the individual strengthened (e.g., Carr et al., 1994; Repp & Singh, 1990; Singh, 1996; Van Houten & Axelrod, 1993). It cannot be overstated that a comprehensive treatment program must include strategies that not only reduce the behavioral excess but also enhance the individual's general quality of life because the reduction of a problem behavior, per se, is only a partial response to a complex problem (Singh, 1995b).

The issue of maintenance and generalization of planned behavior change is important in both community and institutional settings. if the behavioral intervention is comprehensive, undertaken in the natural environment of the individual, and includes behavior reduction, skills training, and other programmed changes that will enhance the individual's quality of life (e.g., vocational training, participation in community activities), it is likely that the new behavior will be "trapped" and maintained by a natural system of reinforcers in the individual's environment (Baer & Wolf, 1970). However, if the behavioral intervention is directed only at reducing the problem behavior in a narrow range of settings, such as those available in an institution, then the lack of an explicit maintenance and generalization program would be a critical omission because the behavior change is unlikely to be maintained or generalized to community settings. Indeed, we question the significance of reducing or treating behavior problems in an institution when the individual continues to be incarcerated in a facility away from the natural rhythm of life in the community. The mere fact that an individual's behavior problem is reduced may not make much of an impact on the person's quality of life because nothing else has changed in his or her life.

Skills Training

All behaviors of the individual, social and antisocial, adaptive and maladaptive, are inextricably interconnected with those of the caretakers and the ecological context. For example, characteristics of the individual, the caretakers (i.e., family members, staff, professionals), and the ecological context in which the individual functions interact with each other over time to produce changes. Thus, there is little reason to believe that caretakers can produce a discrete but meaningful change in an individual's problem behavior independent of the individual's other behaviors, their own behavior, or the environment. One practical implication of this view is that behavior reduction programs and skills training programs must necessarily be integrated to produce lasting and meaningful changes in the individual. Another implication is that skills need to be enhanced within a functional context instead of being taught as a discrete skill independent of the individual's daily living skills (Singh, 1995b).

Traditionally, behavioral skills acquisition programs have emphasized the teaching of new skills derived from a task analysis of the terminal behavior that individuals need to have in their repertoire. Thus, for example, individuals may be taught to discriminate between different colored blocks so that they can know their colors. Typically, one color is taught at a time until mastery is achieved to some predetermined criterion (e.g., 80% correct performance on three consecutive trials). The overall outcome of this type of training is that, if successful, the individual is able to perform a number of isolated skills at given mastery levels, although, often, the skills are not functional because the individual is unable to exhibit the appropriate behavior in the context of daily life. A good example would be an individual who is taught to discriminate between different colors but not in the context of daily living (e.g., to cross the street when the traffic light is green).

Although excellent data can be produced showing the efficacy of training programs in teaching new skills, in these programs efficacy is judged within the context of frequency counts of task performance within a narrowly defined context (e.g., Cindy will discriminate between red, green, and amber on 80% of the trials in three consecutive sessions). These types of programs are no longer acceptable and currently accepted professional standards of care require that training programs produce more comprehensive lifestyle changes than the mere acquisition of isolated skills (Evans & Meyer, 1987; Horner, Sprague, & Flannery, 1993). Although training programs may use discrete steps or skills as the unit of instruction, functional activities or skill clusters are the appropriate units of outcome (Guess & Helmstetter, 1986). In the final analysis, the aim of skills training is not to enable individuals to achieve an arbitrary level of proficiency in isolated skills but to assist them to reach the "criterion of ultimate functioning" (Brown, Neitupski, & Hamre-Neitupski, 1976) so that they are able to use these skills in a functionally acceptable manner within the social norms of the community of their choice.

In summary, behavioral interventions derived through structural and functional analyses of behavior problems are usually more effective than trial-and-error approaches. Skills training has changed in focus from the teaching of isolated skills in sequestered sessions to the teaching of functional tasks within the context of an individual's daily life. Thus, the current emphasis in behavioral treatment is not only on reducing behavioral excesses and remediating skills deficits but also on significantly improving the quality of life of the individual.

Pharmacotherapy

Pharmacotherapy is a common modality for treating the psychiatric disorders and behavior problems of individuals with mental retardation. It is commonly used with individuals who exhibit violent, explosive behavior or engage in life-threatening behaviors, such as self-injury and rumination (Aman & Singh, 1988). In addition, aggression, agitation, property destruction, and stereotypy are other behaviors that may be targeted by pharmacotherapy.

Prevalence of Drug Use

The prevalence of psychotropic drug use in this population depends on whether the individuals live in an institution or in the community (Singh, Ellis, & Wechsler, in press). For example, in institutions it ranges from a low of 19% to a high of 86%, with most studies reporting rates between about 30 and 50%. Medication that is used for controlling seizures ranges from a low of 24% to a high of 56%, although it is typically between 25 and 45%. In general, the use of psychotropic and antiepileptic medication ranges from 50 to 70%, with some individuals being prescribed both types concurrently. For those in the community, the prevalence varies according to their age. For example, for children it ranges from 2 to 7%, and for adults, from 14 to 36%. The use of medication for controlling seizures is between 12 and 31% for children and between 18 and 24% for adults. The combined prevalence of psychotropic and antiepileptic medication is between 19 and 33% for children and between 36 and 48% for adults.

Patterns of Drug Use

A number of factors influence psychotropic drug use by individuals with mental retardation (Singh et al., in press). For example, increasing dosage is highly correlated with increasing age and decreasing intellectual impairment. There is a strong relationship between the type of residential facility and medication use, with more medication being prescribed in larger facilities and in facilities with very restrictive environments. Further, there is a strong positive correlation between the number and severity of the individual's behavioral and psychiatric problems and the use of medication (Aman & Singh, 1988). For example, individuals who exhibit aggression, hyperactivity, self-injury, screaming, or anxiety are more likely to receive drug treatment than those with milder and less disruptive problems (e.g., noncompliance).

Issues in Drug Treatment

Although it is clear that individuals with mental retardation suffer the full range of psychiatric disorders, accurate diagnosis in this population is more of an art than a science. To reach a reliable diagnosis, the active involvement of the client is necessary; however, given the increasingly significant language problems associated with increasing severity of mental retardation, this is often not possible. Thus, the subjective opinions and assumptions of the target individual's caretakers are used to reach a diagnosis. Given that each caretaker is in an interactive relationship with the individual and that the transactions between the two contribute to the psychiatric and behavioral outcomes for the individual, using only caretaker information necessarily provides only a partial view of the nature and cause of the individual's problems. This situation often leads to the identification and treatment of observable behavior problems rather than discrete psychiatric disorders. Thus, for example, intractable self-injury may become the focus of pharmacotherapy even though the self-injury could be the behavioral outcome of any number of factors, including a specific psychiatric disorder (e.g., depression, anxiety), chemical dysfunction (e.g., Lesch–Nyhan syndrome), faulty or incomplete learning, medical illness (e.g., otitis media), or the side effects of medication. However, if a reliable and valid diagnosis of a specific major mental disorder can be made, the clinical decision regarding phar-

macological treatment is clear and follows the same principles as that for an individual without mental retardation. The consideration then is in choosing medication that will provide maximum psychiatric benefits with the least negative effects on the learning and cognition of the individual.

Role of Nonmedical Clinicians. As with all mental health professionals, those who are involved with this population must have some basic knowledge of psychotropic medications and their effects on behavior. Given the limited assistance that individuals with severe and profound mental retardation can provide in self-monitoring the effects of their medication, mental health and other professionals are increasingly asked to monitor and provide feedback to the prescribing physician. Indeed, there is good evidence to show that informed feedback from nonmedical professionals greatly enhances medication-related treatment decisions (Sprague & Gadow, 1976). These findings have led to the development of a number of models of assessment, diagnosis, and treatment of behavioral and psychiatric disorders that rely heavily on informed feedback from parents, clinicians, teachers, and therapists to enhance clinical decision-making regarding drug and other treatments (Singh, Parmelee, Sood, & Katz, 1993; Singh, Sood, Sonenklar, & Ellis, 1991). When compared with the traditional medical method of physician-based treatment decisions, the use of these models typically result in far fewer individuals being placed on medication (Bisconer, Zhang, & Sine, 1995; Briggs, 1989; Findholt & Emmett, 1990).

Psychotropic medication is used as one component of a broad therapeutic approach to help individuals with mental retardation control their behavior and learn alternative, acceptable forms of behavior (Ellis, Singh, & Jackson, 1996). Clearly, medication does *not* teach new skills; it merely acts as a setting event for the occurrence of appropriate behavior when maladaptive behaviors are reduced. Medication provides symptomatic relief for psychiatric disorders, allowing the individual to function more fully at school, work, and home. However, although medication may relieve the individuals' symptoms of psychiatric illness, it does not remove the vulnerability to its recurrence because the environmental and constitutional stresses that gave rise to the illness are not affected by the medication.

Once a decision has been made to initiate psychotropic drug treatment, it is critical to evaluate the drug response using repeated assessment measures, such as rating scales and behavioral observations, and monitor side effects. Standard medication management includes dosage titration at periodic intervals based on continuous evaluation and monitoring of benefits and side effects. Although there is no single assessment instrument that can be used for all disorders and with all individuals, the Aberrant Behavior Checklists (Aman & Singh, 1986, 1994) are the only instruments designed specifically for evaluating the effects of psychotropic drugs in children and adults with mental retardation. These rating scales cover the primary problem behaviors for which antipsychotics and other drugs are usually prescribed as well as a range of other behaviors that may show medication-related changes. In addition, there are a number of assessment instruments that have been designed to record side effects of medication in general as well as instruments designed for measuring side effects of specific medications. Finally, reassessment of the need for continued medication treatment is undertaken at least once every 30 to 90 days to avoid unnecessarily prolonged treatment. In the rare case that an individual is on psychotropic medication for more than a year, it is important that a drug holiday (i.e., a period of time off the medication) be instituted every year to determine the continued need for the medication. In general, it is important to remember that medication, like any other treatment, should be used to improve an individual's general functioning and quality of life rather than strictly for reducing undesirable behaviors (Singh, 1995b).

Effects of Medication

We present only a brief overview of the effects of psychotropic drugs on the behavior and learning of individuals with mental retardation because we have reviewed this area extensively in a number of recent publications (e.g., Ellis et al., 1996; Ellis, Singh, & Singh, 1996; Singh, Ellis, & Singh, 1994). Further, a more detailed introduction to psychotropic drugs in general can be found in other recent publications (e.g., Rosenberg, Holttum, & Gershon, 1994; Schatzberg & Nemeroff, 1995; Wiener, 1996). In Table 3, we present psychotropic drugs by class, generic name, and recommended dosage by age for individuals with mental retardation, and in Table 4, the most common indications and side effects for the different classes of drugs.

Antipsychotics. The antipsychotics are most frequently prescribed to control the behavior of individuals who are aggressive, destructive, self-injurious, hyperactive, and antisocial. However, our knowledge of the behavioral effects of these drugs is rather limited because of the paucity of well-controlled studies in this population. The early enthusiasm for chlorpromazine (Thorazine) was not supported by well-controlled studies of its effects in controlling behavior problems and the drug is not recommended for this use at this time. Thioridazine (Mellaril) is effective in controlling hyperactivity, aggression, and stereotypy in some individuals with mental retardation. Haloperidol (Haldol) is often used instead of chlorpromazine and thioridazine because it is less sedating, but there are very few well-controlled studies attesting to its efficacy with this population (Aman & Singh, 1991). Although used in some institutions, there are very little data to support the use of other antipsychotics, such as fluphenazine (Prolixin), mesoridazine (Serentil), trifluoperazine (Stelazine), thiothixene (Navane), and loxapine (Loxitane), and, in addition, most of these drugs have not been approved by the Food and Drug Administration (FDA) for use in this population. The newer antipsychotics, such

Table 3. Recommended Doses for the Various Classes of Psychotropic Drugs

Drug	Average daily dose		
	Children	Adolescents	Adults
A. Antipsychotics			
Chlorpromazine	30–200 mg	40-400 mg	100–800 mg
(>6 mos of age)*	(2.5–6 mg/kg/day)	(3–6 mg/kg/day)	(max 2000 mg/day)
Thioridazine	75–200 mg	100–200+ mg	150–800 mg
(>2 yrs of age)*	(0.5–3 mg/kg/day)		(max 800 mg/day)
Trifluoperazine	1–15 mg	1–20 mg	15–40 mg
(>6 yrs of age)*			
Thiothixene	2–10 mg	5–30 mg	20–60 mg
(>12 yrs of age)*			
Haloperidol	0.5–4 mg	2–16 mg	2–16+ mg
(>3 yrs of age)*	(0.05–0.15 mg/kg/day)		
Reserpine	0.02–0.25 mg	0.1–1.0 mg	0.1–1.0 mg
Clozapine		50–200 mg	300–450 mg
(>16 yrs of age)*		(3–5 mg/kg/day)	(max 900 mg/day)
Loxapine	5–50 mg	20–100 mg	60–250 mg
(>16 yrs of age)*			
B. Antidepressants			
Amitriptyline	30–100 mg	50–100 mg	75–300 mg
(>12 yrs of age)*	(1–5 mg/kg/day)	(1–5 mg/kg/day)	
Bupropion	25–150 mg	75–300 mg	200–450 mg
(>18 yrs of age)*		(3–6 mg/kg/day)	
Clomipramine	25–100 mg	50–150 mg	100–250 mg
(>10 yrs of age)*		(2–3 mg/kg/day)	
Desipramine	10–150 mg	50–150 mg	100–200 mg
(>12 yrs of age)*	(1–5 mg/kg/day)	(1–5 mg/kg/day)	
Fluoxetine	5–20 mg	10–60 mg	20–80 mg
(>18 yrs of age)*		(0.5–1 mg/kg/day)	
Imipramine	10–150 mg	50–200 mg	75–200 mg
(>6 yrs of age)*	(1–5 mg/kg/day)	(1–5 mg/kg/day)	
Nortriptyline	10–100 mg	50–100 mg	75–200 mg
(>12 yrs of age)*		(1–3 mg/kg/day)	
Phenelzine		15–45 mg	45–90 mg
(>16 yrs of age)*		(0.5–1 mg/kg/day)	
Sertraline	25–100 mg	50–200 mg	50–200 mg
(not in children)*		(1.5–3 mg/kg/day)	
C. Antimanics			
Lithium carbonate**	300–900 mg	900–1200 mg	900–1200 mg
(>12 yrs of age)*		(10–30 mg/kg/day)	
D. Anxiolytics			
Alprazolam	0.25–2 mg	0.75–5 mg	1–8 mg
(>18 yrs of age)*		(0.02–0.06 mg/kg/day)	
Chlordiazepoxide	10–30 mg	20–60 mg	20–100 mg
(>6 yrs of age)*			
Diazepam	1–10 mg	2–20 mg	4–40 mg
(>6 mos of age)*		(max 0.8 mg/kg)	
Lorazepam	0.25–3 mg	0.05–6 mg	1–10 mg
(>12 yrs of age)*		(0.04–0.09 mg/kg/day)	
Diphenhydramine	25–200 mg	50–300 mg	50–400 mg
		(1–5 mg/kg/day)	

(*continued*)

Table 3. (*Continued*)

Drug	Average daily dose		
	Children	Adolescents	Adults
Hydroxyzine	25–100 mg	40–150 mg	75–400 mg
		(2 mg/kg/day)	
Busipirone	2.5–15 mg	5–30 mg	15–60 mg
(>18 yrs of age)*		(0.2–0.6 mg/kg/day)	
E. Stimulants			
Dextroamphetamine	2.5–15 mg	5–40 mg	10–40 mg
(>3 yrs of age)*	(0.15–0.5 mg/kg/dose)	(0.15–0.5 mg/kg/dose)	(0.15–0.5 mg/kg/dose)
Methylphenidate	2.5–30 mg	10–60 mg	20–60 mg
(>6 yrs of age)*	(0.3–1 mg/kg/dose)	(0.3–1 mg/kg/dose)	(0.3–1 mg/kg/dose)
Pemoline	18.75–75 mg	37.5–112.5 mg	37.5–112.5 mg
(>6 yrs of age)*	(1–3 mg/kg/day)	(1–3 mg/kg/day)	(1–3 mg/kg/day)
F. Antiepileptics			
Carbamazepine**	200–800 mg	400–1000 mg	600–1200 mg
(>6 yrs of age)*	(5–20 mg/kg/day)	(10–30 mg/kg/day; max	(max 1200 mg/day)
		1000 mg/day)	
Ethosuximide**	250–800 mg	500–1500 mg	750–1500 mg
	(20–30 mg/kg/day)	(20–40 mg/kg/day)	(max 1500 mg/day)
Phenobarbital**	<250 mg	75–250 mg	150–250 mg
	(4–8 mg/kg/day)	(1–3 mf/kg/day)	
Phenytoin**	<300 mg	300–500 mg	300–400 mg
	(7.5–9 mg/kg/day)	(6–7 mg/kg)	
Primidone	150–750 mg	750–1500 mg	750–2000 mg
Sodium valproate**	250–1000 mg	500–2000 mg	500–2500 mg
			(15–60 mg/kg/day)
G. Others			
Propranolol	5–80 mg	20–140 mg	80–480 mg
		(max 2 mg/kg/day)	
Clonidine	0.25–0.3 mg	0.3–0.4 mg	0.3–0.5 mg
(not in children)*	(3–6 μg/kg/day)	(3–6 μg/kg/day)	
Naltrexone	10–50 mg	40–120 mg	50–150 mg
(>18 yrs of age)*	(0.5–1.5 mg/kg/day)	(1–2 mg/kg/day)	(1–2 mg/kg/day)
Fenfluramine	30–60 mg	40–100 mg	60–120 mg
(>12 yrs of age)*		(1–2 mg/kg/day)	
Benztropine	0.5–4 mg	0.5–6 mg	2–6 mg
(>3 yrs of age)*		(43–86 μg/kg/day)	

Note: From Ellis, Singh, and Singh (1996); reprinted with permission from the authors.
*Recommended FDA guidelines.
**Dosage titrated using serum levels.

as clozapine (Clozaril) and risperidone (Risperdal), appear to show more promise than the traditional antipsychotics but their efficacy remains to be established.

The effects of antipsychotics have been evaluated mainly in terms of behavior reduction rather than learning and performance. Although there are a few studies suggesting that low doses of antipsychotics may actually facilitate learning and performance in some individuals with mental retardation, probably by suppressing incompatible behaviors, there remains concern that antipsychotics may impair cognitive and academic performance, particularly in children with mental retardation (Aman, 1984).

Antidepressants. Despite the absence of scientific evidence to support their efficacy, the an-

Table 4. Psychiatric and Behavioral Indications and Side Effects of Various Classes of Drugs

A. Antipsychotics

Indications	Psychotic states; schizophrenia (exacerbations and maintenance); mania (in conjunction with lithium); behavioral disorders with severe agitation, aggressivity, and self-injury; and dyskinetic movement disorders (e.g., Tourette's disorder and juvenile Huntington's disease)
Side effects	Anticholinergic effects, including dry mouth, constipation, blurred vision, and urinary retention (most common with low-potency phenothiazines); extrapyramidal reactions, including acute dystonia, akathesia, and tremor (particularly with high-potency phenothiazines); neuroleptic malignant syndrome; tardive dyskinesia (lower risk with clozapine); other central nervous system effects, including sedation, fatigue, cognitive blunting, psychotic symptoms, confusion, and excitement; orthostatic hypotension and cardiac conduction abnormalities; endocrine disturbances (e.g., menstrual irregularities and weight gain); gastrointestinal distress; skin photosensitivity; granulocytopenia and agranulocytosis (clozapine); and allergic reactions

B. Antidepressants

Indications	Enuresis; Attention-Deficit/Hyperactivity Disorder; Major Depressive Disorder; and anxiety disorders (including school phobia, separation anxiety disorder, panic disorder, and obsessive-compulsive disorder)
Side effects	*Tricyclics:* anticholinergic effects, including dry mouth, constipation, blurred vision, and urinary retention; cardiac conduction slowing (treatment requires EKG monitoring), mild increases and/or irregularity in pulse rate, and mild decreases or increases in blood pressure; confusion or the induction of psychosis; seizures; rash; and endocrine abnormalities
	Monoamine oxidase inhibitors: Mild decreases or increases in blood pressure; drowsiness; weight gain; insomnia; hypertensive crisis with nonadherence to dietary restrictions (necessary to eliminate high-tyramine foods from diet) or with certain drugs
	Selective serotonin reuptake inhibitors: irritability; gastrointestinal distress; headaches; insomnia
	Other antidepressants: irritability (bupropion, venlafaxine); insomnia (bupropion, venlafaxine); drug-induced seizures (bupropion, with high doses); changes in blood pressure (trazodone, venlafaxine); priapism (trazodone); sedation, sleepiness (trazodone, venlafaxine); gastrointestinal distress (venlafaxine); and headache (venlafaxine)

C. Antimanics

Indications	Manic episodes of Bipolar Disorder; unipolar depression/adjunct treatment in Major Depressive Disorder; behavior disorders with extreme aggression
Side effects	Kidney abnormalities leading to increased urination and thirst; gastrointestinal distress; fine hand tremor, weakness and ataxia; possible thyroid abnormalities (with long-term use), weight gain, and electrolyte imbalances; sedation, confusion, slurred speech, irritability, headache, and subtle cogwheel rigidity; skin abnormalities; orthostatic hypotension and pulse rate irregularities; and allergic reactions

D. Anxiolytics

Indications	Anxiety disorders; seizure control; night terrors; sleepwalking; insomnia and acute management of severe agitation; adjunct treatment in mania and refractory psychosis; Tourette's disorder
Side effects	Headache, sedation, and decreased cognitive performance; behavioral disinhibition, including overexcitement, hyperactivity, increased aggressivity, and irritability; gastrointestinal distress, central nervous system disinhibition resulting in hallucinations, psychoticlike behavior, and depression; physical and psychological dependence (particularly with long-acting benzodiazepines); rebound or withdrawal reactions (particularly with short-acting benzodiazepines); blood abnormalities; anticholinergic effects, including dry mouth, constipation, and blurred vision (antihistamines); and allergic reactions

E. Stimulants

Indications	Attention-Deficit/Hyperactivity Disorder (including those with mental retardation, fragile X-syndrome, Tourette's disorder, head trauma, pervasive developmental disorder, or other comorbid disorders); narcolepsy; adjunctive treatment in refractory depression
Side effects	Decreased appetite; weight loss; abdominal pain; headache, insomnia, irritability; sadness and depression; mild increases in pulse rate and blood pressure; possible temporary suppression of growth (with long-term use); choreoathetosis (pemoline) and, rarely, tic disorders; and elevated liver function tests (pemoline)

(continued)

Table 4. (Continued)

F. Antiepileptics

Indications	Seizure control; Bipolar Disorder; adjunctive treatment in Major Depressive Disorder; severe behavior problems (e.g., aggression, self-injury)
Side effects	Sedation, weakness, dizziness, disturbances of coordination and vision, hallucinations, confusion, abnormal movements, nystagmus, slurred speech, and depression; blood abnormalities; gastrointestinal distress; skin rashes, alterations in pigmentation, and phtosensitivity reactions; increased or decreased blood pressure and congestive heart failure; abnormalities of liver functions [sodium valproate, carbamazepine (rare)]; gentourinary tract dysfunction; coarsening of facial features, enlargement of the lips, gingival hyperplasia, and excessive hair growth (phenytoin); and bone marrow suppression (carbamazepine, sodium valproate)

G. Others

Propranolol	
Indications	Behavior disorders with severe agression, self-injury, or agitation; Tourette's disorder; akathesia
Side effects	Decreased heart rate, peripheral circulation, and blood pressure; fatigue, weakness, insomnia, nightmares, dizziness, hallucinations, and mild symptoms of depression; shortness of breath and wheezing (especially in patients with asthma); gastrointestinal distress; and rebound hypertension on abrupt withdrawal
Clonidine	
Indications	Attention-Deficit/Hyperactivity Disorder; Tourette's disorder; behavior disorders with severe aggression, self-injury, or agitation; adjunctive treatment of schizophrenia and mania; possible use in anxiety disorders
Side effects	Sedation; decrease in blood pressure; rebound hypertension; dry mouth; confusion (with high doses); depression
Guanfacine	
Indications	Attention-Deficit/Hyperactivity Disorder; Tourette's disorder
Side effects	Sedation (less than with clonidine); decrease in blood pressure (less than with clonidine); rebound hypertension; dry mouth; confusion (with high doses); depression
Opiod antagonists	
Indications	Reversal of narcotic depression; self-injury
Side effects	Drowsiness, dizziness, dry mouth, sweating, nausea, abdominal p[ain, and loss of energy
Fenfluramine	
Indications	Management of obesity; possible use in the control of some behavior problems in pervasive development disorder
Side effects	Anorexia, weight loss; drowsiness, dizziness, confusion, headache, incoordination; mood alterations, anxiety, insomnia, weakness, agitation, and slurred speech; gastrointestinal distress; increased or decreased blood pressure and palpitations; skin rashes; dry mouth; eye irritation; and musle aches

Note: From Ellis, Singh, and Singh (1996); reprinted with permission from the authors.

tidepressants are now increasingly being used to manage behavior problems in this population. The MAOIs, which are rarely used with children and adolescents, are ineffective in controlling the behavior problems of adults with mental retardation. The role of tricyclic antidepressants in controlling behavior problems is also not well established. In the two most recent and well-controlled studies, imipramine (Tofranil) increased food consumption, decreased screaming and crying, and stabilized sleep patterns in one study (Field, Aman, White, & Vaithianathan, 1986) and significantly increased irritability, lethargy/social withdrawal, and hyperactivity in the other study (Aman, White, Vaithianathan, & Teehan, 1986). In addition, there is some evidence that second-generation antidepressants (e.g., fluoxetine) may be beneficial in the treatment of self-injury in some individuals with mental retardation (Ricketts, Goza, et al., 1993). We have virtually no knowledge of the effects of antidepressants on the learning, cognition, and adaptive behavior of individuals with mental retardation.

Antimanics. Lithium carbonate is the only important antimanic drug that is used with individuals with mental retardation. It is the drug of choice for treating bipolar disorder and is also used for treating recurrent unipolar depression in this population (Chandler, Gualtieri, & Fahs, 1988). The few studies on lithium in individuals with mental retardation indicate that it may have a modest but clinically significant effect on affective symptoms (i.e., manic and depressive episodes). Also, it increases "adaptability" and reduces aggression, motor activity, restlessness, excitability, and self-injury. Further, lithium is useful in treating those individuals who have nonspecific behavior disorders with a strong family history of bipolar disorder, severe behavior disorders that are cyclic in nature, and uncontrolled, explosive aggressive behavior (Chandler et al., 1988). At present, we have little knowledge of the effects of antimanic drugs on the learning, cognition, and adaptive behavior of individuals with mental retardation.

Anxiolytics. The anxiolytics or antianxiety drugs, such as diazepam (Valium) and chlordiazepoxide (Librium), are used fairly extensively to treat anxiety in the general population, although there are no well-controlled studies attesting to their efficacy for treating this disorder in individuals with mental retardation. These drugs are also used as hypnotics or anticonvulsants (e.g., diazepam) or for their psychotropic effects in controlling such behaviors as hyperactivity, agitation, aggression, and disruption. However, controlled studies have shown that anxiolytics significantly worsen acting-out and hyperactive behaviors in this population (LaVeck & Buckley, 1961; Walters, Singh, & Beale, 1977). More recent studies suggest that buspirone (Buspar), a relatively new serotonergic anxiolytic, may be effective in the management of behavior problems in some individuals with mental retardation (Ricketts et al., 1994). We have

no empirical data on the effects of anxiolytics on the learning or cognition of individuals with mental retardation.

Stimulants. The stimulants, such as methylphenidate (Ritalin), dextroamphetamine (Dexedrine), and pemoline (Cylert), are the drugs of choice for treating attention-deficit hyperactivity disorder but they are not widely used in individuals with mental retardation. The effects of stimulants in this population appear to be related to the severity of mental retardation, decreasing in efficacy with increasing severity. Individuals with mild to moderate mental retardation show a modest but statistically significant improvement in hyperactivity and other behavior problems with stimulant medication (e.g., Varley & Trupin, 1982), whereas they have no effect or worsen the hyperactive behavior of those with severe or profound mental retardation (Aman & Singh, 1982). These and more recent studies suggest that the effects of stimulants on hyperactivity, attention, and impulsivity decrease as the functional level of the individual decreases (Aman, 1996). In one of the few studies reporting the use of a stimulant on a behavior other than those associated with hyperactivity in this population, the frequency of pica decreased in three adolescents with profound mental retardation while on methylphenidate, possibly related to the increased dopaminergic neurotransmission associated with the drug (Singh, Ellis, Crews, & Singh, 1994). Although not well studied, the general findings from the few studies available suggest that stimulants may worsen intellectual performance as measured on the Wechsler Adult Intelligence Scale (Aman & Singh, 1991).

Antiepileptics. Up to 20% of individuals with mental retardation and 50% of those with mental retardation and cerebral palsy have a seizure disorder. The primary mode of treatment for epilepsy is antiepileptic drug treatment and, usually, such treatment is highly effective (Stores, 1988). Antiepileptic drugs also have useful psychotropic properties and are some-times prescribed specifically for the control of problem behaviors. The primary psychiatric use of antiepileptics in individuals with mental re-tardation is for affective disorders (e.g., mania, bipolar disorder, or schizoaffective disorder), particularly if these disturbances have been re-sistant to traditional treatment. Carbamazepine (Tegretol), valproic acid (Depakene, Depakote), and, to a much lesser extent, clonazepam (Klon-opin) are currently being used for this purpose.

Long-term administration of antiepileptic drugs may cause untoward behavioral, cogni-tive, or motoric effects. At high drug concentra-tions, the long-term administration of phe-nobarbital (Luminal), phenytoin (Dilantin), and primidone (Mysoline) is associated with psychomotor deterioration. Deterioration of learning following administration of antiepilep-tics has been noted on tests of intelligence, spe-cialized tests of learning and cognitive style, neuropsychological tests, retrospective clinical judgments, and rating scales (Gay, 1984). Al-though some studies actually indicated an im-provement on some of these measures, judging the research as a whole, the studies show a con-sistent pattern of worsening performance fol-lowing medication (Trimble & Corbett, 1980). Further, phenobarbital has been noted to elicit hyperactivity and aggression in individuals with developmental disabilities, particularly chil-dren (Schain, 1979), and primidone also has been noted to elicit hyperactivity in children.

Novel Agents.   A number of novel psychoac-tive agents are currently being used in this pop-ulation. The rationale for their use has been the discovery of biochemical abnormalities associ-ated with cognitive, behavioral, or motor prob-lems that may be amenable to treatment with specific drugs. Examples of these drugs include fenfluramine (Aman & Kern, 1989), naloxone and naltrexone (Ricketts, Ellis, Singh, & Singh, 1993), propranolol (Singh & Winton, 1989), and various minerals, diets, and vitamins (Sing, Ellis, Mattila, Mulick, & Poling, 1995).

In summary, medication is frequently utilized as one component in the treatment of psychi-atric disorders and severe and refractory behav-ior problems in individuals with mental retarda-tion. Generally, the theoretical rationales, indications, and management principles that drive drug therapy in the general population are consistent with psychotropic medication use in individuals with mental retardation. Clearly, pharmocotherapy in this population should be fully integrated with all other treatment modal-ities so as to maximize both behavioral control and improvement in the individual's quality of life.

CASE STUDY

We present a case illustration of a multi-method assessment and treatment of severe be-havior problems and psychiatric disorder in a young man who had a diagnosis of mental retar-dation and schizophrenia. An interdisciplinary team, including a general physician, consultant psychiatrist, behavioral psychologist, direct care staff, and the young man's parents, were in-volved in the assessment and treatment of his problems.

Referral

Amani, a 22-year-old man, was referred by his community case manager and parents for an interdisciplinary assessment and treat-ment for behavior and psychiatric problems that had worsened dur-ing the previous year despite various interventions. He had been in-stitutionalized at the age of 4 for severe aggressive behaviors that could not be controlled at home. Aggression continued to be a prob-lem for several years at the facility even though he received a number of treatments, including brief physical restraints, timeout, positive re-inforcement for nonaggression, and gentle teaching. These inter-ventions were complemented by adjunctive therapies at various times, including counseling, psychotherapy, play therapy, sensorimo-tor training, and pharmacotherapy. His medication history showed that he had been treated with mesoridazine, trifluoperazine, thioridazine, haloperidol, and trazodone, but no long-term benefit had been evident in terms of the frequency and intensity of Amani's aggressive behaviors. During this time, he also started exhibiting pica behavior for nonspecific items (e.g., cigarette butts, grass, chalk, crayons), which was treated by the institutional staff by relocating him to a "pica unit" where these items were unavailable and he had a one-to-one staffing when he was outside of the unit.

At the age of 14, Amani was transferred to a new facility so that he could be closer to his parents. Fortunately, his therapist at the new facility did not continue the previous treatments and gradually weaned Amani off all medication and used standard behavioral analysis methods, as described in this chapter, to assess the nature of his aggression and pica. She used an informal structural and functional analysis to determine the motivation for his aggression and pica in different settings and matched the new treatments to the motivation of each behavior in different settings. Further, she paired the behavior reduction program with functional skills training, vocational training, and instruction in community living to enhance his quality of life. Within a year, Amani was considered by his Individualized Habilitation Planning team to be ready for reintegration into his local community. Six months later, he was placed in a group home with two others from his facility.

After 2 years in the group home, these three individuals were transferred to a new apartment designed specifically for individuals with mental retardation. Shortly after the transfer, Amani's aggression and pica became a problem. In addition, he appeared to have delusions and auditory hallucinations. These problems gradually affected his work and community placement and he was once again admitted to an institution. Following the failure of behavioral programs to control his aggression and pica, he was treated with thioridazine once again. His aggression decreased to manageable levels but his pica increased slightly in frequency. His pica was controlled by close supervision, such that he was never given the opportunity to place a favored pica item in his mouth. His delusions and hallucinations continued but these were not assessed as significant barriers to his reintegration in the community, which occurred a year later.

His current referral from the community was for aggression, pica, and delusions and hallucinations. He had been maintained on thioridazine and informal positive support programs prior to this admission.

Assessment

The psychologist and physician undertook a structural analysis of Amani's aggression and pica behaviors, and the consultant psychiatrist performed a diagnostic workup in an effort to understand the nature of his delusions and hallucinations. Interviews were conducted with Amani, his work supervisors, parents, and group home staff. The informants were also asked to complete two rating scales, the ABC-Community and the Reiss Screen. This was followed by direct behavioral observations of Amani's behavior, both in the institution and in the community.

The assessment data were discussed with Amani's interdisciplinary treatment team consisting of institutional professionals, the consultant psychiatrist, his parents, group home staff, and workplace staff. The findings indicated that aggression was only partially under the control of learned contingencies. That is, Amani used aggression to escape task demands made by group home and workplace staff. No motivation was apparent for the occurrence of aggression at other times. His pica was unrelated to behavioral motivations. The consultant psychiatrist confirmed the intake diagnosis of schizophrenia.

Clinical Decision-Making

The interdisciplinary team discussed the findings with Amani and his parents and together they came up with a treatment plan: (1) gradually discontinue the thioridazine to assess its role in the maintenance of pica; (2) if pica decreases as a consequence of thioridazine withdrawal but is not eliminated, prescribe a stimulant; (3) if pica persists following the withdrawal of thioridazine, undertake a formal functional analysis of the behavior; (4) institute an escape extinction program to control learned aggression that Amani uses as a way of escaping demand conditions; (5) teach Amani socially acceptable methods of negotiating which tasks he would perform when requested and others that he would complete later; and (6) initiate clozapine treatment for delusions and auditory hallucinations.

The decision to use a pharmacological intervention for pica was based on recent research that suggested that in the absence of a learned motivation, pica may be maintained or exacerbated by use of neuroleptics and reduced by its withdrawal as well as by adjunctive therapy with a dopamine agonist, such as methylphenidate (Singh, Ellis, Crews, et al., 1994). The escape distinction program was based on the finding that Amani engaged in aggression during demand conditions to escape staff demands to work or engage in routine tasks. The team decided to disrupt the escape contingency by teaching the staff not to let Amani escape from completing the tasks as a consequence of his aggression (Singh & Ellis, 1993). The same procedures were taught to Amani's parents so that he would face similar contingencies for his aggression regardless of whether he was at work or visiting his family. The use of clozapine was based on recent findings of its efficacy in treating schizophrenia and aggression in individuals with mild or moderate mental retardation (Cohen & Underwood, 1994). Thus, the interdisciplinary team decided on a multimodal treatment plan using the most recent research as a guide to effective therapy. Further, they decided that there was no reason for continued institutional placement because Amani's problems occurred in the community and that would be the best place to treat them, thus avoiding later problems of maintenance and generalization of behavior change from an institution to the community. By teaching the community staff and parents new ways of handling his behavior, it was hoped that future displays of these behaviors could be effectively controlled by them without additional assistance. Finally, the interdisciplinary team did not want Amani's lifestyle and quality of life compromised during treatment.

Treatment and Outcome

The withdrawal of thioridazine over a period of several weeks resulted in a concomitant reduction in Amani's frequency of pica. However, it was only with the addition of a stimulant that the pica was finally eliminated. The escape extinction program used by the staff and parents was successful although it required persistent effort on their part because there was an initial escalation in Amani's aggression. Further, Amani learned that he could talk to people about the tasks they wanted him to perform and negotiate with them if and when he completed the tasks. The staff and his parents discovered that he was capable of correctly and efficiently completing all of his tasks if he was given the freedom to choose the order in which the tasks were to be completed. The clozapine was effective in controlling his delusions and hallucinations, as well as his residual aggression.

SUMMARY

Mental retardation has had a varied but not very illustrious history in Western culture. However, over the last three decades we have witnessed a change not only in our conceptualization of mental retardation but also in acceptance of the fact that people with mental retardation have the same rights as those in the general population. This has resulted in a major change in the way we structure and deliver services to them. This chapter has highlighted these changes, particularly with regard to multimodal assessment and treatment.

REFERENCES

Aman, M. G. (1984). Drugs and learning in mentally retarded persons. In G. D. Burrows & J. S. Werry (Eds.), *Advances in human psychopharmacology* (Vol. 3, pp. 121–163). Greenwich, CT: JAI Press.

Aman, M. G. (1991). *Assessing psychopathology and behavior problems in persons with mental retardation: A review of available instruments.* Rockville, MD: U.S. Department of Health and Human Services.

Aman, M. G. (1996). Stimulant drugs in the developmental disabilities revisited. *Journal of Developmental and Physical Disabilities, 8,* 347–365.

Aman, M. G., Hammer, D., & Rojahn, J. (1993). Mental retardation. In T. H. Ollendick & M. Hersen (Eds.), *Handbook of child and adolescent assessment* (pp. 321–345). Boston: Allyn & Bacon.

Aman, M.G., & Kern, R. A. (1989). Review of fenfluramine in the treatment of the developmental disabilities. *Journal of the American Academy of Child and Adolescent Psychiatry, 28,* 549–565.

Aman, M. G., & Singh, N. N. (1982). Methylphenidate in severely retarded residents and the clinical significance of stereotypic behavior. *Applied Research in Mental Retardation, 3,* 1–14.

Aman, M. G., & Singh, N. N. (1986). *Aberrant Behavior Checklist—Residential: Manual.* East Aurora, NY: Slosson Educational Publications.

Aman, M. G., & Singh, N. N. (1988). *Psychopharmacology of the developmental disabilities.* Berlin: Springer-Verlag.

Aman, M. G., & Singh, N. N. (1991). Psychopharmacological intervention: An update. In J. L. Matson & J. A. Mulick (Eds.), *Handbook of mental retardation* (2nd ed., pp. 347–372). New York: Pergamon Press.

Aman, M. G., & Singh, N. N. (1994). *The Aberrant Behavior Checklist—Community: Manual.* New York: Slosson Educational Publications.

Aman, M. G., White, A. J., Vaithianathan, D., & Teehan, C. J. (1986). Preliminary study of imipramine in profoundly retarded residents. *Journal of Autism and Developmental Disorders, 16,* 263–273.

American Psychiatric Association. (1980). *Diagnostic and statistical manual of mental disorders* (3rd ed.). Washington, DC: Author.

American Psychiatric Association. (1994). *Diagnostic and statistical manual of mental disorders* (4th ed.). Washington, DC: Author.

Axelrod, S. (1987). Functional and structural analyses of behavior: Approaches leading to reduced use of punishment procedures? *Research in Developmental Disabilities, 8,* 165–178.

Baer, D. M., & Wolf, M. M. (1970). The entry into natural communities of reinforcement. In R. Ulrich, T. Stachnik, & J. Mabry (Eds.), *Control of human behavior* (Vol. 2, pp. 319–324). Glenview, IL: Scott, Foresman.

Baroff, G. S. (1986). *Mental retardation: Nature, cause and management* (2nd ed.). New York: Wiley.

Bisconer, S. W., Zhang, X., & Sine, L. F. (1995). Impact of a psychotropic medication and physical restraint review process on adults with mental retardation, psychiatric diagnoses, and challenging behaviors. *Journal of Developmental and Physical Disabilities, 7,* 123–135.

Briggs, R. (1989). Monitoring and evaluating psychotropic drug use for persons with mental retardation: A follow-up report. *American Journal of Mental Retardation, 93,* 633–639.

Brown, L., Neitupski, J., & Hamre-Neitupski, S. (1976). The criterion of ultimate functioning. In M. A. Thomas (Ed.), *Hey, don't forget about me* (pp. 2–15). Reston, VA: Council for Exceptional Children.

Bruininks, R. H., Hill, B., Weatherman, R., & Woodcock, R. (1986). *Inventory for Client and Agency Planning.* Allen, TX: DLM Teaching Resources.

Bruininks, R. H., Woodcock, R., Weatherman, R., & Hill, B. (1984). *Scales of Independent Behavior: Woodcock–Johnson Psycho-Educational Battery: Part Four.* Allen, TX: DLM Teaching Resources.

Carr, E. G., Levin, L., McConnachie, G., Carlson, J. I., Kemp, D. C., & Smith, C. E. (1994). *Communication-based intervention for problem behavior: A user's guide for producing positive change.* Baltimore: Paul H. Brookes.

Chandler, M., Gualtieri, C. T., & Fahs, J. J. (1988). Other psychotropic drugs. In M. G. Aman & N. N. Singh (Eds.), *Psychopharmacology of the developmental disabilities* (pp. 119–145). New York: Springer-Verlag.

Civil Rights of Institutionalized Persons Act, 42 U.S.C. # 1997 (1981).

Cohen, S. A., & Underwood, M. T. (1994). The use of clozapine in a mentally retarded and aggressive population. *Journal of Clinical Psychiatry, 55,* 440–444.

Doll, E. (1953). *A manual of social competence: A manual for the Vineland Social Maturity Scale.* Minneapolis, MN: Educational Test Bureau.

Ellis, C. R., Singh, N. N., & Jackson, E. V. (1996). Problem behaviors in children with developmental disabilities. In D. X. Parmelee (Ed.), *Child and adolescent psychiatry for the clinician* (pp. 263–275). St. Louis: Mosby.

Ellis, C. R., Singh, Y. N., & Singh, N. N. (1996). Use of behavior modifying drugs. In N. N. Singh (Ed.), *Prevention and treatment of severe behavior problems: Models and methods in developmental disabilities* (pp. 149–176). Pacific Grove, CA: Brooks/Cole.

Evans, I. M., & Meyer, L. H. (1987). Moving to educational validity: A reply to Test, Spooner, and Cooke. *Journal of the Association for Persons with Severe Handicaps, 12,* 103–106.

Felce, D., & Perry, J. (1995). Quality of life: Its definition and measurement. *Research in Developmental Disabilities, 16,* 51–74.

Field, C. J., Aman, M. G., White, A. J., & Vaithianathan, C. (1986). A single-subject study of imipramine in a mentally retarded woman with depressive symptoms. *Journal of Mental Deficiency Research, 30,* 191–198.

Findholt, N. E., & Emmett, C. G. (1990). Impact of interdisciplinary team review on psychotropic drug use with persons who have mental retardation. *Mental Retardation, 25,* 41–46.

Gay, P. E. (1984). Effects of antiepileptic drugs and seizure type on operant responding in mentally retarded persons. *Epilepsia, 25,* 377–386.

Guess, D., & Helmstetter, E. (1986). Skill cluster instruction and the individualized curriculum sequencing model. In R. H. Horner, L. H. Meyer, & H. D. Fredericks (Eds.), *Education of learners with severe handicaps* (pp. 221–248). Baltimore: Paul H. Brookes.

Horner, R. H., Sprague, J. R., & Flannery, K. B. (1993). Building functional curricula for students with severe intellectual disabilities and severe problem behaviors. In R. Van Houten & S. Axelrod (Eds.), *Behavior analysis and treatment* (pp. 47–71). New York: Plenum Press.

Hughes, C., Hwang, B., Kim, J.-H., Eisenman, L. T., & Killian, D. J. (1995). Quality of life in applied research: A review and analysis of empirical measures. *American Journal on Mental Retardation, 99,* 623–641.

Iwata, B. A., Vollmer, T. R., & Zarcone, J. R. (1990). The experimental (functional) analysis of behavior disorders: Methodology, application, and limitations. In A. C. Repp & N. N. Singh (Eds.), *Perspectives on the use of nonaversive and aversive interventions for persons with developmental disabilities* (pp. 301–330). Sycamore, IL: Sycamore Publishing Co.

Lambert, N., Nihira, K., & Leland, H. (1993). *Adaptive Behavior Scale—School: Second edition, examiner's manual.* Austin, TX: Pro-Ed.

LaVeck, G. D., & Buckley, P. (1961). The use of psychopharmacologic agents in retarded children with behavior disorders. *Journal of Chronic Disorders, 13,* 174–183.

Luckasson, R., Coulter, D. L., Polloway, E. A., Reiss, S., Schalock, R. S., Snell, M. E., Spitalnik, D. M., & Stark, J. A. (1992). *Mental retardation: Definition, classification, and systems of supports.* Washington, DC: American Association on Mental Retardation.

Mace, F. C., Lalli, J. S., & Shea, M. C. (1992). Functional analysis and treatment of self-injury. In J. K. Luiselli, J. L. Matson, & N. N. Singh (Eds.), *Self-injurious behavior: Analysis, assessment, and treatment* (pp. 122–152). Berlin: Springer-Verlag.

MacMillan, D. L., Gresham, F. M., & Siperstein, G. N. (1995). Heightened concerns over the 1992 AAMR definition: Advocacy versus precision. *American Journal on Mental Retardation, 100,* 87–97.

Matson, J. L. (1988). *The PIMRA manual.* Orland Park, IL: International Diagnostic Systems, Inc.

McGrew, K. S., Bruininks, R. H., & Thurlow, M. L. (1992). Relationship between measures of adaptive functioning and community adjustment for adults with mental retardation. *Exceptional Children, 58,* 517–529.

McLaren, J., & Bryson, S. E. (1987). Review of recent epidemiological studies of mental retardation: Prevalence, associated disorders, and etiology. *American Journal of Mental Retardation, 92,* 243–254.

Nihira, K., Foster, R., Shellhaas, M., & Leland, H. (1974). *AAMD Adaptive Behavior Scale* (rev. ed.). Washington, DC: American Association on Mental Deficiency.

Ollendick, T. H., & Hersen, M. (Eds.). (1993). *Handbook of child and adolescent assessment.* Boston: Allyn & Bacon.

Pond, D. (1979). Epilepsy and mental retardation. In M. Craft (Ed.), *Tredgold's mental retardation* (12th ed., pp. 331–345). London: Baillière Tindall.

Reiss, S. (1988). *Test manual for the Reiss Screen for Maladaptive Behavior.* Orland Park, IL: International Diagnostic Systems.

Repp, A. C., & Singh, N. N. (1990). *Perspectives on the use of nonaversive and aversive interventions for persons with developmental disabilities.* Sycamore, IL: Sycamore Publishing Co.

Ricketts, R. W., Ellis, C. R., Singh, Y. N., & Singh, N. N. (1993). Opioid antagonists. II: Clinical effects in the treatment of self-injury in individuals with developmental disabilities. *Journal of Developmental and Physical Disabilities, 5,* 17–28.

Ricketts, R. W., Goza, A. B., Ellis, C. R., Singh, Y. N., Chambers, S., Singh, N. N., & Cooke, J. C. (1994). Clinical effects of buspirone on intractable self-injury in adults with mental retardation. *Journal of the American Academy of Child and Adolescent Psychiatry, 33,* 270–276.

Ricketts, R. W., Goza, A. B., Ellis, C. R., Singh, Y. N., Singh, N. N., & Cooke, J. C. (1993). Fluoxetine treatment of severe self-injury in young adults with mental retardation. *Journal of the American Academy of Child and Adolescent Psychiatry, 32,* 865–869.

Rosenberg, D. R., Holttum, J., & Gershon, S. (1994). *Textbook of pharmacology for child and adolescent psychiatric disorders.* New York: Brunner/Mazel.

Rutter, M., Tizard, J., & Whitmore, K. (1970). *Education, health, and behavior.* New York: Wiley.

Sattler, J. M. (1992). *Assessment of children* (3rd ed., rev.). San Diego, CA: Jerome M. Sattler, Publisher, Inc.

Schain, R. J. (1979). Problems with the use of conventional anticonvulsant drugs in mentally retarded individuals. *Brain and Development, 1,* 77–82.

Schatzberg, A. F., & Nemeroff, C. B. (1995). *Textbook of psychopharmacology.* Washington, DC: American Psychiatric Press.

Singh, N. N. (1995a). In search of unity: Some thoughts on family–professional relationships in service delivery systems. *Journal of Child and Family Studies, 4,* 3–18.

Singh, N. N. (1995b). Moving beyond institutional care for individuals with developmental disabilities. *Journal of Child and Family Studies, 4,* 129–145.

Singh, N. N. (1996). *Prevention and treatment of severe behavior problems: Models and methods in developmental disabilities.* Pacific Grove, CA: Brooks/Cole.

Singh, N. N., & Ellis, C. R. (1993, August). *Parents' use of functional analysis to assess and treat severe behavior problems.* Paper presented at the 101st American Psychological Association Convention, Toronto, Canada.

Singh, N. N., Ellis, C. R., Crews, W. D., & Singh, Y. N. (1994). Does diminished dopaminergic neurotransmission increase pica? *Journal of Child and Adolescent Psychopharmacology, 4,* 93–99.

Singh, N. N., Ellis, C. R., Mattila, M. J., Mulick, J. A., & Poling, A. (1995, June). *Vitamin, mineral, and dietary treatments for individuals with developmental disabilities.* Paper presented at the Nisonger-The ARC International Consensus Conference on Psychopharmacology, Columbus, OH.

Singh, N. N., Ellis, C. R., & Singh, Y. N. (1994). Medication management. In E. Cipani & F. Spooner (Eds.), *Curricular and instructional approaches for persons with severe handicaps* (pp. 404–423). Boston: Allyn & Bacon.

Singh, N. N., Ellis, C. R., & Wechsler, H. A. (in press). Psychopharmacoepidemiology in mental retardation. *Journal of Child and Adolescent Psychopharmacology.*

Singh, N. N., Guernsey, T. F., & Ellis, C. R. (1992). Drug therapy for persons with developmental disabilities: Legislation and litigation. *Clinical Psychology Review, 12,* 665–679.

Singh, N. N., Parmelee, D. X., Sood, A. A., & Katz, R. C. (1993). Collaboration of disciplines. In J. L. Matson (Ed.), *Handbook of hyperactivity in children* (pp. 305–322). Boston: Allyn & Bacon.

Singh, N. N., Sood, A. A., Sonenklar, N., & Ellis, C. R. (1991). Assessment and diagnosis of mental illness in persons with mental retardation: Methods and measures. *Behavior Modification, 15,* 419–443.

Singh, N. N., & Winton, A. S. W. (1989). Behavioral pharmacology. In J. K. Luiselli (Ed.), *Behavioral medicine and developmental disabilities* (pp. 152–179). Berlin: Springer-Verlag.

Sparrow, S. S., Balla, D. A., & Cicchetti, D. V. (1984). *Vineland Adaptive Behavior Scales.* Circle Pines, MN: American Guidance Service.

Sprague, R. L., & Gadow, K. D. (1976). The role of the teacher in drug treatment. *School Review, 85,* 109–140.

Stores, G. (1988). Antiepileptic drugs. In M. G. Aman & N. N. Singh (Eds.), *Psychopharmacology of the developmental disabilities* (pp. 101–118). Berlin: Springer-Verlag.

Swiezy, N. B., Matson, J. L., Kirkpatrick-Sanchez, S., & Williams, D. E. (1995). A criterion validity study of the Schizophrenia subscale of the Psychopathology Instrument for Mentally Retarded Adults (PIMRA). *Research in Developmental Disabilities, 16,* 75–80.

Thorndike, R. L., Hagen, E. P., & Sattler, J. M. (1986). *Guide for administering and scoring the Stanford–Binet Intelligence Scale: Fourth Edition.* Chicago: Riverside Publishing.

Trimble, M. R., & Corbett, J. A. (1980). Behavioral and cognitive disturbances in epileptic children. *Irish Medical Journal, 73,* 21–28.

Van Houten, R., & Axelrod, S. (1993). *Behavior analysis and treatment.* New York: Plenum Press.

Varley, C. K., & Trupin, E. W. (1982). Double-blind administration of methylphenidate to mentally retarded children with attention deficit disorder: A preliminary study. *American Journal of Mental Deficiency, 86,* 560–566.

Walters, A., Singh, N. N., & Beale, I. L. (1977). Effects of lorazepam on hyperactivity in retarded children. *New Zealand Medical Journal, 86,* 473–475.

Wechsler, D. (1981). *Manual for the Wechsler Adult Intelligence Scale-Revised.* San Antonio, TX: The Psychological Corporation.

Wechsler, D. (1989). *Manual for the Wechsler Preschool and Primary Scale of Intelligence-Revised.* San Antonio, TX: The Psychological Corporation.

Wechsler, D. (1991). *Manual for the Wechsler Intelligence Scale for Children-Third Edition.* San Antonio, TX: The Psychological Corporation.

Wiener, J. M. (1996). *Diagnosis and psychopharmacology of childhood and adolescent disorders* (2nd ed.). New York: Wiley.

5

Learning Disabilities

JAN L. CULBERTSON

INTRODUCTION

The study of learning disabilities has grown exponentially during the past 30 years, bringing major developments in understanding the etiology, diagnosis, and treatment of this disorder. Learning disabilities formerly were considered an appropriate topic for discussion regarding school-age children, but now we must think of this disorder in terms of the life span. In this chapter, developmental precursors to learning disabilities are discussed, along with issues affecting children and adolescents through the high school years. It is beyond the scope of this chapter to discuss learning disabilities in the adult years, but the interested reader will find a growing literature in this area (e.g., Bigler, 1992; Gajar, 1992; Shafrir & Siegel, 1994). This chapter reviews recent developments in the field of learning disabilities and provides a current overview of the phenomenology, diagnosis, etiology, epidemiology, assessment, and treatment of this disorder.

JAN L. CULBERTSON • Child Study Center, Department of Pediatrics, University of Oklahoma Health Sciences Center, Oklahoma City, Oklahoma 73117.

Handbook of Child Psychopathology, 3rd edition, edited by Ollendick & Hersen. Plenum Press, New York, 1998.

Historical Evolution

Clinical descriptions of learning disabilities were introduced more than 100 years ago with several case reports of patients who were unable to read despite adequate visual acuity. Hinshelwood (1895) described brain-impaired patients who had lost the ability to read following their injury. Morgan (1896) described a 14-year-old boy who was very intelligent but had failed to learn reading and writing in school. Despite many hours of instruction, and memorizing the alphabet, this youngster could not read phonetically. However, he could read numbers well and had age-appropriate mathematical skills. Today, we would recognize such a clinical description as "developmental dyslexia," or a learning disability primarily affecting reading. Morgan referred to the patient has having "congenital word blindness," based on a concept first introduced by Kussmaul in 1877 to describe a patient who, although not blind, was unable to read words. Morgan suggested that the disability may be the result of deficits in the region of the brain's left angular gyrus (a convolution of the left hemisphere cortex near the juncture of the occipital, temporal, and parietal cortex). Hinshelwood (1902) even suggested that children with congenital word blindness be removed from the regular classroom and taught using a kinesthetic modality to help with visual–auditory associative learning.

Subsequent case studies illustrated the variation in symptoms among persons who could not read. Hinshelwood (1900) described an 11-year-old boy who could not read familiar words despite 4 years of instruction, but who had excellent auditory memory. The boy could memorize his lessons by listening to lectures rather than reading. A second child described by Hinshelwood (1900) was a 10-year-boy who could recognize familiar words but could not decode (or use phonetic skills to read) unfamiliar words. A child described by Fisher (1905) displayed poor arithmetic skills, problems with mixing letters, and misnaming musical notes. The child had an uncle who also experienced reading difficulty as a child, and had persistent spelling difficulty as an adult. According to Hynd, Connor, and Nieves (1988),

> by 1905, it was already reasonably well established that 1) severe learning disabilities were manifested in children of normal intelligence (although no standardized measure of IQ was yet generally available), 2) they affected a greater number of boys than girls, 3) the deficits were manifested variably, impacting differentially on each child's ability to read or perform some cognitive task, 4) the disability was not generally responsive to traditional learning opportunities, 5) it seemed to have a genetic component that expressed itself variably, 6) it could be diagnosed using many different informal and formal clinical assessment practices, and 7) it might be related to some neurodevelopmental pathology in the region of the angular gyrus in the left hemisphere. (p. 283)

In the next 60 to 70 years, various researchers attempted to discover the underlying deficient processes that were associated with learning disabilities. Among the most important researchers was Orton (1928, 1937) who hypothesized that a neurodevelopmental failure in establishing cerebral dominance could account for learning disabilities. Subsequent researchers proposed a variety of other underlying processing deficits, including auditory-perceptual and associated

language deficits (de Hirsch, Jansky, & Langford, 1966); visual-perceptual deficits (Frostig, 1964; Kephart, 1971; Lyle & Goyen, 1968, 1975); deficiencies in sensory integration (Birch & Belmont, 1964, 1965; Senf, 1969); and attentional-memory deficits (Lyle & Goyen, 1968, 1975; Thomson & Wilsher, 1978). These researchers approached the study of learning disabilities in a similar fashion by searching for a single underlying processing deficit that could explain this complex disorder. Much of their research focused on reading disorders, to the exclusion of other types of academic learning problems.

During the past 25 years, research has focused on more complex and sophisticated models for conceptualizing learning disabilities, as investigators became aware that the previous single-factor conceptualizations were not broad enough to account for all of the psychoeducational deficits manifested in this disorder. More recent conceptual models have been multifaceted—based on neurocognitive, neurolinguistic, and other neuropsychological factors that are presumed to be associated with the component processes involved in reading (see Leong, 1989), mathematics (see Keller & Sutton, 1991), and written expression (see O'Hare & Brown, 1989a). The more current models have been derived from research paradigms involving dichotic listening and visual-field methods (McKeever & Van Deventer, 1975; Witelson & Rabinovitch, 1972; Yeni-Komshian, Isenberg, & Goldstein, 1975); physiological methods, such as neuroanatomical studies of brain structures and minor cortical malformations (see Galaburda & Livingstone, 1993; Humphreys, Kaufman, & Galaburda, 1990); neuroimaging studies (see Gross-Glenn et al., 1991; Hynd, Semrud-Clikeman, Lorys, Novey, & Eliopulos, 1990; Rumsey et al., 1992); and both clinical-inferential and empirical subtyping methods (see Hooper & Willis, 1989). These various conceptualizations of learning disabilities will be explored later in this chapter. However, it is important to note that the historical evolution of this field has led to better understanding of the nature and etiology of learning disabilities, and in turn has paved the way for more sophisticated diagnostic and intervention methods for children, adolescents, and adults with this disorder.

Terminology and Definitions

The field of learning disabilities has been interdisciplinary from its inception, leading to much debate about terminology and definitions. Professionals from such disciplines as medicine, psychology, speech–language pathology, and education have added to the vast literature. Though the term *learning disability* was coined originally in 1963 by Kirk, many other terms have been used during the 100-year history of this field, such as *congenital word blindness, minimal brain dysfunction, developmental alexia, strephosymbolia, developmental aphasia, perceptual handicaps, dyslexia, dysgraphia,* and *dyscalculia.* For purposes of this chapter, the term *learning disabilities* will be used generically to include disorders affecting reading, mathematics, spelling, writing, listening, thinking, oral language, and social perception. Specific subtypes of learning disabilities to be discussed in this chapter are functionally defined as follows:

Dyslexia is a disorder in one or more of the basic skills involved in reading, including decoding (letter-word recognition and identification, phonetic analysis) and comprehension.

Dyscalculia is a disorder in one or more of the basic skills involved in mathematics, including both computational and reasoning abilities.

Dysgraphia is a disorder of written expression whose deficits may be manifest in (1) knowledge of rules for spelling, grammatic usage, punctuation, and capitalization; (2) the motor production of writing, including letter formation, kinesthetic-motor sequencing of letters to make words, speed of writing production, and spatial organization of written material; (3) semantic abilities that underlie clear expression of ideas in written language; and (4) organization of ideas and themes for written expression.

Social–emotional learning disability is a disorder of social perception and/or expression leading to impairment in adaptation to novel situations, diminished social competence (including judgment, social awareness, social interaction skills), poor pragmatic communication ability, risk for secondary emotional problems of both internalizing and externalizing types, and abnormal activity level, ranging from hypo- to hyperactive (Rourke, 1989). This subtype of learning disability must be distinguished from the common secondary emotional reactions that are experienced by many children related to their primary learning disability. The latter reactions are presumed secondary to stress or frustration associated with the learning disability, whereas the subtype of social–emotional learning disability is presumed to be related to specific patterns of central processing deficits (Rourke, 1989).

The definitions of learning disabilities have been modified over the years to reflect changes in research and advocacy efforts in the field. Although there are five definitions that have been adopted officially by the U.S. government or major professional organizations concerned with learning disabilities (Hooper & Willis, 1989), the most widely used definition is one of the earliest—included in the Rules and Regulations Implementing the Education for All Handicapped Children Act of 1975 (PL 94-142):

> Specific learning disability means a disorder in one or more of the basic psychological processes involved in understanding or using language, spoken or written, in which the disorder may manifest itself in an imperfect ability to listen, think, speak, read, write, spell, or to do mathematical calculations. The term includes such conditions as perceptual handicaps, brain injury, minimal brain dysfunction, dyslexia, and developmental aphasia. The term does not include children who have learning problems which are primarily the result of visual, hearing, or motor handicaps, or mental retardation, or emotional disturbance, or of environmental, cultural, or economic disadvantage. (U.S. Office of Education, 1977, p. 65083)

Despite inclusion of this definition in most state laws that are patterned after the federal law PL 94-142, there is widespread dissatisfaction with its lack of clear operational criteria, being primarily a definition of exclusion, and treating learning disability as a single disorder rather than a heterogeneous disorder (Hooper & Willis, 1989). Subsequent definitions have more specifically acknowledged the presumed neurological basis of learning disabilities and the heterogeneous nature of the disorder (Hammill, Leigh, McNutt, & Larsen, 1981), its chronic course and pervasive impact on an individual's academic and nonacademic functioning (Association for Children and Adults with Learning Disabilities, 1985), and its co-occurrence with other handicapping conditions such as attention-deficit disorder, sensory impairment, emotional disturbance, and sociocultural influences (Interagency Committee on Learning Disabilities, 1987). The lack of a clear consensus on the definition for learning disability has led to many controversies in diagnosis, as will be discussed in more detail in a later section of this chapter.

Federal and State Laws

The conceptualization of learning disabilities has been shaped to some degree by the increased national attention on educational and civil rights of individuals with disabilities over the past 30 years. The focus on educational rights of children with disabilities has forced federal, state, and local education agencies to address issues of definition, diagnosis, and intervention that were heretofore unaddressed. Prior to World War II, there were relatively few laws authorizing special benefits for individuals with disabilities, and public schools were allowed to exclude children who were considered "mentally incapacitated" for schoolwork (National Information Center for Children and Youth with Disabilities [NICHCY], 1991). Since the 1960s, there has been rapid movement toward recognition of the basic rights of persons with disabilities, including the right to a free and appropriate public education.

The earliest legislation providing a foundation for the education of children with disabilities was the Elementary and Secondary Educa-

tion Act of 1965, PL 89-10, which strengthened educational quality and opportunity in elementary and secondary schools (DeStefano & Snauwaert, 1989). This law was soon amended to authorize grants to state agencies for the education of children with disabilities in state-operated schools and institutions (NICHCY, 1991). A further amendment in 1966 (PL 89-750) established the first grant program for education of children with disabilities at the local school level rather than in institutions (NICHCY, 1991). Other amendments followed that ultimately led to passage of the Education of All Handicapped Children Act of 1975 (PL 94-142).

Two precedent-setting court decisions also paved the way for passage of PL 94-142—*the Pennsylvania Association for Retarded Citizens v. Commonwealth of Pennsylvania*, 1972, and *Mills v. Board of Education*, 1972. The Pennsylvania case involved a class-action suit on behalf of 13 children with mental retardation who alleged failure of the state of Pennsylvania to provide a publicly supported education for school-age children with mental retardation. The suit was resolved with the state being required to identify all school-age children with mental retardation who were excluded from the public schools, and provide them with a free and appropriate public education (NICHCY, 1991). In *Mills v. Board of Education*, a class-action suit on behalf of all children with disabilities who were excluded from District of Columbia schools resulted in a judgment against the district school board, who were required to provide a publicly supported education for all children with a disability, regardless of the severity of the disability (NICHCY, 1991). Passage of the Rehabilitation Act of 1973 (PL 93-112) also was critical in strengthening the rights of individuals with disabilities—particularly Section 504, which protected against discrimination of individuals with disabilities under any program receiving federal financial assistance (NICHCY, 1991).

The major purposes of PL 94-142 were to guarantee a free and appropriate public education to all children and youth (age 4 to 21 years) with disabilities, to ensure the rights to due process in decision-making about the provision of special education and related services to these children, and to assist state and local governments financially in providing educational opportunities to children and youth with disabilities (Ballard, Ramirez, & Zantal-Weiner, 1987; DeStefano & Snauwaert, 1989). The Education of the Handicapped Act Amendments of 1983 (PL 98-199) expanded incentives for preschool education, early intervention, and transition programs, whereas the amendments of 1986 (PL 99-457) extended the eligibility for special education and related services to age 3 years. This law also established the Handicapped Infants and Toddlers Program (Part H) to provide early intervention services for children from birth to 3 years and to provide a service plan for their families. Finally, the 1990 amendments (PL 101-476) resulted in significant changes, including a name change to the "Individuals with Disabilities Education Act" (IDEA). These amendments expanded existing discretionary programs to include new programs on transition services for high school children with disabilities who were moving into higher education or vocational arenas; services for children with serious emotional disturbance; a research and information dissemination program on attention-deficit disorder; and expanded services for children with autism and traumatic brain injury (NICHCY, 1991).

Although federal laws have established minimal standards that states must follow for delivery of services in order to receive federal funds, states have flexibility for implementing the program and services established with federal funds. States are required under the due process and equal protection clauses of the 14th Amendment of the U.S. Constitution to provide education to all children on an equal basis, and to provide due process before denying equal education services (NICHCY, 1991). Both federal and state laws provide definitions of each type of disability covered under the laws, and provide rules and regulations for implementing the laws that can affect how children qualify for special services. Practitioners must become familiar

with their state statutes and rules and regulations implementing the educational laws in order to understand special education eligibility criteria in their area for children with learning disabilities.

Subtyping Research with Learning Disabilities

One of the most important developments in recent years has been the understanding that learning disabilities comprise a variety of subtypes that vary in clinical presentation and likely have different etiologies (though the etiologies are not yet fully understood). Much of the early research in the field is flawed by lack of a clear distinction of subtypes among the population of individuals with learning disabilities being studied, thus compromising the generalizability of results. Based on this early research, it was difficult to tie either etiology or intervention techniques to a specific subtype of learning disability, and not surprisingly, many of the results were conflicting. Researchers now have begun to elucidate the different cognitive, linguistic, and neuropsychological processes that underlie the subtypes of learning disabilities, so that research is much more specific and clinically meaningful.

Despite the importance of subtyping research, the current status of the field is confusing because of the sheer number of subtyping models reported to date. Since the early 1960s, over 100 classification studies of learning disabilities have appeared in the literature (Hooper & Willis, 1989). These models have had an important heuristic effect on the field, and have stimulated much additional research into underlying processes. However, from a clinical perspective, it is difficult to evaluate the efficacy of these models to determine which are the most clinically useful. At the current stage of development, the value of subtyping approaches probably lies more in empirical than in clinical use. From a clinical perspective, further validation research is needed to determine which subtypes are more applicable for clinical practice. Regarding an individual client, practitioners can use the subtyping literature as a guide to examining the various cognitive, perceptual, linguistic, and neuropsychological processes that may underlie disorders of learning, while constructing an individualized subtype for each client (Culbertson & Edmonds, 1996). Examples of subtyping models are presented to illustrate ways in which the process has been done.

Many of the early subtyping models were of the clinical-inferential type, in which attempts were made to group individuals into homogeneous clusters by identifying similarities in their performance on either academic achievement tests, neurocognitive (intellectual and neuropsychological) measures, or neurolinguistic measures, or combinations of these types of measures. Boder (1973) provided an early example of a clinical-inferential model based on academic achievement measures (simple word recognition and spelling tasks), from which she described three subtypes of atypical reading–spelling patterns. Children with a *dysphonetic* reading–spelling pattern had deficient auditory sequential processing and phonetic analysis skills, poor auditory memory, and tended to overrely on visual processing strategies. They tended to read using "whole word" strategies in which they focused on the visual gestalt of the printed word. Children with the *dyseidetic* pattern had deficient visuospatial abilities resulting in poor visual gestalt for whole word recognition and poor visual memory skills. They tended to overrely on auditory and phonetic strategies for reading and spelling (e.g., so that "business" might be spelled phonetically as "biznes"). The *mixed* or *alexic* group of children had difficulty with both phonetic analysis and whole word recognition, and had the most difficulty with acquiring reading–spelling skills.

Mattis, French, and Rapin (1975) used a battery of neuropsychological measures to develop a clinical-inferential model in which they isolated three independent dyslexia syndromes that accounted for 90% of the 82 dyslexic children studied. The largest group of dyslexic children (63%) had a language disorder underlying their reading disability, characterized by impair-

ment in naming, verbal comprehension, imitative speech, and speech sound discrimination. The second group (10%) had articulation and graphomotor deficits but normal receptive language and auditory processing abilities. The third group (5%) had visuospatial deficits, characterized by verbal IQ being more than 10 points above nonverbal IQ, along with deficits in abstract nonverbal reasoning and visual memory. However, there were a number of children in this study who did not fit the three subtypes clearly. A subsequent validation study (Mattis, Erenberg, & French, 1978) revealed that 9% of the children presented with two of the three subtypes of dyslexia rather than a single subtype, and there was evidence of a possible fourth subtype involving a sequencing disorder in a small group of children.

Both the Boder and Mattis et al. models are illustrative of the clinical-inferential approach of searching for clinically derived profiles or patterns of performance on a post-hoc basis. However, this approach has been criticized methodologically for limited data reduction strategies and questionable validity of the subtypes (Hooper & Willis, 1989). With the advent of computer technology in the 1980s, subtyping research became more sophisticated through use of statistical procedures such as Q-type factor analysis and cluster analysis; using this methodology, profiles of large numbers of subjects could be compared and analyzed for similarities and differences. However, many of the empirical studies have been criticized for using measures without a specific theoretical rationale for their selection, leading to subtypes that have little clinical utility (Hooper & Willis, 1989).

Petrauskas and Rourke (1979) provided an example of the empirical approach to subtype classification, in which Q-sort factor analysis techniques were used to define profiles of children with learning disabilities. Using a battery of neuropsychological tests that measured tactile-perceptual, motor, sequencing, visuospatial, auditory-verbal, and abstract-conceptual domains, they examined the performance of retarded and normal readers and found four subtypes. The first subtype was characterized by language and auditory processing deficits, in which reading and spelling performance were lower than math. The second subtype had deficits in visual sequencing, bilateral finger agnosia, global deficits in achievement, and the "ACID" pattern (i.e., weaknesses in Arithmetic, Coding, Information, and Digit Span) on the Wechsler Intelligence Scale for Children. The third subtype had right unilateral sensory and motor deficits, with associated impairment in expressive speech and visual-motor coordination. The fourth subtype was not a reliable one, but the pattern of performance in this type was generally normal (Hooper & Willis, 1989; Petrauskas & Rourke, 1979).

It is beyond the scope of this discussion to provide a thorough review of subtyping methodology and models, but the interested reader is referred to Hooper and Willis (1989) for a comprehensive review. In summary, the growing subtyping literature continues to be an important focus of research in the field of learning disabilities. Despite the different classification methods and models described in the literature, the combined evidence would support the existence of at least two major subtypes of children with dyslexia—one associated with disordered linguistic and auditory processing abilities, and the other with fairly intact psycholinguistic skills but deficits in visuospatial or visual-motor abilities. A third, less well-differentiated subtype of dyslexia involves a mixed pattern with both psycholinguistic and visuospatial deficits. Research that delineates subtypes of dyscalculia and dysgraphia has lagged behind research on dyslexia, and less has been reported in this area. However, research supporting the clinical features of these disorders and dyslexia will be reviewed in the next section.

From a clinical perspective, Hynd et al. (1988) suggested that subtypes for individual clients should first be defined clinically through analysis of error patterns in reading, math, and writing performance; these patterns may then reveal potential subprocesses involved in learning within a specific domain. This approach has the advantage of greater ecological validity, allows the practitioner to observe the derived subtype in the clinical setting, and provides direct implications for treatment tied to the subtype of learning disability (Hynd et al., 1988).

PHENOMENOLOGY

Clinical Subtypes of Learning Disabilities

The clinical features of learning disabilities have been described specifically in four major areas: dyslexia, dyscalculia, dysgraphia, and social–emotional learning disabilities. Each of these types of learning disability is further elaborated in terms of its subtypes and presumed underlying processing deficits. This section provides an overview of the clinical features of the major subtypes of learning disabilities.

Dyslexia

Aaron and Simurdak (1991) proposed that poor reading performance could be the result of either weak decoding skills, poor comprehension ability, or a combination of the two. Their classification postulated that words could be decoded through a phonological route—where the pronunciation of a word is possible without intermediary semantic processing—or a semantic route—where the meaning of the word can be determined without intermediary phonological processing (Aaron & Simurdak, 1991). The decoding problems of children with dyslexia are thought to be related in most cases to phonologic processing deficits (Lieberman & Shankweiler, 1985; Snowling, 1980), with errors manifest in slow reading speed, mispronunciations of words in oral reading, and excessive dependence on context for reading. Children with decoding problems may have difficulty remembering phonetic sounds for letters (phoneme–grapheme association), discriminating between similar phonetic sounds (phonemic analysis), blending the phonetic sounds to make words (phonemic synthesis), and breaking words into syllables for pronunciation of the component parts (syllabication). However, decoding problems also can be caused by visual-perceptual deficits in letter recognition and discrimination (visual analysis), sequencing of letters to form words (visual synthesis), and memory for the gestalt (visual pattern) of words. Bakker (1979) suggested that in the early stages of learning to read, children tend to rely more on perceptual strategies mediated by the right hemisphere to help them with visual recognition and discrimination of letters and words. However, as reading becomes more proficient, there is a shift to using linguistic strategies mediated by the left hemisphere. Once reading skills became overlearned and automatic, Bakker felt that children no longer needed to focus on the graphic aspects of reading as much as the linguistic aspects. Bakker's theory was supported by electrophysiological studies that showed differential hemispheric activation during reading, depending on whether right hemisphere or left hemisphere reading strategies were used (Bakker & Vinke, 1985). Bakker's concept of linking cerebral processing to early reading strategies emphasizes the different and conjoint contributions of the two hemispheres, especially when children are learning to read (Leong, 1989).

Children with primary comprehension deficits may make few errors in pronunciation during oral reading, but they have difficulty comprehending the content of the material and are thought to have linguistic deficits involving semantic processing of written language. Deficits may be seen in vocabulary knowledge, knowledge of antonyms and synonyms, and auditory and verbal memory. These children also may have concomitant problems in listening comprehension, which is presumed to share the same cognitive mechanism as reading comprehension (Kintsch & Kozminsky, 1977).

Other children have both decoding and comprehension problems, and Cornwall (1992) illustrated a variety of cognitive and linguistic processes that may determine the severity of these problems. Cornwall demonstrated that verbal memory was a good predictor of word recognition; that phonological awareness was a good predictor of spelling, word attack (phonetic analysis), and reading comprehension; and that rapid naming was a good predictor of reading accuracy, word identification, and reading speed.

Lovett (1984, 1987) suggested that dyslexia also can be classified in terms of accuracy versus rate deficits. Accuracy errors encompass many of the decoding errors already described, whereas rate problems refer to the fluency and speed of reading. Fluency problems, which can result in a slower rate of reading, are caused by such reading errors as repetition of words or phrases, hesitation, mispronunciation, substitution of words that are of the same class or words that are graphically or phonemically similar, omission of letters within words or entire words, and insertion of new words.

In summary, the clinical presentation of dyslexia may involve problems with decoding, comprehension, fluency, rate, or combinations of these problems. Attention to developmental aspects of reading, particularly whether the child is in the early acquisition phase or a more advanced reading phase, is important to understanding potential underlying processes and subsequent intervention strategies.

Dyscalculia

Novick and Arnold (1988) defined dyscalculia as a developmental arithmetic disorder involving deficits in counting, computational skills, ability to solve word problems, and understanding numbers. Kosc (1974) described six types of developmental dyscalculia: (1) the "verbal" type involves problems with naming mathematical amounts, numbers, terms, symbols, and relationships; (2) the "practognostic" type involves an inability to compare, enumerate, and manipulate objects mathematically (pictured or real); (3) the "lexical" type involves difficulty reading mathematics symbols; (4) the "graphical" type involves problems with writing mathematics symbols; (5) the "ideognostical" type involves problems comprehending mathematics concepts and performing mental calculations; and (6) the "operational" type involves deficits in performing computational operations.

O'Hare, Brown, and Aitken (1991) suggested that mathematical skills have their basis in the preschool child's development of language, with understanding of concepts such as size (e.g., larger, smaller) and quantity (e.g., more, less). These authors provided a framework in which to consider a young child's development of mathematical skills. Their framework suggested that children first learn counting (i.e., active counting of objects rather than counting by rote) and then begin to understand the concept of quantity (e.g., concepts such as more and less). After this, children learn to associate the numeric labels with the actual quantity of objects and the graphic symbols (i.e., 1, 2, 3, . . .) for numbers, and learn the operational signs for addition, subtraction, and so forth. The next step is calculation, which involves manipulation of the numbers according to specific rules of operation. At more advanced levels, the calculation system can be further subdivided into such skills as processing of operational symbols, retrieval of basic arithmetic facts (algorithms), and execution of the calculation procedures (O'Hare et al., 1991).

Other investigators have emphasized the importance of sensorimotor processes in the development of mathematics abilities. Rourke and colleagues investigated groups of children with combined reading and mathematics disorders, and those with more severe unitary mathematics disorders, by conducting error analyses of their mathematics performance (Rourke & Finlayson, 1978; Strang & Rourke, 1985). In the group of children with the severe unitary mathematics disorders, they noted a greater degree of mechanical arithmetic errors than errors in judgment and reasoning. Specific error characteristics included spatial organization problems, inadequate attention to visual detail, sequential difficulties in process, problems with mental flexibility, poor graphomotor technique, compromised storage and retrieval of number facts, and poor number logic. Strang and Rourke (1985) suggested that disturbed development in sensorimotor processes may be related to the error pattern displayed by these children.

Cognitive processes also have been studied in relation to mathematics performance. Batchelor, Gray, and Dean (1990) examined the association between visual (computation) and aural (word problem) math tasks and various neurocognitive abilities. They found that mental flexibility, verbal–auditory discrimination ability, long-term memory for general information, and visuospatial processing were related to better mathematics performance on both visual and aural tasks, thus demonstrating that both verbal and nonverbal neurocognitive processes are important in mathematics problem solving.

Keller and Sutton (1991) suggested that additional research is needed to carefully define the cognitive and neuropsychological processes that may be associated with the various subtypes of dyscalculia. On a clinical level, it is important to consider visuospatial and verbal abilities, as well as graphomotor skill, in children suspected of having deficits in mathematics. Children with language-based dyscalculia may have difficulty with comprehension of word problems and instructions, and memorizing facts and the step-by-step procedures for completing math problems; children with spatiotemporal deficits in dyscalculia may have problems such as number reversals, number sequencing errors, and carrying out operations in the wrong sequence (Spreen, Risser, & Edgell, 1995). Most academic measures will tap computational skills, mathematics reasoning ability, and knowledge of numerical concepts. A careful error analysis of the child's performance can provide useful information regarding the type of dyscalculia and possible underlying processes.

Dysgraphia

Writing is considered to be a multidimensional process with several components, including specific handwriting problems (e.g., legibility, fluency); difficulty completing written assignments; poor spelling; and problems with writing composition, such as planning, word choices, sentence construction, and organization of text (Berninger & Hooper, 1993). Chalfant and Scheffelin (1969) distinguished between *writing* (which refers to the commitment of one's thoughts to a written idea, and involves the ideational use of language along with auditory and visual perceptual systems) and *handwriting* (which refers to the motor aspects of writing).

Much has been written about the importance of language as a foundation to later academic skills, including written language. Myklebust (1965) developed a hierarchy for the acquisition of oral language, reading, and writing, in which written language is at the peak of the language hierarchy. At the bottom of the hierarchy is auditory receptive language, which develops around 9 months of age when children begin to understand that words represent objects, experiences, and feelings (Johnson, 1993). This stage is followed by oral expressive language, beginning at age 12 to 18 months and developing through the preschool years. According to Johnson (1993), the rudiments of reading and writing skills are evident when preschool youngsters play with letter tiles or blocks, listen to stories, read logos or signs, or make marks on paper. These experiences build on the child's oral language experiences and skills, and provide a basis for higher levels of learning in the areas of reading, writing, and mathematics. Thus, children who have delayed or disordered receptive or expressive language skills at the preschool level theoretically are at risk for later deficits in written language.

Likewise, children who exhibit delays or disorders in motor development, particularly fine motor and graphomotor (writing–drawing) development, are at risk for dysgraphia. During the preschool years, children are learning how to interpret the world about them spatially, through a developing sense of directionality, using motor planning skills to navigate their environment, and making their hand move in just

the right direction to form an angle while drawing or to reproduce a certain shape. Preschool learning activities help children to refine their coordination, while learning the kinesthetic movement patterns needed to produce written language.

Although clinical and subtyping research with dysgraphia lags far behind that of dyslexia, there have been some attempts to create a classification system related to underlying brain mechanisms. O'Hare and Brown (1989a) described three types of motor dysgraphia: (1) visuospatial (involving recognition of faces, shapes, objects, places, and directions), (2) executive-coordination (involving speed of movement, grip strength, and execution of movements), and (3) dyspraxia (involving motor planning, and sequencing and automaticity of motor movements). They also included a spelling–syntactical category (involving knowledge of rules affecting spelling, punctuation, and sentence structure) and a semantic composition category (involving sentence structure, conceptualization, and understanding of metaphors and analogies). This expanded classification system awaits further validation research, but it offers the practitioner a range of functions that might be examined when assessing for dysgraphia.

Social–Emotional Learning Disabilities

Social–emotional learning disabilities have been the focus of much research and clinical interest in recent years (see Denckla, 1983, 1989; Rourke, 1989; Voeller, 1990), but this disorder was eloquently discussed as early as 1967 by Johnson and Myklebust, who described children with nonverbal disorders of learning who had poor spatial, time, directionality, and social perception. Johnson and Myklebust wrote that these children also had difficulty learning the meaning of other people's actions, were unable to pretend or anticipate, and were unable to understand the implications of gestures, facial expressions, and other nonverbal expressions of attitudes. In much the same way that deficits in visual perception or auditory perception can affect reading, these children were thought to have a disorder of social perception that affected their ability to interpret social cues from others or to understand the effect of their own actions on others (Johnson & Myklebust, 1967). This disorder has been termed *nonverbal perceptual organization output disorder* (Rourke & Finlayson, 1978), *right hemisphere deficit syndrome* (Voeller, 1986), and *nonverbal learning disability* (Rourke, 1989), but the term *social–emotional learning disability* (coined by Denckla, 1983, 1989) will be used for the purposes of this discussion.

Semrud-Clikeman and Hynd (1990) reviewed the major clinical features reported in research on social–emotional learning disabilities, and found several features that were consistent across studies: significantly delayed arithmetic ability, generally good decoding but poor reading comprehension skills, delayed or poorly coordinated motor functioning, poor visuospatial skills, verbal IQ higher than performance IQ, and marked social skills deficits. The most common social characteristics described in the literature include impaired ability to engage in interactive play, abnormal affective expression, difficulty interpreting emotions, poor eye contact, defective use of gesture, problems with interpersonal space, poor pragmatic communication skills, obsession with narrow topics and pursuits, decreased appreciation for metaphor and humor, and poor adaptation to novel situations (Culbertson & Edmonds, 1996). These social deficits often result in peer rejection, social isolation, and development of secondary emotional disorders related to the rejection.

Voeller (1990) described two primary behavioral patterns in children with social–emotional learning disabilities. One group of children tended to be remote, unrelated, withdrawn, have poor eye contact and a limited range of affective expression, and a monotonous quality to their speech. The other group was described as overly friendly and inappropriate in their social actions by invading the space of others, standing too close, touching too much, talking too much,

and using an abundance of cliches and automatic phrases (Voeller, 1990). Voeller also described a characteristic set of neurological factors in patients with social–emotional learning disabilities; many of her patients had left-sided deficits on neurological examination, implicating the right hemisphere. Many also had minor anomalies of the right hemisphere on computed tomography scans, and abnormal medical histories such as premature birth, hypoxic insults, or postnatal neurological injuries.

Rourke (1988) postulated that children with this disorder, which he termed *nonverbal learning disability* (NLD), have primary neuropsychological deficits affecting tactile and visual-perceptual abilities, complex psychomotor skills, and adaptation to novel situations whereas their neuropsychological assets are found in processing information through the auditory modality. Children with NLD have a good verbal rote memory and may become hyperverbal after an initial delay in language. According to Rourke, children with NLD have an early history that is remarkable for their diminished exploration of the environment during the sensorimotor stage of development and their tendency to learn about the environment primarily through verbal means. As these children progress through developmental stages, their primary neuropsychological deficits give way to secondary deficits affecting tactile perception and visual attention; these deficits in turn give way to tertiary neuropsychological deficits affecting tactile and visual memory, concept formation, reasoning, and problem solving, deficient oral-motor praxis, and diminished prosody in verbal expression. The verbal and social deficits are interrelated, in that these children usually are hyperverbal, have a monotonic speech quality, and generally poor pragmatic skills in communication (i.e., poor eye contact, obsessing on narrow topics, superficial quality of verbal content, and poor conversational skills), all of which may be irritating to others. These children are felt to have a poor prognosis for good social adjustment as they get older, and many likely will be diagnosed with one of a variety of psychiatric disorders (e.g., antisocial personality, schizoid or schizotypal personality, Asperger's syndrome, or affective disorders). Many will have difficulty holding a job and problems having meaningful relationships (Rourke, 1988). The broad clinical features of social–emotional learning disabilities require careful assessment of the perceptual, attentional, linguistic, visual-motor, and social–behavioral characteristics that may accompany this disorder.

Developmental Issues

Empirical evidence has supported the importance of preschool developmental skills as predictors of learning disabilities during school age (Hooper, 1988). Several recent reviews of the literature have provided an overview of our current knowledge about which factors consistently predict later functioning, as well as problems encountered in prediction (Horn & Packard, 1985; Tramontana, Hooper, & Selzer, 1988). Horn and Packard (1985) conducted a meta-analysis of 58 studies that attempted to predict reading achievement in Grades 1 and 3. Across these studies, the best single predictors were measures of general intelligence, language, attention–distractibility, and internalizing behavior problems; measures of sensory perceptual functions and soft neurological signs were less effective predictors. However, the studies reviewed by Horn and Packard tended to focus on univariate prediction methods, with less attention given to the effectiveness of combined measures as predictors of later abilities. Also, the studies reviewed did not focus on academic areas other than reading. A review by Tramontana et al. (1988) focused exclusively on studies that examined preschool prediction of later achievement, and found that measures of general cognitive ability, letter naming, language, visual-motor skills, and finger localization were accurate predictors of general reading skills in Grades 1 through 3. However, as Hooper (1988) pointed out, these findings must be viewed as preliminary because few studies examined the component parts of reading (such as decoding

and comprehension). In the Tramontana et al. review, mathematics was found to be predicted about as well as reading, although it was studied less extensively and the component parts of mathematics were rarely considered.

A few exemplary studies have been highlighted by Hooper (1988) in terms of their design and their contributions to understanding developmental factors that influence prediction of later learning disabilities. Jansky and de Hirsch (1972) explored specific language factors that were measured at the end of the kindergarten year and used to predict reading achievement at the end of second grade. The most predictive variables included letter naming, picture naming, word matching, copying, and sentence memory. The Florida Longitudinal Project (Satz, Taylor, Friel, & Fletcher, 1978) represented one of the most comprehensive longitudinal projects conducted; it was distinguished by its multivariate approach to prediction, multiple follow-up points, and numerous cross-validation studies (Hooper, 1988). Their research is important in demonstrating an apparent shift in the predictive power of a set of predictors, with visual perceptual factors being more important in the prediction of early reading acquisition, but verbal abilities being more important in predicting reading achievement at later elementary ages (i.e., Grade 5). These investigators achieved an 84% correct classification rate using variables such as finger localization, recognition-discrimination tasks, and alphabet recitation to predict reading outcomes in second grade. However, a 76% correct classification rate was found in predicting reading achievement in Grade 5, and the best predictors were the Peabody Picture Vocabulary Test, the Developmental Test of Visual-Motor Integration, alphabet recitation, and finger localization ability. The Satz et al. (1978) study demonstrated that the prediction efforts were quite good for designating severely disabled and superior readers (at the extreme ends of the continuum of reading); however, correct classification rates fell significantly for the middle ranges of functioning (Hooper, 1988). Further, there was a problem with false-negative rates, in which as many as 26% of the children who were functioning adequately in kindergarten later developed significant reading problems by Grade 5. This suggests that, in some types of reading disorders, early prediction may not be possible and/or the correct combination of predictors has not yet been discovered.

Two additional studies have been exemplary in isolating a differential set of predictors for reading versus mathematics (Stevenson & Newman, 1986; Stevenson, Parker, Wilkinson, Hegion, & Fish, 1976). These authors found the best kindergarten predictors of reading to be letter naming, visual–auditory paired associates, Horst reversals, and verbal categorization; the best predictors of math included verbal recall, verbal–auditory paired associates, perceptual learning, and coding. The pattern of predictors remained stable from 1st through 10th grade at various follow-up points, and thus provides one of the longest follow-up intervals reported to date (Hooper, 1988).

Investigations of early developmental milestones as possible predictors of later learning deficits have not been useful for clinical application. For example, Shapiro et al. (1990) evaluated whether deviations in infant language and motor milestones would predict later reading delay; when they compared milestones of children who had reading delay at 7½ years with milestones of normal readers, no consistent patterns of difference were evident. These findings suggest that use of infant developmental milestones as markers of later learning disabilities would be unreliable.

The foregoing discussion illustrates that the complex issues in prediction of learning problems during the preschool years have only begun to be addressed, and additional research is needed to clarify the complex set of factors influencing the development of learning disabilities. The existing research suggests that a neuropsychological perspective provides an important theoretical basis to guide the research design of such studies and also could be useful in helping to design new assessment instruments and better criterion measures for prediction of learning disabilities.

Cultural and Environmental Issues

Cultural variables are important determinants of the way children are raised and learning is acquired (Ardila, Rosselli, & Ostrosky-Solis, 1992). Research has shown that cultural background has very critical implications in terms of language, perception, memory, and logical reasoning (Laboratory for Comparative Human Cognition, 1983). For instance, parents with a low socioeconomic level have been observed to use more nonverbal strategies in relating to their children, whereas parents with a higher educational level use verbal strategies more often (Robinson, 1974). Further, the language of parents from lower socioeconomic levels has been described as less fluent with a simpler grammatical structure than language of parents from higher socioeconomic levels (Bernstein, 1974). Perceptual strategies also have been shown to be influenced by cultural variables, e.g., perceptual performance in creating three-dimensional drawings, depth perception in pictures, and recognition of schematized figures (Ardila et al., 1992; Brislin, 1983; Segall, 1986). Disadvantage can occur when children are raised in environments that are impoverished, both in terms of materials or toys available to help them learn, and in terms of the availability, and educational and intellectual resources of the child's primary caregiver(s). Disadvantage can occur also when children are raised in cultures that differ from the majority culture, but are evaluated or confronted with school learning tasks that are founded on the majority culture.

Consideration of cultural influences on test development and theory, children's responses to testing procedures and test content, and the examiners' interpretation of test responses is essential if assessment is to be less biased. A basic premise is that tests are developed to reflect a "universal" standard, usually reflecting the majority culture, to which the child's test responses are compared. Unless a particular test has been locally normed with a culturally homogeneous group, the examiner must acknowledge this universal standard and understand the potential for bias in the way cognitive variables are measured, and also in the way an individual's performance is interpreted (through the idiosyncratic cultural perspective of the examiner). Attention to process variables (e.g., the way in which individuals reason or problem-solve) is at least as important as test scores for guiding diagnostic decisions and development of intervention plans. The relevance of diagnostic information depends on the accuracy with which all test data, including process variables, are interpreted.

When evaluating children for learning disabilities, the practitioner must demonstrate that specific processing deficits (be they cognitive, perceptual, linguistic, or the like) exist and have a bearing on the type of learning disability being diagnosed. At the same time, the practitioner must consider whether these processing deficits are a function of cultural influences that affect the way in which an individual expresses what he or she knows. It is helpful to provide a testing environment in which the child can express his or her knowledge to an examiner who understands the particular cultural background of the child, and it is essential that the child be evaluated in his or her primary language. If issues about cultural influences remain unclear after investigation or evaluation, it may be necessary to defer the diagnostic decision about a possible learning disability until the child has had a greater opportunity for exposure to formal education and/or until the ecology of the testing situation can be more salient for the child.

DIAGNOSIS

Controversies in the Diagnosis of Learning Disabilities

The reliability and validity of diagnostic approaches for learning disabilities have been questioned by many investigators (Adelman & Taylor, 1986; Algozzine & Ysseldyke, 1986; Bryan, Bay, & Donahue, 1988; Heath & Kush, 1991), who argue that the procedures often are inconsistent and unreliable. The basic diagnostic criteria for learning disabilities come from the Rules and Regulations Implementing Education for All Handicapped Children Act of 1975 (1977). According to this document, the diagnosis of learning disability

> is made based on 1) whether a child does not achieve commensurate with his or her age and ability when provided with appropriate educational experience and 2) whether the child has a severe discrepancy between achievement and intellectual ability in one or more of 7 areas relating to communication skills and mathematical abilities.
>
> These concepts are to be interpreted in a case by case basis by the qualified evaluation team members. The team must decide that the discrepancy is not primarily the result of 1) visual, hearing, or motor handicaps; 2) mental retardation; 3) emotional disturbance; or 4) environmental, cultural, or economic disadvantage. (p. 65083)

Although differences in interpreting these guidelines exist from state to state, the most common criteria used across the United States were defined by Chalfant (1984). These criteria require demonstration of: (1) failure to achieve (referring to lack of academic achievement in one or more of the primary areas of academic learning); (2) psychological process disorders (referring to the psychological processes that are believed to underlie academic learning, including understanding and use of oral and written language, attention and concentration, concept formation, and various types of information processing); (3) exclusionary criteria (requiring that the symptoms of learning problems not be related to factors such as sensory deficits, mental retardation, emotional disturbance, or sociocultural or educational disadvantage); (4) etiology of the learning disability (involving review of medical and developmental history to determine if factors are present that might relate to the etiology of the learning disability, such as neurological deficits, delayed speech and language development, perinatal difficulties, or brain injury); and (5) a severe discrepancy between achievement and intellectual ability in one of the seven areas listed in the federal regulations.

These diagnostic criteria for learning disability are not without controversy. For instance, an operational definition of psychological process disorders has been difficult to determine, as has an agreement on what constitutes a "severe" discrepancy between achievement and intellectual abilities. Various models for determining severe discrepancies have been used, ranging from grade level discrepancies using arbitrary grade cutoffs (e.g., performance two grade levels below actual grade placement) to standard score comparison models, requiring that a child's academic achievement test scores fall below their intellectual scores by some predetermined amount (Heath & Kush, 1991). However, grade level discrepancies are problematic in overidentifying children whose intellectual abilities are in the slow learner range, between 70 and 85. Although the grade level achievement of these students falls below their current placement, their achievement is commensurate with their intellectual ability and there is no severe discrepancy (Reynolds, 1990). The standard score comparisons between achievement and intellectual scores are problematic because IQ and achievement tests are not perfectly correlated. In fact, the correlation between most IQ and achievement measures ranges from .50 to .65. Using the straight standard score comparison results in overidentification of underachieving children in the upper IQ range, and underidentification of children in the lower IQ range (Reynolds, 1990).

The current method most commonly used to quantify intelligence–achievement discrepancies is a regression approach, which takes into consideration the regression toward the mean that occurs when achievement scores are predicted from a correlated measure (IQ), as described by Heath and Kush (1991). This method uses a prediction equation that is based on the actual correlation between an IQ test and a specific achievement test, so that the student's actual level of achievement is compared with a predicted achievement score rather than the IQ. Using this approach, only those individuals whose actual level of achievement falls significantly below the predicted level would meet the criterion of having a severe discrepancy (Heath & Kush, 1991). This approach has been used in the development and revisions of many commonly used intelligence–achievement batteries, so that both types of measures are based on the same normative population and have high intertest reliability. Examples include the Kaufman Assessment Battery for Children (Kaufman & Kaufman, 1983) and the Kaufman Test of Educational Achievement (Kaufman & Kaufman, 1985); the Woodcock–Johnson Psychoeducational Battery-Revised Tests of Cognitive Ability and Tests of Achievement (Woodcock & Johnson, 1989); and the Wechsler Intelligence Scale for Children-Third Edition (WISC-III; Wechsler, 1990) and the Wechsler Individual Achievement Test (1992).

By using the regression approach to determine a severe discrepancy between aptitude and achievement, it is possible to assess children across all IQ levels and distinguish between those who have learning disabilities and those who are slow learners (Heath & Kush, 1991). Braden (1987) also suggested that regression methods may produce more proportionate racial representation in learning disabilities classes than do fixed standard-score methods. Finally, IQ remains the best single predictor of academic achievement, and provides a good basis for determining an expected level of achievement (Heath & Kush, 1991; Thorndike & Hagen, 1977). For a more detailed discussion of the conceptual and technical problems in learning disability diagnosis, including use of the regression method for determining severe discrepancy, the reader is referred to Reynolds (1990). It also is important to note that determination of a severe discrepancy is a necessary but not a sufficient condition for the diagnosis of learning disability (Reynolds, 1984). The other components of the definition listed earlier must be considered as well.

Differential Diagnosis

The list of differential diagnoses can be drawn from the exclusionary criteria found in the definition for learning disability, described in an earlier section of this chapter. These exclusionary criteria include sensory deficits, mental retardation, emotional dysfunction, and sociocultural and educational disadvantage. Attentional problems also should be added to the differential list. The practitioner must address each of these potential differential diagnoses in the preassessment interview or as a component of the individual assessment before making a diagnosis of learning disability.

Generally, sensory deficits will be ruled out prior to beginning an assessment for a learning disability. School health screening records or medical records provided by a child's pediatrician can provide useful information on subtle visual and auditory acuity deficits that can be easily mistaken for visual- or auditory-perceptual deficits. Mental retardation is typically ruled out during assessment for learning disabilities through use of cognitive measures.

If symptoms of emotional problems are present, it will be necessary to determine whether these represent a primary or secondary emotional disorder, and whether the child's academic achievement problems could be related to the emotional disturbance. Behavioral ratings obtained from parents and teachers, projective assessment, clinical interview, and behavioral observations can assist in making the differential. Time of onset of the emotional symptoms and their pattern of occurrence with regard to school and academic functioning are helpful in determining primary versus secondary emotional problems. For instance, it is not uncommon for secondary emotional adjustment problems to emerge when children first experience academic difficulty related to their learning disability, or at later stages in their aca-

demic career when major shifts in curriculum occur or the demands imposed by the classroom environment become greater. Examples of such secondary emotional reactions can include withdrawal, regression to a more immature style of behavior, somatic complaints that are likely to occur only on school days, depression associated with feelings of inadequacy, clowning in an attempt to cover feelings of inadequacy or avoid situations that cause distress, and anxiety or fear responses (Silver, 1979). If the child's emotional adjustment problems are determined to be secondary to the learning disability, then the presence of these emotional problems would not preclude diagnosis of the learning disability. This may take some careful explanation to the team charged with determining eligibility and placement within the school system, but generally it is well understood that emotional reactions can be secondary to frustration or stress caused by the primary disorder of learning disability. A more difficult situation occurs when children have a primary emotional disorder (such as depression) and also have evidence of a primary learning disability. In this situation, the practitioner will need to discern, if possible, which aspects of the child's academic and educational problems are related specifically to the learning disability and which are more likely related to the emotional problems. There may be times, particularly in the midst of a major depressive episode, when one must defer evaluation of a learning disability until treatment can be obtained for the primary emotional disorder.

The influences of environmental, cultural, or economic disadvantage on a child's educational functioning are also somewhat difficult to discern, and require a careful history from family members or others familiar with the child's background. The primary concern with disadvantage of these types is the child's diminished exposure to information, experiences, and/or educational opportunities that are important for academic functioning. If environmental, cultural, or economic disadvantages have occurred, and there is concern that these factors may be influencing a child's academic functioning, the best recourse may be to defer assessment for the learning disability until the child has had an opportunity for supportive educational services provided by the school. This is an issue more often with young children who are just entering the school environment than with children who have had several years of formal schooling, which would have provided greater enrichment than was presumably available in their home and family environments. However, one must also carefully assess the quality of the educational environment to determine if there is evidence of educational disadvantage in which the child has not received appropriate placement, instructional methods, or attention to special needs. It is common in many schools for school psychologists and teachers to implement various interventions in the mainstream educational environment and carefully evaluate their effectiveness before referring a child for assessment of a possible learning disability or recommending a placement for special education.

Finally, children with attention deficits often show academic underachievement secondary to their problems with focused attention, persistence on tasks that require sustained effort, organization and study habits, and distractibility. In the past, some professionals have assumed that attention deficits are a type of learning disability, but this is not borne out in the research on the disorders, which clearly sets them apart as separate (Barkley, 1990). A careful evaluation will identify the symptoms specific to each disorder so that each diagnosis can be made or ruled out as appropriate.

Comorbidity

Probably the most prevalent comorbid disorder with learning disabilities is attention-deficit hyperactivity disorder (ADHD). In the research literature, the overlap ranges from as low as 10% (August & Holmes, 1984; Halperin, Gittelman, Klein, & Rudel, 1984) to as high as 92% (Silver, 1981). According to Barkley (1990), the range of overlap is more conservatively between 19 and 26%, with the variability likely relating to differences in selection criteria, sampling, and measurement instruments, as well as inconsistencies in the definitions for both learning disabilities and ADHD over the years. Another confounding variable in determining the overlap between learning disabilities and ADHD is whether the research considered the subtypes of each disorder. ADHD can be subtyped into predominantly inattentive type, predominantly hyperactive–impulsive type, or combined type. The subtypes of learning disabilities have been discussed earlier, and research that takes into consideration the subtypes of both disorders is rare.

Language disorders also are frequently comorbid with learning disabilities. This differential is somewhat confusing because many types of learning disability have underlying phonological processing and/or other linguistic problems. Each of the subtyping studies described in an earlier section (e.g., Boder, 1973; Mattis et al., 1975, 1978; Petrauskas & Rourke, 1979) determined at least one major subtype of learning disabilities to have underlying language deficits. Other neurolinguistic types of learning disabilities have been proposed as part of the subtyping literature, and these are described for the interested reader in Hooper and Willis (1989). However, children with primary language disorders may have problems with fluency, rate, and rhythm of oral expression; articulation or phonological disorders of speech; or problems affecting semantics, syntax, and morphology of receptive and/or expressive language. These deficits, though they most certainly will have an effect on learning, can and should be diagnosed separately from a learning disability by a speech–language pathologist.

There also is a substantial literature that documents the co-occurrence of social deficits and learning disabilities, but much of this research assumes that the social deficits are secondary to the learning disabilities, or more often, secondary to comorbid ADHD and learning disabilities. Flicek and Landau (1985) attempted to sort out the effects of comorbid ADHD on the incidence of social deficits. They found that boys who were learning disabled but not hyperactive were less popular, engaged in significantly lower rates of positive interactions with peers, and experienced more rejection than comparison boys who were not learning disabled. However, the boys with learning disabilities were significantly less symptomatic of social status problems then boys who had comorbid ADHD and learning disabilities. The boys with comorbid disorders were rated by their teachers as significantly more aggressive than boys with pure learning disabilities, and were more frequently rejected by their peers.

Studies of children with pure learning disabilities have examined the behavioral and/or cognitive deficits that might explain their poor interpersonal functioning (Wallander & Hubert, 1987). La Greca (1981) reported that children with learning disabilities who were poorly accepted by peers made fewer positive imitative statements and used more distracting nonverbal behaviors than did poorly accepted nonlearning-disabled peers. Poor communication skills also have been associated with poor peer relations in children with learning disabilities (Donahue & Bryan, 1984; Markoski, 1983). Children with learning disabilities have been shown to display, and to be the recipients of, more negative and rejecting behaviors than nondisabled children (Bryan, Wheeler, Felcan, & Henck, 1976; Sainato, Zigmond, & Strain, 1983). These studies suggest that cognitive and/or linguistic deficits associated with the learning disabilities may contribute to the problems in social skills shown by children with learning disabilities.

ETIOLOGY

The prevailing research on the etiology of learning disabilities has focused on various neurological, immunological, and genetic factors that are presumed to underlie the disorder. As noted earlier in this chapter, most of the research focuses on the etiology of dyslexia, with

less research focused on dyscalculia or dysgraphia. There is an emerging literature on the presumed etiology of social–emotional learning disabilities, but there is continuing debate over the exact mechanisms involved. This section examines major research findings to date on dyslexia, with the hope that it may serve as a prototype for research on other subtypes of learning disabilities.

Neurodevelopmental Conceptualizations of Learning Disabilities

Historically, there have been two major neurodevelopmental conceptualizations to explain how learning disabilities develop. One conceptualization proposes a maturational lag in cortical functioning (Satz & van Nostrand, 1973), and suggests that there are delays in brain maturation that differentially affect higher learning skills associated with reading and math acquisition. Skills that develop during the preschool years, such as visual-perceptual abilities and cross-modal sensory integration, were thought to be delayed because of immaturity in the cortical regions associated with those skills (Hooper, 1988). It was felt that these areas of cortical immaturity would gradually mature, but that other cortical areas affecting skills developed later in childhood would also be developing at a slower rate and would continue to hinder acquisition of reading and math skills. This theory has been questioned from a number of perspectives. First, the concept of a delay in cortical maturation suggests that a child should eventually catch up with chronological age peers rather than continuing to show deficits in achievement. As many children with learning disabilities do not overcome their problems, there is a question about why maturation either does not occur or does not result in improved functioning. Another criticism raised by Hooper (1988) involves the pattern of deficits often noted in learning problems. A developmental delay presumes a relatively normal pattern of skill acquisition that is merely slower than would be expected; however, children with learning disabilities often have disordered or aberrant processing styles as well as delayed abilities. Finally, there are questions as to why some children with learning disabilities do not have apparent problems in early years and only later appear to develop a deficit. The maturational lag theory would not explain this phenomenon (Hooper, 1988).

The second major neurodevelopmental conceptualization involves the notion of a deficiency or dysfunction in brain development that is apparent only when children become old enough for environmental demands to require the specific processing abilities of the involved brain region (Luria, 1980; Rourke, Bakker, Fisk, & Strang, 1983). This theory assumes that deficits are always present, but that they remain "silent" until the affected region of the brain is challenged by demands of the environment. This conceptualization could account for the phenomenon of later-emerging learning disabilities that are not well predicted by preschool-age skills, and would provide an explanation for the broad range of predictors that have been identified during the preschool years (Hooper, 1988). Several recent reviews have supported the conclusion that the abnormal brain development conceptualization is much more likely to be correct than the developmental lag view (Bryden, 1988; Obrzut, 1988; Obrzut, Hynd, & Boliek, 1986).

Anatomical Correlates of Learning Disabilities

Cerebral Lateralization Abnormalities

The notion that disorders of reading are associated with abnormalities in cerebral lateralization has been discussed since the time of Orton (1937). Orton presumed that reversals in reading letters or words occurred because children were delayed in developing cerebral dominance. Orton thought that children who were left-handed or had mixed hand dominance were often deficient readers because of delayed or deficient cerebral dominance. It was believed that only children who were strongly righthanded,

and thus left hemisphere dominant, could be proficient readers (Hynd & Cohen, 1983). According to Orton, this occurs because a given stimulus (e.g., a word such as *saw*) is projected to both hemispheres, but is perceived by the nondominant hemisphere in mirror image (e.g., *was*). Thus, if there is delayed development of left hemisphere dominance, the nondominant hemisphere presumably exerts more influence and the child likely will read the word in mirror image (Corballis & Beale, 1976). Orton's theory was embraced by many clinicians and researchers, partly because of its face validity, as many children with dyslexia were noted to have mixed hand dominance or were left-handed. Children who were left-handed were thought to have language abilities lateralized to the right (or nondominant) hemisphere—which was less suited to subserve language skills—rather than to the left (Hynd & Cohen, 1983). Although Orton's theory fueled a great number of research studies on laterality and cerebral dominance as related to reading disorders, much of the research was frought with conceptual and methodological problems. Subsequent research has established that nearly two-thirds of all left-handed individuals have language skills lateralized to the left (or dominant) hemisphere, as do about 95% of all right-handed individuals (Hynd & Cohen, 1983). Several well-controlled studies have found no evidence to suggest an association between hand dominance and performance on measures of cognitive ability and achievement (Hardyck, Petrinovitch, & Goldman, 1976; Kaufman, Zalma, & Kaufman, 1978; Ullman, 1977). Orton's theory spurred an intense research effort into the possible neurological basis of dyslexia, and thus had a great heuristic effect. However, his theory has now given way to other lines of research into the etiology of learning disabilities that can be better supported anatomically and empirically.

Cerebral Asymmetry Studies

In the study of dyslexia, there is converging evidence for abnormalities in the area of the left hemisphere language cortex—the planum temporale (or temporal plane). Early research (see Geschwind & Levitsky, 1968) documented a normal pattern of brain asymmetry in adults in which the left planum is significantly larger than the right in most nondyslexic individuals; this part of the brain is thought to mediate phonological awareness that is important to reading and thus provides a logical anatomical substrate for linguistic competence. However, in brains of individuals with dyslexia, this normal pattern of asymmetry in the planum often is absent. Brain morphology studies using magnetic resonance (MR) imaging (Hynd et al., 1990; Larsen, Høien, Lundberg, & Ødegaard, 1990) and computed tomography (CT) scans (Hier, LeMay, Rosenberg, & Perlo, 1978) revealed that children with dyslexia often had either equal symmetry or reversed asymmetry of the planum. Larsen et al. (1990) determined that all of the phonological dyslexics in their study had symmetry of the planum, suggesting that normal phonological awareness was dependent on asymmetry of the planum.

Hynd et al. (1995) also investigated asymmetry in the anterior region of the corpus callosum—a band of fibers connecting the two hemispheres of the brain and important in the interhemispheric transfer of information. They found that children with dyslexia had significantly smaller anterior regions of the corpus callosum than controls, implying differences in interhemispheric connections that may affect reading. Other neuroanatomical and imaging studies have documented deviations from the normal asymmetries in such structures as the left anterior speech region, the auditory cortex, the inferior parietal lobe, and the posterior thalamus in individuals with dyslexia (Culbertson & Edmonds, 1996), and research is ongoing.

Minor Cortical Malformations

At the cellular level, there are three areas of cortical dysgenesis (or disorders in development) that have been explored in the brains of individuals with dyslexia: *ectopias,* which are described by Duane (1991) as "superficial clumps of nerve cells left behind in regions from which they should have migrated during fetal development" (p. 15); *dysplasias,* in which there is confused pattern of neuronal organization; and *polymicrogyria,* described by Duane (1991) as "many microscopic in-foldings of the brain trapped beneath the cortical surface" (p. 16). These areas of cortical malformation tend to cluster together in the left hemisphere more than in the right, and are predominantly located along the Sylvian fissure (an infolding of brain tissue that separates the temporal lobe from the frontal and parietal lobes of the brain). They are thought to result from abnormalities in neuronal migration during the second half of fetal brain development, but the factors that trigger this abnormal migration pattern are unclear (Duane, 1991). Geschwind and Galaburda (1985) proposed that the male sex steroid, testosterone, may adversely affect neuronal migration, and therefore could serve as an etiological agent for the cortical malformations that have been described. The anatomical regions in which these cortical malformations are more prevalent are important in mediation of language abilities, and thus could relate to reading disorders.

Immune Disturbances

Immunological mechanisms have been postulated as possible causes of neuronal migration abnormalities and development of learning disabilities. One hypothesis with regard to immunological disturbances suggests that antigens in the maternal circulation cross the placental barrier, attach to neurons in the fetus through fetal circulation to the brain, and thereby influence the organization, migration, and connections of neurons (Duane, 1991). Geschwind and Behan (1982) proposed a positive correlation between left-handedness, immune disturbances, and learning disabilities. They hypothesized that normal development of left hemisphere dominance is suppressed in utero by testosterone, resulting in increased incidence of a pattern of left-handedness, developmental language disorders, and autoimmune diseases (such as asthma, allergies, and migraine headaches). The immune disturbances occur because increased levels of testosterone delay the development of the thymus gland, which controls the immune system. Because males are exposed to higher levels of testosterone, each of these disorders is more pronounced in males. A critical review of the Geschwind theory by McManus and Bryden (1991) pointed out that there are over 30 postulates in this complex theory, and each aspect needs to be thoroughly tested. Those that have been tested to date have not been fully supported, and McManus and Bryden concluded that the theory at present does not provide sufficient theoretical advantage to be useful as part of psychological assessment for learning disorders.

Finally, numerous animal studies have suggested that autoimmune damage to blood vessel walls may damage the developing brain cortex, leading to cortical injury, scars, and malformations (Humphreys, Rosen, Press, Sherman, & Galaburda, 1991; Sherman, Galaburda, & Geschwind, 1985). However, the association among immune disturbances, neurological malformations, and learning disabilities in humans may not be well understood until research is conducted with large populations using standard measures of handedness and diagnostic criteria for learning and immunological dysfunctions (Galaburda, 1993).

Genetic Research on Learning Disabilities

Studies since the 1950s have suggested a familial pattern of dyslexia. Much early genetic research focused on twin studies, as illustrated by the Colorado Reading Project (Decker & Vandenberg, 1985; DeFries, 1985). In this project, an extensive battery of psychometric tests was administered to identical and fraternal twin pairs in which at least one member of each pair was reading disabled, and to twin pairs who were normal readers. Of the 96 identical and fraternal twin pairs who were reading disabled, there was a 71% concordance rate for the identical twins and a 49% concordance rate for the fraternal twins, thus providing strong evidence for a familial pattern of dyslexia, although the exact form of that transmission has remained uncertain.

Some early studies found evidence of an autosomal dominant mode of inheritance for many persons with development dyslexia (Hallgren, 1950; Omenn & Weber, 1978; Smith, Kimberling, Pennington, & Lubs, 1983). Attempts to isolate the specific gene responsible for transmission of familial dyslexia have progressed over the past 10 to 15 years. Smith et al. (1983) were the first researchers to isolate the linkage of a gene on chromosome 15 with a specific dyslexic phenotype. According to Lubs et al. (1991), genetic linkage implies that genes (DNA sequences) at two or more locations on the same chromosome are likely to be coinherited and to segregate together in families. The farther apart two gene locations are on the same chromosome, the less likely that gene markers at these locations will be inherited together. In the Smith et al. (1983) study, linkage analyses were performed between dyslexia and a group of known genetic markers (i.e., chromosomal heteromorphism and polymorphic protein markers). Family members were solicited who had a history of dyslexia in three generations on one side of the family in an autosomal dominant pattern, verbal and performance IQ of at least 90, and no evident external cause of the dyslexia (such as birth injury, head injury, or serious neurological illness). The participating family members were given a battery of neuropsychological and achievement tests to determine if there was consistency of dyslexia subtypes between and within families. The results suggested a tentative linkage of a gene on the short arm of chromosome 15 linked to the dyslexic phenotype. Further molecular genetic studies have shown this gene to be further localized to a small region of the chromosome just below the centromere (Lubs et al., 1991). However, this research has been criticized for its subject selection procedures that resulted in a probable mixture of genetic transmission modes, and therefore clouded the results. Further research is needed to identify the primary gene defect responsible for dyslexia at the level of DNA sequence, and also to identify the corresponding protein that the gene encodes (Lubs et al., 1991). A critical review of the research on familial transmission of dyslexia by Pennington and Smith (1983) concluded that the genetic mode of transmission of dyslexia is likely heterogeneous, with evidence for polygenic inheritance, autosomal dominant inheritance, and autosomal recessive inheritance in female probands.

More recently, Pennington et al. (1991) reported a sex-influenced, additive, major gene transmission of dyslexia in a significant portion of the 204 families in their study. At this point in our understanding of the genetic basis of dyslexia, conclusions about the specific transmission of dyslexia vary widely depending on the methodology and the subject selection procedures; however, the evidence for the existence of forms of familial dyslexia is strong. Evidence for genetic transmission of dyscalculia, dysgraphia, and social–emotional learning disabilities has lagged far behind the research on dyslexia, and certainly has not advanced to the point of designating specific chromosomes linked to these subtypes. Further research is needed to explore the genetic bases of these other subtypes of learning disabilities.

EPIDEMIOLOGY

Children with learning disabilities currently comprise the largest percentage of students aged 6 through 21 who are served under the Individuals with Disabilities Education Act (U.S. Department of Education, 1995). The U.S. Department of Education report documented that in 1993–1994, over 51% of children receiving special services had a primary specific learning disability; this translated to 2,444,020 students. These figures contrast with 21.1% who are being served for speech or language impairments, 11.6% being served for mental retardation, and 8.6% being served for serious emotional disturbance. Other disabilities fall at or below 2% of the total population. For all disabilities together, over 4.7 million children aged 6 through 21 are currently receiving services, and an additional 587,012 children from birth through age 5 are also receiving services. These figures represent an increase of over 1.6 million children receiving services since the program began in 1976.

Children with learning disabilities constitute 7 to 15% of the general school population, according to Gaddes and Edgell (1993). The large number of children diagnosed as having learning disabilities has drawn criticism from some researchers who feel that lack of precision in definition and diagnostic criteria has led to overdiagnosis of this disorder (Algozzine & Ysseldyke, 1986; Heath & Kush, 1991). On the other hand, the economic implications of the high prevalence rate (including need for additional personnel, materials, space, and other costs associated with special education services) generally have led most states to adopt more stringent criteria for diagnosis. Because the prevalence data are confounded by economic considerations at the federal, state, and local educational levels, epidemiological data are difficult to determine exactly (Culbertson & Edmonds, 1996).

Sex distribution in the various subtypes of learning disabilities has been somewhat difficult to discern because of conflicting data, depending on whether the studies involved research-identified or school-identified students. In studies of dyslexia, boys are more prevalent in school-identified samples (Nass, 1992), but some argue that teachers may be biased toward referring more males because they confound behavior with achievement (Shaywitz, Shaywitz, Fletcher, & Escobar, 1990). In contrast, Shaywitz et al. (1990) reported in the Connecticut Longitudinal Study that no differences between males and females were found in the prevalence of dyslexia when the subjects were research-identified.

Estimates of sex-role distribution in dyscalculia are unclear, and even the prevalence of dyscalculia in general is disputed. Semrud-Clikeman and Hynd (1992) reported that the actual incidence of dyscalculia is unknown, and various individual researchers have reported results of small samples. Kosc (1974) identified 6.4% of a group of fifth-grade students as dyscalculic, whereas others described the prevalence of such students among the general population of students with learning disabilities being served as ranging from 8.1% (Norman & Zigmond, 1980) to 26.2% (McLeod & Armstrong, 1982). Prevalence estimates were much higher (ranging from 33 to 40%) when learning disabilities in both reading and math were combined (Carpenter, 1985; McLeod & Armstrong, 1982).

Finally, prevalence estimates in dysgraphia have been estimated at 3 to 4% by Benton (1975), with boys being identified more often than girls (O'Hare & Brown, 1989b). However, the paucity of information on prevalence or sex-role distribution estimates reflects the relatively small amount of attention given to this subtype of learning disability to date (Culbertson & Edmonds, 1996).

ASSESSMENT

Assessment of children and adolescents with learning disabilities involves attention to the definitional and diagnostic criteria set forth in federal and state laws and the guidelines for implementing those laws, attention to the subtype of learning disability (both in terms of the academic/cognitive/social areas in which the symptoms are manifest, and also with regard to the underlying processing deficits), and attention to developmental and cultural issues that influence the expression of the disorder. These issues are discussed in turn, followed by a sug-

gested model for assessment of learning disabilities.

Addressing Definitional and Diagnostic Criteria

As discussed earlier, there are five criteria typically included in the guidelines for diagnosing learning disabilities in most states. The examiner must first demonstrate through history and review of records that the child has failed to achieve in one or more of the primary areas of academic learning despite appropriate educational experiences. Second, the assessment must identify psychological processing disorders that are believed to underlie the learning disability. This implies that the assessment must include evaluation of the child's oral and written language, attention and concentration, concept formation, and various types of information processing through the sensory modalities. Third, a variety of exclusionary criteria must be met, and this requires the examiner to rule out such factors as sensory deficits, mental retardation, emotional disturbance, and sociocultural or educational disadvantage as contributors to the child's failure to achieve. Fourth, the assessment should include some attention to possible etiology of the learning disability, usually obtained from review of medical and developmental records on the child. Finally, the assessment must demonstrate a severe discrepancy between achievement and intellectual ability in at least one of the seven areas listed in the federal regulations, or must demonstrate significant psychological processing disorders that affect both achievement and intelligence so that learning is adversely affected. It is recommended that a regression approach be used to assess intelligence–achievement discrepancies and that the examiner choose intelligence and achievement tests that are highly correlated with each other when making these comparisons.

The assessment for learning disabilities also must rule out other possible comorbid disorders, such as ADHD, language disorders, or social–emotional problems that are not part of the primary learning disability. If another disorder is present, it will be necessary to distinguish the relative effects of this disorder from effects related to the learning disability with regard to academic functioning.

Goals and Components of the Assessment

The assessment of learning disabilities may be organized to allow one to examine a hierarchy of functions that are important in learning, as illustrated in Table 1. These functions range from basic orientation and attention to more sophisticated, higher-order cognitive functioning involving complex linguistic abilities and abstract thinking. A common error in assessment of learning disabilities is the practice of examining only the more complex cognitive or academic functions without attention to more basic skills. With the former approach, one can identify deficient academic skills, but may have little information about the cause of the deficiency. A more systematic examination of basic and higher-level skills along a hierarchy allows for determining the specific processing deficits that underlie the learning disability.

Orientation and Attention

Interview and observational methodology are used along with test performance data to assess a child's orientation and attention. Orientation may include a child's sense of time (e.g., awareness of concepts such as morning versus afternoon, yesterday versus tomorrow, and day/month/year), awareness of order or schedule of events (e.g., what subject is studied first in the school day, or what subject always comes after recess), and place (e.g., awareness of current setting).

Assessment of attention must be conceptualized broadly, to include such functions as the ability to initiate an activity, focus attention and execute a task, sustain attention to task, encode information, and shift the focus of attention flexibly (Denckla, 1991; Mirsky, 1989). The "initiation" dimension of attention may be observed by determining the latency with which the individual begins an activity after being given a prompt, or it may be observed incidentally when the child is given independent work to accomplish (such as math computation problems). The "focus/execute" dimension of attention is often measured via perceptual-motor speed tasks such as the Coding subtest from the Wechsler Intelligence Scale for Children (WISC-III;

Table 1. Components to a Psychological Assessment of Learning Disabilities

Test domain	Functional skils
Orientation/attention	Orientation to time, place, setting; attentional functioning (including ability to sustain attention, flexibility in shifting focus of attention, initiating activity, and freedom from distractibility)
Basic sensory functions	Integrity of child's ability to detect information through visual, auditory, sensory, and motor modalities
Modality-specific learning	Ability to analyze and interpret information through individual modalities (e.g., recognition, discrimination, matching, spatial orientation, motor planning)
Cross-modal sensory integration	Ability to synthesize information simultaneously on tasks requiring more than one modality (e.g., visuomotor, visual-auditory)
Higher-level linguistic and phonological skills	Syntactic, morphological, and vocabulary skills, naming, and verbal concept formation
Higher-order cognitive abilities	Memory (long- and short-term storage, retrieval, delayed recall); concept formation; abstract thinking; problem-solving through different sensory modalities; complex linguistic abilities (e.g., verbal absurdities or malapropisms)

Wechsler, 1990) or letter cancellation tests. The "sustain" dimension of attention refers to vigilance, and is typically assessed via a continuous performance test paradigm, such as that included in the Gordon Diagnostic System (Gordon, 1983). Errors of omission on this task are felt to indicate distractibility and poor vigilance, whereas errors of commission are felt to represent impulsivity. The "encode" dimension of attention refers to numerical–mnemonic abilities that are tapped in such tasks as the WISC-III Arithmetic or Digit Span subtests—both requiring sustained attention and ability to manipulate numerical data. Finally, the "shift" dimension of attention is best measured through such tests as the Trailmaking Test from the Halstead–Reitan Neuropsychological Battery for Children (Reitan, 1979), or the Wisconsin Card Sorting Test (Heaton, 1981). For a more detailed discussion of assessment of attention, including observational and behavior rating scale procedures, refer to Culbertson and Krull (1996).

Information Processing through
the Sensory Modalities

Basic sensory functions may be assessed formally through such measures as the Sensory Perceptual Exam from the Halstead–Reitan Neuropsychological Battery for Children (Reitan, 1979) or informally through observation and screening. The important goal is to assess the child's ability to detect information accurately through the visual, auditory, and tactile sensory modalities, as well as to execute simple motor movements. If a child does not seem aware of auditory stimuli, for instance, one must question auditory acuity or a primary auditory sensory deficit. Referral for medical evaluation would be appropriate in this instance, as well as avoiding those test procedures that require processing of information through the auditory sensory modality.

Modality-specific learning tasks are commonly found in psychological tests during the preschool-age range, and involve such functions as recognition, matching, and discrimination of stimuli; spatial orientation; and motor planning skills—each of which is executed primarily through a single sensory modality or motor function. For example, within the visual modality, children might be asked to match a geometric shape such as a triangle to a similar shape that is placed among an array of geometric shapes. Within the auditory modality, children may be asked to tell if two words are the same or different when spoken by the examiner. Motor planning ability may be observed in the child's ability to move through space without stumbling or falling over obstacles, follow directions to compete "dot-to-dot" drawing tasks, or demonstrate skipping by performing a specific sequence of gross motor movements. Spatial orientation may be observed in children's ability to match similar shapes or copy designs in their correct orientation. These modality-specific skills develop from infancy through the preschool years, and prepare the youngster for multimodality learning experiences during the school-age years.

Cross-modality sensory integration abilities are necessary for execution of most academic tasks during the school-age years. For example, the process of reading aloud involves decoding visual information about the identity and sequence of letters in a word, associating these visual symbols with phonetic sounds, and then using speech (oral motor functioning) and language (semantic knowledge) abilities to produce the sounds in the proper sequence for words and sentences to be read. Taking a spelling test requires a child to process auditorily the spoken word, possibly revisualize the spelling of that word, and then translate the auditory and visual information into a motor response by writing the letters in the proper sequence (using tactile–kinesthetic skills). The ability to integrate and synthesize sensory information from multiple modalities parallels development in cortical regions of the brain during the early school years, and provides the foundation for higher levels of thinking and academic learning. Thus, it is important to present the child with tasks during the evaluation that require cross-modality integration and allow one to assess the child's ability in this area.

Higher-Order Abilities

Higher-order cortical functioning is important in mediating the development of complex linguistic and cognitive abilities in children and adolescents. Linguistic functions of older elementary or adolescent youth involve complex syntactic, morphological, and vocabulary skills; verbal concept formation; and ability to recognize verbal absurdities or malapropisms. These functions develop in conjunction with higher-level cognitive abilities involving abstract reasoning, problem-solving abilities, planning and making use of feedback to change one's behavior, mental flexibility and ability to shift cognitive sets, and various aspects of memory (including long- and short-term storage, retrieval by recognition versus reproduction, and delayed recall).

Social–Emotional Functioning

Although not part of the hierarchy of cognitive abilities just discussed, evaluation of social–emotional functioning is a necessary and important component of an assessment for learning disabilities. One must determine if social–emotional adjustment problems are present, and if they are primary (as in a social–emotional learning disability or a primary emotional disorder) or secondary to the primary learning disability. Secondary adjustment problems often are suspected when parents or teachers express concerns about a child's poor self-concept, psychosomatic or other anxiety symptoms related specifically to academic performance, avoidance of school or academic situations, or acting out and disruptive behavior in the classroom environment. A careful history from parents and teachers often can help one tease out the situational context of the child's adjustment problems.

A social–emotional learning disability is suspected when one hears clinical symptoms involving chronic social rejection and isolation, along with poor pragmatic language abilities, awareness of the nonverbal cues of others, social perception of others' reactions to one's own behavior, adaptation to novel situations, and ability to modulate one's own social reactions. These clinical symptoms must then be supplemented by evaluation data that suggest relatively poor arithmetic, tactile and visuospatial, and abstract problem-solving and reasoning abilities. A pattern of relative sensory and motor deficits on the left side of the body compared with the right may also be found. Children suspected of social–emotional learning disability are good candidates for referral for neuropsychological evaluation so that the specific sensory, motor, and tactile–kinesthetic functions can be assessed more thoroughly in the context of left–right comparisons. The neuropsychological examination also can assess the child's problem-solving capabilities with novel stimuli, along with ability to shift cognitive sets and use feedback to guide performance on tasks.

A primary emotional disorder that is comorbid with learning disability may be diagnosed via careful clinical interview of the child and his or her caregivers (parents, teachers, or others), observation of behavior in various contexts, projective evaluation methods, and/or behavioral rating methods.

Attention to the child's adaptive functioning, including pragmatic self-help and daily living skills, also provides information important to understanding the learning-disabled child. A number of excellent parent and/or teacher rating scales (e.g., the Vineland Adaptive Behavior Scales; Sparrow, Balla, & Cicchetti, 1984) are available to the practitioner.

Integration and Interpretation of Assessment Data

The general procedures just discussed suggest to the practitioner that assessment for learning disabilities be conceptualized through the hierarchy of functional abilities as outlined in Table 1. This approach presumes that one chooses tests and procedures for assessment with a theoretical rationale in mind to guide the selection rather than assuming a standard battery approach to assessment (for a more thorough summary of tests that might be used to assess the various functional areas, the reader is referred to Culbertson & Edmonds, 1996). In our clinic, we often begin the assessment with broad cognitive and achievement batteries, each of which is designed to allow the examiner to profile the child's strengths and weaknesses across a variety of functional areas. Because these cognitive and achievement batteries typically require cross-modal integration and use of higher cortical abilities rather than more basic perceptual and single-modality learning abilities, it is important to supplement these tests with more basic measures assessing simpler cognitive functions. For example, one might choose tasks measuring auditory sound–word discrimination, single-word receptive and expressive vocabulary, and auditory analysis (as in sound–symbol association). Visual modality tasks might involve matching and discrimination of visual stimuli, or visual-motor reproduction of shapes and designs with attention to spatial orientation and directionality. Simple sensory tasks might involve two-point discrimination of touch on the skin, or detection and identification of different visual or auditory stimuli. Motor tasks might involve simple motor planning activities such as walking a line, or moving through an obstacle course. The choice of specific measures is determined after examining the profile of the child's strengths and weaknesses on the more general intellectual and achievement batteries, and then exploring those areas in which deficits are suspected. Errors in interpretation are less likely if the practitioner can determine patterns of similar abilities that are deficient rather than relying excessively on any single deficient test score.

It also is necessary to supplement the learning disabilities evaluation with language measures that assess oral language syntax, morphology, word order, and formulation of sentences and stories from both receptive and expressive perspectives. Although the psychological evaluation is not intended to supplant the important role of speech–language pathologists in the assessment of children with learning disabilities, it is increasingly important for psychologists to include linguistic measures in an assessment battery to determine if phonological processing deficits are present in children with learning disabilities. In our clinic, we also take a language sample to provide a means of analyzing these language functions informally.

As recommended by Hynd et al. (1988), the assessment should be designed so that error patterns in reading, math, spelling, and writing performance can be analyzed to determine the clinical subtype of learning disability. This suggests that the practitioner give as much attention to the process by which a child completes an academic task as to the final score on a test. It is also important to consider the potential underlying processes involved in learning within a specific domain, so that further subtyping can occur at that level as well. For instance, does the child with dyscalculia have underlying problems with spatial reasoning and visual-motor integration? Or does a child with dyslexia have poor auditory discrimination for phonetic sounds, and poor sound–symbol association skills? Answering these questions will involve examination of psychological processes that have been associated with learning disabilities in the various academic areas. Given the heterogeneous nature of learning disabilities, it is important to sample a broad range of information processing abilities to develop a profile of the child's strengths and weaknesses that are important for learning.

Once the assessment is complete, test data are integrated through profiling the child's strengths and weaknesses across the various measures, and analyzing the pattern of results along a variety of dimensions, which are not necessarily mutually exclusive. One level of analysis might contrast the child's verbal and nonverbal abilities, whereas another level might analyze the test data from the perspective of single sensory modalities (e.g., visual, auditory, sensory, motor) to determine where strengths and deficits lie. Another level of analysis includes the error analysis of academic performance, which should then be integrated or compared with data on psychological processing abilities. For instance, if one notes that reading and spelling performance reveals a pattern of visual discrimination errors and poor visual memory along with good phonetic decoding skills, this may relate to other test results that suggest poor visual discrimination and memory abilities, difficulty with visual gestalt analysis, but basically good auditory–verbal discrimination and memory skills. Likewise, deficits in written expression often parallel processing deficits in visual-motor integration abilities. This type of analysis allows the examiner to draw parallels between the psychological processing deficit and the explicit academic deficit so that more practical recommendations for intervention can be made to educators.

Finally, test data should be analyzed from the perspective of higher-order cognitive functions involving complex linguistic ability, memory, conceptualization, and problem-solving, as opposed to the more basic perceptual processes that might underlie learning disorders. The case example presented later in this chapter illustrates the process of profiling the child's strengths and weaknesses in information processing to provide the basis for an intervention.

Once test data are analyzed and integrated, one should have a clear picture of the child's general level of cognitive functioning, academic functioning across several specific areas, and whether there is a severe discrepancy between the child's actual and expected academic functioning. This information will allow one to determine the specific clinical subtype of learning disability, if one exists, as manifest in academic functioning. There should be additional information related to the child's basic orientation and attentional abilities, and their effect on learning; single-modality and cross-modality perceptual processing abilities; linguistic functioning both receptively and expressively; and higher-order thinking abilities. This informa-

tion will provide clues as to the psychological processing abilities that might underlie the learning disability, allowing for subtyping along this dimension as well. Finally, information about the child's adaptive, social, and emotional functioning should be available, and this will help one determine if there are primary or secondary emotional adjustment difficulties present, or if there is a social–emotional learning disability. The profiling of the child's strengths and weaknesses along these several dimensions, and the subtyping of the child's learning disability, provide a basis for making specific recommendations for educational intervention.

TREATMENT

Traditionally, interventions for children with learning disabilities have been provided through special education services in the public school systems, as provided for by federal and state legislation that ensures a free and appropriate education to all children, regardless of disability. Children with secondary social–emotional adjustment problems often are referred for psychotherapy or social skills training programs to ameliorate the distress related to the learning disability and/or to teach the child new social skills that will facilitate peer interaction. However, more recently, attention has been given to learning disabilities in a relational context, examining the effects of this disability on the child's relationship with parents, siblings, peers, teachers, and others in the school environment (Culbertson & Silovsky, 1996). The pervasive impact of this disability on the child's self-concept and position within the family, peer group, and school environment is becoming increasingly apparent. Finally, current intervention strategies with children who have learning disabilities must include transition services beyond the high school level to vocational education, job training, or other types of higher education. Each of these aspects of intervention is discussed in turn.

Special Education Interventions

Special education may vary widely in type, quality, and comprehensiveness. The interventions may vary from total inclusion (in which children are placed full time in the mainstream educational environment with special education personnel serving as monitors and providing consultation to the mainstream teachers), to resource labs (in which children spend time in small-group settings with a special education teacher providing specialized instruction), to self-contained special education classrooms (in which children with learning disabilities obtain instruction for all basic academic subjects in the small-group environment with a special education teacher and other children who have similar disabilities), to special schools for children with disabilities (in which all of the children have disabilities and the teachers are trained in special education). These examples of intervention range from the least to the most restrictive educational environments, and the laws governing education of children with disabilities have clearly mandated that children be educated in the least restrictive environment possible. This requires that, once a learning disability is identified, schools demonstrate efforts to educate the child in the least restrictive environment initially. This may entail such efforts as curriculum modifications in the classroom, special seating arrangements, tutoring from a teacher's aide, or allowing additional time to complete assignments. If such efforts are not successful in ameliorating the effects of the child's learning disability on his or her academic performance, then consideration may be given to a more restrictive environment (such as a resource lab) with more specialized instruction methods. Self-contained classrooms are reserved for those children who have multiple subtypes of learning disabilities with severe consequences for their academic achievement. Special schools for children with disabilities are quite rare at present, as most children with disabilities are well integrated into mainstream schools.

Regardless of the setting in which special education services are provided or the intensity of the services, the common ingredient for children with learning disabilities is an Individualized Educational Program (IEP) that sets specific goals and objectives for instruction, determines methods of evaluating the child's progress toward instructional goals, and sets a timeline for reaching the goals. The child's parents participate in developing the IEP, along with teachers, special education professionals, and those involved in assessment and evaluation. The IEP provides the framework for integrating psychological assessment data (regarding the subtyping of the child's learning disability and its underlying processing deficits) with practical recommendations for instruction directed toward remediation or circumventing the effects of the child's learning disability.

Advocates of special education services for children with learning disabilities note that children are the beneficiaries of highly trained teachers who are skilled in using instructional methods that exploit the child's information processing strengths, while circumventing those areas of information processing deficits that impede learning. Special education interventions also target study skills and organization to enhance the child's general learning ability and assist with completion of assignments. More recent trends in special education have focused on students' self-concept and intrinsic motivation for learning; stimulating organizational frameworks for helping students acquire new information or access information already learned; using cognitive modeling and verbal self-instructional strategies; and promoting the development of strategies, competence, maintenance, and generalization of learned material over tasks and settings (Bos & Van Reusen, 1991). Those who favor special education services for children with learning disabilities point to the importance of teaching these children strategies and self-monitoring techniques that will enable them to acquire new learning and develop competence in academic areas well beyond their school years.

Detractors of special education argue that its

benefits are not readily apparent because (1) the efficacy of special instructional methods is inconclusive, (2) most children continue to have learning disabilities regardless of whether special education is provided, and (3) students receiving special education must contend with the stigma of being segregated from the mainstream educational environment or being treated differently from other students. Indeed, the first criticism has some merit based on the educational literature. Research on the efficacy of special education programs has been limited and inconclusive at best (Council for Exceptional Children, 1993; Martin, 1994). The problem of demonstrating which educational strategies are effective for certain subtypes of learning disabilities has been complicated by poor definitions and inconsistent diagnostic procedures for learning disabilities, as well as changing beliefs about the most useful educational strategies. Wagner (1992–1993) recently completed a large-scale study of 8000 high school students that revealed several shortcomings of the present special education system. In this survey, approximately 65% of students with learning disabilities failed at least one class during high school, and over 33% dropped out of school before graduation. This study is countered by others that have provided a more positive picture of the prognosis for students with learning disabilities, with about 50% of these students pursuing some form of postsecondary education (Mithaug, Horiuchi, & Fanning, 1985; Shaw & Shaw, 1989).

The second criticism—related to the chronic nature of learning disabilities despite intervention—is based on the myth that special education should "cure" the disability. This belief is illogical when one considers the genetic and/or neurological bases of learning disabilities and the fact that these biological factors are not likely to disappear with educational intervention. Perhaps it would be better to conceptualize the benefits of special education by examining factors such as the students' use of compensation strategies that help them learn and achieve despite their learning disability, benefits to their self-esteem through better understanding of their learning disabilities, and opportunities for consultation with teachers who are knowledgeable about resources available to help with academic problems.

Those who would point to the stigmatizing effect of special education often neglect to consider the impact of having a learning disability within a mainstream classroom environment, where students are aware of those who have the most difficulty reading or who often fail to complete assignments. The stigma is present with or without special education intervention, and one of the goals of the educational experience for students with learning disabilities is to help them adapt to the knowledge that they have a disability, but nonetheless can achieve despite their disability. Some combination of educational experiences within the mainstream environment and special education resource programs is ideal for most children with learning disabilities to provide opportunities for socialization and interaction with students who do not have disabilities, and also to provide specialized instruction that is individualized for their needs.

Treatment of Secondary Social–Emotional Adjustment Problems and Relational Problems

Children diagnosed with learning disabilities are at risk for developing secondary emotional reactions or relational problems with significant others. They may benefit from interventions designed to provide information about their disability, address their affective responses, and help them move toward adaptation. The most basic intervention involves providing information to the child and his or her family about the definition and cause of learning disabilities, and the possibility for learning and achievement despite the disability. This intervention addresses the cognitive aspect of adaptation to learning disabilities, and should help to eliminate common misperceptions and confusion regarding the child's abilities. It also helps parents to develop more realistic expectations for their child's academic performance.

Another intervention addresses the affective response of parents and children to the diagnosis of learning disability. Children may react affectively in a variety of ways, ranging from relief at finally understanding the reason for their learning problems, to embarrassment at being different from other students or family members, to feelings of anger related to the difficulties caused by the learning disability (Culbertson & Silovsky, 1996). Parents also experience a variety of affective responses that may include grieving (related to the loss of their idealized child) or development of defenses (such as anger, denial) that can interfere with their adaptation to their child's disability. Helping parents understand their affective responses and examine the possible impact on their relationship with their child is an important goal of intervention.

Children who develop defenses such as acting out, withdrawing, clowning, or avoiding academic situations also can be helped to understand the reasons for their behavior, along with more constructive ways of adapting to their learning disability. Often the knowledge that other people understand the reason for their academic problems, and no longer think of them as "lazy" or "stupid," can ameliorate many of the secondary emotional reactions. Family or peer group sessions that openly discuss issues related to having a learning disability can be useful.

Relational issues also must be explored to better understand the impact on the family system when a child has a learning disability. The impact on the child with the disability may be a lower status within the family hierarchy, perhaps related to the child's deficits in communication, learning, or social skills, or perhaps related to others' perceptions of the child as having diminished abilities. Parental responses to the child with a disability can range from extreme concern, overprotection, and enmeshment to shame, anger, and disengagement. These extreme parental responses are rare, but milder forms of these reactions may occur frequently.

Siblings of children with learning disabilities also need attention to their affective responses and cognitive understanding of the disability. Having a sibling with a disability may set up situations in which the sibling feels he or she is receiving less attention than the child with the disability, or it may create embarrassment over having a sibling who has trouble learning. These examples of relational problems need to be explored, with intervention provided in the form of family therapy as needed (Culbertson & Silovsky, 1996).

Vocational and Career Planning

One of the important provisions included in Public Law 101-476, the Individuals with Disabilities Education Act, is the requirement that "transition services" be provided for students with learning disabilities who are age 16 or older. This legislation requires that a statement regarding the student's transition from high school to vocational training, a job, or postsecondary education be included in the IEP (Culbertson & Edmonds, 1996). Teachers assist students with learning disabilities in making applications for vocational training programs or college, including special provisions needed for taking college entrance exams and providing information about colleges that have special programs for students with disabilities. Transition services are an integral part of planning for the student's adult living adjustment following high school, and they increase the chances for positive postsecondary outcome (O'Leary, 1993).

Alternatives to the transition clauses in the IEP include programs provided by Vocational Rehabilitation, including the Job Training Partnership Act youth program. This program provides job training for youth between ages 16 and 21 who are economically disadvantaged, have a disability, exhibit disruptive behavior, or speak limited English as a second language (Culbertson & Edmonds, 1996).

The Rehabilitation Act of 1975 also provided youth and young adults diagnosed with learning disabilities with legal rights to prevent discrimination in training or employment. This Act has also been used to ensure that college students with learning disabilities receive specialized educational services if needed (Gajar, 1992). Specialized services at the college level are becoming more numerous as students with learning disabilities increasingly seek higher education. Yet, the quality and nature of these services are largely unknown at present, and the field is in need of strong empirical research to document the types of services that are needed and those that are most effective (Mangrum & Strichart, 1988).

CASE STUDY

History and Review of Records

Shane is an 8-year-old boy who is now in first grade and presents with complaints of attention deficit and chronic problems with academic achievement. School history reveals that he attended a structured preschool program beginning at age 3, and was held back from starting kindergarten for 1 year because of his mother's concern about his "immaturity" (this is a frequent descriptor used with children who have learning disabilities and/or attentional disorders in the early grades). Despite having 5 years of structured learning experiences to date, Shane continues to function below grade level in mathematics, reading comprehension, and written expression.

Review of early history reveals that Shane was adopted at birth, and has lived with his adoptive family since that time. There is a younger sister in the family who also is adopted, and the family has provided much enrichment in the form of educational opportunities for Shane. It was reported that his biological mother drank socially (about four or five drinks per week) throughout pregnancy, with occasional binges (five or more drinks per occasion) during the first trimester. Delivery was by Cesarean section following a prolonged labor and failure to progress because of cephalopelvic disproportion. At the time of delivery, Shane had difficulty with respiration and needed to be resuscitated. He responded well, and within five minutes was breathing normally and crying vigorously. There was a suspicion of mild anoxia (or lack of oxygen) during the delivery process, but no other perinatal complications were reported. Shane's developmental history was remarkable for mild delays in motor milestones, with sitting independently at 8 months, crawling at 10 months, and walking independently at 17 months. Speech and language development were complicated by frequent ear infections (serous otitis media) during the first 2 years of life, with intermittent conductive hearing loss secondary to fluid in the ear canals. However, once the ear infections resolved, his language development progressed rapidly with no further problems. Shane had annual audiological evaluations because of his prior history of conductive hearing loss, but his auditory acuity has been normal for the past several years. Likewise, his visual acuity was found to be normal during a school screening 2 months prior to the current examination.

The history obtained thus far reveals a failure to achieve in at least three areas of academic learning, but rules out educational and sociocultural disadvantage as explanations for Shane's poor academic functioning. In addition, Shane's medical history reveals several risk factors that could be related to his present academic problems: prenatal exposure to alcohol during periods of rapid central nervous system development; a possible anoxic episode associated with delivery, suggesting the possibility of a brain insult that could have some bearing on his current problems; and the history of chronic ear infections with conductive hearing loss that placed him at risk for delays in speech–language development and auditory processing abilities.

Formal Assessment

Orientation and Attention

On beginning the formal evaluation, Shane's orientation and motivation were excellent. However, he required frequent redirection to the tasks as the evaluation progressed because of his distractibility and difficulty sustaining attentional focus. His response style was impulsive, in that he often began a task before the instructions were completed, or tried to answer before questions were fully stated. He fidgeted constantly and talked excessively throughout the assessment.

Basic Sensory and Motor Functioning

Shane appeared to understand instructions presented orally, and made good use of visual cues in the test materials, so that he appeared to be stimulable through both the auditory and visual modalities. His motor skills appeared to be slow and poorly coordinated, particularly when using a pencil, and he required additional time to complete all tasks that were written.

Lateral dominance examination revealed a strong preference for right hand, eye, and foot. Motor screening revealed deficient coordination on the nondominant left side compared with normal performance on the right, as evidenced on measures of fine motor speed and dexterity (e.g., finger tapping and pegboard tasks). Cerebellar screening tasks such as finger-to-nose and rapid alternating movements were slow and poorly executed bilaterally. Thus, concerns are evident in gross and fine motor dexterity, particularly on the left side.

General Intellectual and Academic Functioning

On initial cognitive assessment with the WISC-III (Wechsler, 1990), Shane's performance overall was within the borderline range with a Full Scale IQ of 77 (6th percentile). His Verbal IQ of 88 (21st percentile) was within the low average range and his Performance IQ of 71 (3rd percentile) was within the borderline range. These summary scores belied the significant variability among subtest scores. Shane's Verbal Comprehension Index of 95 was within the average range, and reflected average verbal association, vocabulary, and general knowledge abilities. His Perceptual Organization Index of 79 was in the borderline range, and reflected difficulty with such abilities as visuospatial reasoning and construction, awareness of pictorial detail, and sequential arrangement of pictures. Significant deficits were noted on measures that were sensitive to his distractibility (Freedom from Distractibility Index 69) and processing speed (Index 67).

Assessment of academic functioning using the Wechsler Individual Achievement Test (WIAT, 1992) revealed a significant discrepancy between his actual and predicted achievement level in the areas of mathematics reasoning (standard score [SS] 70), numerical operations (SS 65), and written expression (SS 79). His basic reading and reading comprehension scores were congruent with his predicted achievement level, as were spelling, oral expression, and listening comprehension.

Assessment of Modality-Specific and Cross-Modal Sensory Information

Assessment of sensory processing abilities was done to determine factors that might underlie Shane's learning disability in the areas of mathematics reasoning, numerical operations, and written expression. Assessment of phonological processing abilities was accomplished with measures of naming (Expressive One-Word Picture Vocabulary Test; Gardner, 1990), fluency (when asked to generate words that begin with "f," "a," and "s"), and auditory discrimination of similar words (Wepman Auditory Discrimination Test). Shane performed within the average range (25th to 50 percentiles) on these measures of phonological processing, suggesting intact abilities.

Processing of information through the visual modality was assessed through examination of Shane's performance on specific subtests of the WISC-III such as Block Design and Object Assembly (both of which were below average with scaled scores of 6). Cross-modality processing was examined through visual-motor measures such as the Bender Gestalt Test for Young Children (Koppitz, 1975) and the Developmental Test of Visual-Motor Integration (Beery, 1982). Shane performed below average on the Bender with numerous errors of distortion, rotation, and integration, suggesting spatial organization deficits. His Visual-Motor Integration Test score was in the borderline range, but revealed developmental errors and lack of precision in reproduction of geometric shapes and designs. Shane's visual-motor integration abilities were generally deficient relative to his average phonological processing and language abilities.

Measures of information processing speed (Coding, Symbol Search) from the WISC-III revealed that Shane's abilities are deficient for his age.

Assessment of Higher-Order Cognitive Abilities

Shane's memory and learning abilities were assessed with the Wide Range Assessment of Memory and Learning (Sheslow & Adams, 1990). His performance paralleled that of the WISC-III with a significant discrepancy between his average Verbal Memory Index of 100 and his borderline Visual Memory Index of 76. Delayed memory was adequate within both modalities, but mirrored the performance on the immediate memory tasks. Other measures of reasoning and problem-solving ability were obtained from the WISC-III, and suggested generally good verbal reasoning with the exception of arithmetic reasoning abilities, but deficient performance on measures of nonverbal and visuospatial reasoning (such as Picture Arrangement, Block Design, Object Assembly).

Assessment of Social–Emotional Functioning

Clinical interview with Shane's parents revealed that Shane is a very fearful child, who is felt to have excessive fears of clowns, animals, and thunderstorms. He has always had difficulty tolerating new situations or people, or unexpected changes in routine. He has great difficulty remembering the family rules (e.g., remembering not to interrupt when others are talking, and not to take food into the living room). He talks excessively, intrudes on the activities of others, and continually violates others' personal space. He touches inappropriately by clinging to adults, and frequently hugging his peers, much to their annoyment. He never seems to understand jokes, and he laughs inappropriately before the punch line. He also has difficulty understanding the rules of games on the playground, and is rarely chosen to participate in games with peers at school. His mother reported that disciplining Shane is difficult, because she is unsure if he really understands what is expected of him. He is genuinely remorseful when he breaks a rule or makes others unhappy with him, but he seems unable to anticipate others' reactions in time to change his behavior.

Behavioral observations revealed that Shane talked excessively during the evaluation, and did not pick up on nonverbal cues that his talking was inappropriate. Only clear verbal reminders to stop talking and listen to the instructions were heeded, but were soon forgotten as Shane again began talking. He tended to perseverate on a few topics to excess, and he spoke with a monotonic vocal quality while moving about the room. He made fleeting eye contact, hugged the examiner often, but often stepped on the examiner's toes or kicked the examiner under the table without seeming to be aware of his actions. Shane stated that he does not like school because other kids won't play with him.

Integration and Interpretation of Data

Shane's test scores were profiled to illustrate his strengths and weaknesses in cognitive, academic, information processing, and higher cortical functioning, as seen in Figure 1. This profile reveals average verbal cognitive abilities and information processing through the auditory modality, and average verbal memory abilities. His basic reading, reading comprehension, and spelling skills are all congruent with these average abilities. However, Shane has a severe discrepancy between expected and actual achievement in the areas of numerical operations (mathematics computation), mathematics reasoning, and written expression. These academic deficits are likely associated with deficits in visuospatial reasoning, visual-motor integration, and basic fine motor and gross motor skills. The pattern of poorer sensory and motor functioning on the left side compared with the right suggests the possibility of right hemisphere dysfunction. Thus, Shane is felt to have a learning disability involving the clinical subtypes of dyscalculia and dysgraphia, with underlying visuospatial and visual-motor processing deficits. In addition, he exhibits characteristics of a social–emotional learning disability as reflected in his poor social perception, and poor social interaction and pragmatic communication abilities.

Intervention strategies for school involved learning disability resource lab services for two periods per day to address mathematics reasoning and calculation, visuospatial and visual-motor abilities, social interactive skills, and writing. In addition, curriculum modifications were made to address the effects of Shane's dysgraphia in the classroom by abbreviating written assignments, allowing additional time for completion of these assignments, and allowing Shane to take tests orally at times. He also was given access to a computer daily so that he could begin learning keyboard skills to facilitate his written expression. To address the social–emotional concerns, Shane and his family participated in several sessions designed to increase the parents' understanding of the reasons for Shane's disregard of rules

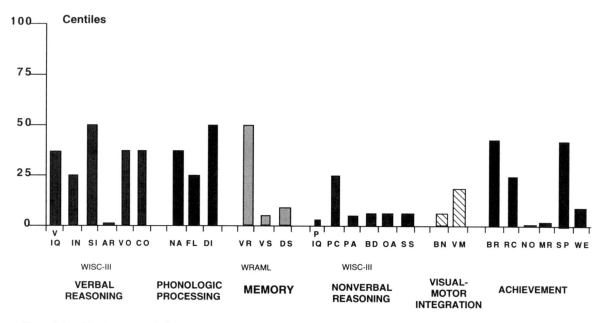

Figure 1. Profile of neuropsychological test results for Shane. VIQ = Wechsler Intelligence Scale for Children: Third Edition (WISC-III) Verbal IQ; IN = WISC-III Information subtest; SI = WISC-III Similarities subtest; AR = WISC-III Arithmetic subtest; VO = WISC-III Vocabulary subtest; CO = WISC-III Comprehension subtest; NA = Expressive One-Word Picture Vocabulary Test; FL = Controlled Oral Word Fluency Test; DI = Wepman Auditory Discrimination Test; VR = Wide Range Assessment of Memory and Learning (WRAML) Verbal Memory Index; VS = WRAML Visual Memory Index; DS = WISC-III Digit Span subtest; PIQ = WISC-III Performance IQ; PC = WISC-III Picture Completion subtest; PA = WISC-III Picture Arrangement subtest; BD = WISC-III block design subtest; OA = WISC-III Object Assembly subtest; SS = WISC-III Symbol Search subtest; BN = Bender Gestalt Test for Young Children; VM = Developmental Test of Visual-Motor Integration; BR = Wechsler Individual Achievement Test (WIAT) Basic Reading subtest; RC = WIAT Reading Comprehension subtest; NO = WIAT Numerical Operations subtest; MR = WIAT Mathematics Reasoning subtest; SP = WIAT Spelling subtest; WE = WIAT Written Expression subtest.

and the persistence of annoying behavior. The sessions also focused on strategies for increasing Shane's self-monitoring of his own social behavior by urging his parents to translate nonverbal social rules and cues into words so that this information could be processed more easily by Shane. They participated in role-play situations with Shane, and devised positive incentive programs for helping Shane remember rules of positive social interaction. Although Shane continued to have difficulty generalizing these rules to new settings (such as the playground at recess), his teachers also participated in the social skills training and this facilitated his behavior at school.

SUMMARY

This chapter has provided an overview of the historical evolution of the field of learning dis-abilities, its clinical features, subtypes, epidemiology, and etiology. Controversies regarding the definition and diagnostic criteria for this disorder have been discussed, along with suggestions for assessment and intervention. The foregoing in many ways raises questions that are yet to be answered empirically—with regard to stable patterns of subtypes, a better understanding of the underlying processing deficits related to subtypes of learning disabilities, and most importantly, effective interventions that are associated with the various subtypes. If the next decade is as productive as the last, many of these questions will undoubtedly be answered.

REFERENCES

Aaron, P. G., & Simurdak, J. (1991). Reading disorders: Their nature and diagnosis. In J. E. Obrzut & G. W. Hynd (Eds.), *Neuropsychological foundations of learning disabilities* (pp. 513–548). San Diego, CA: Academic Press.

Adelman, H. S., & Taylor, L. (1986). The problems of definition and differentiation and the need for a classification system. *Journal of Learning Disabilities, 19,* 514–520.

Algozzine, B., & Ysseldyke, J. (1986). The future of the LD field: Screening and diagnosis. *Journal of Learning Disabilities, 19,* 394–398.

Ardila, A., Rosselli, M., & Ostrosky-Solis, F. (1992). Socioeducational. In A. E. Puente & R. J. McCaffrey (Eds.), *Handbook of neuropsychological assessment: A biopsychosocial perspective* (pp. 181–192). New York: Plenum Press.

Association for Children and Adults with Learning Disabilities. (1985). ACLD offers new definition. *Special Education Today, 2,* 19.

August, G. J., & Holmes, C. S. (1984). Behavior and academic achievement in hyperactive subgroups and learning-disabled boys. *American Journal of Diseases of Children, 138,* 1025–1029.

Bakker, D. J. (1979). Hemispheric differences and reading strategies: Two dyslexias? *Bulletin of the Orton Society, 29,* 84–100.

Bakker, D. J., & Vinke, J. (1985). Effects of hemisphere-specific stimulation on brain activity and reading in dyslexics. *Journal of Clinical and Experimental Neuropsychology, 7,* 503–525.

Ballard, J., Ramirez, B. A., & Zantal-Weiner, K. (1987). *Public Law 94-142, Section 504, and Public Law 99-457: Understanding what they are and are not.* Reston, VA: Council for Exceptional Children.

Barkley, R. A. (1990). *Attention deficit hyperactivity disorder.* New York: Guilford Press.

Batchelor, E. S., Gray, J. W., & Dean, R. S. (1990). Empirical testing of a cognitive model to account for neuropsychological functioning underlying arithmetic problem solving. *Journal of Learning Disabilities, 23,* 38–42.

Beery, K. E. (1982). *Revised administration, scoring, and teaching manual for the Developmental Test of Visual Motor Integration.* Cleveland, OH: Modern Curriculum Press.

Benton, A. L. (1975). Developmental dyslexia: Neurological aspects. In W. J. Friedlander (Ed.), *Advances in neurology.* (Vol. 7, pp. 1–47). New York: Raven Press.

Berninger, V. W., & Hooper, S. R. (1993). Preventing and remediating writing disabilities: Interdisciplinary frameworks for assessment, consultation, and intervention. *School Psychology Review, 22*(4), 590–594.

Bernstein, B. (1974). Language and roles. In R. Huxley & E. Ingram (Eds.), *Language acquisition: Models and methods* (pp. 67–72). New York: Academic Press.

Bigler, E. D. (1992). The neurobiology and neuropsychology of adult learning disorders. *Journal of Learning Disabilities, 25*(8), 488–506.

Birch, H. G., & Belmont, L. (1964). Auditory-visual integration in normal and retarded readers. *American Journal of Orthopsychiatry, 34,* 852–861.

Birch, H. G., & Belmont, L. (1965). Auditory-visual integration, intelligence, and reading ability in school children. *Perceptual and Motor Skills, 20,* 295–305.

Boder, E. (1973). Developmental dyslexia: A diagnostic approach based on three atypical reading–spelling patterns. *Developmental Medicine and Child Neurology, 15,* 663–687.

Bos, C. S., & Van Reusen, A. K. (1991). Academic interventions with learning-disabled students. In J. E. Obrzut & G. W. Hynd (Eds.), *Neuropsychological foundations of learning disabilities: A handbook of issues, methods, and practices* (pp. 659–683). San Diego, CA: Academic Press.

Braden, J. P. (1987). A comparison of regression and standard score discrepancy methods for learning disabilities identification: Effects on racial representation. *Journal of School Psychology, 25,* 23–29.

Brislin, R. W. (1983). Cross-cultural research in psychology. *Annual Review of Psychology, 34,* 363–400.

Bryan, T., Bay, M., & Donahue, M. (1988). Implications of the learning disabilities definition for the regular education initiative. *Journal of Learning Disabilities, 21,* 23–28.

Bryan, T., Wheeler, R., Felcan, J., & Henck, T. (1976). "Come on, Dummy": An observational study of children's communication. *Journal of Learning Disabilities, 9,* 53–61.

Bryden, M. P. (1988). Does laterality make any difference? Thoughts on the relation between cerebral asymmetry and reading. In D. L. Molfese & S. J. Segalowitz (Eds.), *Brain lateralization in children: Developmental implications* (pp. 509–525). New York: Guilford Press.

Carpenter, R. L. (1985). Mathematics instruction in resource rooms: Instruction time and teacher competence. *Learning Disability Quarterly, 8,* 95–100.

Chalfant, J. C. (1984). *Identifying learning disabled students: Guidelines for decision-making.* Burlington, VT: Northeast Regional Resource Center.

Chalfant, J. C., & Scheffelin, M. A. (1969). *Central processing dysfunction in children: A review of research* (NINDS Monograph No. 9). Bethesda, MD: U.S. Department of Health, Education, and Welfare.

Corballis, M. C., & Beale, I. L. (1976). *The psychology of right and left.* Mahwah, NJ: Erlbaum.

Cornwall, A. (1992). The relationship of phonological awareness, rapid naming, and verbal memory to severe reading and spelling disability. *Journal of Learning Disabilities, 25,* 532–538.

Council for Exceptional Children. (1993). *Inclusion: What does it mean for students with learning disabilities?* Reston, VA: Division for Learning Disabilities.

Culbertson, J. L., & Edmonds, J. E. (1996). Learning disabilities. In R. L. Adams, O. A. Parsons, J. L. Culbertson, & S. J. Nixon, *Neuropsychology for clinical practice: Etiology, assessment, and treatment of common neurological disorders* (pp. 331–408). Washington, DC: American Psychological Association.

Culbertson, J. L., & Krull, K. R. (1996). Attention deficit hyperactivity disorder. In R. L. Adams, O. A. Parsons, J. L. Culbertson, & S. J. Nixon, *Neuropsychology for clinical practice: Etiology, assessment, and treatment of common neurological disorders* (pp. 271–330). Washington, DC: American Psychological Association.

Culbertson, J. L., & Silovsky, J. F. (1996). Learning disabilities and attention deficit hyperactivity disorder: Their impact on children's significant others. In F. W. Kaslow (Ed.), *Handbook of relational diagnosis and dysfunctional family patterns* (pp. 186–209). New York: Wiley.

Decker, S. N., & Vandenberg, S. G. (1985). Colorado twin study of reading disability. In D. B. Gray & J. F. Kavanagh (Eds.), *Biobehavioral measures of dyslexia* (pp. 123–135). Parkton, MD: York Press.

DeFries, J. C. (1985). Colorado Reading Project. In D. B. Gray & J. F. Kavanagh (Eds.), *Biobehavioral measures of dyslexia* (pp. 107–122). Parkton, MD: York Press.

de Hirsch, K., Jansky, J., & Langford, W. (1966). *Predicting reading failure.* New York: Harper & Row.

Denckla, M. B. (1983). The neuropsychology of social-emotional learning disability. *Archives of Neurology, 40,* 461–462.

Denckla, M. B. (1989). Social learning disabilities. *International Pediatrics, 4,* 133–136.

Denckla, M. B. (1991). Attention deficit hyperactivity disorder: Residual type. *Journal of Child Neurology, 6*(Suppl.), S44–S50.

DeStefano, L., & Snauwaert, D. (1989). *A value-critical approach to transition policy analysis.* Champaign: University of Illinois, Secondary Transition Intervention Effectiveness Institute. (Available from College of Education, University of Illinois at Urbana–Champaign, 110 Education Bldg., 1310 S. 6th Street, Champaign, IL 61820.)

Donahue, M., & Bryan, T. (1984). Communication skills and peer relations of learning disabled adolescents. *Topics in Language Disorders, 4,* 10–21.

Duane, D. D. (1991). Biological foundations of learning disabilities. In J. E. Obrzut & G. W. Hynd (Eds.), *Neuropsychological foundations of learning disabilities* (pp. 7–27). San Diego, CA: Academic Press.

Education of the Handicapped Act. (1975). 20 U.S.C. Sections 1400–1485.

Fisher, J. H. (1905). Case of congenital word-blindness (inability to learn to read). *Ophthalmic Review, 24,* 315–318.

Flicek, M., & Landau, S. (1985). Social status problems of learning disabled and hyperactive/learning disabled boys. *Journal of Clinical Child Psychology, 14,* 340–344.

Frostig, M. (1964). *Frostig Developmental Test of Visual Perception.* Palo Alto, CA: Consulting Psychologists Press.

Gaddes, W. H., & Edgell, D. (1993). *Learning disabilities and brain function,* 3rd ed. New York: Springer-Verlag.

Gajar, A. (1992). Adults with learning disabilities: Current and future research priorities. *Journal of Learning Disabilities, 25*(8), 507–519.

Galaburda, A. M. (1993). Neurology of developmental dyslexia. *Current Opinion in Neurology, 3,* 237–242.

Galaburda, A., & Livingstone, M. (1993). Evidence for a magnocellular defect in developmental dyslexia. *Annals of the New York Academy of Sciences, 682,* 70–82.

Gardner, M. F. (1990). *Expressive One-Word Picture Vocabulary Test-Revised.* Novato, CA: Academic Therapy Publications.

Geschwind, N., & Behan, P. (1982). Left-handedness: Association with immune disease, migraine, and developmental learning disorder. *Proceedings of the National Academy of Sciences, USA 79,* 5097–5100.

Geschwind, N., & Galaburda, A. M. (1985). Cerebral lateralization: Biological mechanisms, association and pathology. *Archives of Neurology, 42,* 428–459.

Geschwind, N., & Levitsky, W. (1968). Human brain: Left–right asymmetries in temporal speech region. *Science, 161,* 186–187.

Gordon, M. (1983). *The Gordon Diagnostic System.* Boulder, CO: Clinical Diagnostic Systems.

Gross-Glenn, K., Duara, R., Barker, W., Loewenstein, D., Chang, J., Yoshii, F., Apicella, A. M., Pascal, S., Boothe, T., Sevush, S., Jallard, B. J., Novoa, L., & Lubs, H. (1991). Position emission tomographic studies during serial word-reading by normal dyslexia adults. *Journal of Clinical and Experimental Neuropsychology, 13,* 531–544.

Hallgren, B. (1950). Specific dyslexia (congenital word blindness): A clinical and genetic study. *Acta Psychiatrica et Neurologica Scandinavica, 65*(Suppl.), 1–287.

Halperin, J. M., Gittelman, R., Klein, D. F., & Rudel, R. G. (1984). Reading-disabled hyperactive children: A distinct subgroup of attention deficit disorder with hyperactivity? *Journal of Abnormal Child Psychology, 12,* 1–14.

Hammill, D. D., Leigh, J. E., McNutt, G., & Larsen, S. C. (1981). A new definition of learning disabilities. *Learning Disability Quarterly, 4,* 336–342.

Hardyck, C., Petrinovitch, C. F., & Goldman, R. (1976). Left-handedness and cognitive deficit. *Cortex, 12,* 266–278.

Heath, C. P., & Kush, J. C. (1991). Use of discrepancy formulas in the assessment of learning disabilities. In J. E. Obrzut & G. W. Hynd (Eds.), *Neuropsychological foundations of learning disabilities* (pp. 287–307). San Diego, CA: Academic Press.

Heaton, R. K. (1981). *A manual for the Wisconsin Card Sorting Test.* Odessa, FL: Psychological Assessment Resources.

Hier, D. B., LeMay, M., Rosenberg, P. B., & Perlo, V. P. (1978). Developmental dyslexia: Evidence for a subgroup with reverse asymmetry. *Archives of Neurology, 35,* 90–92.

Hinshelwood, J. (1895). Word-blindness and visual memory. *Lancet, 1,* 1506–1508.

Hinshelwood, J. (1900). Congenital word-blindness. *Lancet, 2,* 1564–1570.

Hinshelwood, J. (1902). Congenital word-blindness, with reports of two cases. *Ophthalmic Review, 21,* 91–99.

Hooper, S. R. (1988). The prediction of learning disabilities in the preschool child. In M. G. Tramontana & S. R. Hooper (Eds.), *Assessment issues in child neuropsychology* (pp. 313–335). New York: Plenum Press.

Hooper, S. R., & Willis, W. G. (1989). *Learning disability subtyping: Neuropsychological foundations, conceptual models, and issues in clinical differentiation.* Berlin: Springer-Verlag.

Horn, W. F., & Packard, T. (1985). Early identification of learning problems: A meta-analysis. *Journal of Educational Psychology, 77,* 597–607.

Humphreys, P., Kaufman, W. E., & Galaburda, A. M. (1990). Developmental dyslexia in women: Neuropathological findings in three cases. *Annals of Neurology, 28,* 727–738.

Humphreys, P., Rosen, G. D., Press, D. M., Sherman, G. F., & Galaburda, A. M. (1991). Freezing lesions of the developing rat brain: I. A model for cerebral cortical microgyria. *Journal of Neuropathology and Experimental Neurology, 50,* 145–160.

Hynd, G. W., & Cohen, M. (1983). *Dyslexia: Neuropsychological theory, research, and clinical differentiation.* New York: Grune & Stratton.

Hynd, G. W., Connor, R. T., & Nieves, N. (1988). Learning disability subtypes: Perspectives and methodological issues in clinical assessment. In M. G. Tramontana & S. R. Hooper (Eds.), *Assessment issues in child neuropsychology* (pp. 281–312). New York: Plenum Press.

Hynd, G. W., Hall, J., Novey, E. S., Eliopulos, D., Black, K., Gonzalez, J. J., Edmonds, J. E., Riccio, C., & Cohen, M. (1995). Dyslexia and corpus callosum morphology. *Archives of Neurology, 52,* 32–38.

Hynd, G. W., Semrud-Clikeman, M., Lorys, A. R., Novey, E. S., & Eliopulos, D. (1990). Brain morphology in developmental dyslexia and attention deficit disorder/ hyperactivity. *Archives of Neurology, 47,* 919–926.

Interagency Committee on Learning Disabilities. (1987). *Learning disabilities: A report to the U.S. Congress.* Washington, DC: Author.

Jansky, J. J., & de Hirsch, K. (1972). *Preventing reading failure—Prediction, diagnosis, intervention.* New York: Harper & Row.

Johnson, D. J. (1993). Relationships between oral and written language. *School Psychology Review, 22*(4), 595–609.

Johnson, D. J., & Myklebust, H. R. (1967). Nonverbal disorders of learning. In D. J. Johnson & H. R. Myklebust (Eds.), *Learning disabilities: Educational principles and practices* (pp. 272–306). New York: Grune & Stratton.

Kaufman, A. S., & Kaufman, N. L. (1983). *Kaufman Assessment Battery for Children: Interpretive manual.* Circle Pines, MN: American Guidance Service.

Kaufman, A. S., & Kaufman, N. L. (1985). *Kaufman Test of Educational Achievement.* Circle Pines, MN: American Guidance Service.

Kaufman, A. S., Zalma, R., & Kaufman, N. L. (1978). The relationship of hand dominance to the motor coordination, mental ability, and right–left awareness of young normal children. *Child Development, 49,* 885–888.

Keller, C. E., & Sutton, J. P. (1991). Specific mathematics disorders. In J. E. Obrzut & G. W. Hynd (Eds.), *Neuropsychological foundations of learning disabilities* (pp. 549–571). San Diego, CA: Academic Press.

Kephart, N. C. (1971). *The slow learner in the classroom* (2nd ed.). Columbus, OH: Charles E. Merrill.

Kintsch, W., & Kozminsky, E. (1977). Summarizing stories after reading and listening. *Journal of Educational Psychology, 69,* 491–499.

Kirk, S. A. (1963). Behavioral diagnosis and remediation of learning disabilities. In *Proceedings of the conference on exploration into the problems of the perceptually handicapped child.* Evanston, IL: Fund for the Perceptually Handicapped Child.

Koppitz, E. M. (1975). *The Bender Gestalt Test for Young Children.* New York: Grune & Stratton.

Kosc, L. (1974). Developmental dyscalculia. *Journal of Learning Disabilities, 7,* 164–177.

Kussmaul, A. (1877). Disturbance of speech. *Cyclopedia of Practical Medicine, 14,* 581.

Laboratory for Comparative Human Cognition. (1983). Culture and cognitive development. In P. Mussen (Ed.), *Handbook of child psychology* (Vol. 1, pp. 342–397). New York: Wiley.

LaGreca, A. M. (1981). Social behavior and social perception in learning-disabled children: A review with implication for social skills training. *Journal of Pediatric Psychology, 6,* 395–416.

Larsen, J. P., Høien, T., Lundberg, I., & Ødegaard, H. (1990). MRI evaluation of the size and symmetry of the planum temporale in adolescents with developmental dyslexia. *Brain and Language, 39,* 289–301.

Leong, C. K. (1989). Neuropsychological models of learning disabilities. In C. R. Reynolds & E. Fletcher-Janzen (Eds.), *Handbook of clinical child neuropsychology* (pp. 335–351). New York: Plenum Press.

Lieberman, I. Y., & Shankweiler, D. (1985). Phonology and the problem of learning to read and write. *Remedial and Special Education, 6,* 41–55.

Lovett, M. W. (1984). A developmental perspective on reading dysfunction: Accuracy and rate criteria in the subtyping of dyslexic children. *Brain and Language, 22,* 67–91.

Lovett, M. W. (1987). A developmental approach to reading disability: Accuracy and speed criteria of normal and deficient reading skill. *Child Development, 58,* 234–260.

Lubs, H. A., Rabin, M., Carland-Saucier, K., Wen, X. L., Gross-Glenn, K., Duara, R., Levin, B., & Lubs, M. L. (1991). Genetic bases of developmental dyslexia: Molecular studies. In J. E. Obrzut & G. W. Hynd (Eds.), *Neuropsychological foundations of learning disabilities* (pp. 49–77). San Diego, CA: Academic Press.

Luria, A. R. (1980). *Higher cortical functions in man* (2nd ed.). New York: Basic Books.

Lyle, J. G., & Goyen, J. (1968). Visual recognition, developmental lag and strephosymbolia in reading retardation. *Journal of Abnormal Psychology, 73,* 25–29.

Lyle, J. G., & Goyen, J. (1975). Effects of speed exposure and difficulty of discrimination in visual recognition of retarded readers. *Journal of Abnormal Psychology, 8,* 613–616.

Mangrum, C. T., & Strichart, S. S. (1988). *College and the learning disabled student.* Orlando, FL: Grune & Stratton.

Markoski, B. D. (1983). Conversational interactions of the learning disabled and nondisabled child. *Journal of Learning Disabilities, 16,* 606–609.

Martin, E. W. (1994, April). Inclusion: Rhetoric and reality. *Exceptional Parent,* pp. 39–42.

Mattis, S., Erenberg, G., & French, J. H. (1978, February). *Dyslexia syndromes: A cross validation study.* Paper presented at the sixth annual meeting of the International Neuropsychological Society, Minneapolis, MN.

Mattis, S., French, J. H., & Rapin, I. (1975). Dyslexia in children and young adults: Three independent neuropsychological syndromes. *Developmental Medicine and Child Neurology, 17,* 150–163.

McKeever, W. F., & Van Deventer, A. D. (1975). Dyslexic adolescents: Evidence of impaired visual and auditory language processing. *Cortex, 11,* 361–378.

McLeod, T. M., & Armstrong, S. W. (1982). Learning disabilities in mathematics—skill deficits and remedial approaches at the intermediate and secondary level. *Learning Disability Quarterly, 5,* 305–311.

McManus, I. C., & Bryden, M. P. (1991). Geschwind's theory of lateralization: Developing a formal causal model. *Psychological Bulletin, 110,* 237–253.

Mills v. Board of Education of the District of Columbia, 348 F. Supp. 866 (D.D.C. 1972).

Mirsky, A. F. (1989). The neuropsychology of attention: Elements of a complex behavior. In E. Perecman (Ed.), *Integrating theory and practice in clinical neuropsychology* (pp. 75–91). Hillsdale, NJ: Erlbaum.

Mithaug, D., Horiuchi, C., & Fanning, P. (1985). A report on the Colorado statewide follow-up survey of special education students. *Exceptional Children, 51,* 397–404.

Morgan, W. P. (1896). A case of congenital word-blindness. *British Medical Journal, 2,* 1978.

Myklebust, H. R. (1965). *Development and disorders of written language* (Vol. 1). New York: Grune & Stratton.

Nass, R. (1992). Developmental dyslexia: An update. *Pediatrics in Review, 13*(6), 231–235.

National Information Center for Children and Youth with Disabilities [NICHCY]. (1991). The education of children and youth with special needs: What do the laws say? *NICHCY News Digest, 1*(1), 1–13.

Norman, C. A., & Zigmond, N. (1980). Characteristics of children labeled and served as learning disabled in school systems affiliated with Child Service Demonstration Centers. *Journal of Learning Disabilities, 13,* 542–547.

Novick, B. Z., & Arnold, M. M. (1988). *Fundamentals of clinical child neuropsychology.* New York: Grune & Stratton.

Obrzut, J. E. (1988). Deficient lateralization in learning-disabled children: Developmental lag or abnormal cerebral organization? In D. L. Molfese & S. J. Segalowitz (Eds.), *Brain lateralization in children: Developmental implications* (pp. 567–589). New York: Guilford Press.

Obrzut, J. E., Hynd, G. W., & Boliek, C. A. (1986). Lateralized asymmetries in learning-disabled children's processing. In S. J. Ceci (Ed.), *Handbook of cognitive, social, and neuropsychological aspects of learning disability* (pp. 441–474). Mahwah, NJ: Erlbaum.

O'Hare, A. E., & Brown, J. K. (1989a). Childhood dysgraphia. Part I. An illustrated clinical classification. *Child: Care, Health, and Development, 15,* 79–104.

O'Hare, A. E., & Brown, J. K. (1989b). Childhood dysgraphia. Part 2. A study of hand function. *Child: Care, Health, and Development, 15,* 151–166.

O'Hare, A. E., Brown, J. K., & Aitken, K. (1991). Dyscalculia in children. *Developmental Medicine and Child Neurology, 33,* 356–361.

O'Leary, E. (1993). Transition services and IDEA: Issues for states and local programs. *South Atlantic Regional Resource Center Newsletter, 2,* 1–11.

Omenn, G. S., & Weber, B. A. (1978). Dyslexia: Search for phenotypic and genetic heterogeneity. *American Journal of Medical Genetics, 1,* 333–342.

Orton, S. T. (1928). Specific reading disability—strephosymbolia. *Journal of the American Medical Association, 90,* 1095–1099.

Orton, S. T. (1937). *Reading, writing, and speech problems in children.* New York: Norton.

Pennington, B. F., Gilger, J. W., Pauls, D., Smith, S. A., Smith, S. D., & DeFries, J. C. (1991). Evidence for major gene transmission of developmental dyslexia. *Journal of the American Medical Association, 266,* 1527–1534.

Pennington, B. F., & Smith, S. D. (1983). Genetic influences on learning disabilities and speech and language disorders. *Child Development, 54,* 369–387.

Pennsylvania Association for Retarded Citizens v. Commonwealth of Pennsylvania, 334 F. Supp. 1257 (E.D. Pa. 1972), Consent Agreement.

Petrauskas, R., & Rourke, B. (1979). Identification of subgroups of retarded readers: A neuropsychological multivariate approach. *Journal of Clinical Neuropsychology, 1,* 17–37.

Rehabilitation Act of 1973, 29 U.S.C. Section 701–794.

Reitan, R. M. (1979). *Manual for administration of neuropsychological tests for adults and children.* Tucson, AZ: Neuropsychological Laboratory.

Reynolds, C. R. (1984). Critical measurement issues in learning disabilities. *Journal of Special Education, 18,* 451–476.

Reynolds, C. R. (1990). Conceptual and technical problems in learning disability diagnosis. In C. R. Reynolds & R. W. Kamphaus (Eds.), *Handbook of psychological and educational assessment of children* (pp. 571–592). New York: Guilford Press.

Robinson, W. P. (1974). Social factors and language development in primary school children. In R. Huxley & E. Ingram (Eds.), *Language acquisition: Models and Methods* (pp. 49–63). New York: Academic Press.

Rourke, B. P. (1988). Syndrome of nonverbal learning disabilities: Developmental manifestations in neurological disease, disorder and dysfunction. *The Clinical Neuropsychologist, 2,* 293–330.

Rourke, B. P. (Ed.). (1989). *Nonverbal learning disabilities: The syndrome and the model.* New York: Guilford Press.

Rourke, B. P., Bakker, D. J., Fisk, J. L., & Strang, J. D. (1983). *Child neuropsychology.* New York: Guilford Press.

Rourke, B. P., & Finlayson, M. A. J. (1978). Neuropsychological significance of variations in patterns of academic performance: Verbal and visual-spatial abilities. *Journal of Abnormal Child Psychology, 6,* 121–133.

Rules and Regulations Implementing Education for All Handicapped Children Act of 1975. (1977). Publ. L. No. 94-142, 42 Fed. Reg. 42474.

Rumsey, J. M., Anderson, P., Ametkin, A. J., Aquino, T., King, A. C., Hamburger, S. D., Pikus, A., Rapoport, J. L., & Cohen, R. M. (1992). Failure to activate the left temporoparietal cortex in dyslexia. *Archives of Neurology, 49,* 527–534.

Sainato, D. M., Zigmond, N., & Strain, P. S. (1983). Social status and initiations of interactions by learning disabled students in a regular education setting. *Analysis and Intervention in Developmental Disabilities, 3,* 71–87.

Satz, P., Taylor, H. G., Friel, J., & Fletcher, J. M. (1978). Some developmental and predictive precursors of reading disabilities: A six year follow-up. In A. L. Benton & D. Pearl (Eds.), *Dyslexia: An appraisal of current knowledge* (pp. 315–347). New York: Oxford University Press.

Satz, P., & van Nostrand, G. K. (1973). Developmental dyslexia: An evaluation of a theory. In P. Satz & J. Ross (Eds.), *The disabled learner: Early detection and intervention* (pp. 121–148). Rotterdam: Rotterdam University Press.

Segall, M. H. (1986). Culture and behavior. Psychology in global perspective. *Annual Review of Psychology, 37,* 523–564.

Semrud-Clikeman, M., & Hynd, G. W. (1990). Right hemisphere dysfunction in nonverbal learning disabilities: Social, academic and adaptive functioning in adults and children. *Psychological Bulletin, 107,* 196–209.

Semrud-Clikeman, M., & Hynd, G. W. (1992). Developmental arithmetic disorder. In S. R. Hooper, G. W. Hynd, & R. E. Mattison (Eds.), *Developmental disorders: Diagnostic criteria and clinical assessment* (pp. 97–125). Hillsdale, NJ: Erlbaum.

Senf, G. M. (1969). Development of immediate memory of bisensory stimuli in normal children and children with learning disabilities. *Developmental Psychology, 6,* 28–32.

Shafrir, U., & Siegel, L. S. (1994). Subtypes of learning disabilities in adolescents and adults. *Journal of Learning Disabilities, 27*(2), 123–134.

Shapiro, B. K., Palmer, F. B., Antell, S., Bilker, S., Ross, A., & Capute, A. J. (1990). Precursors of reading delay: Neurodevelopmental milestones. *Pediatrics, 85*(3), 416–420.

Shaw, S. F., & Shaw, S. R. (1989). Learning disability college programming: A bibliography. *Journal of Postsecondary Education and Disability, 6,* 77–85.

Shaywitz, S. E., Shaywitz, B. A., Fletcher, J. M., & Escobar, M. D. (1990). Prevalence of reading disability in boys and girls. *Journal of the American Medical Association, 264,* 998–1002.

Sherman, G. F., Galaburda, A. M., & Geschwind, N. (1985). Cortical anomalies in brains of New Zealand mice: A neuropathologic model of dyslexia? *Proceedings of the National Academy of Sciences USA, 82,* 8072–8074.

Sheslow, D., & Adams, W. (1990). *Wide Range Assessment of Memory and Learning manual.* Wilmington, DE: Jastak Associates.

Silver, L. B. (1979). The minimal brain dysfunction syndrome. In J. D. Noshpitz (Ed.), *Basic handbook of child psychiatry* (Vol. 2, pp. 416–439). New York: Basic Books.

Silver, L. B. (1981). The relationship between learning disabilities, hyperactivity, distractibility, and behavioral problems. *Journal of the American Academy of Child Psychiatry, 20,* 385–397.

Smith, S. D., Kimberling, W. J., Pennington, B. F., & Lubs, H. A. (1983). Specific reading disability: Identification of an inherited form through linkage analysis. *Science, 219,* 1345–1347.

Snowling, M. (1980). The development of grapheme–phoneme correspondence in normal and dyslexic readers. *Journal of Experimental Child Psychology, 29,* 291–305.

Sparrow, S. S., Balla, D. A., & Cicchetti, D. V. (1984). *Vineland Adaptive Behavior Scales.* Circle Pines, MN: American Guidance Service.

Spreen, O., Risser, A. H., & Edgell, D. (1995). In *Developmental neuropsychology* (pp. 489–490). New York: Oxford University Press.

Stevenson, H. W., & Newman, R. S. (1986). Long-term prediction of achievement and attitudes in mathematics and reading. *Child Development, 57,* 646–659.

Stevenson, H. W., Parker, T., Wilkinson, A., Hegion, A., & Fish, E. (1976). Longitudinal study of individual differences in cognitive development and scholastic achievement. *Journal of Educational Psychology, 68,* 377–400.

Strang, J. D., & Rourke, B. P. (1985). Arithmetic disability subtypes: The neuropsychological significance of specific arithmetical impairment in childhood. In B. P. Rourke (Ed.), *Neuropsychology of learning disabilities: Essentials of subtype analysis* (pp. 167–183). New York: Guilford Press.

Thomson, M. E., & Wilsher, C. (1978). Some aspects of memory in dyslexics and controls. In M. M. Gruneberg, P. E. Morris, & R. N. Sykes (Eds.), *Practical aspects of memory* (pp. 545–560). New York: Academic Press.

Thorndike, R. L., & Hagen, E. P. (1977). *Measurement and evaluation in psychology and education* (4th ed.). New York: Wiley.

Tramontana, M. G., Hooper, S. R., & Selzer, S. C. (1988). Research on the preschool prediction of later academic achievement. *Developmental Review, 8,* 89–147.

Ullman, D. G. (1977). Children's lateral preference patterns: Frequency and relationships with achievement and intelligence. *Journal of School Psychology, 15,* 36–43.

U.S. Department of Education. (1995). *To assure the free appropriate public education to all children with disabilities. Seventeenth Annual Report to Congress on the Implementation of the Individuals with Disabilities Education Act.* Washington, DC: Author.

U.S. Office of Education. (1977). *Assistance to states for education of handicapped children: Procedures for evaluating specific learning disabilities.* 42 Fed. Reg. 65082–65085.

Voeller, K. K. S. (1986). Right hemisphere deficit syndrome in children. *American Journal of Psychiatry, 143,* 1004–1009.

Voeller, K. K. S. (1990). Right hemisphere deficit syndrome in children: A neurological perspective. *International Pediatrics, 5,* 163–170.

Wagner, M. (1992–1993). *National longitudinal transition study of special education students.* Menlo Park, CA: SRI International.

Wallander, J. L., & Hubert, N. C. (1987). Peer social dysfunction in children with developmental disabilities: Empirical basis and a conceptual model. *Clinical Psychology Review, 7,* 205–221.

Wechsler, D. (1990). *Wechsler Intelligence Scale for Children-Third Edition manual.* San Antonio, TX: Psychological Corporation.

Wechsler Individual Achievement Test. (1992). *Manual.* San Antonio, TX: Psychological Corporation.

Witelson, S. F., & Rabinovitch, M. S. (1972). Hemispheric speech lateralization in children with auditory-linguistic defects. *Cortex, 8,* 412–426.

Woodcock, R. W., & Johnson, M. B. (1989). *Woodcock Johnson Psychoeducational Battery-Revised.* Allen, TX: DLM Teaching Resources.

Yeni-Komshian, G. H., Isenberg, P., & Goldstein, H. (1975). Cerebral dominance and reading disability: Left visual-field deficit in poor readers. *Neuropsychologia, 8,* 83–94.

6

Autistic Disorder

LAURA SCHREIBMAN AND MARJORIE H. CHARLOP-CHRISTY

INTRODUCTION

Autistic disorder is a severe form of psychopathology evidenced early in childhood and characterized by severe, pervasive behavioral deficits and bizarre behavioral patterns. Although the disorder is relatively rare, the severity and nature of the children's behavior have attracted the attention of researchers and clinicians for decades. This interest no doubt relates to the profound impact such a child has on the family, school, community, and society. Autism has challenged professionals in every field relating to child development. What follows is a discussion of this unique disorder.

The first identification of autism as a specific syndrome, then called *early infantile autism*, was by Dr. Leo Kanner in 1943. In his original paper, he described 11 children who differed qualitatively from other recognized child clinical populations. The characteristics of these chil-

dren included the inability to develop relationships with other people ("autistic aloneness"), a delay in the acquisition of speech, the noncommunicative nature of speech if it did develop, echolalia, pronominal reversal (e.g., substituting *you* for *I*), repetitive and stereotyped play activities, a compulsive desire for the maintenance of sameness in the environment, lack of imagination, good rote memory, and normal physical appearance. Many of the abnormalities appeared during infancy.

In the decades since Kanner first described what he considered the seminal features of autism, there has been a good deal of argument and controversy about which symptoms are essential for the diagnosis. (For more detailed discussions of this literature the reader is directed to American Psychiatric Association, 1994; Ritvo & Freeman, 1978; Rutter, 1966, 1968, 1971, 1978; Schreibman, 1988; Schreibman & Charlop, 1987; J. K. Wing, 1976.) Kanner later identified two symptoms he felt were essential for the diagnosis: "extreme aloneness" and "preoccupation with the preservation of sameness" (Eisenberg & Kanner, 1956). Others, however, felt that the focus on these two behaviors obscured the importance of other symptoms, particularly language deficits, which, interestingly, Kanner omitted as part of the essential behav-

LAURA SCHREIBMAN • Department of Psychology, University of California, San Diego, La Jolla, California 92093-0109. MARJORIE H. CHARLOP-CHRISTY • Department of Psychology, Claremont McKenna College, Claremont, California 91711.

Handbook of Child Psychopathology, 3rd edition, edited by Ollendick & Hersen. Plenum Press, New York, 1998.

ioral characteristics. Rutter (1978), in his review of the diagnosis of autism, pointed out that to determine the essential features of the disorder, one needed to identify those symptoms universal among and specific to children with autism. To this end, Rutter and his colleagues (Rutter, 1966; Rutter & Lockyer, 1967) conducted a research program to determine the symptoms specific to autism. Their results indicated that three broad groups of symptoms were found in all (or almost all) of those children diagnosed as autistic (or infantile psychotic); moreover, the symptoms were much less frequent in children with other psychiatric disorders. These symptoms included: (1) a profound and general failure to develop social relationships; (2) a delay in the acquisition of language, accompanied by impaired comprehension, echolalia, and pronominal reversal; and (3) ritualistic, compulsive behaviors.

Although the controversy over the identification of the "true" combination of symptoms will no doubt continue for some time, one can describe the behavioral characteristics most commonly associated with autism today. The reader will note that the basic symptoms of the disorder follow closely the original descriptions of Kanner (1943) and Rutter (1978).

PHENOMENOLOGY

Social Behavior

The failure to develop normal social relationships is a characteristic of autism consistently emphasized in the literature as one of the most profound and pervasive deficits of the syndrome (Rimland, 1964; Rutter, 1978; Schreibman, 1988; Wing, 1976). Children with autism generally prefer to be alone. They do not bond with their parents nor seek affection from them. To various degrees (Borden & Ollendick, 1994; Wing & Attwood, 1987) they may avoid people, resist affectionate overtures of others, fail to make eye contact, and seldom seek comfort from others. This is in sharp contrast to intense interest in, and attachment to, inanimate objects (e.g., Volkmar & Cohen, 1994).

As infants, autistic children lack attachment behavior and may not mold to their parent's body when held. Unlike typical infants, autistic children may either become stiff and rigid or "go limp" when held. True affective attachment to parents and others may occur but it is typically limited, not reflecting the rich range of attachment shown by typical children (Volkmar & Cohen, 1994). Social impairment is also seen in their failure to make friends or to play with peers. Their toy play is also inappropriate in that it tends to be self-stimulatory or ritualized (e.g., Stahmer, 1995). Deviant and/or deficient social behavior and attachment may be shown in the child's failure to socially reference, utilize joint attention to involve another person, direct the attention of others, or attend to the emotional distress of others (Lord, Rutter, & LeCouteur, 1994). In short, one may be struck by the true insularity of these children.

Speech and Language

Another hallmark feature of autistic children is their severe deficit in all aspects of communication (Paul, 1987; Rimland, 1964; Schreibman, 1988). Approximately 50% of autistic children are nonverbal. Many of these may eventually learn some appropriate speech (or alternative form of communication such as signing or use of a communication board) but only after intensive therapy. Those autistic children who do acquire speech (before training) usually exhibit speech that is noncommunicative. Often the speech takes the form of echolalia, wherein children merely repeat what they have heard with little or no comprehension. The speech may be deviant in other ways as well. The speech may involve pronoun reversals (e.g., substitute *you* for *I*, refer to themselves by name), dysprosody (e.g., incorrect intonation, inflection, rhythm), extreme literalness, neologisms, and/or idiosyncratic word use. Even individuals with autism who are very high functioning (i.e., normal or above-normal intelligence) and have relatively sophisticated language skills typically have problems with more subtle areas of communication. They may have difficulties integrating affective cues and the literal content of the speech (Volkmar & Cohen, 1994), may perseverate on topics, by unresponsive to cues of the listener, have difficulties integrating the social flow of conversation, and so forth. Thus, they may be considered "eccentric" or "odd" in their conversation speech (Schreibman, 1988).

Ritualistic Behavior and Insistence on Sameness

Rutter (1978) proposed that this category includes four characteristics commonly seen in autistic children. First, their play is very limited and rigid. They tend to play in an inappropriate, ritualistic manner such as lining up objects by shape or color, forming collections of objects of a particular shape or texture. For example, one child had a ritual in which he would sleep only on the den floor with the TV on, after he had lined up, in a semicircle, pegs from a pegboard game, grouped according to color.

Second, the child may become attached to a particular object and will seek it out, demand to have it at all times, talk about it, and tantrum if it is not accessible. Such "obsessions" may involve unusual or very specific types of items. Examples known to the authors include fiberglass, specific plastic alphabet letters, Honda Civics, gasoline credit cards, and newsman Dan Rather. Third, children with autism may have unusual preoccupations with concepts such as numbers, geometric shapes, schedules, and colors. One child known to the authors insisted on counting the number of songs on the car radio during the trip from home to school; another child was preoccupied with shapes and yelled "hexagon" on noticing the shape of a classroom table. Fourth, children with autism often demonstrate an intense insistence on sameness and a marked resistance to change in their environment. If a change in the environment is made, the child may become very agitated and upset. Typically, changes in the physical environment (e.g., familiar furniture arrangements), routes of travel, and daily routing are the most disruptive.

Abnormalities in Response to the Sensory Environment

Typically, autistic children appear to have a sensory deficit and are generally unresponsive to their environment (Schreibman, 1988). The children act, at times, as if they do not hear, even loud noises, or do not see, even when an object is displayed right in front of their eyes. However, their vision and audition are typically intact, and those same children who do not respond to loud noises may orient to the crinkling of a candy wrapper or the presence of a cookie. Also, some autistic children overreact to certain environmental stimuli; for example, they may cover their ears when a rattle is shaken. This abnormal responsiveness is associated with the tactile sensory as well (Ritvo & Freeman, 1978) such that a child may be oversensitive to a tickle and undersensitive to pain. In fact, the same child may at different times be under- or overresponsive to the same form of sensory stimulation.

Research has indicated that many children with autism have a characteristic attentional deficit wherein only a very restricted portion of available cues acquire control over their behavior. This attentional deficit, called *stimulus over-selectivity,* means that the children often do not learn about all of the necessary cues in a learning situation (e.g., the word *dog* presented with a picture of a dog). This attentional deficit has been implicated in the difficulty these children have learning new behaviors, generalizing newly acquired behaviors, social recognition, using prompts in teaching situations, and other areas requiring attention to compound stimuli (see Lovaas, Koegel, & Schreibman, 1979; Schreibman, 1988, for discussions of this literature).

Self-Stimulatory Behavior

Many individuals with autism display disturbances of motility typically referred to as *self-stimulation* or *stereotypy*. Such behavior is commonly defined as repetitive behavior that seems to serve no other purpose than to provide sensory input (e.g., Lovaas, Litrownik, & Mann, 1971; Lovaas, Newsom, & Hickman, 1987). These motor movements include flapping hands or arms or waving objects, rhythmic rocking and head rolling, toe walking, body posturing, and jumping, darting, or pacing. In addition to such gross motor examples, more subtle forms include the child's staring at lights out of the corners of her or his eyes, rubbing hands along surfaces, saliva swishing, and sniffing. Some self-stimulatory behavior may be verbal as when the child repeats the same sounds or words in rapid succession or driven by visual or auditory stimulation as when the child gazes at lights, intently fixates on spinning objects, or taps a table repeatedly. Although self-stimulation appears to be a highly preferred behavior, it remains the case that such behavior may have serious deleterious effects. These include stigmatizing the individual because of the bizarre nature of the behavior, making the person unresponsive to other environmental stimulation (e.g., Lovaas et al., 1971), and interfering with learning of new behaviors (e.g., Koegel & Covert, 1972). However, other literature is more hopeful in showing that some children can learn even when self-stimulation is present (e.g., Runco, Charlop, & Schreibman, 1986), and that self-stimulation may be used as a reinforcer to motivate the children to learn (e.g., Charlop, Kurtz, & Casey, 1990; Wolery, Kirk, & Gast, 1985). Finally, research has suggested that the children may not always be oblivious to their surroundings and the behavior may have social functions in that it is used to escape work demands (Durand & Carr, 1987).

Self-Injurious Behavior

No behavior seen in autism is as dramatic as self-injurious behavior (SIB). SIB is defined as behavior in which the child inflicts physical damage on his or her own body (Tate & Baroff, 1966). SIB includes a wide variety of behaviors such as hair pulling, face scratching, slapping, eye gouging, and arm and leg banging (Schreibman & Mills, 1983). The most common forms of SIB are head banging and biting of hands or wrists (Rutter & Lockyer, 1967). Although intensities vary across children, there is no doubt that SIB causes a great deal of damage, ranging from bruises and calluses, to broken bones, fractured skulls, detached retinas, and the removal of large portions of skin (Carr, 1977; Lovaas & Simmons, 1969). To protect the child, restraints may be necessary. However, prolonged use of restraints has been associated with structural changes, such as demineralization of the bones, shortening of the tendons, and arrested motor development (Lovaas & Simmons, 1969). Thus, there has been an emphasis on finding other approaches to decreasing SIB. Fortunately, research in the functional analysis of behavior has suggested that SIB may be maintained by several sources of reinforcement (e.g., Carr, 1977) and an analysis of these in a specific individual may lead to successful treatment (Carr & Durand, 1985; Iwata, Dorsey, Slifer, Bauman, & Richman, 1982).

Inappropriate Affect

It is common for autistic children to display emotions that are contextually inappropriate. For example, they may laugh in situations where others would be sad and they may cry inconsolably for no apparent reason. Some children have tremendous mood swings, with cheerfulness at one moment followed unpredictably by a screaming tantrum. Others display a flattened affect, "coasting" through a variety of emotional situations (Rimland, 1964). Additionally, some autistic children show inappropriate fears. Some children are extremely afraid of commonplace items or situations and become terrified when confronted with them (L. Wing, 1976). Examples of irrational fears include tortillas, ferns, Bill Cosby, pictures of yellow ducks, and white bread. Other children display no fear at all, even when there is a real danger; they may run out into the middle of a busy street, climb on the roof, or grab a hot curling iron.

Intellectual Functioning

Initially, it was thought that autistic children were intelligent (Kanner, 1943) and that their poor performance in a variety of areas was secondary to their social deficits. Kanner noted the children's serious facial expressions, their "clever" manipulative behavior, their good performance on certain tasks such as puzzles, and their excellent rote memories (Eisenberg & Kanner, 1956; Kanner, 1943). However, normal or above-normal intelligence is not associated with autism today. In fact, current estimates suggest that cognitive impairment is common with approximately 80% exhibiting some degree of mental retardation (e.g., Schreibman, 1988; Volkmar & Cohen, 1994). Interestingly, although full-scale IQ scores are typically low, there is often a scatter of abilities in which performance on visuospatial subtests may be much higher than performance on verbal, conceptual, and abstract reasoning tasks (e.g., Schreibman, 1988). Sometimes an individual with autism will exhibit superior skills, typically in the areas of memory, mechanical ability, music, or calculation (numerical or calendar). These abilities, sometimes at the "savant" level, may be quite dramatic (e.g., Rimland, 1978; Schreibman, 1988). The same properties of IQ seen in normal children apply to autistic children as well (Rutter, 1978). Their IQ tends to remain stable during middle childhood and adolescence (Lockyer & Rutter, 1969) and tends to be predictive of educational performance (Rutter & Bartak, 1973).

DIAGNOSIS

A major result of the evolutionary process in diagnosis, of the appearance of different sets of diagnostic criteria, and of different motivations for diagnosis (e.g., research, education, and funding considerations) is that the diagnostic criteria are not universally accepted or consistently applied. The result is a tremendous amount of heterogeneity in the population of children diagnosed as having autism.

One major problem associated with the heterogeneity in the population is that it has led to confusion both in diagnosing the children and in choosing suitable comparison groups for research purposes. Sometimes it has been suggested that autism is a by-product of a specific known pathology, such as rubella or phenylketonuria (Coleman, 1976). In some instances, autism is known to coexist with another disorder, such as Down syndrome (e.g., Wakabayashi, 1979). Additionally, it is now known that many children with autism develop seizures in adolescence, suggesting the presence of a neurological disorder (e.g., Rutter, 1978). Another factor resulting in group heterogeneity is that autism shares central features with other disorders. Thus, impaired cognitive ability is a characteristic of both mental retardation and autism. Language deficits are characteristic of autism, mental retardation, and other forms of developmental delay. In this sense, the question is not whether a particular child is autistic or retarded or aphasic, but whether it is useful for researchers and practitioners to distinguish between these disorders. Many are of the opinion that precision in diagnosis is necessary both for the advancement of research and for the development of effective treatments.

In the United States the most widely used and accepted set of diagnostic criteria have been developed for the *Diagnostic and Statistical Manual of Mental Disorders, Fourth Edition* (DSM-IV; American Psychiatric Association, 1994). Within the diagnostic category of "Pervasive Developmental Disorders" the DSM-IV includes five subcategories: Autistic Disorder, Rett's Disorder, Childhood Disintegrative Disorder, Asperger's Disorder, and Pervasive Developmental Disorder Not Otherwise Specified.

According to the DSM-IV, in addition to onset

of the disorder prior to 3 years of age, the essential features of autistic disorder are the following: (1) a qualitative impairment in social interaction, (2) qualitative impairments in communication, and (3) restricted repetitive and stereotyped behaviors, interests, and activities.

Differential Diagnoses

According to the DSM-IV, autistic disorder is distinguished from other forms of pervasive developmental disorder. Children with autistic disorder differ from children with *Rett's Disorder* in that the latter has been diagnosed only in females, is indicated by a characteristic pattern of head growth deceleration, loss of previously acquired purposeful hand skills, poorly coordinated gait and trunk movement, and lack of the consistent deficits in social interaction. These are not features associated with autistic disorder. Autistic disorder differs from *childhood disintegrative disorder* in that the latter is characterized by a distinctive pattern of developmental regression following a minimum of 2 years of normal development. This is in contrast to autistic disorder where the developmental abnormalities are typically apparent from the beginning of life (or at least within the first year). *Asperger's Disorder* has in the past often been referred to as *high-functioning autism*. Asperger's cases are distinguished from autistic disorder primarily by their lack of delay in language development. They do, however, share the deficits in social interaction and the presence of restricted, repetitive, and stereotyped patterns of behavior. Further, whereas many individuals with autism also are cognitively impaired, individuals with Asperger's Disorder are not. The diagnosis of pervasive developmental disorder not otherwise specified is made when the diagnostic criteria for autistic disorder or other subcategories of pervasive developmental disorder are not met but rather some of the above-mentioned characteristics such as severe and pervasive impairment in the development of reciprocal social interaction, deficits in communication, or re-stricted, repetitive, stereotyped patterns of behaviors are present.

ETIOLOGY

Although the precise basic pathology underlying autistic disorder has yet to be determined, a number of theories have been advanced to account for the development of the disorder. Researchers and theorists have focused their attention on three fundamental mechanisms: (1) the relation between autistic children and their surrounding social environment, (2) cognitive deficits and abnormalities, and (3) basic biological factors.

Perhaps the most emotionally charged theory of the cause of autism is the idea that the disorder is caused by the parents and the social environment they provide. This psychogenic theory of etiology was first proposed by Kanner (1943) and Eisenberg and Kanner (1956). Parents were described as well-educated upper-class individuals, involved in careers and intellectual pursuits, who were aloof, obsessive, and emotionally cold. The general idea was that some parental psychopathology prevented the parents from providing the warm, nurturing, and accepting environment so essential for healthy development. As a consequence, the children interpreted the world as a dangerous place and "withdrew" into autism (e.g., Bettelheim, 1967). This "parent-causation" hypothesis has never been supported by systematic investigations and in fact there are several findings that point away from such a cause (see Rimland, 1964; Schreibman, 1988), including the early onset of the condition (i.e., evident from birth in many cases), indications of organic involvement (e.g., seizures, various neurological "soft" signs, abnormalities in MRI and EEM tests), and findings suggesting no psychopathology in the parents (e.g., Koegel, Schreibman, O'Neill, & Burke, 1983). In essence, there is no empirical support for the psychogenic hypothesis of etiology and few subscribe to this theory today.

A growing body of literature views many characteristic autistic behaviors as resulting from a fundamental cognitive deficit and/or abnormality. Although a specific basic cognitive defect has not been identified, several theories have been put forward. This work is wide-ranging, including focus on perceptual and attentional processes, cognitive impairment, and language processes. With normal academic, language, and social functioning depending on the ability to accurately perceive stimuli in the environment and to have one's attention directed in an appropriate manner, it is reasonable to speculate that deficits in the ability to apprehend and utilize important environmental stimulation would lead to many of the deficits so characteristic of autism. These would include failure to learn new behaviors, failure to generalize, and deviant response to the environment. In fact, there are findings consistent with such deficits, such as the literature on "stimulus overselectivity" (e.g., Lovaas et al., 1979; Schreibman, 1988) mentioned earlier. Further, work by Courchesne and his colleagues suggests that at a more basic level these children may have neurological abnormalities associated with deficits in shifting attention (Akshoomoff & Courchesne, 1994) and, in work related to overselectivity, in apprehending a broad array of cues (Townsend & Courchesne, 1994). Although important and intriguing, work in this area to date has not shown a specific pattern peculiar to autism. In addition, it is important to remember that these are correlational data, and that we cannot be certain of a causal etiological relationship. In the domain of cognitive processes, recent work has put forward the hypothesis that autistic disorder is characterized by a basic cognitive deficit wherein these individuals have difficulty attributing mental states to others (e.g., Baron-Cohen, 1989; Leslie & Frith, 1988). The cognitive theory suggests that individuals with autism are unable to form mental representations of the perceptions and/or beliefs of others and thus are unable to accurately predict the behavior of others. Thus, it is hypothesized that these children do not have a "theory of mind" and

that this cognitive deficit underlines a good deal of the behaviors we see in the disorder. The findings in this are are somewhat inconsistent, however (e.g., Leslie & Frith, 1988; Lewis & Boucher, 1988). Thus, although the specific characteristics of a cognitive basis to autistic disorder may as yet be unidentified, it is certainly reasonable that such deficits are associated with many autistic behaviors.

At present, the most widely accepted view of the etiology of autism is that it is an organically based disorder. However, we do not as yet know the precise nature of the organic deficit or deficits. Specific biological factors that have been suggested as causative are genetic, neurochemical, and neuroanatomical.

Recent evidence suggests the possible role of genetic mechanisms in the etiology of at least some cases of autism. Siblings of individuals with autism are at increased risk for a range of developmental problems as well as for autism, and the concordance risk among monozygotic twins is high (e.g., Folstein & Rutter, 1977; Pauls, 1987). Further, there is evidence that the genetic effects may not necessarily take the form of autism as investigators have found a significantly high proportion of twins and other relatives with problems such as learning disabilities, language delays, and mental retardation (Folstein & Rutter, 1977; Ritvo, 1981). Neurochemical and metabolic factors have generated quite a bit of interest in the area of autism etiology. Of particular interest has been research in the neurotransmitter serotonin. The level of blood serotonin appears to be age related such that higher levels are found in normal infants, decrease throughout childhood, and stabilize at a lower level in adulthood. However, approximately 30 to 40% of individuals with autism fail to show this age-related decrease and remain hyperserotonemic throughout life (Freeman & Ritvo, 1984). Some have viewed this as indicative of the immaturity in the autistic neurological system. With other studies (Campbell, Deutsch, Perry, Wolsky, & Palij, 1986) indicating that higher serotonin levels are most clearly related to low intellectual functioning, it is not surprising that researchers have attempted to reduce serotonin levels (e.g., via fenfluramine or other serotonin inhibitor) and note any changes in autistic symptomology. Very early studies supported the view that reducing serotonin levels led to improvement in intellectual functioning and behavior, but later reports did not consistently support this finding (Schreibman, 1988). Another line of interest has focused on the role of opioid antagonists. This line of reasoning speculates that individuals with autism have an abnormally high level of opioid activity in the brain that serves to reduce the reinforcing effects of affection and comfort. Opioid inhibitors such as naltrexone have been administered, but, like with fenfluramine, the results have been inconclusive (e.g., Panksepp, Lensing, Leboyer, & Bouvard, 1991). Thus, there has been no confirmed finding to date on the role of a specific neurochemical etiological agent.

More consistent findings seem to be coming from research in neuroanatomical studies. To date, specific neuroanatomical abnormalities have been reported in the vermis of the cerebellum (e.g., Bauman & Kemper, 1985; Courchesne, Saitoh, et al., 1994), limbic structures (Bauman & Kemper, 1994; Courchesne, Hesselink, Jernigan, & Yeung-Courchesne, 1987), and parietal lobes (Courchesne, Press, & Yeung-Courchesne, 1993). Although researchers have been studying the potential function of, and etiology of, such neuroanatomical abnormalities, there have been no findings to date that suggest a specific etiology for the disorder. However, some researchers have begun to try to relate specific neuroanatomical findings to particular areas of functioning. Thus, Courchesne and his colleagues have provided findings suggesting that abnormality in the cerebellum may relate to deficiencies in shifting attention (Courchesne, Townsend, et al., 1994). Such a finding suggests that the well-documented attentional abnormalities noted in this population may have a basis in a specific neuroanatomical abnormality. This type of research holds potential for understanding possible etiological factors for some specific behaviors.

One conclusion about etiology that seems to be widely held is that a single etiology is unlikely. Autism is a behaviorally defined disorder and probably one with multiple etiologies, courses, and prognoses. We are dealing with a disorder with multiple subtypes, and although this may make the task of finding the etiology or the etiologies more complex, the ultimate identification of these factors will surely lead to more specific and individualized treatments.

EPIDEMIOLOGY

Autistic disorder is a relatively infrequent occurrence with most estimates suggesting its incidence to be 2–5 cases per 10,000 individuals (APA, 1994; Schreibman, 1988). The disorder is consistently reported to be more frequent in males, with the ratio typically reported in the range of 3–5:1 (e.g., Ando & Tsuda, 1975; APA, 1994; Schreibman, 1988). It is also reported that girls with the disorder are more likely to exhibit severe mental retardation.

ASSESSMENT

There are two main approaches to assessment of children with autism, nomothetic and idiographic (Harris, Belchic, Blum, & Celiberti, 1994). The nomothetic approach focuses on norm-based measures and standardized tools. In the case of autism, a comprehensive assessment battery typically includes measures such as IQ and achievement tests, social maturity, and perceptual-motor ability along with specific diagnostic assessments. This approach is important in that it places the individual child in relation to a larger comparison group, usually that of typical children the same age or, in the case of diagnostic assessments, of the general population of children with autism. The other approach to assessment, idiographic, enables the child to be individually assessed and his or her behavior analyzed. This approach includes clinical interview, direct observation, and behavioral assessment. Although it is beyond the scope of this chapter to discuss the merits and uses of all standardized assessment procedures, we will focus below on those specific to the assessment and diagnosis of autism.

Diagnostic Assessments

The general purpose of these assessments is to determine whether autism is an appropriate diagnosis for a child and, in some cases, to assess the severity of the disorder. The most commonly used include those described below.

The Autism Diagnostic Interview-Revised (ADI-R; Lord et al., 1994) is a semistructured, investigator-based interview for caregivers (usually parents) of children and adults for whom autism or pervasive developmental disorder is a possible diagnosis. During the interview, which may last from $1\frac{1}{2}$ hours (for very young children) to significantly longer (for older children and adults), the caregiver is asked a number of questions grouped into five sections: opening questions, questions on communication (both early and current), questions on the child's social development and play, questions about repetitive and restrictive behaviors, and questions concerning general behavior problems. The interviewer follows strict scoring procedures while administering the ADI-R. An algorithm for diagnosis has been generated by selecting ADI-R items that most closely depict the specific abnormalities described in the clinical descriptions and diagnostic guidelines from the DSM-IV (APA, 1994) and the *International Classification of Diseases* (ICD-10; WHO, 1993). The ADI-R is appropriate for children with mental ages from about 18 months to adulthood (Lord et al., 1994).

Although the ADI-R provides very useful information regarding the child's history and behavioral profile, it is important to obtain information directly from the affected individual. The Autism Diagnostic Observation Scale (ADOS; Lord et al., 1989) is a standardized interview/observational assessment in which the interviewer provides a social–communicative sequence of activities that combines a series of unstructured and structured situations that serve to provide a variety of situations designed to assess particular kinds of social and communicative behavior. Such activities range from providing a situation in which the child can/should ask the adult for play materials, to advanced conversational activities where the adult engages the child in discussion regarding emotions and social awareness. As with the ADI-R, the interviewer follows strict scoring procedures and applies the diagnostic algorithm developed for the ADOS. The ADOS is appropriate for children of chronological age from 6 to adulthood and mental age from 3 to maturity. Recently, a version of this assessment has been developed appropriate for children younger than 6 who do not have phrase speech and are suspected of having autism. This instrument is called the Pre-Linguistic Autism Diagnostic Observation Schedule (PL-ADOS; DiLavore, Lord, & Rutter, 1995). Whereas the ADI-R, the ADOS, and the PL-ADOS are relatively new instruments, the Childhood Autism Rating Scale (CARS; Schopler, Reichlef, DeVellis, & Daly, 1980) has been used for many years. This is a checklist instrument wherein an examiner observes a child and then completes a rating scale that allows for a rating for each of several behaviors deemed important in the diagnosis of autism (e.g., relating to people, adaptation to change, verbal communication). The scores for these rating areas are tallied and range from 15 to 60 with scores between 30 and 60 leading to a diagnosis of autism.

Another frequently used behavior checklist is Rimland's Diagnostic Checklist for Behavior-Disturbed Children, revised form E-2 (Rimland, 1971). This checklist contains questions about the child's behavior and development to be answered by the parents. Both behavior and language scores are derived from the checklist.

The limitations of the use of checklists, as with other nomoethic data, include the inability to directly prescribe treatment. Thus, although information in terms of diagnosis and symptomatology can be obtained, it does not lend itself to prescriptive treatment for the individual case. For this reason, we recommend that checklists be used as a complement to behavioral assessment.

Behavioral Assessment

Behavioral assessment addresses the limitations inherent with the use of checklists. First, it is an idiographic approach in which the individual child, with his or her specific behaviors, is the focus. Because autism is heterogeneous, diagnosis itself may not present specific symptomatology for a given child. Second, as noted above, the diagnosis of autism does not directly imply the specifics of a treatment protocol. Although professionals may agree on a general treatment approach, such as behavior therapy, specific treatment techniques are used for specific symptoms or behaviors, not for the syndrome as a whole. Finally, a label of autism does not provide a specific prognosis, whereas the presence or absence of specific symptoms is more helpful in suggesting a prognosis than the diagnosis per se.

Behavioral assessment circumvents the problems discussed above and provides a functional definition of the syndrome of autism as it is specific to an individual child. Schreibman and Koegel (1981) suggested three steps in the behavioral assessment of autism. First, specific behaviors displayed by an individual child are operationally defined. Broad categories (i.e., stereotypy) are deemphasized and specific behaviors (i.e., hand flapping, body rocking) are delineated. Second, the environmental variables that control the specific behaviors are identified. For example, a child may engage in tantrums only when demands are made as an attempt to escape the demands. More recently, this has been referred to as functional analysis, and various new methodologies have been presented for it. (Functional analysis will be discussed later in this chapter.) Finally, specific behaviors are grouped according to common controlling variables. For example, for a particular child, stereotypy behaviors and self-injurious behaviors may be controlled by the same variables. Part and parcel with behavioral assessment is behavioral observation. This is generally a structured or semistructured setting in which the child's specific behaviors are carefully observed. The reader is referred to Lovaas, Koegel, Simmons, and Long (1973) and Schreibman and Charlop (1987) for a more detailed account of structured observations. At the conclusion of the observation, a specific profile emerges for each child. Specific behavioral excesses and deficits are thus identified for the individual child, which directly prescribes treatment. For example, if the specific child is mute, engages in high frequencies of stereotypic behaviors such as hand flapping and body rocking, lacks eye contact, and bites his hand, then this is suggestive of necessary treatments. The behavioral excesses of hand flapping, body rocking, and hand biting need to be decreased, while the behavioral deficits of communication and eye contact (and other social skills) need to be taught. There is an arsenal of behavioral procedures available, many of which will be discussed in the following section, to treat these behaviors.

TREATMENT

Behavioral Deficits

Speech and Language

As noted earlier, approximately half of children with autism are functionally mute. Of the programs that teach speech to nonverbal children, two stand out in the literature as having the most success.

The first treatment program is a verbal imitation paradigm designed by Lovaas and his colleagues and consisting of a systematic discrimination training paradigm. Specifically, this treatment regimen involves intensive one-to-one, repetitive practice, discrete-trial training wherein the trainer identifies the task to be taught and using systematic discrimination training teaches the language task. The training typically involves teaching individual target behaviors, sequentially, so as to build up a more comprehensive response repertoire. The reader is referred to Lovaas (1981) for a detailed account of these procedures. This work has been important as it was the first to establish speech and language in this population. It has served as the basis for the development of subsequent programs (including those described below) that have helped to resolve some of the limitations of these earlier methods, e.g., limited generalization of treatment effects. The second program designed to teach speech is discussed here because it includes provisions to ameliorate two problems of children with autism, motivation and generalization of acquired behavior. This procedure has been called the Natural Language Paradigm (NLP) (Koegel, O'Dell, & Koegel, 1987; Laski, Charlop, & Schreibman, 1988). NLP is conducted during short sessions in which the therapist (or parent) presents several toys and allows the child to choose one. Then the therapist models a variety of appropriate responses, specific to the chosen toy, for the child to imitate. All attempts and approximations to verbally communicate are reinforced with access to the toy and with praise. NLP closely approximates normal language interactions (e.g., turn taking, sharing, natural consequences). It includes variables that facilitate motivation to respond (e.g., reinforcement of attempts to respond, novel stimuli, task variation, direct reinforcers). NLP also incorporates facilitators of generalization to extratherapy settings (common stimuli, parents as therapists, natural environment, loose structure).

Many children with autism do speak, although their speech predominantly consists of echolalia. Procedures for teaching speech to echolalic children generally differ from those described for teaching mute children, although NLP has been effective for echolalic children as well (Laski et al., 1988). Many earlier procedures had focused on eliminating echolalic speech (e.g., Schreibman & Carr, 1978). More recently, it has been suggested that echolalia serves a language function and perhaps should not be eliminated in all circumstances (Charlop, 1983; Freeman, Ritvo, & Miller, 1975; Prizant, 1983). Charlop (1983) used echolalia to advantage by designing a procedure to teach receptive labeling wherein the child was allowed to echo the name of the correct choice in a discrimination task. Charlop (1983) suggested that by echoing the stimulus the children may have provided their own self-imposed discriminative stimulus, thus facilitating acquisition and generalization of receptive labeling. Using echolalia to facilitate acquisition has been replicated in additional language tasks (Charlop-Christy, Gershater, & Ball, 1995). In addition to focusing on functional uses of behaviors (i.e., echolalia) present in the children's repertoires, recent research has focused on teaching language under more natural conditions, to promote spontaneous, generalized language use. One such procedure, time delay, has been quite effective in teaching more naturalized speech, specifically spontaneous speech (e.g., Charlop, Schreibman, & Thibodeau, 1985). This procedure consists of transferring stimulus control of an appropriate verbal response from the therapist's prompt (e.g., saying *Cookie*) to the presentation of a stimulus (i.e., a cookie) (Halle, Marshall, & Spradlin, 1979). Generally, this is accomplished by presenting the stimulus and modeling the correct verbal response, then gradually delaying the presentation of the modeled response in small time increments, until the child anticipates the prompt and speaks spontaneously before any prompt to do so.

The transfer of stimulus control to less obvious cues such as certain actions, settings, or temporal cues has also been studied (Charlop & Trasowech, 1991; Charlop & Walsh, 1986). Time delay has also been effective in teaching spontaneous speech during play and other naturally occurring situations (Ingenmey & Van Houten, 1991; Matson, Sevin, Fridley, & Love, 1990). Another promising line of research has investigated the effects of peer modeling in facilitating autistic children's speech and language (e.g., Charlop, Schreibman, & Tryon, 1983; Coleman & Stedman, 1974). This line of research has been extended by Charlop and Milstein (1989) who investigated a more cost-efficient modeling procedure, video modeling.

Incidental teaching involves teaching functional speech and language within naturally occurring context, such as free-play (Hart & Risley, 1980) or meal preparation (McGee, Krantz, Mason, & McClannahan, 1983). In other words, one waits for the naturally occurring situation to arise, and then models, prompts, and reinforces appropriate speech in the situation it needs to occur. This approach facilitates acquisition, generalization, and maintenance of speech and language (Halle, 1984) and bodes well for the child's future communication skills.

Social Skills

Many studies have focused on the acquisition and generalization of social skills. Charlop-Christy and Kelso (in press) suggested a scheme to organize this literature, and the reader is referred to this article as well as to Matson and Swiezy (1994) for more detailed discussion. According to Charlop-Christy and Kelso (in press), the social skills literature on autism may be viewed as fitting into four broad categories or levels of instruction: peer level (peers are taught to initiate social responses with children with autism), individual level (direct training of the child with autism), combination peer and individual level, and family level (training of parents and/or siblings to improve skills of the child with autism). Each level has its advantages and disadvantages.

The peer level of research originated with Strain and his colleagues, who in their seminal article (Strain, Kerr, & Ragland, 1979) taught a nonhandicapped peer to initiate social responses with children with autism. The peer was taught to deliver instructions (e.g., say "Let's play" and give the child a toy) as well as provide feedback (say "very good"). Many other studies

confirmed the positive findings of this approach (e.g., Goldstein, Kaczmarek, Pennington, & Shafer, 1992; Pierce & Schreibman, 1995; Sainato, Goldstein, & Strain, 1992; Sainato, Strain, Lefebvre, & Rapp, 1987). However, a disadvantage of this approach is the lack of generalization. Typically, in the absence of the trained peer, the child with autism fails to engage in the behavior. For this reason, researchers have proposed the approach be used at the combination level, where both peers and children with autism are trained (e.g., Goldstein & Cisar, 1992; Kamps, Leonard, Vernon, & Dugan, 1992). Treatment at this level promotes positive peer attitudes while enhancing generalization of social skills by the children with autism.

These treatments typically involve prompting, modeling, and reinforcement, whereas treatment at the individual level has added the use of preferred activities (Koegel, Dyer, & Bell, 1987), video modeling (Charlop, Milstein, & Moore, 1989; Charlop, Spitzer, & Kurtz, 1990; Oke & Schreibman, 1990), self-management (Stahmer & Schreibman, 1992), and language training (Gaylord-Ross, Haring, Breen, & Pitts-Conway, 1984; Krantz & McClannahan, 1993). Finally, approaches included in the family level have the dual benefit of improving the acquisition and generalization of social skills in the child and also improving familial attitudes toward the child. Much of this work has focused on teaching siblings techniques to teach social skills to their autistic brother or sister (Clark, Cunningham, & Cunningham, 1989; Coe, Matson, Graigie, & Gossen, 1991). Additionally, Krantz, MacDuff, and McClannahan (1993) taught parents to use photographic activity schedules consisting of separate photographs representing various daily social activities. Parents and siblings effectively used this procedure in the home.

Attention

As discussed earlier, many autistic children display unique attentional deficits such that their behavior comes under the control of an overly restricted range of environmental stimulation and/or under the control of unusual or irrelevant stimuli. To date, treatment procedures have addressed the issue of overselective attention by designing procedures to either allow for learning even if the child is responding in an overselective manner, or eliminating the overselective attention by broadening the range of cues utilized in learning.

Schreibman (1975) developed a "within stimulus" prompting procedure that allows for the learning of a discrimination task despite the child's overselectivity. This procedure involves the exaggeration and gradual fading of a prompt that is a relevant feature of the stimuli to be discriminated. (This differs from the more traditional "extrastimulus" prompt, which involves adding another stimulus to guide the child to the correct response.) In this procedure the relevant feature of the training stimulus, the one necessary to make the discrimination, is initially exaggerated (made bigger, darker). That is, the child's attention is directed to the cue necessary to focus on in order to learn the task. Once responding occurs to the exaggerated version of the relevant cue, it is gradually faded out until the child is responding correctly to the stimuli in their original form. For descriptions of the use of this procedure the reader is referred to Schreibman (1975) and Rincover (1978).

Although the within-stimulus prompting procedure is effective for teaching many discriminations, it is limited in that there are many discriminations that do not lend themselves to the use of the procedure (e.g., cross-modality tasks). To address this limitation a second approach has been developed to directly remediate overselectivity by teaching the children to respond to multiple cues (Koegel & Schreibman, 1977). Schreibman, Charlop, and Koegel (1982) demonstrated that autistic children who failed to learn difficult discrimination tasks when provided with an extrastimulus pointing prompt could learn to respond to multiple cues after training on several successive conditional discriminations. (A conditional discrimination is

one requiring response to multiple cues, such as choosing a blue toothbrush from among a blue toothbrush, a red toothbrush, and a blue comb.) Further, after this training to eliminate overselectivity, the children could now utilize the previously unsuccessful prompt. Importantly, these findings suggested that the children could learn from a more traditional teaching technique and may now be able to respond to their environment in a manner more similar to that of typical children.

Motivation

Unlike typical children, autistic children are usually not motivated by achievements, praise, success, or other social reinforcers. When presented with difficult tasks, these children frequently engage in inappropriate behaviors (e.g., tantrums, SIB) to escape the learning environments or may cease responding altogether. Thus, increasing motivation is crucial to the child's continued improvement and to overall treatment success. Because of this, a number of studies have addressed strategies to increase motivation to learn.

One line of research has focused on interspersing trials of previously learned, or "maintenance," tasks with trials of a new, "acquisition," task. Dunlap and Koegel (1980) demonstrated superior motivation (as measured by attempts to respond and lack of avoidance and escape behaviors) using this procedure. As few correct responses are typically made during initial learning of a task, procedures that include the interspersal of maintenance tasks ensure that the child receives a high density of reinforcement during the learning session. Attention and responsiveness are thus maintained, resulting in increased learning.

Other manipulations of reinforcer delivery have increased motivation for these children. For example, Koegel, Dyer, and Bell (1987) demonstrated that social responsiveness may be improved greatly by giving the child the opportunity to choose the nature of the learning task and the reinforcer. Such increases in motivation have also been demonstrated when children with autism receive reinforcement for attempts at correct responses, instead of only for specific correct responses (Koegel, O'Dell, & Dunlap, 1988).

Other researchers have approached the motivation problem by identifying new reinforcers. In one study, Charlop, Kurtz, and Casey (1990) assessed the effectiveness of using autistic children's aberrant behaviors as reinforcers to increase appropriate responding. In a series of three experiments, reinforcer conditions of self-stimulation, delayed echolalia, and obsessive behavior were compared with food reinforcer and varied (food/aberrant behavior) reinforcer conditions. For example, during sessions of the delayed echolalia condition, each child was permitted to utter a favored delayed echo (e.g., say "Eat your beef stew") after each correct response. Similarly, the child was allowed 3 to 5 seconds to engage in self-stimulation (e.g., tap the table) as a reinforcer during the self-stimulation condition. Finally, during the observation as reinforcer condition, the child was given the opportunity to briefly interact with an item she or he was preoccupied with (e.g., picture of Honda Civic cars). Results indicated that task performance was best when brief opportunities to engage in an aberrant behavior were provided as reinforcers as opposed to traditional food reinforcers. Importantly, no negative side effects (i.e., increase in aberrant behavior) were observed. Research into the nature of reinforcers, variables relating to their method of delivery, and other aspects of the learning environment have allowed behavior therapists to increase the repertoire of effective reinforcers for children with autism.

Generalization

The procedures described in this chapter have greatly increased our ability to effect encouraging gains in the behavioral repertoires of children with autism. However, treatment gains do not always generalize to nontreatment environments (stimulus generalization), across untreated behaviors (response generalization), or over time (maintenance). Treatment is of little value if generalization does not occur, and this has led researchers to place an increasing emphasis on the occurrence and assessment of generalization effects.

Stokes and Baer (1977) described strategies to promote generalization of behavior change, several of which have been added to the treatment of children with autism. One approach to facilitating generalization is to make the treatment environment more similar to the natural environment. This can be done in several ways. One way is to use intermittent schedules of reinforcement during treatment to provide a learning environment that more closely approximates the natural environment. Several studies (e.g., Charlop et al., 1983; Koegel & Rincover, 1977) have suggested that intermittent schedules increase the durability of treatment gains by reducing the discriminability of the reinforcement schedules used in the treatment and nontreatment settings.

Another strategy is to use naturally maintaining contingencies (natural reinforcers) during training, which will further reduce the differences between the treatment and nontreatment environments (Stokes & Baer, 1977). Thus, reinforcers should be like those found in the individual's natural environment such as social reinforcers or preferred activities. Also, behaviors taught should be those that will access these reinforcers. To illustrate, Carr, Binkoff, Kologinsky, and Eddy (1978) taught children with autism to use sign language to request items that were likely to be found in the natural environment. The children were taught to spontaneously request (via signing) their favorite toys as opposed to specific educational stimuli. This led to generalized spontaneous signing. In addition, this procedure incorporates another of the generalization strategies identified by Stokes and Baer (1977): the use of common stimuli (those found in treatment and nontreatment settings).

Behavior therapy often incorporates procedures that directly train generalization. Sequential modification occurs when generalization is programmed by teaching the targeted behavior in every nongeneralized condition (e.g., across people, settings, behaviors). However, it may be impractical to train a behavior in every potential situation. An alternative approach is to merely train sufficient exemplars (Stokes & Baer, 1977). This technique may also be difficult because it is usually impossible to determine beforehand the necessary number of situations or exemplars that will be required before generalization is achieved. To reduce this problem, Stokes and Baer (1977) suggested using mediated generalization. This procedure focuses on teaching a target response that is likely to occur in both treatment and nontreatment situations. The most common mediator is language. Children giving self-instructions in different environments are using this generalization strategy. Few studies have addressed the use of mediated generalization with children with autism. However, as discussed earlier, Charlop (1983) demonstrated that children with autism might be able to use their echolalia as a verbal mediator.

Self-management procedures may also be considered mediated generalization because the target behavior (self-management) can be taken from the training environment to other settings. It has been only relatively recently that researchers have successfully taught this procedure to children with autism (e.g., Koegel & Koegel, 1990; Pierce & Schreibman, 1994; Stahmer & Schreibman, 1992). Teaching self-management procedures contains several steps (Koegel, Koegel, & Parks, 1989). First, both appropriate and inappropriate target behaviors are operationally defined. Second, functional reinforcers, chosen by the child, are identified and an appropriate period of time, or unit of behavior small enough to ensure success on the child's part, is determined. Next, the child learns to self-monitor. During this stage of the training, the child is taught to discriminate between correct and incorrect behavior. Following this, the child is taught to self-observe, self-evaluate, and then record the presence of the target behavior. After the child has demonstrated the ability to perform the self-management in the training setting, he or she is prompted to do so in the natural environment.

It should be apparent that research into achieving generalization of treatment effects has become a top priority. In addition to these specific strategies, generalization has been enhanced by extending the treatment environment. Thus, the incorporation of parent training programs (Koegel, Schreibman, Britten, Burke, & O'Neill, 1982; Sloane, Endo, Hawkes, & Jenson, 1991), teacher training programs (Koegel, Rincover, & Egel, 1982), and sibling training programs (Schreibman, O'Neill, & Koegel, 1983) have all been used to extend treatment delivery into those environments in which the child lives.

Behavioral Excesses

Behavioral excesses demonstrated by children with autism include SIB, self-stimulatory behavior, perseverative behaviors, noncompliance, tantrums, aggression, and a multitude of other unwanted behaviors. Over the past three decades, behavioral researchers have developed a rather vast arsenal of specific techniques to decrease behavioral excesses by increasing competing behaviors (e.g., differential reinforcement of other behavior [DRO] and related procedures), and by the use of various punishment procedures such as time out, overcorrection, application of aversive stimuli, and withdrawal of positive stimuli. Although punishment procedures have a long history of use and efficacy (e.g., Azrin, Hake, Holz, & Hutchinson, 1965; Dorsey, Iwata, Ong, & McSween, 1980; Lovaas & Simmons, 1969), negative side effects, limited generalization of treatment effects, and our increased ability to effect significant improvement via positive procedures have led the field to explore other strategies to reduce severe inappropriate behaviors. Probably the most important addition to our arsenal of effective treatment procedures is the emphasis on functional analysis.

Functional analysis identifies a relationship between contextual events and behaviors. This can be done in a variety of ways including observing the children in the natural environment, paper-and-pencil assessments, and by creating analog settings in which environmental variables may be systematically altered to assess the relationship with the target behavioral excess. In a seminal study, Iwata et al. (1982) studied the effects of specific environmental conditions on SIB. Four analog conditions were used that had been suggested in the literature to be the most likely to occasion SIB. The conditions were social disapproval, being alone, academic demand, and unstructured play (control condition). Each condition was associated with a specific function that the SIB was serving. For example, if SIB occurred for one child only in the academic demand condition, then it would be clear that escape was the motivation for the SIB. Thus, a treatment preventing escape would be indicated. Or, if the child maintained a high frequency of SIB in all conditions, then the function of the behavior was self-stimulatory and treatment would likely consist of a reductive procedure. The function of SIB for each child varies and treatment must be designed based on these individual results.

Durand and Carr (1987) found that for some children disruptive behaviors serve a communicative function. In this study, children engaged in self-stimulation when difficult demands were presented; thus, the behavior was escape motivated. However, by teaching the children an alternative behavior, to say "help me," the stereotypy decreased. Thus, understanding the complex relationships between behavior and environmental variables is of paramount importance in determining appropriate treatment for behavioral excesses.

Naturalistic Teaching Strategies

Incorporating many of the treatment strategies described above, more naturalistic training programs have been developed. These pro-grams share an emphasis on teaching language and other skills in the situations and environments in which they naturally occur, providing naturalistic contingencies, and allowing the individual to have more control over the training situation. All of these strategies also share an emphasis on incorporating training within the ongoing activities of the individual, as opposed to the setting up of artificial, highly structured teaching situations as has been the case in prior years. Also, these strategies are all associated with rapid behavior gains (Schreibman & Koegel, 1996), generalized treatment effects (Schreibman & Koegel, 1996), and positive reception by the treatment providers (Schreibman, Kaneko, & Koegel, 1991). We will describe one of these naturalistic strategies, pivotal response training (PRT; Koegel, Schreibman, et al., 1989). In traditional discrete-trial, repetitive practice training, the focus is on training individual target behaviors in sequences and the trainer determines the task to be taught, the stimuli to be used, the nature of the training interaction, and the reinforcer to be used. In contrast, PRT incorporates specific strategies to increase the "pivotal" responses of motivation and responsivity to multiple cues. These are considered to be "pivotal" in that changes in each of these behaviors are assumed to lead to changes in an array of other behaviors. To enhance motivation, PRT utilizes the following strategies: (1) allowing the child to have significant control over the nature of the training task, stimuli, and reinforcer; (2) interspersal of maintenance tasks; (3) direct reinforcement, which means the reinforcer is directly associated with the response (e.g., the reinforcer for saying *car* is access to a toy car, rather than a piece of candy for "good talking"); and (4) reinforcement of the child's attempts to respond rather than only providing reinforcement for correct responses. To increase responsivity to multiple cues, tasks are chosen that require responding to conditional discriminations. For example, the child is asked to go get her "red sweater," which requires her to respond on the basis of color and subject. For a complete description of PRT the reader is referred to Koegel, Schreibman, et al. (1989).

As with another naturalistic treatment, "incidental teaching," PRT enhances generalization by embedding teaching trials within the child's daily activities. Using this strategy, the therapist or teacher is vigilant for teaching opportunities signaled by the child and can thus use natural stimuli and reinforcers during the trial. For example, a child reaching for an apple might be required to say *apple* (or some approximation) before receiving the apple. The child is clearly motivated for the fruit and the teacher can take advantage of the naturally occurring stimulus and subsequent reinforcer (i.e., apple). McGee et al. (1985) taught autistic children to receptively learn labels of objects used in meal preparation (e.g., knife, sandwich). The training occurred in the kitchen during the daily lunch preparation. This "loose structure" in the teaching situation also helps promote generalization (Stokes & Baer, 1977).

CASE STUDY

Greg was 6 years old when he was referred to our behaviorally oriented treatment and research center. He looked as if he had just stepped out of a Norman Rockwell painting, with his blond hair, sparkling blue eyes, pug nose, and freckles across the bridge of his nose. Greg's early history was "textbook" in terms of his symptomatology. His mother had a normal pregnancy and delivery, and described Greg as an "easy" child because he did not demand the attention of others. Indeed, Greg seemed disinterested in his mother's attention and was content to lie in his crib by himself. As he grew, his developmental milestones were by and large normal, although a few were advanced. Because of this his mother was not worried about his "loner" attitude or disinterest in being hugged or cuddled. However, he began to appear so unresponsive to his environment that his mother suspected he might be deaf. Hearing tests revealed no impairment, but concern grew as Greg failed to talk and understand language. As he grew older, Greg's delay in speech became more obvious. Other symptoms also became striking. He remained disinterested in interacting with his family and peers, avoiding eye contact and touch. He did not play with toys appropriately; instead he waved them in front of his eyes in a self-stimulatory manner. Finally, at around the age of 4, Greg began to speak. However, his speech was predominantly echolalic, repeating others' words and expressions he heard on TV. Behavioral assessment led to a treatment individually designed for Greg based on his specific behaviors and their functions. Below is a brief description of Greg's treatment.

Behavioral Deficits

Speech and Language

When Greg entered treatment, the majority of his speech was echolalic and obsessional. He displayed both immediate and delayed echolalia. Greg's delayed echolalia is best illustrated by the following examples. Greg approached the second author and said, "The Dow Jones Industrial Averages dropped 10 points today." He also lacked contextually appropriate spontaneous speech, and would only speak when spoken to. The only time Greg would initiate speech was when it was obsessional in nature. He was preoccupied with his next activity in his daily schedule, and would frequently repeat "Where are we going next?" or "What are we going to do?"

Greg's speech and language deficits were a main focal point of his treatment. Speech improvement would not only help Greg communicate, but would also help improve his social skills as he lacked verbal social interaction skills. Speech improvement would also likely decrease his tantrums as the majority of these occurred because he could not adequately communicate his needs. Greg's immediate echolalia was used to increase his appropriate speech and language. The echo procedure described by Charlop (1983) served to increase Greg's vocabulary. As his vocabulary grew, and his understanding of language concomitantly increased, his immediate echolalia decreased. The NLP was also used to increase appropriate speech and decrease echolalia. As his speech and language improved, Greg's lack of spontaneous speech was next targeted. The time delay procedure, described earlier in this chapter, was instrumental in helping Greg acquire spontaneous speech. His mother was taught these procedures, so his speech began to generalize to a variety of environments. Conversational speech was taught via video modeling, which had the added positive side effect of improving his social interaction with peers. As his speech thus became more naturalized and functional, his inappropriate speech (echolalia) decreased. It is important to note that, as with other children with autism, although Greg's speech and language has improved dramatically, it is still characterized by inappropriate intonation and pronominal reversal. Also, although his conversational skills have improved to the point where he can maintain a conversation with a nonhandicapped peer, he still prefers to converse about his own (typically obsessional) interests.

Motivation

At the start of treatment, Greg was disinterested in learning. He failed to pay attention and often engaged in self-stimulatory behaviors instead of working on educational tasks. He expressed boredom and frustration by throwing tantrums, whining, noncompliance, and disruptive behavior. Motivation was improved by several procedures, which ultimately led to improved learning and a decrease in inappropriate behaviors. First, choice was introduced into Greg's treatment in several ways. First, he was allowed choice in terms of what educational stimuli he wanted to work with. As in NLP, Greg was encouraged to choose his favorite toys and activities. Second, Greg was allowed choice in his reinforcers. A variety of Greg's favorite snacks and activities were available on completion of his task.

Along with choice of reinforcer, selection of reinforcers was an essential part of increasing motivation. Initial assessments were performed to determine specifically what items and activities would serve as reinforcers. Here, some of Greg's aberrant behaviors were used to advantage to motivate him. He was allowed to briefly engage in self-stimulatory behaviors (e.g., 2 seconds of twirling a twig) and obsessional behaviors (i.e., reading a Honda Civic catalog) as a reinforcer for appropriate responding. Greg's family members were taught to employ these motivating procedures to improve generalization and maintenance.

Finally, Greg's motivation was improved by interspersing maintenance (previously mastered) tasks with new tasks. In this way, the overall frequency of reinforcement was kept high and frustration was kept low. This helped keep him motivated to continue to learn.

Social Skills

Prior to treatment, Greg showed little interest in peers, his eye contact was poor, and he did not play appropriately or independently with toys. His leisure time was spent pacing throughout his house or engaging in self-stimulation or rituals.

The acquisition of social skills was a key to successful treatment. Not only would appropriate behaviors such as toy play, independence, and peer interaction increase, but these behaviors would serve to partially replace some of the existing inappropriate behaviors in Greg's repertoire and behavior problems resulting from lack of anything better to do (e.g., running away, throwing sand in the pool, closing all doors and windows). Additionally, appropriate social behavior, such as speech, would be instrumental in accessing information from the environment. Prompting and reinforcement were used to increase eye contact. Once the frequency of eye contact increased, it was required during all learning sessions and tasks in order to obtain reinforcement. Eventually, eye contact was naturally reinforced by an increase in attention from others in various environments (e.g., school, supermarkets, neighborhood children).

More complex social skills such as verbal interactions and play were taught at the combination peer and individual level, and at the family level. Video modeling was used to teach independent play behaviors with toys and cooperative play skills with peers. Greg was taught directly, and once skills were acquired, peers were recruited to join in the games. Once Greg acquired the skills to play appropriately, he derived pleasure from his interactions with peers. Peers also enjoyed playing with him because he was now able to keep a game going.

An important aspect of Greg's social skills training was the involvement of his mother and brother. Of particular concern at home was his preference to engage in self-stimulatory behaviors as opposed to playing appropriately and independently. His family took advantage of his self-stimulatory behavior and other aberrant behaviors and used them effectively as reinforcers for appropriate leisure activities. For example, he enjoyed twisting a blade of grass and would spend much of his day doing so. His mother made a list of appropriate play activities (swimming, riding bikes, playing basketball with a neighbor) and initially requested Greg to engage in these activities for 10 minutes. At the conclusion of the 10-minute session, he would then be entitled to 2 minutes of twisting the blade of grass. Sessions of leisure activities were systematically increased until he played all afternoon for only 2 minutes with his blade of grass. His blade of grass was soon replaced with more appropriate behavior. Importantly, frequency of inappropriate behaviors decreased as Greg learned to enjoy more appropriate kinds of activities.

Attention

Although Greg did not display stimulus overselectivity, he had difficulties paying attention. For Greg, improving motivation improved attention to the learning situation, and subsequently led to treatment gains. The motivation-enhancing procedures discussed above in the section on PRT were employed. Accordingly, Greg was given control in his treatment by being given choice, task variation procedures were used as well as direct reinforcement. Also, by reinforcing general on-task behaviors in addition to specific correct responses, attempts at learning were reinforced. Finally, utilization of PRT helped Greg with his responsiveness to the various cues in his environment by presenting multiple-cue tasks.

Generalization

Throughout treatment, provisions to facilitate generalization and maintenance of treatment gains were incorporated into the treatment plan. Differences in the treatment environment and the natural environment were minimized by using intermittent schedules of reinforcement and natural reinforcers (e.g., social attention and preferred activities) found in the natural environment. Treatment was also presented in the settings in which generalization needed to occur, such as home, school, and the community (market, mall). Greg's parents and older brother were trained to provide treatment and further facilitate generalization. Additionally, target behaviors to enhance mediated generalization (i.e., speech and language) were chosen. In addition, he was taught self-management procedures wherein he learned to monitor and record incidences of self-stimulation. He self-reinforced for low rates of the behavior.

Incidental teaching was also used by embedding teaching trials within Greg's daily activities. This strategy was taught to his mother and teacher to easily implement learning directly in the natural environment.

Behavioral Excesses

Greg displayed tantrum and self-stimulatory behaviors. Functional analyses were performed for these two classes of behaviors. For tantrums, it appeared that the function of this behavior was to express boredom, frustration, and dislike. As Greg's speech was severely impaired at the start of treatment, he could not communicate these emotions verbally. With speech training, he learned how to use words to communicate and the tantrums decreased without any direct intervention. Also, as provisions for motivation were incorporated into his therapy sessions, he had less occasion to be bored or frustrated.

A functional analysis of self-stimulatory behaviors suggested that Greg engaged in such behavior because it was reinforcing to do so. His self-stimulation occurred in most settings, throughout the day and night, although it increased during unstructured times (e.g., at home after school). As described earlier, Greg's mother implemented a program to allow him brief opportunities to engage in self-stimulation contingent on longer periods in which none occurred. Additionally, as his acquisition of appropriate leisure skills increased, self-stimulation decreased. Finally, he was taught a self-management program to control his own self-stimulation.

Outcome

At the time of this writing, Greg is 15 years old. He lives at home with his mother and brother and attends high school in a class for students with communication handicaps. He has chores around the house, which he diligently does daily, and then is free to engage in leisure activities of swimming, bike riding, and watching TV. He functions well in the community, able to order his own meals at restaurants and pay for himself. He demonstrates few behavior problems and reserves self-stimulation for times when he is alone in his room. He communicates his needs well with speech, but his intonation is still incorrect, and he usually does not initiate conversations unless the topic is one of his special interests. We anticipate that Greg will live at home for the immediate future and ultimately live in an adult group living situation.

SUMMARY

This chapter has been an overview of the puzzling and fascinating syndrome of autism. A description of the disorder, a discussion of the etiology, and a brief presentation of assessment and treatment have been provided. Finally, the reader was introduced to Greg, our case study, to bring to life some of the symptoms and courses of treatment discussed in the text. It is hoped that the reader has a greater understanding of this enigmatic disorder, an appreciation of treatment, and an optimism for the future of these children.

ACKNOWLEDGMENT

Preparation of this chapter was facilitated by USPHS Research Grants MH 39434 and MH 28210 from the National Institute of Mental Health.

REFERENCES

Akshoomoff, N. A., & Courchesne, E. (1994). ERP evidence for a shifting attention deficit in patients with damage to the cerebellum. *Journal of Cognitive Neuroscience, 6,* 388–399.

American Psychiatric Association (1994). *Diagnostic and statistical manual of mental disorders* (4th ed.). Washington, DC: Author.

Ando, H., & Tsuda, K. (1975). Intrafamilial incidence of autism, cerebral palsy, and mongolism. *Journal of Autism and Childhood Schizophrenia, 5,* 267–274.

Azrin, N. H., Hake, D. F., Holz, W. C., & Hutchinson, R. R. (1965). Motivational aspects of escape from punishment. *Journal of the Experimental Analysis of Behavior, 8,* 31–44.

Baron-Cohen, S. (1989). The autistic child's theory of mind: A case of specific developmental delay. *Journal of Child Psychology and Psychiatry, 30,* 285–297.

Bauman, M. L., & Kemper, T. L. (1985). Histoanatomic observations of the brain in early infantile autism. *Neurology, 35,* 866–874.

Bauman, M. L., & Kemper, T. L. (1985). Histoanatomic observations of the brain in early infantile autism. *Neurology, 35,* 866–874.

Bauman, M. M., & Kemper, T. L. (1994). Neuroanatomic observations of the brain in autism. In M. L. Bauman & T. L. Kemper (Eds.), *The neurobiology of autism* (pp. 119–145). Baltimore: Johns Hopkins University Press.

Bettelheim, B. (1967). *The empty fortress.* New York: Free Press.

Borden, M. C., & Ollendick, T. H. (1994). An examination of the validity of social subtypes in autism. *Journal of Autism and Developmental Disorders, 24,* 23–37.

Campbell, M., Deutsch, S. I., Perry, R., Wolsky, B. B., & Palij, M. (1986). Short-term efficacy and safety of fenfluramine in hospitalized preschool-age autistic children: An open study. *Psychopharmacology Bulletin, 22,* 141–147.

Carr, E. G. (1977). The motivation of self-injurious behavior. A review of some hypotheses. *Psychological Bulletin, 81,* 800–816.

Carr, E. G., Binkoff, J. A., Kologinsky, E., & Eddy, M. (1978). Acquisition of sign language by autistic children. I. Expressive labeling. *Journal of Applied Behavior Analysis, 11,* 489–501.

Carr, E. G., & Durand, V. M. (1985). Reducing behavior problems through functional communication training. *Journal of Applied Behavior Analysis, 18,* 111–126.

Charlop, M. H. (1983). The effects of echolalia on acquisition and generalization of receptive labeling in autistic children. *Journal of Applied Behavior Analysis, 16,* 111–126.

Charlop, M. H., Kurtz, P. F., & Casey, F. G. (1990). Using aberrant behaviors as reinforcers for autistic children. *Journal of Applied Behavior Analysis, 23,* 163–181.

Charlop, M. H., & Milstein, J. P. (1989). Teaching autistic children conversational speech through video modeling. *Journal of Applied Behavior Analysis, 22,* 275–285.

Charlop, M. H., Milstein, J. P., & Moore, M. (1989, May). *Teaching autistic children cooperative play.* Paper presented at the Annual Convention for the Association for Behavior Analysis, Milwaukee.

Charlop, M. H., Schreibman, L., & Thibodeau, M. G. (1985). Increasing spontaneous verbal responding in autistic children using a time delay procedure. *Journal of Applied Behavior Analysis, 18,* 155–166.

Charlop, M. H., Schreibman, L., & Tryon, A. S. (1983). Learning through observation: The effects of peer modeling on acquisition and generalization in autistic children. *Journal of Abnormal Child Psychology, 11,* 355–366.

Charlop, M. H., Spitzser, S., & Kurtz, P. F. (1990, May). *Teaching autistic children independent play through video modeling*. Paper presented at the Annual Convention for the Association for Behavior Analysis, Nashville, TN.

Charlop, M. H., & Trasowech, J. B. (1991). Increasing autistic children's daily spontaneous speech. *Journal of Applied Behavior Analysis, 24,* 247–261.

Charlop, M. H., & Walsh, M. (1986). Increasing autistic children's spontaneous verbalizations of affection through time delay and modeling. *Journal of Applied Behavior Analysis, 19,* 307–314.

Charlop-Christy, M. H., Gershater, R., & Ball, K. (1995). *Using autistic children's immediate echolalia to facilitate acquisition of abstract concepts.* Working paper.

Charlop-Christy, M. H., & Kelso, S. (in press). Autism. In V. L. Schwean & D. H. Saklofse (Eds.), *The psychological correlates of exceptionality.* Newark, NJ: Harwood Academic Publishers.

Clark, M. L., Cunningham, L. H., & Cunningham, C. E. (1989). Improving the social behavior of siblings of autistic children using a group problem solving approach. *Child and Family Behavior Therapy, 11,* 19–33.

Coe, D., Matson, J. L., Craigie, C. J., & Gossen, M. A. (1991). Play skills of autistic children: Assessment and instruction. *Child and Family Behavior Therapy, 13,* 13–40.

Coleman, M. (1976). Introduction. In M. Coleman (Ed.), *The autistic syndromes* (pp. 1–10). New York: American Elsevier.

Coleman, S. L., & Stedman, J. M. (1974). Use of a peer model in language training in an echolalic child. *Journal of Behavior Therapy and Experimental Psychiatry, 5,* 275–279.

Courchesne, E., Hesselink, J. R., Jernigan, T. L., & Yeung-Courchesne, R. (1987). Abnormal neuroanatomy in a nonretarded person with autism: Unusual findings with magnetic resonance imaging. *Archives of Neurology, 44,* 335–340.

Courchesne, E., Press, G. A., & Yeung-Courchesne, R. (1993). Parietal lobe abnormalities detected on magnetic resonance images of patients with infantile autism. *American Journal of Roentgenology, 160,* 387–393.

Courchesne, E., Saitoh, O., Townsend, J. P., Yeung-Courchesne, R., Press, G. A., Lincoln, A. J., Haas, R. H., & Schreibman, L. (1994). Abnormality of cerebellar vermian lobules VI and VII in patients with infantile autism: Identification of hypoplastic and hyperplastic subgroups by MR imaging. *American Journal of Roentgenology, 162,* 123–130.

Courchesne, E., Townsend, J., Akshoomoff, N. A., Saitoh, O., Yeung-Courchesne, R., Lincoln, A. J., James, H. E., Haas, R. H., Schreibman, L., & Lau, L. (1994). Impairment in shifting attention in autistic and cerebellar patients. *Behavioral Neuroscience, 108,* 848–865.

DiLavore, P. C., Lord, C., & Rutter, M. (1995). The Pre-Linguistic Autism Diagnostic Observation Schedule (PL-ADOS). *Journal of Autism and Developmental Disorders.*

Dorsey, M. F., Iwata, B. A., Ong, P., & McSween, T. E. (1980).

Treatment of self-injurious behavior using a water mist: Initial response suppression and generalization. *Journal of Applied Behavior Analysis, 13,* 343–353.

Dunlap, G., & Koegel, R. L. (1980). Motivating autistic children through stimulus variation. *Journal of Applied Behavior Analysis, 13,* 619–627.

Durand, V. M., & Carr, E. G. (1987). Social influences of self-stimulatory behavior: Analysis and treatment application. *Journal of Applied Behavior Analysis, 20,* 119–132.

Eisenberg, L., & Kanner, L. (1956). Early infantile autism: 1943–1955. *American Journal of Orthopsychiatry, 26,* 55–65.

Folstein, S., & Rutter, M. (1977). Genetic influences and infantile autism. *Nature, 265,* 726–728.

Freeman, B. J., & Ritvo, E. R. (1984). The syndrome of autism: Establishing the diagnosis and principles of management. *Pediatric Annals, 13,* 284–305.

Freeman, B. J., Ritvo, E., & Miller, R. (1975). An operant procedure to teach an echolalic autistic child to answer questions appropriately. *Journal of Autism and Childhood Schizophrenia, 5,* 169–176.

Gaylord-Ross, R. J., Haring, T. G., Breen, C., & Pitts-Conway, V. (1984). The training and generalization of social interaction skills with autistic youth. *Journal of Applied Behavior Analysis, 17,* 229–247.

Goldstein, H., & Cisar, C. L. (1992). Promoting interaction during sociodramatic play: Teaching scripts to typical preschoolers and classmates with disabilities. *Journal of Applied Behavior Analysis, 25,* 265–280.

Goldstein, H., Kaczmarek, L., Pennington, R., & Shafer, K. (1992). Peer-mediated intervention: Attending to, commenting on, and acknowledging the behavior of preschoolers with autism. *Journal of Applied Behavior Analysis, 25,* 289–305.

Halle, J. (1984). Natural environment language assessment and intervention with severely impaired preschoolers. *Topics in Early Childhood Special Education, 4,* 36–56.

Halle, J., Marshall, A. M., & Spradlin, J. E. (1979). Time delay: A technique to increase language use and facilitate generalization in retarded children. *Journal of Applied Behavior Analysis, 12,* 431–439.

Harris, S. L., Belchic, J., Blum, L., & Celiberti, D. (1994). Behavioral assessment of autistic disorder. In J. L. Matson (Ed.), *Autism in children and adults: Etiology, assessment, and intervention* (pp. 127–146). Pacific Grove, CA: Brooks/Cole.

Hart, B., & Risley, T. R. (1980). In vivo language intervention: Unanticipated general effects. *Applied Behavior Analysis, 13,* 407–432.

Ingenmey, R., & Van Houten, R. (1991). Using time delay to promote spontaneous speech in an autistic child. *Journal of Applied Behavior Analysis, 24,* 591–596.

Iwata, B. A., Dorsey, M. F., Slifer, K. J., Bauman, K. E., & Richman, G. E. (1982). Toward a functional analysis of self-injury. *Analysis and Intervention in Developmental Disabilities, 2,* 3–20.

Kamps, D. K., Leonard, B. R., Vernon, S., & Dugan, E. P. (1992). Teaching social skills to students with autism to increase peer interactions in an integrated first-grade classroom. *Journal of Applied Behavior Analysis, 25,* 281–288.

Kanner, L. (1943). Autistic disturbances of affective contact. *Nervous Child, 2,* 217–250.

Koegel, L. K., Koegel, R. L., & Parks, D. R. (1989). *How to teach self-management skills to people with severe disabilities: A training manual.* University of California, Santa Barbara.

Koegel, R. L., & Covert, A. (1972). The relationship of self-stimulation to learning in autistic children. *Journal of Applied Behavior Analysis, 5,* 381–387.

Koegel, R. L., Dyer, K., & Bell, L. K. (1987). The influence of child preferred activities on autistic children's social behavior. *Journal of Applied Behavior Analysis, 20,* 243–252.

Koegel, R. L., & Koegel, L. K. (1990). Extended reductions in stereotypic behaviors through self-management in multiple community settings. *Journal of Applied Behavior Analysis, 23,* 119–127.

Koegel, R. L., O'Dell, M. C., & Dunlap, G. (1988). Producing speech use in nonverbal autistic children by reinforcing attempts. *Journal of Autism and Developmental Disorders, 18,* 525–538.

Koegel, R. L., O'Dell, M. C., & Koegel, L. K. (1987). A natural language paradigm for teaching non-verbal autistic children. *Journal of Autism and Developmental Disorders, 17,* 187–199.

Koegel, R. L., & Rincover, A. (1977). Research on the difference between generalization and maintenance in extra-therapy responding. *Journal of Applied Behavior Analysis, 10,* 1–12.

Koegel, R. L., Rincover, A., & Egel, A. L. (1982). *Educating and understanding autistic children.* Houston, TX: College Hill Press.

Koegel, R. L., & Schreibman, L. (1977). Teaching autistic children to respond to simultaneous multiple cues. *Journal of Experimental Child Psychology, 24,* 299–311.

Koegel, R. L., Schreibman, L., Britten, K. R., Burke, J. C., & O'Neill, R. E. (1982). A comparison of parent training to direct clinic treatment. In R. L. Koegel, A. Rincover, & A. L. Egel (Eds.), *Educating and understanding autistic children* (pp. 260–279). Houston, TX: College Hill Press.

Koegel, R. L., Schreibman, L., Good, A. B., Cerniglia, L., Murphy, C., & Koegel, L. K. (1989). *How to teach pivotal behaviors to autistic children: A training manual.* University of California, Santa Barbara.

Koegel, R. L., Schreibman, L., O'Neill, R. E., & Burke, J. C. (1983). The personality and family-interaction characteristics of parents of autistic children. *Journal of Consulting and Clinical Psychology, 51,* 683–692.

Krantz, P. J., MacDuff, M. T., & McClannahan, L. E. (1993). Programming participation in family activities for children with autism: Parents' use of photographic activity schedules. *Journal of Applied Behavior Analysis, 26,* 137–148.

Krantz, P. J., & McClannahan, L. E. (1993). Teaching children with autism to initiate to peers: Effects of a script-fading procedure. *Journal of Applied Behavior Analysis, 26,* 121–132.

Laski, K. E., Charlop, M. H., & Schreibman, L. (1988). Training parents to use the Natural Language Paradigm to increase their autistic children's speech. *Journal of Applied Behavior Analysis, 21,* 391–400.

Leslie, A. M., & Frith, U. (1988). Autistic children's understanding of seeing, knowing, and believing. *British Journal of Developmental Psychology, 6,* 315–324.

Lewis, V., & Boucher, J. (1988). Spontaneous, instructed and elicited play in relatively able autistic children. *British Journal of Developmental Psychology, 6,* 325–339.

Lockyer, L., & Rutter, M. (1969). A five to fifteen year follow-up study of infantile psychosis: 3. Psychological aspects. *British Journal of Psychology, 115,* 865–882.

Lord, C., Rutter, M., Goode, S., Heemsbergen, J., Jordan, H., Mawhood, L., & Schopler, E. (1989). Autism Diagnostic Observation Schedule: A standardized observation of communicative and social behavior. *Journal of Autism and Developmental Disorders, 19,* 185–212.

Lord, C., Rutter, M., & Le Couteur, A. (1994). Autism Diagnostic Interview-Revised: A revised version of a diagnostic interview for caregivers of individuals with possible pervasive developmental disorders. *Journal of Autism and Developmental Disorders, 24,* 659–686.

Lovaas, O. I. (1981). *Teaching developmentally disabled children: The me book.* Austin, TX: Pro-Ed.

Lovaas, O. I., Koegel, R. L., & Schreibman, L. (1979). Stimulus overselectivity in autism. A review of research. *Psychological Bulletin, 86,* 1236–1254.

Lovaas, O. I., Koegel, R. L., Simmons, J. Q., & Long, J. S. (1973). Some generalization and follow-up measures on autistic children in behavior therapy. *Journal of Applied Behavior Analysis, 6,* 131–166.

Lovaas, O. I., Litrownik, A., & Mann, R. (1971). Response latencies to auditory stimuli in autistic children engaged in self-stimulatory behavior. *Behaviour Research and Therapy, 9,* 39–49.

Lovaas, O. I., Newsom, C. D., & Hickman, C. (1987). Self-stimulatory behavior and perceptual development. *Journal of Applied Behavior Analysis, 20,* 45–68.

Lovaas, O. I., & Simmons, J. Q. (1969). Manipulation of self-destruction in three retarded children. *Journal of Applied Behavior Analysis, 2,* 143–157.

Matson, J. L., Sevin, J. A., Fridley, P., & Love, S. R. (1990). Increasing spontaneous language in three autistic children. *Journal of Applied Behavior Analysis, 23,* 227–233.

Matson, J. L., & Swiezy, N. (1994). Social skills: Training with autistic children. In J. L. Matson (Ed.), *Autism in children and adults: Etiology, assessment, and intervention* (pp. 241–260). Pacific Grove, CA: Brooks/Cole.

McGee, G. G., Krantz, P. J., Mason, D., & McClannahan, L. E. (1983). The facilitative effects of incidental teaching on preposition use by autistic children. *Journal of Applied Behavior Analysis, 18,* 17–31.

Oke, N. J., & Schreibman, L. (1990). Training social initiations to a high-functioning autistic child: Assessment of collateral change and generalization in a case study. *Journal of Autism and Developmental Disorders, 20,* 479–497.

Panksepp, J., Lensing, P., Leboyer, M., & Bouvard, M. P. (1991). Naltrexone and other potential new pharmacological treatments of autism. *Brain Dysfunction, 4,* 281–300.

Paul, R. (1987). Communication in autism. In D. Cohen & A. Donnellan (Eds.), *Handbook of autism and pervasive developmental disorders* (pp. 61–84). New York: Wiley.

Pauls, D. (1987). The familiarity of autism and related disorders: A review of the evidence. In D. Cohen & A. Donnellan (Eds.), *Handbook of autism and pervasive developmental disorders* (pp. 192–198). New York: Wiley.

Pierce, K., & Schreibman, L. (1994). Teaching children with autism daily living skills in unsupervised settings through pictorial self-management. *Journal of Applied Behavior Analysis, 27,* 471–481.

Pierce, K., & Schreibman, L. (1995). Increasing complex social behaviors in children with autism: Effects of peer-implemented pivotal response training. *Journal of Applied Behavior Analysis, 28,* 285–295.

Prizant, B. M. (1983). Language acquisition and communicative behavior: Toward an understanding of the "whole" of it. *Journal of Speech and Hearing Disorders, 48,* 296–307.

Rimland, B. (1964). *Infantile autism.* New York: Appleton–Century–Crofts.

Rimland, B. (1971). The differentiation of childhood psychoses: An analysis of checklists for 2,218 psychotic children. *Journal of Autism and Childhood Schizophrenia, 1,* 161–174.

Rimland, B. (1978). Inside the mind of the autistic savant. *Psychology Today, 12,* 68–80.

Rincover, A. (1978). Variables affecting stimulus-fading and discriminative responding in psychotic children. *Journal of Abnormal Psychology, 87,* 541–553.

Ritvo, E. R. (1981). *Genetic and immuno-hematologic studies on the syndrome of autism.* Paper presented at the International Conference on Autism, Boston.

Ritvo, E. R., & Freeman, B. J. (1978). National Society for Autistic Children definition of the syndrome of autism. *Journal of Autism and Childhood Schizophrenia, 8,* 162–167.

Runco, M. A., Charlop, M. H., & Schreibman, L. (1986). The occurrence of autistic self-stimulation as a function of novel versus familiar setting, persons, and tasks. *Journal of Autism and Developmental Disorders, 16,* 31–44.

Rutter, M. (1966). Behavioural and cognitive characteristics of a series of psychotic children. In J. Wing (Ed.), *Early childhood autism* (pp. 51–81). Elmsford, NY: Pergamon Press.

Rutter, M. (1968). Concepts of autism: A review of research. *Journal of Child Psychology and Psychiatry, 9,* 1–25.

Rutter, M. (1971). The description and classification of infantile autism. In D. W. Churchill, G. D. Alpern, & M. K. DeMyer (Eds.), *Infantile autism* (pp. 8–28). Springfield, IL: Thomas.

Rutter, M. (1978). Diagnosis and definition of childhood autism. *Journal of Autism and Childhood Schizophrenia, 8,* 139–161.

Rutter, M., & Bartak, L. (1973). Special educational treatment of autistic children: A comparative study. II. Follow-up findings and implications of services. *Journal of Child Psychology and Psychiatry, 14,* 241–270.

Rutter, M., & Lockyer, L. (1967). A five to fifteen year follow-up study of infantile psychosis. I. Description of sample. *British Journal of Psychiatry, 113,* 1169–1182.

Sainato, D. M., Goldstein, H., & Strain, P. S. (1992). Effects of self-evaluation on preschool children's use of social interaction strategies with their classmates with autism. *Journal of Applied Behavior Analysis, 25,* 127–141.

Sainato, D. M., Strain, P. S., Lefebvre, D., & Rapp, N. (1987). Facilitating transition times with handicapped preschool children: A comparison between peer-mediated and antecedent prompt procedures. *Journal of Applied Behavior Analysis, 20,* 285–291.

Schopler, E., Reichler, R. J., DeVellis, R. F., & Daly, K. (1980). Toward objective classification of childhood autism: Childhood Autism Rating Scale (CARS). *Journal of Autism and Developmental Disorders, 10,* 91–103.

Schreibman, L. (1975). Effects of within-stimulus and extra-stimulus prompting on discrimination learning in autistic children. *Journal of Applied Behavior Analysis, 8,* 91–112.

Schreibman, L. (1988). *Autism.* Newbury Park, CA: Sage Publishing Co.

Schreibman, L., & Carr, E. G. (1978). Elimination of echolalic responding to questions through the training of a generalized verbal response. *Journal of Applied Behavior Analysis, 11,* 453–463.

Schreibman, L., & Charlop, M. H. (1987). Autism. In V. B. Van Hasselt & M. Hersen (Eds.), *Psychological evaluation of the developmentally and physically disabled* (pp. 155–177). New York: Plenum Press.

Schreibman, L., Charlop, M. H., & Koegel, R. L. (1982). Teaching autistic children to use extra-stimulus prompts. *Journal of Experimental Child Psychology, 33,* 475–491.

Schreibman, L., Kaneko, W. M., & Koegel, R. L. (1991). Positive affect of parents of autistic children: A comparison across two teaching techniques. *Behavior Therapy, 22,* 479–490.

Schreibman, L., & Koegel, R. L. (1981). A guideline for planning behavior modification programs for autistic children. In S. Turner, K. Calhoun, & H. Adams (Eds.),

Handbook of clinical behavior therapy (pp. 500–526). New York: Wiley.

Schreibman, L., & Koegel, R. L. (1997). Fostering self-management: Parent-delivered pivotal response training for children with autistic disorder. In E. D. Hibbs & P. S. Jensen (Eds.), *Psychosocial treatments for child and adolescent disorders: Empirically based strategies for clinical practice*. Washington, DC: American Psychological Association.

Schreibman, L., & Mills, J. I. (1983). Infantile autism. In T. H. Ollendick & M. Hersen (Eds.), *Handbook of child psychopathology* (pp. 123–149). New York: Plenum Press.

Schreibman, L., O'Neill, R. E., & Koegel, R. L. (1983). Behavioral training for siblings of autistic children. *Journal of Applied Behavior Analysis, 16,* 129–138.

Sloane, H. N., Endo, G. T., Hawkes, T. W., & Jenson, W. R. (1991). Reducing children's interrupting through self-instructional parent training materials. *Education and Treatment of Children, 14,* 38–52.

Stahmer, A. C. (1995). Teaching symbolic play skills to children with autism using Pivotal Response Training. *Journal of Autism and Developmental Disorders, 25,* 123–141.

Stahmer, A. C., & Schreibman, L. (1992). Teaching children with autism appropriate play in unsupervised environments using a self-management treatment package. *Journal of Applied Behavior Analysis, 25,* 447–459.

Stokes, T. F., & Baer, D. M. (1977). An implicit technology of generalization. *Journal of Applied Behavior Analysis, 10,* 349–368.

Strain, P. S., Kerr, M. M., & Ragland, E. U. (1979). Effects of peer-mediated social initiations and prompting/reinforcement procedures on the social behavior of autistic children. *Journal of Autism and Developmental Disorders, 9,* 41–54.

Tate, B. G., & Baroff, G. S. (1966). Aversive control of self-injurious behavior in a psychotic boy. *Behaviour Research and Therapy, 4,* 281–287.

Townsend, J., & Courchesne, E. (1994). Parietal damage and narrow "spotlight" spatial attention. *Journal of Cognitive Neuroscience, 6,* 218–230.

Volkmar, F. R., & Cohen, D. J. (1994). Autism: Current concepts. *Psychoses and Pervasive Developmental Disorders, 3,* 43–52.

Wakabayashi, S. (1979). A case of infantile autism associated with Down's syndrome. *Journal of Autism and Developmental Disorders, 9,* 31–36.

Wing, J. K. (1976). Kanner's syndrome: A historical introduction. In L. Wing (Ed.), *Early childhood autism: Clinical, educational and social aspects* (2nd ed, pp. 3–14). Elmsford, NY: Pergamon Press.

Wing, L. (1976). Diagnosis, clinical description, and prognosis. In L. Wing (Ed.), *Early childhood autism: Clinical, educational and social aspects* (2nd ed., pp. 15–48). Elmsford, NY: Pergamon Press.

Wing, L. (1988). The continuum of autistic characteristics. In E. Schopler & A. Mesibov (Eds.), *Diagnosis and assessment in autism: Current issues in autism* (pp. 91–110). New York: Plenum.

Wolery, M., Kirk, K., & Gast, D. L. (1985). Stereotypic behavior as a reinforcer: Effects and side effects. *Journal of Autism and Developmental Disorders, 15,* 149–161.

World Health Organization. (1993). *Mental disorders: Glossary and guide to their classification in accordance with the tenth revision of the International Classification of Diseases.* Geneva: Author.

7

Attention-Deficit / Hyperactivity Disorders

Carol K. Whalen and Barbara Henker

INTRODUCTION

On first meeting a hyperactive boy, you are likely to be charmed by his outgoing and enthusiastic nature. He looks and behaves like any other child and may even seem especially bright and responsive. It will often take some time to realize that there are serious problems. Some of these children have difficulty settling into or completing tasks and assignments, and they appear dreamy, distractible, and disorganized. Others are forever seeking and exploring, confronting their environments in ways that violate social conventions and place them in harm's way. Often but not always, defiance and aggression are part of this behavioral brew. The current diagnostic term for this constellation of problems is attention-deficit/hyperactivity disorder, and the core characteristics are inattention, impulsivity, and excessive motor activity. The behavioral profiles are highly heterogeneous, however, and there is an ongoing search for subgroups that can be identified on the basis of characteristics, correlates, and course.

The decades of research synthesized in this chapter span an array of diagnostic labels and criteria. Some investigators use categorical selection and others use dimensional procedures; some focus on community samples and others on clinical samples. As well, the studies were conducted during the tenure of three different versions of the *Diagnostic and Statistical Manual* (DSM) of the American Psychiatric Association. For convenience, the terms *hyperactivity, attention-deficit disorder with hyperactivity* (ADDH), and *attention-deficit/hyperactivity disorder* (ADHD) are used interchangeably, but readers should be aware of the diversity of diagnostic methods and subject selection criteria. When findings converge, this diversity increases our confidence in the conclusions. But when contradictory results emerge, it is difficult to separate substance from artifact.

CAROL K. WHALEN • Department of Psychology and Social Behavior, University of California, Irvine, Irvine, California 92697. BARBARA HENKER • Department of Psychology, University of California, Los Angeles, Los Angeles, California 90095.

Handbook of Child Psychopathology, 3rd edition, edited by Ollendick & Hersen. Plenum Press, New York, 1998.

CHARACTERISTICS, CORRELATES, AND COURSE

ADHD is both a heterogeneous and a pervasive disorder. Each child has a unique constellation of problems, but in all cases multiple domains of functioning are affected. Typically, difficulties surface in any or all of the domains of attention and cognition, impulsivity and response inhibition, activity level, and social interaction. As an organizing schema, this extensive empirical and theoretical literature will be summarized by examining in turn two spheres of functioning: the ADHD child as an individual, and the ADHD child as a social being.

The ADHD Child as an Individual: Thinking and Doing

Natural (Social Ecological) Indicators

Inattention has been well documented in a number of ways. On questionnaires, items such as "difficulty concentrating" and "fails to finish things s/he starts" are frequently endorsed. When behaviors are observed directly, the child with ADHD is often found to be "off task," perhaps looking out the window while the teacher gives instructions, or examining the contents of his desk while classmates work on the math assignment. If one had to select the single most reliable indicator for distinguishing between ADHD and normal children and also for demonstrating treatment-related improvement, it would probably be direct observations of the frequency or duration of task attention during structured activities, especially those in classroom settings (Abikoff, Gittelman, & Klein, 1980; Whalen, Henker, Collins, Finck, & Dotemoto, 1979). These attentional patterns are often linked to performance deficits in the cognitive realm, and many children with ADHD experience serious learning problems and school failure (Faraone, Biederman, Lehman, Spencer, et al., 1993; Frick et al., 1991; Hinshaw, 1992; Semrud-Clikeman et al., 1992).

It is somewhat ironic that the problem domain that generated the initial names for this disorder, hyperkinesis and hyperactivity, is no longer seen as a defining or even a necessary ingredient. Even so, there is clear evidence that many children with ADHD show high and poorly modulated levels of motor activity. Buitelaar, Swinkels, de Vries, van der Gaag, and van Hooff (1994) demonstrated that, during dyadic activities with an adult, hyperactive children show elevated rates of squirming and manipulating objects and decreased duration of sitting when compared with either aggressive or normal agemates. Using diverse measures, other investigators have documented high levels of motor activity, most consistently in structured school settings, but also on weekends and while sleeping (Porrino et al., 1983).

Direct observations and reports from significant others (primarily parents and teachers) provide important information that has obvious ecological validity. For the clinician, this type of information is critical for functional diagnosis and effective treatment. For the research investigator who is attempting to understand the nature of ADHD, however, this information is quite limited. First, the problems that are pinpointed in this manner are not specific to ADHD. Second, what remains unclear is the relative contribution of definable deficits (e.g., in cognitive processing or disinhibition), motivational difficulties, or other nonspecific interference factors such as distractibility, disorganization, or noncompliance. For these reasons, researchers continue to bring both the child and the processes into the laboratory where they can be subjected to detailed scrutiny. Laboratory procedures enable precise task definition and manipulation of potentially relevant parameters such as rate of stimulus presentation, duration of task, cognitive load or difficulty, context or ambient stimulation, and reinforcement or payoff.

Laboratory and Quasinaturalistic Indicators

One traditional laboratory approach to assessing attention uses variants of the Continuous Performance Task (CPT). The objective is to respond when and only when a particular target stimulus occurs, for example, the letter *X* when it follows the letter *A*. Because targets appear infrequently, often only 10% of the time, successful performance requires "protected" attention as well as response inhibition. Halperin and colleagues are taking a new look at this traditional paradigm by conducting fine-grained analyses of the types and timing of errors. Children may make omission errors, failing to respond to a true signal, or they may make different kinds of commission errors, for example, responding to an *A* before another letter appears, or to an *X* that was not preceded by an *A*. CPT performance may be useful not only in distinguishing between ADHD and normal children, but also in differentiating "pure" ADHD children from those with conduct and anxiety problems (Halperin et al., 1993), as well as in distinguishing between inattentive and impulsive subgroups of ADHD (Halperin et al., 1990).

Sergeant and van der Meere (1990, 1994) have also used these types of tasks, combined with the logic of Sternberg's (1969) Additive Factor Method (AFM), to show that the undisputed attentional difficulties of ADHD children on purportedly simple vigilance tasks are attributable, in large part, to strategic factors and effort allocation on the output side rather than to central stages of search and decision. These difficulties are heightened at slow event rates (van der Meere, Vreeling, & Sergeant, 1992), thus appearing to rule out attentional processing deficits per se. Also revealing are analyses of what children do after making an error on a challenging task: Normal children tend to slow down, whereas children with ADHD fail to adjust their response speed. This pattern provides further evidence of the role of temporal parameters and output or motor-related processes in the performance deficits associated with ADHD (van der Meere, van Baal, & Sergeant, 1989).

There are large numbers of studies that relate laboratory task performance to diagnostic group membership, and thus some degree of external validity for tasks such as CPTs can be in-ferred. If diagnoses reflect symptoms, then it follows that the laboratory tasks that discriminate diagnostic categories will probably predict those same symptoms. For many reasons, however, such relationships may be weak, and the external validity of laboratory tasks, or the applicability of their findings to the child's everyday world, is far from established.

Clinicians often hear parents ask, "If he really has an attention deficit, how can he stay glued to the TV for hours at a time?" Such queries may be followed with, "I wonder how much of it he really gets." Partly in answer to such questions and partly in response to the limited appeal that laboratory tasks have for subjects and critics alike, Lorch and Milich and their colleagues have adapted television viewing as a paradigm to test attentional efficiency and comprehension in youngsters with ADHD (Milich & Lorch, 1994). Salient among their intriguing findings is that attention in ADHD and control boys did not differ in the absence of a competing activity (a no-toy condition), and the presence of toys sharply reduced the ADHD boys' attending to TV but not their cued recall of its factual content. In another study, boys with ADHD did have more difficulty than control boys in free recall of information from situational comedies and action shows but not from a more structured educational TV program. In several studies, the number of looks at the TV screen, but not the time spent looking, was higher in the ADHD boys, supporting Ceci and Tishman's (1984) description of diffuse attentional patterns that seem to be effective as long as processing demands are low. Several empirical strands are converging on the conclusion that boys with ADHD are more likely to show performance deficits when cognitive demands increase, as in free-recall versus cued-recall tests. A second example is the contrast between TV programs that require integrative processing and those with a simpler focus on discrete facts. Whether these deficits stem from problems with information processing (e.g., retrieval inadequacy), energy allocation (e.g., effort), or a combination of the two is a key question for ongoing inquiry.

Integrative Theories of the Nature of ADHD

The ingenuity and diversity displayed in these several strands of research may belie a common thread: Current approaches are blurring the traditional distinctions among attention, cognition, impulsivity, and motor activity, and contemporary studies focus on interdependent processes rather than domain-specific functions. The increasing recognition of domain interdependence is generating overarching constructs that at least describe and at some future point may help explain both the panoply of findings and the nature of ADHD.

One example is the notion of inhibitory failure. It has been said by more than one sage that the essence of the socialized being lies in knowing what *not* to do. The ability to withhold or delay one's prepotent response is just as essential to overall adaptation as the ability to emit an adaptive response on demand. In the past decade, a number of theorists have been drawn to an examination of inhibitory failure as the mechanism central to the numerous difficulties that ADHD children show in modulating their attention, their choices, and their energies.

Salient among these, Quay (1988, 1993) took Gray's (1991) model of limbic system functioning in anxiety disorders and extended it to children, focusing on impulse control in disruptive and aggressive children (see also McBurnett, 1992). Quay attributed ADHD to underactivation of the behavioral inhibition system, resulting in failures to interrupt or withhold responses in the face of cues for nonreward, punishment, or novelty. Newman and Wallace (1993) provided a thorough explication of Gray's theory applied to disinhibition in adults and considered its extension to children with ADHD.

A somewhat different view of inhibitory failure, and one aligned more closely to cognitive than conditioning models, is the race model (Logan & Cowan, 1984) and the stop signal paradigm used to test its predictions (Chee, Logan, Schachar, Lindsay, & Wachsmuth, 1989; Schachar, Tannock, & Logan, 1993). According

to the model, the outcome of everyday situations requiring inhibition, such as looking before running into a street, results from a race between a primary goal process and the inhibitory or stop process. The two processes are independent and their relative speeds determine the outcome. The stop signal task brings this race into the laboratory in the form of a forced-choice, reaction-time task in which a fixed but unpredictable percentage of the trials (usually 25%) contain a stop signal. The task permits separate assessment of the efficiency of inhibitory control processes and the primary task reaction processes.

Results from this research group have been persuasive in demonstrating that children with ADHD show deficits in inhibitory control but not in attentional resources. Importantly, the deficits appear more pronounced in pervasive ADHD than in situational ADHD, conduct disorder (CD), or mixed CD + ADHD.

Still others seek a purchase on disinhibition through a focus not on signaled response withholding but on the maintenance of delay. According to Barkley (1994), the hallmark of ADHD may be a fundamental dysfunction in the ability to delay responding. For Sonuga-Barke (1995), on the other hand, the well-known difficulties that ADHD children have with delay-of-gratification tasks, as well as their impulsive or commission errors on match-to-sample tasks, may be motivational in nature. It isn't that the children can't delay but that they are delay *averse* and choose not to. The contrast between Barkley's position of reduced ability and Sonuga-Barke's hypothesis of delay aversion is reminiscent of the "can't, don't, or won't" question posed by Douglas (1983) about ADHD children's structured task performance.

Perhaps the most widely cited theory of ADHD is that of Douglas (1983, 1988, 1989), who proposed defective self-regulation as an umbrella construct under which are grouped four domains of problematic functioning. In addition to dysfunctional inhibitory control, Douglas designated difficulties in modulating arousal to meet situational demands, atypical responses to reinforcers and response consequences, and failures to deploy and maintain attention over time as the central interrelated deficits. In contrast to Barkley's view of disinhibition as the failure to delay reward, Douglas's emphasis is on the failure to withhold inappropriate responses. In contrast to Schachar and Logan's use of precisely timed choice tasks, Douglas's empirical tests focus on higher-level cognitive tasks requiring strategic planning and effortful processing. As the studies continue, however, the implications begin to converge. For example, Schachar, Tannock, Marriott, and Logan (1995) documented a separate deficit in changing or reengaging a new response following an inhibited action, a pattern that lends further support to Douglas's framing of a fundamental dysfunction in executive processing.

The view that one overarching construct, even one so broad as inhibitory failure, will carry enough explanatory power to be considered the heart of ADHD children's difficulties is probably unrealistic. Yet, testing these grounded theories is one of the most active and promising research directions in the contemporary ADHD arena. The search is fueled not only by advances in our understanding of cognition and disinhibition, but also by the increasing technological sophistication of neurophysiological probes. Particularly exciting are recent integrations of cognitive, behavioral, and neurophysiological findings such as the schema proposed by Malone, Kershner, and Swanson (1994; see below).

The ADHD Child as a Social Being: Interpersonal Dysfunction and Peer Relations

Interpersonal difficulties are a hallmark of the disorder and often the "last straw" that leads to clinical referral, despite the fact that social dysfunction is not a defining characteristic of ADHD. Some children with ADHD are aggressive and disruptive, some are socially clumsy and ineffective, and still others may seem disengaged or isolated. The common thread is unsatisfying interpersonal relations, often despite (or perhaps because of) a high level of social activity and interest. Whalen and Henker (1992) described a social profile consisting of the five fundamental facets that follow.

Social Response Patterns

As a group, children with ADHD exhibit an excess of inappropriate and aversive behavior and difficulties maintaining the give-and-take of social exchange. Many are as impulsive and inattentive in their social transactions as in their schoolwork. They barge right in rather than waiting their turn. They attempt to dominate and redirect rather than to join ongoing activities and follow accepted routines. They respond immaturely when peers disagree or refuse. In brief, their actions are more likely to disrupt the flow of social exchange than to facilitate it. Also common, but far from universal, is serious aggression, especially the reactive or explosive type, rather than the more instrumental, planful, or goal-oriented variant.

In contrast to the multiplicity of studies of disruptive and aggressive behavior, there is a paucity of research on prosocial activity. The jury is still out on whether children with ADHD have deficiencies in the positive as well as the negative realms of social intercourse (Buhrmester, Whalen, Henker, MacDonald, & Hinshaw, 1992).

Style of Approach

In many instances, the social clumsiness may be a function of high levels of intensity, an overzealous quality that others may experience as aversive. There are indications of affective dysregulation, a bountiful emotionality that may be difficult to direct or constrain. These youngsters also have difficulties shifting behaviors in accord with changing situational or role demands (Landau & Milich, 1988; Whalen, Henker, Collins, McAuliffe, & Vaux, 1979), often missing the subtle cues and signals that guide social exchange.

Social Information Processing

The search for a cognitive explanation for the interpersonal difficulties of ADHD children has not been notably productive to date. Although many studies have demonstrated dysfunctional social cue utilization, appraisal, and problem-solving processes in aggressive boys (Lochman & Dodge, 1994), the empirical literature on ADHD is not as clear. These youngsters do not seem to be deficient in their knowledge of social scripts or in their abilities to evaluate social acts (Whalen, Henker, & Granger, 1990). They seem as able as their peers to think through the basic steps of interpersonal encounter, but less competent at enactment, especially when excited, frustrated, or provoked. This pattern suggests that the differences may be more motivational than cognitive, more a function of social preferences and agendas than of social knowledge per se.

Some children with ADHD may have subtle problems with social attention. Hyperactive children seem to spend less time than their normal counterparts observing the ongoing behaviors of their peers (Cunningham, Siegel, & Offord, 1985), and the temporal associations between an adult's conversational speech and the child's behavior seem to be weaker with hyperactive children than with either aggressive or normal agemates (Buitelaar et al., 1994).

Peer Appeal and Social Standing

Negative peer regard is the rule rather than the exception for children with ADHD. Even those who are not actively disliked have difficulty establishing friendships. Pope, Bierman, and Mumma (1989) distinguished between high rejection and low acceptance, demonstrating that both aggression and hyperactivity are linked to the former, but that hyperactivity was the more important determinant of the latter. Although it can be assumed that the aversive behaviors of ADHD children earn them much of their negative reputation, inattention without impulsivity may also have pervasive social conse-

quences, especially when children are mutually dependent such as during team sports or group projects (e.g., Pelham et al., 1990). The mere expectation that a child is hyperactive, in the absence of confirmatory evidence, decreases the friendliness and involvement of normal youngsters and has a negative impact on social status (Harris, Milich, Corbitt, Hoover, & Brady, 1992).

Social Impact and Influence

ADHD has social ramifications that extend far beyond the children themselves. People respond differently when in the presence of a child with ADHD. Hubbard and Newcomb (1991) found that dyads consisting of one normal and one hyperactive boy, versus those with two normal boys, engaged in more solitary play, were less likely to return to constructive play after a disruption, and also showed lower levels of verbal reciprocity and affective expression. Such bidirectional effects can, of course, further constrict the social learning opportunities of children with ADHD and prevent the corrective exchanges that facilitate interpersonal skill development.

Elevated rates of negative and controlling behaviors have been documented also in parents and teachers, as have withdrawal and decreased responsiveness (Cunningham & Siegel, 1987; Hubbard & Newcomb, 1991; Johnston, 1996; Whalen, Henker, & Dotemoto, 1981). Although it is difficult to establish direction of causality, children with ADHD may also contribute to diminished parenting self-efficacy and satisfaction as well as heightened parenting stress (Anastopoulos, Guevremont, Shelton, & DuPaul, 1992; Fischer, 1990; Mash & Johnston, 1990). Even increased alcohol consumption in adults has been associated with ADHD-type behaviors in children, a connection apparently mediated by child-induced stress (Pelham & Lang, 1993). It seems clear that children with ADHD have negative catalytic effects, changing the social ecologies of family, school, and peer cultures.

Patterns of Comorbidity (Coexisting Conditions)

One ineluctable conclusion from recent epidemiological studies of childhood disorders is that comorbidity is the rule and "pure" or single disorders the exception. Bird, Gould, and Staghezza (1993) found that 62.9% of youngsters who met DSM-III diagnostic criteria for any disorder met these criteria for two or more disorders. This high rate is especially noteworthy because disorders were grouped into four supraordinate domains (attention deficit, conduct/oppositional, anxiety, and depression), and thus the high comorbidity rates could not be attributed to links between similar disorders such as two subtypes of anxiety. When we focus specifically on ADHD, we find consistently high comorbidity rates, especially for learning problems and oppositional/conduct disorders. We are also learning that comorbidity crosses the line between externalizing and internalizing domains; 20 to 50% of children with ADHD may also have severe problems with anxiety or depression (Angold & Costello, 1993; Bird et al., 1993; Hammen & Compas, 1994; Verhulst & van der Ende, 1993). ADHD is also found in a substantial proportion of cases of Tourette's syndrome (TS), a disorder characterized by motor and vocal tics that may include the involuntary and inappropriate uttering of obscenities known as coprolalia (Robertson, 1994).

As Caron and Rutter (1991) explicated, there are many potential sources of artifactual comorbidity, including overlapping diagnostic criteria, artificial subdivision of syndromes, and developmental progressions in which one disorder is an early version of another. Negative expectancies or halo effects may also contribute to high comorbidity rates (Abikoff, Courtney, Pelham, & Koplewicz, 1993). There are also instances of true comorbidity, however, when the comorbid pattern constitutes a meaningful syndrome that can be differentiated from single disorders on the basis of etiology, characteristics, course, or treatment response. For example, children with comorbid anxiety and ADHD display less impulsivity and fewer behavior problems than children who show ADHD without anxiety, and these two groups also appear to differ in catecholamine response to mentally stressful tasks (Pliszka, 1989, 1992; Pliszka, Maas, Javors, Rogeness, & Baker, 1994). Importantly, stimulant treatment is markedly less beneficial for children with combined ADHD and anxiety problems than for those with ADHD only; in contrast, the co-occurrence of CD and ADHD does not seem to influence stimulant responsiveness (Pliszka, 1989; Taylor et al., 1987).

Comorbidity appears to be more common in younger than in older children (Bird et al., 1993; Russo & Beidel, 1994) and in clinical than in community samples (McConaughy & Achenbach, 1994). As would be expected, comorbidity relates positively to both degree of clinical impairment and utilization of mental health services (Bird et al., 1993; Russo & Beidel, 1994) and inversely to prognosis (Verhulst & van der Ende, 1993). Compared with either disorder alone, the co-occurrence of ADHD and CD is associated with the heaviest dose of biological and environmental adversity as well as the poorest prognosis throughout the life span (Loeber & Keenan, 1994).

Developmental Progressions and Extensions

Age of Onset

The peak period for the diagnosis of ADHD is between the ages of 7 and 9, but problems are apparent often before the age of 3 (Cohen et al., 1993). The relatively high rate of diagnosis during the early school years probably reflects the fact that academic settings and routines, in contrast to home environments, tend to be more demanding, less flexible, and less likely to accommodate individual differences. An intriguing analysis by McGee, Williams, and Feehan (1992) suggests that age of onset may distinguish between pervasive (onset by age 5–6) and situational ADHD (onset between ages 6 and 7). Those with earlier onset were more likely to have comorbid disorders, cognitive deficits, family disadvantage, and persistence of problems at least into adolescence, whereas later-onset difficulties seemed to be secondary to reading failure and to have a markedly better prognosis. Delineations of alternate developmental pathways promise not only to elucidate etiological chains, but also to help us predict outcome and design optimal intervention packages.

Developmental Course and Long-Term Outcomes

The developmental course of ADHD is characterized by what has been called *heterotypic continuity*—changes in the form though not necessarily the severity or extensity of problems. For example, the excessive gross motor activity of childhood may be transformed into less salient—but still dysfunctional—fidgetiness and restlessness. In many cases, there is significant improvement as the child matures, with symptom amelioration more likely to be seen in the realm of hyperactivity-impulsivity than inattention (Hart, Lahey, Loeber, Applegate, & Frick, 1995). In other cases, problem severity increases with age as early difficulties create later disadvantages that have cumulative consequences on learning, social relations, and self-esteem.

In the past it was assumed that, whatever the childhood course, ADHD virtually disappeared with the onset of puberty. This assumption has been disproved by mounting evidence, from both clinical and epidemiological studies, of moderate continuity of ADHD-type problems into the adult years (Ferdinand, Verhulst, & Wiznitzer, 1995). Longitudinal studies indicate that ADHD persists at least until midadolescence in 40 to 70% of individuals diagnosed during childhood (Klein & Mannuzza, 1991; Weiss & Hechtman, 1993). The outlook may be somewhat more positive by young adulthood, but significant proportions continue to meet diagnostic criteria for ADHD into and perhaps beyond their 30s (Klein & Mannuzza, 1991; Mannuzza, Klein, Bessler, Malloy, & LaPadula, 1993). Antisocial and substance use disorders

are also likely during adolescence and adulthood, especially when (1) aggression was problematic during the early years or (2) ADHD persists beyond childhood (Barkley, Fischer, Edelbrock, & Smallish, 1990; Mannuzza et al., 1991). There is no compelling evidence that children with ADHD are at elevated risk for later mood or anxiety disorders (Mannuzza et al., 1991).

When we move from formal diagnoses to everyday functioning, we find multiple indicators of continuing educational and vocational disadvantage such as lower scores on standardized achievement tests, more failed grades and school suspensions, and poorer job performance. As a group, adults who were diagnosed with ADHD during childhood tend to complete fewer years of education, change jobs more frequently, and stop at lower rungs on the occupational ladder (e.g., Barkley, Fischer, et al., 1990; Mannuzza et al., 1993). Continuing problems with social relationships and self-esteem have also been documented, as have elevated rates of unintentional injuries, physical violence, and criminal activity (Hellgren, Gillberg, Gillberg, & Enerskog, 1993; Weiss & Hechtman, 1993). Even mundane activities such as automobile driving are affected, with ADHD adolescents and young adults more likely than their peers to receive traffic citations (especially for speeding and failing to stop), to have their driver's licenses revoked, to have multiple crashes, to be deemed at fault for these crashes, and to sustain crash-related injuries (Barkley, Guevremont, Anastopoulos, DuPaul, & Shelton, 1993). Interestingly, Barkley et al. (1993) found no group differences in the proportion who had had a single crash, suggesting that during this high-risk period, normal youth are more able than their ADHD counterparts to learn from experience.

One intriguing hypothesis is that there are two distinctive subtypes of ADHD, a "maturational lag" subgroup, about a third to a half of those diagnosed ADHD, whose adjustment normalizes by the age of 15–16, and a "persistent" subgroup who continue to show multiple problems, perhaps throughout the life span (Klein & Mannuzza, 1989). Whether or not this subtyping relates to the situational–pervasive distinction posed by others such as Campbell and colleagues (e.g., Campbell, Pierce, March, Ewing, & Szumowski, 1994) and McGee et al. (1992) is a topic for further inquiry. The search continues for reliable predictors of outcome, a literature that is replete with methodological pitfalls and contradictory findings. To date, the sturdiest predictor seems to be childhood aggression. Associations between long-term adjustment and other obvious factors such as social adversity, parental psychopathology, low IQ, or neurological involvement surface in scattered studies and for specific outcome variables, but in a far from consistent or pervasive pattern (Klein & Mannuzza, 1991; Weiss & Hechtman, 1993). Important questions for future research include whether there are qualitatively distinctive subtypes that can be defined by persistence and, if so, whether these differences in outcome are associated with differences in the mix of etiological agents, symptom patterns, and treatment responsiveness.

Adult ADHD

The validity of adult ADHD remains a controversial issue. First, the diagnosis is based on a childhood history of ADHD, which typically requires retrospective reporting that is subject to memory lapses and recall biases. Second, symptoms such as distractibility and impulsivity lack diagnostic specificity and may accompany other disorders such as substance abuse or depression. Third, there is concern that adult ADHD is becoming a ready excuse for chronic academic, occupational, and interpersonal difficulties or even a vehicle for obtaining restricted (stimulant) drugs (Shaffer, 1994).

Despite these caveats, evidence is growing that there is an adult variant of ADHD, as suggested by Wender's pioneering studies over the past two decades (e.g., Wender, Reimherr, Wood, & Ward, 1985). These individuals, who may not come to clinical attention until their adult years, have developmental profiles similar to those diagnosed during childhood. In a re-

view of studies that included over 1700 adults with a history of ADHD, Spencer, Biederman, Wilens, and Faraone (1994) provided convincing arguments for the validity of ADHD in adults, demonstrating patterns of dysfunction, comorbidity, familial aggregation, and response to stimulant treatment that, with some important exceptions, generally mirror those found for ADHD children.

Adults who are newly diagnosed with ADHD often express a pervasive sense of relief, as illustrated by the comments of a psychiatrist who, at the age of 31, first learned that he might have this disorder:

> At least there was a term to explain the conversations I tuned out of, involuntarily, for no apparent reason. . . . For forgetting the task at hand as I go off on the wings of a new thought or off in search of what I forgot. For the love of the chase, the new project, the hot idea, for the love of, the need for, something highly stimulating and riveting. . . . Now with a name rooted in neurobiology I could begin to make sense of, in a forgiving way, parts of myself that had often frustrated or scared me. (Hallowell & Ratey, 1994, p. x)

Much remains to be learned about the nature and treatment of adult ADHD. Given the clinical and methodological challenges, investigators have been warned to proceed with caution, but proceeding they are.

DIAGNOSIS

In the United States, the *Diagnostic and Statistical Manual* of the American Psychiatric Association (APA) provides the "official" diagnostic nomenclature. Since 1968, there have been four sets of diagnostic criteria for the problem constellation now identified as ADHD. First identified in the second edition of the DSM (DSM-II; APA, 1968) and labeled *Hyperkinetic Reaction of Childhood,* the disorder was defined primarily on the basis of overactivity, restlessness, distractibility, and short attention span. The syndrome was renamed *Attention Deficit Disorder*

(ADD) in the third edition (DSM-III; APA, 1980) to reflect a growing consensus that attentional dysfunction was more fundamental and consequential than excessive motoric activity. Three symptom clusters and two diagnostic subgroups were identified. When problems were apparent in all three areas—inattention, impulsivity, and motoric overactivity—the child was diagnosed attention deficit with hyperactivity (ADDH). When activity level did not seem to be problematic, the diagnosis was attention deficit without hyperactivity (ADD/WO). Investigators encountered difficulties in their early attempts to validate this new schema, however, especially in establishing the validity and reliability of the ADD/WO subtype.

A revision of the third edition—DSM-III-R, published in 1987—seemed to reverse the previous refinements by recombining all symptoms into a single, undifferentiated listing and again renaming the disorder, this time to *attention-deficit/hyperactivity disorder* (ADHD) (APA, 1987). But just as the new, unidimensional revision was taking hold, studies that distinguished empirically between ADDH and ADD/WO on a number of important dimensions were appearing in print (Barkley, DuPaul, & McMurray, 1990; Bauermeister, Alegria, Bird, Rubio-Stipec, & Canino, 1992; Cantwell & Baker, 1992; Goodyear & Hynd, 1992). These new data were providing more support for the diagnostic dichotomy identified in DSM-III than for the polythetic approach that was in the process of replacing it (Goodyear & Hynd, 1992). Although this temporal juxtaposition seems somewhat ironic, it is not surprising, given the lengthy preparation time and publication lag for empirical research studies.

With the fourth and most recent revision of DSM (APA, 1994), the face of attention deficit/hyperactivity has been altered once again. The subtype approach that was attempted in DSM-III and discarded in DSM-III-R has resurfaced but in a new form and on firmer empirical ground. The new version again distinguishes between inattention and hyperactivity, but this time impulsivity is combined with the latter rather than with the former, yielding a better match with the empirical literature. The current nomenclature delineates three subtypes, one that is predominantly inattentive (ADHD-PI), one that is predominantly hyperactive-impulsive (ADHD-PH), and one that combines both domains (ADHD-C). The diagnosis cannot be made on the basis of the symptom picture alone; age of onset, persistence, evidence of clinically significant impairment, and cross-setting generality must also be considered, as can be seen in Table 1.

To date, the results of systematic field trials of DSM-IV have been promising. Especially encouraging is the improved reliability and validity for the predominantly inattentive subtype (compared with ADD/WO in DSM-III). The PI subgroup is distinguished by having a higher proportion of girls, a later age of onset, and greater impairment in academic performance (Lahey et al., 1994). Preliminary evidence suggests that this is a distinct subgroup with elevated rates of internalizing symptoms (e.g., anxiety, shyness, withdrawal), cognitive deficits, and motivational problems. Another group, probably the vast majority and those who will now be labeled ADHD-C, are more likely to show problems with conduct and oppositionality as well as attentional dysfunction and impulsivity.

In systematic comparisons of who gets diagnosed by the three most recent systems, Baumgaertel, Wolraich, and Dietrich (1995) found a 64% increase in ADHD prevalence when they shifted from DSM-III-R to DSM-IV. Lahey et al. (1994) also reported increased prevalence using DSM-IV, although the difference was not as dramatic. In the Lahey et al. study, the added cases identified by DSM-IV were more than twice as likely to be girls, and most met criteria for the inattentive subtype. In addition, the newly identified cases that met criteria for ADHD-PH were, on the average, 3–5 years younger than those in the other two categories, a pattern suggesting that ADHD-PH may be the developmental precursor to ADHD-C rather than a distinct subtype (Lahey et al., 1994). Thus, DSM-IV may identify some children earlier and other

Table 1. Attention-Deficit/Hyperactivity Disorder (DSM-IV)

A. For either (1) or (2), six (or more) symptoms have persisted for at least 6 months to a degree that is maladaptive and inconsistent with developmental level:

(1) Inattention
    (a) often fails to give close attention to details or makes careless mistakes in schoolwork, work, or other activities
    (b) often has difficulty sustaining attention in tasks or play activities
    (c) often does not seem to listen when spoken to directly
    (d) often does not follow through on instructions and fails to finish schoolwork, chores, or duties in the workplace (not due to oppositional behavior or failure to understand instructions)
    (e) often has difficulty organizing tasks and activities
    (f) often avoids, dislikes, or is reluctant to engage in tasks that require sustained mental effort (such as schoolwork or homework)
    (g) often loses things necessary for tasks or activities (e.g., toys, school assignments, pencils, books, or tools)
    (h) is often easily distracted by extraneous stimuli
    (i) is often forgetful in daily activities

(2) Hyperactivity-Impulsivity
    (a) often fidgets with hands or feet or squirms in seat
    (b) often leaves seat in classroom or in other situations in which remaining seated is expected
    (c) often runs about or climbs excessively in situations in which it is inappropriate (in adolescents or adults, may be limited to subjective feelings of restlessness)
    (d) often has difficulty playing or engaging in leisure activities quietly
    (e) is often "on the go" or often acts as if "driven by a motor"
    (f) often talks excessively
    (g) often blurts out answers before questions have been completed
    (h) often has difficulty awaiting turn
    (i) often interrupts or intrudes on others (e.g., butts into conversations or games)

B. Some hyperactive-impulsive or inattention symptoms that caused impairment were present before age 7 years.
C. Some impairment from the symptoms is present in two or more settings.
D. There must be clear evidence of clinically significant impairment in social, academic, or occupational functioning.

Note: Adapted from American Psychiatric Association. (1994). *Diagnostic and statistical manual of mental disorders* (4th ed.). Washington, DC: Author.

children who may have escaped diagnosis entirely with DSM-III or DSM-III-R. Whether or not these additional and earlier diagnoses are beneficial in the sense of facilitating better treatments and outcomes—or in uncovering alternate etiological or developmental pathways—is an important question for future research.

The evolutionary history of diagnostic labels and criteria is a direct reflection of progressive gains in knowledge and methodological sophistication, providing assurance that we are getting closer to a functional understanding of ADHD phenomena. The nature and number of changes over the past 25 years also remind us, however, that diagnostic systems—even those that are systematic and scientific—are basically subjective constructions.

ETIOLOGICAL INFLUENCES

Family-Genetic Risk Factors

Familial aggregation of ADHD is well documented, with rates of ADHD as high as 25 to 30% in first-degree relatives of probands (i.e., diagnosed ADHD cases). Family members also show elevated rates of hostility, antisocial behavior, and drug dependence, especially when the ADHD child also has conduct problems (Barkley et al., 1991; Faraone, Biederman, Keenan, & Tsuang, 1991b), and an analogous pattern seems to obtain for anxiety disorders (Biederman, Faraone, Keenan, Steingard, & Tsuang, 1991). Biederman, Faraone, Keenan, Knee, and

Tsuang (1990) reported familial aggregations in the first-degree relatives of children with ADD but not in relatives of a psychiatric control group, indicating that the patterns are specific to ADD and not attributable to more general aspects of psychopathology.

As family-genetic studies benefit from progressively more sophisticated methodologies, the data supporting genetic transmission become increasingly compelling (Faraone et al., 1992), and twin and sibling studies provide further support for such hypotheses (Goodman & Stevenson, 1989; Levy, Hay, Waldman, McLaughlin, & Wood, 1994). These biological mechanisms do not, however, preclude environmental influences. For example, family members who display antisocial behaviors often function as negative role models and create unsalutary environments for children with ADHD. To cite another example, the stress generated by a hyperactive child's behavior problems can contribute substantially to maternal depression, independently of any genetic linkage between the two disorders. A final example can be taken from indications that ADHD and learning disabilities are genetically independent, with patterns of comorbidity and familial aggregation resulting from nonrandom mating rather than from shared genetic risk (Faraone, Biederman, Lehman, Keenan, et al., 1993).

Neurobiological Patterns

Another active area of research is the delineation of the neuroanatomical, neurochemical, and neurophysiological correlates of ADHD. A multiplicity of studies using diverse methods and measures have supported involvement of the frontal lobes, the caudate nucleus within the basal ganglia, the corpus callosum which connects the two lobes, and related "circuitry" or pathways between these structures (Giedd et al., 1994; Hynd et al., 1993; Semrud-Clikeman et al., 1994; Zametkin et al., 1990). At present, the neurochemical focus is on the catecholamines dopamine and norepinephrine, neurotransmitters that are known to affect diverse behavioral realms. There is consensus that catecholamine dysfunction is central to ADHD and that the dysfunction most likely involves more than a single neurotransmitter system (Zametkin & Rapoport, 1987). In one provocative analysis, Malone et al. (1994) proposed a bihemispheric imbalance involving underactivation of the left-hemisphere dopaminergic system combined with overarousal of the right-hemisphere noradrenergic system. Progress in the delineation of specific mechanisms is slow, however, and the difficulties are amplified by the fact that several different classes of drugs, with heterogeneous modes of action, produce similar behavioral changes.

Over the past few years, exciting findings have been emerging from the use of positron emission tomographic (PET) scans to measure cerebral glucose metabolism. Zametkin et al. (1990) documented decreased metabolic activity in a group of 25 adults with childhood histories of ADHD, and the largest reductions were in areas involved in the control of attention and motor activity, the premotor and superior prefrontal cortex. More recent studies have only partially replicated these results and have also suggested that the reduced brain metabolism may be more apparent in girls than in boys with ADHD, although the reasons for such differences are unknown (Ernst et al., 1994).

There are several methodological factors that cloud interpretation of these preliminary findings, and the difficulty of establishing consistent links between neurochemical and behavioral indicators continues. Nevertheless, diverse findings implicate neurobiological dysfunction. The continuing search for biological markers and pathways is being facilitated by technological developments that make assessments not only less invasive and cumbersome, but also more reliable.

Physical Environmental Influences

Dietary Contributions

Hypotheses about diet–behavior interactions are alluring, both because they match everyday notions about health and the environment and because they promise workable solutions to childhood problems. In the 1970s, concerns were expressed about widespread harmful effects of food dyes and additives as well as natural salicylates, which are present in a wide array of everyday foods such as tomatoes and oranges (Feingold, 1976). Controlled studies have not supported these vivid claims, but a sprinkling of findings suggest that some children may have food sensitivities or allergies that lead to adverse behavioral responses, perhaps mediated by physical discomfort or other physiological symptoms (Carter et al., 1993; Egger, Carter, Graham, Gumley, & Soothill, 1985; Kaplan, McNicol, Conte, & Moghadam, 1989). These effects appear to be rare and are more likely to occur in preschool than in school-age children.

More recently, attention has been focused on sugar and the artificial sweetener aspartame. Studies such as the one conducted by Wolraich et al. (1994) have used creative methods to neutralize expectancy or placebo effects and ensure compliance with experimental and control diets. Moreover, the investigators enrolled children who, according to parental report, were especially sensitive to sugar, thereby stacking the deck in favor of finding deleterious effects. But even in these instances, such effects could not be demonstrated. The number of times that rigorous methodologies have yielded null findings suggests the wisdom of shifting research energies away from studies of sweetener effects per se and toward examination of psychological processes that produce such strong parental beliefs. On the other hand, there appears to be enough evidence of idiosyncratic food sensitivities (e.g., to chocolate, wheat, or oranges) to merit clinical evaluation when parents report such effects (Carter et al., 1993).

Environmental Toxins

As an environmental toxin, lead is both pervasive and enduring. As a potential contributor to ADHD, lead is both extensively studied and highly controversial. There are widespread concerns that even slightly elevated body lead levels may result in cognitive impairment and perhaps behavior problems as well, problems that may be mild but persistent (Bellinger, Stiles, & Needleman, 1992; Fergusson, Horwood, & Lynskey, 1993). Although lead-based paint has been banned and leaded gasolines discontinued, lead continues to permeate dust and soil from products and practices of the recent and distant past. According to the Environmental Protection Agency, approximately 3 million children in 1990 had blood lead levels high enough to have a negative impact on intelligence and development (Binder & Matte, 1993). The empirical literature remains contradictory and inconclusive, however, with some studies demonstrating toxic effects on behavior or cognitive competence and others showing no effects when potential confounding factors are controlled. Particularly pertinent are recent findings that treatment-induced decreases in blood lead levels are followed by small but reliable cognitive improvements (Ruff, Bijur, Markowitz, Ma, & Rosen, 1993), although practice effects may have contributed to this finding. There is no basis for hypothesizing that lead in environmentally available doses is linked specifically with ADHD, but there is sufficient evidence of potentially harmful effects to justify attempts to limit exposure to this toxin. No level of lead in the body is viewed as safe, and protection is especially critical during childhood because of the increased vulnerability of developing organisms (Binder & Matte, 1993; Kruesi, 1990; Tesman & Hills, 1994).

Psychosocial Influences and Nature–Nurture Interactions

Although there is no conclusive evidence of psychosocial causation, social and environmental factors play important roles in shaping and modulating ADHD, influencing the range and severity of problems as well as treatment response and long-term outcomes. Several sets of findings converge to indicate that persistent externalizing problems in children are associated with family adversity and stressful life events, marital distress, parental symptomatology (especially maternal depression), disturbed parent–child relationships, and negative parental control tactics (Campbell, 1995; Haapasalo & Tremblay, 1994). Psychosocial adversity appears to play a greater etiological role in aggression and CD than in ADHD (Schachar, 1991) and is thus more apparent in children who are comorbid for the two disorders than in those with "pure" ADHD (Bauermeister, Canino, & Bird, 1994; Sanson, Smart, Prior, & Oberklaid, 1993). Comprehensive clinical studies are suggesting that psychosocial factors may do more than modulate severity or course; there may in fact be a nonfamilial or psychogenic form of ADHD that is especially responsive to environmental adversity (e.g., Bauermeister et al., 1992; Biederman et al., 1990).

We have seen that ADHD is a highly heterogeneous disorder in terms of characteristics, concomitants, and course. This is also the case regarding etiology. Multiple causal agents have been implicated, but none has been associated with ADHD specifically, exclusively, or definitively. For any one child diagnosed with ADHD, there is likely to be a complex web of interacting causal influences. As our techniques and knowledge increase, it can be predicted that distinct etiological subgroups will emerge that reflect alternative pathogenic pathways ending in the array of discordant behaviors that characterize ADHD.

EPIDEMIOLOGY

Prevalence

ADHD is one of the most frequent diagnoses given to referred children, and prevalence rates in clinical or special education samples often hover around 50 to 60% (Forness, Swanson, Cantwell, Guthrie, & Sena, 1992). Rates are much lower, of course, in community epidemiological samples, varying from a low of about 2% to a high of 10% (Bauermeister et al., 1994). A reasonable summary estimate is 5% of school-age children.

Gender

There are several basic findings in the field of ADHD that can be counted on to replicate in study after study despite widely varying sites, samples, objectives, and methods. One of these findings is that boys will outnumber girls, often by 2:1 and at times by as much as 9:1 (e.g., Anderson, Williams, McGee, & Silva, 1987; Bird et al., 1988). Because of the relative rarity of girls in this diagnostic group, many seminal studies have restricted their samples to boys, and thus there are gaps in our knowledge about gender differences and similarities. In the past few years, investigators have attempted to rectify this situation by expanding their recruitment efforts and combining across samples to achieve the needed number of girls with ADHD. Recent family studies indicate that relatives of ADHD boys and girls show similar patterns of elevated risk of psychopathology (Faraone, Biederman, Keenan, & Tsuang, 1991a); treatment studies indicate similar responsiveness to stimulant therapy (Pelham, Walker, Sturges, & Hoza, 1989); and follow-up data suggest similar long-term outcomes (Klein & Mannuzza, 1989). The evidence regarding behavioral and academic profiles is more mixed. Some studies yield markedly similar behavioral and academic profiles in boys and girls with ADHD (Breen, 1989; McGee & Feehan, 1991). As noted earlier, others indicate that girls with ADHD are more likely to have cognitive and academic impairments and less likely to show severely disruptive behaviors than are their male counterparts (Brown, Madan-Swain, & Baldwin, 1991; Gaub & Carlson, 1997). In fact, McGee and Feehan (1991) suggested that ADHD may be underrecognized in girls precisely because girls tend not to present the management difficulties found in boys. Many treatment decisions are based more on how much adult discomfort the child's behavior engenders than on how severe the child's level of dysfunction is (Costello & Janiszewski, 1990). This contention is buttressed by the fact that gender disparities tend to be greater in clinic-referred than in community samples. McGee and Feehan (1991) recommended that sex-specific norms and diagnostic criteria be used to ensure appropriate identification of girls with ADHD.

Cross-Cultural Patterns

The cluster of problem behaviors currently labeled ADHD has been found in all countries and cultures studied thus far, including diverse Western societies such as Australia, New Zealand, Germany, and Great Britain, as well as non-Western cultures in Japan, Ethiopia, Uganda, and China (Mann et al., 1992; Mulatu, 1995; Tao, 1992). Moreover, the disproportionate male/female ratios appear across cultures, as do the associations with aggressive behavior patterns and learning difficulties. Thus, there is no support for claims that ADHD is a product of Western cultural practices. There are, however, broad variations in prevalence rates across cultures, with estimates ranging from 1 to 13%, but such broad variations also emerge across studies within the United States. It is impossible at this time to disentangle the effects of cultural norms or diagnostic practices from those of actual differences in child behavior patterns. Clinicians in Great Britain, for example, tend to follow the stringent International Classification of Diseases (ICD) criteria for hyperkinetic disorder, a syndrome that is less common and more severe than ADHD and usually involves neurological impairment; many of the children diagnosed with ADHD in the United States would probably be diagnosed with CD in Great Britain. Comparing prevalence rates of hyperkinetic disorder and ADHD in a community sample of 6- to 7-year-old boys in London, Taylor, Sandberg, Thorley, and Giles (1991) reported that the former was 1/10th of the latter. Also noteworthy is the

fact that U.S./British differences are more apparent in judgments made by clinicians in the two countries than in judgments made by research investigators trained to apply the same criteria (Prendergast et al., 1988). Thus, there seems to be more evidence of differential diagnostic practices than of differential prevalence rates in the two countries.

Divergent cultural norms and behavioral standards may also contribute to varying prevalence rates. In an interesting study of rater perceptions, Mann et al. (1992) had mental health professionals from China, Indonesia, Japan, and the United States independently evaluate the same videotapes of four boys engaged in individual and social activities. The differences were striking: Specialists from China and Indonesia gave higher hyperactivity ratings than did those from Japan and the United States. Tao (1992) suggested that there may be an over-inclusive use of ADHD labels in China, perhaps because of the newness of the construct in combination with the high premium many Chinese adults place on academic excellence and orderly, obedient behavior. When standard diagnostic criteria are applied, prevalence rates appear comparable to those reported in the United States. In summary, the evidence indicates that ADHD-type problems occur in all societies, but that cultural perceptions and practices play important roles in the identification of children who are deviant and in need of treatment.

ASSESSMENT

Questionnaires and structured interviews continue to be the primary assessment instruments for children with ADHD. Each has important advantages and limitations. Typically, questionnaires are simpler, more cost-effective, more portable, and easier to analyze. Interviews can be more interactive and responsive to the individual and provide richer, more personalized information over broader areas of functioning. Information source is a critical consideration when using either type of instrument. Mothers, fathers, teachers, and peers all have different "snapshots" and cumulative impressions. Each sees the child in different settings and situations, has different agendas, experiences different consequences when interacting with the child, and processes observations through unique psychological filters. Thus, it is not surprising that there is often little correspondence in evaluations from different sources. In fact, the correlations for different traits assessed by the same rater are often higher than the correlations for the same trait measured by different raters (Stanger & Lewis, 1993). Despite cross-source discrepancies and lack of consensus on how to combine discrepant information, most experts agree that information from more than one source enables the clinician to construct a more articulated picture of the child's functioning. Diagnoses based on a single informant provide a partial picture at best and yield prevalence rates that can be so high as to suggest overdiagnosis.

Before a useful assessment strategy can be outlined, we must ask "assessment for what?" There are several alternative answers to this question, including (1) population screening, (2) diagnosing individual cases, (3) ruling out medical conditions (e.g., mental retardation, neurological disease, HIV infection), (4) pinpointing strengths and problem domains, (5) identifying environmental contributors (e.g., marital discord, unrealistic parental expectations or incompetent parenting, schoolyard bullying), and (6) evaluating treatments. These assessment goals raise different issues and dictate different strategies and measures. For example, when the goal is population screening for ADHD, the consensus recommendation is for the use of multistage–multimethod approaches, beginning with screening instruments (usually questionnaires) that can be administered economically to large numbers of children, and then proceeding to more fine-gauged assessments, often using structured interview protocols, of the subgroup of children who reach a specified cutoff level on the screening instru-

ment. This strategy has the advantages of maximizing information while minimizing cost, but there is always a risk of false negatives during the screening phase. Examples of this methodology can be found in Bird et al. (1988) and Cohen et al. (1993).

When evaluation of an individual child is the goal, an assessment should involve, at a minimum, three information sources: parents, teacher, and child. Although it is important that the child receive a thorough medical evaluation, there is no medical test that is pathognomic for ADHD. For parents, an entire psychiatric interview may not be necessary, but both a careful history and standardized behavioral ratings should be obtained. Ratings from the teacher are also important, whereas a teacher interview is desirable but not always feasible. Several widely used rating scales can be completed by both parents and teachers, enabling important comparisons. Examples of brief ADHD checklists are the 10-item Conners Abbreviated Symptom Questionnaire or Hyperkinesis Index (Goyette, Conners, & Ulrich, 1978) and the IOWA Conners Scale, which has the advantage of distinguishing between inattention-overactivity and aggression (Loney & Milich, 1982). An instrument has been in use for rating specific DSM-III-R criteria (DuPaul, 1992), and an analogous scale for DSM-IV can be constructed easily. Longer scales such as the Child Behavior Checklist (Achenbach, 1991) that cover broader aspects of psychopathology may also be useful.

Child self-reports are of limited utility. A more informative approach is to observe the child in a setting that will provoke problematic behavior (e.g., a classroom or structured playroom session in which the child is asked to perform specific tasks). It is preferable to observe the child on at least two occasions, because initial encounters often benefit from novelty effects. Comprehensive coverage of assessment modes and instruments can be found in Barkley (1990), Conners, March, Erhardt, Butcher, & Epstein (1993), DuPaul (1992), and Klein et al. (1994).

TREATMENT

Of all child therapies, stimulant treatment of ADHD is both the most efficacious and the most rigorously studied (Whalen & Henker, 1997). Although the use of a stimulant to "calm" a hyperactive child still appears enigmatic to many, there is little disagreement about the effectiveness of this treatment mode. However, stimulant treatment cannot address the full range of a child's problems, even when the medication response is considered ideal. We have seen that ADHD is a multiproblem disorder, and stimulant treatment is limited in extent, range, and duration. Pills do not teach skills, but rather alter the frequencies and intensities of behaviors already in a child's repertoire (Werry & Aman, 1993). Optimal intervention requires domain-specific skill building for the child and coordinated consultation with the family, school, and others with whom the child interacts. In the following paragraphs we summarize accepted conclusions and ongoing issues surrounding stimulant treatment and then describe the current status of psychosocial interventions.

Stimulant Pharmacotherapy

Prevalence

Most children diagnosed with ADHD receive stimulant treatment, often for many years (Copeland, Wolraich, Lindgren, Milich, & Woolson, 1987; Wolraich et al., 1990), and there is evidence that its use is increasing (Safer & Krager, 1988). Just under 1 million patients made, collectively, 1.7 million visits to physicians for evaluation and treatment of ADHD in 1990 (Williams, Lerner, & Swanson, 1994). The dramatic nature of the increase is illustrated by the corresponding numbers for 1994: 2.5 million patients made approximately 5 million visits. About 90% of physician visits result in a prescription, the vast majority for the stimulant methylphenidate.

Short-Term Gains

In the short-term, stimulant-related improvement occurs in 70 to 85% of those treated (Wilens & Biederman, 1992). Gains have been documented across settings and measures and in multiple problem domains. Smoother day-to-day transactions are the most salient changes. The core symptoms of inattention, impulsivity, and excessive motor activity improve, as do associated problems with task performance, social relations, aggression, and oppositionality (Forness et al., 1992; Gadow, Nolan, Sverd, Sprafkin, & Paolicelli, 1990; Rapport, Denney, DuPaul, & Gardner, 1994; Swanson, McBurnett, Christian, & Wigal, 1995; Whalen & Henker, 1991a). Although the effects on academic performance are somewhat variable, several studies have documented medication-related gains in the quantity and accuracy of academic work, especially when attentional resources are taxed (Carlson & Bunner, 1993; Douglas, Barr, Amin, O'Neill, & Britton, 1988; Elia, Welsh, Gullotta, & Rapoport, 1993). For example, medication–placebo differences are more likely to emerge with problems requiring combinations of mathematical manipulations than with simple addition or subtraction problems (Elia et al., 1993). Stimulant treatment also seems to improve consistency or reduce the variability in classroom functioning (DuPaul & Rapport, 1993).

Normalization

Although the degree of improvement is clinically significant in the majority of cases, the gains often fall short of "normalization." Many children who are positive medication responders can still be distinguished from their peers on the basis of dysfunctional behavior patterns and academic performance (DuPaul & Rapport, 1993; Rapport et al., 1994).

Choice of Medication and Dosage

In clinical practice, methylphenidate is clearly the preferred stimulant (Safer & Krager, 1988), and the typical dose is quite often 10 mg in the morning and again at midday. This dosage extends across a surprising range of ages and body sizes, and there is seldom a need to adjust upward as the child grows. Doses as low as 2.5 mg, or half of the smallest available tablet, have occasionally been found effective. It is not uncommon for physicians to prescribe higher doses, even exceeding the accepted single-dose limit of 20 to 25 mg.

Nonresponse and Adverse Reactions

Although the majority of children with ADHD improve with stimulant treatment, a subgroup appear not to benefit, and a small minority may show adverse responses (Rapport et al., 1994; Solanto & Wender, 1989; Werry & Aman, 1993). Elia, Borcherding, Rapoport, and Keysor (1991) examined the effects of methylphenidate versus dextroamphetamine on cognitive and behavior ratings. On the group level, the two drugs seemed similarly safe and effective. For any individual child, one was often superior, and adverse effects that occurred with one drug were unlikely to occur with the other. These investigators concluded that, if responsiveness is evaluated in the context of the two drugs and a wide dosage range, true nonresponders or adverse responders are rare (4%). There is an important caution here, however: Dosages used in this study were higher than those often used in clinical practice (e.g., 2.5 mg/kg methylphenidate), and 40% of the youngsters required dosage adjustments because of severe side effects.

Because of the multiplicity of domains affected by stimulants, and the fact that there is no single index of response, questions about adverse reactions are better construed in relative than in absolute terms. At times there may be trade-offs and the need to decide, for example, whether to accept mild social disengagement, affective flattening, or overpersistence in order to achieve more adaptive behavior.

Side Effects

Sleep disturbances and diminished appetite are the most frequently reported side effects.

Also relatively common are cardiovascular changes (mild elevations in heart rate and diastolic blood pressure), stomachaches, headaches, irritability, tics and other nervous mannerisms, unhappiness, and withdrawal (Barkley, McMurray, Edelbrock, & Robbins, 1990; Klein & Bessler, 1992). Also noteworthy are reports of behavioral rebound (e.g., increased activity, irritability, or impulsivity) when the effects of stimulants wear off or treatment is discontinued. Serious problems such as stimulant-related psychosis or movement disorders are rare. It is important to note that relatively high rates of "side effects" are also reported when placebos are given (Barkley, McMurray, et al., 1990; Klein & Bessler, 1992), raising questions about the extent to which such effects are attributable to preexisting conditions or even expectancy biases. In general, side effects are relatively mild, definitely dose related, and readily reversible through adjustments in amount or timing of medication (Wilens & Biederman, 1992).

Reductions in growth velocity have also been reported during extended treatment periods, but there is evidence of compensatory growth during drug holidays or after discontinuation. When stimulant treatment terminates before the growth spurt, no long-term height or weight reductions have been found, and effects on growth velocity during adolescence are as yet unknown (Klein & Bessler, 1992). Growth studies of treated teenagers are critically needed, given the increasing practice of initiating or continuing stimulant treatment during adolescence. In summary, the evidence underscores the relative safety of stimulant medications in recommended dosages, but the wide range of possible effects coupled with broad individual differences mandate careful monitoring. As Werry sagely counseled, "enthusiasm for stimulants must be tempered by what we do not yet know" (1994, p. 327).

Domain Specificity and Individual Differences

Some problem areas are more resistant to change than others. Decreases in negative behaviors (e.g., disruptiveness) are more likely than increases in positive activities, particularly where specific skills are involved (e.g., prosocial behavior). In fact, problems with peer relations and reputations may be especially intractable (Whalen & Henker, 1992; Whalen et al., 1991). Improvements in daily classroom work and on laboratory tasks are found consistently, whereas enduring gains in academic achievement remain elusive (Carlson & Bunner, 1993). There are also broad individual differences in stimulant response. It is difficult to know which domains will improve in a particular child, and gains in one area do not predict gains in another. As noted above, children with combined ADHD and anxiety are less likely to respond positively to stimulant treatment and may in fact show adverse effects (DuPaul, Barkley, & McMurray, 1994; Pliszka, 1989).

Dose–Response Relationships

Early concerns that moderate to high doses may cause deterioration in cognitive performance, especially a cognitive constriction and perseveration, have not been well substantiated. In fact, the opposite may be the case, at least within typical dosage ranges. Douglas, Barr, Desilets, and Sherman (1995) reported increasingly positive effects on several cognitive measures, including tests of mental flexibility, with dosages ranging from 0.3 to 0.9 mg/kg methylphenidate. In several other studies, performance on complex cognitive tasks and classroom behavior improved rather than deteriorated as a function of increasing dose, especially in the low to moderate ranges (Douglas et al., 1988; Solanto & Wender, 1989). There is some evidence of a law of diminishing returns, reflected in a leveling off of improvement above a certain dosage threshold, e.g., 10 mg (Rapport, Denney, DuPaul, & Gardner, 1994) or 0.6 mg/kg methylphenidate (Douglas et al., 1995).

Despite these reassuring findings, the question of cognitive toxicity is not yet settled, and the answers may depend on a complex blend of child characteristics, specific cognitive functions, dosing practices, and task parameters. Suggesting that medication-related improvements in cognitive functioning may result from enhanced persistence, Douglas et al. (1995) warned that, at high doses, persistence may be increased beyond an optimal level. The nagging possibility of adverse cognitive effects underscores the merit of using the lowest effective dose for any individual child and carefully monitoring across a broad array of performance measures.

Behavioral Tolerance

Although concerns have been raised about the development of tolerance, there has been markedly little evidence of diminution of behavioral improvements over time. In some cases when treatment continues over the years of rapid growth, body weight corrections in dosage may be necessary (Wilens & Biederman, 1992). Drug holidays or a switch to a different stimulant may be useful in cases of true tolerance (Elia et al., 1991).

Maintenance and Long-Term Gains

Whereas few would question the conclusion that stimulants result in marked behavioral improvement, most would agree that such gains are more temporary than enduring, dissipating rapidly after treatment cessation (Jacobvitz, Sroufe, Stewart, & Leffert, 1990; Swanson, McBurnett et al., 1995; Werry & Aman, 1993). Evidence to date suggests that stimulants dampen problematic behaviors on a day-to-day basis without facilitating the acquisition of either complex skills or enduring self-regulation competencies that the child with ADHD can apply across settings and domains. It is important to note, however, that follow-up studies pose multiple methodological hurdles, and the most fundamental questions about long-term outcomes are still to be answered (Schachar & Tannock, 1993).

Nonpharmacological Approaches

Stimulant pharmacotherapy for ADHD has a stronger track record than almost any other therapy for any child disorder. Although stimulant therapy is considered the treatment of choice, few specialists are sanguine about exclusive reliance on any single modality. The multiproblem nature of ADHD dictates multimodal therapies (Whalen & Henker, 1997).

On a relatively small scale, diverse psychosocial and behavioral treatments have been applied to ADHD. Included in this list are parent training and family counseling, social skills training, academic remediation, cognitive-behavior modification, biofeedback, insight therapy and psychoanalysis, and even exercise regimens. Cognitive-behavioral approaches that emphasize self-regulation training appeared especially promising, given the pervasive self-regulatory deficits of ADHD children, but the outcome data have been disappointing (Abikoff & Klein, 1992; Whalen & Henker, 1986). In the vast majority of controlled studies, nonpharmacological approaches pale relative to stimulant treatment, and the question of whether any psychosocial treatment makes an additive contribution remains open (Abikoff & Klein, 1992; Ialongo et al., 1993). It is important to consider drug dosage when making these determinations, however, given the possibility that the addition of a behavioral program may enable a lower dose of medication (Carlson, Pelham, Milich, & Dixon, 1992). Nonpharmacological treatment may also help sustain treatment-related gains once medication is discontinued or perhaps enable a shorter course of stimulant treatment.

In the first major clinical trial to focus on a childhood disorder, the National Institute of Mental Health (NIMH) has initiated a study comparing stimulant pharmacotherapy and a broad-based package of psychosocial treatments. The project spans six treatment sites and assesses multiple domains of functioning (Richters et al., 1995). Called the Multisite Multimodal Treatment Study of Children with ADHD (MTA), this ambitious investigation seeks important information about an array of critical issues, including the comparative efficacy of single and combined treatments, the durability of therapeutic gains, and the optimal match of child and treatment characteristics. In the meantime, there are sound arguments to support multimodal treatments that combine pharmacological and psychosocial approaches (Whalen & Henker, 1991b). Information about the techniques and efficacy of these therapeutic approaches can be found in Abikoff & Hechtman (1996), Barkley, Guevremont, Anastopoulos, and Fletcher (1992), Conners et al. (1994), Hinshaw and Erhardt (1993), Kazdin (1994), and Kendall and Braswell (1993).

CASE STUDY

Taylor, who will be 9 next month, has had difficulties at school from the outset. Seven prior placements in regular classes have all failed. His teachers consistently report that, one on one, he is challenging but manageable. In a full classroom, however, he is out of his seat, disruptive, and, when challenged, obnoxiously defiant. Sometimes Taylor will work on class assignments, such as art or science projects, but he refuses most academic tasks and has never been known to complete one. He clowns habitually and competes with the teacher for the class's attention. He is a frequent visitor to both the principal's office and the school's time-out room.

Taylor's IQ scores on the WISC III place him in the high average range, with Verbal scores significantly elevated and Performance scores just below the mean. His achievement test scores indicate that he can read and comprehend at a level 3 years beyond other third graders at his school, yet Taylor spends all day in a special class. The others in the class are either younger autistic children or much older children with severe underachievement and histories of truancy, theft, and assault. Taylor seeks the company of the three older boys in his class, but they exclude him. They do, however, often ask him to help them plan future thefts and shoplifting expeditions.

When he is with peers, Taylor is bossy and verbally bullying. He often joins ongoing groups and intrudes on others with the apparent purpose of sidetracking their activities or just messing things up. When others don't follow his suggestions, he is likely to lose his temper and shout obscenities. He does not initiate physical aggression, although he unflinchingly stands his ground or fights back when his taunts and insults provoke attacks from others. He is the last one to be chosen for teams at school and is openly scorned by other boys his age. Highly self-critical, Taylor repeatedly expresses deep regret over being out of control, but his promises of reform seen short-lived.

His mother, who had "always" planned to become and remain a single parent, is a struggling filmmaker who easily admits that she has been overindulgent, "partly to make it up to him that he doesn't have a father." Frequently unemployed, Taylor's mother spends a lot of time with him, often in educational enrichment or science activities. She describes herself as caving in to his demands, hastily adding, "because that's the only solution. Getting him to do anything he dislikes is simply impossible and has been all his life. It seems he was born running and yelling, and it never stops." If it were economically feasible she would quit working and spend her time on home schooling for Taylor.

The family doctor first prescribed medication for Taylor when he was 4, beginning with a week's trial of methylphenidate. The medication was discontinued because it seemed to make his incessant talking even worse, although he was calmer overall. he has been on a combination of clonidine and an MAO inhibitor for the last 4 years. He was recently switched back to methylphenidate, because of low blood pressure when he took the other medications. This time, methylphenidate seems to be helping, but those who work with him note that it certainly is no miracle.

His mother was pleased to learn about a study being done by the local university that involved a cognitive-behavioral approach to teaching children self-regulation strategies. Taylor was enrolled in the program and participated in group sessions at school three times each week. Systematic behavior observations done by the university research team confirmed the informal impression that there were decided improvements. These gains were more noticeable in the classroom than on the playground or at home. When one of his trainers wasn't around, Taylor just didn't use the new skills he had learned, lamenting after each incident that he "just forgot." When the treatment study was over, the gains he had made began to erode, indicating a need for "booster" treatments, continued consultation, or both.

Taylor's mother also joined two parent groups, one focused on mutual support and the other on parenting skills. She worked hard to learn the parenting techniques and she readily volunteers that they are often effective. She confesses, though, that it is difficult for her to follow through systematically and often easier for her to yield to Taylor's preferences. She found it equally difficult to reliably record assessment data. On balance, the improvements are definite and welcome—but far from complete—and it is difficult to divide the credit between medication and psychosocial treatments, or to determine the role played by developmental maturation. Taylor's mother now sees his problems as enduring ones and feels that the various therapies are all helpful, but there is neither a quick nor a lasting "fix." When asked about her most important hope for the future, she replied, "Well, he's creative and he'll find his niche in life, in spite of the school system, not because of it. I guess what I hope for him most is just one friend."

RESEARCH NEEDS AND TRENDS

We have seen that ADHD is not a rare disorder, nor is it circumscribed or self-limiting. ADHD involves such serious and enduring difficulties in so many areas of functioning that it is now viewed as a chronic public health problem (Spencer et al., 1994). The research energies that are being devoted to understanding ADHD promise not only to benefit individual children and families, but also to yield discoveries that will be useful in preventing and treating other pervasive problems and increasing the well-being of society at large. By way of summary, ongoing trends and research needs are delineated below.

Risk and Resilience

How do patterns of temperament, genetic makeup, social adversity, and other traits and environmental stressors interact to increase the probability that a child will develop ADHD? Which combinations of factors increase the risk for comorbid disorders such as learning and conduct problems, and which serve protective functions? Are there environmental resources that mediate the effects and improve the outcomes?

Gender Patterns

Is ADHD a different disorder in girls than in boys? As noted earlier, glimmers of intriguing gender differences are emerging across a broad range of domains, including associated cognitive impairments, the course and severity of comorbid disorders, and even brain metabolism. Girls are an understudied group and may also be underrecognized when it comes to ADHD.

Comorbidity

Is the increasing rate of comorbid disorders a function of recent changes in diagnostic and assessment procedures or a reflection of actual changes in the phenomenology of childhood disorders? Do subtypes established on the basis of comorbid disorders differ in etiology, course, or outcome?

Task Performance and Cognitive Competencies

To what extent are the performance deficiencies seen in many children with ADHD a result of specific cognitive deficits, ineffective information-processing strategies, or dysfunctional regulation of motivation and affect?

Adult ADHD

Further information is needed to confirm the validity of adult ADHD. We still do not know whether there is overzealous diagnosing, especially of parents whose children have ADHD, nor do we know the extent to which adults with ADHD are underidentified and undertreated. Also needed is more extensive information on the interpersonal functioning of adults with ADHD and on the changes in social behaviors that attend treatment (Shaffer, 1994). Delineation of developmental trajectories is another need, including comparisons of adults with ADHD who were diagnosed during childhood and those who escaped clinical referral until adulthood.

Multimodal Treatments

Are multimodal treatment strategies that combine psychosocial and psychopharmacological approaches superior to stimulant treatment alone? Also critically needed is information about how to optimize treatment packages for individual children. What are the most effective therapeutic approaches for specific problem domains and subtypes of ADHD, and how should these components be sequenced or patterned? Despite continuing optimism about the superiority of combined treatments in comparison to any unimodal approach, empirical substantiation has only just begun.

Nonstimulant Medications and Combined Pharmacotherapy

An array of antidepressants and other drugs such as the antihypertensive clonidine have been used in the treatment of ADHD, either singly or in combination with stimulants (Barrick-

man et al., 1995; Pataki, Carlson, Kelly, Rapport, & Biancaniello, 1993; Rapport, Carlson, Kelly, & Pataki, 1993). One hope is that a second medication may lower the required dose of stimulants or produce synergistic effects that enhance ultimate outcomes; thus far there is little empirical documentation of such effects, however. At times, a second drug is prescribed to combat the side effects of the first drug, but this is a risky practice at best. Despite the potential benefits, use of multiple agents should proceed cautiously because of the lack of knowledge about dosing parameters and the risks of serious, even possibly fatal, drug interactions (Cantwell, Swanson, & Connor, 1997; Wilens, Spencer, Biederman, Wozniak, & Connor, 1995).

Extended versus Acute Stimulant Treatment Effects

Although stimulant treatment typically extends over years, most of the scientific information is based on studies that span only days or weeks. There are, of course, important methodological and ethical reasons for this imbalance. Given the prevalence of stimulant treatment and its documented short-term efficacy, it is important to develop procedures for studying longer-term issues such as those related to maintaining gains and to identifying potential adverse effects.

Emanative Effects of Treatment

Two decades ago, we raised the possibility that the positive effects of stimulant treatment may be accompanied, under some unknown conditions, by a negative impact on the child's perceptions of self-efficacy (Whalen & Henker, 1976). The concern was that there may be an implicit message of medication, one that confirms for the child and his significant others that his behavior is not under his own control, but rather results from a "good-behavior pill." While peers are building their competencies and gaining increasing control over their actions and outcomes, children with ADHD must rely on pills to get along and meet others' expectations. The recommendation was not that stimulant treatment be abandoned, but rather that attributional messages be considered as a component of multimodal treatment.

To date, there has been only limited evidence of such negative psychological effects on children with ADHD or their parents (e.g., Borden & Brown, 1989; Whalen, Henker, Hinshaw, Heller, & Huber-Dressler, 1991), and there are in fact indications that the behavioral successes that attend stimulant treatment may have positive attributional outcomes (Milich, Carlson, Pelham, & Licht, 1991). When behavior improves, children are likely to feel better about themselves and their abilities. The jury is still out on whether these desirable changes in self-perceptions are diluted if the improvement is attributed to medication. Accurate assessments of children's causal reasoning processes and self-perceptions are notoriously difficult, partly because of social desirability biases, and the hypothesized negative effects on self-perceptions are subtle and much more difficult to detect than are the salient changes in overt behaviors. It is important to continue to refine measures of children's self-perceptions and to monitor covert consequences of all child therapies, whether pharmacological or psychosocial.

Contextual Facets of Treatments and Compatibility Issues

Identifying the most efficacious treatment is only one component of a clinical investigator's task. No matter how potent and convenient the intervention, there are often problems with acceptance, adherence, and satisfaction. Drug treatments have a unique advantage when it comes to cost, time, and ease of administration, but they also carry a special attitudinal burden, given that many people resist using pharmacological modes of behavioral control (Whalen & Henker, 1991b). There is a paucity of informa-

tion on the attitudinal and contextual factors that enhance or impede treatment delivery, although the empirical literature is beginning to grow (Brown, Dingle, & Landau, 1994; Rostain, Power, & Atkins, 1993). Also needed are more refined studies of the goodness of fit between specific treatments, individual children, and social ecologies, including physical settings as well as parent and teacher characteristics (Greene, 1995; Jensen et al., 1993).

SUMMARY

As we approach the twenty-first century, the face of mental health services for children is undergoing dramatic transformation. In theory, the increasing recognition that ADHD is a public health problem should help ensure access to needed interventions. But in practice, in these tense and troubled times, the dollars for both health care and research are shrinking dramatically. We have entered the era of managed care in which only empirically validated treatments are likely to be available. The empirical documentation underlying stimulant treatment for ADHD is compelling, but we also know that the needs of these multiproblem children extend beyond the scope of any unimodal treatment. The challenge for researchers and practitioners alike is to find ways of validating and delivering the array of services needed by children diagnosed with ADHD.

ACKNOWLEDGMENT

We gratefully acknowledge the competent and congenial assistance of Suzanne D. Gates in the preparation of this chapter.

REFERENCES

Abikoff, H., Courtney, M., Pelham, W. E., Jr., & Koplewicz, H. S. (1993). Teachers' ratings of disruptive behaviors: The influence of halo effects. *Journal of Abnormal Child Psychology, 21,* 519–533.

Abikoff, H., Gittelman, R., & Klein, D. F. (1980). A class-room observation code for hyperactive children: A replication of validity. *Journal of Consulting and Clinical Psychology, 48,* 555–565.

Abikoff, H., & Hechtman, L. (1996). Multimodal therapy and stimulants in the treatment of children with ADHD. In E. D. Hibbs & P. S. Jensen (Eds.), *Psychosocial treatments for child and adolescent disorders: Empirically based strategies for clinical practice* (pp. 341–369). Washington, DC: American Psychological Association.

Abikoff, H., & Klein, R. G. (1992). Attention-deficit hyperactivity and conduct disorder: Comorbidity and implications for treatment. *Journal of Consulting and Clinical Psychology, 60,* 881–892.

Achenbach, T. M. (1991). *Manual for the Child Behavior Checklist and 1991 Child Behavior Profile.* Burlington: University of Vermont, Department of Psychiatry.

American Psychiatric Association. (1968). *Diagnostic and statistical manual of mental disorders* (2nd ed.). Washington, DC: Author.

American Psychiatric Association. (1980). *Diagnostic and statistical manual of mental disorders* (3rd ed.). Washington, DC: Author.

American Psychiatric Association. (1987). *Diagnostic and statistical manual of mental disorders* (3rd ed.-rev.). Washington, DC: Author.

American Psychiatric Association. (1994). *Diagnostic and statistical manual of mental disorders* (4th ed.). Washington, DC: Author.

Anastopoulos, A. D., Guevremont, D. C., Shelton, T. L., & DuPaul, G. J. (1992). Parenting stress among families of children with attention deficit hyperactivity disorder. *Journal of Abnormal Child Psychology, 20,* 503–520.

Anderson, J. C., Williams, S., McGee, R., & Silva, P. A. (1987). DSM-III disorders in preadolescent children: Prevalence in a large sample from the general population. *Archives of General Psychiatry, 44,* 69–76.

Angold, A., & Costello, E. J. (1993). Depressive comorbidity in children and adolescents: Empirical, theoretical, and methodological issues. *American Journal of Psychiatry, 150,* 1779–1791.

Barkley, R. A. (1990). *Attention-deficit hyperactivity disorder: A handbook for diagnosis and treatment.* New York: Guilford Press.

Barkley, R. A. (1994). Impaired delayed responding: A unified theory of attention-deficit hyperactivity disorder. In D. K. Routh (Ed.), *Disruptive behavior disorders in childhood* (pp. 11–57). New York: Plenum Press.

Barkley, R. A., DuPaul, G. J., & McMurray, M. B. (1990). Comprehensive evaluation of attention deficit disorder with and without hyperactivity as defined by research criteria. *Journal of Consulting and Clinical Psychology, 58,* 775–789.

Barkley, R. A., Fischer, M., Edelbrock, C. S., & Smallish, L. (1990). The adolescent outcome of hyperactive children diagnosed by research criteria: I. An 8-year pro-spective follow-up study. *Journal of the American Academy of Child and Adolescent Psychiatry, 29,* 546–557.

Barkley, R. A., Fischer, M., Edelbrock, C., & Smallish, L. (1991). The adolescent outcome of hyperactive children diagnosed by research criteria: III. Mother–child interactions, family conflicts and maternal psychopathology. *Journal of Child Psychology and Psychiatry, 32,* 233–255.

Barkley, R. A., Guevremont, D. C., Anastopoulos, A. D., DuPaul, G. J., & Shelton, T. L. (1993). Driving-related risks and outcomes of attention deficit hyperactivity disorder in adolescents and young adults: A 3- to 5-year follow-up survey. *Pediatrics, 92,* 212–218.

Barkley, R. A., Guevremont, D. C., Anastopoulos, A. D., & Fletcher, K. E. (1992). A comparison of three family therapy programs for treating family conflicts in adolescents with attention-deficit hyperactivity disorder. *Journal of Consulting and Clinical Psychology, 60,* 450–462.

Barkley, R. A., McMurray, M. B., Edelbrock, C. S., & Robbins, K. (1990). Side effects of methylphenidate in children with attention deficit hyperactivity disorder: A systematic, placebo-controlled evaluation. *Pediatrics, 86,* 184–192.

Barrickman, L. L., Perry, P. J., Allen, A. J., Kuperman, S., Arndt, S. V., Herrmann, K. J., & Schumacher, E. (1995). Bupropion versus methylphenidate in the treatment of attention-deficit hyperactivity disorder. *Journal of the American Academy of Child and Adolescent Psychiatry, 34,* 649–657.

Bauermeister, J. J., Alegria, M., Bird, H. R., Rubio-Stipec, M., & Canino, G. (1992). Are attentional-hyperactivity deficits unidimensional or multidimensional syndromes? Empirical findings from a community survey. *Journal of the American Academy of Child and Adolescent Psychiatry, 31,* 423–431.

Bauermeister, J. J., Canino, G., & Bird, H. (1994). Epidemiology of disruptive behavior disorders. *Child and Adolescent Psychiatric Clinics of North America, 3,* 177–194.

Baumgaertel, A., Wolraich, M. L., & Dietrich, M. (1995). Comparison of diagnostic criteria for attention deficit disorders in a German elementary school sample. *Journal of the American Academy of Child and Adolescent Psychiatry, 34,* 629–638.

Bellinger, D. C., Stiles, K. M., & Needleman, H. L. (1992). Low-level lead exposure, intelligence and academic achievement: A long-term follow-up study. *Pediatrics, 90,* 855–861.

Biederman, J., Faraone, S. V., Keenan, K., Knee, D., & Tsuang, M. T. (1990). Family-genetic and psychosocial risk factors in DSM-III attention deficit disorder. *Journal of the American Academy of Child and Adolescent Psychiatry, 29,* 526–533.

Biederman, J., Faraone, S. V., Keenan, K., Steingard, R., & Tsuang, M. T. (1991). Familial association between attention deficit disorder and anxiety disorders. *American Journal of Psychiatry, 148,* 251–256.

Binder, S., & Matte, T. (1993). Childhood lead poisoning.

The impact of prevention. *Journal of the American Medical Association, 269,* 1679–1681.

Bird, H. R., Canino, G., Rubio-Stipec, M., Gould, M. S., Ribera, J., Sesman, M., Woodbury, M., Huertas-Goldman, S., Pagan, A., Sanchez-Lacay, A., & Moscoso, M. (1988). Estimates of the prevalence of childhood maladjustment in a community survey in Puerto Rico. *Archives of General Psychiatry, 45,* 1120–1126.

Bird, H. R., Gould, M. S., & Staghezza, B. M. (1993). Patterns of diagnostic comorbidity in a community sample of children aged 9 through 16 years. *Journal of the American Academy of Child and Adolescent Psychiatry, 32,* 361–368.

Borden, K. A., & Brown, R. T. (1989). Attributional outcomes: The subtle messages of treatments for attention deficit disorder. *Cognitive Therapy and Research, 13,* 147–160.

Breen, M. J. (1989). Cognitive and behavioral differences in ADHD boys and girls. *Journal of Child Psychology and Psychiatry,* 711–716.

Brown, R. T., Dingle, A., & Landau, S. (1994). Overview of psychopharmacology in children and adolescents. *School Psychology Quarterly, 9,* 4–25.

Brown, R. T., Madan-Swain, A., & Baldwin, K. (1991). Gender differences in a clinic-referred sample of attention-deficit-disordered children. *Child Psychiatry and Human Development, 22,* 111–128.

Buhrmester, D., Whalen, C. K., Henker, B., MacDonald, V., & Hinshaw, S. P. (1992). Prosocial behavior in hyperactive boys: Effects of stimulant medication and comparison with normal boys. *Journal of Abnormal Child Psychology, 20,* 103–121.

Buitelaar, J. K., Swinkels, S. H. N., de Vries, H., van der Gaag, R. J., & van Hooff, J. A. R. A. M. (1994). An ethological study on behavioural differences between hyperactive, aggressive, combined hyperactive/aggressive and control children. *Journal of Child Psychology and Psychiatry, 35,* 1437–1446.

Campbell, S. B. (1995). Behavior problems in preschool children: A review of recent research. *Journal of Child Psychology and Psychiatry, 36,* 113–149.

Campbell, S. B., Pierce, E. W., March, C. L., Ewing, L. J., & Szumowski, E. K. (1994). Hard-to-manage preschool boys: Symptomatic behavior across contexts and time. *Child Development, 65,* 836–851.

Cantwell, D. P., & Baker, L. (1992). Attention deficit disorder with and without hyperactivity: A review and comparison of matched groups. *Journal of the American Academy of Child and Adolescent Psychiatry, 31,* 432–438.

Cantwell, D. P., Swanson, J., & Connor, D. F. (1997). Case study: Adverse response to clonidine. *Journal of the American Academy of Child and Adolescent Psychiatry, 36,* 539–544.

Carlson, C. L., & Bunner, M. R. (1993). Effects of methylphenidate on the academic performance of children with attention-deficit hyperactivity disorder and learning disabilities. *School Psychology Review, 22,* 184–198.

Carlson, C. L., Pelham, W. E., Milich, R., & Dixon, J. (1992). Single and combined effects of methylphenidate and behavior therapy on the classroom performance of children with attention-deficit hyperactivity disorder. *Journal of Abnormal Child Psychology, 20,* 213–231.

Caron, C., & Rutter, M. (1991). Comorbidity in child psychopathology: Concepts, issues and research strategies. *Journal of Child Psychology and Psychiatry, 32,* 1063–1080.

Carter, C. M., Urbanowicz, M., Hemsley, R., Mantilla, L. Strobel, S., Graham, P. J., & Taylor, E. (1993). Effects of a few food diet in attention deficit disorder. *Archives of Disease in Childhood, 69,* 564–568.

Ceci, S. J., & Tishman, J. (1984). Hyperactivity and incidental memory: Evidence for attentional diffusion. *Child Development, 55,* 2192–2203.

Chee, P., Logan, G., Schachar, R., Lindsay, P., & Wachsmuth, R. (1989). Effects of event rate and display time on sustained attention in hyperactive, normal, and control children. *Journal of Abnormal Child Psychology, 17,* 371–391.

Cohen, P., Cohen, J., Kasen, S., Velez, C. N., Hartmark, C., Johnson, J., Rojas, M., Brook, J., & Streuning, E. L. (1993). An epidemiological study of disorders in late childhood and adolescence—I. Age- and gender-specific prevalence. *Journal of Child Psychology and Psychiatry, 34,* 851–867.

Conners, C. K., March, J. S., Erhardt, D., Butcher, T., & Epstein, J. (1995). Assessment of attention deficit disorders (ADHD): Conceptual issues and future trends. *Journal of Psychoeducational Assessment* (monograph series, special ADHD issue), *13,* 185–204.

Conners, C. K., Wells, K. C., Erhardt, D., March, J. S., Schulte, A., Osborne, S., Fiore, C., & Butcher, A. T. (1994). Multimodality therapies. Methodologic issues in research and practice. *Child and Adolescent Psychiatric Clinics of North America, 3,* 361–377.

Copeland, L., Wolraich, M., Lindgren, S., Milich, R., & Woolson, R. (1987). Pediatricians' reported practices in the assessment and treatment of attention deficit disorders. *Developmental and Behavioral Pediatrics, 8,* 191–197.

Costello, E. J., & Janiszewski, S. (1990). Who gets treated? Factors associated with referral in children with psychiatric disorders. *Acta Psychiatrica Scandinavica, 81,* 523–529.

Cunningham, C. E., & Siegel, L. S. (1987). Peer interactions of normal and attention-deficit-disordered boys during free-play, cooperative task, and simulated classroom situations. *Journal of Abnormal Child Psychology, 15,* 247–268.

Cunningham, C. E., Siegel, L. S., & Offord, D. R. (1985). A developmental dose-response analysis of the effects of methylphenidate on the peer interactions of attention deficit disordered boys. *Journal of Child Psychology and Psychiatry, 26,* 955–971.

Douglas, V. I. (1983). Attentional and cognitive problems.

In M. Rutter (Ed.), *Developmental neuropsychiatry* (pp. 280–328). New York: Guilford Press.

Douglas, V. I. (1988). Cognitive deficits in children with attention deficit disorder with hyperactivity. In L. M. Bloomingdale & J. Sergeant (Eds.), *Attention deficit disorder: Criteria, cognition, intervention* (pp. 65–81). Elmsford, NY: Pergamon.

Douglas, V. I. (1989). Can Skinnerian theory explain attention deficit disorder?—A reply to Barkley. In L. M. Bloomingdale & J. Swanson (Eds.), *Attention deficit disorder: Current concepts and emerging trends in attentional and behavioral disorders of childhood* (pp. 235–254). Elmsford, NY: Pergamon Press.

Douglas, V. I., Barr, R. G., Amin, K., O'Neill, M. E., & Britton, B. G. (1988). Dosage effects and individual responsivity to methylphenidate in attention deficit disorder. *Journal of Child Psychology and Psychiatry, 29,* 453–475.

Douglas, V. I., Barr, R. G., Desilets, J., & Sherman, E. (1995). Do high doses of stimulants impair flexible thinking in attention-deficit hyperactivity disorder? *Journal of the American Academy of Child and Adolescent Psychiatry, 34,* 877–885.

DuPaul, G. J. (1992). How to assess attention-deficit hyperactivity disorder within school settings. *School Psychology Quarterly, 7,* 60–74.

DuPaul, G. J., Barkley, R. A., & McMurray, M. B. (1994). Response of children with ADHD to methylphenidate: Interaction with internalizing symptoms. *Journal of the American Academy of Child and Adolescent Psychiatry, 33,* 894–903.

DuPaul, G. J., & Rapport, M. D. (1993). Does methylphenidate normalize the classroom performance of children with attention deficit disorder? *Journal of the American Academy of Child and Adolescent Psychiatry, 32,* 190–198.

Egger, J., Carter, C. M., Graham, P. J., Gumley, D., & Soothill, J. F. (1985). Controlled trial of oligoantigenic treatment in the hyperkinetic syndrome. *Lancet, 1,* 540–545.

Elia, J., Borcherding, B. G., Rapoport, J. L., & Keysor, C. S. (1991). Methylphenidate and dextroamphetamine treatments of hyperactivity: Are there true nonresponders? *Psychiatry Research, 36,* 141–155.

Elia, J., Welsh, P. A., Gullotta, C. S., & Rapoport, J. L. (1993). Classroom academic performance: Improvement with both methylphenidate and dextroamphetamine in ADHD boys. *Journal of Child Psychology and Psychiatry, 34,* 785–804.

Ernst, M., Liebenauer, L. L., King, A. C., Fitzgerald, G. A., Cohen, R. M., & Zametkin, A. J. (1994). Reduced brain metabolism in hyperactive girls. *Journal of the American Academy of Child and Adolescent Psychiatry, 33,* 858–868.

Faraone, S. V., Biederman, J., Chen, W. J., Krifcher, B., Keenan, K., Moore, C., Sprich, S., & Tsuang, M. T. (1992). Segregation analysis of attention deficit hyperactivity disorder. *Psychiatric Genetics, 2,* 257–275.

Faraone, S. V., Biederman, J., Keenan, K., & Tsuang, M. T. (1991a). A family-genetic study of girls with DSM-III at-

tention deficit disorder. *American Journal of Psychiatry, 148,* 112–117.

Faraone, S. V., Biederman, J., Keenan, K., & Tsuang, M. T. (1991b). Separation of DSM-III attention deficit disorder and conduct disorder: Evidence from a family-genetic study of American child psychiatric patients. *Psychological Medicine, 21,* 109–121.

Faraone, S. V., Biederman, J., Lehman, B. K., Keenan, K., Norman, D., Seidman, L. J., Kolodny, R., Kraus, I., Perrin, J., & Chen, W. J. (1993). Evidence for the independent familial transmission of attention deficit hyperactivity disorder and learning disabilities: Results from a family genetic study. *American Journal of Psychiatry, 150,* 891–895.

Faraone, S. V., Biederman, J., Lehman, B. K., Spencer, T., Norman, D., Seidman, L. J., Kraus, I., Perrin, J., Chen, W. J., & Tsuang, M. T. (1993). Intellectual performance and school failure in children with attention deficit hyperactivity disorder and in their siblings. *Journal of Abnormal Psychology, 102,* 616–623.

Feingold, B. F. (1976). Hyperkinesis and learning disabilities linked to the ingestion of artificial food colors and flavors. *Journal of Learning Disabilities, 9,* 551–559.

Ferdinand, R. F., Verhulst, F. C., & Wiznitzer, M. (1995). Continuity and change of self-reported problem behaviors from adolescence into young adulthood. *Journal of the American Academy of Child and Adolescent Psychiatry, 34,* 680–690.

Fergusson, D. M., Horwood, L. J., & Lynskey, M. T. (1993). Early dentine lead levels and subsequent cognitive and behavioural development. *Journal of Child Psychology and Psychiatry, 34,* 215–227.

Fischer, M. (1990). Parenting stress and the child with attention deficit hyperactivity disorder. *Journal of Clinical Child Psychology, 19,* 337–346.

Forness, S. R., Swanson, J. M., Cantwell, D. P., Guthrie, D., & Sena, R. (1992). Response to stimulant medication across six measures of school-related performance in children with ADHD and disruptive behavior. *Behavioral Disorders, 18,* 42–53.

Frick, P. J., Kamphaus, R. W., Lahey, B. B., Loeber, R., Christ, M. A., Hart, E. L., & Tannenbaum, L. E. (1991). Academic underachievement and the disruptive behavior disorders. *Journal of Consulting and Clinical Psychology, 59,* 289–294.

Gadow, K. D., Nolan, E. E., Sverd, J., Sprafkin, J., & Paolicelli, L. (1990). Methylphenidate in aggressive-hyperactive boys: I. Effects on peer aggression in public school settings. *Journal of the Academy of Child and Adolescent Psychiatry, 29,* 710–718.

Gaub, M., & Carlson, C. L. (1997). Gender differences in ADHD: A meta-analysis and critical review. *Journal of the American Academy of Child and Adolescent Psychiatry, 36,* 1036–1045.

Giedd, J. N., Castellanos, F. X., Casey, B. J., Kozuch, P., King, A. C., Hamburger, S. D., & Rapoport, J. L. (1994).

Quantitative morphology of the corpus callosum in attention deficit hyperactivity disorder. *American Journal of Psychiatry, 151,* 665–669.

Goodman, R., & Stevenson, J. (1989). A twin study of hyperactivity—II. The aetiological role of genes, family relationships and perinatal adversity. *Journal of Child Psychology and Psychiatry, 30,* 691–709.

Goodyear, P., & Hynd, G. W. (1992). Attention-deficit disorder with (ADD/H) and without (ADD/WO) hyperactivity: Behavioral and neuropsychological differentiation. *Journal of Clinical Child Psychology, 21,* 273–305.

Goyette, C. H., Conners, C. K., & Ulrich, R. F. (1978). Normative data on revised Conners Parent and Teacher Rating Scales. *Journal of Abnormal Child Psychology, 6,* 221–236.

Gray, J. A. (1991). Neural systems, emotion and personality. In J. Madden (Ed.), *Neurobiology of learning, emotion and affect* (pp. 273–306). New York: Raven Press.

Greene, R. W. (1995). Students with ADHD in school classrooms: Teacher factors related to compatibility, assessment, and intervention. *School Psychology Review, 24,* 81–93.

Haapasalo, J., & Tremblay, R. E. (1994). Physically aggressive boys from age 6 to 12: Family background, parenting behavior, and prediction of delinquency. *Journal of Consulting and Clinical Psychology, 62,* 1044–1052.

Hallowell, E. M., & Ratey, J. J. (1994). *Driven to distraction.* New York: Pantheon.

Halperin, J. M., Newcorn, J. H., Matier, K., Sharma, V., McKay, K. E., & Schwartz, S. (1993). Discriminant validity of attention-deficit hyperactivity disorder. *Journal of the American Academy of Child and Adolescent Psychiatry, 32,* 1038–1043.

Halperin, J. M., O'Brien, J. D., Newcorn, J. H., Healey, J. M., Pascualvaca, D. M., Wolf, L. E., & Young, J. G. (1990). Validation of hyperactive, aggressive, and mixed hyperactive/aggressive childhood disorders: A research note. *Journal of Child Psychology and Psychiatry, 31,* 455–459.

Hammen, C., & Compas, B. E. (1994). Unmasking unmasked depression in children and adolescents: The problem of comorbidity. *Clinical Psychology Review, 14,* 585–603.

Harris, M. J., Milich, R., Corbitt, E. M., Hoover, D. W., & Brady, M. (1992). Self-fulfilling effects of stigmatizing information on children's social interactions. *Journal of Personality and Social Psychology, 63,* 41–50.

Hart, E. L., Lahey, B. B., Loeber, R., Applegate, B., & Frick, P. J. (1995). Developmental change in attention-deficit hyperactivity disorder in boys: A four-year longitudinal study. *Journal of Abnormal Child Psychology, 23,* 731–751.

Hellgren, L., Gillberg, C., Gillberg, I. C., & Enerskog, I. (1993). Children with deficits in attention, motor control and perception (DAMP) almost grown up: General health at 16 years. *Developmental Medicine and Child Neurology, 35,* 881–892.

Hinshaw, S. P. (1992). Externalizing behavior problems and academic underachievement in childhood and adolescence: Causal relationships and underlying mechanisms. *Psychological Bulletin, 111,* 127–155.

Hinshaw, S. P., & Erhardt, D. (1993). Behavioral treatment. In V. B. Van Hasselt & M. Hersen (Eds.), *Handbook of behavior therapy and pharmacotherapy for children: A comparative analysis* (pp. 233–250). Boston: Allyn & Bacon.

Hubbard, J. A., & Newcomb, A. F. (1991). Initial dyadic peer interaction of attention deficit–hyperactivity disorder and normal boys. *Journal of Abnormal Child Psychology, 19,* 179–195.

Hynd, G. W., Hern, K. L., Novey, E. S., Eliopulos, D., Marshall, R., Gonzalez, J. J., & Voeller, K. K. (1993). Attention deficit–hyperactivity disorder and asymmetry of the caudate nucleus. *Journal of Child Neurology, 8,* 339–347.

Ialongo, N. S., Horn, W. F., Pascoe, J. M., Greenberg, G., Packard, T., Lopez, M., Wagner, A., & Puttler, L. (1993). The effects of a multimodal intervention with attention-deficit hyperactivity disorder children: A 9-month follow-up. *Journal of the American Academy of Child and Adolescent Psychiatry, 32,* 182–189.

Jacobvitz, D., Sroufe, L. A., Stewart, M., & Leffert, N. (1990). Treatment of attentional and hyperactivity problems in children with sympathomimetic drugs: A comprehensive review. *Journal of the American Academy of Child and Adolescent Psychiatry, 29,* 677–688.

Jensen, P. S., Koretz, D., Locke, B. Z., Schneider, S., Radke-Yarrow, M., Richters, J. E., & Rumsey, J. M. (1993). Child and adolescent psychopathology research: Problems and prospects for the 1990s. *Journal of Abnormal Child Psychology, 21,* 551–580.

Johnston, C. (1996). Parent characteristics and parent–child interactions in families of nonproblem children and ADHD children with higher and lower levels of oppositional-defiant behavior. *Journal of Abnormal Child Psychology, 24,* 85–104.

Kaplan, B. J., McNicol, J., Conte, R. A., & Moghadam, H. K. (1989). Dietary replacement in preschool-aged hyperactive boys. *Pediatrics, 83,* 7–17.

Kazdin, A. E. (1994). Psychotherapy for children and adolescents. In A. E. Bergin & S. L. Garfield (Eds.), *Handbook of psychotherapy and behavior change* (4th ed., pp. 543–594). New York: Wiley.

Kendall, P. C., & Braswell, L. (1993). *Cognitive-behavioral therapy for impulsive children* (2nd ed.). New York: Guilford Press.

Klein, R. G., Abikoff, H., Barkley, R. A., Campbell, M., Leckman, J. F., Ryan, N. D., Solanto, M. V., & Whalen, C. K. (1994). Clinical trials in children and adolescents. In R. F. Prien & D. S. Robinson (Eds.), *Clinical evaluation of psychotropic drugs: Principles and guidelines* (pp. 501–546). New York: Raven Press.

Klein, R. G., & Bessler, A. W. (1992). Stimulant side effects in children. In J. M. Kane & J. A. Lieberman (Eds.), *Ad-

verse effects of psychotropic drugs (pp. 470–496). New York: Guilford Press.

Klein, R. G., & Mannuzza, S. (1989). The long-term outcome of the attention deficit disorder/hyperkinetic syndrome. In T. Sagvolden & T. Archer (Eds.), *Attention deficit disorder* (pp. 71–91). Hillsdale, NJ: Erlbaum.

Klein, R. G., & Mannuzza, S. (1991). Long-term outcome of hyperactive children: A review. *Journal of the American Academy of Child and Adolescent Psychiatry, 30,* 383–387.

Kruesi, M. J. P. (1990). Biological risk factors in the aetiology of childhood psychiatric disorders. In B. Tonge, G. D. Burrows, & J. S. Werry (Eds.), *Handbook of studies on child psychiatry* (pp. 13–28). Amsterdam: Elsevier Science Publishers.

Lahey, B. B., Applegate, B., McBurnett, K., Biederman, J., Greenhill, L., Hynd, G. W., Barkley, R. A., Newcorn, J., Jensen, P., Richters, J., Garfinkel, B., Kerdyk, L., Frick, P. J., Ollendick, T., Perez, D., Hart, E. L., Waldman, I., & Shaffer, D. (1994). DSM-IV field trials for attention-deficit/hyperactivity disorder in children and adolescents. *American Journal of Psychiatry, 151,* 1673–1685.

Landau, S., & Milich, R. (1988). Social communication patterns of attention-deficit-disordered boys. *Journal of Abnormal Child Psychology, 16,* 69–81.

Levy, F., Hay, D., Waldman, I., McLaughlin, M., & Wood, K. (1994, July). *Attention deficit disorder speech and reading in twins: A large-scale study.* Paper presented at the Behavior Genetics Associates Annual Meeting, Barcelona.

Lochman, J. E., & Dodge, K. A. (1994). Social-cognitive processes of severely violent, moderately aggressive, and nonaggressive boys. *Journal of Consulting and Clinical Psychology, 62,* 366–374.

Loeber, R., & Keenan, K. (1994). Interaction between conduct disorder and its comorbid conditions: Effects of age and gender. *Clinical Psychology Review, 14,* 497–523.

Logan, G. D., & Cowan, W. B. (1984). On the ability to inhibit thought and action: A theory of an act of control. *Psychological Review, 91,* 295–327.

Loney, J., & Milich, R. (1982). Hyperactivity, inattention, and aggression in clinical practice. In M. Wolraich & D. Routh (Eds.), *Advances in developmental and behavioral pediatrics* (Vol. 3, pp. 113–147). Greenwich, CT: JAI Press.

Malone, M. A., Kershner, J. R., & Swanson, J. M. (1994). Hemispheric processing and methylphenidate effects in attention-deficit hyperactivity disorder. *Journal of Child Neurology, 9,* 181–189.

Mann, E. M., Ikeda, Y., Mueller, C. W., Takahashi, A., Tao, K. T., Humris, E., Li, B. L., & Chin, D. (1992). Cross-cultural differences in rating hyperactive-disruptive behaviors in children. *American Journal of Psychiatry, 149,* 1539–1542.

Mannuzza, S., Klein, R. G., Bessler, A., Malloy, P., & LaPadula, M. (1993). Adult outcome of hyperactive boys. *Archives of General Psychiatry, 50,* 565–576.

Mannuzza, S., Klein, R. G., Bonagura, N., Malloy, P., Giampino, T. L., & Addalli, K. A. (1991). Hyperactive boys almost grown up. V. Replication of psychiatric status. *Archives of General Psychiatry, 48,* 77–83.

Mash, E. J., & Johnston, C. (1990). Determinants of parenting stress: Illustrations from families of hyperactive children and families of physically abused children. *Journal of Clinical Child Psychology, 19,* 313–328.

McBurnett, K. (1992). Psychobiological approaches to personality and their applications to child psychopathology. In B. B. Lahey & A. E. Kazdin (Eds.), *Advances in clinical child psychology* (Vol. 14, pp. 107–164). New York: Plenum Press.

McConaughy, S. H., & Achenbach, T. M. (1994). Comorbidity of empirically based syndromes in matched general population and clinical samples. *Journal of Child Psychology and Psychiatry, 35,* 1141–1157.

McGee, R., & Feehan, M. (1991). Are girls with problems of attention underrecognized? *Journal of Psychopathology and Behavioral Assessment, 13,* 187–198.

McGee, R., Williams, S., & Feehan, M. (1992). Attention deficit disorder and age of onset of problem behaviors. *Journal of Abnormal Child Psychology, 20,* 487–502.

Milich, R., Carlson, C. K., Pelham, W. E., & Licht, B. G. (1991). Effects of methylphenidate on the persistence of ADHD boys following failure experiences. *Journal of Abnormal Child Psychology, 19,* 519–536.

Milich, R., & Lorch, E. P. (1994). Television viewing methodology to understand cognitive processing of ADHD children. In T. H. Ollendick & R. J. Prinz (Eds.), *Advances in clinical child psychology* (Vol. 16, pp. 177–201). New York: Plenum Press.

Mulatu, M. S. (1995). Prevalence and risk factors of psychopathology in Ethiopian children. *Journal of the American Academy of Child and Adolescent Psychiatry, 34,* 100–109.

Newman, J. P., & Wallace, J. F. (1993). Diverse pathways to deficient self-regulation: Implications for disinhibitory psychopathology in children. *Clinical Psychology Review, 13,* 699–720.

Pataki, C. S., Carlson, G. A., Kelly, K. L., Rapport, M. D., & Biancaniello, T. M. (1993). Side effects of methylphenidate and desipramine alone and in combination in children. *Journal of the American Academy of Child and Adolescent Psychiatry, 32,* 1065–1072.

Pelham, W. E., & Lang, A. R. (1993). Parental alcohol consumption and deviant child behavior: Laboratory studies of reciprocal effects. *Clinical Psychology Review, 13,* 763–784.

Pelham, W. E., McBurnett, K., Harper, G. W., Milich, R., Murphy, D. A., Clinton, J., & Thiele, C. (1990). Methylphenidate and baseball playing in ADHD children: Who's on first? *Journal of Consulting and Clinical Psychology, 58,* 130–133.

Pelham, W. E., Walker, J. L., Sturges, J., & Hoza, B. (1989). The comparative effects of methylphenidate on ADD girls and boys. *Journal of the American Academy of Child and Adolescent Psychiatry, 28,* 773–776.

Pliszka, S. R. (1989). Effect of anxiety on cognition, behavior, and stimulant response in ADHD. *Journal of the American Academy of Child and Adolescent Psychiatry, 28,* 882–887.

Pliszka, S. R. (1992). Comorbidity of attention deficit hyperactivity disorder and overanxious disorder. *Journal of the American Academy of Child and Adolescent Psychiatry, 31,* 197–203.

Pliszka, S. R., Maas, J. W., Javors, M. A., Rogeness, G. A., & Baker, J. (1994). Urinary catecholamines in attention-deficit hyperactivity disorder with and without comorbid anxiety. *Journal of the American Academy of Child and Adolescent Psychiatry, 33,* 1165–1173.

Pope, A. W., Bierman, K. L., & Mumma, G. H. (1989). Relations between hyperactive and aggressive behavior and peer relations at three elementary grade levels. *Journal of Abnormal Child Psychology, 17,* 253–267.

Porrino, L. J., Rapoport, J. L., Behar, D., Sceery, W., Ismond, D. R., & Bunney, W. E., Jr. (1983). A naturalistic assessment of the motor activity of hyperactive boys. I. Comparison with normal controls. *Archives of General Psychiatry, 40,* 681–687.

Prendergast, M., Taylor, E., Rapoport, J. L., Bartko, J., Donnelly, M., Zametkin, A., Ahearn, M. B., Dunn, G., & Wieselberg, H. M. (1988). The diagnosis of childhood hyperactivity: A US-UK cross-national study of DSM-III and ICD-9. *Journal of Child Psychology and Psychiatry, 29,* 289–300.

Quay, H. C. (1988). The behavioral reward and inhibition system in childhood behavior disorder. In L. M. Bloomingdale (Ed.), *Attention deficit disorder* (Vol. 3, pp. 176–186). New York: Spectrum.

Quay, H. C. (1993). The psychobiology of undersocialized aggressive conduct disorder. *Development and Psychopathology, 5,* 165–180.

Rapport, M. D., Carlson, G. A., Kelly, K. L., & Pataki, C. (1993). Methylphenidate and desipramine in hospitalized children: I. Separate and combined effects on cognitive function. *Journal of the American Academy of Child and Adolescent Psychiatry, 32,* 333–342.

Rapport, M. D., Denney, C., DuPaul, G. J., & Gardner, M. J. (1994). Attention deficit disorder and methylphenidate: Normalization rates, clinical effectiveness, and response prediction in 76 children. *Journal of the American Academy of Child and Adolescent Psychiatry, 33,* 882–893.

Richters, J. E., Arnold, E., Jensen, P. S., Abikoff, H., Conners, C. K., Greenhill, L. L., Hechtman, L., Hinshaw, S. P., Pelham, W. E., & Swanson, J. M. (1995). National Institute of Mental Health collaborative multisite multimodal treatment study of children with attention-deficit hyperactivity disorder (MTA): I. Background and rationale. *Journal of the American Academy of Child and Adolescent Psychiatry, 34,* 1–14.

Robertson, M. M. (1994). Gilles de la Tourette syndrome—An update. *Journal of Child Psychology and Psychiatry, 35,* 597–611.

Rostain, A. L., Power, T. J., & Atkins, M. S. (1993). Assessing parents' willingness to pursue treatment for children with attention-deficit hyperactivity disorder. *Journal of the American Academy of Child and Adolescent Psychiatry, 32,* 175–181.

Ruff, H. A., Bijur, P. E., Markowitz, M., Ma, Y.-C., & Rosen, J. F. (1993). Declining blood lead levels and cognitive changes in moderately lead-poisoned children. *Journal of the American Medical Association, 269,* 1641–1646.

Russo, M. F., & Beidel, D. C. (1994). Comorbidity of childhood anxiety and externalizing disorders: Prevalence, associated characteristics, and validation issues. *Clinical Psychology Review, 14,* 199–221.

Safer, D. J., & Krager, J. M. (1988). A survey of medication treatment for hyperactive/inattentive students. *Journal of the American Medical Association, 260,* 2256–2258.

Sanson, A., Smart, D., Prior, M., & Oberklaid, F. (1993). Precursors of hyperactivity and aggression. *Journal of the American Academy of Child and Adolescent Psychiatry, 32,* 1207–1216.

Schachar, R. (1991). Childhood hyperactivity. *Journal of Child Psychology and Psychiatry, 32,* 155–191.

Schachar, R., & Tannock, R. (1993). Childhood hyperactivity and psychostimulants: A review of extended treatment studies. *Journal of Child and Adolescent Psychopharmacology, 3,* 81–97.

Schachar, R. J., Tannock, R., & Logan, G. (1993). Inhibitory control, impulsiveness, and attention deficit hyperactivity disorder. *Clinical Psychology Review, 13,* 721–739.

Schachar, R., Tannock, R., Marriott, M., & Logan, G. (1995). Deficient inhibitory control in attention deficit hyperactivity disorder. *Journal of Abnormal Child Psychology, 23,* 411–437.

Semrud-Clikeman, M., Biederman, J., Sprich-Buckminster, S., Lehman, B. K., Faraone, S. V., & Norman, D. (1992). Comorbidity between ADDH and learning disability: A review and report in a clinically referred sample. *Journal of the American Academy of Child and Adolescent Psychiatry, 31,* 439–448.

Semrud-Clikeman, M., Filipek, P. A., Biederman, J., Steingard, R., Kennedy, D., Renshaw, P., & Bekken, K. (1994). Attention-deficit hyperactivity disorder: Magnetic resonance imaging morphometric analysis of the corpus callosum. *Journal of the American Academy of Child and Adolescent Psychiatry, 33,* 875–881.

Sergeant, J., & van der Meere, J. (1990). Convergence of approaches in localizing the hyperactivity deficit. In B. B. Lahey & A. E. Kazdin (Eds.), *Advances in clinical child psychology* (Vol. 13, pp. 207–245). New York: Plenum Press.

Sergeant, J. A., & van der Meere, J. (1994). Toward an empirical child psychopathology. In D. K. Routh (Ed.), *Disruptive behavior disorders in childhood* (pp. 59–85). New York: Plenum Press.

Shaffer, D. (1994). Attention deficit hyperactivity disorder in adults. *American Journal of Psychiatry, 151,* 633–638.

Solanto, M. V., & Wender, E. H. (1989). Does methylphenidate constrict cognitive functioning? *Journal of the American Academy of Child and Adolescent Psychiatry, 28,* 897–902.

Sonuga-Barke, E. J. S. (1995). Disambiguating inhibitory dysfunction in childhood hyperactivity. In J. Sergeant (Ed.), *Eunethydis: European approaches to hyperkinetic disorder* (pp. 209–223). Amsterdam: University of Amsterdam.

Spencer, T., Biederman, J., Wilens, T., & Faraone, S. V. (1994). Is attention-deficit hyperactivity disorder in adults a valid disorder? *Harvard Review of Psychiatry, 1,* 326–335.

Stanger, C., & Lewis, M. (1993). Agreement among parents, teachers, and children on internalizing and externalizing behavior problems. *Journal of Clinical Child Psychology, 22,* 107–115.

Sternberg, S. (1969). Discovery of processing stages: Extensions of Donders' method. In W. G. Koster (Ed.), *Attention and performance* (Vol. 2, pp. 276–315). Amsterdam: North-Holland.

Swanson, J. M., McBurnett, K., Christian, D. L., & Wigal, T. (1995). Stimulant medications and the treatment of children with ADHD. In T. H. Ollendick & R. J. Prinz (Eds.), *Advances in clinical child psychology* (Vol. 17, pp. 265–322). New York: Plenum Press.

Tao, K. T. (1992). Hyperactivity and attention deficit disorder syndromes in China. *Journal of the American Academy of Child and Adolescent Psychiatry, 31,* 1165–1166.

Taylor, E., Sandberg, S., Thorley, B. A., & Giles, S. (1991). *The epidemiology of childhood hyperactivity.* London: Oxford University Press.

Taylor, E., Schachar, R., Thorley, G., Weiselberg, H. M., Everitt, B., & Rutter, M. (1987). Which boys respond to stimulant medication? A controlled trial of methylphenidate in boys with disruptive behaviours. *Psychological Medicine, 17,* 121–143.

Tesman, R. J., & Hills, A. (1994). Developmental effects of lead exposure in children. *Social Policy Report, VIII,* 1–16.

van der Meere, J., van Baal, M., & Sergeant, J. (1989). The additive factor method: A differential diagnostic tool in hyperactivity and learning disability. *Journal of Abnormal Child Psychology, 17,* 409–422.

van der Meere, J., Vreeling, H. J., & Sergeant, J. (1992). A motor presetting study in hyperactive, learning disabled and control children. *Journal of Child Psychology and Psychiatry, 33,* 1347–1354.

Verhulst, F. C., & van der Ende, J. (1993). "Comorbidity" in an epidemiological sample: A longitudinal perspective. *Journal of Child Psychology and Psychiatry, 34,* 767–783.

Weiss, G., & Hechtman, L. T. (1993). *Hyperactive children grown up. ADHD in children, adolescents, and adults* (2nd ed.). New York: Guilford Press.

Wender, P. H., Reimherr, F. W., Wood, D., & Ward, M. (1985). A controlled study of methylphenidate in the treatment of attention deficit disorder, residual type, in adults. *American Journal of Psychiatry, 142,* 547–552.

Werry, J. S. (1994). Pharmacotherapy of disruptive behavior disorders. *Child and Adolescent Psychiatric Clinics of North America, 3,* 321–341.

Werry, J. S., & Aman, M. G. (Eds.) (1993). *Practitioner's guide to psychoactive drugs for children and adolescents.* New York: Plenum Medical.

Whalen, C. K., & Henker, B. (1976). Psychostimulants and children: A review and analysis. *Psychological Bulletin, 83,* 1113–1130.

Whalen, C. K., & Henker, B. (1986). Cognitive behavior therapy for hyperactive children: What do we know? *Journal of Children in Contemporary Society, 19,* 123–141.

Whalen, C. K., & Henker, B. (1991a). The social impact of stimulant treatment for hyperactive children. *Journal of Learning Disabilities, 24,* 231–241.

Whalen, C. K., & Henker, B. (1991b). Therapies for hyperactive children: Comparisons, combinations, and compromises. *Journal of Consulting and Clinical Psychology, 59,* 126–137.

Whalen, C. K., & Henker, B. (1992). The social profile of attention-deficit hyperactivity disorder: Five fundamental facets. *Child and Adolescent Psychiatric Clinics of North America, 1,* 395–410.

Whalen, C. K., & Henker, B. (1997). Stimulant pharmacotherapy for attention-deficit/hyperactivity disorders: An analysis of progress, problems, and prospects. In S. Fisher & R. Greenberg (Eds.), *From placebo to panacea: Putting psychiatric drugs to the test* (pp. 323–355). New York: Wiley.

Whalen, C. K., Henker, B., Buhrmester, D., Hinshaw, S. P., Huber, A., & Laski, K. (1989). Does stimulant medication improve the peer status of hyperactive children? *Journal of Consulting and Clinical Psychology, 57,* 545–549.

Whalen, C. K., Henker, B., Collins, B. E., Finck, D., & Dotemoto, S. (1979). A social ecology of hyperactive boys: Medication effects in structured classroom environments. *Journal of Applied Behavior Analysis, 12,* 65–81.

Whalen, C. K., Henker, B., Collins, B. E., McAuliffe, S., & Vaux, A. (1979). Peer interaction in a structured communication task: Comparisons of normal and hyperactive boys and of methylphenidate (Ritalin) and placebo effects. *Child Development, 50,* 388–401.

Whalen, C. K., Henker, B., & Dotemoto, S. (1981). Teacher response to the methylphenidate (Ritalin) versus placebo status of hyperactive boys in the classroom. *Child Development, 52,* 1005–1014.

Whalen, C. K., Henker, B., & Granger, D. A. (1990). Social judgment processes in hyperactive boys: Effects of methylphenidate and comparisons with normal peers. *Journal of Abnormal Child Psychology, 18,* 297–316.

Whalen, C. K., Henker, B., Hinshaw, S. P., Heller, T., & Huber-Dressler, A. (1991). The messages of medication:

Effects of actual versus informed medication status on hyperactive boys' expectancies and self-evaluations. *Journal of Consulting and Clinical Psychology, 59,* 602–606.

Wilens, T. E., & Biederman, J. (1992). The stimulants. *Pediatric Psychopharmacology, 15,* 191–222.

Wilens, T. E., Spencer, T., Biederman, J., Wozniak, J., & Connor, D. (1995). Combined pharmacotherapy: An emerging trend in pediatric psychopharmacology. *Journal of the American Academy of Child and Adolescent Psychiatry, 34,* 110–112.

Williams, L., Lerner, M., & Swanson, J. (1994, November). *Prevalence of office visits for ADD: Gender differences over the past five years (1990–1994).* Paper presented at the NIMH Conference on Sex Differences in ADHD. Rockville, MD.

Wolraich, M. L., Lindgren, S., Stromquist, A., Milich, R., Davis, C., & Watson, D. (1990). Stimulant medication use by primary care physicians in the treatment of attention deficit hyperactivity disorder. *Pediatrics, 86,* 95–101.

Wolraich, M. L., Lindgren, S. D., Stumbo, P. J., Stegink, L. D., Appelbaum, M. I., & Kiritsy, M. C. (1994). Effects of diets high in sucrose or aspartame on the behavior and cognitive performance of children. *New England Journal of Medicine, 330,* 301–307.

Zametkin, A. J., Nordahl, T. E., Gross, M., King, A. C., Semple, W. E., Rumsey, J., Hamburger, S., & Cohen, R. M. (1990). Cerebral glucose metabolism in adults with hyperactivity of childhood onset. *New England Journal of Medicine, 323,* 1361–1366.

Zametkin, A. J., & Rapoport, J. L. (1987). Neurobiology of attention deficit disorder with hyperactivity: Where have we come in 50 years? *Journal of the American Academy of Child and Adolescent Psychiatry, 26,* 676–686.

8

Conduct Disorders

PAUL J. FRICK

INTRODUCTION

Antisocial behavior in children and adolescents has long been a major societal concern. This societal concern seems justified given the high cost at which antisocial behavior operates to society including the cost of incarceration of juvenile offenders, the cost associated with vandalism of public property, and the cost to the victims of youth crime and their families (Zigler, Taussig, & Black, 1992). Reflecting societal concerns, researchers from a host of scientific disciplines have spent decades investigating the causes, the course, and the methods of preventing and treating severe antisocial behavior, or what is referred to in psychiatric terminology as conduct disorders. It is arguably one of the most intensively studied of all forms of childhood psychopathology. However, there is still great debate over "how the accumulated facts should be interpreted, such as why antisocial trajectories develop, why they broaden and deepen with development in some children yet taper off in others, and why they are so difficult to deflect once

stabilized" (Richters & Cicchetti, 1993, p. 2). Although the field is far from reaching a consensus on these questions, there are several promising theories based on the available research and the goal of this chapter is to provide a brief overview of these promising approaches.

To appropriately interpret the research on conduct disorders, one must accept two basic assumptions about the nature of conduct disorders. First, children with conduct disorders represent a very heterogeneous group of children in terms of the types of conduct problems being exhibited, the causal factors involved, the developmental course of the problems, and the response to treatment. Therefore, one must approach this area of research recognizing this heterogeneity. For example, rather than seeking to find a single causal theory to explain the development of conduct problems in all children, one should seek to delineate which causal theories might apply best to certain subgroups of children with conduct disorders. Second, even within more homogeneous subgroups, one must recognize that multiple factors operating at different levels of analysis (e.g., physiological, psychological, and sociological) interact to lead to the development and continuation of conduct disorders. As a result, any theory or treatment that focuses on only one level of anal-

PAUL J. FRICK • Department of Psychology, University of Alabama, Tuscaloosa, Alabama 35487.

Handbook of Child Psychopathology, 3rd edition, edited by Ollendick & Hersen. Plenum Press, New York, 1998.

lysis will be inadequate to fully explain or to effectively prevent the development of conduct disorders. These two issues will be revisited throughout this chapter.

PHENOMENOLOGY

Conduct problems and *antisocial behavior* are terms used interchangeably in this chapter. Both terms refer to a heterogeneous dimension of behavior with the common theme of a failure of the individual to conform his or her behavior to expectations of some authority (e.g., parent or teacher) or to societal norms. The behaviors can range from chronic conflicts with authority (e.g., noncompliance, defiance, argumentativeness) to violations of societal norms (e.g., truancy, running away from home) to serious violations of the rights of others (e.g., aggression, vandalism, firesetting, stealing). These behaviors are considered to be indicative of a clinical syndrome (i.e., a conduct disorder) when they are severe, persistent, and lead to significant impairment in a child's psychosocial functioning.

Developmental Progression of Conduct Problems

From this description of conduct problems, it is evident that conduct problems can range greatly in severity (e.g., argumentativeness and physical assault) and type (e.g., fighting and stealing). Some of the variations can be explained by a hierarchical and developmental sequencing of conduct problem behavior. For example, research has found that preadolescent children rarely begin showing conduct problem behaviors by exhibiting the more severe conduct problems. Instead, there seems to be a typical developmental progression in which children start to show oppositional and argumentative behaviors early in life (e.g., between the ages of 3 and 8) and then gradually progress into increasingly more severe patterns of con-

duct problem behavior (Loeber, Green, Lahey, Christ, & Frick, 1992). This developmental progression is visually represented in Figure 1.

There are two other important aspects of the developmental progression of conduct problem behaviors that are represented in Figure 1. First, although most children who show the more severe conduct problems start by showing the less severe oppositional behaviors, a large number of children who show the less severe oppositional symptoms do not go on to show the more severe conduct problems (Lahey & Loeber, 1994). This is why the pyramid, with the large base and smaller peak, is used to illustrate this asymmetrical relationship. Second, most children who move on to display the more severe types of conduct problems do not *change* the types of behaviors they display but instead *add* the more severe conduct problem behaviors (Lahey & Loeber, 1994). That is, most children who show the more severe behaviors at the top of the pyramid in Figure 1 continue to show conduct problems from the lower levels.

Childhood-Onset and Adolescent-Limited Distinctions

The developmental progression described in the previous section is typical of children who begin showing conduct problems prior to adolescence, which is referred to as the *childhood-onset* pattern of conduct disorder. However, there are a substantial number of youth who begin showing antisocial behavior as they approach adolescence, with no history of oppositional behavior during childhood (Hinshaw, Lahey, & Hart, 1993). Moffitt (1993a) coined the term *adolescence-limited* to reflect the findings from many longitudinal studies that youth who begin showing conduct problems in adolescence are much less likely to persist in their antisocial behavior into adulthood. Also, boys revealing childhood-onset conduct problem behavior are more aggressive and have more neuropsychological deficits than boys with the adolescent-limited pattern (Lahey, Hart, Pliszka, Apple-

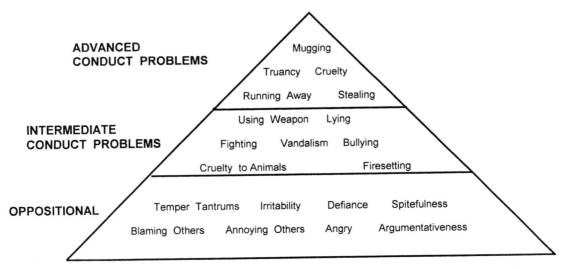

Figure 1. A visual heuristic describing the developmental progression of conduct problems. Problems at the lower levels of the pyramid tend to emerge earlier in development and are predictive of the emergence of the more severe problems at the upper levels of the pyramid later in development. Adapted with permission from Lahey and Loeber (1994).

gate, & McBurnett, 1993; Moffitt, 1993a). It would seem from these findings that onset in childhood represents a much more severe pattern of dysfunction, whereas the adolescent-limited pattern may be better considered an exaggeration of a normal developmental process.

Developmental Progressions and Gender

Much of the research on the developmental progressions of conduct problems and the influence on the timing of onset has been conducted on male samples. In the few studies that have explored gender differences, there appear to be several differences in the developmental trajectories for girls with conduct disorders. Epidemiological studies have found that boys are more likely to show conduct disorders than girls throughout childhood and adolescence, but this ratio decreases dramatically in samples of adolescents (Offord et al., 1987). Therefore, a greater proportion of girls with conduct disorders show the adolescent-onset pattern. Also, such girls seem to show a severe type of disturbance that is similar in many respects to boys

with the childhood-onset pattern. That is, irrespective of the timing of onset, girls with conduct disorders tend to have high rates of neuropsychological dysfunction and are at high risk for having significantly impaired adult functioning (Moffitt, 1993a). Therefore, in contrast to the findings for boys, the adolescent-onset pattern in girls does not seem to represent a less severe and less chronic type of disturbance.

The Stability of Conduct Disorders

There has been a great debate over the degree of stability in childhood conduct problems, despite the fact that there have been numerous longitudinal studies investigating both the short- and long-term stability of conduct disorders. The debate often centers around four key issues. First, some research focuses on the stability of only one type of behavior (e.g., aggression) and other research focuses on the stability of a range of antisocial behavior. Focusing on a single antisocial behavior ignores the highly changeable manifestations in antisocial behavior over time and, therefore, may underestimate the stability of conduct disorders (Loeber, 1991).

Second, confusion over the stability of conduct disorders may be partly a function of differing temporal perspectives for studying stability. For example, retrospective studies suggest that most antisocial adults have childhood histories of antisocial behavior (Robins, Tipp, & Pryzbeck, 1991). In contrast, estimates from prospective studies suggest that around 40% of children with conduct disorders will exhibit antisocial personality disorder as adults (Robins, 1966; Zoccolillo, Pickles, Quinton, & Rutter, 1992). Therefore, most antisocial adults have childhood histories of conduct disorders, but over half of the children with conduct disorders will not show antisocial disorders as adults.

Third, stability estimates in longitudinal study could be influenced by fluctuations in the severity of conduct problems over time. For example, Lahey et al. (1995) found that 50% of children with a conduct disorder were rediagnosed at any single follow-up point in their 4-year longitudinal study. However, they also found that few children with conduct disorders were ever completely free of conduct problem behaviors, even if they were not "rediagnosed" during the study. Also, 88% of those diagnosed with a conduct disorder at year 1 were diagnosed in at least one yearly assessment over the 4-year study period. Therefore, estimates of continuity that do not consider a range of conduct problem behavior and that rely on a single assessment point may underestimate the stability of conduct problem behavior.

Fourth, and perhaps most importantly, there seem to be certain subgroups of children with conduct disorders who show more stable patterns of antisocial behavior than others. One variable that has already been discussed is the age at initiation of conduct problem behavior. Other indicators of more stable conduct disorders include showing a high rate of multiple types of conduct problems (Loeber, 1991), having an attention-deficit disorder (Farrington, 1991), being of lower intelligence (Farrington, 1991; Lahey et al., 1995; Stattin & Magnusson,

1989), and having a parent with an antisocial disorder (Lahey et al., 1995).

DIAGNOSIS

Despite the general consensus regarding the basic nature of conduct disorders, there is great debate over what specific behaviors should be used to identify conduct disorders, what criteria should be used to define subgroups of children with conduct problems, and how one should determine whether a child's conduct problems are severe enough to be considered "pathological" or not. As a result, there have been many different approaches to classifying children with conduct disorders.

DSM-IV

Criteria in the fourth edition of the *Diagnostic and Statistical Manual of Mental Disorders* (American Psychiatric Association, 1994) for the Disruptive Behavior Disorders are one of the most influential and widely used systems for classifying children with conduct disorders. The criteria specify two conduct disorders with very explicit symptom lists for making the diagnosis. Oppositional Defiant Disorder (ODD) is defined as:

> a recurrent pattern of negativistic, defiant, disobedient and hostile behavior toward authority figures that persists for at least 6 months and is characterized by the frequent occurrence of at least four of the following behaviors: losing temper, arguing with adults, actively defying or refusing to comply with requests or rules of adults, deliberately doing things that will annoy other people, blaming others for his or her own mistakes or misbehavior, being touchy or easily annoyed by others, being angry and resentful, or being spiteful or vindictive. (p. 91)

Conduct Disorder (CD) is defined as:

> a repetitive and persistent pattern of behavior which violates the rights of others or major

age appropriate societal norms or rules. These behaviors fall into four main groupings: aggressive conduct that threatens physical harm to other people or animals, nonaggressive conduct that causes property loss or damage, deceitfulness and theft, and serious violations of rules. Three or more characteristic behaviors must have been present during the past 12 months. (p. 85)

As discussed previously, the less severe ODD symptoms seem to be linked to the more severe CD symptoms both hierarchically and developmentally in preadolescent children. Also supporting the notion that CD is simply a developmentally advanced form of ODD, research has fairly consistently linked ODD and CD to similar correlates. That is, both children with ODD and children with CD differ from other clinic-referred children by: being from families of lower socioeconomic status (Faraone, Biederman, Keenan, & Tsuang, 1991; Frick et al., 1992; Rey et al., 1988), being more likely to have a parental history of antisocial personality disorder (Faraone et al., 1991; Frick et al., 1992), and having parents who use ineffective discipline practices (Frick et al., 1992). The difference between the two disorders on each of these variables seems to be one of degree, with CD children being somewhat more divergent from control children on these variables than children with ODD.

In addition to distinguishing between ODD and CD, the DSM-IV system recognizes the important distinction between children who begin showing conduct problems in early childhood and those who begin showing problems only as they approach adolescence. Those children who meet criteria for CD and who had any of the symptoms present prior to age 10 are classified as Childhood-Onset Type. Those children who meet criteria for CD and who had no symptoms present prior to age 10 are classified as Adolescent-Onset Type.

Explicit in the DSM-IV criteria is the use of number of symptoms (four for ODD and three for CD) as a primary means of making a diagnosis and thereby designating pathological from nonpathological levels of conduct prob-

lem behavior. These diagnostic thresholds were developed by comparing children at different levels of symptom severity on several clinically important criteria. Prior to publication of the DSM-IV, a large multisite field trial was conducted using a sample of 440 clinic-referred children between the ages of 4 and 17 (Lahey et al., 1994). The results of this field trial indicated that using the threshold of four symptoms of ODD designated children who were judged by parents and clinicians as showing significant impairments in psychosocial functioning and it led to optimal agreement with independent diagnoses made by trained clinicians. In similar analyses using the CD symptoms, children with only one symptom were judged by parents and clinicians to have significant impairments in their psychosocial functioning. However, a diagnostic threshold of three symptoms led to optimal correspondence with clinician diagnoses of CD. Also, there was a nonlinear relationship between number of CD symptoms and number of police contacts (adjusted for age of the child) with children who had less than three symptoms rarely having police contacts and children with three or more symptoms having a high rate of police contact.

Subtypes Based on Patterns of Behavioral Covariation

Predating the recent revisions of the DSM in which explicit diagnostic criteria were provided for conduct disorders, many researchers attempted to define conduct disorders and important subgroups within this dimension based on the patterns of covariation among conduct problem behaviors (see Quay, 1986, for a review). These classification systems often relied on multivariate statistical analyses, such as factor analysis, to determine whether there were distinct clusters or "factors" of interrelated conduct problem behaviors. As a way of summarizing this literature, Frick et al. (1993) conducted a quantitative meta-analysis of 60 factor analyses of conduct problem behaviors with a combined sample of 28,401 children and adolescents. The results indicated that conduct problem behaviors could be summarized by two bipolar dimensions. One dimension divided behaviors into overt behaviors involving direct confrontation with others and covert behaviors not involving direct confrontation. The second orthogonal dimension was a destructive–nondestructive dimension of behavior. The intersection of these two bipolar dimensions resulted in a division of conduct problem behavior into four quadrants, illustrated in Figure 2.

Based on this meta-analysis, one cluster of behaviors (Overt–Nondestructive) corresponds quite well to the DSM-IV definition of ODD. However, the CD symptoms were divided among the other three quadrants. Frick et al. (1993) tested the results of the meta-analysis in a sample of 177 clinic-referred boys between the ages of 6 and 13 and found that these clusters of behavior were strongly related to age. That is, the oppositional behaviors tended to emerge first (median age of onset 6.0 years) followed by the aggressive behaviors (median age of onset 6.75 years), the covert–property destructive behaviors (median age of onset 7.25), and the status violations (median age of onset 9.0 years). This supports the developmental progression of conduct problem behavior in preadolescent children that was discussed in an earlier section of this chapter.

Undersocialized and Aggressive Subtypes

In the two versions of the DSM that predated the DSM-IV (DSM-III, American Psychiatric Association, 1980; DSM-III-R, American Psychiatric Association, 1987), there were several subtypes of CD related to a child's status on two dimensions. First, there was a distinction made between those youth with CD who are able to form and maintain social relationships and who primarily commit antisocial acts with other antisocial peers (socialized or group type) and those youths with CD who are not able to form and maintain social relationships and who primarily

commit antisocial acts alone (undersocialized or solitary type). Second, there were distinctions made between children with CD who exhibited aggressive behaviors as part of their pattern of antisocial behavior and those who displayed no aggressive behaviors.

Research has supported the use of these dimensions for subtyping children with conduct problems, especially for delineating children who are both undersocialized and aggressive. This undersocialized–aggressive group seems to show a very persistent form of conduct disorder that is quite resistant to treatment (see Quay, 1987). Also, Lahey et al. (1993) reviewed studies on the neurophysiological correlates of conduct disorders and concluded that the neurophysiological variables (e.g., neurochemical abnormalities, indices of aberrant autonomic reactivity) that have been linked to adult antisocial behavior seem to be characteristic only of the undersocialized–aggressive children. Therefore, this undersocialized and aggressive distinction seems to designate an especially severe form of conduct disorder and one that has unique neurophysiological correlates.

Comorbid Conditions

Comorbidity refers to the co-occurrence of two or more pathological conditions in the same child. In children with conduct disorders, as with other children who have severe emotional or behavior disturbances, comorbidity is the rule rather than the exception. Understanding common comorbid conditions is crucial because the presence of specific types of co-occurring problems can affect the manifestation, course, and treatment of the disorder. There is no better illustration of this fact than the comorbidity between attention-deficit/hyperactivity disorder (ADHD) and conduct disorders. In samples of children with conduct disorders, the proportion of children with ADHD ranges from 65% (Stewart, Cummings, Singer, & deBlois, 1981; Trites & Laprade, 1983) to 90% (Abikoff & Klein, 1992; Prinz, Connor, & Wil-

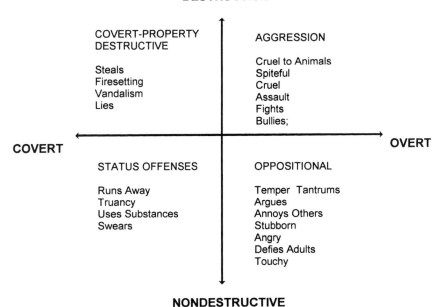

Figure 2. These clusters of behaviors are based on the meta-analysis of 60 factor analyses conducted by Frick et al. (1993). The clusters are formed from the intersection of two dimensions of behavior covariation. The horizontal dimension captures a bipolar dimension ranging from overt to covert patterns of behavior, and the vertical dimension captures a dimension ranging from destructive to nondestructive types of behavior.

son, 1981). Importantly, the comorbidity with ADHD seems to affect the manifestation and course of conduct disorders. As summarized by Abikoff and Klein (1992), the presence of ADHD leads to more severe and aggressive conduct problems, more persistent conduct problems, and more peer rejection in children with conduct disorders.

A second common comorbidity with conduct disorders is anxiety. In community samples, between 22 and 33% of children with conduct problems also have an anxiety disorder, whereas the rates range from 60 to 75% in clinic-referred samples (Russo & Beidel, 1994). However, in contrast to the research on ADHD, the presence of anxiety in children with conduct problems seems to delineate a less severe disturbance, at least in prepubertal children. For example, Walker et al. (1991) reported that children with CD who also had an anxiety disorder had fewer police contacts, fewer school suspensions, and

were rated as less aggressive by peers than children with CD who did not show elevated levels of anxiety. However, this moderating influence of anxiety may not hold for adolescents with conduct disorders (Zoccolillo, 1992).

One additional comorbidity that has been the focus of research is the comorbidity of conduct disorders and depression. Unlike ADHD or anxiety, the co-occurrence of depression does not seem to alter the course of conduct disorders (Capaldi, 1992; Harrington, Fudge, Rutter, Pickles, & Hill, 1991). Also, the presence of conduct problems generally seems to predate the onset of depressive symptoms (Capaldi, 1992). As a result, depressive symptoms are often viewed as secondary to conduct disorders with depression resulting from the conflict and rejection from others and frequent failure experiences (e.g., with peers and in school) that children with conduct disorders often have to face (Capaldi, 1992; Panak & Garber, 1992). However, it appears that the presence of depression may be a clinically important consideration in children with conduct disorders because it signals an increased risk for suicidal ideation. For example, in a community sample of seventh and eighth graders, 31% of the children with both conduct problems had depression reported suicidal ideation ($n = 26$) compared with 12% of the children with only conduct problems ($n = 34$) (Capaldi, 1992).

Callous–Unemotional Traits in Classification

Most methods of classifying children with conduct disorders do not consider a child's affective and interpersonal style. However, some children with conduct problems show a callous (e.g., lack of empathy, use of other for own gain) and unemotional (e.g., constricted affect, lack of remorse and guilt) interpersonal style that seems to be analogous to the concept of "psychopathy" that has been applied to antisocial adults (Frick, O'Brien, Wootton, & McBurnett, 1994). When the callous–unemotional traits accompany conduct disorders, the children engage in a greater number of conduct problem behaviors, they engage in a greater variety of conduct problem behaviors (especially more covert/property-destructive conduct problems), they have more police contacts, and they have stronger parental histories of antisocial personality disorder as compared with children with conduct disorders who do not show the callous–unemotional traits (Christian, Frick, Hill, Tyler, & Frazer, 1997). These differences are important because they have proven to be predictive of a more severe and chronic pattern of antisocial behavior in longitudinal research (see section entitled "The Stability of Conduct Disorders").

ETIOLOGY

The focus of this section is on several types of causal factors that seem to play an important

role in the development of conduct disorders. The main division is between dispositional and environmental factors. Dispositional factors are factors within the individual that predispose him or her to act in antisocial ways. Environmental factors are factors within a child's social ecology that may promote conduct problem behavior. This should not be viewed as a simple "nature versus nurture" distinction, as many dispositional factors are often shaped by the child's psychosocial environment, and the child's dispositional tendencies can have a dramatic effect on his or her environment. Also, given the multiply determined nature of conduct disorders, one must continually recognize that any causal factor or any one set of causal factors provides only one piece to a very complex puzzle.

Dispositional Factors

Genetic and Neurophysiological Predispositions

Several studies have linked several types of neurochemical abnormalities to conduct disorders in children, including low levels of serotonin (Kreusi et al., 1990), low levels of epinephrine (Magnusson, 1988; Olweus, Mattesson, Schalling, & Low, 1988), and high levels of testosterone (Olweus et al., 1988; Scerbo & Kolko, 1994). Also, several studies have found abnormalities in the autonomic nervous system functioning in children with conduct disorders; more specifically, children with conduct disorders have been shown to have decreased autonomic reactivity on skin conductance measures (Delameter & Lahey, 1983; Schmidt, Solanto, & Bridger, 1985), heart rate measures (Delameter & Lahey, 1983; Raine, Venables, & Williams, 1990), and event-related electroencephalographic potentials (Raine et al., 1990). However, findings in each of these areas have not been consistent, especially in comparison with research on antisocial adults (Raine, 1993). Many studies have failed to find neurochemical or autonomic differences between children with conduct disorders and controls (e.g., Constantino et al., 1993; Gerralda, Connell, & Taylor, 1991). These inconsistent findings on specific neurophysiological correlates mirror the great variability in heritability estimates for child and adolescent antisocial behavior found in twin and adoption studies, which also are in contrast to more consistent findings in the adult literature (Mason & Frick, 1994; Rutter et al., 1990).

There are several factors that could lead to these weak and often inconsistent findings on genetic and biological underpinnings to childhood conduct disorders. First, it is possible that this variability reflects the fact that conduct problems in children are less strongly related to biological and genetic factors than is the case for antisocial behavior in adults. Second, it is possible that the variability in findings is related to the weak methodology used in many studies of the neurophysiological correlates to childhood conduct disorders and in the behavior genetic studies on childhood antisocial behavior (Lahey et al., 1993; Mason & Frick, 1994). Third, it is possible that children with conduct disorders constitute a more heterogeneous group than adults with antisocial disorders. As a result, genetic and neurophysiological factors may only be related to specific subgroups of children with conduct disorders.

There are several lines of evidence in support of this third possibility. Mason and Frick (1994) conducted a meta-analysis of twin and adoption studies of antisocial behavior and found that heritability estimates were generally lower in samples of children and adolescents relative to estimates obtained in adult samples. However, when the analyses were limited only to severe manifestations of antisocial behavior (e.g., physical aggression toward persons versus hits to a toy doll), the heritability estimates in children were much higher and comparable to those found for adult samples (see also Ghodsian-Carpey & Baker, 1987). Also, Lahey et al. (1993) reviewed studies on the neurophysiological correlates to conduct disorder and concluded that neurochemical and autonomic abnormalities were "only characteristic of those youths with

CD who are characterized as aggressive, undersocialized, and psychopathic" (p. 150). Therefore, there seem to be specific subgroups of children with conduct disorders in which genetic and neurophysiological factors may play a greater causal role.

Responsiveness to Rewards and Punishments

Several authors have suggested that a specific learning style, one that leads to an overfocus on rewards at the expense of ignoring cues to punishment, may underlie disinhibitory syndromes such as conduct disorders (Newman & Wallace, 1993; Quay, 1993). This learning style could prevent a child from inhibiting antisocial behavior in the face of potential punishment. Consistent with this possibility, several studies have shown that children with conduct disorders perseverate with a previously rewarded response in the face of increasing rates of punishment, a learning style that has been labeled *reward dominant* (Daugherty & Quay, 1991; O'Brien, Frick, & Lyman, 1994; Shapiro, Quay, Hogan, & Schwartz, 1988). Again, there is evidence that this reward-dominant response style is not characteristic of all children with conduct disorders. Instead, this response style seems to only be characteristic of children with conduct disorders who are not also anxious (O'Brien et al., 1994; O'Brien & Frick, 1996) or who show the callous–unemotional traits discussed previously (O'Brien & Frick, 1996).

Intelligence and Academic Underachievement

Children with conduct disorders tend to have low intellectual levels, especially in the area of verbal intelligence (Hinshaw, 1992; Moffitt, 1993b). Moffitt (1993b) summarized several of the major theories that have been used to explain this association. First, language deficits could affect the development of self-control strategies and the child's ability to delay gratification and anticipate consequences. Second, low verbal intelligence may influence a child's ability to generalize learning, such as what behaviors are acceptable and unacceptable. Third, lower intelligence may affect a child's ability to understand the emotions of others, either victims or adversaries. Fourth, children with low verbal intelligence may elicit more negative reactions from others, contributing to their negative interactional style. Fifth, the behavior of children with conduct disorders could hamper their ability to benefit from formal education, by affecting their ability to learn in traditional school classrooms or by leading to early withdrawal from school.

In addition to intellectual deficits, children with conduct disorders tend to perform poorly in academics even after controlling for differences in their intellectual ability. Approximately 20 to 25% of children with conduct disorders have at least one academic area in which they are achieving significantly below a level predicted by their intellectual level (Frick et al., 1991). As was the case for intellectual deficits, there are numerous possible reasons for this link with academic underachievement. Hinshaw (1992), in an excellent review of the research, suggested that the mechanisms involved in this link may vary depending on the age of the child studied. That is, in elementary schoolchildren the link between conduct disorders and academic underachievement seems to be largely accounted for by the comorbidity with ADHD (see also Frick et al., 1991). However, academic deficits seem to predate antisocial behavior in some adolescent samples. Therefore, it is possible that learning difficulties play a causal role in some children with the adolescent-onset pattern of conduct disorders. For example, academic deficits could lead to high levels of frustration, alienation, and truancy and thus lead an adolescent to withdraw from school, increasing his or her exposure to a deviant peer group.

Deficits in Social Cognition

Another important area of research has found that children with conduct disorders have deficits in social cognition and informa-tion processing that could play a causal role in the development of conduct disorders. For example, aggressive children tend to overattribute hostile intent to others (Dodge, Murphy, & Buchsbaum, 1984; Lochman, 1987) and in general tend to miss important social cues in their interactions with others (Dodge & Frame, 1982). Also, aggressive children are less able to access and use nonaggressive problem-solving strategies (Asarnow & Callan, 1985) and they tend to see aggression as an effective way of obtaining positive outcomes (Perry, Perry, & Rasmussen, 1986). It is unclear how these cognitive processing biases originate (e.g., Dodge, Bates, & Pettit, 1990) but it is clear that these biases tend to result in a behavioral repertoire that is limited and overly focused on aggressive responding.

Callous–Unemotional Traits

As mentioned previously, a callous and unemotional interpersonal style seems to designate a group of children with conduct disorders who show a more severe type of disturbance (Christian et al., 1997). However, these traits could also be viewed as a dispositional risk factor for the development of conduct disorders, with children who lack empathy and guilt being more likely to act in an antisocial manner. As a result, the presence of callous and unemotional traits may designate one pathway to the development of conduct disorders. By conceptualizing this pattern of interpersonal responding in this way, it leaves open the possibility that some causal factors to conduct disorders may be mediated by the presence of the callous and unemotional traits. This possibility is consistent with several lines of research.

First, many of the neurophysiological indicators of constricted autonomic reactivity seem to be characteristic only of children with conduct disorders who show this interpersonal style (see Lahey et al., 1993). Second, Frick et al. (1994) found that the callous–unemotional traits were inversely correlated with measures of anxiety and positively correlated with sensation-seeking behavior, whereas conduct disorders were positively associated with anxiety and uncorrelated with sensation-seeking behaviors after controlling for the presence of callous–unemotional traits. Third, O'Brien and Frick (1996) found that the reward-dominant response style was more specifically associated with the callous–unemotional traits and not with conduct problems in the absence of these traits. The common thread to all of these findings is that factors related directly (e.g., skin conductance) or theoretically (e.g., sensation seeking, reward dominance) with low emotional reactivity seem to be associated with conduct disorders largely through the presence of the callous and unemotional interpersonal style.

Environmental Factors

Family Dysfunction

There is an enormous body of research that has consistently linked several aspects of the child's family environment to antisocial behavior. These aspects of family functioning are summarized in Table 1. Given the size and consistency of this literature, any theory of conduct disorders must account for these factors. However, the next generation of research in this area, one that has already begun to emerge, needs to go beyond documenting *what* family factors are related to conduct problems and focus on *how* these family factors are related to conduct problems in children. The following discussion focuses on some examples of research in this area.

Several studies have tested the potential mediating role of family functioning in the development of conduct problems. That is, certain aspects of the family environment are viewed as primary causal agents (e.g., socialization practices) and other risk factors, either within the family (e.g., maternal depression) or outside the family (e.g., poverty), are viewed as being related to conduct problems only through their effects on the primary causal agent. For example, Forehand, Lautenschlager, Faust, and Graziano (1986) reported that maternal depression was associated with child conduct problems only indirectly through its effect on the parent's disciplinary practices. Similarly, Laub and Sampson (1988) reported that parental criminality and alcohol abuse were related to delinquency in their children primarily through the disruptions they caused on the parents' discipline practices, the parents' ability to supervise their child, and the attachment between parent and child.

Other authors have studied how a child's behavior contributes to disruptions in family functioning (see Bell, 1968; Lytton, 1990). For example, in a classic longitudinal study of the effects of divorce on child behavior, children with difficult temperaments were found to have parents who were more likely to divorce *at a later date* (Hetherington, 1991). One interpretation of this finding would be that stressors in the family that preceded the divorce (e.g., high parental conflict), also caused the difficult temperament in the child. However, it is also possible that children with difficult temperaments place an additional stressor on the marriage, making divorce more likely.

Although the effects of a child's behavior on the family context are important to consider, research also suggests that any unidirectional model is insufficient. Instead, bidirectional or "transactional" models, in which the child's family context both shapes and is shaped by a child's behavior, seem most appropriate (see Lytton, 1990). One of the best examples of a transactional model comes from Patterson's laboratory (Patterson, Reid, & Dishion, 1992). Through rigorous observations of parent and child interactions, these authors documented a pattern of interactions that they have labeled the *coercive cycle*. This cycle describes a pattern of interactions that develops in families of children with conduct problems in which parental behavior inadvertently reinforces negative behavior in their children (e.g., parent does not force compliance because of a child's temper tantrum) and a child's negative behavior rein-

Table 1. Familial Factors Consistently Associated with Conduct Disorders

General type of dysfunction	Specific aspects of dysfunction	Summary of key findings
Parental Psychopathology	Parental Depression Parental Substance Abuse Parental Antisocial/Criminal Behavior	Parental depression and substance use have nonspecific associations with child psychopathology. That is, they are associated with many types of child problems including conduct disorders (Downey & Coyne, 1990; West & Prinz, 1987). Parental antisocial behavior shows a more specific relationship with conduct disorders (Frick et al., 1992), one that may have a genetic component (Jarey & Stewart, 1985).
Parental Marital Relationship	Divorce Marital Satisfaction Marital Conflict	The key variable on child adjustment seems to be the degree of overt conflict witnessed by the child (Amato & Keith, 1991).
Parental Socialization Practices	Lack of Parental Involvement Poor Parental Supervision and Monitoring Ineffective Discipline Practices Inconsistency Failure to use positive change strategies Harsh discipline	In a meta-analysis of several hundred studies, Loeber and Stouthamer-Loeber (1986) found that parental involvement in their child's activities and parental supervision and monitoring of their child showed the strongest and most consistent association with conduct disorders across all areas of family dysfunction studied. Parental discipline exhibited a less consistent relationship across studies but seems to be a critical focus of some of the most successful interventions for conduct disorders (Kazdin, 1987, 1993).

Note: This summary is based on a review of the research by Frick (1993).

forces inappropriate parenting behavior (e.g., a child complies with parental requests only after the parent uses harsh discipline). Therefore, parent and child behavior are mutually dependent and this mutual dependence defines a transactional system.

Another possibility that has been tested in research is that some of the correlations between family functioning and childhood conduct problems are spurious. That is, the correlation is related to some other variable(s) that causes both family dysfunction and child conduct problems. For example, it is possible that antisocial behavior in parents is causally related to some forms of conduct disorders in their offspring through a mechanism that is independent of the family environment (e.g., biological predispositions). As antisocial adults tend to have problems in marital adjustment and in using appropriate socialization strategies with their children, it is possible that marital adjustment and inappropriate socialization strategies are only correlated with child conduct problems because of the common cause of having an antisocial parent (Frick & Jackson, 1993). Consistent with this possibility, Frick et al. (1992) found that poor parenting was not associated with child CD *independent* of parental antisocial personality disorder.

Researchers have also tested how a child's family context may interact with factors outside the family, or how several factors within the family context may interact, to lead to the development of conduct problems. That is, several aspects of a child's family environment may act conjointly and result in the development of child conduct problems. Alternatively, some aspects of the family environment may not cause conduct problems but still could "moderate" the effects of other causal factors. For example, a positive family context could protect or buffer a child from stressors in the child's social ecology (e.g., poor housing, high crime rate in the neighborhood) or could help to channel the behavior of a child with a difficult temperament into more socially acceptable behaviors. As an illustration of the potential protective effects of a child's family environment, McCord (1991) reported that for sons who had a criminal father (who were at higher risk for delinquency than sons of noncriminal fathers) the presence of a mother who was affectionate or confident in her parenting abilities led to a decrease in the risk for criminality. Therefore, the quality of the mother–son relationship appeared to be "protective" for sons with criminal fathers.

Peer Rejection and Association with a Deviant Peer Group

There is a well-established relationship between a child's antisocial behavior and antisocial behavior in the child's peer group (Keenan, Loeber, Zhang, Stouthamer-Loeber, & van Kammen, 1995; Patterson et al., 1992; Roff & Wirt, 1984). This association has largely been studied in boys but it may be even stronger for girls with conduct disorders (Emler, Reicher, & Ross, 1987). What is unclear from this research is whether association with a deviant peer group leads to conduct disorders or whether children with conduct disorders tend to select an antisocial peer group. Patterson et al. (1992) proposed a model in which conduct disorders lead to high rates of rejection from prosocial peers. This rejection increases a child's likelihood of associating with a deviant peer group, leading to an increase in the frequency and severity of the child's antisocial behavior.

Poverty and Neighborhood

Another set of environmental factors that have long been associated with the development of conduct problems is economic deprivation and the quality of a child's neighborhood (e.g., Shaw & McKay, 1972). That is, conduct disorders tend to be more prevalent in economically disadvantaged families (e.g., Farrington, 1991; Frick, Lahey, Hartdagen, & Hynd, 1989) and in certain neighborhoods (Peeples & Loeber, 1994). These are not independent causal factors in that the level of poverty is one aspect of the neighborhood that seems to result in high rates of youth with conduct problems. However, there are other aspects of the neighborhood that seem to predict high rates of youth with conduct disorders *within impoverished neighborhoods*. These variables include physical deterioration in housing, high rates of unemployment, high rates of population mobility, and high rates of births to unmarried parents (Peeples & Loeber, 1994; Shaw & McKay, 1972). Also, there are several pieces of evidence to suggest that many, if not all, of the effects of living under these stressful conditions are mediated by the disruptions they cause on family functioning (Larzelere & Patterson, 1990; Wahler & Sansbury, 1990).

EPIDEMIOLOGY

Prevalence estimates for conduct disorders in community samples of youth generally range between 6 and 10% (Anderson, Williams, McGee, & Silva, 1987; Costello et al., 1988; Offord et al., 1987). When broken down by type of conduct disorder diagnoses using DSM-III diagnoses (American Psychiatric Association, 1980), Oppositional Disorder (OPP) seems to be present in about 5–7% of the population and CD seems to be present in about 2–4% of the population (Anderson et al., 1987; Offord et al., 1987). It is important to note that these figures are based on the older DSM-III definitions of conduct disorders and likely overestimate the prevalence of the more restrictive DSM-IV criteria, especially for the revised category of ODD (Lahey et al., 1994).

Besides diagnostic criteria, there are several other sources of variability in estimating the prevalence of conduct disorders. First, the prevalence rate varies according to the informants used to assess the disorders. For example, in a community sample of children aged 7 to 11, Costello et al. (1988) found a prevalence rate of 4.7% for parent report of OPP, 2.1% for child report, and 6.6% for a combination of parent and child report. Similar estimates for CD were 1% for parent report, 1.6% for child report, and 2% for a combination of parent and child report. Second, conduct disorders vary by gender. For all conduct disorders, there is a clear male predominance of the disorder with the male/female ratio ranging from about 2:1 to 4:1 (Anderson et al., 1987; Offord et al., 1987). Third, conduct disorders seem to vary by age with about 4% of children aged 4 to 11 having conduct disorders and 7% of children aged 12 to 16 having conduct disorders (Offord et al., 1987).

Earlier in this chapter, there was a discussion of a gender by age interaction on the prevalence rates of conduct disorders. Offord et al. (1987) studied the 6-month prevalence of conduct disorders in 2674 children between the ages of 4 and 16. For boys there was a 6-month prevalence of conduct disorders of 6.5% in the 4 to 11 age range and of 10.4% in the 12 to 16 age range. For girls the corresponding prevalence estimates were 1.8 and 4.1%. Therefore, whereas the prevalence of conduct disorders increased in adolescence for both sexes, this increase was more dramatic for girls.

ASSESSMENT

A General Framework for Assessment

Up to this point, the focus of the chapter has been on research investigating the nature, course, and causes of conduct disorders. The focus of the remainder of the chapter is on applying this basic research to the assessment and treatment of conduct disorders. Table 2 summarizes several issues that have emerged in this research that have particular relevance to the assessment process. These issues lead to a general framework for the assessment of children with conduct disorders that is organized around three goals:

1.   To assess the type and severity of conduct problem behaviors and other psychological dimensions (e.g., age of onset, affective and motivational style) related to important subtypes of conduct disorders

2.   To assess multiple aspects of a child's emotional and behavioral functioning, especially the most common co-occurring types of problems

3.   To obtain a comprehensive evaluation of the child's individual vulnerabilities (e.g., social-cognitive style) and important aspects of his or her environmental context (e.g., parental socialization practices) that may have contributed to the development of conduct disorders and should be targeted in treatment

It is evident from these goals that, because of the complex and pervasive nature of conduct disorders, clinical assessments often involve assessing many aspects of the child's functioning and many aspects of his or her psychosocial environment.

To add to the complexity of the assessment process, each domain assessed should be assessed using multiple informants (e.g., parent, child, and teacher) and using multiple assessment modalities (e.g., rating scales, structured interviews). The need for a multi-informant and multimethod assessment process is dictated by the fact that any single source of information is limited and imperfect. For example, behavior rating scales often provide very reliable information on the presence and severity of conduct problems and often provide some of the best information on how a child's behavior compares with the behavior of other children. However,

Table 2. Major Findings from Research and Their Implications for Assessment of Conduct Disorders

Research findings	General goal	Specific goals
1. Conduct disorders represent a heterogeneous category with many important subtypes	1. Assess the type and severity of conduct problem behaviors and other psychological dimensions related to important subtypes	1a. Assess wide range of conduct problem behaviors 1b. Assess other factors related to subtypes, such as the presence of callous and unemotional features 1c. Assess developmental progressions of conduct problems and the timing of onset of conduct problem behaviors
2. Conduct disorders are often accompanied by several co-morbid types of problems that can influence the manifestation of conduct disorders	2. Assess multiple aspects of child's emotional and behavioral functioning	2a. Assess for the presence of ADHD 2b. Assess for the presence of anxiety and depression 2c. If depression is present, assess suicidal ideation
3. The development of conduct disorders is the result of an interaction of numerous factors within the child and within his or her psychosocial environment	3. Obtain a comprehensive evaluation of the child's individual vulnerabilities and aspects of his or her environmental context that may have contributed to the development of the conduct disorder and should be targeted in treatment	3a. Assess child's intellectual level and level of academic achievement 3b. Assess child's cognitive/attributional style in interpersonal situations 3c. Assess important aspects of child's family environment (see Table 1) 3d. Assess important aspects of child's social ecology (e.g., living conditions) 3e. Assess peer relations and association with deviant peer group

Note: Adapted from Frick and O'Brien (1995).

they often do not provide information on other important parameters of a child's behavior, such as the duration and onset of the problem behaviors or the developmental progression of problem behaviors.

Similarly, any single informant, whether providing information on a rating scale or clinical interview, will also be imperfect. There is a large body of evidence that a child's behavior, both problematic and normal, varies from setting to setting (see Achenbach, McConaughy, & Howell, 1987). Therefore, information from various people who see the child in different settings is necessary to obtain a complete picture of the child's behavioral functioning. Second, self-re-

ports from the child and reports from others are *perceptions* of a child's behavior. These perceptions can be influenced by a number of factors, such as the mood and motivations of the informant. Third, some behaviors are evident only in certain settings or to certain people. For example, the child's display of covert conduct problems (e.g., stealing, lying, substance use) may not be apparent to a parent or teacher and can only be reported by the child.

Given the imperfection inherent in any one source and method of obtaining information, a combination of sources and methods is the only way to obtain the assessment information needed to accomplish the goals outlined in Table 2. In subsequent sections, the primary methods for obtaining this information are discussed. Although several examples of specific instruments are provided, an exhaustive summary of the available techniques is beyond the scope of this chapter (see Kamphaus & Frick, 1996).

Behavior Rating Scales

Behavior rating scales have several important characteristics that make them indispensable to the assessment process. First, they allow for the collection of information in a reliable and time-efficient format. Second, many rating scales have forms for parents, teachers, and children, so that analogous information on a child's functioning can be obtained from multiple informants. Third, many behavior rating scales allow for a comparison of a child's score on a rating scale with the scores of a large representative sample of children. This information allows one to compare the degree and severity of a child's behavior with those of a normative group. Fourth, rating scales often assess many aspects of a child's emotional and behavioral functioning, thereby aiding in the assessment of potential comorbid problems. Fifth, many rating scales assess important contextual factors that could be related to a child's problem behaviors, such as peer relationships and family functioning. How well a specific rating scale accomplishes each of these five objectives varies considerably. These five criteria provide a good basis for evaluating individual scales for use in the assessment of conduct disorders.

One example of a comprehensive behavior rating scale that seems to do well when evaluated against these five criteria is the Behavior Assessment System for Children (BASC; Reynolds & Kamphaus, 1992). The BASC is an objective behavior rating that has proven to be highly reliable. It has analogous forms to be completed by parents, teachers, and the child. Further, the BASC was standardized on a large representative nationwide sample of children, which al-

lows one to compare a child's score to a normative group. The BASC covers many dimensions of a child's emotional and behavioral functioning, including two scales that assess both overt (Aggression Scale) and covert (Conduct Problems Scale) types of conduct problems, as well as scales assessing many of the more common comorbid conditions (ADHD, anxiety, and depression). Also, the BASC provides a screener for learning problems on the parent and teacher forms and assesses a preference for sensation-seeking behavior on the child's self-report form. The self-report version of the BASC assesses a child's attitudes toward school and teachers and the child's perceptions of his or her relations with parents, thereby providing information on important dimensions of a child's individual vulnerabilities and his or her psychosocial context.

Clinical Interviews

Like behavior rating scales, clinical interviews can be used to assess for the presence and severity of emotional and behavior problems, including conduct problems and the many common comorbidities, using multiple informants. However, there are several important pieces of information that are more readily obtained in an interview format. First, interviews can assess for the duration and age of onset of problem behaviors, two parameters that are crucial in the assessment of conduct problems. Second, interviews can provide information on the temporal relationship of behaviors, so that one can understand the developmental progression of problem behaviors. Third, interviews allow for an assessment of the degree of impairment (e.g., impairments in social and academic functioning) associated with a child's conduct disturbance.

One criticism of unstructured clinical interviews that allow the assessor to determine the method of obtaining information (e.g., what questions to ask, how to word the questions) has been their unreliability. In response to this criticism, a number of structured interview schedules were developed that provide the assessor with a standard format for obtaining information and with specific rules for rating the information obtained. The length and content of these interview schedules differ, as do the availability of analogous forms to obtain information from different informants. Most of the interview schedules were designed to correspond to the DSM system of classification. For example, the National Institute of Mental Health Diagnostic Interview Schedule for Children (DISC; Shaffer, Fisher, Piacentini, Schwab-Stone, & Wicks, 1992) has been continually updated to correspond to changes in the DSM system.

Behavioral Observations

Another method for assessing a child's behavioral and emotional functioning is by directly observing his or her behavior, either in naturalistic settings (e.g., home or school) or in an analogue setting (e.g., clinic). There are several observational systems available that define specific target behaviors to be observed, define the situations in which the behavior is to be observed, define the observational method (e.g., frequency counts of behavior), and establish training procedures for the observers. These observational systems make many unique contributions to the assessment process. First, they allow for an assessment of a child's behavior that is not "filtered" through the perceptions of an informant. Second, observational systems allow for an assessment of the environmental context of a child's behavior, such as assessing the antecedents and consequences of a child's conduct problem behavior or assessing a parent's response to the child's behavior.

For example, Patterson and colleagues (Patterson et al., 1992) developed a direct observational system to assess children's conduct problems in the home and to assess the interactional patterns in which the conduct problems are often embedded. The Family Interaction Coding System (FICS) is composed of 29 code categories that include both child behaviors and the response of others to this behavior. The FICS was designed to have data coded continuously and to provide a sequential account of the interactions between a child and other family members.

Unfortunately, behavioral observation systems, like the FICS also, have several limitations that have prevented their widespread use in the assessment of conduct problems. First, conducting behavioral observations is time-consuming and costly, making it impossible in many research and clinical settings. Second, designing observational situations with ecological validity is difficult, either because the observational situations are so artificial that they do not actually mirror a child's typical environmental context or because the process of observation leads to changes in a child's behavior or the behavior of others in his or her environment. Third, many types of conduct problems are difficult to assess through observations, either because of their covert nature (e.g., lying and stealing) or because of their infrequent occurrence (e.g., fighting).

Other Aspects of a Comprehensive Assessment

Given the association between conduct problems, intellectual deficits, and learning disabilities, a psychoeducational evaluation that includes a standardized intelligence test and an academic achievement screening should be a part of most evaluations of children with conduct problems. Also, each of the areas of family dysfunction that research has consistently linked to conduct disorders (see Table 1) should be assessed to understand the context in which the conduct disorder may have developed and to document potential targets of intervention. Finally, because peer rejection is predictive of the development of conduct problems and is associated with an adolescent's association with a deviant peer group, assessing a child's peer relationships is a critical assessment goal.

TREATMENT

A General Framework for Treatment

As was the case for assessment, treatment approaches should be driven by our knowledge of the basic nature and causes of conduct disorders. As Dodge (1993) pointed out, "short term symptom relief (for conduct disorders) is possible through theory-guided environmental interventions" (p. 311). In this section, two such theory-driven approaches to treating conduct disorders are discussed, one that is based on changing several family contextual factors believed to be involved in the development of conduct disorders and another focusing on changing the cognitive biases and problem-solving deficits exhibited by children with conduct disorders.

Unfortunately, even the most promising approaches to intervention, such as the ones reviewed in this chapter, have generally showed only modest long-term effects (Kazdin, 1993). This is likely related to the fact that most past treatment efforts have focused on changing a single type of causal factor. This ignores the heterogeneity of children with conduct disorders, many with different causal factors leading to the development of conduct disorders, and it ignores the multiply determined nature of conduct problems. Also, conduct problems seem to be most changeable when the child is young and early in the developmental sequence of conduct problem behaviors (Kazdin, 1987, 1993). As a result, treatment of conduct disorders is most likely to advance if (1) treatments target multiple factors leading to a child's conduct problem behavior, (2) treatments are flexible enough to encompass the variability in the needs of the individual child, and (3) treatments are prevention-oriented in which high-risk children are treated prior to their advance into more severe and stable forms of antisocial behavior (Dodge, 1993). Therefore, this section on treatment concludes with a description of a "state-of-the-art" treatment model that addresses each of these three crucial factors.

Parent Management Training

Parent Management Training (PMT) refers to a set of interventions in which parents are taught methods of interacting with their children in ways that enhance their children's functioning. Most PMT approaches were designed to target parenting skills that are critical to the socialization of the child. They focus on parents being more involved with their child, using positive contingencies to increase prosocial child behaviors, using consistent noncorporal discipline to reduce conduct problems, and being better able to monitor their child's behavior. These are all aspects of family functioning that research has consistently linked to the development of conduct disorders (see Table 1 and Loeber & Stouthamer-Loeber, 1986). There are numerous PMT treatment packages available for use with children (e.g., Forehand & McMahon, 1981) and adolescents (e.g., Patterson & Forgatch, 1987) and most of these can be used in both individual and group formats.

There seem to be several critical considerations in implementing a successful PMT program for families of children with conduct disorders. First, the intervention must help the parent to learn methods of *both* increasing their child's positive behaviors and decreasing their child's negative behaviors. Second, teaching the parents general social learning principles, in addition to specific child management techniques, appears to enhance treatment effectiveness (McMahon, Forehand, & Griest, 1981). Third, involving both parents when possible seems to be critical in enhancing treatment effectiveness, especially in maintaining treatment effects over time (Webster-Stratton, 1985). Fourth, PMT interventions can be enhanced by including long-term follow-up sessions, often termed *booster sessions,* in which families are seen periodically on a long-term basis and the PMT interventions are reviewed and modified as needed (Kazdin, 1987).

In comparing PMT interventions to other interventions for conduct disorders, PMT may be one of the most effective approaches (Kazdin, 1987, 1993). Outcome research has consistently shown that (1) PMT programs lead to significant changes in child behavior when compared with control groups, (2) PMT approaches generally are more effective than other approaches to treatment, (3) PMT often brings the behavior of the treated children into a normative range, (4) changes brought about by PMT tend to generalize to multiple children in a family, and (5) the changes last from 1 to 5 years following treatment (Kazdin, 1987, 1993). Unfortunately, these positive treatment outcomes, although clearly surpassing most other types of intervention, must be placed in a realistic context. The most favorable outcomes are generally found for younger children (8 and under) who exhibit mild conduct problems (oppositional, noncompliant, and mild aggressive behaviors), and who come from families without severe dysfunction (e.g., without economic disadvantage, severe parental psychopathology, high levels of marital conflict, or low levels of social support).

Given the several limitations to the effectiveness of PMT programs, Miller and Prinz (1990) recommended expanding the skills taught to parents beyond those included in most PMT programs. For example, teaching parents conflict-resolution skills (e.g., expressing feelings, reflective listening, and negotiation) and self-control strategies (e.g., goal setting, self-monitoring, and self-reinforcement) could increase the maintenance of newly acquired parenting skills. These authors also highlight the need to incorporate into the PMT model a more broad-based approach to family intervention by intervening into areas of family functioning that transcend parenting behaviors. For example, directly intervening into areas of parental psychiatric adjustment (e.g., depression, substance abuse), marital discord, and extrafamilial stressors (e.g., unemployment, lack of social support) may be required if PMT interventions are to be more successful.

Cognitive Problem-Solving Training

Although PMT seems to be a critical component to the treatment of conduct disorders, for some children in certain settings (e.g., in residential treatment centers, in very dysfunctional families) the parents are either unwilling or unable to participate in PMT. This has led to a continuing search for effective treatment modalities that do not require family participation. Cognitive Problem-solving Training (CPT) is one promising child-focused approach. It is based on the assumption that aggressive and hostile behaviors are the result of cognitive and attributional biases that a child uses in social situations (see section entitled "Deficits in Social Cognition"). CPT programs are designed to teach children ways to modify these biases (e.g., Kazdin, Esveldt-Dawson, French, & Unis, 1987; Lochman & Curry, 1986). Children are taught to (1) recognize problem situations, (2) use self-statements to reduce impulsive responses, (3) generate multiple solutions to problems, (4) evaluate possible consequences of actions, and (5) take the perspective of others. These skills are taught using either a group (Lochman & Curry, 1986) or an individual (Kazdin et al., 1987) format.

The outcome research on the use of CPT for children with conduct disorders suggests that it is a promising approach to treatment because (1) it has had positive effects on child adjustment relative to control groups and to alternative treatments and (2) its effects have been durable at up to 1-year follow-up. Unfortunately, these studies also found that CPT did not typically change a child's behavior sufficiently to bring the level of functioning into a normative range. For example, Kazdin et al. (1987) documented the superiority of their individually administered CPT in treating antisocial children on a psychiatric inpatient unit, in comparison with antisocial children receiving relationship therapy and a treatment-contact control group. Immediately following treatment, however, only 17.6% of the children receiving CPT had scores on rating scales that were below what is typically considered clinically deviant.

The Family and Schools Together Program

The Family and Schools Together Program (FAST Track Program) is a multisite collaborative program supported by the National Institute of Mental Health (Conduct Problems Prevention Research Group, 1992). This program was designed to provide a comprehensive intervention to young children (kindergarten) who show disruptive behavior and poor peer relations both at home and at school. The FAST Track program was designed to be "multi-faceted, involving multiple agents who have an impact on child socialization (i.e., parents, teachers, and peers), and to be cross-situational, targeting improvements in home and school contexts and augmenting the synchrony between the two contexts" (Conduct Problems Prevention Research Group, 1992, p. 515).

The FAST Track Program involves five component interventions. The first component is a 22-session *PMT program* that is conducted in a group format. In addition to the typical focus on parenting skills and positive parent–child interactions found in most PMT programs, the FAST Track PMT Program also focuses on ways in which parents can foster their children's learning and develop positive family–school relationships. This PMT program is supplemented by *home visits* in which parents are aided in applying the concepts learned in PMT to their individual family context. The home visits also provide a context for the parents to learn problem-solving skills and to enhance family organization. The third component is a *cognitive problem-solving training* program designed to improve a child's social problem-solving ability and to develop other social skills necessary to make and maintain friendships. The fourth component focuses on *academic tutoring* in reading skills. The fifth component is a *classroom intervention* in which the child's teacher is taught effective management of disruptive behavior in the classroom and taught to implement a curriculum that teaches children how to control their anger, to communicate more effectively, to develop friendships, and to use effective problem-solving strategies.

Each component of the FAST Track Program has been tested individually and has proven to have some moderate level of success. The important aspect of this program, however, is its attempt to target multiple risk factors in a comprehensive and coordinated intervention program. There are no data available yet on the effectiveness of the program and its most crucial test will be its long-term effectiveness, as this is where the individual components have generally fallen short. However, this program illustrates the several important aspects in the treatment of conduct disorders that were outlined previously. It attempts to intervene with children early in their development of conduct problem behavior and it intervenes on multiple levels in a variety of settings. Each component of the intervention is also based on a sound theoretical model in which processes believed to be critical to the development of conduct problems are targeted for change. This prevention-oriented, comprehensive, theory-driven approach to the treatment of conduct disorders serves as an excellent model for future intervention efforts to follow.

CASE STUDY

Many of the basic characteristics of conduct disorders, the interplay of multiple etiological factors, and several issues in the clinical management of conduct disorders can be found in the following case study. Patrick was 15 years old when his mother requested a comprehensive psychological evaluation from a university-based outpatient psychological clinic. She was concerned about Patrick's poor grades in school and his frequent lying, and also expressed concerns about his frequent fights both at school and in his neighborhood.

A history provided by Patrick's mother indicated that Patrick was initially seen at a community mental health center at age 8 because of behavior problems, which included being very oppositional and defiant both at home and at school, and being involved in several physical fights. In addition to these conduct problems, Patrick displayed many symptoms of an attention-deficit disorder and was started on a trial of stimulant medication. The medication seemed to be effective but his parents discontinued it after about 8 months because his father lost his job and they "could no longer afford the medication."

At age 8, Patrick was also seen in individual therapy at the community mental health center with the goal of helping him to cope with his parent's ongoing marital conflict. They had separated three times, and frequently had very heated arguments that were witnessed by Patrick. They subsequently divorced when Patrick was 11, following his father's arrest for selling drugs. Patrick remained in individual therapy for only three sessions. No other mental health treatment had been sought until the current referral, although Patrick had been suspended an average of two times a year for fighting and had once been brought to juvenile court (at age 11) for shoplifting.

The assessment at age 15, using a combination of behavior rating scales and a structured clinical interview, revealed the presence of numerous severe conduct problems. Both Patrick and his mother reported that Patrick had engaged in repeated instances of lying, repeated instances of stealing items from other family members and stores, and numerous physical fights. His mother also reported several instances of truancy and Patrick admitted to breaking into a neighbor's house to steal things, to vandalizing several buildings, and to using a knife in a fight. Patrick further admitted to occasional use of marijuana. Also, both Patrick and his mother reported that Patrick experiences frequent periods of depression, often lasting for as long as a month. At the time of the assessment, Patrick had been experiencing significant periods of sadness over the past 3 weeks. Patrick reported that he had twice in the past 2 years thought of killing himself by cutting his wrist and on one occasion had actually started to use a knife but was reportedly "stopped by a classmate." Both Patrick and his mother reported that the episodes of depression seemed to coincide with disciplinary confrontations, such as being grounded for a school suspension.

A psychoeducational assessment at age 15 also revealed that Patrick was functioning in the "low average" range of intellectual abilities and he scored in a range commensurate with this intellectual level on an academic achievement screener. However, Patrick expressed no intention of remaining in school after age 16 when schooling was no longer compulsory. In a clinical interview, his mother reported that she had great difficulty monitoring and supervising Patrick and she often did not know where he was and when he would be home. Patrick's behavior was reportedly a source of frequent arguments between his mother and stepfather. His mother had remarried when Patrick was 14 years old.

As a result of the assessment, Patrick's family started attending family therapy sessions in which components of the PMT programs described previously were implemented. The family also participated in a case manager program at the local community mental health center, in which a team of case managers made periodic home visits to help the family implement the behavior management techniques discussed in family therapy and to help improve family communication patterns and problem-solving skills. Patrick was also seen in individual therapy that focused on a cognitive problem-solving approach to dealing with interpersonal situations. Patrick was very uncomfortable in social situations and tended to be easily angered, which led to many of his fights. Also in individual therapy, Patrick's depression and suicide ideation was continuously monitored and issues involving his lack of contact with his biological father were also discussed. Patrick's individual therapist also consulted with his teacher on developing effective behavior management strategies in the classroom and on developing ways of motivating Patrick to complete work. Patrick started in an intensive vocational training program that involved work at a local community college one afternoon each week, where he was trained to work on computer hardware.

SUMMARY

Conduct disorders represent a serious form of child psychopathology that operates at high cost to society. Although there has been a substantial amount of research conducted on conduct disorders in children, the complex nature of the disturbance has led to little consensus on how to interpret this large body of research. The first aspect of this complex nature is the fact that children with conduct disorders represent a very heterogeneous group. Children with conduct disorders vary greatly as to type, severity, and course of their conduct disturbance. Therefore, a substantial portion of this chapter focused on various methods of defining or classifying more homogeneous groups of children with conduct disorders. This issue of classifying more homogeneous groups of children with conduct disorders pervades all aspects of understanding and treating the disorder. For example, the importance of different causal factors seems to vary across subgroups of children with conduct disorders and, therefore, the specific focus of treatment also must vary across subgroups.

The second aspect of the complex nature of conduct disorders is that, even within more homogeneous subgroups of children with conduct problems, the development of conduct disorders is a result of a complex interaction of multiple causal factors operating at many different levels. In this chapter, there was a focus on several types of dispositional variables that seem to place a child at risk for developing conduct problems, as well as numerous factors within a child's social ecology that seem to promote and/or maintain antisocial behavior. Theories on the development of conduct disorders must not only identify which causal factors seem to be important for certain children with conduct disorders but also specify how these factors interact to lead to the development of conduct problem behavior.

This multiply determined nature of conduct disorders also is important for guiding the treatment of conduct disorders. Several types of treatments have focused on changing specific causal factors that are theoretically important in explaining the development of conduct problems, such as enhancing family functioning and enhancing a child's social problem-solving skills. However, even the most promising of these approaches to treatment have shown only short-term improvements in some children. To be effective for a greater number of children with conduct disorders and to show a more sustained effect on a child's behavior, interventions need to recognize the multiply determined nature of conduct disorders. In this chapter, an intervention model that intervenes early in a child's development of conduct problems and intervenes on multiple levels and in multiple contexts in a coherent and integrated treatment approach was described. This type of prevention-oriented and comprehensive approach to intervention seems to have the greatest chance of success in bringing about long-term changes in children's conduct problem behavior. As a result, the old maxim seems to hold true for the treatment of conduct disorders: complex problems require complex solutions.

REFERENCES

Abikoff, H., & Klein, R. G. (1992). Attention-deficit hyperactivity and conduct disorder: Co-morbidity and implications for treatment. *Journal of Consulting and Clinical Psychology, 60,* 881–892.

Achenbach, T. M., McConaughy, S. H., & Howell, C. T. (1987). Child/adolescent behavioral and emotional problems: Implications of cross-informant correlations for situational specificity. *Psychological Bulletin, 101,* 213–232.

Amato, P. R., & Keith, B. (1991). Parental divorce and the well-being of children: A meta-analysis. *Psychological Bulletin, 110,* 26–46.

American Psychiatric Association. (1980). *The diagnostic and statistical manual of mental disorders* (3rd ed.). Washington, DC: Author.

American Psychiatric Association. (1987). *The diagnostic and statistical manual of mental disorders* (3rd ed. rev.). Washington, DC: Author.

American Psychiatric Association. (1994). *The diagnostic and statistical manual of mental disorders* (4th ed.). Washington, DC: Author.

Anderson, J. C., Williams, S., McGee, R., & Silva, P. A. (1987). DSM-III disorders in preadolescent children. *Archives of General Psychiatry, 44,* 69–76.

Asarnow, J., & Callan, J. (1985). Boys with peer adjustment problems: Social cognitive processes. *Journal of Consulting and Clinical Psychology, 53,* 80–87.

Bell, R. Q. (1968). A reinterpretation of the direction of effects in studies of socialization. *Psychological Review, 75,* 81–95.

Capaldi, D. M. (1992). Co-occurrence of conduct problems and depressive symptoms in early adolescent boys: II. A 2-year follow-up at Grade 8. *Development and Psychopathology, 4,* 125–144.

Christian, R. E., Frick, P. J., Hill, N. J., Tyler, L., & Frazer, D. (1997). Psychopathy and conduct problems in children: II. Subtyping children with conduct problems based on their interpersonal and affective style. *Journal of the American Academy of Child and Adolescent Psychiatry, 36,* 233–241.

Conduct Problems Prevention Research Group. (1992). A developmental and clinical model for the prevention of conduct disorder: The FAST Track Program. *Development and Psychopathology, 4,* 509–527.

Constantino, J. N., Grosz, D., Saenger, P., Chandler, D. W., Nandi, R., & Earls, F. J. (1993). Testosterone and aggression in children. *Journal of the American Academy of Child and Adolescent Psychiatry, 32,* 1217–1222.

Costello, E. J., Costello, A. J., Edelbrock, C., Burns, B. J., Dulcan, M. K., Brent, D., & Janiszewski, S. (1988). Psychiatric disorders in pediatric primary care. *Archives of General Psychiatry, 45,* 1107–1116.

Daugherty, T. K., & Quay, H. C. (1991). Response perseveration and delayed responding in childhood behavior disorders. *Journal of Child Psychology and Psychiatry, 32,* 453–461.

Delamater, A. M., & Lahey, B. B. (1983). Physiological correlates of conduct problems in hyperactive and learning disabled children. *Journal of Abnormal Child Psychology, 11,* 85–100.

Dodge, K. A. (1993). The future of research on the treatment of conduct disorder. *Development and Psychopathology, 5,* 311–320.

Dodge, K. A., Bates, J. E., & Pettit, G. S. (1990). Mechanisms in the cycle of violence. *Science, 250,* 1678–1683.

Dodge, K. A., & Frame, C. L. (1982). Social cognitive biases and deficits in aggressive boys. *Child Development, 53,* 620–635.

Dodge, K. A., Murphy, R. R., & Buchsbaum, K. (1984). The assessment of intention–cue detection skills in children: Implications for developmental psychopathology. *Child Development, 55,* 163–173.

Downey, G., & Coyne, J. C. (1990). Children of depressed parents: An integrated review. *Psychological Bulletin, 108,* 50–76.

Emler, N., Reicher, S., & Ross, A. (1987). The social context of delinquent context. *Journal of Child Psychology and Psychiatry, 28,* 99–109.

Faraone, S. V., Biederman, J., Keenan, K., & Tsuang, M. T. (1991). Separation of DSM-III attention deficit disorder and conduct disorder: Evidence from a family genetic study of American child psychiatry patients. *Psychological Medicine, 21,* 109–121.

Farrington, D. P. (1991). Childhood aggression and adult violence: Early precursors and later-life outcomes. In D. J. Pepler & K. H. Rubin (Eds.), *The development and treatment of childhood aggression* (pp. 5–29). Hillsdale, NJ: Erlbaum.

Forehand, R., Lautenschlager, G. J., Faust, J., & Graziano, W. G. (1986). Parent perceptions and parent–child interactions in clinic-referred children: A preliminary investigation of the effects of maternal depressive moods. *Behavioral Research and Theory, 24,* 73–75.

Forehand, R., & McMahon, R. J. (1981). *Helping the noncompliant child: A clinician's guide to parent training.* New York: Guilford Press.

Frick, P. J. (1993). Childhood conduct problems in a family context. *School Psychology Review, 22,* 376–385.

Frick, P. J., & Jackson, Y. K. (1993). Family functioning and childhood antisocial behavior: Yet another reinterpretation. *Journal of Clinical Child Psychology, 22,* 410–419.

Frick, P. J., Kamphaus, R. W., Lahey, B. B., Loeber, R., Christ, M. A. G., Hart, E. L., & Tannenbaum, L. E. (1991). Academic underachievement and the disruptive behavior disorders. *Journal of Consulting and Clinical Psychology, 59,* 289–294.

Frick, P. J., Lahey, B. B., Hartdagen, S., & Hynd, G. W. (1989). Conduct problems in boys: Relations to maternal personality, marital satisfaction, and socioeconomic status. *Journal of Clinical Child Psychology, 18,* 114–120.

Frick, P. J., Lahey, B. B., Loeber, R., Stouthamer-Loeber, M., Christ, M. A. G., & Hanson, K. (1992). Familial risk factors to oppositional defiant disorder and conduct disorder: Parental psychopathology and maternal parenting. *Journal of Consulting and Clinical Psychology, 60,* 49–55.

Frick, P. J., Lahey, B. B., Loeber, R., Tannenbaum, L. E., Van Horn, Y., Christ, M. A. G., Hart, E. L., & Hanson, K. (1993). Oppositional defiant disorder and conduct disorder: A meta-analytic review of factor analyses and cross-validation in a clinic sample. *Clinical Psychology Review, 13* 319–340.

Frick, P. J., & O'Brien, B. S. (1995). Conduct disorders. In R. T. Ammerman & M. Hersen (Eds.), *Handbook of child behavior therapy in the psychiatric setting* (pp. 199–216). New York: Wiley.

Frick, P. J., O'Brien, B. S., Wootton, J. M., & McBurnett, K. (1994). Psychopathy and conduct problems in children. *Journal of Abnormal Psychology, 103,* 700–707.

Gerralda, M. E., Connell, J., & Taylor, D. C. (1991). Psychophysiological anomalies in children with emotional and conduct disorders. *Psychological Medicine, 21,* 947–957.

Ghodsian-Carpey, J., & Baker, L. A. (1987). Genetic and environmental influences on aggression in 4- to 7-year old twins. *Aggressive Behavior, 13,* 173–186.

Harrington, R., Fudge, H., Rutter, M., Pickles, A., & Hill, J. (1991). Adult outcomes of childhood and adolescent depression: II. Links with antisocial disorders. *Journal of the American Academy of Child and Adolescent Psychiatry, 30,* 434–439.

Hetherington, E. M. (1991). Role of individual differences and family relationships in children's coping with divorce and remarriage. In P. A. Cowan & E. M. Hetherington (Eds.), *Family transitions* (pp. 165–197). Hillsdale, NJ: Erlbaum.

Hinshaw, S. P. (1992). Externalizing behavior problems and academic underachievement in childhood and adolescence: Causal relationships and underlying mechanisms. *Psychological Bulletin, 111,* 127–155.

Hinshaw, S. P., Lahey, B. B., & Hart, E. L. (1993). Issues of taxonomy and co-morbidity in the development of conduct disorder. *Development and Psychopathology, 5,* 31–50.

Jarey, M. L., & Stewart, M. A. (1985). Psychiatric disorder in the parents of adopted children with aggressive conduct disorder. *Neuropsychobiology, 13,* 7–11.

Kamphaus, R. W., & Frick, P. J. (1996). *The clinical assessment of children's emotion, behavior, and personality.* Boston: Allyn & Bacon.

Kazdin, A. E. (1987). Treatment of antisocial behavior in children: Current status and future directions. *Psychological Bulletin, 102,* 187–203.

Kazdin, A. E. (1993). Treatment of conduct disorder: Progress and directions in psychotherapy research. *Development and Psychopathology, 5,* 277–310.

Kazdin, A. E., Esveldt-Dawson, K., French, N. H., & Unis, A. S. (1987). Problem-solving skills training and relationship therapy in the treatment of antisocial child behavior. *Journal of Consulting and Clinical Psychology, 55,* 76–85.

Keenan, K., Loeber, R., Zhang, Q., Stouthamer-Loeber, M., & van Kammen, W. B. (1995). The influence of deviant peers on the development of boys' disruptive and delinquent behavior: A temporal analysis. *Development and Psychopathology, 7,* 715–726.

Kreusi, M. J. P., Rapoport, J. L., Hamburger, S., Hibbs, E., Potter, W. Z., Lenane, M., & Brown, G. L. (1990). Cerebrospinal fluid monamine metabolites, aggression, and impulsivity in disruptive behavior disorders of children and adolescents. *Archives of General Psychiatry, 47,* 419–426.

Lahey, B. B., Applegate, B., Barkley, R. A., Garfinkel, B., McBurnett, K., Kerdyk, L., Greenhill, L., Hynd, G. W., Frick, P. J., Newcorn, J., Biederman, J., Ollendick, T., Hart, E. L., Perez, D., Waldman, I., & Shaffer, D. (1994). DSM-IV field trials for oppositional defiant disorder and conduct disorder in children and adolescents. *American Journal of Psychiatry, 151,* 1163–1171.

Lahey, B. B., Hart, E. L., Pliszka, S., Applegate, B., & McBurnett, K. (1993). Neurophysiological correlates of conduct disorder: A rationale and a review of research. *Journal of Clinical Child Psychology, 22,* 141–153.

Lahey, B. B., & Loeber, R. (1994). Framework for a developmental model of oppositional defiant disorder and conduct disorder. In D. K. Routh (Ed.), *Disruptive behavior disorders in childhood* (pp. 139–180). New York: Plenum Press.

Lahey, B. B., Loeber, R., Hart, E. L., Frick, P. J., Applegate, B.

Zhang, Q., Green, S. M., & Russo, M. F. (1995). Four-year longitudinal study of conduct disorder in boys: Patterns of predictors of persistence. *Journal of Abnormal Psychology, 104,* 83–93.

Larzelere, R. E., & Patterson, G. R. (1990). Parental management: Mediator of the effect of socioeconomic status on early delinquency. *Criminology, 18,* 301–323.

Laub, J. H., & Sampson, R. J. (1988). Unraveling families and delinquency: A reanalysis of the Gluecks' data. *Criminology, 26,* 355–380.

Lochman, J. E. (1987). Self and peer perceptions and attributional biases of aggressive and non-aggressive boys in dyadic interactions. *Journal of Consulting and Clinical Psychology, 55,* 404–410.

Lochman, J. E., & Curry, J. F. (1986). Effects of social problem-solving training and self-instruction training with aggressive boys. *Journal of Clinical Child Psychology, 15,* 159–164.

Loeber, R. (1991). Antisocial behavior: More enduring than changeable? *Journal of the American Academy of Child and Adolescent Psychiatry, 30,* 393–397.

Loeber, R., Green, S. M., Lahey, B. B., Christ, M. A. G., & Frick, P. J. (1992). Developmental sequences in the age of onset of disruptive child behaviors. *Journal of Child and Family Studies, 1,* 21–41.

Loeber, R., & Stouthamer-Loeber, M. (1986). Family factors as correlates and predictors of juvenile conduct problems and delinquency. In M. Tonry & N. Morris (Eds.), *Crime and justice* (Vol. 7, pp. 29–149). Chicago: University of Chicago Press.

Lytton, H. (1990). Child and parent effects in boys' conduct disorder: A reinterpretation. *Developmental Psychology, 26,* 683–697.

Magnusson, D. (1988). Aggressiveness, hyperactivity, and autonomic activity/reactivity in the development of social maladjustment. In D. Magnusson (Ed.), *Individual development from an interactional perspective: A longitudinal study* (pp. 153–172). Hillsdale, NJ: Erlbaum.

Mason, D. A., & Frick, P. J. (1994). The heritability of antisocial behavior: A meta-analysis of twin and adoption studies. *Journal of Psychopathology and Behavioral Assessment, 16,* 301–323.

McCord, J. (1991). The cycle of crime and socialization practices. *The Journal of Criminal Law and Criminality, 82,* 211–228.

McMahon, R. J., Forehand, R., & Griest, D. L. (1981). Effects of knowledge of social learning principles on enhancing treatment outcome and generalization in a parent training program. *Journal of Consulting and Clinical Psychology, 49,* 526–532.

Miller, G. E., & Prinz, R. J. (1990). Enhancement of social learning family interventions for childhood conduct disorder. *Psychological Bulletin, 108,* 291–307.

Moffitt, T. E. (1993a). Adolescence-limited and life-course persistent antisocial behavior: A developmental taxonomy. *Psychological Review, 100,* 674–701.

Moffitt, T. E. (1993b). The neuropsychology of conduct disorder. *Development and Psychopathology, 5,* 135–152.

Newman, J. P., & Wallace, J. F. (1993). Diverse pathways to deficient self-regulation: Implications for disinhibitory psychopathology in children. *Clinical Psychology Review, 13,* 699–720.

O'Brien, B. S., & Frick, P. J. (1996). Reward dominance: Associations with anxiety, conduct problems, and psychopathy in children. *Journal of Abnormal Child Psychology, 24,* 223–240.

O'Brien, B. S., Frick, P. J., & Lyman, R. D. (1994). Reward dominance among children with disruptive behavior disorders. *Journal of Psychopathology and Behavioral Assessment, 16,* 131–145.

Offord, D. R., Boyle, M. H., Szatmari, P., Rae-Grant, N. I., Links, P. S., Cadman, D. T., Byles, J. A., Crawford, J. W., Blum, H. M., Byrne, C., Thomas, H., & Woodward, C. A. (1987). Ontario Child Health Study: II. Six-month prevalence of disorder and rates of service utilization. *Archives of General Psychiatry, 44,* 832–836.

Olweus, D., Mattesson, A., Schalling, D., & Low, H. (1988). Circulating testosterone levels and aggression in adolescent males: A causal analysis. *Psychosomatic Medicine, 50,* 261–272.

Panak, W. F., & Garber, J. (1992). Role of aggression, rejection, and attributions in the prediction of depression in children. *Development and Psychopathology, 4,* 145–166.

Patterson, G. R., & Forgatch, M. S. (1987). *Parents and adolescents living together.* Eugene, OR: Castalia.

Patterson, G. R., Reid, J. B., & Dishion, T. J. (1992). *Antisocial boys.* Eugene, OR: Castalia.

Peeples, F., & Loeber, R. (1994). Do individual factors and neighborhood context explain ethnic differences in juvenile delinquency? *Journal of Quantitative Criminology, 10,* 141–157.

Perry, D. G., Perry, L. C., & Rasmussen, P. (1986). Cognitive social learning mediators of aggression. *Child Development, 57,* 700–711.

Prinz, R. J., Connor, P. A., & Wilson, C. C. (1981). Hyperactive and aggressive behaviors in childhood: Intertwined dimensions. *Journal of Abnormal Child Psychology, 9,* 191–202.

Quay, H. C. (1986). Classification. In H. C. Quay & J. S. Werry (Eds.), *Psychopathological disorders of childhood* (3rd ed., pp. 1–42). New York: Wiley.

Quay, H. C. (1987). Patterns of delinquent behavior. In H. C. Quay (Ed.), *Handbook of juvenile delinquency* (pp. 118–138). New York: Wiley.

Quay, H. C. (1993). The psychobiology of undersocialized aggressive conduct disorder. *Development and Psychopathology, 5,* 165–180.

Raine, A. (1993). *The psychopathology of crime: Criminal behavior as a clinical disorder.* New York: Academic Press.

Raine, A., Venables, P. H., & Williams, M. (1990). Relationships between central and autonomic measures of arousal at age 15 and criminality at age 24 years. *Archives of General Psychiatry, 47,* 1003–1007.

Rey, J. M., Bashir, M. R., Schwarz, M., Richards, I. N., Plapp, J. M., & Stewart, G. W. (1988). Oppositional disorder: Fact or fiction? *Journal of the American Academy of Child and Adolescent Psychiatry, 27,* 157–162.

Reynolds, C. R., & Kamphaus, R. W. (1992). *The Behavior Assessment System for Children.* Circle Pines, MN: American Guidance Service.

Richters, J. E., & Cicchetti, D. (1993). Toward a developmental perspective on conduct disorder. *Development and Psychopathology, 5,* 1–4.

Robins, L. N. (1966). *Deviant children grown up: A sociological and psychiatric study of sociopathic personality.* Baltimore: Williams & Wilkins.

Robins, L. N., Tipp, J., & Pryzbeck, T. (1991). Antisocial personality. In L. N. Robins & D. A. Regier (Eds.), *Psychiatric disorders in America* (pp. 224–271). New York: Free Press.

Roff, J. D., & Wirt, R. D. (1984). Childhood aggression and social adjustments as antecedents of delinquency. *Journal of Abnormal Child Psychology, 12,* 111–126.

Russo, M. F., & Beidel, D. C. (1994). Co-morbidity of childhood anxiety and externalizing disorders: Prevalence, associated characteristics, and validation issues. *Clinical Psychology Review, 14,* 199–221.

Rutter, M., Macdonald, H., Le Couteur, A. Harrington, F. R., Bolton, P., & Abiley, A. (1990). Genetic factors in child psychiatric disorders: II. Empirical findings. *Journal of Child Psychology and Psychiatry, 31,* 39–83.

Scerbo, A., & Kolko, D. J. (1994). Salivary testosterone and cortisol in disruptive children: Relationship to aggressive, hyperactive, and internalizing behavior. *Journal of the American Academy of Child and Adolescent Psychiatry, 33,* 1174–1184.

Schmidt, K., Solanto, M. V., & Bridger, W. H. (1985). Electrodermal activity of undersocialized aggressive children. *Journal of Child Psychology and Psychiatry, 26,* 653–660.

Shaffer, D., Fisher, P., Piacentini, J., Schwab-Stone, M., & Wicks, J. (1992). *NIMH Diagnostic Interview Schedule for Children—Version 2.3.* New York State Psychiatric Institute.

Shapiro, S. K., Quay, H. C., Hogan, A. E., & Schwartz, K. P. (1988). Response perseveration and delayed responding in undersocialized aggressive conduct disorder. *Journal of Abnormal Psychology, 97,* 317–373.

Shaw, C. R., & McKay, H. D. (1972). *Juvenile delinquency and urban areas: A study of rates of delinquency in relation to differential characteristics of local communities in American cities.* Chicago: University of Chicago Press.

Stattin, H., & Magnusson, D. (1989). The role of early aggressive behavior in the frequency, seriousness, and types of later crime. *Journal of Consulting and Clinical Psychology, 57,* 710–718.

Stewart, M. A., Cummings, C., Singer, S., & deBlois, C. S. (1981). The overlap between hyperactive and unsocialized aggressive children. *Journal of Child Psychology and Psychiatry, 22,* 35–45.

Trites, R. L., & Laprade, K. (1983). Evidence of an independent syndrome of hyperactivity. *Journal of Child Psychology and Psychiatry, 24,* 573–586.

Wahler, R. G., & Sansbury, L. E. (1990). The monitoring skills of troubled mothers: Their problems in defining child deviance. *Journal of Abnormal Child Psychology, 18,* 577–589.

Walker, J. L., Lahey, B. B., Russo, M. F., Frick, P. J., Christ, M. A. G., McBurnett, K., Loeber, R., Stouthamer-Loeber, M., & Green, S. M. (1991). Anxiety, inhibition, and conduct disorder in children: I. Relations to social impairment. *Journal of the American Academy of Child and Adolescent Psychiatry, 30,* 187–191.

Webster-Stratton, C. (1985). The effects of father involvement in parent training for conduct problem children. *Journal of Child Psychology and Psychiatry, 26,* 801–810.

West, M. O., & Prinz, R. J. (1987). Parental alcoholism and childhood psychopathology. *Psychological Bulletin, 102,* 204–218.

Zigler, E., Taussig, C., & Black, K. (1992). Early childhood intervention: A promising preventative for juvenile delinquency. *American Psychologist, 47,* 997–1006.

Zoccolillo, M. (1992). Co-occurrence of conduct disorder and its adult outcomes with depressive and anxiety disorders: A review. *Journal of the American Academy of Child and Adolescent Psychiatry, 31,* 547–556.

Zoccolillo, M., Pickles, A., Quinton, D., & Rutter, M. (1992). The outcome of childhood conduct disorder: Implications for defining antisocial disorder and conduct disorder. *Psychological Medicine, 22,* 971–986.

9

Anxiety Disorders

WENDY K. SILVERMAN AND GOLDA S. GINSBURG

INTRODUCTION

Because children with externalizing disorders, such as those discussed in Chapters 7 and 8 in this volume, have a direct and disruptive effect on other individuals and institutions, these are the children who are most frequently referred to mental health clinics and who have been the primary focus of research attention. Consequently, conceptual and practical knowledge pertaining to children with internalizing problems, particularly anxiety, have lagged behind. However, research interest in anxiety in youth burgeoned with the establishment of the broad diagnostic category, Anxiety Disorders of Childhood and Adolescence, in the third edition of the Diagnostic and Statistical Manual (DSM-III; American Psychiatric Association, 1980).

In the latest edition of the DSM (DSM-IV; American Psychiatric Association, 1994), major changes were made in the classification of anxiety disorders in youth. Most significant was the elimination of the broad diagnostic category, i.e., Anxiety Disorders of Childhood and Adolescence. Within this diagnostic category, Avoidant Disorder (AVD) was eliminated and Overanxious Disorder was subsumed under the adult disorder Generalized Anxiety Disorder (GAD). The only childhood anxiety disorder that remained was Separation Anxiety Disorder (SAD), which was reclassified under the broad category Other Disorders of Childhood and Adolescence. The changes made in the classification of the so-called adult disorders were relatively minor, and were more cosmetic than substantive (e.g., Simple Phobia was renamed Specific Phobia). A summary of the classification of the anxiety disorders in DSM-III-R versus DSM-IV is presented in Table 1.

These disorders are the focus of this chapter. The chapter begins with a description of the phenomenology of anxiety disorders in children, followed by a discussion of differential diagnosis, etiology, and epidemiology. Assessment and treatment are covered next. An illustrative case concludes the chapter.

WENDY K. SILVERMAN • Child and Family Psychosocial Research Center, Department of Psychology, Florida International University, Miami, Florida 33199.   GOLDA S. GINSBURG • Division of Applied Psychology and Quantitative Methods, University of Baltimore, Baltimore, Maryland 21201.

Handbook of Child Psychopathology, 3rd edition, edited by Ollendick & Hersen. Plenum Press, New York, 1998.

Table 1. Classification of Anxiety Disorders in DSM-III-R and DSM-IV

DSM-III-R	DSM-IV
Anxiety Disorders of Childhood or Adolescence	Other Disorders of Infancy, Childhood, or Adolescence
Separation Anxiety Disorder	Separation Anxiety Disorder
Avoidant Disorder	
Overanxious Disorder	
Anxiety Disorders	Anxiety Disorders
Panic Disorder with Agoraphobia	Panic Disorder with Agoraphobia
Panic Disorder without Agoraphobia	Panic Disorder without Agoraphobia
	Agoraphobia without History of Panic Disorder
Simple Phobia	Specific Phobia
Social Phobia	Social Phobia (Social Anxiety Disorder)
Obsessive Compulsive Disorder	Obsessive-Compulsive Disorder
Post-traumatic Stress Disorders	Posttraumatic Stress Disorder
	Acute Stress Disorder
Generalized Anxiety Disorder	Generalized Anxiety Disorder (includes Overanxious Disorder of Childhood)
	Anxiety Disorder Due to a General Medical Condition
	Substance-Induced Anxiety Disorder
Anxiety Disorder Not Otherwise Specified	Anxiety Disorder Not Otherwise Specified

PHENOMENOLOGY

> I have awakened in the night, being slightly unwell and felt so much afraid. The sensation of fear is accompanied by troubled beating of heart, sweat, trembling of muscles—Charles Darwin

> He who is afraid of leaves must not come in the woods—French proverb

> Sometimes the objects of my fear changes, and sometimes the quality of my fear changes—but I find too much fear, in a way. I can't go to sleep in a hotel without thinking, "Who is in the room underneath me, dead drunk and smoking a cigarette and about to fall asleep so that the room catches fire?"—Stephen King

Listening to the voices of others[1] (and to our own sensations) is a useful way to appreciate the phenomenology of anxiety/fear. For example, Darwin is describing the bodily or physiological

responses that are experienced when one is frightened or anxious, the French proverb is describing the behavioral avoidant response, and Stephen King, the popular novelist who made a fortune by scaring the wits out of readers, is describing the related thoughts and cognitions. And in fact, researchers and practitioners have described phenomenology in precisely these ways, referring to the physiological, the behavioral, and the cognitive as the three-response system (e.g., Lang, 1977). Methods and procedures have been developed for assessing each system (described under Assessment).

We should note that we are skeptical whether these methods and procedures (e.g., a score of 16 on an anxiety questionnaire) fully capture the richness of phenomenology. Investigators working in other areas in psychology, such as psychotherapy process and gender research, have found qualitative research methods useful for pushing forward the boundaries of knowledge (e.g., Belenky, Clinchy, Goldberger, & Tarule, 1986; Gilligan, 1982), and we believe this would be true as well in research on phenomenology. In lieu of this type of work, what is

---

[1]To hear more voices we recommend *The Little Book of Phobias* by Joe Kohut, a delightful compilation of more than 250 quotations about phobias.

known about the phenomenology of anxiety in children? The answer is not much. What is known is summarized below.

Developmental Variations

A couple of studies have examined "symptom expression" in children who presented to a childhood anxiety specialty clinic (e.g., Francis, Last, & Strauss, 1987; Strauss, Lease, Last, & Francis, 1988). Based on children's and parents' responses to a structured interview schedule, Francis et al. (1987) compared symptoms in children across three age groups: young (age 5 to 8), middle (age 9 to 12), and older (age 13 to 16). Findings revealed that young children diagnosed with SAD (described below) were more likely than older children to present with the symptom Nightmares about Separation. Middle children were more likely than older children to present with the symptom Excessive Distress upon Separation. A significantly greater proportion of children in the younger age group (100%) than in the middle (but not older) age group (69%) received a diagnosis of SAD on the basis of having met four or more of the nine symptoms that comprise the diagnostic criteria.

In another clinical study comparing developmental differences in the symptom expression of overanxious disorder (OAD), older children (age 12 to 19) were more likely to present with the symptom Unrealistic Concern about the Appropriateness of Past Behavior relative to younger children (age 5 to 11) (Strauss, Lease, et al., 1988). The older children also presented with a higher total number of OAD symptoms than younger children; 28% of older children met all seven DSM criteria for the disorder whereas only 4% of younger children presented with all of the criteria.

Gender Variations

Research on gender variations in anxiety disorders has been conducted primarily with respect to prevalence rates (see Epidemiology section below). We could not locate research on gender variations in the phenomenology of anxiety in clinical samples of children. There has been research conducted, however, on gender variations in fear in nonclinical samples of children: Across a variety of rating forms (self-, parent-, teacher-, and peer-), girls obtain higher ratings of fears than boys (in terms of both frequency and intensity) (e.g., Croake, 1969; Ollendick, Yang, Dong, Xia, & Lin, 1995; Silverman & Nelles, 1988a). These findings have been explained, in part, by gender role expectations (i.e., it is more acceptable for girls to admit to fear than boys, and for others, including girls, to ascribe more fear to girls than to boys; Maccoby, 1980). However, this explanation remains tentative until children's gender role expectations are directly measured and examined in relation to fear ratings.

Racial and Cultural Variations

As with gender variations, investigators have examined race and cultural variations in fears in nonclinical samples of children. For example, fears have been found to be more frequent and intense in African-American children than in white children (Neal, Lilly, & Zakis, 1993). Little research has been conducted, however, on how phenomenology may vary with race or culture in clinical samples. One recent example of such a study was conducted by Last and Perrin (1993), who compared the sociodemographic background, clinical characteristics, and lifetime prevalence rates of specific DSM-III-R disorders of African-American ($n = 30$) and white children ($n = 139$). The children (age 5 to 17) presented to a childhood anxiety clinic, and met DSM-III-R diagnoses for anxiety disorders. Overall, the children were found to be more similar than different on the variables examined. However, although not statistically significant, clinicians' rating of severity for the primary diagnosis were higher for the white children than for the African-American children, and more of the white children were school refusers. The African-American children, on the other hand, scored higher than the white children on a fear inventory and showed a higher lifetime prevalence rate of Posttraumatic Stress Disorder (PTSD) (2.2% for whites versus 13.3% for African Americans).

The present authors conducted a similar study comparing Hispanic ($n = 99$) and white children ($n = 143$) who presented at a childhood anxiety disorders clinic (Ginsburg & Silverman, 1996). Like Last and Perrin, the children were more similar than different on the variables examined. However, one significant difference was that Hispanic parents rated their children as having more fears than did parents of white children (using a parent version of a child fear inventory).

Although the studies reviewed in this section require replication in both clinical and community samples, they represent an important beginning. Hopefully they will serve as a springboard for future, theory-driven research on developmental, gender, racial, and cultural variations in the phenomenology of anxiety disorders in children.

Stability of Anxiety Disorders

Support for the stability of some types of anxiety problems comes from retrospective studies of phobic adults who report that age of onset ranges between age 5 and 10 (e.g., Abe, 1972; Ost, 1987). Although research on the stability of anxiety disorders using prospective methods is sparse, reviews suggest that approximately 20 to 30% of anxiety disorders diagnosed in childhood are stable over time (approximately 2 to 5 years) (see Costello & Angold, 1995; Ollendick & King, 1994). However, the studies that have been conducted have methodological limitations, such as small sample sizes and the absence of formal diagnoses, and in many cases, the children being followed had undergone treatment (e.g., Hampe, Noble, Miller, & Barrett, 1973).

One of the most frequently cited studies is Agras, Chapin, and Oliveau (1972) who fol-

lowed a community sample of 30 untreated phobic individuals (10 children under the age of 20 years and 20 adults) over a 5-year period. After 5 years, 100% of the children were viewed as "improved" compared to 43% of the adults. Although the conclusion drawn was that many phobic conditions improve without treatment, particularly in children, Ollendick's (1979) reinterpretation of this study was that the improved children were not symptom-free, and most continued to exhibit symptoms of sufficient intensity to be rated between "no disability" and "maximum disability" at the follow-up assessment. This reinterpretation suggests that some types of phobias persist over time for a proportion of youngsters.

Cantwell and Baker (1989) examined a sample of 151 children (age 2.3 to 15.9 years) who presented at a speech and hearing clinic over a 4- to 5-year period. Of 31 children initially diagnosed with a DSM-III childhood anxiety disorder (SAD, OAD, and AVD), the percentage of children who retained the same diagnosis at the follow-up was 11% for SAD, 25% for OAD, and 29% for AVD. The percentage of children considered "well" was 44, 25, and 36% for SAD, OAD, and AVD, respectively. OAD was the least stable diagnosis as the remaining 50% of children who initially received this diagnosis received an alternative diagnosis at follow-up. Findings such as these led to the suggestion that OAD may be a prodromal form of other anxiety disorders, and contributed to the decision to eliminate OAD as a distinct childhood anxiety disorder subcategory in the DSM-IV, although this decision was viewed by some investigators as premature (e.g., Silverman, 1992; Werry, 1991). The stability of DSM-IV GAD diagnoses in youth awaits determination.

Of all of the anxiety disorders, Obsessive-Compulsive Disorder (OCD) is considered to be the most stable or chronic (March, Leonard, & Swedo, 1995). Follow-up investigations generally indicate that approximately 30–40% of children who receive an initial diagnosis of OCD continue to receive the diagnosis at 2- to 7-year follow-up assessments (Berg et al., 1989; Flament et al., 1988).

In sum, although some of the anxiety disorders appear to show stability over time (e.g., some types of phobias), the pattern of stability for each specific subcategory of anxiety disorders varies, and has not been studied in others (e.g., GAD).

DIAGNOSIS

Separation Anxiety Disorder

The predominant feature displayed by children with SAD is excessive anxiety or distress on separation or on threat of separation from a primary attachment figure or from home. Children with SAD often worry that harm (e.g., being kidnapped or being involved in an accident) will befall either themselves or a parent. When separation is imminent, they may cry, cling to the parent, scream, or beg the parent not to leave. They may act aggressively to avoid separation, and may also report somatic complaints (e.g., stomachaches) when separation is anticipated. To receive a diagnosis of SAD, the symptoms must be present for 4 consecutive weeks and be non-age-appropriate.

The types of situations that children with SAD may avoid or attempt to avoid include school, camp, social activities, and being left alone. However, although children with SAD may avoid school, not all children who avoid school are children with SAD (see reviews by Atkinson, Quarrington, Cyr, & Atkinson, 1989; Burke & Silverman, 1987; Kearney, Eisen, & Silverman, 1995). Children who refuse school are heterogeneous: Although a proportion refuse school because of difficulties with SAD, a proportion also refuse because of other problems, such as Social and Specific Phobia or GAD.

Social Phobia (Social Anxiety Disorder)

The predominant feature of children with Social Phobia (SOP) is persistent and irrational fears of social or performance situations, particularly situations in which they might be scrutinized by others. Children with SOP fear that when they are in such situations, they may behave in certain ways, or display certain symptoms, that will lead to humiliation or embarrassment. As a consequence, they avoid or attempt to avoid social or performance situations. When in these situations, they experience marked distress, and may shrink from contact with others, cling to their parent, or "freeze up." To receive a diagnosis of SOP, the symptoms must be present for 6 consecutive months, be non-age-appropriate, and interfere in the child's functioning.

SOP may be of a generalized type (i.e., fear across most social situations—public and interpersonal) or a specific type, i.e., fear in specific situations, such as parties or club meetings. Although SOP has been documented in young children (Beidel & Turner, 1988), the average age of onset (based on reports of children who present for treatment) reportedly ranges from 11.3 to 12.3 years (Last, Perrin, Hersen, & Kazdin, 1992; Strauss & Last, 1993).

Specific Phobia

Children with Specific Phobia (SP) display excessive fear in the presence of, or in anticipation of, a circumscribed object or event. The fear is out of proportion to reality; however, unlike adults, children may not view their fear as excessive or unreasonable. Children with SP show marked avoidance of the feared object or event, or experience severe distress on confrontation. To receive a diagnosis of SP, the symptoms must be present for 6 consecutive months, be non-age-appropriate, and interfere in the child's functioning. Although in some cases the fear may be age-appropriate, it may be so excessive and impairing that treatment might nonetheless be considered.

In the differential diagnosis of SP, the fear must be focused on specific objects or situations, i.e., not situations that involve separation, as in SAD, or that are social, as in SOP. It is also essential that the fear not be a part of a larger reaction to a traumatic event, as in PTSD, or a fear of contamination, as in OCD. Although SP has been documented in young children, it appears to peak between ages 10 and 13 (Beidel & Turner, 1988; Strauss & Last, 1993), with the average age of onset ranging from 7.8 to 8.4 years (based on reports of children who present for treatment) (Last et al., 1992; Strauss & Last, 1993).

Generalized Anxiety Disorder (Including Overanxious Disorder of Childhood)

The predominant feature displayed by children with GAD is excessive and preoccupying worry that is not focused on a specific situation or object, that is not related to a recent stressor, and that is difficult to control. Areas of worry can include performance, health, family, and seemingly trivial things. These difficulties must have been ongoing for at least 6 months. In addition, one of the following physical symptoms must be present: restlessness, fatigue, concentration difficulties, irritability, muscle tension, or sleep disturbances. Because all children worry (Silverman, La Greca, & Wasserstein, 1995), a diagnosis of GAD is only appropriate if the worry is clearly deemed excessive and uncontrollable.

In the differential diagnosis of GAD, as noted, the anxieties and worries must not be focused on specific objects as in SP, on separation situations as in SAD, or on social scrutiny as in SOP; and must not occur during the course of PTSD. In addition, the intrusive thoughts of GAD differ from those in OCD in that in the latter the thoughts are usually in the form of "egodystonic intrusions" that take the form of urges, impulses, and images, and are usually accompanied by compulsions (American Psychiatric Association, 1994). The average age of onset for GAD/OAD (based on reports of children who present for treatment) is 8.8 years (Last et al., 1992); the mean age of children who presented for treatment ranges between 10.8 and 13.4 years (Last, Hersen, Kazdin, Finkelstein, & Strauss, 1987; Last, Strauss, & Francis, 1987).

Panic Disorder with and without Agoraphobia and Agoraphobia without Panic

The predominant feature displayed by youth with panic disorder (PD) is discrete periods of intense fear or discomfort, manifested by a variety of somatic/psychological symptoms, i.e., panic attacks. The most common symptoms of panic reported by children and adolescents include trembling, shaking, palpitations, dizziness/faintness, dyspnea, and sweating (Moreau & Follet, 1993). Panic symptoms must not be under direct control, and must not be related to the physiological effects of a substance or medical condition or better accounted for by another mental disorders (American Psychiatric Association, 1994). To be diagnosable, at least one of the panic attacks must be followed by 1 month (or more) of one or more of the following: (1) persistent concern about having additional attacks, (2) worry about the implications of the attack or its consequences (e.g., losing control, having a heart attack), and (3) significant change in behavior related to the attacks. Panic may be accompanied by agoraphobia, which is characterized by either marked avoidance of situations in which escape may be difficult or embarrassing (if symptoms occurred), or the situation is endured only with severe distress, or with a companion. Examples of situations avoided include school, movies, malls, and being alone.

Although the existence of panic attacks and panic disorder is well established in adults, controversy exists regarding their prevalence in children and adolescents. It has been hypothesized that children cannot experience panic because they lack the ability for "catastrophic misinterpretation" of the somatic symptoms associated with panic; that is, children's cognitive reactions are thought to be dominated by notions of external causation, and only in adolescence do the internal attributions characteristic of panic (e.g., "Oh, oh, I am going to die") develop (Nelles & Barlow, 1988). Although an interesting hypothesis, there is no direct evidence that children's thinking about panic symptoms changes in this way. On the contrary, a recent study conducted by Mattis and Ollendick (1997) found that a nonclinical sample of school-age children reported these types of internal attributions while engaging in panic imagery.

Because adolescents are thought to have the cognitive capabilities to experience panic, and because studies have documented the presence of panic in adolescent samples (see Epidemiology section), investigators have concluded that panic attacks are common in adolescents and that PD occurs "not infrequently" (Ollendick, Mattis, & King, 1994). However, methodological problems with these studies, such as the failure to use structured interview techniques, have led others to remain cautious about the prevalence of PD in adolescence (at least as described in the DSM), until more rigorous studies are conducted (Kearney & Silverman, 1992).

Obsessive-Compulsive Disorder

The predominant feature of OCD is persistent obsessions (ideas, thoughts, or images) and/or compulsions (repetitive, purposeful behaviors usually engaged in response to obsessions) that are intrusive, time consuming (more than 1 hour daily), and significantly interfere with daily functioning (American Psychiatric Association, 1994). Unlike adults, children may not recognize that their obsessions or compulsions are excessive or unreasonable. The most common obsessions of youth include fears of contamination (such as getting AIDS, cancer, or other life-threatening illness) and thoughts of harm to self and familiar figures (Flament et al., 1988). The most common compulsions of children include washing and cleansing rituals and repeating and checking behaviors (Flament et al., 1988). The mean age of onset of OCD for youth seeking treatment is approximately 10 (e.g., Albano, Knox, & Barlow, 1995; Leonard & Rapoport, 1991), although OCD has been diagnosed in children as young as 6 (Swedo, Rapoport, Leonard, Lenane, & Cheslow, 1989).

Comorbid Conditions

Clinical and community studies indicate that up to one-half of all children present with more than one comorbid disorder (see Caron & Rutter, 1991, for review). Last and colleagues have conducted several studies documenting the comorbid patterns among samples of clinic-referred children with anxiety disorders. For example, in a sample of 73 children (age 5 to 18), 57 of whom met four major primary diagnostic groups, specifically, diagnoses of SAD ($n = 24$), SOP ($n = 11$), OAD ($n = 11$), and major depression (MD; $n = 11$), Last, Strauss, and Francis (1987) found that the majority of children in each of the four groups currently met criteria for one or more additional disorder (ranging from 64% for the SP group to 100% for the MD group). The most common comorbid anxiety disorder diagnosis for children in the SAD group was OAD (33%); for children in the OAD group it was SOP (36.4%).

In a subsequent study, Last et al. (1992) examined history of comorbid diagnoses (as opposed to current rates) in children ($n = 188$; age 5 to 18). A majority (62.5 to 96%) of children in each of the diagnostic categories were found to have a history of more than one anxiety disorder diagnosis. Children with OAD and AVD displayed the highest rates of comorbid anxiety disorder diagnoses (90 and 96.1%, respectively).

Hammond-Laurence and Silverman (submitted) examined current rates of comorbid diagnoses in a large sample of children referred to an anxiety specialty clinic ($N = 310$; age 6 to 17). Similar to the work of Last and her colleagues, the majority of children in each of the diagnostic categories displayed comorbid diagnoses (77 to 96%), with over one-half of the children in each group receiving two or more additional diagnoses. Further, almost one-third of the children met criteria for an additional externalizing disorder, usually attention-deficit/hyperactivity disorder (ADHD) or oppositional defiant disorder.

Although the high comorbid rates reported in the studies above could be related in part to the Berkson effects—i.e., both the Last et al. (1987, 1992) and the Hammond-Laurence and Silverman (submitted) studies were conducted at anxiety specialty clinics that attract the most severely anxious youth—these findings are in accord with the growing body of literature concerned with comorbidity (see Caron & Rutter, 1991). However, a great deal more work is needed to understand the meaning and implications of comorbidity—not only in terms of clinical presentation, but also in terms of prognosis and treatment.

ETIOLOGY

Genetic and Neurobiology

The evidence for the role of genetic and neurobiological dispositional factors is based largely on findings from family studies (see reviews by Ginsburg, Silverman, & Kurtines, 1995a; Klein & Last, 1989; Silverman, Cerny, & Nelles, 1988), twin studies (e.g., see review by Torgersen, 1990), and studies on behavioral inhibition (see review by Biederman, Rosenbaum, Chaloff, & Kagan, 1995). These are briefly summarized below.

Family studies document familial aggregation and can therefore provide evidence that a disorder is familial. There are two types of family studies: top down and bottom up. Top-down studies examine the prevalence of psychopathology in children whose parents have received an anxiety diagnosis; bottom-up studies examine the prevalence of psychopathology in parents of children who have received an anxiety diagnosis. However, if familial risk is found to significantly exceed lifetime prevalence rates of the general population in such studies, this is necessary but not sufficient evidence of genetic transmission: Such findings can result from either shared genes or common family environmental factors or their interaction (Foley & Hay, 1992; Silverman et al., 1988). With this caveat in mind, what do the results of family studies suggest regarding the familial contribution to anxiety disorders in children?

Findings from top-down studies generally reveal that children whose parents have an anxiety disorder are at risk for developing an anxiety disorder themselves (e.g., Berg, 1976; Fyer et al., 1990; Moran & Andrews, 1985; Reich & Yates, 1988; Silverman, Cerny, Nelles, & Burke, 1988; Solyom, Beck, Solyom, & Hugel, 1974; Turner, Beidel, & Costello, 1987; Weissman, Leckman, Merikangas, Gammon, & Prusoff, 1984). For example, Turner et al. (1987) examined the prevalence of anxiety disorders (via semistructured interview and self-report measures) in the offspring (age 7 to 12) of parents with an anxiety disorder (agoraphobia or OCD) ($n = 16$), dysthymic disorder ($n = 14$), and normal controls ($n = 13$). Findings revealed that the offspring whose parents were diagnosed with an anxiety disorder were over two times as likely to meet DSM-III criteria for an anxiety disorder themselves relative to the offspring of parents who were diagnosed with dysthymic disorder and seven times more likely than the offspring of the normal controls.

Similarly, findings from bottom-up studies generally reveal that parents whose children have an anxiety disorder are likely to show anxiety disorders or symptoms (Berg, Butler, & Pritchard, 1974; Bernstein & Garfinkel, 1988; Kashani et al., 1990; Last, Hersen, Kazdin, Francis, & Grubb, 1987; Last, Hersen, Kazdin, Orvaschel, & Perrin, 1991; Last, Phillips, & Statfeld, 1987; Livingston, Nugent, Rader, & Smith, 1985; Messer & Beidel, 1994; Rosenbaum et al., 1992). For example, Last et al. (1991) examined rates of anxiety and other psychiatric disorders in the first- and second-degree relatives of 94 children with anxiety disorders, 58 children with ADHD, and 87 children who were never psychiatrically ill (NPI). Available family members (usually mothers) were interviewed directly using the family history method. Information about unavailable family members was obtained by interviewing the available family members. The results indicated that parents (both mothers and fathers combined) of children with anxiety disorders had significantly higher rates of anxiety diagnoses compared with parents of children with ADHD and NPI children.

As noted, because family studies can only demonstrate familiality and not heritability, it is also important to use methods that disrupt the environmental and genetic relationships found within the family. The twin studies of Torgersen (1985, 1990) are exemplary of such methods. Briefly, Torgersen interviewed all twin pairs born in Norway between 1910 and 1955, where one or both had received inpatient or outpatient care for "neurotic" or "borderline psychotic states." Discriminant function analysis of Present State Examination symptoms was used to identify three groups of disorders, namely, Pure Anxiety Neurosis, Mixed Anxiety-Depression, and Pure Neurotic Depression. The different monozygotic and dizygotic concordance rates found across the three groups led Torgersen to conclude that only pure anxiety has a genetic basis.

Overall, despite methodological variations across both family and twin studies, such as in the data-gathering procedures used (e.g., structured diagnostic interview versus unstructured clinical interview), the samples used (e.g., community versus clinic), and the types of problems studied ("pure" diagnostic groups versus groups with comorbid diagnoses), and despite methodological limitations (e.g., small sample sizes, reliance on retrospective reports, the use of volunteer registries in twin studies), the evidence from these studies is suggestive of a genetic or familial contribution. However, the specific nature of this contribution remains unclear. That is, is it specific or is it general to all of the anxiety disorders or even more general to a wider range of disorders (Foley & Hay, 1992)? Resolving this issue will be an important challenge for future researchers.

In addition to family and twin studies, recent research on the interface between neurobiology and anxiety in children has provided important insights regarding the correlates and possible etiologies of anxiety disorders (Sallee & Greenawald, 1995). Perhaps the most useful heuristic in examining the neurobiology of childhood anxiety has been the construct of behavioral inhibition provided by Kagan and colleagues. Behavioral inhibition (BI; Biederman et al., 1990, 1993a,b; Hirshfeld et al., 1992; Kagan, Reznick, & Gibbons, 1989; Kagan, Reznick, & Snidman, 1987, 1988; Rosenbaum et al., 1988) refers to the temperament of approximately 10–15% of white infants (as far as we can discern, the samples in BI studies have all been white) who are predisposed to being irritable, shy, and fearful as toddlers, and cautious, quiet, and introverted as school-age children (e.g., Kagan, 1989). Primate work with monkeys, rats, cats and dogs similarly supports the hypothesis of early behavioral, and physiological characteristics akin to BI (e.g., Adamec & Stark-Adamec, 1989; Suomi, 1984, 1986).

Of particular relevance to this chapter is the observation that children with BI display many of the same behavioral, affective, and physiological characteristics as children with anxiety disorders. These characteristics include avoidance and withdrawal from novel situations, clinging or dependence on parents, fearfulness, and physiological arousal (e.g., increased heart rate) when exposed to unfamiliar settings, people, and objects (e.g., Kagan et al., 1987). Moreover, similar to findings from the top-down studies cited above, significantly more children whose parents present with an anxiety disorder (i.e., PD/AG [agoraphobia]) display BI compared with children whose parents present with a psychiatric disorder other than anxiety or depression (Rosenbaum et al., 1988). Most tantalizing is the emerging evidence that BI in infancy may be a risk factor for later anxiety disorders in childhood (e.g., Biederman et al., 1990, 1993a). For example, Biederman et al. (1990), using a structured interview (administered to parents), examined the prevalence of DSM-III internalizing (major depression, SAD, OAD, AVD, phobic disorders, and OCD) and externalizing disorders (oppositional, conduct, and attention deficit) in three groups of children. The first group, examined cross-sectionally, was comprised of offspring of parents with psychiatric diagnoses. Children in this cohort were classified as either inhibited ($n = 18$; mean age 5.9 years) or uninhibited ($n = 12$; mean age 4.9 years). The second group was an epidemiologically derived sample of children who, at age 21 months, had been classified as either inhibited ($n = 22$) or uninhibited ($n = 19$) (see Kagan et al., 1987). The mean age of the children at the time of the reassessment was 8 years. The third group of children had no medical or psychiatric disorders ($n = 20$; mean age 7.8 years) and were obtained from primary pediatric care referrals.

Overall, the results indicated that the inhibited children had higher rates of each of the anxiety disorders compared with the uninhibited and healthy controls (although not all comparisons reached statistical significance; Biederman et al., 1990). For example, 27.8% of children with BI met criteria for four or more anxiety disorders compared with 0% of uninhibited children and 0% of the healthy control children. Despite these findings, the authors noted that not all children with early BI developed an anxiety disorder (approximately 70% did not), and consequently, they concluded that future research should focus on identifying "risk factors that can influence the evolution of behavioral inhibition to manifest anxiety disorders" (Biederman et al., 1990, p. 26).

In summary, although investigations support genetic/familial contributions and neurobiology as dispositional factors in the etiology of anxiety disorders in children, specific mechanisms of transmission remain unknown. Also, although BI in infants may be an important dispositional factor, not all children with early BI later develop anxiety disorders. These findings underscore the importance of psychosocial factors as well.

Psychosocial Factors

In thinking about psychosocial factors that contribute to the etiology of anxiety disorders in children, researchers and practitioners are likely to fall back on the therapeutic traditions to which they may ascribe (e.g., psychoanalytic, behavioral, cognitive, familial, group). And there are psychosocial explanations that stem from each of these traditions. They are briefly summarized below.

Psychoanalytic

Based on Freud's psychoanalytic conceptualization of Little Hans's phobia of horses (Freud, 1909/1955), phobias reflect the child's attempt to defend against or avoid anxiety aroused by unconscious forbidden thoughts or impulses (e.g., Hans's sexual desire for his mother and his wish to do away with his father, the competitor). The child's defense against this internal conflict is to displace the anxiety onto an external object that can be avoided (e.g., horses). Avoidance was thus viewed as protecting the child from situations in which these aggressive or erotic impulses might be aroused.

It has been difficult to empirically verify the psychoanalytic conceptualization of childhood phobia because of the unconscious nature of the main, hypothesized processes (e.g., displacement). Wolpe and Rachman (1960), in their critique of the Little Hans case, reported that they could find no direct evidence for Hans's wish to sleep with his mother, for his hatred or fear of his father, or for the supposed relationship between horses and Hans's father. Wolpe and Rachman (1960) provided an alternative conceptualization of Hans's phobia, namely, a behavioral conceptualization, discussed next.

Behavioral

Wolpe and Rachman (1960) noted that in Freud's case description Hans was described as having experienced a traumatic event involving horses (a horse pulling a bus had fallen), and according to Hans's mother, the phobia developed immediately after this event. Hence, Wolpe and Rachman argued that Hans's phobia was the result of traumatic Pavlovian conditioning. In the case of Hans, horses (CS) had acquired the capacity to elicit fear (CR) after being involved in the accident (UCS) that had caused the initial startle and distress (UCR). Earlier case reports, such as Little Peter (Jones, 1924a,b) and Little Albert (Watson & Rayner, 1920), had similarly argued for a Pavlovian account of the acquisition or instruction. Support for these pathways has been provided in the subclinical fears of adults (e.g., Hekmat, 1987; Murray & Foote, 1979; Ost, 1985; Rimm, Janda, Lancaster, Nahl, & Dittmar, 1977), as well as in the fears of non-clinic-referred children (Ollendick & King, 1991).

Although the Pavlovian account of fear acquisition has received support from laboratory and clinical studies (e.g., Liddell & Lyons, 1978; Merckelbach, De Ruiter, Van De Hout, & Hoekstra, 1989), the research findings have been generally inconsistent, leading many researchers and theorists to question its adequacy (see Menzies & Clark, 1995, for a review of these arguments). This has led to extensions of conditioning theory—or to "neoconditioning" theory—reflected by the writings of Rescorla (1988), Reiss (1991), and Davey (1992), to name just a few. For example, in Rescorla's and Davey's reformulation of conditioning the emphasis is not on contiguous pairing of stimuli, but on UCS revaluation. Reiss (1991) delineated a cognitive expectancy account that involves certain individual personality differences such as anxiety sensitivity.

Also representing an important extension of the Pavlovian conditioning model was Mowrer's (1939) two-factor model that endorsed Pavlovian conditioning in the initial acquisition of fear, but also argued that fear could serve as an acquired source of motivation or drive, i.e., behaviors that reduced fear would be reinforced. However, the adequacy of Mowrer's model in explaining the persistence of phobic fear and avoidance also has been questioned because many individuals with phobias can confront the phobic stimulus without either covert avoidance or a subsequent aversive UCS (Menzies & Clark, 1995). According to Mowrer, this should lead to reductions in fear and avoidant behavior but this does not necessarily always occur (Clarke & Jackson, 1983). Modified conditioning explanations were consequently developed to account for this, such as the partial irreversibility of fear account (Solomon & Wynne, 1954), the preparedness account (Seligman, 1970, 1971), the incubation account (Eysenck, 1979), the safety signal account (Rachman, 1983), and the serial CS account (Stampfl, 1991).

Rachman's (1977) highly influential article also espoused the importance of additional pathways in "indirect" fear acquisition, namely, vicarious exposure and the transmission of information or instruction. Support for these pathways has been provided in the subclinical fears of adults (e.g., Hekmat, 1987; Murray & Foote, 1979; Ost, 1985; Rimm, Janda, Lancaster, Nahl, & Dittmar, 1977), as well as in the fears of non-clinic-referred children (Ollendick & King, 1991).

Taken together, however, empirical support for the various conditioning reformulations and extensions has been uneven across laboratories, samples, and disorders. This unevenness helped to spur the "cognitive revolution" that occurred in behavioral psychology in the 1970s, which emphasized the role of cognitions. The cognitive view is presented next.

Cognitive

Although controversies about whether the cognitions of children with anxiety disorders are causes or consequences of the fear/anxiety response, there is consensus that these children display distorted and maladaptive thoughts (e.g., Kendall, Howard, & Epps, 1988). For example, highly test-anxious children are more likely than non-test-anxious children to engage in task-debilitating thoughts (e.g., those that are off-task and focusing on negative evaluations or unfavorable social comparisons, and few positive self-evaluations; Francis, 1988; Kendall & Chansky, 1991; Zatz & Chassin, 1985). Highly test-anxious children also report more on-task and coping thoughts, but these thoughts have no task-facilitating role (Fox & Houston, 1981; Prins, 1986; Prins, Matti, Groot, & Hanewald, 1994; Zatz & Chassin, 1985). These findings are consistent with the idea that nonnegative thinking may be more strongly related to adjustment than the presence of positive cognition, or with Kendall's notion of the "power of nonnegative thinking."

Factors that influence the thinking of anxious children are beginning to be studied, such as the role of causal attributions (see Bell-Dolan & Wessler, 1994) and information processing (Vasey, Daleiden, Williams, & Brown, 1995). However, we note that these do not occur in a vacuum in children. Families are likely to have an important influence. This thus leads us to familial explanations.

Family

Familial explanations are defined broadly here to include parenting style, family functioning, family environment, and parent–child attachment patterns (see Ginsburg et al., 1995a). Parents of anxious children have long been described as "overprotecting," "ambivalent," "rejecting," and "hostile" (e.g., Berg & McGuire, 1974; Berg, Nichols, & Pritchard, 1969). Retrospective reports of adults who suffer from anxiety disorders show that these adults view their parents, and their relationship with them, in similar ways (e.g., overcontrolling and less affectionate) (see Gerslma, Emmelkamp, & Arrindell, 1990, for review).

As noted earlier, many children with school refusal behavior are likely to meet criteria for some type of anxiety disorder diagnosis. Thus, relevant is research indicating that the families of these children score lower on indices of child independence and participation in recreational activities, and higher on indices of hostility/conflict (see Kearney & Silverman, 1995, for review). These families have also been found to be more overprotective and more disturbed in role performance, communication, affective expression, and control relative to families of children with nonanxiety psychiatric disorders (e.g., Bernstein & Garfinkel, 1986, 1988).

Direct observations of parent–child interactions have recently shed some light on such patterns in the families of clinical samples of children with anxiety disorders (Barrett, Rapee, Dadds, & Ryan, 1996; Dadds, Barrett, Rapee, & Ryan, 1996). Dadds and colleagues in a series of studies classified children (age 7–14) into the following three groups using a structured interview: (1) anxiety disorders ($n = 152$; diagnoses included OAD, SAD, SOP, and SP), (2) oppositional defiant disorder (ODD; $n = 27$), and (3) normal controls ($n = 26$), and observed the children and their parents interpret and develop a plan of action for a series of ambiguous, hypothetical situations. Results indicated that following a family discussion of the hypothetical situations, children with anxiety disorders were more likely to generate avoidance solutions compared with children with ODD or the normal controls. According to the authors, such findings suggest that there might be family processes that are specific to families of children with anxiety disorders, and that these processes might serve to either bring out and/or maintain these disorders in children (Dadds et al., 1996). The results of a recent study by Chorpita, Albano, and Barlow (1996) provide additional support for this view.

Another familial influence that is likely to be important but to date has been insufficiently studied is the role of caregiver–infant attachment patterns (Bowlby, 1973). Using the strange situation to assess attachment patterns (Ainsworth, Blehar, Waters, & Wall, 1978), three major patterns have been described: (1) secure, (2) insecure–avoidant, and (3) insecure–anxious/ambivalent. These early attachment patterns are viewed as persisting over time, and to be important in influencing children's sense of trust in others and their feelings of self-efficacy, among other things (e.g., Main, Kaplan, & Cassidy, 1985; Waters, 1978). Although direct links between attachment and anxiety disorders have not been documented, attachment theorists hypothesize that the internal working models of insecurely attached infants predispose them to engage in distorted ways of thinking, selective encoding of threatening information, interpersonal difficulties, and behavioral avoidance—all of which may be precursors to anxiety and other internalizing disorders (e.g., Rubin & Mills, 1991; Sroufe, 1983). Research findings have been recently reported that provide preliminary support for a link between attachment and childhood anxiety (e.g., Manassis, Bradley, Goldberg, Hood, & Swinson, 1994).

Peer Influence

Like cognitions, it is unclear whether peer problems of children with anxiety disorders are causes or consequences of their anxious and avoidant behaviors. However, there is growing evidence that anxiety symptoms and/or disorders co-occur with social deficits and poor peer relationships (e.g., Asher & Cole, 1990; Parker & Asher, 1987). For instance, research using nonclinical samples has shown that in comparison with accepted and well-liked children, children with peer problems (either rejected and/or neglected) have higher levels of social anxiety and other forms of internal distress such as loneliness, depression, and feelings of inadequacy (e.g., La Greca & Stone, 1993; Rubin & Mills, 1991).

Studies examining the peer social status of anxious children have reached similar conclusions (Strauss, Frame, & Forehand, 1987). Strauss et al. (1987) classified 48 elementary school children as "highly anxious" or "nonanxious" using teachers' ratings on Quay and Peterson's (1983) Revised Behavior Rating Scale. Classmates provided peer nominations of three children whom they "liked the most" and "liked the least." Peer nominations of the most shy, aggressive, and socially withdrawn, and peer nominations of three children they most and least liked to play with in the class were obtained. Overall, children in the highly anxious group were more likely to be nominated as shy and socially withdrawn than their nonanxious counterparts and received more "least liked" and fewer "liked most" nominations.

As far as we are aware, Strauss and colleagues have been the only investigators to also examine the peer social status of clinical samples of children with anxiety disorders (Strauss, Lahey, Frick, Frame, & Hynd, 1988). Studying children 6 to 13 years of age, Strauss, Lahey, et al. (1988) compared the peer social status of children with anxiety disorders (SAD, OCD, or OAD; $n = 16$), conduct disorder (CD; $n = 26$), and a nonreferred control group ($n = 45$). Diagnoses were obtained using structured interviews with the children, and the investigators also obtained classroom peer nominations of social status, i.e., three children liked the most, the least, and who fought the most, respectively. Findings revealed that children with anxiety disorders were less likely to be nominated as "most liked" relative to their nonreferred peers; no differences were

found in the "most liked" nominations between the children with anxiety disorders and CD. In addition, relative to children with CD or to the nonreferred group, a significantly higher proportion of children with anxiety disorders were classified as "neglected."

Strauss, Lease, Kazdin, Dulcan, and Last (1989), in another study using a clinical sample of children with anxiety disorders, assessed children's social competence using a variety of child-, parent-, and teacher-rating scales. The anxiety-disordered group was comprised of 55 children (SAD, OAD, SP; mean age 10.8 years) and the comparison groups consisted of a nonanxious clinical group (ADHD, CD, ODD, and adjustment disorder; $n = 18$; mean age 9.6 years) and a nonreferred group of children ($n = 20$; mean age 9.4 years). The results revealed that children with anxiety disorders were less socially competent than the nonreferred children. Specifically, they were rated as more shy, socially withdrawn, lonely, and lacking in appropriate social skills. Although the nonanxious clinical group also evidenced social deficits (e.g., low rates of appropriate social skills, high rates of inappropriate assertiveness, feelings of loneliness), the children with anxiety disorders were rated as more shy and socially withdrawn.

Interestingly, however, not all children with anxiety disorders display problematic peer relationships. Strauss, Lahey, et al. (1988) noted that 63% of the children with anxiety disorders in their study showed no significant deficits in their peer social status. Post hoc analyses suggested that the presence of comorbid depression may be an important contributing factor. Ginsburg, Alonso, Hammond-Laurence, and Silverman (1995) recently provided additional empirical support for this suggestion. In a clinical sample of children with anxiety disorders ($n = 45$; age 7 to 17; mean age 10.4), depressive symptoms significantly added to the prediction of poor peer relationships, over and above levels of anxiety. Further research is needed to determine additional factors that may put children with anxiety disorders at risk for peer difficulties or that may buffer children from such risk. Also, as noted at the beginning of this section, research is needed to disentangle the role of peers in the development and maintenance of anxiety disorders, i.e., are peer problems causes or consequences of childhood anxiety? Research using longitudinal designs is needed to answer such questions.

EPIDEMIOLOGY

Efforts to understand the epidemiology of psychiatric disorders in youth, including the anxiety disorders, as defined by the DSM-IV were under way at the time of writing this chapter with the National Institute of Mental Health's childhood catchment area studies. What is known about the epidemiology of anxiety disorders in youth using DSM-III and DSM-III-R criteria is summarized in Table 2. As is apparent, the data vary considerably as a result of methodological differences across studies. These differences include the informant, the assessment method, the sample, the age of the participants, the specific disorder assessed, and whether an impairment index was included as part of the definition. These differences not withstanding, estimated prevalence rates of "any anxiety disorder" appear to range between

5.78 and 17.7%, with the most prevalent disorders being OAD/GAD, SAD, and SP.

Although several community- and clinic-based studies have examined prevalence in relation to sociodemographic variables, such as socioeconomic status (SES), race, gender, and age, no consistent findings have emerged (e.g., Bird et al., 1988; Bird, Gould, Yager, Staghezza, & Canino, 1989; Velez, Johnson, & Cohen, 1989). For example, in terms of SES, although children who presented to anxiety specialty clinics have been found to generally come from middle- to upper-income families (Last et al., 1992; Silverman & Nelles, 1988b), other studies have found variations across specific anxiety disorders: Low SES has been found to be associated with SAD but not OAD (Velez et al., 1989); low and middle SES have been found to be associated with SP and SOP (Strauss & Last, 1993).

Epidemiological studies of anxiety disorders in children have rarely been conducted using diverse ethnic or racial groups. An exception is the work of Bird and colleagues (Bird et al., 1988) who conducted a community study of behavioral and emotional problems in youth aged 4 to 16 in Puerto Rico. Using a multistage assessment procedure consisting of the parent and teacher versions of the Child Behavior Checklist (CBCL; Achenbach & Edelbrock, 1983) at the first stage (for screening), and a structured in-

Table 2. Prevalence of Anxiety Disorders in Recent Epidemiological Studies

Study	N	Age	Disorder					
			SAD	OAD/GAD	SP	SOP	PD/AG	AVD
Anderson et al. (1987)	792	11	3.5	2.9	2.4	2.4	—	—
McGee et al. (1990)	943	15	2.3	5.9	3.6	1.1	—	—
Bird et al. (1988)	777	4–16	4.7	—	2.6	—	—	—
Costello et al. (1988)	789	7–11	4.1	4.6	9.1	1.0	1.2	1.6
Fergusson et al. (1993)	961	15	0.5	6.3	5.1	1.7	—	—
Kashani et al. (1987)	150	14–16	4.1	—	9.1	—	—	—
Kashani et al. (1990)	210	8, 12, 17	12.9	12.4	3.3	1.0	—	—
Velez et al. (1989)	776	11–20	5.1	2.7	—	—	—	—
Cohen et al. (1993)	1495	10–20	6.1	11.3	—	—	—	—
Bowen et al. (1990)	1221	12–16	2.4	3.6	—	—	—	—

Note: Adapted from Anderson (1994).

terview at the second stage (for diagnosing), prevalence rates for the most common anxiety disorders were 2.6% for SP and 4.7% for SAD.

Prevalence rates of anxiety disorders have also rarely been examined in diverse ethnic or racial groups in clinic-based studies. Canino, Gould, Prupis, and Schaffer (1986) compared rates of anxiety symptoms (not diagnoses) in an outpatient clinic sample of African-American (n = 53) and Hispanic (n = 96) youth (age 5 to 14). Based on the children's intake information, the Hispanic children were found to present with more symptoms of fears, phobias, anxiety, panic, school refusal, and disturbed peer relationships than the African-American children.

In Last and Perrin's (1993) study comparing clinic-referred African-American and white children, rates of anxiety diagnoses were examined. No significant differences were observed between the two groups in the lifetime prevalence rates of these diagnoses. Interestingly, the top four diagnoses were the same for both groups: SP (50% in the African Americans, 40.3% in the whites), SAD (36.7 and 41%), SOP (26.7 and 36.7%), and OAD (23.3 and 28.1%). Similarly, in the authors' comparison of Hispanic and white children with anxiety disorders (Ginsburg & Silverman, 1996), the top primary diagnoses were also the same for both groups: SP (38.4% in the Hispanics and 47.6% in the whites), OAD (20.2 and 17.5%, respectively), SAD (20.2 and 10.5%), and SOP (15.2 and 9.8%).

In terms of gender, although findings in the adult area document clearly that anxiety disorders are more prevalent in women than men (Kessler et al., 1994), no clear and consistent pattern has emerged with children. In a recent review of the research literature, Costello and Angold (1995) suggested that girls may be more likely than boys to present with some type of anxiety disorder. However, the authors further noted that when specific disorders are examined, gender ratios vary and/or become inconsistent. These differences and inconsistencies

are probably related to the methodological differences noted earlier that exist across studies, as well as the different referral rates of boys and girls to mental health clinics.

In terms of age, several studies have found that, with the exception of SAD, the prevalence of anxiety disorders generally increases with age. However, inconsistencies have been reported and appear to depend on the specific disorder (e.g., Anderson, Williams, McGee, & Silva, 1987; Cohen, Cohen, & Brook, 1993; Costello et al., 1988; McGee, Feehan, Williams, & Anderson, 1992; Velez et al., 1989).

ASSESSMENT

In this section the most widely used methods for assessing anxiety disorders in children are briefly summarized. We note that there is no "best" method of assessment, as the "best" depends largely on one's specific goal or desired outcome: Different methods are better suited to attain certain goals or outcomes than others (e.g., self-rating scales for screening; interview schedules for diagnosing) (Silverman & Kurtines, 1996a). Overall, however, the prototypic assessment involves eliciting information from multiple perspectives (child, parent, teacher) and examining the three response systems—the subjective, the behavioral, and the physiological.

Clinical Interviews

The most widely used assessment method of the cognitive/subjective system is the clinical interview. Interviews are most useful for diagnosis and treatment planning. Clinical interviews are characterized as either unstructured (or nonstandardized) or structured (or standardized) (Richardson, Dohrenwend, & Klein, 1965). In the unstructured interview, different questions are asked across respondents, and the questioning proceeds in different ways depending on the respondents' presenting problems and on the interviewers' subjective judgments/training. Because of problems with the reliability of diagnoses derived from unstructured interviews (Edelbrock & Costello, 1984), the use of structured (or standardized) and semi-structured interview schedules has increased through the years. Each of these interview schedules contains its own specific series of questions that are asked of all respondents (see Silverman, 1991, 1994, for reviews).

Of the interview schedules available (e.g., the Schedule for Affective Disorders and Schizophrenia for School-Aged Children, Puig-Antich & Chambers, 1978; the Diagnostic Interview for Children and Adolescents, Herjanic & Reich, 1982; the Diagnostic Interview Schedule for Children, Costello, Edelbrock, Dulcan, Kalas, & Klaric, 1984), the Anxiety Disorders Interview Schedule for Children (ADIS-C/P; Silverman & Nelles, 1988b) was specifically designed for use with children with anxiety disorders, and its utility for diagnosing anxiety disorders in youth has been extensively studied (Rapee, Barrett, Dadds, & Evans, 1994; Silverman & Eisen, 1992; Silverman & Nelles, 1988b; Silverman & Rabian, 1995).

Self-Rating Scales

Another frequently used method for assessing the cognitive/subjective system are child self-rating scales. These scales are especially useful for screening and for identifying and quantifying symptoms. The most widely used scales for assessing general anxiety in children are the Revised Children's Manifest Anxiety Scale (Reynolds & Richmond, 1978) and the State Trait Anxiety Inventory for Children (Spielberger, 1973). Scales to assess social anxiety in children have also been developed including the Social Anxiety Scale for Children - Revised (La Greca & Stone, 1993) and the Social Phobia and Anxiety Inventory for Children (Beidel, Turner, & Morris, 1995). Measures have also been developed to assess other types of anxiety such as test

anxiety (Sarason, Davidson, Lighthall, Waite, & Ruebush, 1960), as well as to assess other specific dimensions of anxiety (e.g., anxiety sensitivity, Silverman, Fleisig, Rabian, & Peterson, 1991; school refusal behavior, Kearney & Silverman, 1993). Ollendick (1983) revised the Fear Survey Schedule for Children, a widely used measure that is useful for assessing the objects and events that children fear.

Despite the advantages of children's self-rating scales, including their ease in administration and objective scoring procedures, as well as their apparent face validity, groups defined as anxious via these rating scales are not necessarily defined this way via diagnoses. Studies comparing diagnoses with presentation on various rating scales demonstrate that optimal cutoff scores produce a high rate of false positives and false negatives (e.g., Mattison, Bagnato, & Brubaker, 1988). And declines in scores have been found to occur irrespective of treatment (e.g., Finch, Saylor, Edwards, & McIntosh, 1987; Nelson & Politano, 1990; see Silverman & Rabian, in press, for review).

In addition, these scales' discriminant and construct validity have not been sufficiently established. Specifically, it is not clear that these scales can differentiate children with anxiety disorders from children with other types of disorders (either internalizing or externalizing) (e.g., Hodges, Kline, Stern, Cytryn, & McKnew, 1982; Perrin & Last, 1992). Also, recent reviews of the research literature suggest that these scales assess the diffuse global state of "negative affectivity" (Finch, Lipovsky, & Casat, 1989; King, Ollendick, & Gullone, 1991). However, one factor that appears to distinguish between anxiety and depression is positive affectivity (e.g., Lonigan, Carey, & Finch, 1994; Watson, Clark, & Carey, 1988): Negative affectivity appears to be related to *both* anxiety and depression; the absence of positive affectivity appears to be related *only* to depression. Discriminant validity of anxiety (and depression) self-rating scales might thereby be improved by assessing the degree to which respondents report high positive affective states and to infer depression from the relative absence of such experiences (Watson & Kendall, 1989).

Self-Monitoring Procedures

Self-monitoring requires a child to self-observe and systematically record the occurrence of behavior. In working with children with anxiety disorders, self-monitoring is a useful way to assess the frequency and severity of anxiety symptoms and their antecedents and consequences. In our work, we have found it clinically useful to have children self-monitor via a "Daily Diary." The Daily Diary requires the child to keep a record of the situations in which fear/anxiety was experienced, whether she or he confronted or avoided the situation, accompanying cognitions, and a rating of fear.

Some children may have difficulty in completing the Daily Diary, however, and may thus benefit from more structured procedures. One such procedure is the self-monitoring form described by Beidel, Neal, and Lederer (1991) in which children mark on a checklist whether certain events occurred and whether they experienced certain feelings. In a community sample of elementary schoolchildren involved in an investigation of test anxiety, Beidel et al. (1991) examined the reliability of the children's self-monitoring, and also compared the frequency and severity of anxiety-producing events during a 2-week period for a test-anxious ($n = 17$) and non-test-anxious ($n = 17$) subsample. Compliance was also evaluated.

As Beidel et al. pointed out, assessing reliability for an event-oriented assessment procedure is difficult as events are variable and fluctuating. Not surprisingly, therefore, the resulting reliability coefficient (based on $N = 13$) was relatively modest and not significant ($r = .50$). As preliminary support for validity, however, the test-anxious children reported significantly more emotional distress and more negative behaviors (e.g., crying, somatic complaints) than the non-test-anxious children. In terms of compliance, Beidel et al. found compliance to be mixed, with 56% of the test-anxious children completing the forms 10 of the 14 days, and with the percentage of children completing the forms for all 14 days dropping to 31%.

In sum, although self-monitoring assessment data are clinically useful, their psychometrics require further verification. Reactivity effects and whether self-monitoring data are sensitive regarding clinical change from pre- to posttreatment also warrant investigation. Methods to increase children's compliance with and accuracy of self-monitoring should also be studied. As Beidel et al. noted, one possible way might be to present the self-monitoring task as an endeavor for the entire family (see Israel, Silverman, & Solotar, 1987, for example).

Observational Procedures

Similar to self-monitoring procedures, observational procedures are useful methods for assessing the frequency and severity of anxiety symptoms as well as their antecedents and consequences. However, rather than relying on children as self-observers, others (e.g., trained raters, parents, teachers, clinicians) serve as observers. Observational procedures also can provide researchers and clinicians with rich information about how children may behaviorally manifest the experience of fear or anxiety. Several behavior observation coding schemes have been developed to assess this manifestation (e.g., Glennon & Weisz, 1978), and they can be adapted for use in naturalistic and analogue situations.

Most clinicians are likely to find that using an analogue observational procedure is more feasible than conducting a naturalistic observation in practice. A procedure we find useful involves asking the children to confront or approach the feared object or situation. Examples of tasks might include asking children to talk about themselves for 5 minutes in front of a small audience (for SOP), to approach a dog (for SP), and to leave the clinic with the examiner without the parent (for SAD). We assess whether the child can engage in the task, for how long, and if relevant, the distance approach. These indices have also been found to be useful for evaluating change at pre- and posttreatment, in outcome research (Kendall, 1994). The reliability and validity of observational procedures in clinical samples of children with anxiety disorders have been insufficiently studied, however. The precise effects of reactivity and low- and high-demand instructions also have not been compared (e.g., "stop as soon as you begin to feel scared" versus "keep trying as hard as you can").

Psychophysiological Procedures

Assessment of the psychophysiological system typically involves measuring a child's heart rate and electrodermal activity (e.g., finger or palm sweat; see King, Hamilton, & Ollendick, 1988). There is a paucity of data on the assessment of autonomic reactivity in clinical samples of anxious children using these types of measures. An exception is Beidel (1988) who compared the pulse rate responses of children with SOP, children with OAD, and normal controls when taking a test or reading aloud in front of a small group. Children with SOP were found to have higher increases in pulse rates in both of these situations relative to children with OAD and normal controls. Although these findings suggest the potential utility of psychophysiological assessment in working with children with anxiety disorders, the complexities of this type of assessment, individual differences in arousal patterns, and the instruments' sensitivity to nonanxiety influences have served to hinder the full establishment of their psychometric properties. This remains to be done in future research.

TREATMENT

Of the various treatment approaches that have been used (e.g., psychodynamic, family systems, cognitive, behavioral, and pharmacological), the cognitive and behavioral have been studied the most systematically. However, even these procedures have been insufficiently evaluated via controlled clinical trials designs, multimethod–multisource assessments, and systematic follow-up procedures. In addition, our knowledge about potential predictors of treatment outcome (e.g., comorbidity, parental anxiety symptoms) remains elusive. Also notably absent from the literature is a framework to help guide clinicians' and researchers' thinking in how to go about developing and implementing intervention approaches for children with anxiety disorders. In this section we provide a brief overview of the research literature on each of these treatment approaches. We then present our evolving "transfer of control" model, which may serve as a useful framework for developing and implementing psychosocial interventions.

Psychodynamic

Most of the literature using psychodynamic approaches is characterized by case reports (e.g., Le Roy & Derdeyn, 1976). The absence of experimental studies is related, in part, to difficulties in defining the constructs of psychodynamic theory and the long duration of psychodynamic treatment (see King et al., 1988). Thus, although the published case reports generally demonstrate success, documentation of the effectiveness of psychodynamic treatment for childhood anxiety awaits controlled testing (Bemporad, Beresin, & Rauch, 1993).

A recent study provided some preliminary support, however (Fonagy & Target, 1994). Although the focus of this study was on the effectiveness of treatment for children with disruptive disorders, the investigators used a comparison group of children with "emotional disorders." Sixty-eight percent of the children in this group presented with some type of anxiety disorder. Specifically, the study examined treatment outcome, based on chart reviews, of 135 children (age 3.2 to 17.6 years) with disruptive disorders and 135 children (age 2.7 to 18 years) with "emotional disorders." Treatment outcome was assessed via clinician-determined diagnostic status and two measures of clinically significant change (improvement or return to normal functioning). Relevant here is the finding that 52.6% of the 135 children in the emotional disorder group no longer met diagnostic criteria at the end of treatment and 72.6% showed reliable improvement. Interestingly, children with disruptive disorders who presented with a comorbid anxiety disorder showed greater improvement than children with disruptive disorders who had no comorbid anxiety disorder. Despite methodological limitations of this study (e.g., method and timing of assessments, lack of random assignment and control group), it represents an initial step in identifying the types of child problems that may improve from psychodynamic treatment.

Cognitive Behavioral

A variety of procedures fall within the cognitive-behavioral approach including systematic desensitization, flooding, modeling, contingency management, modeling, and self-control. Descriptions of each of these procedures along with evidence supporting their effectiveness have been presented elsewhere (e.g., see King et al., 1988; Silverman & Eisen, 1993). Although this evidence has been viewed as promising, as noted, there is a paucity of controlled clinical trials.

Recently, however, Kendall (1994) reported the results of a controlled clinical trials study designed to evaluate the effectiveness of a cognitive-behavioral treatment program for children diagnosed with DSM-III-R anxiety disorders (except SP). The program was 16 weeks in duration and involved cognitive (i.e., recognizing and clarifying distorted cognitions and attributions, devising coping plans, evaluating performance, and administering self-reinforcement) and behavioral (i.e., in vivo exposures, relaxation training, contingent reinforcement) components. The children (age 9–13) were randomly assigned to the cognitive-behavioral condition (n = 27) or a wait-list control condition (n = 20). A multimethod approach to assessing treatment outcome was used, including diagnosis (via the ADIS-C/P), several self-, parent-, and teacher-rating scales, and behavioral observations. Overall, findings revealed that the treatment group displayed significantly greater improvement compared with the wait-list control group on most measures at posttreatment. Further, 1- and 3.35-year follow-up assessments were conducted (Kendall & Southam-Gerow, 1996). The significant improvements found on the diagnostic changes, self-report measures, parent-report measures, and behavioral observations were maintained.

The authors have recently completed a controlled clinical trials study for children with phobic disorders. This study compared the relative effectiveness of an exposure-based contingency management (CM) condition, an exposure-based self-control (SC) condition, and an education support (ES) condition in which exposure was discussed but was not directly prescribed (such as in CM or SC). A total of 99 children (age 6–16 years, mean age = 9.9 years) and their parents participated in the study. Fifty-two were boys and 47 were girls. All children met criteria for a primary DSM-III-R diagnosis for phobic disorder, including SP (n = 82), SOP (n = 10), or AG (n = 7), based on a structured interview administered separately to the child and parent.

Each of the 99 children and their parents were randomly assigned to one of the three conditions. There were 37 children in the CM condition, 40 in the SC condition, and 22 in ES. Each condition was a 10-week treatment program in which the children and parents were seen in separate treatment sessions with the therapist, followed by a brief conjoint meeting. Results indicated that all the procedures that were used to facilitate the occurrence of exposure—the CM condition, the SC condition, and the ES condition, produced effective therapeutic change on all of the main outcome measures (child, parent, and clinicians), including the indices of clinically significant change (i.e., percentage of children who no longer met diagnostic criteria). Even more impressive, these gains were maintained at 3-, 6-, and 12-months follow-up.

In addition, the authors recently examined the effectiveness of a group format for treating children with OAD/GAD and SOP relative to a wait-list control condition. A total of 56 children (34 boys, 22 girls) and their parents participated in this study: The children were 6–17 years old, with an average age of 9.96 years. Using proportional random assignment, 37 (66%) of the participants were assigned to the group treatment format and 19 (33%) to the wait-list condition.

The results of this clinical trials outcome study provided strong evidence for the group treatment format's efficacy. Differences in the recovery rates for participants in group treatment versus the wait-list control condition were dramatic. This was observed first with respect to diagnosis: 63% of the children in the group treatment were recovered at posttreatment (i.e., no longer met diagnostic criteria) compared to only 20% in the control condition. Treatment maintenance was equally impressive: There was a consistent trend for treatment gains to continue well after treatment ended. For example, there was no evidence at any of the follow-up points (3, 6, and 12 months) for the occurrence of relapse among any of the recovered participants. And even the children who had continued to meet diagnostic criteria at posttreatment showed a pattern of improvement in terms of severity and interference ratings.

This pattern of improvement in terms of diagnosis and clinical severity and interference (at posttreatment and throughout the follow-ups) was evident as well by both the child- and parent-completed measures. Specifically, there was a pattern of significant condition by time interactions. This was observed on the most important child self-report measure of anxious symptomatology, the RCMAS. This pattern of the differential effectiveness of group treatment (i.e., significant condition by time interactions) was even more dramatic for the various parent-completed measures, such as the parent-completed version of the RCMAS, the CBCL subscales and total scale, and parents' global ratings of severi-

ty. In addition, not only did parents in the group treatment report gains for their children, but parents in the wait-list control condition also reported that their children were worse, or had deteriorated, at the postwait assessment.

Finally, the pattern for all the child- and parent-completed measures indicated a continued reduction in degree and severity of anxious symptomatology from posttreatment to 3 months' follow-up, with improvement leveling off at that time but still being maintained at 6- and 12-month follow-up.

The authors and colleagues (e.g., Silverman & Kurtines, 1996a,b) have incorporated the research findings from these two clinical trial studies in developing a model or framework to help conceptualize the treatment of anxiety disorders in children. This model, referred to as the transfer-of-control, is discussed subsequently.

Family

There is very little in the treatment research literature on reducing fear and anxiety in children using family systems intervention approaches. Interestingly, the case reports and few controlled studies that do exist frequently include the concepts and procedures of cognitive-behavioral therapy (as opposed to the concepts and procedures of family systems therapy). For example, Dadds and colleagues have been involved in evaluating the effectiveness of a family intervention approach that emanates from cognitive-behavioral theory and therapy. In a preliminary study, Dadds, Heard, and Rapee (1992) randomly assigned 14 children (age 7–14) diagnosed with an anxiety disorder to either a cognitive-behavioral therapy plus family management treatment condition (which focused on how parents interact with their child during displays of anxiety, their management of emotional upsets, and family communication and problem-solving skills), or to a wait-list control condition. At posttreatment, 5 of the 7 children in the family treatment no longer met diagnostic criteria. No changes were found in the diagnostic status of the children in the wait-list condition. Children in the family treatment also showed significant improvement relative to the wait-list controls on anxiety and behavior rating scales.

In a larger randomized clinical trial study, Barrett, Dadds, & Rapee (1996) recently compared the effectiveness of this cognitive-behavioral therapy plus family management intervention ($n = 25$) to a cognitive-behavioral therapy condition (without the family management component; $n = 28$) and to a wait-list control condition ($n = 26$). The results indicated that across treatment conditions, 69.8% of children no longer fulfilled diagnostic criteria for an anxiety disorder in comparison with 26% of children in the wait-list. At 12-month follow-up, however, 70.3% of children in the cognitive-behavioral therapy condition no longer met criteria for diagnostic status, in comparison with 95.6% of children in the cognitive-behavioral therapy plus family management intervention condition. Children in the latter condition also showed greater improvement on self-rating scales and clinician ratings.

Pharmacological

Reviews of the pharmacological treatment literature reveal that a variety of pharmacological agents such as antidepressants, antihistamines, stimulants, and anxiolytics have been used in the treatment of childhood anxiety disorders. Much of this work predates DSM-III and ambiguous terms such as *neurosis, phobic neurosis, anxious,* or *school phobic* were used to describe the child participants limiting the generalizability of these studies. Although more recent studies have employed DSM-III or DSM-III-R criteria (e.g., Kranzler, 1988; Leonard et al., 1989; Simeon et al., 1992), the number of studies are small and few have used double-blind placebo controls.

Recent literature reviews have concluded that, with the exception of clomipramine and fluoxetine for the treatment of OCD and ben-

zodiazepines for PD, the efficacy of psychopharmacological treatments for anxiety disorders in children is unclear. Moreover, although some medications appear helpful, it is generally recommended that they be used in combination with other therapies, particularly cognitive and behavioral (Kutcher, Reiter, & Gardner, 1995; Kutcher, Reiter, Gardner, & Klein, 1992).

A Framework for Treatment: Transfer of Control

As indicated in the introduction to this section, absent from the literature is a model or framework to guide clinicians' and researchers' thinking about how to go about developing and implementing intervention approaches for children with anxiety disorders. In this section we briefly summarize our evolving transfer of control model, which may be useful for such purposes (Silverman, Ginsburg, & Kurtines, 1995; Silverman & Kurtines, 1996a,b). According to the transfer-of-control model, the therapist is viewed as an expert consultant who possesses knowledge of the skills and methods necessary to produce long-term child therapeutic change. Effective change involves a gradual transfer of the knowledge, skills and methods from the therapist to the parent to the child (Silverman & Kurtines, 1996). In treating children with anxiety disorders, the focus of treatment is on controlling the occurrence and successful implementation of exposure to the feared object or situation.

Based on our findings from our treatment outcome studies reviewed here, we have come to believe that there are several pathways that might be used to facilitate an adequate transfer of control and, consequently, there are several strategies and formats that might be used. These include a parent-focused strategy, such as CM; a child-focused strategy, such as SC; a combination of a parent- and child-focused strategy (CM followed by SC); a less prescriptive strategy, such as ES; and a group treatment strategy (Ginsburg, Silverman, & Kurtines, 1995b). The task that the authors see ahead for clinicians and researchers is to delineate the particular pathway, and thus, treatment strategy or format, that might be most useful for a child who suffers from anxiety disorders.

Our experiences have also led us to think about how treatment strategies or formats might need to be modified to try to remove "blocks" in the transfer of control. For example, elsewhere we have detailed how certain maladaptive family factors, such as parental anxiety and problematic parent-child interactions, may serve as blocks. Thus, we have suggested, and we are beginning to study, the utility of a dyadic format in which children and parents are both seen together in treatment and simultaneously work on reducing their anxious symptomatology and maladaptive interactional patterns (Ginsburg et al., 1995a). Although the transfer of control model awaits further testing and refinement, the authors are hopeful that it will serve as a useful starting point that will guide researchers' and clinicians' thinking about intervening with children with anxiety disorders.

CASE STUDY

Presenting Problems

Louis Marks, a 12-year-old white male, was referred to our Center by a school counselor because of periodic episodes of school refusal, excessive social withdrawal, and an extreme need for reassurance. Almost daily Louis would tell the teacher that he could no longer stay in the classroom, and would ask to be excused. Louis would generally be sent to the school nurse or counselor office, until his mother picked him up early from school. The counselor felt this was not a good practice, and was concerned about Louis's extreme social withdrawal and avoidance.

Assessment and Diagnosis

Louis and his mother were administered respective child and parent versions of the ADIS-C and ADIS-P. Louis also completed several self-rating scales, and was administered an in vivo behavioral task during which time his heart rate was monitored. During the interview, both Louis and his mother reported that Louis had few friends and that he hardly ever went to social activities that involved other chil-

dren. Activities that were particularly difficult for Louis included parties, eating in public, and going to public bathrooms. In school, Spanish was especially troublesome because a regular assignment was to read aloud in class and to carry on conversations with his classmates. Louis's mother described him as being "scared of everything." She said that for as long as she could remember, Louis was excessively fearful, timid, and needed constant reassurance.

Ms. Marks, a single parent, also told us that she had received psychotherapy and medication herself for panic attacks 2 years ago. She felt the treatment was generally successful, but she reported having occasional panic episodes and experiences of anxiety. Ms. Marks also told us that she was afraid to meet new people and that she had little to do with other people; stating "it's basically just Louis and me."

Based on Louis and his mothers' responses to the interview, Louis was assigned a diagnosis of SOP and GAD. His scores on the questionnaire were also elevated. Louis's in vivo behavioral exposure test, which required him to talk about himself for 5 minutes in front of a small audience, was terminated after 3 minutes on his request that the task be discontinued.

Treatment

Louis was enrolled in a 10-week exposure-based treatment program in which parent and child were seen individually and then briefly together. The program, based on the transfer of control model, involved first teaching Louis's mother the principles of contingency management and then teaching both Louis and his mother child self-control strategies. These strategies were then applied in gradual exposure tasks that involved Louis staying for increasingly longer periods of time in Spanish class as well as using the public bathrooms in school. In planning these exposures we consulted with both the Spanish teacher and the school counselor and enlisted their cooperation and assistance.

Initial exposure tasks were successful, but as the tasks became more difficult, there was increased noncompliance. For example, the day that Louis was supposed to speak in Spanish class for 5 minutes, he spent the day running errands with his mother. In discussing this incident with Louis's mother at the next treatment session, she indicated that she thought the task too hard and was worried that her son might get a panic attack while attempting it. Thus, related in part to Ms. Marks's own history of anxiety, the transfer of control pathway from mother to child was "blocked" in this particular incident.

In subsequent treatment sessions, emphasis was placed on "unblocking" the mother–child pathway of transfer of control. This was accomplished by first pointing out to Ms. Marks how her behaviors were working against the program's main goals of increasing Louis's approach behavior, and she was helped to see distinctions between herself and her son (e.g., "because you panic doesn't mean Louis will"). Ms. Marks was encouraged to discuss her discomfort in seeing her son anxious and her "instinct" to reassure and protect him. The role that her own social anxiety played in this incident was also discussed. Alternative solutions to such "protective behaviors" were generated. After discussing these issues, Ms. Marks signed up for an adult community education class—something she always wanted to do. Ms. Marks also received additional training in the use and application of appropriate contingencies, followed by more explicit instruction in how to encourage Louis to use his newly acquired self-control skills.

All of these methods were helpful in unblocking the pathway between Ms. Marks and Louis; their subsequent contracts were all successfully carried out, including the one that had previously given

Louis trouble, namely, speaking about himself in Spanish for 5 minutes in front of the class.

In the final phase of the transfer of control, wherein self-control strategies were used (including self-reward to replace parental rewards), Louis practiced examining the specific cognitions that played a role in maintaining his fear of social situations (e.g., "the kids will laugh at me"). Louis learned to recognize when he was afraid or worried, to employ more adaptive coping thoughts and behaviors, and to praise himself for doing so.

Posttreatment and Follow-up

At posttreatment assessment, readministration of the relevant sections of the ADIS-C and ADIS-P revealed that Louis no longer met criteria for SOP and GAD, and there was no longer any interference in his daily functioning. In addition, his scores on the questionnaires decreased markedly and Louis was able to talk about himself in front of a small audience for the full 5 minutes of the in vivo behavioral exposure test. These gains were maintained at 3-, 6-, and 12-month follow-up assessment points.

SUMMARY

This chapter presented an overview of what is currently known about anxiety disorders in children, beginning with a discussion about phenomenology and differential diagnosis. Current thinking about etiology—both genetic/neurobiological and psychosocial perspectives—was presented next. This was followed by a summary of the epidemiological data, which indicate an average prevalence rate of about 5% (based primarily on Caucasian community samples), with higher rates in clinical samples. The chapter discussed assessment and treatment procedures that have been found useful for working with children with anxiety disorders, including our evolving transfer of control model as a possible framework to help guide clinicians' and researchers' thinking in how to develop and implement interventions. A case study was presented to illustrate the treatment model. Overall, this chapter illustrates the strides made by recent research pertaining to children with anxiety disorders. We are confident that further strides will continue into the next century and significantly advance conceptual and practical knowledge.

REFERENCES

Abe, K. (1972). Phobias and nervous symptoms in childhood and maturity: Persistence and associations. *British Journal of Psychiatry, 120,* 275–283.

Achenbach, T. M., & Edelbrock, C. (1983). *Manual for the Child Behavior Checklist and Revised Child Behavior Profile.* Burlington: University of Vermont, Department of Psychology.

Adamec, R. E., & Stark-Adamec, C. S. (1989). Behavioral inhibition and anxiety: Dispositional, developmental, and neural aspects of the anxious personality of the domestic cat. In J. S. Reznick (Ed.), *Perspective on behavioral inhibition* (pp. 93–124). Chicago: University of Chicago Press.

Agras, W. S., Chapin, H. N., & Oliveau, D. C. (1972). The natural history of phobia, *Archives of General Psychiatry, 26,* 315–317.

Ainsworth, M. D. S., Blehar, M., Waters, E., & Wall, S. (1978). *Patterns of attachment.* Hillsdale, NJ: Erlbaum.

Albano, A. M., Knox, L. S., & Barlow, D. H. (1995). Obsessive-compulsive disorder. In A. R. Eisen, C. A. Kearney, & C. A. Schafer (Eds.), *Clinical handbook of anxiety disorders in children and adolescents* (pp. 282–316). Northvale, NJ: Jason Aronson, Inc.

American Psychiatric Association. (1980). *Diagnostic and statistical manual of mental disorders* (3rd ed.). Washington, DC: Author.

American Psychiatric Association. (1994). *Diagnostic and statistical manual of mental disorders* (4th ed.). Washington, DC: Author.

Anderson, J. C. (1994). Epidemiology. In T. H. Ollendick, N. J. King, & W. Yule (Eds.), *International handbook of phobic and anxiety disorders in children and adolescents* (pp. 293–315). New York: Plenum Press.

Anderson, J. C., Williams, S., McGee, R., & Silva, P. A. (1987). DSM-III disorders in preadolescent children. *Archives of General Psychiatry, 44,* 69–76.

Asher, S. R., & Coie, J. D. (1990). *Peer rejection in childhood.* London: Cambridge University Press.

Atkinson, L., Quarrington, B., Cyr, J. J., & Atkinson, F. V. (1989). Differential classification in school refusal. *British Journal of Psychiatry, 155,* 191–195.

Barlow, D. H. (1988). *Anxiety and its disorders: The nature and treatment of anxiety and panic.* New York: Guilford Press.

Barrett, P. M., Dadds, M. R., & Rapee, R. M. (1996). Family treatment of childhood anxiety: A controlled trial. *Journal of Consulting and Clinical Psychology, 64,* 333–342.

Barrett, P. M., Rapee, R. M., Dadds, M. M., & Ryan, S. M. (1996). Family enhancement of cognitive style in anxious and aggressive children. *Journal of Abnormal Child Psychology, 24,* 187–203.

Beidel, D. C. (1988). Psychophysiological assessment of anxious emotional states in children. *Journal of Abnormal Child Psychology, 97,* 80–82.

Beidel, D. C., Neal, A. M., & Lederer, A. S. (1991). The feasibility and validity of a daily diary for the assessment of anxiety in children. *Behavior Therapy, 22,* 505–517.

Beidel, D. C., & Turner, S. M. (1988). Comorbidity of test anxiety and other anxiety disorders in children. *Journal of Abnormal Child Psychology, 16,* 275–287.

Beidel, D. C., Turner, S. M., & Morris, T. L. (1995). A new inventory to assess childhood social anxiety and phobia: The Social Phobia and Anxiety Inventory for Children. *Psychological Assessment, 7,* 73–79.

Belenky, M. F., Clinchy, B. M., Goldberger, N. R., & Tarule, J. M. (1986). *Women's ways of knowing.* New York: Basic Books.

Bell-Dolan, D., & Wessler, A. E. (1994). Attributional style of anxious children: Extensions from cognitive theory and research on adult anxiety. *Journal of Anxiety Disorders, 8,* 79–96.

Bemporad, J. R., Beresin, E., & Rauch, P. (1993). Psychodynamic theories and treatment of childhood anxiety disorders. *Child and Adolescent Psychiatric Clinics of North America, 2,* 763–777.

Berg, C., Rapoport, J. L., Whitaker, A., Davies, M., Leonard, H., Swedo, S., Braiman, S., & Lenane, M. (1989). Childhood obsessive compulsive disorder: A two-year prospective follow-up of a community sample. *Journal of the American Academy of Child and Adolescent Psychiatry, 28,* 528–533.

Berg, I. (1976). School phobia in the children of agoraphobic women. *British Journal of Psychiatry, 128,* 86–89.

Berg, I., Butler, A., & Pritchard, J. (1974). Psychiatric illness in the mothers of school phobic adolescents. *British Journal of Psychiatry, 125,* 466–467.

Berg, I., & McGuire, R. (1974). Are mothers of school phobic adolescents over protective? *British Journal of Psychiatry, 124,* 10–13.

Berg, I., Nichols, K., & Pritchard, C. (1969). School-phobia—Its classification and relationship to dependency. *Journal of Child Psychology and Psychiatry, 10,* 123–141.

Bernstein, G. A., & Garfinkel, B. D. (1986). School phobia: The overlap of affective and anxiety disorders. *Journal of the American Academy of Child and Adolescent Psychiatry, 25,* 235–241.

Bernstein, G. A., & Garfinkel, B. D. (1988). Pedigrees, functioning, and psychopathology in families of school phobic children. *Journal of the American Academy of Child and Adolescent Psychiatry, 27,* 70–74.

Biederman, J., Rosenbaum, J. F., Bolduc-Murphy, E. A., Faraone, S. V., Chaloff, J., Hirshfeld, D. R., & Kagan, J. (1993a). A three year follow-up of children with and without behavioral inhibition. *Journal of the American Academy of Child and Adolescent Psychiatry, 32,* 814–821.

Biederman, J., Rosenbaum, J. F., Bolduc-Murphy, E. A., Faraone, S. V., Chaloff, J., Hirshfeld, D. R., & Kagan, J. (1993b). Behavioral inhibition as a temperamental risk factor for anxiety disorders. *Child and Adolescent Psychiatric Clinics of North America, 2,* 667–684.

Biederman, J., Rosenbaum, J. F., Chaloff, J., & Kagan, J. (1995). Behavioral inhibition as a risk factor. In J. S. March (Ed.), *Anxiety disorders in children and adolescents* (pp. 61–81). New York: Guilford Press.

Biederman, J., Rosenbaum, J. F., Hirshfeld, D. R., Faraone, V., Bolduc, E., Gersten, M., Meminger, S., & Reznick, S. (1990). Psychiatric correlates of behavioral inhibition in young children of parents with and without psychiatric disorders. *Archives of General Psychiatry, 47,* 21–26.

Bird, H. R., Canino, G., Rubio-Stipec, M., Gould, M. S., Ribera J., Sesman, M., Woodbury, M., Huertas-Goldman, S., Pagan, A., Sanches-Lacay, A., & Moscoso, M. (1988). Estimates of the prevalence of childhood maladjustment in a community survey in Puerto Rico. *Archives of General Psychiatry, 45,* 1120–1126.

Bird, H. R., Gould, M. S., Yager, T., Staghezza, B., & Canino, G. (1989). Risk factors for maladjustment in Puerto Rican children. *Journal of the American Academy of Child and Adolescent Psychiatry, 28,* 847–850.

Bowen, R. C., Offord, D. R., & Boyle, M. H. (1990). The prevalence of overanxious disorder and separation disorder in the community results from the Ontario Mental Health Study. *Journal of the American Academy of Child and Adolescent Psychiatry, 29,* 753–758.

Bowlby, J. (1973). *Attachment and loss: Vol. 2. Separation.* New York: Basic Books.

Burke, A. E., & Silverman, W. K. (1987). The prescriptive treatment of school refusal. *Clinical Psychology Review, 29,* 570–574.

Canino, I. A., Gould, M. S., Prupis, S., & Shaffer, D. (1986). A comparison of symptoms and diagnosis in Hispanic and black children in an outpatient mental health clinic. *Journal of the American Academy of Child Psychiatry, 25,* 254–259.

Cantwell, D. P., & Baker, L. (1989). Stability and natural history of DSM-III childhood diagnoses. *Journal of the American Academy of Child and Adolescent Psychiatry, 29,* 691–700.

Caron, C., & Rutter, M. (1991). Comorbidity in child psychopathology: Concepts, issues, and research. *Journal of Child Psychology and Psychiatry, 32,* 1063–1080.

Chorpita, B. F., Albano, A. M., & Barlow, D. H. (1996). Cognitive processing in children: Relationship to anxiety and family influences. *Journal of Clinical Child Psychology, 25,* 170–176.

Clarke, J. C., & Jackson, J. A. (1983). *Hypnosis and behavior therapy: The treatment of anxiety and phobias.* Berlin: Springer.

Cohen, P., Cohen, J., & Brook, J. S. (1993). An epidemiological study of disorders in late childhood and adolescence: II. Persistence of disorders. *Journal of Child Psychology and Psychiatry, 34,* 867–875.

Costello, A. J., Edelbrock, C. S., Dulcan, M. K., Kalas, R., & Klaric, S. H. (1984). *Report to NIMH on the NIMH Diagnostic Interview Schedule for Children (DISC).* Washington, DC: National Institute of Mental Health.

Costello, E. J., & Angold, A. (1995). Epidemiology. In J. S. March (Ed.), *Anxiety disorders in children and adolescents* (pp. 109–122). New York: Guilford Press.

Costello, E. J., Costello, A. J., Edelbrock, C. S., Burns, B. J., Dulcan, M. J., Brent, D., & Janiszewski, S. (1988). DSM-III disorders in pediatric primary care: Prevalence and risk factors. *Archives of General Psychology, 45,* 1107–1116.

Croake, J. W. (1969). Fears of children. *Human Development, 12,* 239–247.

Dadds, M. R., Barrett, P. M., Rapee, R. M., & Ryan, S. (1996). Family process and child anxiety and aggression: An observational analysis. *Journal of Abnormal Child Psychology, 24,* 715–734.

Dadds, M. R., Heard, P. M., & Rapee, R. M. (1992). The role of family intervention in the treatment of childhood anxiety disorders: Some preliminary findings. *Behaviour Change, 9,* 171–177.

Davey, G. C. L. (1992). Classical conditioning and the acquisition of human fears and phobias: A review and synthesis of the literature. *Advances in Behaviour Research and Therapy, 14,* 29–66.

Edelbrock, C., & Costello, A. (1984). Structured psychiatric interviews for children and adolescents. In G. Goldstein & M. Hersen (Eds.), *Handbook of psychological assessment* (pp. 276–290). New York: Pergamon Press.

Eysenck, H. J. (1979). The conditioning model of neurosis. *Behavioral and Brain Sciences, 2,* 155–199.

Fergusson, D. M., Horwood, L. J., & Lynskey, M. T. (1993). Prevalence and comorbidity of DSM-III-R diagnoses in a birth cohort of 15 year-olds. *Journal of the American Academy of Child and Adolescent Psychiatry, 32,* 1127–1134.

Finch, A. J., Jr., Lipovsky, J. A., & Casat, C. D. (1989). Anxiety and depression in children and adolescents: Negative affectivity or separate constructs? In P. C. Kendall & D. Watson (Eds.), *Anxiety and depression: Distinctive and overlapping features* (pp. 171–196). San Diego, CA: Academic Press.

Finch, A. J., Saylor, C. F., Edwards, G. L., & McIntosh, J. A. (1987). Children's Depression Inventory: Reliability over repeated administrations. *Journal of Clinical Child Psychology, 16,* 339–341.

Flament, M. F., Whitaker, A., Rapoport, J. L., Davies, M., Zeremba-Berg, C., Kalikow, K. S., Sceery, W., & Shaffer, D. (1988). Obsessive compulsive disorder in adolescence: An epidemiological study. *Journal of the American Academy of Child and Adolescent Psychiatry, 27,* 764–771.

Foley, D., & Hay, D. A. (1992). Genetics and the nature of anxiety disorders. In G. F. Burrows, M. Roth, & R. Noyes, Jr. (Eds.), *Handbook of anxiety: Contemporary issues and prospects for research in anxiety disorders* (pp. 21–56). Amsterdam: Elsevier.

Fonagy, P., & Target, M. (1994). The efficacy of psychoanalysis for children with disruptive disorders. *Journal of the American Academy of Child and Adolescent Psychiatry, 33,* 45–55.

Fox, J. E., & Houston, B. K. (1981). Efficacy of self-instructional training for reducing children's anxiety in an evaluative situation. *Behavior Research and Therapy, 19,* 509–515.

Francis, G. (1988). Assessing cognitions in anxious children. *Behavior Modification, 12,* 267–280.

Francis, G., Last, C. G., & Strauss, C. C. (1987). Expression of separation anxiety disorder: The roles of age and gender. *Child Psychiatry and Human Development, 18,* 82–89.

Freud, S. (1909/1955). Analysis of a phobia in a five-year-old boy. In J. Strachey (Ed. and Trans.), *Standard edition of the complete psychological works of Sigmund Freud* (Vol. 10, pp. 3–149). London: Hogarth Press.

Fyer, A. J., Mannuzza, S., Gallops, M. P., Martin, L. Y., Aaronson, C., Gorman, J. M., Liebowitz, M. R., & Klein, D. F. (1990). Familial transmission of simple phobias and fears. *Archives of General Psychiatry, 47,* 252–256.

Gerslma, C., Emmelkamp, P. M. G., & Arrindell, W. A. (1990). Anxiety, depression, and perception of early parenting: A meta-analysis. *Clinical Psychology Review, 10,* 251–277.

Gilligan, C. (1982). *In a different voice.* Cambridge, MA: Harvard University Press.

Ginsburg, G. S., Alonso E., Hammond-Laurence, K., & Silverman, W. K. (1995, November). *Depressive symptoms as a predictor of impaired peer relationships in youth with anxiety disorders.* Poster session presented at the 29th Annual Association for the Advancement of Behavior Therapy, Washington, DC.

Ginsburg, G. S., & Silverman, W. K. (1996). Phobic and anxiety disorders in Hispanic and Caucasian youth. *Journal of Anxiety Disorders, 10,* 517–528.

Ginsburg, G. S., Silverman, W. K., & Kurtines, W. M. (1995a). Family involvement in treating children with anxiety and phobic disorders: A look ahead. *Clinical Psychology Review, 15,* 457–473.

Ginsburg, G. S., Silverman, W. K., & Kurtines, W. M. (1995b). Cognitive-behavioral group therapy. In A. R. Eisen, C. A. Kearney, & C. E. Schaefer (Eds.), *Clinical handbook of anxiety disorders in children* (pp. 521–549). Northvale, NJ: Jason Aronson.

Glennon, B., & Weisz, J. R. (1978). An observational approach to the assessment of anxiety in young children. *Journal of Consulting and Clinical Psychology, 46,* 1246–1257.

Hammond-Laurence, K., & Silverman, W. K. (submitted). Comorbidity among childhood psychiatric disorders in clinic-referred children and adolescents with anxiety disorders.

Hampe, E., Noble, M., Miller, L. C., & Barrett, C. L. (1973). Phobic children at two years post-treatment. *Journal of Abnormal Psychology, 82,* 446–453.

Hekmat, H. (1987). Origins and development of human fear reactions. *Journal of Anxiety Disorders, 1,* 197–218.

Herjanic, B., & Reich, W. (1982). Development of a structured psychiatric interview for children: Agreement between child and parent on individual symptoms. *Journal of Abnormal Child Psychiatry, 10,* 307–324.

Hirshfeld, D. R., Rosenbaum, J. F., Biederman, J., Bolduc, E. A., Faraone, S. V., Snidman, N., Reznick, J. S., & Kagan, J. (1992). Stable behavioral inhibition and its association with anxiety disorder. *Journal of the American Academy of Child and Adolescent Psychiatry, 31,* 103–111.

Hodges, K., Kline, J., Stern, L., Cytryn, L., & McKnew, D. (1982). The development of a child assessment interview for research and clinical use. *Journal of Abnormal Child Psychology, 10,* 173–189.

Israel, A. C., Silverman, W. K., & Solotar, L. C. (1987). Baseline adherence as a predictor of dropout in a children's weight-reduction program. *Journal of Consulting and Clinical Psychology, 55,* 791–793.

Jones, M. C. (1924a). The elimination of children's fears. *Journal of Experimental Psychology, 1,* 383–390.

Jones, M. C. (1924b). A laboratory study of fear: The case of Peter. *Pedagogical Seminar, 31,* 308–315.

Kagan, J. (1989). Temperamental contributions to social behavior. *American Psychologist, 44,* 668–674.

Kagan, J., Reznick, J. S., & Gibbons, J. (1989). Inhibited and uninhibited types of children. *Child Development, 60,* 838–845.

Kagan, J., Reznick, J. S., & Snidman, N. (1987). The physiology and psychology of behavioral inhibition. *Child Development, 58,* 1459–1473.

Kagan, J., Reznick, J. S., & Snidman, N. (1988). Biological bases of childhood shyness. *Science, 240,* 167–171.

Kashani, J. H., Beck, N. C., Hoeper, E. W., Fallahi, C., Corcoran, C. M., McAllister, J. A., Rosenberg, T. K., & Reid, J. C. (1987). Psychiatric disorders in a community sample of adolescents. *American Journal of Psychiatry, 144,* 584–589.

Kashani, J. H., Vaidya, A. F., Soltys, S. M., Dandoy, A. C., Katz, L. M., & Reid, J. C. (1990). Correlates of anxiety in psychiatrically hospitalized children and their parents. *Journal of Psychiatry, 143,* 319–323.

Kearney, C. A., Eisen, A. R., & Silverman, W. K. (1995). The legend and myth of school phobia. *School Psychology Quarterly, 10,* 65–85.

Kearney, C. A., & Silverman, W. K. (1992). Let's not push the "panic button": A cautionary analysis of panic disorder in adolescents. *Clinical Psychology Review, 12,* 293–302.

Kearney, C. A., & Silverman, W. K. (1993). Measuring the function of school refusal behavior: The School Refusal Assessment Scale. *Journal of Clinical Child Psychology, 22,* 85–96.

Kearney, C. A., & Silverman, W. K. (1995). Family environment of youngsters with school refusal behavior: A synopsis with implications for assessment and treatment. *American Journal of Family Therapy, 23,* 59–72.

Kendall, P. C. (1994). Treating anxiety disorders in children: Results of a randomized clinical trial. *Journal of Consulting and Clinical Psychology, 62,* 200–210.

Kendall, P. C., & Chansky, T. E. (1991). Considering cogni-

tion in anxiety-disordered children. *Journal of Anxiety Disorders, 5,* 167–185.

Kendall, P. C., Howard, B. L., & Epps, J. (1988). The anxious child: Cognitive behavioral treatment strategies. *Behavior Modification, 12,* 281–310.

Kendall, P. C., & Southam-Gerow, M. A. (1996). Long-term follow-up of a cognitive-behavioral therapy for anxiety-disordered youths. *Journal of Consulting and Clinical Psychology, 64,* 724–730.

Kessler, R. C., McGonagle, K. A., Zhao, S., Nelson, C. B., Hughes, M., Eshleman, S., Wittchen, H. U., & Kendler, K. S. (1994). Lifetime and 12-month prevalence of DSM-III-R psychiatric disorders in the United States. *Archives of General Psychiatry, 51,* 8–19.

King, N. J., Hamilton, D. I., & Ollendick, T. H. (1988). *Children's phobias: A behavioural perspective.* New York: Wiley.

King, N. J., Ollendick, T. H., & Gullone, E. (1991). Negative affectivity in children and adolescents: Relations between anxiety and depression. *Clinical Psychology Review, 11,* 441–459.

Klein, G. K., & Last, C. G. (1989). *Anxiety disorders in children.* Newbury Park, CA: Sage.

Kohut, J. (1994). *The little book of phobias.* Running Press: Philadelphia, PA.

Kranzler, H. (1988). Use of buspirone in an adolescent with overanxious disorder. *Journal of the American Academy of Child and Adolescent Psychiatry, 27,* 789–790.

Kutcher, S. P., Reiter, S., & Gardner, D. M. (1995). Pharmacotherapy: Approaches and applications. In J. S. March (Ed.), *Anxiety disorders in children and adolescents* (pp. 341–385). New York: Guilford Press.

Kutcher, S. P., Reiter, S., Gardner, D. M., & Klein, R. G. (1992). The pharmacotherapy of anxiety disorders in children and adolescents. *Child and Adolescent Psychiatric Clinics of North America, 15,* 41–67.

La Greca, A. M., & Stone, W. L. (1993). The Social Anxiety Scale for Children-Revised. Factor structure and concurrent validity. *Journal of Clinical Child Psychology, 22,* 17–27.

Lang, P. J. (1977). Imagery in therapy: An information processing analysis of fear. *Behavior Therapy, 8,* 862–886.

Last, C. G., Hersen, M., Kazdin, A. E., Finkelstein, R., & Strauss, C. C. (1987). Comparison of DSM-III separation anxiety and overanxious disorder: Demographic characteristics and patterns of comorbidity. *Journal of the American Academy of Child and Adolescent Psychiatry, 26,* 527–531.

Last, C. G., Hersen, M., Kazdin, A. E., Francis, G., & Grubb, H. J. (1987). Psychiatric illness in the mothers of anxious children. *American Journal of Psychiatry, 144,* 1580–1583.

Last, C. G., Hersen, M., Kazdin, A., Orvaschel, H., & Perrin, S. (1991). Anxiety disorders and their families. *Archives of General Psychiatry, 48,* 928–934.

Last, C. G., & Perrin, S. (1993). Anxiety disorders in African-American and white children. *Journal of Abnormal Child Psychology, 2*, 153–164.

Last, C. G., Perrin, S., Hersen, M., & Kazdin, A. E. (1992). DSM-III-R anxiety disorders in children: Sociodemographic and clinical characteristics. *Journal of the American Academy of Child and Adolescent Psychiatry, 31*, 1070–1076.

Last, C. G., Phillips, J. E., & Statfeld, A. (1987). Childhood anxiety disorders in mothers and their children. *Child Psychiatry and Human Development, 18*, 103–110.

Last, C. G., Strauss, C. C., & Francis, G. (1987). Comorbidity among childhood anxiety disorders. *Journal of Nervous and Mental Disease, 175*, 726–730.

Leonard, H. L., & Rapoport, J. (1991). Obsessive compulsive disorder. In J. M. Wiener (Ed.), *Textbook of child and adolescent psychiatry* (pp. 323–329). Washington, DC: American Psychiatric Press.

Leonard, H. L., Swedo, S. E., Rapoport, J. L., Koby, E. V., Lenane, M. C., Cheslow, D. L., & Hamburger, S. D. (1989). Treatment of obsessive-compulsive disorder with clomipramine and desipramine in children and adolescents. A double-blind crossover comparison. *Archives of General Psychiatry, 46*, 1088–1092.

Le Roy, J. B., & Derdeyn, A. (1976). Drawings as a therapeutic medium: The treatment of separation anxiety in a four-year-old boy. *Child Psychiatry and Human Development, 6*, 155–169.

Liddell, A., & Lyons, M. (1978). Thunderstorm phobias. *Behaviour Research and Therapy, 16*, 306–308.

Livingston, R., Nugent, H., Rader, L., & Smith, G. R. (1985). Family histories of depressed and severely anxious children. *Journal of the American Academy of Child and Adolescent Psychiatry, 142*, 1497–1499.

Lonigan, C. J., Carey, M. P., & Finch, A. J. (1994). Anxiety and depression in children and adolescents: Negative affectivity and the utility of self-reports. *Journal of Consulting and Clinical Psychology, 62*, 1000–1008.

Maccoby, E. E. (1980). *Social development: Psychological growth and the parent–child relationship.* New York: Harcourt Brace Jovanovich.

Main, M., Kaplan, N., & Cassidy, J. (1985). Security in infancy, childhood and adulthood: A move to the level of representation. In I. Bretherton & E. Waters (Eds.), Growing points of attachment theory and research. *Monographs of the Society for Research in Child Development, 50*(1–2, Serial No. 209), 66–104.

Manassis, K., Bradley, S., Goldberg, S., Hood, J., & Swinson, R. P. (1994). Attachment in mothers with anxiety disorders and their children. *Journal of the American Academy of Child and Adolescent Psychiatry, 33*, 1106–1113.

March, J. S., Leonard, H. L., & Swedo, S. E. (1995). Obsessive-compulsive disorder. In J. S. March (Ed.), *Anxiety disorders in children and adolescents* (pp. 251–275). New York: Guilford Press.

Mattis, S. G., & Ollendick, T. H. (1997). Children's cognitive responses to the somatic symptoms of panic. *Journal of Abnormal Child Psychology, 25*, 47–57.

Mattison, R. E., Bagnato, S. J., & Brubaker, B. M. (1988). Diagnostic utility of the Revised Children's Manifest Anxiety Scale in children with DSM-III anxiety disorders. *Journal of Anxiety Disorders, 2*, 147–155.

McGee, R., Feehan, M., Williams, S., & Anderson, J. (1992). DSM-III disorders from age 11 to age 15 years. *Journal of the American Academy of Child and Adolescent Psychiatry, 31*, 50–59.

McGee, R., Feehan, M., Williams, S., Partridge, F., Silva, P. A., & Kelly, J. (1990). DSM-III disorders in a large sample of adolescents. *Journal of the American Academy of Child and Adolescent Psychiatry, 29*, 611–619.

Menzies, R. G., & Clarke, J. C. (1995). The etiology of phobias: A nonassociative account. *Clinical Psychology Review, 15*, 23–48.

Merckelbach, H., De Ruiter, C., Van De Hout, M. A., & Hoekstra, R. (1989). Conditioning experiences and phobias. *Behaviour Research and Therapy, 27*, 657–662.

Messer, S. C., & Beidel, D. C. (1994). Psychosocial correlates of childhood anxiety disorders. *Journal of the American Academy of Child and Adolescent Psychiatry, 33*, 975–983.

Moran, C., & Andrews, G. (1985). The familial occurrence of agoraphobia. *British Journal of Psychiatry, 146*, 262–267.

Moreau, D., & Follet, C. (1993). Panic disorder in children and adolescents. *Child and Adolescent Psychiatric Clinics of North America, 2*, 581–602.

Mowrer, O. H. (1939). A stimulus–response theory of anxiety and its role as reinforcing agent. *Psychological Review, 46*, 553–565.

Murray, E. J., & Foote, F. (1979). The origins of fear of snakes. *Behaviour Research and Therapy, 17*, 489–493.

Neal, A. M., Lilly, R. S., & Zakis, S. (1993). What are African American children afraid of? A preliminary study. *Journal of Anxiety Disorders, 7*, 129–139.

Nelles, W. B., & Barlow, D. H. (1988). Do children panic? *Clinical Psychology Review, 8*, 359–372.

Nelson, W. M., III, & Politano, P. M. (1990). Children's Depression Inventory: Stability over repeated administrations in psychiatric inpatient children. *Journal of Clinical Child Psychology, 19*, 254–256.

Ollendick, T. H. (1979). Fear reduction techniques with children. In M. Hersen, R. M. Eisler, & P. M. Miller (Eds.), *Progress in behavior modification* (Vol. 8, pp. 127–168). New York: Academic Press.

Ollendick, T. H. (1983). Reliability and validity of the revised Fear Survey Schedule for Children (FSSC-R). *Behaviour Research and Therapy, 21*, 395–399.

Ollendick, T. H., & King, N. J. (1991). Origins of childhood fears: An evaluation of Rachman's theory of fear acquisition. *Behaviour Research and Therapy, 29*, 117–123.

Ollendick, T. H., & King, N. J. (1994). Diagnosis, assessment, and treatment of internalizing problems in children: The role of longitudinal data. *Journal of Consulting and Clinical Psychology, 62*, 918–927.

Ollendick, T. H., Mattis, S. G., & King, N. J. (1994). Panic in children and adolescents: A review. *Journal of Child Psychology and Psychiatry, 35,* 113–134.

Ollendick, T. H., Yang, B., Dong, Q., Xia, Y., & Lin, L. (1995). Perceptions of fear in other children and adolescents: The role of gender and friendship status. *Journal of Abnormal Child Psychology, 23,* 439–452.

Ost, L. G. (1985). Ways of acquiring phobias and outcome of behavioral treatments. *Behaviour Research and Therapy, 23,* 683–689.

Ost, L. (1987). Age of onset in different phobias. *Journal of Abnormal Psychology, 96,* 123–145.

Parker, J. G., & Asher, S. R. (1987). Peer relations and later personal adjustment: Are low-accepted children at risk? *Psychological Bulletin, 102,* 357–389.

Perrin, S., & Last, C. G. (1992). Do childhood anxiety measures measure anxiety? *Journal of Abnormal Child Psychology, 20,* 567–578.

Prins, P. J. M. (1986). Children's self-speech and self-regulation during a fear-provoking behavioral test. *Behaviour Research and Therapy, 24,* 181–191.

Prins, P. J. M., Groot, M. J. M., & Hanewald, G. J. F. P. (1994). Cognition in test-anxious children: The role of on-task and coping cognition reconsidered. *Journal of Consulting and Clinical Psychology, 62,* 404–409.

Puig-Antich, J., & Chambers, W. (1978). *The Schedule for Affective Disorders and Schizophrenia for School-Aged Children.* New York: New York State Psychiatric Institute.

Quay, H. C., & Peterson, D. R. (1983). Interim manual for the Revised Behavior Problem Checklist. (Available from Herbert C. Quay, Box 248074, University of Miami, Coral Gables, FL 33124.)

Rachman, S. (1977). The conditioning therapy of fear acquisition: A critical examination. *Behaviour Research and Therapy, 15,* 375–387.

Rachman, S. (1983). Irrational thinking, with special reference to cognitive therapy. *Advances in Behaviour Research and Therapy, 5,* 63–68.

Rapee, R. M., Barrett, P. M., Dadds, M. R., & Evans, L. (1994). Reliability of the DSM-III-R childhood anxiety disorders using structured interview: Interrater and parent–child agreement. *Journal of the American Academy of Child and Adolescent Psychiatry, 33,* 984–992.

Reich, J., & Yates, W. (1988). Family history of psychiatric disorders in social phobia. *Comprehensive Psychiatry, 29,* 72–75.

Reiss, S. (1991). Expectancy model of fear, anxiety and panic. *Clinical Psychology Review, 11,* 141–154.

Rescorla, R. A. (1988). Pavlovian conditioning: It's not what you think it is. *American Psychologist, 43,* 151–160.

Reynolds, C. R., & Richmond, B. O. (1978). What I think and feel: A revised measure of children's manifest anxiety. *Journal of Abnormal Child Psychology, 6,* 271–280.

Richardson, S. A., Dohrenwend, B. S., & Klein, D. (1965). *Interviewing: Its forms and functions.* New York: Basic Books.

Rimm, D. C., Janda, H. L., Lancaster, D. W., Nahl, M., & Ditt-mar, K. (1977). An exploratory investigation of the origin and maintenance of phobias. *Behaviour Research and Therapy, 15,* 231–238.

Rosenbaum, J. F., Biederman, J., Bolduc, E. A., Hirshfeld, D. R., Faraone, S. V., & Kagan, J. (1992). Comorbidity of parental anxiety disorders as risk for childhood-onset anxiety in inhibited children. *American Journal of Psychiatry, 149,* 475–481.

Rosenbaum, J. F., Biederman, J., Gersten, M., Hirshfeld, D. R., Meminger, S. R., Herman, J. B., Kagan, J., Reznick, J. S., & Snidman, N. (1988). Behavioral inhibition in children of parents with panic disorder and agoraphobia. A controlled study. *Archives of General Psychiatry, 45,* 463–470.

Rubin, K. H., & Mills, R. S. L. (1991). Conceptualizing developmental pathways to internalizing disorders in childhood. *Canadian Journal of Behavioral Science, 23,* 300–317.

Sallee, R., & Greenawald, J. (1995). Neurobiology. In J. S. March (Ed.), *Anxiety disorders in children and adolescents* (pp. 3–34). New York: Guilford Press.

Sarason, S. B., Davidson, K. S., Lighthall, F. F., Waite, R. R., & Ruebush, B. K. (1960). *Anxiety in elementary school children.* New York: Wiley.

Seligman, M. E. P. (1970). On the generality of the laws of learning. *Psychological Review, 77,* 406–418.

Seligman, M. E. P. (1971). Phobias and preparedness. *Behavior Therapy, 2,* 307–320.

Silverman, W. K. (1991). Diagnostic reliability of anxiety disorders in children using structured interviews. *Journal of Anxiety Disorders, 5,* 105–124.

Silverman, W. K. (1992). Taxonomy of anxiety disorders in children. In G. D. Burrows, R. Noyes, & S. M. Roth (Eds.), *Handbook of anxiety* (Vol. 5, pp. 281–308). Amsterdam: Elsevier.

Silverman, W. K. (1993, June). Behavioral treatment of childhood phobias: An update and preliminary research findings. In E. Hibbs (Chair), *Psychosocial and combined treatment for childhood disorders: Development and issues.* Symposium conducted at the meeting of the New Clinical Drug Evaluation Unit program, Boca Raton, FL.

Silverman, W. K. (1994). Structured diagnostic interviews. In T. H. Ollendick, N. J. King, & W. Yule (Eds.), *International handbook of phobic and anxiety disorders in children and adolescents* (pp. 293–315). New York: Plenum Press.

Silverman, W. K., Cerny, J. A., & Nelles, W. B. (1988). The familial influence in anxiety disorders: Studies on the offspring of patients with anxiety disorders. In B. B. Lahey & A. E. Kazdin (Eds.), *Advances in clinical child psychology* (Vol. 11, pp. 223–248). New York: Plenum Press.

Silverman, W. K., Cerny, J. A., Nelles, W. B., & Burke, A. E. (1988). Behavior problems in children of parents with anxiety disorders. *Journal of the American Academy of Child and Adolescent Psychiatry, 27,* 779–784.

Silverman, W. K., & Eisen, A. R. (1992). Age differences in the reliability of parent and child reports of child anxious symptomatology using a structured interview. *Journal of American Academy of Child and Adolescent Psychiatry, 31,* 117–124.

Silverman, W. K.,& Eisen, A. R. (1993). Phobic disorders. In R. T. Ammerman, C. G. Last, & M. Hersen (Eds.), *Handbook of prescriptive treatments for children and adolescents* (pp. 17–197). Boston: Allyn & Bacon.

Silverman, W. K., Fleisig, W., Rabian, B., & Peterson, R. A. (1991). Childhood anxiety sensitivity index. *Journal of Clinical Child Psychology, 20,* 162–168.

Silverman, W. K., Ginsburg, G. S., & Kurtines, W. M. (1995). Clinical issues in the treatment of children with anxiety and phobic disorders. *Cognitive and Behavioral Practice, 2,* 93–117.

Silverman, W. K., & Kurtines, W. K. (1996a). *Anxiety and phobic disorders: A pragmatic approach.* New York: Plenum Press.

Silverman, W. K., & Kurtines, W. K. (1996b). Treating internalizing disorders in youth: The evolution of a transfer of control psychosocial treatment approach. In E. D. Hibbs & P. Jensen (Eds.), *Psychosocial treatment of child and adolescent disorders: Empirically based strategies for clinical practice* (pp. 63–82). Washington, DC: American Psychological Association.

Silverman, W. K., La Greca, A. M., & Wasserstein, S. (1995). What do children worry about? Worry and its relation to anxiety. *Child Development, 66,* 671–686.

Silverman, W. K., & Nelles, W. B. (1988a). The influence of gender on children's ratings of fear in self and same-aged peers. *Journal of Genetic Psychology, 149,* 17–22.

Silverman, W. K., & Nelles, W. B. (1988b). The Anxiety Disorders Interview Schedule for Children. *Journal of the American Academy of Child and Adolescent Psychiatry, 27,* 772–778.

Silverman, W. K., & Rabian, B. (1995). Test–retest reliability of the DSM-III-R anxiety disorders symptoms using the Anxiety Disorders Interview Schedule for Children. *Journal of Anxiety Disorders, 9,* 1–12.

Silverman, W. K., & Rabian, B. (in press). Rating scales for anxiety and mood disorders. In D. Shaffer & J. Richters (Eds.), *Assessment in child psychopathology.* New York: Guilford Press.

Simeon, J. G., Ferguson, H. B., Knott, V., Roberts, N., Gauthier, B., Dubois, C., & Wiggins, D. (1992). Clinical, cognitive and neurophysiological effects of alprazolam in children and adolescents with overanxious and avoidant disorders. *Journal of the American Academy of Child and Adolescent Psychiatry, 31,* 29–33.

Solomon, R. L., & Wynne, L. C. (1954). Traumatic avoidance learning: The principles of anxiety conservation and partial irreversibility. *Psychological Review, 61,* 358–385.

Solyom, L., Beck, P., Solyom, C., & Hugel, R. (1974). Some etiological factors in phobic neurosis. *Canadian Psychiatric Association Journal, 19,* 69–78.

Spielberger, C. D. (1973). *Manual for the State-Trait Anxiety In-*

ventory for Children. Palo Alto, CA: Consulting Psychologists Press.

Sroufe, L. A. (1983). Infant–caregiver attachment and patterns of adaptation in preschool: Roots of maladaptation and competence. *Minnesota Symposia on Child Psychology, 16.* Hillsdale, NJ: Erlbaum.

Stampfl, T. G. (1991). Analysis of aversive events in human psychopathology: Fear and avoidance. In M. R. Denny (Ed.), *Fear, avoidance, and phobias: A fundamental analysis* (pp.363–393). Hillsdale, NJ: Erlbaum.

Strauss, C. C., Frame, C. L., & Forehand, R. (1987). Psychosocial impairment associated with anxiety in children. *Journal of Clinical Child Psychology, 16,* 235–239.

Strauss, C. C., Lahey, B. B., Frick, P., Frame, C. L., & Hynd, G. W. (1988). Peer social status of children with anxiety disorders. *Journal of Consulting and Clinical Psychology, 56,* 137–141.

Strauss, C. C., & Last, C. G. (1993). Social and simple phobias in children. *Journal of Anxiety Disorders, 2,* 141–152.

Strauss, C. C., Lease, C. A., Kazdin, A. E., Dulcan, M. K., & Last, C. G. (1989). Multimethod assessment of the social competence of children with anxiety disorders. *Journal of Clinical Child Psychology, 18,* 184–189.

Strauss, C. C., Lease, C. A., Last, C. G., & Francis, G. (1988). Overanxious disorder: An examination of developmental differences. *Journal of Abnormal Child Psychology, 16,* 433–443.

Suomi, S. J. (1984). The development of affect in rhesus monkeys. In N. Fox & R. Davidson (Eds.), *The psychobiology of affective disorders* (pp. 119–159). Hillsdale, NJ: Erlbaum.

Suomi, S. J. (1986). Anxiety-like disorders in young nonhuman primates. In R. Gittleman (Ed.), *Anxiety disorders of childhood* (pp. 1–23). New York: Guilford Press.

Swedo, S. E., Rapoport, J. L., Leonard, H., Lenane, M., & Cheslow, D. (1989). Obsessive-compulsive disorder in children and adolescents. *Archives of General Psychiatry, 46,* 335–341.

Torgersen, S. (1985). Heredity differentiation of anxiety and affective neuroses. *British Journal of Psychiatry, 146,* 530–534.

Torgersen, S. (1990). Comorbidity of major depression and anxiety disorders in twin pairs. *American Journal of Psychiatry, 147,* 1199–1202.

Turner, S. M., Beidel, D. C., & Costello, A. (1987). Psychopathology in the offspring of anxiety disorders patients. *Journal of Consulting and Clinical Psychology, 55,* 229–235.

Vasey, M. W., Daleiden, E. L., Williams, L. L., & Brown, L. (1995). Biased attention in childhood anxiety disorders: A preliminary study. *Journal of Abnormal Child Psychology, 23,* 267–279.

Velez, C. N., Johnson, J., & Cohen, P. (1989). A longitudinal analysis of selected risk factors for childhood psychopathology. *Journal of the American Academy of Child and Adolescent Psychiatry, 28,* 861–864.

Waters, E. (1978). The stability of individual differences in infant–mother attachment. *Child Development, 49,* 483–494.

Watson, D., Clark, L. A., & Carey, G. (1988). Positive and negative affectivity and their relation to anxiety and depressive disorders. *Journal of Abnormal Psychology, 97,* 346–353.

Watson, D., & Kendall, P. C. (1989). Common and differentiating features of anxiety and depression: Current findings and future directions. In P. C. Kendall & D. Watson (Eds.), *Anxiety and depression: Distinctive and overlapping features* (pp. 493–508). New York: Academic Press.

Watson, J. B., & Rayner, R. (1920). Conditioned emotional reactions. *Journal of Experimental Psychology, 3,* 1–14.

Weissman, M. M., Leckman, J. F., Merikangas, K. R., Gammon, G. D., & Prusoff, B. A. (1984). Depression and anxiety disorders in parents and children. *Archives of General Psychiatry, 41,* 845–852.

Werry, J. S. (1991). Overanxious disorder: A review of its taxonomic properties. *Journal of the American Academy of Child and Adolescent Psychiatry, 30,* 533–544.

Wolpe, J., & Rachman, S. (1960). Psychoanalytic "evidence": A critique based on Freud's case of Little Hans. *Journal of Nervous and Mental Disease, 131,* 135–147.

Zatz, S., & Chassin, L. (1985). Cognitions of test-anxious children under naturalistic test-taking conditions. *Journal of Consulting and Clinical Psychology, 53,* 393–401.

10

Depressive Disorders

JENNIFER A. J. SCHWARTZ, TRACY R. G. GLADSTONE, AND NADINE J. KASLOW

INTRODUCTION

Several myths characterized the literature on childhood depression: (1) if depression exists in children, it is rare or occurs in "masked" form; (2) depression in youth is a transitory developmental phenomenon; and (3) childhood depression reflects a normal developmental stage. Clinical and empirical observations counter these myths, suggesting that youth depression is a major problem that interferes with development across functional domains.

This chapter uses a developmental psychopathology framework, emphasizing cognitive and interpersonal processes, to review the phenomenology, diagnosis, etiology, epidemiology, assessment, and treatment of childhood depression. Developmental psychopathologists attend to continuities and discontinuities of development, focus on the parallels between normal or abnormal processes of adaptation to stress, and suggest a bidirectional association between developmental capacities and the expression of psychopathology. The developmental psychopathology rubric guiding this chapter incorporates knowledge of normal development in understanding the expression of depression across the life span (Cicchetti & Schneider-Rosen, 1986), and emphasizes cognitive and interpersonal processes to address the depressed youth's inner experiences and transactions with the environment (Gotlib & Hammen, 1992). An illustrative case vignette and directions for future research are provided.

PHENOMENOLOGY

The historical dearth of research on childhood depression may be attributed to conflicting views regarding the existence and nature of depression in youth. For example, classical psychoanalysts maintained that depression cannot exist in children because of their immature superego development and lack of stable self-representation (e.g., Rie, 1966). Advocates of the "masked depression" perspective argued that

JENNIFER A. J. SCHWARTZ AND NADINE J. KASLOW • Department of Psychiatry and Behavioral Sciences, Emory University School of Medicine, Atlanta, Georgia 30335. TRACY R. G. GLADSTONE • Judge Baker Children's Center, Boston, Massachusetts 02115.

Handbook of Child Psychopathology, 3rd edition, edited by Ollendick & Hersen. Plenum Press, New York, 1998.

depression exists in children, but is manifested via depressive equivalents (e.g., elimination disorders, antisocial behavior, somatization) (Glaser, 1968). The most commonly held position presented in the fourth edition of the *Diagnostic and Statistical Manual* (DSM-IV; APA, 1994) is that child and adult depression present with similar affective, cognitive, motivational, and vegetative symptoms, although there may be age-specific features of mood disorders. In contrast to these conceptualizations, developmental psychopathologists suggest that depression manifests distinctly at each developmental phase (Digdon & Gotlib, 1985). They argue that in understanding depressive phenomena, it is important to consider the cognitive, affective, and interpersonal competencies associated with normal development from infancy through adolescence. To this end, the phenomenology of depression across developmental stages will be reviewed.

Infancy and Toddlerhood (0–24 Months)

The study of depressive phenomena in infancy presents a challenge, as infants lack the cognitive and language skills necessary to self-reflect and report depressive thoughts and symptoms. As a result, many caution that depressive behavior in infants may not be equivalent to adult depressive symptoms (Kovacs & Beck, 1977). However, observation of distressed infants reveals symptoms commonly associated with depression including: lethargy; feeding and sleep problems; irritability; sad or expressionless faces; decreased affective responsivity, attentive behavior, and curiosity; and increased frowning and crying (Carlson & Kashani, 1988; Field, 1984). These symptoms mimic deprivation reactions noted in infants separated from their primary caretakers (Bowlby, 1981; Spitz, 1946).

Preschool Years (2–5 Years)

Research identifies several symptoms associated with depressive behavior in preschoolers, including anger and irritability, sad facial expres-

sion, labile mood, somatic complaints, feeding and sleep problems, lethargy, excessive crying, hyper- or hypoactivity, decreased socialization, tantrums, separation anxiety, and anhedonia (Carlson & Kashani, 1988; Kashani, Holcomb, & Orvaschel, 1986). Depression in preschoolers is difficult to assess, as these children have difficulty verbalizing and reflecting on their inner experiences. Parents who observe mood and vegetative disturbances in their children typically present to pediatricians, rather than mental health professionals. Thus, clinical reports of preschool depression are rare and may underestimate the true prevalence of depressive symptoms (Trad, 1994).

Middle Childhood (6–12 Years)

In examining depression in children aged 6 and older, speculation is replaced by empirical investigation. There is a relatively stable pattern of depressive symptoms in 6- to 8-year-olds that includes prolonged unhappiness, decreased socialization, sleep problems, irritability, lethargy, poor school performance, accident-proneness, phobias, separation anxiety, and attention-seeking behaviors (Carlson & Kashani, 1988; Edelsohn, Ialongo, Werthamer-Larsson, Crockett, & Kellam, 1992). Children at this age typically do not verbalize hopelessness and self-deprecation; rather, they express their inner experiences through behavioral problems. In contrast, 9- to 12-year-olds, who are more self-aware, often verbalize feelings of low self-esteem and helplessness when depressed. They also evidence irritability, depressed mood, sad expression, aggression, lethargy, guilt, poor school performance, phobias, and separation anxiety (Carlson & Kashani, 1988; Weiss et al., 1992). More severe symptoms may emerge at this time, such as suicidal ideation (Poznanski, 1982), hallucinations (Ryan et al., 1987), and self-destructive behaviors (Bemporad & Lee, 1984).

Although these symptoms are similar to those observed in adults, there are developmental differences in the epidemiology and correlates of depressive symptoms in middle childhood.

First, depressive symptoms in children may not represent a unique syndrome, but may overlap with other disorders (for review, see Angold, 1988). Second, some of the biological correlates of childhood depression differ from those in adults. For example, sleep patterns noted in depressed adolescents and adults are less evident in depressed children (Emslie, Weinberg, Kennard, & Kowatch, 1994; Puig-Antich, 1987).

Adolescence

In contrast to the study of childhood depression, research on adolescent depression has been conducted from a developmental perspective. Studies comparing the phenomenology of depression in child and adolescent samples indicate that the similarities in symptom expression exceed the differences (Mitchell, McCauley, Burke, & Moss, 1988; Ryan et al., 1987). Both groups evidence somatic complaints, social withdrawal, hopelessness, and irritability. However, as a result of the cognitive developmental shift that accompanies formal operations, relative to depressed elementary school children, depressed adolescents report more concern about the future and pessimism, worthlessness, and apathy (Weiss et al., 1992). Increased autonomy and peer comparison contribute to depressed adolescents' tendency to engage in more lethal suicide attempts, substance abuse, eating disorders, and antisocial behavior (Reinherz, Frost, & Pakiz, 1991; Ryan et al., 1987).

Cultural Perspective

It is important to examine cultural differences and similarities in the etiology, expression, and phenomenology of depressive disorders (Marsella, Sartorius, Jablensky, & Fenton, 1985). Research questions the universality of the expression of depression, and suggests that culture influences the manifestation of depressive symptoms in youth. For example, somatic complaints and interpersonal difficulties are common in de-

pressed Native American children, whereas cognitive and affective complaints characterize depressed European children (Manson, Ackerson, Dick, Baron, & Fleming, 1990).

In contrast to the idea that the expression of depressive symptoms varies across cultures, Schwab and Schwab (1978) argued that measures used in Western societies are adequate for assessing depression in many cultures. Some cross-cultural research supports this assertion. For example, similar to children in North America, 40–50% of Mexican children report significant depressive symptoms (CES-D $\geq$ 16) (Swanson, Linskey, Quintero-Salinas, Pumariega, & Holzer, 1992). Research using the Beck Depression Inventory (BDI) with Arabic and Swedish youth indicates that, similar to other countries, depressive symptoms are common (Ghareeb & Beshai, 1989; Larsson & Melin, 1990).

DIAGNOSIS

Depression may be considered a mood, syndrome, or disorder (Angold, 1988; Hammen & Compas, 1994; Petersen et al., 1993). Each approach to diagnosis and conceptualization represents a different level of the phenomena and set of assumptions about the nature of psychopathology and the purpose of classification. Because of the high rates of co-occurrence with other psychiatric conditions, which often complicates the diagnosis of depression in youth, the phenomenon of comorbidity will be presented.

Depressed Mood

Research on depressed mood is concerned with the presence of sadness or dysphoria for an unspecified time period. This approach emerged from developmental research in which depressed feelings are understood within the context of the normal range of human emotions. No assumptions are made about coinciding emotions, cognitions, or behaviors. Depressed mood typically is measured with self-report scales or subscales of general inventories (e.g., affect subscale of the Children's Depression Inventory) (Reynolds, 1994).

Depressive Syndromes

Research on depressive syndromes, conducted primarily by Achenbach (1991a), defines depression as a set of behaviors that occur together more often than is expected by chance. The behaviors that comprise the syndrome are derived statistically, and are based on multivariate empirical methods for analyzing reports of youth, parents, and teachers. The cluster of symptoms that emerges from this statistical procedure does not imply a particular model or etiological pathway. For children (age 4–11), the depressive syndrome is based on parent report. The cluster, which differs somewhat according to age and gender, involves the following behaviors: feels lonely; cries; fears doing bad things; feels the need to be perfect; feels unloved; believes others are out to get him/her; feels worthless, nervous, fearful, guilty, self-conscious, suspicious, sad, and worried. For adolescents (age 11–18), the syndrome is based on a similar cluster of complaints reported by the youth, parent, and/or teacher. For youth of all ages, the depressive syndrome contains both depression and anxiety symptoms.

Depressive Disorders

The depressive disorders approach uses categorical diagnostic systems, such as the DSM-IV (APA, 1994). The following sections review the commonly diagnosed forms of depressive phenomena in children and adolescents contained in the DSM-IV. It should be noted that the DSM-IV may have limited applicability to youth depression. There are no diagnostic criteria listed in the section on "Disorders Usually First Diagnosed in Infancy, Childhood, or Adolescence," and the criteria listed in the mood disorders section suggest that when diagnosing a child or adolescent as depressed, the adult criteria should

be used with only minimal modifications. Moreover, the current criteria lack attention to the cognitive, emotional, and interpersonal competencies of children.

Major Depressive Disorder (MDD)

MDD is characterized by a history of one or more major depressive episodes in the absence of manic, hypomanic, or mixed episodes of mood disturbance. To meet criteria for a major depressive episode, a child's symptoms must cause distress or impairment and reflect a change from baseline functioning. Symptoms may not be related to uncomplicated bereavement, a general medical condition, or substance induced.

A major depressive episode is characterized by five or more of the following symptoms present for the same 2-week period: (1) depressed or irritable mood, (2) anhedonia, (3) significant changes in weight or appetite or failure to make expected weight gains, (4) sleep disturbance, (5) psychomotor retardation or agitation, (6) fatigue or loss of energy, (7) feelings of worthlessness or inappropriate guilt, (8) concentration difficulties or indecisiveness, and (9) thoughts of death or suicide. One symptom must be depressed/irritable mood or anhedonia. Although the criteria for a major depressive episode are almost identical for children and adults, the DSM-IV indicates that psychomotor retardation, hypersomnia, and delusions are rare in prepubertal children, whereas somatic complaints, irritability, and social withdrawal may be prominent. The DSM-IV also notes that during adolescence, psychomotor retardation, hypersomnia, and delusions are relatively common, and major depressive episodes often co-occur with other disorders (e.g., disruptive behavior, attention-deficit, anxiety, substance-related, eating).

Dysthymic Disorder (DD)

DD in youth is characterized by chronically depressed or irritable mood for at least 1 year, plus two of the following: (1) appetite disturbance, (2) sleep disturbance, (3) decreased energy, (4) low self-esteem, (5) concentration problems, and (6) feelings of helplessness. One of the only differences between the criteria for DD in youth versus adults is that the duration of symptoms is 2 years in adults and 1 year in children. When DD occurs before age 21, it is specified as early onset.

Adjustment Disorder with Depressed Mood (ADDM)

This diagnosis is characterized by depressive symptoms reflecting a maladaptive reaction to an identifiable psychosocial stressor. Symptoms must occur within 3 months of the onset of the stressor, and cannot persist longer than 6 months after the stressor has resolved. ADDM is diagnosed when a child's symptoms do not meet criteria for MDD or DD, but are of significant concern to warrant treatment. When depressive symptoms occur in conjunction with anxiety, a diagnosis of Adjustment Disorder with Mixed Anxiety and Depressed Mood is warranted. Adjustment Disorder with Mixed Disturbance of Emotion and Conduct is diagnosed when depressive symptoms occur with a behavioral disturbance. Criteria for adjustment disorders are identical for children, adolescents, and adults.

Mood Disorder Related to a General Medical Condition

This diagnosis is made when there is evidence from a child's medical history, physical examination, or laboratory findings that a mood disturbance is the result of the direct physiological effects of a medical condition. Differential diagnosis between depressive symptoms related to a general medical condition and MDD or DD is based on whether or not the youth's symptoms are the direct physiological consequence of a medical condition.

Substance-Induced Mood Disorder

Given the high incidence of alcohol/drug abuse among adolescents, substance-induced mood disorders should be ruled out when evaluating mood disturbance in youth. When a youth develops a mood disturbance during or within a month of alcohol or drug intoxication or withdrawal, Substance Induced Mood Disorder is diagnosed if there is evidence that the substance use is related etiologically to the mood disorder.

Depressive Disorder Not Otherwise Specified

This diagnosis is made when depressive symptoms do not meet criteria for MDD, DD, or ADDM. Examples include minor depressions, depressions superimposed on schizophrenia spectrum disorders, and conditions in which it is unclear if the etiology is a general medical condition or substance induced.

Comorbidity

Children are more likely than adults to exhibit depression comorbid with other disorders (Cantwell, 1992), and depressed youth are 20 to 80 times more likely to experience another internalizing or externalizing disorder (Angold & Costello, 1993). A review of studies of clinic-referred children revealed that 30 to 75% of clinically depressed youth had a diagnosable anxiety disorder (Kovacs, 1989). Puig-Antich (1982) reported rates of comorbid depression and conduct disorder among his clinical sample to be 33%. Empirical evidence suggests that comorbid diagnoses exist in community as well as clinical samples. Kashani, Carlson, et al. (1987) found that in a community sample of depressed adolescents, 75% had concurrent anxiety disorders, 33% received a conduct disorder diagnosis, and 50% had oppositional defiant disorder. Depression co-occurs with many other disorders, notably attention-deficit disorder, substance use disorders, and eating disorders (Angold & Costello, 1993; Kashani, Carlson, et al., 1987).

ETIOLOGY

Neurobiological and psychological correlates of depression in youth have been identified, including genetic factors (Downey & Coyne, 1990; Tambs & Moum, 1993), neurobiological markers (Emslie, Weinberg, Kennard, & Kowatch, 1994; Puig-Antich, 1987), personality vulnerabilities (Block, Gjerde, & Block, 1991; Luthar & Blatt, 1993), disruptions in attachment (Bowlby, 1981; Kobak, Sudler, & Gamble, 1992), family and peer functioning (Kaslow, Deering, & Racusin, 1994; Marton, Connolly, Kutcher, & Korenblum, 1993), cognitive processes (e.g., Garber & Hilsman, 1992; Kaslow, Brown, & Mee, 1994), and life stress (e.g., Garber & Hilsman, 1992). Research on these correlates has led to the development of a number of etiological models of mood disorders in youth.

Although there are biological vulnerabilities for depression in youth, this chapter addresses the psychosocial aspects of depression onset and maintenance. Because the bulk of the psychosocial research on etiological factors examines cognitive and interpersonal theories, these models will be the focus of the present review. Hammen's (1992) etiological model, which highlights the complex transactions among interpersonal variables, cognitive processes, and life stress using a developmental psychopathology framework, will assist in organizing and integrating the data on these psychosocial correlates of depression. According to Hammen (1992), maladaptive attachment patterns with parents are reinforced by later difficulties in familial and peer interactions. In the context of impaired early social functioning, individuals develop unhealthy cognitive styles, including maladaptive models of self and others, and ineffective coping skills. These cognitive styles increase the likelihood that stressful life events will occur, and are associated with difficulty managing stressful events. The presence of stressful life events and impaired coping skills contributes to the development and maintenance of depressive reactions. Because Hammen (1992) posits that the origin of depressive conditions involves early relationships, interpersonal theories of youth depression will be discussed first, followed by supporting data. Then, consistent with Hammen's notion that mal-

adaptive cognitive styles of life stress both cause and result from early relationships, the role of cognitive and life stress variables in childhood depression will be presented.

Interpersonal Factors

According to interpersonal theories, depressed individuals and people in their environment engage in a cycle of depressive symptoms and reactions (Coyne, 1976). Depressive symptoms and their interpersonal manifestations are aversive and arouse guilt in others, thereby causing them to avoid the depressed person while simultaneously providing ingenuine forms of support (Coyne, 1976). As a result, the depressed person's negative self-views are confirmed, and further depressive behaviors are elicited. Coyne's model focuses on transactional patterns between the depressed individual and primary figures in his or her social environment. According to the developmental psychopathology perspective, the primary people in one's environment shift with development. Thus, depression may originate in the context of maladaptive attachment patterns with primary caregivers that are reinforced by later difficulties in familial and peer interactions (Hammen, 1992).

Attachment and Family Functioning

According to attachment theories, early relationships with caregivers play a crucial role in predisposing individuals to depression and sensitizing them to later loss experiences or threats (Bowlby, 1981). Individuals with an early history of disrupted attachment bonds, either through actual separation and loss or through parental emotional unresponsivity or inaccessibility, are vulnerable to depression (Bowlby, 1981). Thus, depression emerges in children and adolescents who fail to form stable, secure attachments with their parents, or lose such attachments. Data supporting this model indicate that: (1) human and primate infants abruptly separated from their mothers evidence depressivelike states (McKinney, 1986), (2) depressed youth report less secure attachment to their parents than do nondepressed psychiatric patients and nonpsychiatric controls (Armsden, McCauley, Greenberg, Burke, & Mitchell, 1990), (3) there is a negative correlation between severity of depression and security of attachment to parents (Armsden et al., 1990; Kubak et al., 1992), and (4) children who lose key attachment figures through divorce or death evidence elevated depression rates (Wallerstein & Corbin, 1991; Weller, Weller, Fristad, & Boews, 1991).

Relationships within the family during childhood also influence the development and maintenance of depressive conditions. First, depression in youth is related to parental psychopathology in general (Puig-Antich et al., 1989), and parental affective disorders in particular (Downey & Coyne, 1990). Moreover, there is a relation between the timing of depressive episodes in depressed mothers and their children (Hammen, Bruge, & Adrian, 1991). Second, children of divorced, single-parent, and low-socioeconomic-status families are at particularly high risk for depression (Garrison, Schlucter, Schoenbach, & Kaplan, 1989; Gibbs, 1985; Warner, Weissman, Fendrich, Wickramaratne, & Moreau, 1992). Third, depressed youths' families are characterized by hostile, tense, and punitive communication patterns (Puig-Antich et al., 1985, 1993). In addition, depressed children and adolescents describe their family environments as less cohesive, supportive, and adaptable, and more controlling and conflictual, than do their nondepressed counterparts (Barrera & Garrison-Jones, 1992; Cumsille & Epstein, 1994; Messer & Gross, 1995).

Peer Relationships

The transactional patterns that characterize peer relationships often mimic those observed within the family. In fact, those depressed youths most likely to evidence peer problems are those with problematic relationships with their parents (Puig-Antich et al., 1993). Myriad interpersonal difficulties have been associated with peer relationships among depressed youths. Relative to their nondepressed counterparts, depressed children are more rejected by peers, rated by their peers to have more negative social behaviors, perceived as less likable and attractive, and thought to be in greater need of psychological help (Bell-Dolan, Reaven, & Peterson, 1993; Cole, 1991; Cole & Carpentieri, 1990; Peterson, Mullins, & Ridley-Johnson, 1985; Rudolph, Hammen, & Burge, 1994). Children, particularly girls, who are neglected by their peers are at risk for developing depressive symptoms (Kupersmidt & Patterson, 1991).

Concluding Comments

Attachment difficulties, parental psychiatric illness, disruptions in family composition, and negative family environments both may produce and result from childhood depression. Similarly, peer-related difficulties contribute to, and reflect, the development of depressive symptoms in youth. Although the mechanisms by which disturbed relationships influence depression remain unclear, one possibility involves the youth's cognitive interpretations of these interactions (Hammem, 1992). Thus, cognitive and life stress theories are now reviewed.

Cognitive Factors

Widespread attention has focused on adult cognitive models of depression as they pertain to children. These models include Beck's cognitive theory (Beck, 1967), the twice-revised learned helplessness theory (Abramson, Metalsky, & Alloy, 1989; Abramson, Seligman, & Teasdale, 1978; Seligman, 1975), and the self-control model (Rehm, 1977). Despite their unique characteristics, these models each focus on the interplay between cognitive styles and stressful life events. Although these models have not been adapted sufficiently to accommodate the cognitive competencies of children, this review focuses on those researchers who have examined these constructs in young populations (for review, see Garber & Hilsman, 1992; Kaslow, Brown, & Mee, 1994).

Beck's Cognitive Theory

The central tenet of Beck's (1967) cognitive theory is the negative cognitive triad, consisting of negative schemata that result in distorted processing of information about self, others, and the future. These negative views typically are manifested in low self-esteem, self-criticism, underestimation of one's abilities, hopelessness, and pessimism. As a diathesis-stress model, Beck's theory suggests that the negative self-schema (diathesis) and the experience of a negative life event (stress) lead to cognitive distortions and subsequent depression. Although there is inconsistent support for the presence of more negative schemata in depressed than in nondepressed children (Hammen & Zupan, 1984; Prieto, Cole, & Tageson, 1992; Whitman & Leitenberg, 1990), depressed youth have low self-esteem, rate themselves as less competent than others, feel hopeless, and report more negatively distorted cognitions on self-report measures (e.g., Cognitive Biases Questionnaire for Children) (Asarnow & Bates, 1988; Haley, Fine, Marriage, Moretta, & Freeman, 1985; Kendall, Stark, & Adam, 1990; King, Naylor, Segal, Evans, & Shain, 1993; Worchel et al., 1990).

Self-Control Theory

Rehm's (1977) self-control theory posits that depressives have deficits in self-monitoring, evaluation, and/or -reinforcement in response to stress. They may attend to negative events to the exclusion of positive ones, monitor immediate versus delayed consequences of behavior, set stringent self-evaluative criteria, provide insufficient positive self-reinforcement, and/or be excessively self-punishing. Research indicates that depressed children evidence impaired self-monitoring, -evaluation, and -reinforcement (Kaslow, Rehm, & Siegel, 1984; Kaslow, Rehm, Pollack, & Siegel, 1988). Myer, Dyck, and Petrinack (1989) found that, despite similar perfor-

mance, depressed youth provided lower evaluations of their performance and punished themselves more than nondepressed youth, although there were no between-group differences in reward. Finally, depressed clinic children reported more overall self-control difficulties as measured by the Usually That's Me (Kaslow et al., 1988) control measure than did the nondepressed clinic children and normal controls.

Learned Helplessness Theory and Revisions

According to the original learned helplessness model (Seligman, 1975), individuals become helpless and depressed when they perceive environmental events as uncontrollable. After several empirical investigations with humans, the model was revised, and the attributional reformulation was proposed (Abramson et al., 1978). According to the revised theory, the manner in which a person explains the causes of life events is the cognitive process by which learned helplessness is modulated. Individuals whose explanatory styles are characterized by internal, stable, and global attributions for negative events are at greater risk for developing depressive symptoms than are those who make external, unstable, and specific attributions for these same events. More recently, the model has been revised further and presented as the hopelessness theory of depression (Abramson et al., 1989). In this revision, attributional style (diathesis) serves as a moderator between negative life events perceived to be important (stress) and the development of hopelessness. Hopelessness, in turn, is thought to lead directly to the experience of depression. Thus, depression is thought to result from a state of hopelessness engendered by the attribution of negative life events to internal, stable, and global factors.

Research supports learned helplessness theory's application to depression in youth. Regarding the original formulation, a series of studies indicate that depressive symptoms in youth are associated with "personal helplessness" (i.e., perceived incompetence) and "universal helplessness" (i.e., perceived noncontingency) (Weisz,

Sweeney, Proffitt, & Carr, 1993). With respect to the attributional reformulation, the large body of research on attributional patterns yields contradictory findings. However, the bulk of this work reveals that, relative to their nondepressed counterparts, depressed youngsters evidence a more internal, stable, and global attributional pattern for negative events, and a more external, unstable, and specific attributional style for positive events according to their responses on the Children's Attributional Style Questionnaire (CASQ; Seligman et al., 1984) (Gladstone & Kaslow, 1995; Nolen-Hoeksema, Girgus, & Seligman, 1986). Finally, although no published study has tested thoroughly the hopelessness revision, some researchers (e.g., Garber & Hilsman, 1992; Nolen-Hoeksema, Girgus, & Seligman, 1992) provide data supporting the diathesis-stress component of the theory. For example, Garber and Hilsman (1992) found that students who attributed poor grades to internal, stable, and global factors were more distressed after receiving their report cards than were students without such an attributional style.

Concluding Comments

Research on the cognitive, self-control, and learned helplessness theories indicates that negative self-views, distorted cognitions, errors in self-evaluation and self-reinforcement, maladaptive attributional styles, and the presence of negative life events all are associated with depressive conditions in youth. Unfortunately, the diathesis-stress components of these theories have not been investigated adequately in children and adolescents, and future longitudinal research is needed in this area.

Hammen's (1992) developmental psychopathology model highlights the interactive roles of interpersonal, cognitive, and life stress variables in the etiology and maintenance of depression in children. However, most of the research to date has focused on these factors in isolation. Longitudinal research is needed to examine the interactions between these variables, and their relative importance at different developmental stages.

EPIDEMIOLOGY

There are no nationally representative epidemiological studies of depressive phenomena in youth, perhaps reflecting the variability in diagnostic criteria, assessment devices, and populations sampled (for review, see Fleming & Offord, 1990; Kaslow, Celano, & McCarthy, 1993). Available research indicates that prevalence rates for mood disorders in youth range from 2 to 5% in community samples and from 10 to 50% in psychiatric settings (Fleming & Offord, 1990; McCracken, 1992; Petersen et al., 1993). Despite differences in prevalence rates across age, sex, and sociocultural background (Fleming & Offord, 1990), most concur that depressive episodes in youth persist and recur (Kovacs, 1989).

Research on the development of depression indicates that rates of depressive disorders increase with age (Angold & Rutter, 1992). Depressive disorders are rare in preschool children, regardless of whether or not they are receiving psychiatric treatment (e.g., Kashani et al., 1986). For elementary schoolchildren, depression rates range from 2–4% among community samples (Angold & Rutter, 1992) to 8–15% among children admitted to a psychiatric facility (Kashani, Cantwell, Shekim, & Reid, 1982). During adolescence, prevalence rates increase dramatically, such that 7% of adolescents in community samples are depressed (Petersen et al., 1993), and 57% of a clinical sample meet criteria for depression (Kovacs, 1989).

Research on sex differences in depression indicates a sex and age interaction. Among prepubertal children, some researchers report higher rates of depression in prepubertal boys than girls (Anderson, Williams, McGee, & Silva, 1987), whereas others report an absence of sex differences in depression (Fleming, Offord, & Boyle, 1989). However, studies consistently reveal that, by age 15, females are twice as likely as males to receive a depressive diagnosis (Angold & Rutter, 1992; Kandel & Davies, 1986; Nolen-Hoeksema & Girgus, 1994). Explanations for sex differences in depression among adolescents include differences in sex-role socialization, cognitive styles, the presence and timing of negative life events during early adolescence, and differential hormonal changes associated with puberty (e.g., Brooks-Gunn & Warren, 1989; Petersen et al., 1993).

There are limited data on the impact of sociocultural variables on the prevalence of depression in youth. Some research indicates that low socioeconomic status is associated with higher rates of depression (e.g., Kandel & Davies, 1982 Roa et al., 1995). Research on ethnicity and childhood depression is inconsistent, with some studies revealing higher rates of depressive disorders in African-American than Caucasian young males, and others indicating no relation between race and depression (e.g., Harrington, 1993).

Depressive disorders in children and adolescents persist and influence the course of future episodes of depression (Hanna, 1992; Harrington, 1992). In a longitudinal study of clinic-referred youth, Kovacs and colleagues (for review see Kovacs, 1989) found that the average length of episode for ADDM, MDD, and DD is 6 months, 8 months, and 3 years, respectively. Moreover, children with intake diagnoses of MDD or DD are at increased risk for future episodes of MDD. Finally, early depression is associated with a range of psychiatric, psychosocial, and physical health problems in adulthood (e.g., Fleming, Boyle, & Offord, 1993; Kandel & Davies, 1986; Rao et al., 1995). However, not all individuals who become depressed during childhood evidence recurring psychological and social difficulties (Rao et al., 1995).

ASSESSMENT

Accurate assessment is important to evaluate the presence of depressive symptoms, and to examine treatment efficacy (Reynolds, 1994). Techniques have been refined to aid in the assessment of depression in youth based on a multimethod, multi-informant approach. This section reviews the methods by which childhood depression may be assessed and the importance of using multiple informants. A modification of Reynolds's (1986a) multistage assessment procedure for identifying youth depression will be presented as a way of integrating these multiple sources of data into a meaningful diagnostic impression.

Methods of Assessment

Self-Report Measures

Self-report measures of depression for children and adolescents include the Children's Depression Inventory (CDI) (Kovacs & Beck, 1977; Kovacs, 1992), Children's Depression Scale (CDS) (Lang & Tisher, 1978), Reynolds Adolescent Depression Scale (RADS) (Reynolds, 1986b), and Center for Epidemiologic Studies–Depression Scale (CES-D) (Radloff, 1977). Self-report measures are useful for evaluating the severity of depressive symptoms, but are not appropriate for diagnosing the presence or absence of a depressive syndrome. Advantages of self-report methods include: (1) assessment of the child's perceptions of his or her internal states that frequently are unobservable to others, (2) rapid assessment of the severity of symptoms, (3) facilitation of large-scale screening, (4) ease of administration by nonprofessionals, and (5) well-documented psychometric properties (e.g., the CDI; Kovacs, 1992). Despite these advantages, self-report measures are limited because they require cognitive, language, and reading skills that may exceed the abilities of many children (Stark, 1990). They do not assess the etiology of symptoms and so may lead to inaccurate diagnostic impressions (e.g., sleep disturbance related to depression versus a loud sibling), and they may emphasize recent experiences over more general behaviors. Moreover, children and adolescents tend to score higher on initial than on subsequent administrations of self-report measures, resulting in false-positive caseness (Tharinger & Stark, 1990).

Diagnostic Interviews

Structured diagnostic interviews are used commonly for the diagnosis of depressive syndromes in youth. Examples of structured diagnostic interviews are the Schedule of Affective Disorders and Schizophrenia in School-Aged Children (K-SADS; Puig-Antich & Chambers, 1978), Diagnostic Interview Schedule for Children (DISC; Costello, Edelbrock, Dulcan, Kalas, & Klaric, 1984), and Child Assessment Scale (CAS; Hodges, Cools, & McKnew, 1989). Advantages of structured diagnostic interviews include: (1) providing a consensus diagnosis based on multiple informants; (2) enabling interviewers to adapt questions to the child's developmental level; (3) allowing interviewers to observe the child's behavioral, emotional, and cognitive functioning; and (4) providing a means of assessing symptoms of comorbid disorders (Puig-Antich et al., 1989). However, diagnostic interviews are time-consuming and thus may be taxing to those being interviewed. Structured interviews also are cumbersome to administer to groups and require interviewers to be trained extensively. Finally, children below age 10 may not be reliable informants when reporting certain symptoms (e.g., fears); thus, diagnostic interviews must include a lengthy parent interview as well as a child report (Edelbrock, Costello, Dukan, Kalas, & Conover, 1985).

Informants

When assessing depression, members of the child's social world (parents, teachers, peers) provide an important source of information. The most commonly used parent and teacher measures include the Child Behavior Checklist (CBCL) and the CBCL-Teacher Report Form (CBCL-TRF) (Achenbach, 1991b,c, respectively). The Peer Nomination Inventory of Depression (PNID; Lefkowitz, Tesiny, & Solodrow, 1989) is the most widely used peer measure. Clarizio (1994) outlines several advantages of parent, teacher, and peer ratings. First, these measures capitalize on others' substantial previous experience with the child over time and across settings. Second, parents and teachers have access to normative information about same-aged peers in social and school settings, and thus can evaluate behavior in comparison with others. Third, these measures have ecological validity (i.e., they gather information from outside the clinical setting). Finally, parent and teacher measures (e.g., CBCL, CBCL-TRF) have strong psychometric properties. The disadvantages include: (1) the inability of parents, teachers, and peers to evaluate the internal aspects of depression (e.g., suicidal ideation, guilt); (2) the ambiguity in the meaning of the symptoms evaluated (e.g., depressed mood); (3) the differences among raters in what constitutes impairment, and (4) the failure to ascertain antecedents and consequences of the child's behavior.

Although many researchers agree that multiple respondents provide for a comprehensive assessment of depression in youth, informants do vary in their views of the child. For example, children and parents evidence low agreement on individual symptoms as well as overall ratings of depression (Ivens & Rehm, 1988). Moreover, peer and teacher reports yield low correlations with children's self-reports of depression (Jacobson, Lahey, & Strauss, 1983; Lefkowitz & Tesiny, 1984). Thus, clinicians frequently must integrate discrepant information in arriving at diagnoses. Research suggests that parent reports be given more credence when externalizing behaviors are in question, and that child report may be more accurate regarding internalizing behaviors (Kolko & Kazdin, 1993).

Integrative Multistage, Multimethod, Multi-Informant Assessment Approach

Because of the limitations of current assessment methods and informant sources, researchers have called for a multistage, multimethod, multi-informant approach to the assessment of depression in youth (Reynolds, 1994). Reynolds (1986a) outlined a multistage assessment procedure for screening and identifying depression in youth. In this three-stage procedure, children are screened first in large groups with self-report questionnaires of depressive symptoms. Those whose scores meet criteria for clinical levels of depressive symptomatology are retested with questionnaires in smaller groups to control for overendorsement of depressive symptoms on the initial assessment. Finally, youth who report depressive symptoms at Stages 1 and 2 are assessed with semistructured diagnostic interviews. This procedure has been implemented in several school systems, both for identifying children in need of psychological services and for selecting research participants (Stark, 1990). Despite its strengths, this model is limited by its reliance on self-report measures and clinician interviews. If modified to include data from teachers, parents, and peers, perhaps during Stage 3, the model's utility would be enhanced.

TREATMENT

Research on treating depression in youth primarily has been based on downward extensions of adult interventions (Stark, Rouse, & Kurowski, (1994). Although adult models provide helpful guidelines in designing intervention programs for youngsters, differences between children's and adults' cognitive, affective, and interpersonal functioning require corresponding variations in treatment procedures. Thus, prior to reviewing the treatment outcome data for children and adolescents, issues unique to treating each age group will be introduced.

Child Treatment

Treatment Considerations

Developmental literature highlights several challenges associated with treating depressed children. First, children have limited memory and attentional capacities (Siegler, 1986). As such, they may benefit from short and repetitious treatment sessions. Second, because of children's limited verbal capacities, they may be engaged most effectively when games, activities, and stories are incorporated into treatment protocols (Stark et al., 1994). Finally, because children are dependent on, and influenced by, their families, family involvement in treatment may be beneficial and even necessary (Kaslow & Racusin, 1994).

Treatment Outcome Research

Research on the psychosocial treatment of childhood depression has been limited. However, a handful of treatment outcome studies have been conducted using a control condition and random assignment of subjects (e.g., Butler, Miezitis, Friedman, & Cole, 1980; Liddle & Spence, 1990; Stark, Reynolds, & Kaslow, 1987; Stark, Rouse, & Livingston, 1991).

Butler et al. (1980) conducted the first empirical treatment study with fifth and sixth graders evidencing depressive symptoms. Treatment involved ten 1-hour weekly group sessions. Children were assigned randomly to one of four conditions: cognitive restructuring, role-play, attention placebo, or no-treatment control. In the cognitive-restructuring condition, participants learned to recognize self-deprecating thoughts, generate adaptive cognitions, and develop better social skills. The role-play condition involved enacting personal problems to enhance interpersonal problem-solving skills. Youth in both the cognitive-restructuring and role-play conditions improved in their self-reported ratings of depression, relative to individuals in the attention placebo and control conditions. Moreover, relative to their peers in the cognitive-restructuring condition, participants in the role-playing condition improved more across outcome measures (measures of depression and related constructs).

More recently, Stark et al. (1991) evaluated self-control therapy for depressed fourth through seventh graders. This 24- to 26-session cognitive-behavioral treatment consisted of self-control and social skills training, cognitive restructuring, and problem-solving. This treatment was compared with a traditional counseling condition designed to control for nonspecific intervention elements. For the cognitive-behavioral groups, monthly family meetings encouraged parents to assist their children in applying new skills learned in the treatment sessions, and increase the frequency of positive family activities. In the traditional counseling condition, monthly family sessions addressed improving communication and increasing pleasant family events. Postintervention and 7-month follow-up assessments revealed decreased self-reported depressive symptoms for both groups of youth, although children in the cognitive-behavioral group reported fewer depressive symptoms on a semistructured interview and endorsed fewer depressive cognitions than did those in the control condition.

Taken together, treatment studies conducted with nonreferred children evidencing depressive symptoms indicate that, relative to nontreatment controls, a variety of intervention approaches (typically with a cognitive-behavioral orientation) are helpful in decreasing depressive symptoms. However, few differences have been found between treatment conditions. Although recent studies reflect greater developmental sensitivity than earlier studies, the treatment outcome literature for childhood depression remains limited in several ways. First, as most studies involved nonreferred children, it is unclear whether or not these findings generalize to clinical populations (Asarnow, 1990; Harrington, 1992). Second, many intervention approaches consist of multiple components; however, there are limited data regarding which specific component(s) may be most beneficial (Asarnow, 1990). Third, although these studies appropriately examine depressive symptoms as the outcome variable, they fail to investigate changes in the target behaviors and cognitions (e.g., social skills, depressive cognitions). Finally, these outcome studies fail to assess the effectiveness of intervention strategies for youth at different developmental levels. Thus, research may benefit from continued efforts to incorporate a developmental perspective in designing and implementing psychosocial treatments for depressed children.

Adolescent Treatment

Treatment Considerations

As with children, in evaluating treatment procedures for use in adolescence, it is important to consider the challenges associated with this developmental stage. First, adolescence is characterized by the transition from concrete to formal operational thought (Piaget, 1946), and adolescents often are excited by their newly developing abilities for metacognition. As a result, therapies that exercise these new abilities may be met with less resistance than is found with many adults (Rush & Nowels, 1994). In addition, adolescence is characterized by biological, psychological, and social developmental changes that occur during puberty (Rutter & Hersov, 1985; Wilkes, 1994). According to Petersen and colleagues (Petersen & Crockett, 1985), when multiple life changes occur simultaneously (e.g., changes in school and pubertal status), individuals increasingly are vulnerable to depressive symptomatology. Thus, treatment approaches must consider not only the adolescent's cognitive and internal psychological processes, but also his or her psychosocial environment (e.g., peers, family, social activities).

Treatment Outcome Research

Few studies have explored empirically the treatment of adolescent depression (e.g., Brent, Poling, McKain, & Baugher, 1993; Fine, Forth, Gilbert, & Haley, 1991; Kahn, Kehle, Jenson, & Clark, 1990; Mufson et al., 1994; Reynolds & Coates, 1986; Robbins, Alessi, & Colfer, 1989). These intervention studies have incorporated cognitive-behavioral, interpersonal, psychodynamic, and psychoeducational perspectives. Below, a representative subset of studies is reviewed.

The most methodologically sophisticated treatment outcome research has been conducted by Lewinsohn, Clarke, Hops, and Andrews (1990). Adolescents aged 14 to 18 who met diagnostic criteria for depressive disorders were assigned randomly to: (1) a 14-session cognitive-behavioral group treatment for the adolescent only, (2) cognitive-behavioral treatment groups for the depressed adolescent (14 sessions) and separate sessions for his or her parents (7 sessions), and (3) a wait-list control. The cognitive-behavioral intervention focused on experiential learning and skills training (e.g., mood monitoring, relaxation), and targeted improving communication and negotiation/conflict resolution skills. The complementary parent intervention was aimed at enhancing parents' capacities to reinforce and promote the adolescent's adaptive changes. Results revealed that fewer adolescents in the active treatment conditions met diagnostic criteria for depression posttreatment than did the wait-list controls. Treatment gains were maintained at 2-year follow-up. Although a trend indicated that the adolescent-and-parent condition was more effective than the adolescent-only condition, few between-group differences reached statistical significance.

Another treatment approach currently under investigation is Interpersonal Therapy (IPT; Klerman, Weissman, Rounsaville, & Chevron, 1984), recently modified for use with adolescents (IPT-A; Mufson et al., 1994). The two main goals of the original IPT include identifying and treating both the patient's depressive symptoms and his or her associated problem area(s) (e.g., grief, interpersonal role disputes, role transitions, interpersonal deficits). The overall goals and problem areas of IPT-A are similar to those of IPT. However, a fifth problem area, the single-parent family, is added because of its frequent occurrence and the problems it engenders for adolescents. Results of a 12-week course of individual psychotherapy revealed that adolescents reported decreases in depressive symptoms (Mufson et al., 1994). Improvements were noted in other psychological symptoms and physical distress.

Overall, the treatment outcome literature for adolescent depression indicates that short-term therapies, regardless of their theoretical underpinnings, are efficacious in decreasing depressive symptoms. As with the child studies, however, it is premature to conclude that any given intervention is the most effective. Future research is needed as adolescents are less likely than adults to improve without treatment (Lewinsohn et al., 1990).

Summary

Longitudinal research indicates that once depressed, youth are likely to continue to struggle with depressive symptoms and other problematic behaviors throughout the life span (Kandel & Davies, 1986; Kovacs, 1989; Lewinsohn, Hops, Roberts, Seeley, & Andrews, 1993). This research underscores the importance of treating child and adolescent depression. Additionally, these findings highlight the need for preventive intervention approaches to youth depression. Specifically, current advancements in treatment outcome research may be particularly useful in directing future efforts to intervene with high-risk youth before they become depressed (Beardslee et al., 1988).

CASE STUDY

Debbie, an 8-year-old Caucasian female, was brought for evaluation by her biological parents, the Bakers. Debbie and her family resided in a suburban upper-middle-class neighborhood. Her mother, age 37, was employed as a psychiatric social worker. Her father, age 39, worked as an engineer. The couple had an adopted son, Brian, age 9, who had been diagnosed and treated successfully for Attention-Deficit/Hyperactivity Disorder.

Debbie, an attractive and verbally precocious child, presented with depressive symptoms and functional difficulties. In terms of psychological symptomatology, she exhibited irritability, anhedonia, lack of energy, feelings of worthlessness, and a diminished ability to concentrate in school. She denied any neurovegetative symptoms or suicidal ideation. Cognitively, she revealed an impaired sense of self-esteem and diminished academic performance, despite her high level of assessed cognitive ability. Underlying her tendency to externalize blame for her difficulties, she harbored a depressive attributional style in which she considered herself at fault for family difficulties.

Debbie also experienced problems modulating her negative affect, resulting in tantrums and irritability. In her interpersonal relationships, despite relating in an age-appropriate manner with the therapist, according to teachers, parents, and the child herself she had few friends and did not seek out peer relationships. Her relationships with authority figures were characterized by excessive deference and avoidance. Her family functioning was marked by frequent arguing with her parents and brother, an absence of feelings of emotional warmth, and an impaired ability to discuss problems with a sense that such discussion would prove beneficial. Finally, in her adaptive behavior, her irritability at home compromised her acquisition of age-appropriate daily living skills, and her interpersonal skills also were deficient, as noted above.

Over the course of the evaluation, the family revealed more systemic family dysfunction. First, depressive symptoms were evident in both parents. Mrs. Baker evidenced obesity, alcohol abuse, and Borderline Personality Disorder, and Mr. Baker was obese and met diagnostic criteria for Avoidant Personality Disorder. Second, a pervasive cognitive style was evident in which family members felt negatively about themselves, the world, and the future, and blamed themselves for negative events. Third, the family exhibited difficulty regulating negative affect, particularly sadness and anger. Fourth, all family members displayed difficulty negotiating age-appropriate interpersonal relationships. Fifth, family members demonstrated adaptive behavior deficits in daily living skills (e.g., limited frustration tolerance) and socialization skills. Finally, parent–child relationships were characterized by the parents' alternating overinvolvement and rejection of their children as evidenced, for example, in their adversarial encounters with school personnel on behalf of their daughter, interspersed with their condemnation of her for failure to perform academically. Substantial marital dysfunction was observed, characterized by reciprocal verbal abuse and minimal sexual involvement.

Based on data gleaned from the evaluation, concurrent individual and family treatment was recommended. Pharmacological intervention was not deemed necessary, reflecting her lack of vegetative symptomatology. In individual sessions, initial interventions employed cognitive-behavioral techniques in which Debbie was taught more adaptive causal attributions of responsibility for positive and negative events. She was helped to identify maladaptive automatic thoughts and beliefs and later the therapist began to help her challenge these depressive cognitions. To address her difficulties with affect regulation, strategies were used to assist Debbie in increasing her awareness of her emotional variability and the interpersonal and cognitive precipitants of these mood changes. As a result of these interventions, Debbie began to make more favorable self-appraisals and more balanced attributions about positive and negative life events, and was more able to regulate her distressing affects.

Concurrent family sessions using an interpersonal family therapy model (Kaslow & Racusin, 1994) were conducted. The family was educated concerning the irrational beliefs, cognitive distortions, and depressogenic attributions associated with both Debbie's depression as well as the depressive symptoms manifested by her parents. Cognitive distortions were challenged and alternative explanations were generated. To address the interpersonal deficits noted in all family members, effective interpersonal problem-solving strategies were taught, and family members were encouraged to help one another utilize these techniques. Family members as a unit and appropriate subsystems (e.g., marital dyad, sibship) were urged to engage in pleasurable activities. These family-based cognitive and interpersonal interventions served to ameliorate Debbie's depressive symptoms and alter those parent–child interactions that appeared to be reinforcing Debbie's depression. Unfortunately, however, after 6 months of this combined intervention, Debbie's peer interaction difficulties persisted. To address these problems, she was referred to a group that focused on social skills training.

SUMMARY

There has been a plethora of empirical research regarding the symptom presentation, assessment, and diagnosis of depressive disorders in youth. However, research from a developmental perspective regarding the phenomenology of depressive disorders, as well as the epidemiology of these disorders in children and adolescents has been relatively sparse. Further, the limited number of longitudinal investigations of depressive disorders in childhood, as well as in children at risk for depression, has resulted in myriad theoretical conceptualizations but a dearth of conclusive empirical evidence regarding the validity of these etiological models. Additionally, although treatment outcome studies indicate that short-term therapies, regardless of their theoretical underpinnings, are efficacious in decreasing depressive symptoms in children and adolescents, it is premature to conclude that any given intervention, or specific component thereof, is superior.

To address these limitations, a number of avenues of research may prove fruitful. First, we encourage large-scale epidemiological studies of childhood symptoms and disorders. Findings from this kind of research will shed some additional light on the epidemiology of depressive and comorbid conditions in children and adolescents. The utility of these kinds of studies can be increased by using developmentally sensitive diagnostic criteria and associated assessment strategies. Second, longitudinal investigations spanning infancy, childhood, and adolescence and focusing on the cognitive and interpersonal processes associated with depression risk and course will enhance our understanding of the causes and consequences of depressive phenomena across the life span. Third, to facilitate the implementation of effective psychosocial interventions for depressed children and adolescents, it behooves clinical researchers to conduct larger scale and more methodologically rigorous studies utilizing a developmental psychopathology framework. It is important that these research endeavors focus on ascertaining which treatment interventions are most effective for particular children given their developmental phase, psychological symptomatology, cognitive and interpersonal competencies, and the social context within which they are embedded. Finally, as research accumulates regarding those factors that place children and adolescents at risk for depression, more targeted preventive intervention programs can be developed and implemented.

REFERENCES

Abramson, L. Y., Metalsky, G. I., & Alloy, L. B. (1989). Hopelessness depression: A theory-based subtype of depression. *Psychological Bulletin, 96,* 358–372.

Abramson, L. Y., Seligman, M. E. P., & Teasdale, J. (1978). Learned helplessness in humans: Critique and reformulation. *Journal of Abnormal Psychology, 87,* 49–74.

Achenbach, T. M. (1991a). *Integrative guide for the 1991 CBCL/4–18, YSR, and TRF profiles.* Burlington: University of Vermont Department of Psychiatry.

Achenbach, T. M. (1991b). *Manual for the Child Behavior Checklist/4–18 and 1991 profile.* Burlington: University of Vermont Department of Psychiatry.

Achenbach, T. M. (1991c). *Manual for the Teacher's Report Form and 1991 profile.* Burlington: University of Vermont Department of Psychiatry.

American Psychiatric Association. (1994). *Diagnostic and statistical manual of mental disorders* (4th ed.). Washington, DC: Author.

Anderson, J. C., Williams, S., McGee, R., & Silva, P. A. (1987). DSM-III disorders in preadolescent children. *Archives of General Psychiatry, 44,* 69–76.

Angold, A. (1988). Childhood and adolescent depression: I. Epidemiological and aetiological aspects. *British Journal of Psychiatry, 152,* 601–617.

Angold, A., & Costello, E. J. (1993). Depressive comorbidity in children and adolescents: Empirical, theoretical, and methodological issues. *American Journal of Psychiatry, 150,* 1779–1791.

Angold, A., & Rutter, M. (1992). Effects of age and pubertal status in a large clinical sample. *Development and Psychopathology, 4,* 5–28.

Armsden, G. C., McCauley, E., Greenberg, M. T., Burke, P. M., & Mitchell, J. R. (1990). Parent and peer attachment in early adolescent depression. *Journal of Abnormal Child Psychology, 18,* 683–697.

Asarnow, J. R. (1990). Psychosocial intervention strategies for the depressed child: Approaches to treatment and prevention. *Child and Adolescent Psychiatric Clinics of North America, 1,* 257–283.

Asarnow, J. R., & Bates, S. (1988). Depression in child psychiatric inpatients: Cognitive and attributional patterns. *Journal of Abnormal Child Psychology, 16,* 601–615.

Barrera, M., & Garrison-Jones, C. (1992). Family and peer social support as specific correlates of adolescent depressive symptoms. *Journal of Abnormal Child Psychology, 20,* 1–16.

Beardslee, W. R., Keller, M. B., Lavori, P. W., Klerman, G. L., Dorer, D. J., & Samuelson, H. (1988). Psychiatric disorder in adolescent offspring of parents with affective disorders in a non-referred sample. *Journal of Affective Disorders, 15,* 313–322.

Beck, A. T. (1967). *Depression: Clinical, experimental, and theoretical.* New York: Hoeber.

Bell-Dolan, D. J., Reaven, N. M., & Peterson, L. (1993). Depression and social functioning: A multidimensional study of the linkages. *Journal of Clinical Child Psychology, 22,* 306–315.

Bemporad, J. R., & Lee, K. W. (1984). Developmental and psychodynamic aspects of childhood depression. *Child Psychiatry and Human Development, 14,* 145–157.

Block, J., Gjerde, P. F., & Block, J. H. (1991). Personality antecedents of depressive tendencies in 18-year olds: A prospective study. *Journal of Personality and Social Psychology, 60,* 726–738.

Bowlby, J. (1981). *Attachment and loss: Vol. 3. Sadness and depression.* Harmondsworth, Middlesex: Penguin.

Brent, D. A., Poling, K., McKain, B., & Baugher, N. (1993). A psychoeducational program for families of affectively ill children and adolescents. *Journal of the American Academy of Child and Adolescent Psychiatry, 32,* 770–774.

Brooks-Gunn, J., & Warren, M. P. (1989). Biological and social contributions to negative affect in young adolescent girls. *Child Development, 60,* 40–55.

Butler, L., Miezitis, S., Friedman, R., & Cole, E. (1980). The effect of two school-based intervention programs on depressive symptoms in preadolescents. *American Educational Research Journal, 17,* 111–119.

Cantwell, D. P. (1992). Clinical phenomenology and nosology. *Child and Adolescent Psychiatric Clinics of North America, 1,* 1–11.

Carlson, G. A., & Kashani, J. H. (1988). Phenomenology of major depression from childhood through adulthood: Analysis of three studies. *American Journal of Psychiatry, 145,* 1222–1225.

Cicchetti, D., & Schneider-Rosen, K. (1986). An organizational approach to childhood depression. In M. Rutter,

C. E. Izard, & P. B. Read (Eds.), *Depression in young people: Developmental and clinical perspectives* (pp. 71–134). New York: Guilford Press.

Clarizio, H. F. (1994). *Assessment and treatment of depression in children and adolescents*. Brandon, VT: Clinical Psychology Publishing.

Cole, D. A. (1991). Preliminary support for a competency-based model of depression in children. *Journal of Abnormal Psychology, 100,* 181–190.

Cole, D. A., & Carpentieri, S. (1990). Social status and the comorbidity of child depression and conduct disorder. *Journal of Consulting and Clinical Psychology, 58,* 748–757.

Costello, A. J., Edelbrock, L. S., Dulcan, M. K., Kalas, R., & Klaric, S. H. (1984). *Report on the NIMH Diagnostic Interview Schedule for Children (DISC)*. Washington, DC: National Institute of Mental Health.

Coyne, J. C. (1976). Toward an interactional description of depression. *Psychiatry, 39,* 28–40.

Cumsille, P. E., & Epstein, N. (1994). Family cohesion, family adaptability, social support, and adolescent depressive symptoms in outpatient clinic families. *Journal of Family Psychology, 8,* 202–214.

Digdon, N., & Gotlib, I. H. (1985). Developmental considerations in the study of childhood depression. *Developmental Reviews, 5,* 162–199.

Downey, G., & Coyne, J. C. (1990). Children of depressed parents. An integrative review. *Psychological Bulletin, 108,* 50–76.

Edelbrock, C., Costello, A. J., Dulcan, M., Kalas, R., & Conover, N. C. (1985). Age differences in the reliability of the psychiatric interview of the child. *Child Development, 56,* 265–275.

Edelsohn, G., Ialongo, N., Werthamer-Larsson, L., Crockett, I., & Kellam, S. (1992). Self-reported depressive symptoms in first-grade children: Developmentally transient phenomena? *Journal of the American Academy of Child and Adolescent Psychiatry, 31,* 282–290.

Emslie, G. J., Weinberg, W. A., Kennard, B. D., & Kowatch, R. A. (1994). Neurobiological aspects of depression in children and adolescents. In W. M. Reynolds & H. F. Johnston (Eds.), *Handbook of depression in children and adolescents* (pp. 143–165). New York: Plenum Press.

Field, T. (1984). Perinatal risk factors for infant depression. In J. D. Call, E. Galenson, & R. L. Tyson (Eds.), *Frontiers of infant psychiatry* (Vol. II, pp. 152–159). New York: Basic Books.

Fine, S., Forth, A., Gilbert, M., & Haley, G. (1991). Group therapy for adolescent depressive disorder: A comparison of social skills and therapeutic support. *Journal of the American Academy of Child and Adolescent Psychiatry, 30,* 79–85.

Fleming, J. E., Boyle, M. H., & Offord, D. R. (1993). The outcome of adolescent depression in the Ontario Child Health Study follow-up. *Journal of the American Academy of Child and Adolescent Psychiatry, 32,* 28–33.

Fleming, J. E., & Offord, D. R. (1990). Epidemiology of childhood depressive disorders: A critical review. *Journal of the American Academy of Child and Adolescent Psychiatry, 29,* 571–580.

Fleming, J. E., Offord, D. R., & Boyle, M. H. (1989). Prevalence of childhood and adolescent depression in the community: Ontario Child Health Study. *British Journal of Psychiatry, 155,* 647–654.

Garber, J., & Hilsman, R. (1992). Cognitions, stress, and depression in children and adolescents. *Child and Adolescent Psychiatric Clinics of North America, 1,* 129–167.

Garrison, C. Z., Schlucter, M. D., Schoenbach, V. J., & Kaplan, B. K. (1989). Epidemiology of depressive symptoms in young adolescents. *Journal of the American Academy of Child and Adolescent Psychiatry, 28,* 343–351.

Ghareeb, G. A., & Beshai, J. A. (1989). Arabic version of the Children's Depression Inventory: Reliability and validity. *Journal of Clinical Child Psychology, 18,* 323–326.

Gibbs, J. T. (1985). Psychosocial factors associated with depression in urban adolescent females: Implications for assessment. *Journal of Youth and Adolescence, 14,* 47–60.

Gladstone, T. R. G., & Kaslow, N. J. (1995). Depression and attributions in children and adolescents: A meta-analytic review. *Journal of Abnormal Child Psychology, 23,* 597–606.

Glaser, K. (1968). Masked depression in children and adolescents. *Annual Progress in Child Psychiatry and Child Development, 1,* 345–355.

Gotlib, I. H., & Hammen, C. L. (1992). *Psychological aspects of depression: Toward a cognitive-interpersonal integration*. New York: Wiley.

Haley, G. M. T., Fine, S., Marriage, K., Moretti, M. M., & Freeman, R. J. (1985). Cognitive bias and depression in psychiatrically disturbed children and adolescents. *Journal of Consulting and Clinical Psychology, 53,* 535–537.

Hammen, C. (1992). Cognitive, life stress, and interpersonal approaches to a developmental psychopathology model of depression. *Development and Psychopathology, 4,* 189–206.

Hammen, C., Burge, D., & Adrian, C. (1991). The timing of mother and child depression in a longitudinal study of children at risk. *Journal of Consulting and Clinical Psychology, 59,* 341–345.

Hammen, C., & Compas, B. E. (1994). Unmasking unmasked depression in children and adolescents: The problem of comorbidity. *Clinical Psychology Review, 14,* 585–603.

Hammen, C., & Zupan, B. A. (1984). Self-schemas, depression, and the processing of personal information in children. *Journal of Experimental Child Psychology, 37,* 598–608.

Hanna, G. L. (1992). Natural history of mood disorders. *Child and Adolescent Psychiatric Clinics of North America, 1,* 169–181.

Harrington, R. (1992). Annotation: The natural history and treatment of child and adolescent affective disorders. *Journal of Child Psychology and Psychiatry, 33,* 1287–1302.

Harrington, R. (1993). *Depressive disorder in childhood and adolescence.* New York: Wiley.

Hodges, K., Cools, J., & McKnew, D. (1989). Test–retest reliability of a clinical research interview for children: The Child Assessment Schedule (CAS). *Psychological Assessment: A Journal of Consulting and Clinical Psychology, 1,* 317–322.

Ivens, C., & Rehm, L. P. (1988). Assessment of childhood depression: Correspondence between reports by child, mother, and father. *Journal of the American Academy of Child and Adolescent Psychiatry, 27,* 738–741.

Jacobson, R., Lahey, B. B., & Strauss, C. C. (1983). Correlates of depressed mood in normal children. *Journal of Abnormal Child Psychology, 11,* 29–39.

Kahn, J. S., Kehle, T. J., Jenson, W. R., & Clark, E. (1990). Comparison of cognitive-behavioral, relaxation, and self-modeling interventions for depression among middle-school students. *School Psychology Review, 19,* 196–211.

Kandel, D. B., & Davies, M. (1982). Epidemiology of depressive mood in adolescents. *Archives of General Psychiatry, 39,* 1205–1212.

Kandel, D. B., & Davies, M. (1986). Adult sequelae of adolescent depressive symptoms. *Archives of General Psychiatry, 43,* 255–262.

Kashani, J. H., Cantwell, D. P., Shekim, W. O., & Reid, J. C. (1982). Major depressive disorder in children admitted to an inpatient community mental health center. *American Journal of Psychiatry, 139,* 671–672.

Kashani, J. H., Carlson, G. A., Beck, N. C., Hoeper, E. W., Corcoran, C. M., McAllister, J. A., Fallahi, C., Rosenberg, T. K., & Reid, J. C. (1987). Depression, depressive symptoms, and depressed mood among a community sample of adolescents. *American Journal of Psychiatry, 144,* 931–934.

Kashani, J. H., Holcomb, W. R., & Orvaschel, H. (1986). Depression and depressive symptoms in preschool children from the general population. *American Journal of Psychiatry, 143,* 1138–1143.

Kaslow, N. J., Brown, R. T., & Mee, L. L. (1994). Cognitive and behavioral correlates of childhood depression: A developmental perspective. In W. M. Reynolds & H. F. Johnston (Eds.), *Handbook of depression in children and adolescents* (pp. 97–121). New York: Plenum Press.

Kaslow, N. J., Celano, M. P., & McCarthy, S. M. (1993). Cognitive-behavioral perspectives on childhood depression: A developmental and contextual model. In V. B. Van Hasselt & M. Hersen (Eds.), *Handbook of behavioral therapy and pharmacotherapy with children: A comparative analysis* (pp. 71–87). Boston: Allyn & Bacon.

Kaslow, N. J., Deering, C. G., & Racusin, G. R. (1994). Depressed children and their families. *Clinical Psychology Review, 14,* 39–59.

Kaslow, N. J., & Racusin, G. R. (1994). Family therapy for depression in young people. In W. M. Reynolds & H. F. Johnston (Eds.), *Handbook of depression in children and adolescents* (pp. 345–363). New York: Plenum Press.

Kaslow, N. J., Rehm, L. P., Pollack, S., & Siegel, A. W. (1988). Attributional style and self-control behavior in depressed and nondepressed children and their parents. *Journal of Abnormal Child Psychology, 16,* 163–177.

Kaslow, N. J., Rehm, L. P., & Siegel, A. W. (1984). Social cognitive and cognitive correlates of depression in children. *Journal of Abnormal Child Psychology, 12,* 605–620.

Kendall, P. C., Stark, K. D., & Adam, T. (1990). Cognitive deficit or cognitive distortion in childhood depression. *Journal of Abnormal Child Psychology, 18,* 255–270.

King, C. A., Naylor, M. W., Segal, H. G., Evans, T., & Shain, B. N. (1993). Global self-worth, specific self-perceptions of competence, and depression in adolescents. *Journal of the American Academy of Child and Adolescent Psychiatry, 32,* 745–752.

Klerman, G. L., Weissman, M. M., Rounsaville, B. J., & Chevron, E. S. (1984). *Interpersonal psychotherapy of depression.* New York: Basic Books.

Kobak, R. R., Sudler, N., & Gamble, W. (1992). Attachment and depressive symptoms during adolescence: A developmental pathways analysis. *Development and Psychopathology, 3,* 461–474.

Kolko, D. J., & Kazdin, A. E. (1993). Emotional/behavioral problems in a clinic and nonclinic children: Correspondence among child, parent, and teacher reports. *Journal of Child Psychology and Psychiatry, 34,* 991–1006.

Kovacs, M. (1989). Affective disorder in children and adolescents. *American Psychologist, 44,* 209–215.

Kovacs, M. (1992). *Children's Depression Inventory Manual.* North Tonawanda, NY: Multi-Health Systems.

Kovacs, M., & Beck, A. T. (1977). An empirical-clinical approach toward a definition of childhood depression. In J. G. Schulterbrandt & A. Raskin (Eds.), *Depression in childhood: Diagnosis, treatment, and conceptual models* (pp. 1–25). New York: Raven Press.

Kupersmidt, J. B., & Patterson, C. J. (1991). Childhood peer rejection, aggression, withdrawal, and perceived competence as predictors of self-reported behavior problems in preadolescence. *Journal of Abnormal Child Psychology, 19,* 427–449.

Lang, M., & Tisher, M. (1978). *Children's Depression Scale.* Victoria: Australian Council for Educational Research.

Larsson, B., & Melin, I. (1990). Depressive symptoms in Swedish adolescents. *Journal of Abnormal Child Psychology, 18,* 91–103.

Lefkowitz, M. M., & Tesiny, E. P. (1984). Rejection and depression: Prospective and contemporaneous analyses. *Developmental Psychology, 20,* 776–785.

Lefkowitz, M. M., Tesiny, E. P., & Solodow, W. (1989). A rating scale for assessing dysphoria in youth. *Journal of Abnormal Child Psychology, 17,* 337–347.

Lewinsohn, P. M., Clarke, G. N., Hops, H., & Andrews, J. (1990). Cognitive-behavioral treatment for depressed adolescents. *Behavior Therapy, 21,* 385–401.

Lewinsohn, P. M., Hops, H., Roberts, R. E., Seeley, J. R., & Andrews, J. A. (1993). Adolescent psychopathology: I.

Prevalence and incidence of depression and other DSM-III-R disorders in high school students. *Journal of Abnormal Psychology, 102,* 133–144.

Liddle, B., & Spence, S. H. (1990). Cognitive-behaviour therapy with depressed primary school children: A cautionary note. *Behavioural Psychotherapy, 18,* 85–102.

Luthar, S. S., & Blatt, S. J. (1993). Dependent and self-critical depressive experiences among inner city adolescents. *Journal of Personality, 61,* 365–386.

Manson, S. M., Ackerson, L. M., Dick, R. W., Baron, A. E., & Fleming, C. M. (1990). Depressive symptoms among American Indian adolescents: Psychometric characteristics of the Center for Epidemiologic Studies–Depression Scale (CES-D). *Psychological Assessment: A Journal of Consulting and Clinical Psychology, 2,* 231–237.

Marsella, A. J., Sartorius, N., Jablensky, A., & Fenton, F. R. (1985). Cross-cultural studies of depressive disorders: An overview. In A. Kleinman & B. Good (Eds.), *Culture and depression* (pp. 299–324). Berkeley: University of California Press.

Marton, P., Connolly, J., Kutcher, S., & Korenblum, M. (1993). Cognitive social skills and social self-appraisal in depressed adolescents. *Journal of the American Academy of Child and Adolescent Psychiatry, 32,* 739–744.

McCracken, J. T. (1992). The epidemiology of child and adolescent mood disorders. *Child and Adolescent Psychiatric Clinics of North America, 1,* 53–72.

McKinney, W. T. (1986). Primate separation studies: Relevance to bereavement. *Psychiatric Annals, 16,* 281–287.

Messer, S. C., & Gross, A. M. (1995). Childhood depression and family interaction: A naturalistic observation study. *Journal of Clinical Child Psychology, 24,* 77–88.

Mitchell, J., McCauley, E., Burke, P. M., & Moss, S. J. (1988). Phenomenology of depression in children and adolescents. *Journal of the American Academy of Child and Adolescent Psychiatry, 27,* 12–20.

Mufson, L., Moreau, D., Weissman, M., Wickramaratne, P., Martin, J., & Samoilov, A. (1994). Modification of interpersonal psychotherapy with depressed adolescents (IPT-A): Phase I and II studies. *Journal of the American Academy of Child and Adolescent Psychiatry, 33,* 695–705.

Myer, N. E., Dyck, D. G., & Petrinack, R. J. (1989). Cognitive appraisal and attributional correlates of depressive symptoms in children. *Journal of Abnormal Child Psychology, 17,* 325–336.

Nolen-Hoeksema, S., & Girgus, J. S. (1994). The emergence of gender differences in depression during adolescence. *Psychological Bulletin, 115,* 424–443.

Nolen-Hoeksema, S., Girgus, J. S., & Seligman, M. E. P. (1986). Learned helplessness in children: A longitudinal study of depression, achievement, and explanatory style. *Journal of Personality and Social Psychology, 51,* 435–442.

Nolen-Hoeksema, S., Girgus, J. S., & Seligman, M. E. P. (1992). Predictors and consequences of childhood depressive symptoms: A 5-year longitudinal study. *Journal of Abnormal Psychology, 101,* 405–422.

Petersen, A. C., Compas, B. E., Brooks-Gunn, J., Stemmler, M., Ey, S., & Grant, K. E. (1993). Depression in adolescence. *American Psychologist, 48,* 155–168.

Petersen, A. C., & Crockett, L. (1985). Pubertal timing and grade effects on adjustment. *Journal of Youth and Adolescence, 14,* 101–106.

Peterson, L., Mullins, L. L., & Ridley-Johnson, R. (1985). Childhood depression: Peer reactions to depression and life stress. *Journal of Abnormal Child Psychology, 13,* 597–609.

Piaget, J. (1946). *The development of children's concept of time.* Paris: Presses Universitaires de France.

Poznanski, E. O. (1982). The clinical phenomenology of childhood depression. *American Journal of Orthopsychiatry, 52,* 308–313.

Prieto, S. L., Cole, D. A., & Tageson, C. W. (1992). Depressive self-schemas in clinic and nonclinic children. *Cognitive Therapy and Research, 16,* 521–534.

Puig-Antich, J. (1982). Major depression and conduct disorder in prepuberty. *Journal of the American Academy of Child Psychiatry, 21,* 118–128.

Puig-Antich, J. (1987). Sleep and neuroendocrine correlates of affective illness in childhood and adolescence. *Journal of Adolescent Health Care, 8,* 505–529.

Puig-Antich, J., & Chambers, W. (1978). *The Schedule for Affective Disorders and Schizophrenia for School-Aged Children (Kiddie-SADS).* New York: New York State Psychiatric Institute.

Puig-Antich, J., Goetz, D., Davies, M., Kaplan, T., Davies, S., Ostrow, L., Asnis, L., Twomey, J., Iyengar, S., & Ryan, N. (1989). A controlled family history study of prepubertal major depressive disorder. *Archives of General Psychiatry, 46,* 406–418.

Puig-Antich, J., Kaufman, J., Ryan, N. D., Williamson, D., Dahl, R. E., Lukens, E., Todak, G., Ambrosini, P., Rabinovich, H., & Nelson, B. (1993). The psychosocial functioning and family environment of depressed adolescents. *Journal of the American Academy of Child and Adolescent Psychiatry, 32,* 244–253.

Puig-Antich, J., Lukens, E., Davies, M., Goetz, D., Brennan-Quattrock, J., & Todak, G. (1985). Psychosocial functioning in prepubertal major depressive disorder. *Archives of General Psychiatry, 42,* 500–507.

Radloff, L. S. (1977). A CES-D Scale: A self-report depression scale for research in the general population. *Applied Psychological Measurement, 1,* 358–401.

Rao, U., Ryan, N. D., Birmaher, B., Dahl, R. E., Williamson, D. E., Kaufman, J., Rao, R., & Nelson, G. (1995). Unipolar depression in adolescents: Clinical outcome in adulthood. *Journal of the American Academy of Child and Adolescent Psychiatry, 34,* 566–578.

Rehm, L. P. (1977). A self-control model of depression. *Behavior Therapy, 8,* 787–804.

Reinherz, H. Z., Frost, A. K., & Pakiz, B. (1991). Changing

faces: Correlates of depressive symptoms in late adolescence. *Family and Community Health, 14*, 52–63.

Reynolds, W. M. (1986a). A model for the screening and identification of depressed children and adolescents in school settings. *Professional School Psychology, 1*, 117–129.

Reynolds, W. M. (1986b). *Assessment of depression in adolescents: Manual for Reynolds Adolescent Depression Scale.* Odessa, FL: Psychological Assessment Resources.

Reynolds, W. M. (1994). Assessment of depression in children and adolescents by self-report questionnaires. In W. M. Reynolds & H. F. Johnston (Eds.), *Handbook of depression in children and adolescents* (pp. 209–234). New York: Plenum Press.

Reynolds, W. M., & Coates, K. I. (1986). A comparison of cognitive-behavioral therapy and relaxation training for the treatment of depression in adolescents. *Journal of Consulting and Clinical Psychology, 54*, 653–660.

Rie, H. E. (1966). Depression in childhood: A survey of some pertinent contributions. *Journal of the American Academy of Child Psychiatry, 5*, 653–685.

Robbins, D. R., Alessi, N. E., & Colfer, M. V. (1989). Treatment of adolescents with major depressive disorder: Implications of the DST and the melancholic subtype. *Journal of Affective Disorders, 17*, 99–104.

Rudolph, K. D., Hammen, C., & Burge, D. (1994). Interpersonal functioning and depressive symptoms in childhood: Addressing the issues of specificity and comorbidity. *Journal of Abnormal Child Psychology, 22*, 355–371.

Rush, A. J., & Nowels, A. (1994). Adaptation of cognitive therapy for depressed adolescents. In T. C. R. Wilkes, G. Belsher, A. J. Rush, & E. Frank (Eds.), *Cognitive therapy for depressed adolescents* (pp. 3–21). New York: Guilford Press.

Rutter, M., & Hersov, L. (Eds.). (1985). *Child and adolescent psychiatry.* London: Blackwell.

Ryan, N. D., Puig-Antich, J., Ambrosini, B., Rabinovich, H., Robinson, D., Nelson, B., Iyengar, S., & Twomey, J. (1987). The clinical picture of major depression in children and adolescents. *Archives of General Psychiatry, 44*, 854–861.

Schwab, J. J., & Schwab, M. E. (1978). *Sociocultural roots of mental illness.* New York: Plenum Press.

Seligman, M. E. P. (1975). *Helplessness: On depression, development, and death.* San Francisco: Freeman.

Seligman, M. E. P., Peterson, C., Kaslow, N. J., Tanenbaum, R. L., Alloy, L. B., & Abramson, L. Y. (1984). Attributional style and depressive symptoms among children. *Journal of Abnormal Psychology, 93*, 235–238.

Siegler, R. S. (1986). *Children's thinking.* Englewood Cliffs, NJ: Prentice–Hall.

Spitz, R. (1946). Anaclitic depression. *Psychoanalytic Study of the Child, 5*, 113–177.

Stark, K. D. (1990). *Childhood depression: School-based intervention.* New York: Guilford Press.

Stark, K. D., Reynolds, W. R., & Kaslow, N. J. (1987). A comparison of the relative efficacy of self-control therapy and a behavioral problem-solving therapy for depression in children. *Journal of Abnormal Child Psychology, 15*, 91–113.

Stark, K. D., Rouse, L. W., & Kurowski, C. (1994). Psychological treatment approaches for depression in children. In W. M. Reynolds & H. F. Johnston (Eds.), *Handbook of depression in children and adolescents* (pp. 275–307). New York: Plenum Press.

Stark, K. D., Rouse, L. W., & Livingston, R. (1991). Treatment of depression during childhood and adolescence: Cognitive-behavioral procedures for the individual and family. In P. Kendall (Ed.), *Child and adolescent therapy* (pp. 165–206). New York: Guilford Press.

Swanson, J. W., Linskey, A. O., Quintero-Salinas, R., Pumariega, A. J., & Holzer, C. E. (1992). A binational school survey of depressive symptoms, drug use, and suicidal ideation. *Journal of the American Academy of Child and Adolescent Psychiatry, 31*, 669–678.

Tambs, K., & Moum, T. (1993). Low genetic effect and age-specific family effect for symptoms of anxiety and depression in nuclear families, halfsibs, and twins. *Journal of Affective Disorders, 27*, 183–195.

Tharinger, D. J., & Stark, K. (1990). A qualitative versus quantitative approach to evaluating the Draw-A-Person and Kinetic Family Drawing: A study of mood- and anxiety-disorder children. *Psychological Assessment: A Journal of Consulting and Clinical Psychology, 2*, 365–375.

Trad, P. V. (1994). Depression in infants. In W. M. Reynolds & H. F. Johnston (Eds.), *Handbook of depression in children and adolescents* (pp. 401–426). New York: Plenum Press.

Wallerstein, J. S., & Corbin, S. B. (1991). The child and the vicissitudes of divorce. In M. Lewis (Ed.), *Child and adolescent psychiatry: A comprehensive textbook* (pp. 1108–1117). Baltimore: Williams & Wilkins.

Warner, V., Weissman, M., Fendrich, M., Wickramaratne, P., & Moreau, D. (1992). The course of major depression in the offspring of depressed parents: Incidence, recurrence, and recovery. *Archives of General Psychiatry, 49*, 795–801.

Weiss, B., Weisz, J. R., Politano, M., Carey, M., Nelson, W. M., & Finch, A. J. (1992). Relations among self-reported depressive symptoms in clinic-referred children versus adolescents. *Journal of Abnormal Psychology, 101*, 391–387.

Weisz, J. R., Sweeney, L., Proffitt, V., & Carr, T. (1993). Control-related beliefs and self-reported depressive symptoms in late childhood. *Journal of Abnormal Psychology, 102*, 411–418.

Weller, R., Weller, E., Fristad, M., & Bowes, J. (1991). Depression in recently bereaved prepubertal children. *American Journal of Psychiatry, 148*, 1536–1540.

Whitman, P. B., & Leitenberg, H. (1990). Negatively biased recall in children with self-report symptoms of depression. *Journal of Abnormal Child Psychology, 18,* 15–27.

Wilkes, T. C. R. (1994). Developmental considerations. In T. C. R. Wilkes, G. Belsher, A. J. Rush, & E. Frank (Eds.), *Cognitive therapy for depressed adolescents* (pp. 69–79). New York: Guilford Press.

Worchel, F. F., Hughes, J. N., Hall, B. M., Stanton, S. B., Stanton, S., & Little, V. Z. (1990). Evaluation of subclinical depression in children using self-, peer-, and teacher-report measures. *Journal of Abnormal Child Psychology, 18,* 271–282.

11

Eating Disorders

DONALD A. WILLIAMSON, BRET G. BENTZ, AND JODIE Y. RABALAIS

INTRODUCTION

Anorexia nervosa was first described as a psychiatric syndrome by Gull (1874) and Lasegue (1873). There were other reports of patients with symptoms resembling anorexia and bulimia nervosa prior to 1873, however. In 1694, Morton described a young woman with the symptoms of anorexia nervosa, e.g., starvation, absence of menstrual cycle, and exhaustion (Yates, 1989). She eventually died after refusing treatment. Morton called this woman's disorder "nervous consumption." James (1743) described patients with voracious appetites. Some of these patients terminated their binges with vomiting. In a recent historical review of these early reports, Stunkard (1993) concluded that the modern clinical syndromes of anorexia and bulimia nervosa, in which overconcern with body size is a primary determining factor, probably emerged only in the past 150 years. The origins of Western society's obsession with thinness can be traced back to Banting's (1864) *Letter on Corpulence*. Pri-

or to Banting's book, excessive adiposity was not considered to be of serious medical concern. Yet, since the mid-1800s, social derogation of obesity has gradually emerged as normative. By the 1990s, no one even questions the negative attitudes pertaining to obesity and the positive attitudes pertaining to thinness. From these sociocultural changes, both healthy habits (e.g., increased fitness and reduced consumption of dietary fat) and unhealthy habits (e.g., extreme dieting, purging, and obligatory exercise) have emerged (Brownell, 1991). Changes in attitudes about body weight have been more dramatic in developed countries, resulting in a higher prevalence rate of eating disorders in these societies (Fairburn, Hay, & Welch, 1993). Thus, in the modern world, anorexia and bulimia nervosa are regarded as having the essential characteristics of fear of fatness and overconcern with body size and shape. This chapter will review research evidence concerning the diagnosis, assessment, and treatment of these eating disorders.

DONALD A. WILLIAMSON, BRET G. BENTZ, AND JODIE Y. RABALAIS • Department of Psychology, Louisiana State University, Baton Rouge, Louisiana 70803.

Handbook of Child Psychopathology, 3rd edition, edited by Ollendick & Hersen. Plenum Press, New York, 1998.

PHENOMENOLOGY

The essential characteristics of anorexia nervosa are a refusal to maintain a minimal normal body weight, an intense fear of gaining weight, a distorted perception of body image, and amenorrhea in females. The anorexic patient commonly engages in restrictive eating and excessive exercise to attain and maintain a low body weight, which in extreme cases can be life threatening. In addition, patients with anorexia nervosa may binge episodically and use purgative methods to control weight gain (Garfinkel, Moldofsky, & Garner, 1979; Halmi & Falk, 1982).

Epidemiological surveys of the incidence of anorexia nervosa have generally reported a significant increase since the 1950s and 1960s (Jones, Fox, Babigian, & Hutton, 1980; Willi & Grossman, 1983). Anorexia nervosa is a psychiatric disorder associated with young, white females from upper socioeconomic status (Kinder, 1991). The usual age of onset is during the adolescent years and the early 20s. Anorexia nervosa is found to be far less prevalent in nonindustrialized cultures (Nasser, 1988) where adiposity is associated with wealth, fertility, or womanhood. It has been suggested that this difference in prevalence may be related to the impact of Western society on women's idealization of thinness which leads to body-image dissatisfaction (Polivy & Herman, 1993).

Clinically, anorexic patients report feeling fat even though they may be significantly underweight (Williamson, Barker, & Norris, 1993). In addition, they often experience obsessional thoughts of thinness, which motivates extreme methods of attaining and maintaining low body weight. To the clinician, this fear of weight gain and obsession with thinness may be manifested as resistance to treatment.

The central feature of bulimia nervosa is recurrent episodes of uncontrolled binge eating. These binge episodes are often followed by the use of purgative methods to control weight gain. These methods of weight control often take the form of self-induced vomiting, excessive exercise, restrictive eating, and the use of laxatives and diuretics. It is generally believed that these behaviors are motivated by an intense fear of weight gain and a distorted perception of body size similar to that seen in anorexia nervosa. However, unlike the anorexic, bulimic patients are usually within the normal weight range as a result of binge eating.

Estimates of the incidence of bulimia nervosa have ranged from 1 to 3% (Fairburn & Beglin, 1990). Similar to the anorexic, the bulimic patient is often young, white, and female (Powell & Kahn, 1995; Striegel-Moore, Silberstein, & Rodin, 1986). As will be presented later, bulimia nervosa is also frequently associated with other forms of psychopathology, including depression, anxiety, and substance abuse (Wilson & Pike, 1993).

Clinically, the bulimic patient presents with an obsessive concern with body weight, shape/size, and "fattening" foods. Binge eating often occurs after the patient's efforts to diet have been disrupted (Williamson, 1990). Binge eating causes increased anxiety and obsessional thinking about weight gain. Purgative methods are used to reduce this anxiety and worry. The bulimic patient is often difficult to treat because of a denial of the problems caused by their obsession with thinness. Also, they fear that modification of their eating and purgative habits will result in weight gain, a consequence that they abhor.

DIAGNOSTIC CONSIDERATIONS

Over the past 25 years, overconcern with body size and shape has come to be seen as a central diagnostic feature of anorexia and bulimia nervosa. As recently as 1960, diagnostic descriptions of anorexia nervosa focused solely on low weight status without regard to a fear of being fat (Stunkard, 1993). In recent years, clinical researchers have focused on fear of fatness and body image disturbances as a fundamental motivational component of the eating disorders (Williamson, 1990). These theories have hypothesized that the development of an eating disorder usually occurs in adolescence or early adulthood. Typically, the person will begin to focus on thinness as the secret to happiness and self-esteem and/or will use binge eating as a method for coping with stress. If restrictive eating and/or purgative habits predominate, the syndrome of anorexia nervosa usually emerges. If binge eating and subsequent compensatory behaviors (such as self-induced vomiting) predominate, then the syndrome of bulimia nervosa usually develops. Very frequently, a person with an eating disorder will change from a predominantly bulimic pattern to a predominantly anorexic one, or vice versa, over time (Williamson, 1990). If binge eating predominates without purgative habits, binge eating disorder or nonpurging bulimia nervosa typically emerges (Fairburn & Wilson, 1993).

TYPES OF EATING DISORDERS

Delineation of different types of eating disorders has been a source of controversy for many years. At present, there is general agreement between the descriptions of anorexia and bulimia nervosa provided by the World Health Organization (1992) and the American Psychiatric Association (1994). A summary of the central features of these two eating disorders is provided in Tables 1 and 2.

Anorexia Nervosa

DSM-IV Description

A summary of the fourth edition of the *Diagnostic and Statistical Manual of Mental Disorders* (DSM-IV; American Psychiatric Association, 1994) diagnostic criteria for anorexia nervosa is presented in Table 1. The diagnostic criteria for anorexia nervosa have changed little from the 1987 DSM-III-R description of anorexia nervosa (American Psychiatric Association, 1987). Four symptoms must be present for the diagnosis of anorexia nervosa. First, the patient must exhibit a refusal to maintain a minimal normal body weight, defined as 85% of the expected normal body weight. Second, a fear of gaining weight or becoming fat must be evident even though the patient may be severely underweight. Third, the patient must have a distorted perception of his or her body weight or body shape. Finally, in females there must be an absence of at least three consecutive menstrual cycles.

In DSM-IV, two subtypes of anorexia nervosa are described, restricting and binge eating/purging types. The restricting subtype is characterized by classic starvation and low body weight indicative of anorexia in the absence of binge eating and purging behavior. In contrast, the binge eating/purging subtype of anorexia nervosa is characterized by episodes of binge eating and purging in addition to low body weight, amenorrhea, and so forth.

Differential Diagnosis

Anorexia nervosa is often comorbid with disorders such as depression, obsessive-compulsive disorder, and personality disorders. One study found a high frequency of lifetime affective disorders among anorexics, with 42.8% receiving a diagnosis of major depression (Piran, Kennedy, Garfinkel, & Owners, 1985). Characteristics shared by the two syndromes are weight loss,

Table 1. Summary of DSM-IV Diagnostic Criteria for Anorexia Nervosa

A. Refusal to maintain minimal normal body weight.
B. Intense fear of gaining weight or becoming fat.
C. Body image disturbances.
D. Amenorrhea, for at least three consecutive menstrual cycles.
  Restricting type: The person does not regularly engage in binge eating or purging behavior.
  Binge eating/purging type: The person regularly engages in binge eating or purging behavior.

Table 2. Summary of DSM-IV Diagnostic Criteria for Bulimia Nervosa

A. Recurrent binge eating, characterized by both of the following:
    (1)   Eating an amount of food that is larger than what most people would eat.
    (2)   A sense of lack of control over eating during the binge episode.
B. Inappropriate compensatory behavior to prevent weight gain, such as vomiting, misuse of laxatives or diuretics, fasting, or excessive exercise.
C. Binge eating and compensatory behavior both occur at least twice a week for 3 months.
D. Overconcern with body size strongly influences self-evaluation.
E. Disturbance does not occur during episodes of Anorexia Nervosa.
    Purging type: The person engages in vomiting or the misuse of laxatives or diuretics.
    Nonpurging type: The person uses other compensatory behaviors, such as fasting or excessive exercise.

sleep disturbance, and poor concentration. A central distinguishing feature between the two syndromes is that in anorexia nervosa, weight loss results from fear of fatness, whereas in depression, weight loss is caused by loss of appetite.

Obsessive-compulsive disorder has also been found in a significant percentage of anorexics (Kasvikis, Tsakiris, Marks, Basoglu, & Noshirvani, 1986). The obsession with body size in anorexia is often just one of several obsessions (e.g., contamination, doubt) in such cases. Also, personality disorders often accompany anorexia nervosa. Personality research has found that cluster C personality disorders (avoidant, dependent, compulsive, and passive-aggressive) are most commonly associated with anorexia nervosa (Johnson & Wonderlich, 1992).

Bulimia Nervosa

DSM-IV Description

A summary of the DSM-IV (American Psychiatric Association, 1994) diagnostic criteria for bulimia nervosa is presented in Table 2. It is important to note that bulimia is a disorder of binge eating and that purging via vomiting or laxative abuse is not specifically required for the diagnosis. Binge eating episodes are characterized by eating an amount of food that is larger than what most people would eat and by a lack of control over eating during the episode. In addition, the frequency of binge eating and compensatory behavior must average at least twice per week for 3 months to meet diagnostic criteria.

Two subtypes of bulimia nervosa have been described in DSM-IV, purging and nonpurging types. The purging subtype is defined by regular episodes of self-induced vomiting or the misuse of laxatives or diuretics. In contrast, the nonpurging subtype binges, but uses other compensatory behavior such as fasting or excessive exercise and does not regularly engage in episodes of self-induced vomiting or the misuse of laxatives or diuretics to control body weight. Recent research (Williamson, Gleaves, & Savin, 1992) has found that nonpurging bulimics are usually overweight, probably reflecting the relative inefficiency of fasting and exercise to compensate for the foods consumed during binges. A final diagnostic criterion is that the disturbance must not occur exclusively during episodes of anorexia nervosa. Thus, a diagnosis of anorexia nervosa supersedes a diagnosis of bulimia nervosa.

Differential Diagnosis

Bulimia nervosa has been found to be associated with a wide range of other psychopathology including depression, anxiety, and personality disorders. For example, Lewinsohn, Hops, Roberts, Seeley, and Andrews (1993) reported that among the eating disorder diagnoses, 69.2% of the sample were also diagnosed with depression.

The cluster B personality disorders (borderline, histrionic, narcissistic, and antisocial) have been associated with bulimia nervosa (Johnson & Wonderlich, 1992). Prevalence rates for histrionic personality disorder in bulimic samples have been found to be higher than in anorexic samples, and similar but conflicting evidence supports higher rates of borderline personality disorder among bulimics. Anxiety and obsessive-compulsive disorders have often been found to frequently coexist with bulimia nervosa. Bulik, Beidel, Duchmann, Weltzin, and Kaye (1991) reported lifetime prevalence rates of obsessive-compulsive disorder to be about 20% in women diagnosed with bulimia nervosa. In addition, high rates of panic disorder, simple phobia, and social phobia have been reported in surveys of bulimia nervosa (Williamson et al., 1993).

Eating Disorder Not Otherwise Specified (NOS)

DSM-IV Description

As can be seen in Table 3, DSM-IV (American Psychiatric Association, 1994) has provided several examples of eating disorder NOS. These variants of eating disorders do not meet DSM-IV criteria for anorexia or bulimia, yet in many cases the patient exhibits a mixture of anorexic and bulimic symptoms. In addition, it has been found that many of the defining characteristics of atypical eating disorders are similar to anorexia and bulimia. For example, descriptive reports (Mitchell, Pyle, Hatsukami, & Eckert, 1986; Norvell & Cooley, 1987; Williamson, Gleaves, & Sav-

in, 1992) have suggested that the central characteristics of eating disorder NOS are: (1) intense fear of weight gain, (2) overconcern with body size and shape, and (3) use of extreme methods for weight control. Generally, these symptoms of eating disorder NOS are quite similar in severity to those found in anorexia and bulimia nervosa (Williamson, Gleaves, & Savin, 1992).

Differential Diagnosis

There are many variants of anorexia and bulimia nervosa that do not meet all of the DSM-IV diagnostic criteria for anorexia or bulimia nervosa. As can be seen in Table 3, these atypical eating disorders are often subthreshold cases, cases that lack one specific criterion (e.g., no loss of menses in anorexia).

In anorexia, it is critical that sufficient weight loss and the absence of menses (in females) be present for the diagnosis. In bulimia, the patient must engage in episodes of binge eating and express persistent overconcern with body shape and weight.

Depression, obsessive-compulsive disorder, and conversion disorder must be ruled out before a diagnosis of eating disorder NOS is assigned (Williamson, 1990). The differential diagnosis of subclinical anorexia nervosa and depression, which can cause a loss of appetite and weight loss, is based on the presence of body image disturbance, preference for thinness, and a fear of weight gain that is associated with an eating disorder, but is not generally associated with depression. An eating disorder can

---

Table 3. Examples of the DSM-IV Diagnosis of Eating Disorder Not Otherwise Specified

1. A patient who has met all of the cirteria for Anorexia Nervosa except the patient has regular menses.
2. A patient who has met all of the criteria for Anoirexia Nervosa except the patient's current weight is normal.
3. A patient who has met all of the criteria for Bulimia Nervosa except binges occur at a frequency of less than twice a week.
4. A patient who does engage in recurrent episodes of binge eating, but does not engagte in the inappropriate compensatory behaviors such as vomiting and the misuse of laxatives or diuretics.
5. Tasting food by chewing and then spitting the food out.
6. Binge eating disorder, which is associated with frequent binge eating, obesity, and the absence of extreme weight regulation methods such as purging or excessive exercise.

be distinguished from obsessive-compulsive disorder on the basis of the content of the obsessive thoughts and the nature of the person's compulsive behavior. If an obsession is related to food or poisoning, but not to a fear of fatness, the diagnosis of an eating disorder is usually inappropriate. Finally, the differential diagnosis of conversion disorder is typically based on the presence or absence of body image disturbance and the nature of the self-induced physical symptoms. For example, in conversion disorder, laxatives may be taken to produce a medical symptom, diarrhea; whereas in bulimia nervosa, laxatives are taken to compensate for binges and to lose body weight.

ETIOLOGY

Biological Theories

Although the physiological underpinnings of eating disorders have not been definitively discovered, several biological and psychobiological theories of eating disorders have been proposed. Disturbance in neurotransmitter (Kaye, 1992) and hormone regulation (Geracioti & Liddle, 1988) are among the biological mechanisms that have been associated with eating disorder symptoms. The regulation of appetite has been described as a complex process involving psychological events (hunger perceptions, cravings, taste sensations), behavioral events (macronutrient intake, meals, snacks), metabolic events, and neurotransmitter activity (Blundell & Hill, 1993). When one or more of these events are deficient or excessive, appetite can become dysregulated, and eating disorders may be more likely to develop. Restrictive eating, for example, may result in decreased carbohydrate consumption and increased hunger motivation (Blundell & Hill, 1993), and this hunger may increase the likelihood of binge eating and the subsequent development of an eating disorder.

Relative to normal subjects, women diagnosed with bulimia nervosa were found to have lower levels of cholecystokinin, a hormone that

is released by the gastrointestinal tract into the plasma and functions to produce satiety (Geracioti & Liddle, 1988). Another line of evidence from animal studies indicates that severe dietary restriction, as seen in anorexia nervosa, may be maintained by endogenous opiates (Marrazzi & Luby, 1986). It has been hypothesized that increased levels of endogenous opiates produced during starvation and following periods of excessive exercise may create a sense of analgesic euphoria or "high" (Marrazzi & Luby, 1986). Thus, anorexia nervosa may in part reflect a physiological and psychological addiction to an elevated mood state. If, however, endogenous opiate "addiction" were responsible for the maintenance of eating disorders, a reduction in endorphin production should result in decreased features of the disorders. Opiate antagonists, however, have not been effective in alleviating fear of weight gain or preoccupation with dieting (Yates, 1989).

Additional research suggests that binge eating and purging can be favorably reduced by antidepressant pharmacotherapy (Fairburn, Agras, & Wilson, 1992). In fact, bulimia nervosa has been conceptualized as having the same biological basis as depression (Pope & Hudson, 1988). This theory is based on the finding that bulimics often have a personal and family history of affective disorders and that bulimics have shown positive responses to antidepressant medications. Such data, however, are largely correlational, and the theory that bulimia is a form of depression has not been strongly supported (Hinz & Williamson, 1987). Rather, eating disorders appear to commonly co-occur with other affective disorders.

Psychosocial Theories

Eating disorders represent a complex interplay of several variables, and researchers have developed models that incorporate biological, psychological, and sociocultural factors in the development of eating disorders (Attie & Brooks-Gunn, 1992; Striegel-Moore et al., 1986; Williamson, 1990). Specific risk factors include female gender, high socioeconomic status, specific environmental contexts (competitive schools, appearance-related sports such as ballet), and a family history of eating disorders (Attie & Brooks-Gunn, 1992). Sociocultural factors such as societal emphasis on feminine beauty and thinness, centrality of beauty in the female sex-role stereotype, and specific subcultural pressures for thinness have also been implicated (see Striegel-Moore et al., 1986, for a discussion of these factors). Given the sociocultural determinants of eating disorder pathology, one would expect eating disorders to be rare or nonexistent in cultures in which excessive adiposity is valued rather than criticized. Indeed, cross-cultural research has indicated that eating disorders are relatively rare in non-Western cultures in which plumpness is regarded as a sign of wealth, beauty, or womanhood (Nasser, 1988). Further, specific subcultural groups are considered to be at increased risk for developing eating disorders. Female athletes, for example, may have a greater likelihood of developing eating disorders than nonathletes as a result of pressures to maintain a thin body shape in sports such as gymnastics and ballet (Streigel-Moore et al., 1986).

Etiological models have also highlighted the role of developmental factors (Attie & Brooks-Gunn, 1989; Levine & Smolak, 1992) in the emergence of eating disorder symptoms in adolescent girls. Specifically, the development of body image, sexuality, self-esteem, and body esteem, and the interaction of these factors with family and peer relationships are proposed to be critical determinants of healthy or pathological eating attitudes and behaviors (Attie & Brooks-Gunn, 1992). Other researchers have focused on normal developmental stressors, such as weight gain and changes in peer and family relationships during adolescence, that may lead to increased body dissatisfaction and dieting (Levine & Smolak, 1992). Additionally, research has examined factors during childhood that may be related to later eating disorder pathology. These include: childhood obesity (Fairburn & Cooper, 1982), teasing related to body size (Fabian & Thompson, 1989), early physical maturation (Thompson, 1990), conflicts over

food preferences (see Thelen, Lawrence, & Powell, 1992), low self-esteem, and depression (Veron-Guidry, Williamson, & Netemeyer, in press). In addition, physical or sexual trauma may also be related to excessive concern about body image (Finn, Hartman, Leon, & Lawson, 1986), though the incidence of abuse among persons with eating disorders is comparable to that in other clinical populations.

Although integrative models of eating disorders are useful because they point to the complex relationships among several variables, such models have been criticized because they generally do not specify the importance of each factor (Polivy & Herman, 1993). Recently, models of eating disorders have been developed based on structural modeling analysis that allows researchers to compare the influence of several factors (Williamson et al., 1995).

We shall discuss each of the factors reported by Netemeyer et al. (in press) that were found to be significantly associated with eating disorder symptoms. The model was based on four samples of female elementary, middle school, high school, and college students ranging in age from 8 to 24. One of the four samples was a sample of female college athletes. The model is depicted in Figure 1. Williamson, Netemeyer, and Barker (1995) found three exogenous risk factors to be associated with eating disorder symptoms: sociocultural pressures for thinness, overconcern with physical appearance, and negative evaluation of one's physical appearance. These exogenous risk factors and pathological eating behaviors such as restrictive eating, purging, and binge eating were found to be mediated by body dissatisfaction or "body dysphoria" and depression. From these findings we have depicted how specific DSM-IV diagnoses correspond to different patterns of pathological eating behaviors.

Sociocultural Pressure for Thinness

As mentioned earlier, social and cultural variables have been viewed as important determinants of eating disorders (Attie & Brooks-Gunn, 1989; Striegel-Moore et al., 1986; Williamson, 1990). Stereotypes of the "thin ideal" body size

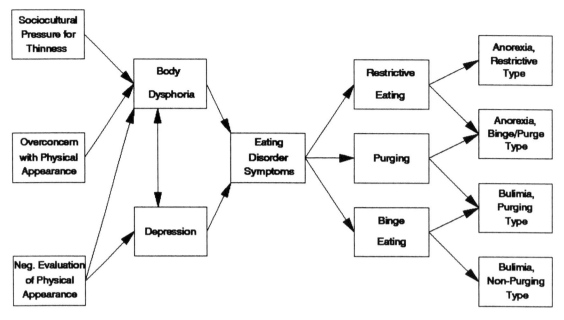

Figure 1. Psychosocial risk factor model for anorexia and bulimia nervosa.

have been promoted by the media (Richins, 1991), and research has indicated that cultural expectations of thinness have grown stronger in recent decades. In a study of Miss America contestants and Playboy centerfolds from 1959 to 1978, Garner, Garfinkel, Schwartz, and Thompson (1980) noted a trend toward thinner body shapes. In actuality, the average body weight of women under age 30 during the same time period increased (Striegel-Moore et al., 1986), starkly illustrating the growing disparity between cultural "ideal" body size and actual body size for U.S. women in recent decades. Also, women's magazines have been noted to contain considerably greater numbers of advertisements and articles promoting dieting than do men's magazines (Anderson & DiDomenico, 1992). Williamson et al. (1995) found pressure from coaches and sports competition to be a significant risk factor for the development of body dysphoria and eating disorder symptoms. As noted in Figure 1, sociocultural pressure for

thinness was found to be associated with the development of body dissatisfaction.

Overconcern with Physical Appearance

Excessive concern with physical appearance is also associated with the development of eating disorders (American Psychiatric Association, 1994). Overconcern with appearance is presumed to lead to increased body dissatisfaction because of overreactivity to minor changes in physical appearance (Williamson et al., 1993). A labile relationship between overconcern with physical appearance, perception of body size, and body dissatisfaction has been reported in two recent studies (Baker, Williamson, & Sylve, 1995; McKenzie, Williamson, & Cubic, 1993). In the Williamson et al. (1995) study, overconcern with physical appearance was associated with body dysphoria, although this relationship was not as strong as that between other variables in the model (i.e., sociocultural pressure for thinness, negative evaluation of physical appearance) and body dysphoria. This finding suggests that concern about physical appearance is necessary but not always sufficient to result in dissatisfaction with one's body.

Negative Evaluation of Physical Appearance

Negative evaluation of physical appearance refers to an individual's perception that he or she is unattractive, regardless of actual physical appearance (Williamson et al., 1995). This factor was found to be highly associated with body dysphoria, as indicated in Figure 1. Also, positive evaluation of one's physical appearance was found to be associated with a decreased likelihood of depression.

Body Dysphoria

It appears that eating disorders are as much disorders of thinking about body shape and weight as they are disorders of eating behavior. Body dysphoria, which refers to dissatisfaction and preoccupation with body size and shape, is generally viewed as a precursor to the development of eating disorders (Rosen, 1992; Slade, 1994; Williamson, 1990). Empirical investigations have supported this idea (Attie & Brooks-Gunn, 1989; Williamson et al., 1995). In the Netemeyer study, body dysphoria was strongly associated with depression and with the development of eating disorder symptoms.

Depression

The relationships between depression and other variables in the model depicted in Figure 1 are consistent with other research on the development of eating disorders. Depression has been found to be closely associated with body dysphoria (Allgood-Merton, Lewinsohn, & Hops, 1990; Rodin, Silberstein, & Striegel-Moore, 1985) and negatively associated with perceptions of physical attractiveness (Noles, Cash, & Winstead, 1985). In other words, being dissatisfied with one's appearance was associated with

depression, whereas having a positive view of one's physical appearance was associated with a low likelihood of depression. Further, depression has been found to be a strong predictor of negative affect related to eating disorders (Striegel-Moore et al., 1986; Williamson, Kelley, Davis, Ruggiero, & Blovin, 1985). In the Netemeyer study the relationship between depression and body dysphoria was quite strong. Further, depression was negatively associated with negative evaluation of physical appearance and was positively associated with the development of eating disorder symptoms.

Finally, the model includes three pathological eating behaviors, restrictive eating, purging, and binge eating, which may occur in sufficient severity to warrant DSM-IV diagnoses. As indicated in Figure 1, a pattern of restrictive eating may be termed "anorexia nervosa, restrictive subtype." Dietary restraint may alternate with episodes of binging and purging to meet the DSM-IV diagnosis "anorexia nervosa, binge/purge subtype." If binge eating is followed by compensatory behaviors (such as self-induced vomiting or laxative abuse), then the syndrome of "bulimia nervosa, purging subtype" usually develops. Binge eating, however, may occur without attempts to rid excess calories. In such cases, "bulimia nervosa, nonpurging subtype" may develop.

EPIDEMIOLOGY

Prevalence

Prevalence rates of eating disorders have varied by population. Among females in late adolescence and early adulthood, 0.5 to 1.0% have been found to meet full diagnostic criteria for anorexia nervosa and 1 to 3% for bulimia nervosa (American Psychiatric Association, 1994). It should be noted that the prevalence of eating disorders fluctuates with age and development. The risk for developing anorexia nervosa has been reported to peak during adolescence, and the most common developmental period for women to develop bulimia extends into early adulthood (Attie & Brooks-Gunn, 1992).

Sex Distribution

Eating disorders overwhelmingly affect females. Over 90% of cases of anorexia nervosa occur in females, and the risk for developing bulimia nervosa is approximately ten times greater for females (American Psychiatric Association, 1994). Males, however, are not immune to eating disorders. The sociocultural environments of some male athletes, male models (Eller, 1993), and homosexual males (Siever, 1994) emphasize thinness and physical appearance for social acceptance or for a competitive "edge," and, thus, these men are at increased risk for developing an eating disorder.

ASSESSMENT

Evaluation of persons with an eating disorder requires a multidisciplinary team, usually a physician, a psychiatrist, a psychologist, and a dietitian. We believe that it is best for the person to be evaluated by health care professionals who are very familiar with the eating disorders. The different types of examinations and tests conducted by each member of the team are summarized below.

Medical Examination

Medical problems are often associated with eating disorders (Williamson, Davis, & Ruggiero, 1987). A complete medical evaluation is recommended for all persons with an eating disorder. Anorexia nervosa is especially dangerous, with a mortality rate of approximately 5%. Common problems associated with both anorexia and bulimia nervosa are: endocrine abnormalities, electrolyte, and fluid disturbances, and metabolic abnormalities (Williamson et al., 1987). Most of the medical problems associated

with eating disorders are reversible by refeeding and restoration of normal weight. Renal disease and loss of bone density are two nonreversible medical conditions that are associated with the chronic malnutrition of anorexia nervosa.

Diagnosis

Diagnostic interviews are the best method for establishing a diagnosis of anorexia nervosa, bulimia nervosa, or eating disorder NOS. Two structured interview formats that have been developed most extensively are the Eating Disorder Examination (Fairburn & Cooper, 1993) and the Interview for Diagnosis of Eating Disorders (Williamson, 1990).

Psychological Evaluation

The eating disorders are associated with primary psychopathology, e.g., abnormal eating habits and body image disturbances, as well as secondary psychopathology, e.g., depression, obsessive-compulsive habits, and personality disorders. Psychological testing, direct behavioral observation, and self-monitoring of eating behavior are commonly used to assess these problem areas. The most commonly used psychological tests for the eating disorders are the Eating Disorder Inventory-2 (Garner, 1991), the Eating Attitudes Test (Garner & Garfinkel, 1979), and the Bulimia Test-Revised (Thelen, Farmer, Wonderlich, & Smith, 1991). For a more complete description of the methods used to evaluate these psychological disturbances, the reader may refer to Williamson (1990) and Allison (1995).

Dietary Assessment

Measurement of caloric intake and macronutrient intake is very important in the overall treatment plan for eating disorders. Self-report of food intake is the most common method for dietary assessment. With inpatients, hospital staff can directly observe food intake, which substantially increases reliability and accuracy of this method of assessment (Williamson, 1990).

TREATMENT

Cognitive-Behavior Therapy

Over the past 10 years cognitive-behavior therapy for the eating disorders has been tested in many controlled outcome studies (Agras, 1993). The principal components of this form of treatment are: modification of irrational thinking about eating and body size, gradual introduction of three nutritionally balanced meals per day, and exposure to the consumption of forbidden foods without purging. Bulimia nervosa can usually be treated in an outpatient setting, but anorexia nervosa usually can only be treated in an inpatient setting (Williamson, Davis, & Duchmann, 1992). Refeeding and weight restoration are typically the first goals of treatment for anorexia nervosa. The anxiety and body image disturbances caused by refeeding and weight gain are usually so intense that most anorexics are unable to comply with the treatment program without professional supervision. Bulimia nervosa has been treated in group and individual therapy. Most often treatment programs are conducted over a 3- to 6-month period. In a recent review of cognitive-behavior therapy for bulimia, Agras (1993) concluded that the average dropout rate was 16% and the average rate of abstinence from binge eating was 40%. Kennedy and Garfinkel (1989) followed a large number of anorexic patients treated with cognitive-behavior therapy. Follow-up periods ranged from 1 to 5 years. They reported a good to intermediate outcome in 83% of the cases.

Interpersonal Therapy

In recent years, structured short-term psychotherapy has been evaluated as a treatment for bulimia nervosa. The psychotherapeutic approach most extensively studied is interpersonal therapy. This type of therapy emphasizes interpersonal problems that are associated with the development and maintenance of disordered eating and body concerns (Agras, 1993). Eating behaviors and distorted cognitions related to body size are not directly addressed in this approach. Dropout rates for short-term psychotherapies are about 17% and abstinence from binge eating is about 24%, which is significantly lower than the 40% abstinence rate found for cognitive-behavior therapy (Agras, 1993). Only one long-term follow-up study for interpersonal therapy has been reported (Fairburn, Jones, Peveler, Hope, & O'Connor, 1993). In this investigation, interpersonal therapy and cognitive-behavior therapy were found to be equally effective 12 months after the termination of therapy.

Pharmacotherapy

Antidepressant medications have most frequently been used in controlled studies of drug therapy for anorexia and bulimia nervosa (Williamson, Sebastian, & Varnado, 1995). Other types of medications that have been tested include: anticonvulsants, opiate antagonists, appetite suppressants, and lithium carbonate (Mitchell & de Zwaan, 1993). Most of the antidepressant medications evaluated as a treatment for bulimia nervosa have been found to be more effective than placebo. Pharmacotherapy for anorexia nervosa has generally proved to be unsuccessful, however (Williamson et al., 1995). Several studies have examined pharmacotherapy and cognitive-behavior therapy and found the latter to be more effective, leading Mitchell and de Zwaan (1993) to conclude that antidepressant medications should primarily be used in cases with a coexisting affective disorder or in cases who do not respond to psychological therapies.

ASSESSMENT × TREATMENT MATCHING

The eating disorders are a very serious psychiatric problem. Dangerous medical conditions may result from anorexia and bulimia nervosa, including death. Also, depression and other psychiatric syndromes frequently coexist with an eating disorder. In recent years, considerable research has been conducted on the psychopathology of the eating disorders. An important finding is that fear of weight gain and body image dysphoria are primary features of both anorexia and bulimia nervosa. From this research, improved diagnostic procedures and improved treatment procedures have emerged. Also, we are much more informed about how to match treatment to diagnosis and level of severity. At present, outpatient cognitive-behavior therapy approaches appear to be most effective for bulimia nervosa and multidisciplinary inpatient treatment is most effective in treating anorexia nervosa. When affective disorders are comorbid, current research suggests that a trial of antidepressant medications should be initiated concurrently with other therapies. A general consensus has emerged that a comorbid personality disorder can negatively impact the normal course of treatment for anorexia and bulimia nervosa. In such cases, the problems caused by the personality disorder must be treated first or concurrently with problems associated with the eating disorder. Alcoholism/drug dependence is sometimes diagnosed in patients with an eating disorder. Our treatment strategy with these cases has generally been to treat the alcohol and drug problems first and then to address the eating problems.

CASE STUDY

Presenting Problems

Cindy was a 15-year-old Caucasian female, referred by a school counselor. Her parents were recently divorced. Her father was a physician and her mother worked at home. Three months prior to her first appointment, she weighed 105 lb. Her height was 4 feet 11 inches. She denied the presence of symptoms associated with anorexia or bulimia nervosa. This report was not consistent with observations reported by her mother who had discovered that Cindy was purging via self-induced vomiting and laxative use. Cindy's mother also suspected secretive binge eating. Over the course of 3 months,

Cindy lost 18 lb. At this point, Cindy acknowledged that she was purging and restricting her eating so as to lose weight.

In addition to problems related to restrictive eating and purging, Cindy expressed a strong drive for thinness and was reluctant to gain weight. Her menstrual period had been absent for at least 3 months.

Cindy and her mother reported considerable conflict resulting in Cindy residing with her father. Also, Cindy reported strained relationships with most of her peers. She had only two close friends. Both had expressed great concern related to her eating and weight loss.

Psychological Assessment

Psychological testing and clinical interviews indicated that Cindy was attempting to minimize problems with eating. Her mother presented a picture of much more severe behavior problems than her father. Personality testing suggested primary problems related to social relationships. Cindy was very suspicious and did not easily trust others. The family environment was described as low in cohesion and freedom of expression and high in conflict and control. Self-monitoring of eating indicated a pattern of eating three meals per day with a variety of foods. Analysis of nutrition indicated average caloric intake was about 1300 kcal/day, which was about 500 kcal/day below her caloric needs.

Case Formulation

Cindy had gradually developed the symptoms of anorexia nervosa. She lost weight at a rate of 6 lb/month. She acknowledged purging in the past, but denied purging at the initiation of assessment. She was resistant to gaining weight. It appeared that she was in the early stages of anorexia nervosa and had very limited insight about the problem. Her parents began to recognize the extent of her eating problems and were supportive of treatment.

Diagnosis

Axis I:	Anorexia Nervosa (307.10)
Axis II:	None
Axis III:	Amenorrhea and low body weight
Axis IV:	Social and Family Problems
Axis V:	Global Assessment of Functioning: Moderate (65)

Treatment Recommendations

Based on the initial evaluation, the following recommendations for treatment were made.

1. Outpatient individual and family therapy
2. Referral to an outpatient eating disorders program including: (a) adolescent group therapy, (b) family group therapy, and (c) dietary consultation
3. Consultation with Cindy's pediatrician to rule out medical reasons for recent weight loss

4. Program to stabilize and then regain weight up to 95–100 lb
5. Hospitalization if the outpatient program failed

Course of Treatment

During the first 2 months of outpatient therapy, Cindy continued to deny the presence of anorexia nervosa and was resistant to therapy and especially to weight gain. She was hospitalized during the third month of treatment and gained weight to 100 lb. Her eating behavior was improved and purging ceased. She is currently being followed in outpatient therapy.

SUMMARY

Research on the diagnosis of anorexia and bulimia nervosa has progressed considerably over the past 15 years. Also, a diversity of assessment methods have been developed. Treatment methods have been tested in a number of controlled investigations and have been empirically validated. As a result of these efforts, the eating disorders, once viewed as very recalcitrant, can usually be effectively treated. This treatment is often quite lengthy and intense. Relapse occurs, unfortunately, all too often. The next logical step in our efforts to manage these problems is the development of prevention programs in our schools and communities. If prevention can reduce the incidence of the eating disorders in our society, then the economic and emotional costs of these problems can be substantially reduced.

REFERENCES

Agras, W. S. (1993). Short-term psychological treatments for binge eating. In C. G. Fairburn & G. T. Wilson (Eds.), *Binge eating: Nature, assessment, and treatment* (pp. 270–286). New York: Guilford Press.

Allgood-Merton, B., Lewinsohn, P., & Hops, H. (1990). Sex differences and adolescent depression. *Journal of Abnormal Psychology, 99,* 55–63.

Allison, D. B. (1995). *Handbook of assessment methods for eating behaviors and weight-related problems: Measures, theory, and research.* Beverly Hills, CA: Sage Publications.

American Psychiatric Association. (1987). *Diagnostic and statistical manual of mental disorders* (3rd ed.-rev.). Washington, DC: Author.

American Psychiatric Association. (1994). *Diagnostic and statistical manual of mental disorders* (4th ed.). Washington, DC: Author.

Anderson, A. E., & DiDomenico, L. (1992). Diet vs. shape content of popular male and female magazines: A dose–response relationship to the incidence of eating disorders. *International Journal of Eating Disorders, 11,* 283–287.

Attie, I., & Brooks-Gunn, J. (1989). Development of eating problems in adolescent girls. *Developmental Psychology, 25,* 70–79.

Attie, I., & Brooks-Gunn, J. (1992). Developmental issues in the study of eating problems and disorders. In J. H. Crowther, D. L. Tennenbaum, S. E. Hobfoll, & M. A. P. Stephens (Eds.), *The etiology of bulimia nervosa: The individual and familial context* (pp. 35–58). Washington, DC: Hemisphere.

Baker, J. D., Williamson, D. A., & Sylve, C. (1995). Body image disturbance, memory bias, and body dysphoria: Effects of negative mood induction. *Behavior Therapy, 26,* 747–759.

Banting, W. (1864). *Letter on corpulence* (3rd ed.). London: Harrison.

Blundell, J. E., & Hill, A. J. (1993). Binge eating: Psychobiological mechanisms. In C. G. Fairburn & G. T. Wilson (Eds.), *Binge eating: Nature, assessment, and treatment* (pp. 206–224). New York: Guilford Press.

Brownell, K. D. (1991). Dieting and the search for the perfect body: Where physiology and culture collide. *Behavior Therapy, 22,* 1–12.

Brownell, K. D., Rodin, J., & Wilmore, J. H. (1992). *Eating, body weight, and performance in athletes: Disorders of modern society.* Philadelphia: Lea & Febiger.

Bulik, C. M., Beidel, D. C., Duchmann, E., Weltzin, T. E., & Kaye, W. H. (1991). An analysis of social anxiety in anorexic, bulimic, social phobia, and control women. *Journal of Psychopathology and Behavioral Assessment, 13*(3), 199–211.

Eller, B. (1993). Males with eating disorders. In A. J. Giannini & A. E. Slaby (Eds.), *The eating disorders* (pp. 133–146). Berlin: Springer-Verlag.

Fabian, L. J., & Thompson, J. K. (1989). Body image and eating disturbance in young females. *International Journal of Eating Disorders, 8,* 63–74.

Fairburn, C. G., Agras, S., & Wilson, G. T. (1992). The research on the treatment of bulimia nervosa: Practical and theoretical implications. In G. H. Anderson & S. H. Kennedy (Eds.), *The biology of feast and famine: Relevance to eating disorders* (pp. 318–340). San Diego: Academic Press.

Fairburn, C. G., Beglin, S. J. (1990). Studies in the epidemiology of bulimia nervosa. *American Journal of Psychiatry, 147,* 401–408.

Fairburn, C. G., & Cooper, P. J. (1982). Self induced vomiting and bulimia nervosa: An undetected problem. *British Medical Journal, 284,* 1153–1155.

Fairburn, C. G., & Cooper, Z. (1993). The Eating Disorder Examination (12th ed.). In C. G. Fairburn & G. T. Wilson (Eds.), *Binge eating: Nature, assessment, and treatment* (pp. 317–360). New York: Guilford Press.

Fairburn, C. G., Hay, P. J., & Welch, S. L. (1993). Binge eating and bulimia nervosa: Distribution and determinants. In C. G. Fairburn & G. T. Wilson (Eds.), *Binge eating: Nature, assessment, and treatment* (pp. 123–143). New York: Guilford Press.

Fairburn, C. G., Jones, R., Peveler, R. C., Hope, R. A., & O'Connor, M. (1993). Psychotherapy and bulimia nervosa: Longer-term effects of interpersonal psychotherapy, behavior therapy, and cognitive behavior therapy. *Archives of General Psychiatry, 50,* 419–428.

Fairburn, C. G., & Wilson, G. T. (1993). Binge eating: Definition and classification. In C. G. Fairburn & G. T. Wilson (Eds.), *Binge eating: Nature, assessment, and treatment* (pp. 3–14). New York: Guilford Press.

Finn, S. E., Hartman, M., Leon, G. R., & Lawson, O. (1986). Eating disorders and sexual abuse: Lack of confirmation for a clinical hypothesis. *International Journal of Eating Disorders, 5,* 1051–1060.

Garfinkel, P. E., Moldofsky, H., & Garner, D. M. (1979). The heterogeneity of anorexia nervosa: Bulimia as a distinct subgroup. *Archives of General Psychiatry, 37,* 1036–1040.

Garner, D. M. (1991). *Eating Disorder Inventory-2 manual.* Odessa, FL: Psychological Assessment Resources.

Garner, D. M., & Garfinkel, P. E. (1979). The Eating Attitudes Test: An index of the symptoms of anorexia nervosa. *Psychological Medicine, 9,* 273–279.

Garner, D. M., Garfinkel, P. E., Schwartz, D., & Thompson, M. (1980). Cultural expectations of thinness in women. *Psychological Reports, 47,* 483–491.

Geracioti, T. D., & Liddle, R. A. (1988). Impaired cholecystokinin secretion in bulimia nervosa. *New England Journal of Medicine, 319,* 683–688.

Gull, W. W. (1874). Anorexia nervosa. *Transactions of the Clinical Society of London, 7,* 22–28.

Halmi, K. A., & Falk, J. R. (1982). Anorexia nervosa: A study of outcome discriminators in exclusive dieters and bulimics. *Journal of the American Academy of Child Psychiatry, 21,* 369–375.

Hinz, L. D., & Williamson, D. A. (1987). Bulimia and depression: A review of the affective variant hypothesis. *Psychological Bulletin, 102,* 150–158.

James, R. (1743). *A medical dictionary.* London: T. Osborne.

Johnson, C., & Wonderlich, S. (1992). Personality characteristics as a risk factor in the development of eating disorders. In J. Crowther, D. Tennenbaum, S. Hobfoll, & M. Stephens (Eds.), *The etiology of bulimia nervosa: The individual and familial context* (pp. 179–196). Washington, DC: Hemisphere.

Jones, D. J., Fox, M. M., Babigian, H. M., & Hutton, H. E. (1980). Epidemiology of anorexia nervosa in Monroe County, New York: 1960–1976. *Psychological Medicine, 42,* 551–558.

Kasvikis, Y. G., Tsakiris, F., Marks, I. M., Basoglu, M., & Noshirvani, H. F. (1986). Past history of anorexia nervosa in women with obsessive-compulsive disorder. *International Journal of Eating Disorders, 5,* 1069–1075.

Kaye, W. H. (1992). Neurotransmitter abnormalities in anorexia nervosa and bulimia nervosa. In G. H. Anderson & S. H. Kennedy (Eds.), *The biology of feast and famine: Relevance to eating disorders* (pp. 105–134). San Diego: Academic Press.

Kennedy, S. H., & Garfinkel, P. E. (1989). Patients admitted to a hospital with anorexia nervosa and bulimia nervosa: Psychopathology, weight gain, and attitudes toward treatment. *International Journal of Eating Disorders, 8,* 181–190.

Kinder, B. N. (1991). Eating disorders: Anorexia nervosa and bulimia nervosa. In M. Hersen & S. M. Turner (Eds.), *Adult psychopathology and diagnosis* (2nd ed., pp. 392–409). New York: Wiley.

Lasegue, E. C. (1873). De l'anorexie hysterique. *Archives of General Medicine, 21,* 385–403.

Levine, M., & Smolak, L. (1992). Toward a model of the developmental psychopathology of eating disorders: The example of early adolescence. In J. H. Crowther, D. L. Tennenbaum, S. E. Hobfoll, & M. A. P. Stephens (Eds.), *The etiology of bulimia nervosa: The individual and familial context* (pp. 59–80). Washington, DC: Hemisphere.

Lewinsohn, P. M., Hops, H., Roberts, R. E., Seeley, J. R., & Andrews, J. A. (1993). Adolescent psychopathology: I. Prevalence and incidence of depression and other DSM-III-R disorders in high school students. *Journal of Abnormal Psychology, 102*(3), 133–144.

Marrazzi, M. A., & Luby, E. D. (1986). An auto-addiction model of chronic anorexia nervosa. *International Journal of Eating Disorders, 5,* 191–208.

McKenzie, S. J., Williamson, D. A., & Cubic, B. A. (1993). Stable and reactive body image disturbances in bulimia nervosa. *Behavior Therapy, 24,* 195–207.

Mitchell, J. E., & de Zwaan, M. (1993). Pharmacological treatments of binge eating. In C. G. Fairburn & G. T. Wilson (Eds.), *Binge eating: Nature, assessment, and treatment* (pp. 250–269). New York: Guilford Press.

Mitchell, J. E., Pyle, R. L., Hatsukami, D., & Eckert, E. D. (1986). What are the atypical eating disorders? *Psychosomatics, 27,* 21–25.

Nasser, M. (1988). Culture and weight consciousness. *Journal of Psychosomatic Research, 32,* 573–577.

Noles, S. W., Cash, T. F., & Winstead, B. A. (1985). Body image, physical attractiveness, and depression. *Journal of Consulting and Clinical Psychology, 53,* 88–94.

Norvell, N., & Cooley, E. (1987). Diagnostic issues in eating disorders: Two cases of atypical eating disorder. *International Journal of Psychiatry in Medicine, 16,* 317–323.

Piran, N., Kennedy, S., Garfinkel, P. E., & Owners, M. (1985). Affective disturbance in eating disorders. *Journal of Nervous and Mental Disease, 173,* 395–400.

Polivy, J., & Herman, C. P. (1993). Etiology of binge eating:

Psychological mechanisms. In C. G. Fairburn & G. T. Wilson (Eds.), *Binge eating: Nature, assessment, and treatment* (pp. 173–205). New York: Guilford Press.

Pope, H. G., & Hudson, J. I. (1988). Is bulimia nervosa a heterogeneous disorder? Lessons from the history of medicine. *International Journal of Eating Disorders, 7,* 155–166.

Powell, A. D., & Kahn, A. S. (1995). Racial differences in women's desires to be thin. *International Journal of Eating Disorders, 17,* 191–195.

Richins, M. A. (1991). Social comparison and the idealized images of advertising. *Journal of Consumer Research, 18,* 71–83.

Rodin, J., Silberstein, L. R., & Striegel-Moore, R. H. (1985). Women and weight: A normative discontent. In T. B. Sondregger (Ed.), *Nebraska Symposium on Motivation: Vol. 32. Psychology and Gender* (pp. 267–307). Lincoln: University of Nebraska Press.

Rosen, J. C. (1992). Body image disorder: Definition, development, and contribution to eating disorders. In J. H. Crowther, D. L. Tennenbaum, S. E. Hobfoll, & M. A. P. Stephens (Eds.), *The etiology of bulimia: The individual and family context* (pp. 157–177). Washington, DC: Hemisphere.

Siever, M. D. (1994). Sexual orientation and gender as factors in socioculturally acquired vulnerability to body dissatisfaction and eating disorders. *Journal of Consulting and Clinical Psychology, 62*(2), 252–260.

Slade, P. D. (1994). What is body image? *Behavior Research and Therapy, 32,* 497–502.

Striegel-Moore, R. H., Silberstein, L. R., & Rodin, J. (1986). Toward an understanding of risk factors for bulimia. *American Psychologist, 41,* 246–263.

Stunkard, A. J. (1993). A history of binge eating. In C. G. Fairburn & G. T. Wilson (Eds.), *Binge eating: Nature, assessment, and treatment* (pp. 15–34). New York: Guilford Press.

Thelen, M. H., Farmer, J., Wonderlich, S., & Smith, M. (1991). A revision of the Bulimia Test: The BULIT-R. *Psychological Assessment, 3,* 119–124.

Thelen, M. H., Lawrence, C. M., & Powell, A. L. (1992). Body image, weight control, and eating disorders among children. In J. H. Crowther, S. E. Hobfoll, M. A. P. Stephens, & D. L. Tennenbaum (Eds.), *The etiology of bulimia: The individual and family context* (pp. 81–102). Washington, DC: Hemisphere.

Thompson, J. K. (1990). *Body image disturbances: Assessment and treatment.* Elmsford, NY: Pergamon Press.

Veron-Guidry, S., Williamson, D. A., & Netemeyer, R. G. (in press). Structural modeling analysis of risk factors for eating disorders in children and preadolescents. *Eating Disorders: The Journal of Treatment and Prevention.*

Willi, J., & Grossman, S. (1983). Epidemiology of anorexia nervosa in a defined region of Switzerland. *American Journal of Psychiatry, 140,* 564–567.

Williamson, D. A. (1990). *Assessment of eating disorders: Obesity, anorexia, and bulimia nervosa.* Elmsford, NY: Pergamon Press.

Williamson, D. A., Barker, S. E., & Norris, L. E. (1993). Etiology and management of eating disorders. In P. B. Sutker & H. E. Adams (Eds.), *Comprehensive handbook of psychopathology* (2nd ed., pp. 505–530). New York: Plenum Press.

Williamson, D. A., Davis, C. J., & Duchmann, E. G. (1992). Anorexia and bulimia nervosa. In V. B. Van Hasselt & D. J. Kolko (Eds.), *Inpatient behavior therapy for children and adolescents* (pp. 341–364). New York: Plenum Press.

Williamson, D. A., Davis, C. J., & Ruggiero, L. (1987). Eating disorders. In R. L. Morrison & A. S. Bellack (Eds.), *Medical factors and psychological disorders: A handbook for psychologists* (pp. 351–370). New York: Plenum Press.

Williamson, D. A., Gleaves, D. H., & Savin, S. M. (1992). Empirical classification of eating disorder NOS: Support for DSM-IV changes. *Journal of Psychopathology and Behavioral Assessment, 14*(2), 201–216.

Williamson, D. A., Kelley, M. L., Davis, C. J., Ruggiero, L., & Blouin, D. C. (1985). Psychopathology of eating disorders: A controlled comparison of bulimic, obese, and normal subjects. *Journal of Consulting and Clinical Psychology, 53,* 161–166.

Williamson, D. A., Netemeyer, R. G., & Barker, S. E. (1995). Psychosocial and cognitive factors associated with unhealthy responses to healthy messages. In M. Ruwe & H. Spotts (Eds.), *Advances in health care research* (pp. 50–55). Madison, WI: American Association for advances in Health Care Research, Omni Press.

Williamson, D. A., Netemeyer, R. G., Jackman, L. P., Anderson, D. A., Funsch, C. L., & Rabalais, J. Y. (1995). Structural equation modeling of risk factors for the development of eating disorder symptoms in female athletes. *International Journal of Eating Disorders, 17*(4), 387–393.

Williamson, D. A., Sebastian, S. B., & Varnado, P. J. (1995). Anorexia and bulimia nervosa. In A. J. Goreczny (Ed.), *Handbook of health and rehabilitation psychology* (pp. 175–196). New York: Plenum Press.

Wilson, G. T., & Pike, K. M. (1993). Eating disorders. In D. H. Barlow (Ed.), *Clinical handbook of psychological disorders* (pp. 278–317). New York: Guilford Press.

World Health Organization. (1992). *The ICD-10 Classification of mental and behavioral disorders.* Geneva: Author.

Yates, A. (1989). Current perspectives on the eating disorders: I. History, psychological, and biological aspects. *Journal of the American Academy of Child and Adolescent Psychiatry, 28,* 813–828.

12

Self-Injurious Behavior and Stereotypies

JOHANNES ROJAHN, MARC J. TASSÉ, AND DIANE MORIN

INTRODUCTION

Mental retardation is characterized by significant intellectual limitations and poor adaptive behavior appearing before the age of 18 (Aman, Hammer, & Rojahn, 1993; Luckasson et al., 1992; Tassé, Aman, Rojahn, & Kern, in press). It is a persistent condition caused by a variety of biological and psychosocial determinants. Mental retardation manifests on a continuum of severity with a rapidly decelerating rate of occurrence as the behavioral and intellectual limitations increase. Neurological illnesses such as cerebral palsy, spina bifida, and seizure disorders frequently accompany mental retardation but

without causal connection. In addition, individuals with mental retardation are highly vulnerable for psychopathology. Ever since the landmark Isle of Wight epidemiological studies conducted between 1964 and 1974 (Rutter, Tizard, Yule, Graham, & Whitmore, 1976), we have known that individuals with mental retardation have an elevated risk for psychiatric disorders such as schizophrenia and depression. Besides, many develop severe behavior disorders during their lives, such as aggressive and destructive behavior, violent tantrum behavior, or stereotyped and self-injurious behaviors.

Neither self-injury nor stereotypies are specific to mental retardation. They occur in people with schizophrenia, autism, and other conditions as well. Some mental retardation researchers have thought of self-injurious behavior (SIB) and stereotyped behaviors as etiologically related (e.g., Matson, 1989). The few data we have to date that address this relationship in mental retardation show statistically significant, but not particularly high correlations between these two global groups of behavior, namely, .10 and .27, respectively (Rojahn, Borthwick-Duffy, & Jacobson, 1993). Rojahn (1986) found that individuals with SIB are twice

This text is based in part on a chapter by Rojahn and Sisson (1990).

JOHANNES ROJAHN • Nisonger Center for Developmental Disabilities and Department of Psychology, Ohio State University, Columbus, Ohio 43210.   MARC J. TASSÉ • Départment de psychologie, Université du Quebéc à Montréal, Montréal, Quebéc, Canada. DIANE MORIN • Centre de Consultation Psychologique et Éducationnelle, Montréal, Quebec, Canada.

Handbook of Child Psychopathology, 3rd edition, edited by Ollendick & Hersen. Plenum Press, New York, 1998.

as likely to have concurrent stereotyped behavior than those without SIB. Some hypothesized that stereotyped behavior was a benign developmental precursor of SIB (Baumeister & Rollings, 1976), and also believed that stereotypies were rudimentary behaviors rooted in repetitive motor movements common among healthy infants (Lourie, 1949). Early in life repetitive behavior may assume an important neurodevelopmental function. Some children with mental retardation and other conditions fail to outgrow these behaviors, and instead keep them in their repertoire for a long time, sometimes throughout their life (Berkson, 1983; Thelen, 1981). SIB and stereotypic behavior have received a great deal of attention in the clinical research literature during the past 35 years. Most notably these behaviors have been studied intensively by applied behavior analysts since the first carefully conducted single-case studies showed successful control of previously all but unmanageable behavior problems.

PHENOMENOLOGY

The global categories of SIB and stereotypic behavior consist of a large variety of response topographies. LaGrow and Repp (1984) listed 66 different stereotyped behavior topographies when they reviewed the treatment literature. Similarly, Rojahn (1994) identified 38 distinguishable SIB topographies in scanning the epidemiological SIB literature.

Behavioral researchers define SIB often as behavior that leads immediately or cumulatively to self-inflicted tissue damage. This definition, which dates back to Tate and Barroff (1966), uses *outcomes* rather than behavior topography as the constituting characteristic. Such a functional definition intends to enhance objectivity by curtailing implicit but unproven assumptions about underlying motives of the behavior concealed in terms like *self-punitive, self-aggressive,* or *driven.* Yet still, despite this functional definition, inconsistency exists among researchers

with respect to which behaviors are legitimate forms of SIB. For instance, opinions vary on pica (ingestion of inedible objects), teeth grinding, self-induced vomiting and rumination, aerophagia (swallowing air), or polydipsia (excessive drinking). Occasionally these discrepancies may be related to variations in how the definition is interpreted (e.g., one can disagree whether pica causes "tissue damage" or not, because the effect depends on the types of objects swallowed). Other inconsistencies may exist because of the extreme rarity of the behavior; for example, tearing out fingernails, which Oliver, Murphy, and Corbett (1987) included in an SIB survey, or burning self and self-choking, which appeared in an SIB checklist by Maurice and Trudel (1982). Researchers typically exclude behaviors such as nail biting, substance abuse, or suicide from SIB in mental retardation although they clearly fit the functional definition of SIB. In other words, we still do not know for certain whether SIB represents more than a loose descriptive term. In any case, the most common forms of SIB discussed in the mental retardation literature are self-biting, head banging, striking oneself, and scratching (Rojahn, 1994). These behaviors can vary greatly in intensity and ensuing harm. Head banging, for instance, can range from soft tapping of the head to ferocious, full-force blows that can lead to reddening of the skin, lacerations, and to the formation of callus. In some individuals head banging causes blindness as a result of detachment of the retinas, and in some cases even death. Biting, which is particularly fierce in the X-linked genetically transmitted Lesch-Nyhan syndrome, usually results in deep cuts and scarring. In this syndrome, if the person is not physically prevented, biting is so severe that it leads to the loss of digits of the hands and chewed off lips and oral tissue. SIB can also vary in its conspicuousness. For instance, biting or head banging are often so dramatic that they are difficult to ignore by caretakers. However, other perilous behaviors, such as pica, can go unnoticed for a long time, only to become recognized when serious medical complications occur.

Stereotypies are repetitive, voluntary, and often idiosyncratic behaviors perceived as "strange" or "bizarre." Contrary to the SIB definition, this is a descriptive rather than a functional definition. In an attempt to empirically classify different forms of stereotyped and other unusual behaviors, Berkson, Gutermuth, and Baranek (1995) assessed 246 individuals with mental retardation. Their 45-item scale included the common topographies such as body rocking and twirling. It also contained phenomena such as unusual motivational patterns (labeled *Abnormal Focused Affections*), rituals, sensory defensiveness, savant skills, behavioral rigidities, and others that we typically do not call *stereotypic* in mental retardation. Factor analysis revealed seven orthogonal factors. They labeled these factors "Rigidity," "Visual Stereotypies," "Stereotypical Vocalizations," "Motor Stereotypies," and "Food Preference." Two factors remained unnamed. In another classification study, Rojahn, Tassé, and Sturmey (1997) developed a 26-item scale (Stereotyped Behavior Scale) with a sample of 599 adults with mental retardation. In this case, factor analysis led to a single factor. Thus, both of these studies found support for the notion of a general stereotypic behavior factor.

DIAGNOSIS

The fourth edition of the *Diagnostic and Statistical Manual of Mental Disorders* (DSM-IV; American Psychiatric Association, 1994) contains the diagnostic category of *Stereotypic Movement Disorder* (code 307.3) under *Other Disorders of Infancy, Childhood, and Adolescents*. It is an umbrella category for benign stereotyped behavior and SIB and uses the following criteria: (1) motor behavior that is repetitive, seemingly driven, and nonfunctional; (2) that markedly interferes with normal activities (or results in self-inflicted bodily injury that requires medical treatment); (3) that is repetitive and cannot be better accounted for by an Obsessive-Compulsive Disor-

der, a Tic Disorder, or a Pervasive Developmental Disorder (hair pulling or trichotillomania is excluded from the diagnosis of Stereotypic Movement Disorder); (4) that is not related to a substance or a medical condition; and (5) that persists for more than 4 weeks. The DSM-IV Stereotypic Movement Disorder diagnosis requires that the clinician specify whether the behavior causes physical injury or not.

This diagnostic category still needs clinical and scientific validation because the concept remains vague. As we pointed out before, it is still ambiguous whether stereotyped behavior and SIB represent meaningful categories, nor do we know whether they belong in one category. The data we have suggest that stronger relationships exist between *some* forms of stereotypy and *some* forms of SIB, but that this is not the case for all topographies. For instance, Rojahn (1986) found body rocking to be significantly correlated with head banging; yet it did not correlate with self-biting, scratching, or pinching. Multivariate analyses on large numbers of individuals with mental retardation and SIB alone, with stereotypies alone, and with both SIB and stereotypies would clarify this issue.

ETIOLOGY

Researchers have been interested in unusual repetitive behavior for more than 30 years. Consequently, large amounts of etiologically relevant data in both humans and animals have been reported. Many factors have been associated with repetitive behavior. Complex, yet only partly substantiated, theories of the origin of stereotyped behavior have been proposed. The current state of our knowledge suggests that SIB and stereotyped behaviors are determined by multiple interdependent biological and environmental factors, and that these factors have a strong developmental component. We will discuss etiological models that have at least partial empirical support and present them under the headings of physiological, neurochemical, behavioral, psychopathological, and social/ environmental theories. This organization should not mislead the reader to assume that these models are mutually exclusive. On the contrary, it is our belief that different combinations of some or all of these factors play a role in the development of stereotyped behavior and SIB.

Developmental Theory

As mentioned before, some researchers have explored the possibility that stereotyped behavior may be a rudimentary behavior that is neuro-developmentally useful to children at a certain stage (Berkson, 1983; Thelen, 1981). For unknown reasons, some children with disabilities fail to outgrow them.

Genetic Syndromes Associated with Stereotypies and SIB

Several genetic syndromes are known to be associated with mental retardation and repetitive movement disorders. For instance, in *Lesch-Nyhan syndrome,* which is characterized by abnormalities on the long arm of the X chromosome and hyperuricemia, the best-known manifestation is severe self-biting, which is displayed by almost all patients (Nyhan, 1994). Targeted areas are primarily the lips and fingers. Individuals with *Cornelia DeLange syndrome,* which has distinct physical features (such as hirsutism), are at high risk for developing self-hitting or self-biting (Johnson, Ekman, Friesen, Nyhan, & Shear, 1976). A third syndrome associated with SIB is *Smith-Magenis syndrome.* A variety of SIB topographies such as head banging, wrist biting, and pulling out fingernails and toenails have been observed in this syndrome, which is chromosomally characterized by a partial deletion of chromosome 17 but for which no genetic etiology has been reported (Greenberg et al., 1991). *Rett syndrome,* which affects almost exclusively females, is associated with hand-to-hand patting and tongue grasping (Hagberg, 1993). The link

between genetic disorders and behavior problems suggests a biological determinant of behavioral manifestations and holds the promise that advances in molecular genetics will greatly assist us in the identification of these determinants.

Physiological Theories

Physiological theories are based on the assumption that internal mechanisms maintain repetitive behavior in relative absence of external antecedents or consequences. This independence from direct external control may explain in part the difficulty behavioral interventions have had in achieving lasting treatment effects. The two most prominent physiological theories of aberrant repetitive behavior are the homeostasis theory and the central oscillator theory.

Homeostasis Theory

The organism strives for the maintenance of a balanced arousal level of the central nervous system (CNS). Many individuals with mental retardation are believed to have arousal levels that are off balance, and the monotonous stereotyped movements function to block external stimulation, thus modulating the arousal (Lovaas, Newsom, & Hickman, 1987). Overall, the empirical evidence related to the arousal hypothesis in humans is limited.

Central Oscillator Theory

The rhythmical nature of some stereotyped topographies led to the proposition that stereotyped movement might be controlled by a neural oscillator mechanism in the CNS. Support for this assumption was found in biorhythm research on temporal patterns of rhythmic stereotyped topographies in children and adolescents with mental retardation (e.g., Lewis et al., 1984; Lewis, MacLean, Johnson, & Baumeister, 1981; Lewis, Silva, & Silva, 1995; Pohl, 1977). The central oscillator theory of repetitive behavior has been mostly of heuristic value.

Neurotransmitter Theories

Neurotransmitters are neurochemical substances necessary for the flow of activity from one brain cell to the next. Transmission of activity occurs by the flow of these neurochemical substances from one cell terminus (synapse) into the next cell. Different types of neurotransmitters are concentrated in specific locations of the cerebrum and are responsible for different types of activity.

Dopamine Theory

The dopamine hypothesis, also known as dopaminergic supersensitivity hypothesis, suggests that chronically low levels of the neurotransmitter dopamine in postsynaptic cells of the basal ganglia cause repetitive behavior such as biting and head banging. Because of this state of depletion, the postsynaptic cells become supersensitive to dopamine, and even a low dose of dopamine transmission causes extremely strong reactions. In other words, this supersensitivity causes overcompensation. It is believed that depletion of dopamine at postsynaptic receptor sites can be produced by: a blockage of dopamine receptor sites caused by chronic administration of neuroleptic medication; by denervation of dopamine pathways; and by stress. Lewis and Baumeister (1982) hypothesized that such supersensitivity in persons with mental retardation is most plausibly caused by lesions and/or disuse of dopaminergic pathways. In support of this hypothesis, dopamine antagonists (such as neuroleptic drugs) have proven to reduce repetitive behavior, whereas dopamine agonists (such as L-dopa and amphetamines) have been shown to exacerbate preexisting stereotypies and even produce new forms. Conventional neuroleptics (such as chlorpromazine, thioridazine, and haloperidol) were found to reduce stereotyped behavior and to a lesser degree SIB. Research has begun on a new generation of neuroleptic drugs that selectively target specific dopamine receptor subtypes. Preliminary results have been promising (e.g., Schroeder et al., 1995).

Endorphin Theory

Endorphins or endogenous opioids are substances produced in the brain that are chemically related to substances derived from opium. Endorphin release in the brain is a natural response triggered by several forms of stimulation, including vigorous motor activity. Its effect is analgesic, reducing the intensity of pain sensation. It also results in a mildly euphoric state (Lewis & Baumeister, 1982). The endorphin hypothesis explains how internal reinforcement maintains repetitive behavior (euphoric effect) even if the behavior ought to be painful under ordinary circumstances (analgesic effect). Most important for treatment considerations, the endorphin theory has led to promising research on opiate antagonistic medication such as naloxone and naltrexone, substances that counteract the endorphin action in the brain (see further below).

Conditioned Response Theories

We distinguish four operant models for the explanation of repetitive behavior in mental retardation, depending on whether the target behavior is maintained by positive reinforcement (behavior produces a positive stimulus) or negative reinforcement (behavior serves to escape or avoid an aversive stimulus), and whether the critical stimulus is external or internal. In addition, we will describe schedule-induced behavior as a model of aberrant repetitive behavior.

Positive External Reinforcement Theory

The positive external reinforcement theory states that external positive reinforcement motivates repetitive behavior. Conspicuous behaviors such as some forms of SIB are not easy to ignore and are therefore likely to elicit some response from parents or teachers trying to calm down the child or simply to prevent injury. The irony is that this sympathetic reaction has the potential to aggravate this behavior in frequency and intensity because it can have unintentional reinforcing properties. Lovaas and Simmons (1969) were the first to produce compelling evidence for the positive social reinforcement explanation in a classic study, showing that SIB could be increased by systematic attention of an adult provided contingent upon the behavior. Whenever the boy exhibited SIB, the adult approached the boy, held his hands and pleaded with him not to hurt himself. The rate of SIB rapidly and immediately increased. We can assume that care giver attention is less likely to be a motivating contingency for benign stereotyped behavior than for more dramatic self-injury.

Positive Internal Reinforcement Theory

Functionally related to the positive reinforcement model, the positive internal reinforcement or automatic reinforcement theory holds that repetitive behaviors are operants maintained by reinforcement produced by the behavior itself (Lovaas et al., 1987). These reinforcing stimuli can be exteroceptive (e.g., lights, sounds), interoceptive (e.g., vestibular stimulation, endorphin release, homeostatic balance), or both. As mentioned before, repetitive movement is widespread among infants during the first year of life, which led some theorists to posit that rhythmic movements are innate substrates of more complex motor behavior. Berkson (1983) argued that rhythmic movement may have internal reinforcing properties. Stereotyped behavior is often a highly preferred activity, and in accordance with the Premack principle of reinforcement the opportunity to engage in stereotyped behavior can have reinforcing effects. Selective permission to engage in stereotyped behavior has been used to increase the rate of low probability but desirable behaviors (e.g., Hung, 1978; Wolery, Kirk, & Gast, 1985), and to eliminate inappropriate behavior (Foxx, McMorrow, Fenlon, & Bittle, 1986).

Negative External Reinforcement Theory

The negative reinforcement theory, also known as "escape/avoidance theory" assumes a learning history where the behavior allows the individual to escape or avoid unpleasant conditions. Durand and Carr (1987) found evidence in support of the escape/avoidance hypothesis of stereotyped behavior. They showed that hand-flapping and body rocking in four children with developmental disabilities increased with the introduction of difficult academic tasks. They also showed that removal of these tasks contingent upon stereotyped behavior resulted in increased rates of these stereotyped behaviors.

Negative Internal Reinforcement Theory

It has long been suggested that some forms of self-injury may be maintained by their pain masking effects. DeLissevoy's (1963) early clinical observations that some children exhibit head banging to alleviate pain caused by otitis media has found modern day support in the previously mentioned endorphin hypothesis.

Schedule-Induced Behavior Theory

Another behavioral model is based on the observation that repetitive *collateral* behaviors appear in laboratory animals when placed under conditions of low rates of reinforcement for a different behavior (DRL). This schedule-induced repetitive behavior is seemingly independent of external consequences and therefore reminiscent of stereotyped behavior in individuals with developmental disabilities (Lewis & Baumeister, 1982). If such a DRL condition is equivalent to understimulating environments, cage pacing of feral animals in captivity might be an example of schedule-induced behavior.

Communication Hypothesis

The communication hypothesis suggests these problem behaviors serve as an attempt to communicate personal needs (Carr & Durand, 1985a,b). A bout of head-banging, for instance, is likely to attract some form of social attention. Underlying this hypothesis is the assumption that the individual has developed problematic behavior because of the lack of socially more acceptable forms of communication. Consequently, treatment ought to be focused on the establishment of *functionally equivalent* communication behavior. Etiologically, the communication hypothesis is a learning hypothesis, in which the lack of acceptable communication skills represents a prerequisite condition (establishing operation) for a learning process of SIB, stereotypies, and other undesirable behaviors.

Integrated Bio-Psycho-Social Model

In an attempt to integrate different findings about the origin and maintenance of stereotyped behavior and SIB into a coherent model, Guess and Carr (1991) proposed a three-stage bio-psycho-social hypothesis. In the first stage, internally regulated rhythmic behaviors appear in most infants, both in those who develop normally and in those with disabilities (*developmental theory*). The second stage assumes that repetitive behaviors are used to modulate environmental over- or understimulation (*homeostasis theory*). In the third stage, social contingencies shape these regulatory behaviors into their definitive appearance (*conditioned response theories*).

Repetitive Behavior as a Manifestation of Mental Illness

An alternate view of aberrant repetitive behaviors in mental retardation is that they could be symptoms of some forms of mental illness, which manifest themselves differently in this population as a result of cognitive and emotional limitations. King (1993), for instance, suggested that some forms of SIB and stereotypy may be symptoms of an obsessive-compulsive disorder. Two independent findings have supported the compulsive behavior theory of repetitive behavior. First, Bodfish, Crawford, Powell, Golden, & Lewis (1995) found an association between the presence of compulsive symptoms and SIB and stereotypy. Second, several studies have reported successful treatment of repetitive

behavior in mental retardation with medication that is typically prescribed for individuals with obsessive-compulsive disorders and depression (Bodfish & Madison, 1993; Garber, McGonigle, Slomka, & Monteverde, 1992; Sovner, Foxx, Lowry, & Lowry, 1993).

The Impact of Early Social Conditions on Repetitive Behavior

Berkson and Mason (1964) and Davenport and Berkson (1963) noticed similarities between repetitive behavior in humans with mental retardation and pathological behavior in isolation-reared monkeys. This has led to the hypothesis that stereotypic behavior is in fact pathological, caused by deprived conditions in early childhood. Recent primate research suggests, however, that the relationship between rearing conditions and repetitive behavior is more complicated, and that there are strong interindividual differences (Kraemer, Ebert, Schmidt, & McKinney, 1991).

It was also found that different forms of stereotyped behavior may reflect different psychological reactions. For example, Kraemer et al. (1991) conducted a longitudinal study on a group of rhesus monkeys. These workers took repeated behavioral measures of mother-reared versus surrogate-reared animals and monitored their behavioral reaction to environmental stressors. Exposure to stress that occurred in the form of separation from the mother or the surrogate at 6 to 7 months of age, caused significant differences between the two groups. In the mother-reared monkeys, behaviors indicative of protest, such as vocalization, locomotion, and motor stereotype, increased; the surrogate-reared monkeys showed an increase in despair behavior, such as huddling, body rocking, and other self-directed behavior.

Environmental Factors

Stereotyped behavior and SIB can be influenced by a variety of environmental conditions.

For instance, researchers have observed that repetitive behavior increased with novel restrictive environments (Berkson & Mason, 1963), unfamiliar therapists (Runco, Charlop, & Schreibman, 1986), television turned on (Gary, Tallon, & Stangl, 1980), prior movement restraint (Forehand & Baumeister, 1970), or the removal of a preferred toy (Greer, Becker, Saxe, & Mirabella, 1985). Wolery et al. (1985) reported that stereotypies by one individual can trigger stereotypic behavior in others. Decreases in repetitive behavior are often related to opportunities for alternative behavior (Berkson & Mason, 1963; Goodall & Corbett, 1982), the availability of toys (Davenport & Berkson, 1963) particularly in combination with staff interaction (Berkson & Mason, 1964; Moseley, Faust, & Reardon, 1970), training in how to engage in toy play (Greer et al., 1985; Mulick, Hoyt, Rojahn, & Schroeder, 1978), and prior to rigorous physical exercise (Allen, 1980; Kern, Koegel, & Dunlap, 1984; Kern, Koegel, Dyer, Blew, & Fenton, 1982; Watters & Watters, 1980). In the classroom, short intertrial intervals during teaching procedures were also associated with lower rates of stereotypies as compared with long intervals (Dunlap, Dyer, & Koegel, 1983).

The same environmental stimuli can have different effects in different individuals. For instance, it was reported that popular music increased stereotyped behaviors in 12 adults with mental retardation who engaged in body rocking (Tierney, McGuire, & Walton, 1978), whereas normal easy-listening radio also played at "normal volume" did not increase the rate of stereotyped behaviors in four other individuals (Adams, Tallon, & Stangl, 1980). Similar contradiction exists about the rate effect of rhythmic cuing on the tempo of stereotyped behavior (Christopher & Lewis, 1984; Soraci, Deckner, McDaniel, & Blanton, 1982; Stevens, 1971).

Many studies cited above used few subjects and manipulated only a small number of ecological variables at a time. However, there is probably a higher order of complexity in the relationship between environmental events and different repetitive behavior. For instance, Win-

nega and Berkson (1986) found that in a group of 10 clients non-object-related stereotypies were more frequent during a music condition as compared with meal times. This difference was not found for stereotyped object manipulations. In another example, Frankel, Freeman, Ritvo, and Pardo (1978) found that the degree with which the level of environmental stimulation affected the stereotyped behavior of children with autism was dependent on their level of functioning.

EPIDEMIOLOGY

Two important parameters used in descriptive epidemiology are prevalence and incidence. Prevalence refers to the proportion of afflicted cases in the entire population. Incidence is the rate of newly emerging afflicted cases within a defined period. Incidence data of SIB and stereotyped behavior in persons with mental retardation are very rare, probably because of the overwhelming expense in collecting good longitudinal data of that sort and the difficulty in ensuring participant cooperation over time. One of the few incidence statistics we have today is that abnormal repetitive behavior generally does not appear before the second year of life (Berkson, McQuiston, Jacobson, Eyman, & Borthwick, 1985).

Prevalence

Prevalence is generally easier to obtain than incidence, but even that is complicated to estimate reliably. Prevalence statistics of repetitive behavior vary widely depending on the surveyed population, case identification methods, and the data collection method employed. Prevalence of stereotyped behaviors ranges from 5 to more than 60% of the population with mental retardation (Berkson & Davenport, 1962; Dura, Mulick, & Rasnake, 1987; Jacobson, 1982; Kaufman & Levitt, 1965; Rojahn, 1986), whereas SIB prevalence ranges from approximately 4 to 15% (Rojahn, 1994).

For this chapter we will present prevalence statistics for children through adults up to age 45. Estimates were based on all individuals who received state-funded mental retardation services in the states of New York and California.[2] These databases are actuarial rather than scientific and may therefore contain certain biases reflecting the specific populations served in these two states rather than the population in general. However, none of the other published SIB and stereotyped behavior data sets are without a flaw. The advantage of the present data is that they reflect conditions in two entire populations of well-defined cases in a system of mandatory reporting on behavior problems. As of the time at which these data were obtained (1993), California had almost 90,000 individuals in the desired age range, and New York had more than 45,000. Among the approximately 135,000 individuals with developmental disabilities in both states combined, the *overall prevalence rates* (i.e., prevalence across all age groups and all levels of mental retardation) of stereotyped behavior and SIB were 6.5 and 8.5%, respectively. As we will show, both stereotyped behavior and SIB are strongly associated with several characteristics. Therefore, global prevalence rates reveal only little about these phenomena.

Level of Intellectual Functioning

The prevalence of problem behaviors, including aggressive behavior and destruction of inanimate objects, is higher in persons with more severe levels of intellectual impairment. The same is true for stereotyped behavior and SIB (Eyman & Call, 1977; Jacobson, 1982; Thompson & Berkson, 1985). The data in Figure 1 from California and New York databases show the same linear negative relationship between rates of oc-

[2]We thank Sharon Borthwick-Duffy and John W. Jacobson for their generous permission to use these data for this chapter.

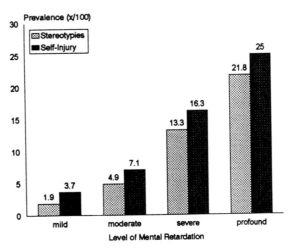

Figure 1. The prevalence of self-injurious and stereotyped behavior as a function of mental retardation level.

currence and level of mental retardation. Stereotyped behavior ranges from 1.9% in mild mental retardation to 21.8% in profound mental retardation. SIB prevalence ranges from 3.7% in mild to 25% in profound mental retardation.

Sex

Figure 2 contains data from the California population only. It shows that 8.4% of the women and 8.9% of the men with developmental disabilities in this state exhibit SIB, and 5.8 and 7.0% respectively show stereotyped behavior. In other words, repetitive behaviors are slightly more common among men than among women with mental retardation, particularly stereotypies.

Communication

As previously discussed, several researchers have argued that problem behaviors may be attempts to communicate with others (Carr & Durand, 1985a; Carr et al., 1994). If so, we would

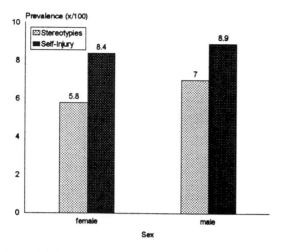

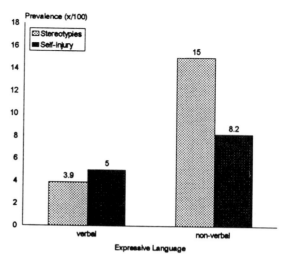

Figure 2. The prevalence of self-injurious and stereotyped behavior as a function of sex (i.e., rate of occurence within the population of males and females).

Figure 3. The prevalence of self-injurious and stereotyped behavior as a function of the presence or absence of verbal communication skills.

expect individuals without verbal communication skills to be more likely to exhibit stereotypies and SIB than individuals with verbal communication skills. Figure 3 confirms this. We must caution the reader against taking this finding as anything more than being supportive of the communication hypothesis. These data do not show to what extent the variable of interest *itself,* in this case verbal communication skills, has a causal relationship with problem behavior. It is possible that this effect is better explained by intellectual functioning, for instance, which itself is correlated with communication skills.

Chronological Age

Previous studies have suggested that SIB and stereotyped behavior are related to chronological age in an inverse U-shaped function (Berkson et al., 1985; Murphy et al., 1993; Rojahn, 1994). Prevalence of stereotyped behaviors increases until the teenage years and then slowly diminishes. In the population with profound mental retardation the peak prevalence rates occur relatively later in life as compared with people with less severe retardation (Berkson et

al., 1985). Interestingly, Thompson and Berkson (1985) reported that stereotyped behaviors in children and young adolescents without object involvement (e.g., body rocking, head rolling, postures) did correlate positively with age, whereas stereotyped behaviors involving objects (e.g., shaking, twirling, or patting objects) did not. Figure 4 shows slightly different results, namely, that prevalence of stereotypies and SIB steadily increases into middle adulthood.

Residential Setting

SIB and stereotyped behaviors become more prevalent with increasing restrictiveness of residential conditions. Many sources confirm this trend (Borthwick, Meyers, & Eyman, 1981; Eyman & Call, 1977; Jacobson, 1982) and concerns were raised that restrictive residential facilities may contribute to behavioral deterioration. However, whether restrictive environments "cause" the development of SIB and stereotyped behaviors is difficult to establish with prevalence data. Problem behaviors are a major reason why individuals with developmental dis-

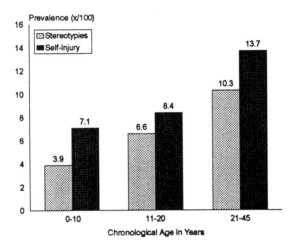

Figure 4. The prevalence of self-injurious and stereotyped behavior as a function of chronological age.

abilities fail to adjust in nonrestrictive community settings. At the same time, there is a strong push to empty out the restrictive "institutions." It is therefore likely that restrictive residential facilities are becoming increasingly last-resort options for people with severe behavior problems, including SIB.

Mental Illness

As previously mentioned, children and adolescents with mental retardation are at a much higher risk for emotional and behavioral disturbances than the nondisabled population. Until recently very little was known about psychiatric disorders in mental retardation, and their diagnosis still presents considerable problems (Reiss, 1994). The question has been raised whether stereotyped behaviors are associated with common psychiatric disorders such as mood disorders, schizophrenia, and personality disorders, or whether they represent a separate, population-specific form of psychopathology.

Reid, Ballinger, and Heather (1978) developed a diagnostic framework for individuals with severe and profound mental retardation by investigating the natural relationships of gener-

al psychiatric symptoms and behavioral disturbances associated with mental retardation. The data were collected via nursing staff ratings, record searches, and a standardized psychiatric patient interview (Goldberg, Cooper, Eastwood, Kedward, & Shephard, 1970). The data of 100 hospitalized adults with severe and profound mental retardation were analyzed by cluster analysis. They distinguished eight types of individuals. Stereotyped behavior especially characterized one cluster of individuals, whereas the other one represented the most severely disturbed subgroup of patients with multiple behavioral abnormalities. Fraser, Leudar, Gray, and Campbell (1986) related psychiatric diagnoses to behavior problems by stepwise multiple regression, including idiosyncratic mannerisms. No significant relationships between any of the eight factors of psychiatric disturbance and idiosyncratic mannerisms were found. Neither stereotyped behavior nor SIB appeared to predict mental illness. A very similar finding was reported by Rojahn et al. (1993). In summary, to date we have little empirical evidence in support of the assumption that stereotypies and SIB are linked to special forms of psychiatric illness. This is consistent with DSM-IV (APA, 1994) keeping a separate psychiatric category for these behaviors. However, with the advent of more sophisticated diagnostic and assessment procedures, more reliable data will be collected in this very important area of research.

ASSESSMENT

Assessment of challenging behaviors typically has one of three major functions: (1) to survey the presence of behavior problems within a population; (2) to discover the motivation or the functional properties of the behavior (*functional analysis*), which is important for the selection of the proper behavioral intervention strategy (*treatment indication*); and (3) to quantify behavior for *treatment evaluation*. Surveys usually rely on checklists and behavior rating scales. In addition to behavior checklists and behavior rating scales, treatment outcome evaluation and functional analysis also rely on behavioral interviews, focused behavior observations, and experimentation.

Survey Assessment

For surveys, the most useful methods of data collection are symptom checklists or behavior rating scales.

Behavior Checklists

There are a few new behavior or symptom checklists available for SIB with good psychometric properties. For instance, the *Self-Injury Checklist* (Bodfish et al., 1995), a seven-item instrument adapted from a survey instrument by Maurice and Trudel (1982), has a mean 89% interobserver agreement, 91.6% mean stability, and 90.2% congruence with observational data. Another type of instrument is the *Self-Injury Trauma* (SIT) scale (Iwata, Pace, Kissel, Nau, & Farber, 1990). For stereotyped behavior, the *Stereotypy Checklist* (Bodfish et al. 1995) should be mentioned, an instrument adapted from the *Timed Stereotypies Checklist* (Campbell, 1985). The Stereotypy Checklist has a mean interobserver reliability of 81.3% occurrence agreement, a mean test–retest stability of 78.7%, and a 94.3% congruence with observational data. Another recent checklist for stereotypies was published by Berkson et al. (1995).

Behavior Rating Scales

As far as behavior rating scales are concerned, there are several broad-spectrum instruments, such as the *Aberrant Behavior Checklist* (Aman, Singh, Stewart, & Field, 1985), the *Strohmer-Prout Behavior Rating Scale* (Strohmer & Prout, 1989), the *Vineland Adaptive Behavior Scales* (Sparrow, Balla, & Cicchetti, 1984), and the *Nisonger Child Behavior Rating Form* (Aman, Tassé, Rojahn, & Hammer, 1996; Tassé, Aman, Hammer, & Ro-

jahn, 1996), that contain SIB and stereotypy items or subscales. Instruments specifically designed for SIB topographies are the *Behavior Problem Inventory* (Rojahn, 1986; Rojahn, Polster, Mulick, & Wisniewski, 1989) and the *Self-Injurious Behavior Questionnaire* (Gualtieri & Schroeder, 1989; Schroeder, Rojahn, & Reese, 1997). For stereotyped behavior the 26-item factor-analytically derived *Stereotyped Behavior Scale* (Rojahn, Tassé, & Sturmey, 1997) should be mentioned.

Functional Analysis

The purpose of functional analysis is to reveal whether challenging behavior is motivated by external or internal positive reinforcement (social attention, communication, self-stimulation), external or internal negative reinforcement (escape/avoidance), or whether other variables are responsible for the target behavior. As Table 1 shows, each of these functions has functionally commensurate treatment options. For instance, if we were to treat a target behavior motivated by positive social reinforcement, a social extinction procedure or teaching appropriate requesting for attention may be two of several possible options to choose from. Table 1 is an attempt to link certain functional properties of the behavior with some appropriate treatment choices.

A concise functional analysis is an important basis for treatment selection (Carr, 1977; Day, Horner, & O'Neill, 1994; Derby et al., 1994; Smith, Iwata, Vollmer, & Zarcone, 1993). It has long been accepted that the potential efficacy of a treatment intervention of maladaptive behaviors is closely related to an a priori analysis of the variables regulating the target behaviors (Favell, Azrin, et al., 1982; Iwata, Dorsey, Slifer, Bauman, & Richman, 1982; Repp, Felce, & Barton, 1988; Wieseler, Hanson, Chamberlain, & Thompson, 1985).

Two studies provided estimates of the proportions of motivational conditions in cases with repetitive behavior. Iwata et al. (1994) conducted

Table 1. Treatment Indication Based on Functional Property of the Target Behavior

Functional property of the behavior		Rational intervention alternatives
Functional stimulus	Functional intent of the behavior	
External stimulus External positive stimulus	Behavior produces external positive stimulus	A. *Social rewards* • Social extinction • Use social rewards to reinforce appropriate behavior (DRO, DRI, DRA) • Teach appropriate request for attention • Increase the rate of noncontingent attention • Increase opportunities for social interaction • Increase interactive activities • Nonexclusionary time-out B. *Tangible rewards* • Tangible reward extinction • Satiation • Teach appropriate request for tangible rewards • Use tangible rewards to reinforce appropriate behavior (DRO, DRI, DRA) • Increase rate of noncontingent access to tangible rewards
External negative stimulus	Behavior avoids or escapes external negative stimulus	• Extinction (e.g., guided compliance, continued instruction) • Teach appropriate escape response (e.g., request assistance, request breaks) • Reduce task difficulty (e.g., schedule frequent breaks) • Increase reinforcement for task engagement
Internal stimulus Positive internal stimulus	Behavior produces positive internal stimulus	• Sensory extinction • Environmental enrichment (e.g., increase noncontingent social interaction, introduce interesting activities and materials) • Teach appropriate request for stimulation
Negative internal stimulus	Behavior avoids or escapes negative internal stimulus	• If discomfort is related to pain: request comprehensive medical checkup and treatment and/or analgesics (medication, TENS) • If discomfort is related to hunger, thirst; provide food or liquids

functional analyses with 152 SIB cases and found that functional properties were indeed detectable in the majority of SIB cases (90%). Approximately 40% of them were clearly escape or avoidance motivated (38.1%), roughly one-quarter each by positive external reinforcement (26.3%) and sensory reinforcement (25.7%), and about 5% had more than one type of motivation. The rest showed inconsistent patterns of responding. A decade earlier, Wieseler et al. (1985) estimated functional properties of SIB and stereotyped behavior. The results of the Iwata et al. and the Wieseler et al. studies are summarized in Table 2. The proportions of motivational conditions for SIB were remarkably similar across studies, particularly the estimate for the SIB cases motivated by escape/avoidance. It also shows that quite in contrast to

Table 2. Estimates of the Percentage of Functional Properties of Stereotyped and Self-Injurious Behaviors from Two Studies

	Iwata et al. (1994) $n = 152$	Wieseler et al. (1985) $n = 60$	
	SIB	SIB	Stereotypy
Positive external reinforcement	26%	30%	3%
Negative external reinforcement (escape/avoidance)	38%	38%	4%
No environmental consequence (positive internal reinforcement)	26%	32%	92%
Multiple functions	5%	—	—
Uncertain	5%	—	—

SIB, stereotypy has a very different motivational profile with the vast majority of cases being reinforced by self-stimulatory consequences.

Functional analysis usually begins by interviewing people who are most familiar with the person. Questions will center on gathering information on the individual's behavior and the circumstances under which it typically occurs. This should be supplemented by focused observations of the behavior, its antecedents and consequences in critical situations in the natural environment (O'Neill, Horner, Albin, Storey, & Sprague, 1990). Such interviews will often lead to good initial hypotheses. However, detecting functional properties from staff interviews or from mere observation is often difficult because of reliability problems. This has been the problem with rating instruments based on staff interviews, such as the *Motivational Assessment Scale* (MAS; Durand & Crimmins, 1983, 1988). The MAS, a 16-item informant rating scale, has been found to have poor reliability (Newton & Sturmey, 1991; Zarcone, Rodgers, Iwata, Rourke, & Dorsey, 1991). Therefore, it will frequently be necessary to conduct an analogue experiment to test the functional hypotheses (Iwata et al., 1982; Iwata, Vollmer, & Zarcone, 1990). One must also realize that the methodology of functional analysis has evolved since its early conception of looking solely at positive and negative reinforcement, and now encompasses contextual considerations, biological factors, or group interactions, to name only a few

cited by Carr (1994). Readers interested in a more detailed practical guide and assessment forms for conducting a functional analysis in children with mental retardation and SIB or stereotypies may consult Carr et al. (1994) or O'Neill et al. (1990) for details.

Treatment Evaluation

In the tradition of operant behavioral research, the most common treatment evaluation method is repeated systematic behavior observation prior to and during intervention within a single-subject experimental design. A variety of observational data collection methods exist. One can distinguish between event-based (event sampling) and time-based (time sampling) techniques, and for each several different methods are available. In *event sampling* the observer records all events within a designated observation period. To enhance data objectivity, the targeted behaviors ought to be defined by concrete and observable features. Behavior definitions for observation systems are usually customized to a particular individual's behaviors. Occasionally, however, observation packages consisting of predetermined behavior categories have been developed for certain clinical phenomena. One of those, which has been used extensively with SIB and stereotyped behavior, is the 24-behavior *Ecobehavioral Assessment System* (Rojahn & Schroeder, 1979; Schroeder, Rojahn,

& Mulick, 1978). For a more detailed discussion of behavior observation techniques in the field of mental retardation, see Rojahn and Schroeder (1991). In addition to systematic behavior observation, checklists and rating scales can also be used for treatment evaluation. Unfortunately, only very few stereotypy and SIB assessment instruments have been scrutinized for their sensitivity to treatment. One of those instruments is the *Aberrant Behavior Checklist* (Aman et al., 1985), which has been shown to be sensitive to behavioral change in response to psychopharmacological interventions.

TREATMENT

Several treatment modalities are available when attempting to modify the occurrence of SIB and stereotypy. This section will present the different approaches available. As previously mentioned, because no one existing etiological or motivational hypothesis of SIB and stereotypy can account for all cases, any treatment intervention should be derived from a concise analysis of the target behaviors' antecedent and consequent stimuli (Repp et al., 1988). Specific functional properties of the target behavior lead to rational treatment alternatives (see Table 1).

Behavioral Treatment Procedures

Behavioral approaches are considered the treatment strategies of choice for SIB and stereotypic behavior (Matson, 1989; Reiss, 1994; Rojahn & Sisson, 1990). A meta-analysis of studies reporting the use of behavioral treatment strategies for SIB published between 1967 and 1986 indicated maintenance of treatment effect in 70% of cases at an average 9-month follow-up (Morin, 1987). In this section we will present the following behavioral treatment approaches: differential reinforcement procedures, functional communication training, extinction and time-out manipulation, environmental changes, sensory extinction, alternate sensory activities, and punishment.

Differential Reinforcement Procedures

The purpose of differential reinforcement procedures is to reduce maladaptive behavior. This is accomplished by withholding reinforcement when the client emits the target maladaptive behaviors and by concurrently reinforcing other, more appropriate behaviors. Three variants of differential reinforcement can be found in the literature on problem behaviors in mental retardation: differential reinforcement of other behaviors (DRO), differential reinforcement of incompatible behaviors (DRI), and differential reinforcement of alternative behaviors (DRA). The choice of an appropriate reinforcer (i.e., preference, salience) is an important variable in the success of differential reinforcement procedures (Mazaleski, Iwata, Vollmer, Zarcone, & Smith, 1993; O'Brien & Repp, 1990). The differential reinforcement procedures are among the most frequently used nonaversive techniques in the treatment of SIB (Lennox, Miltenberger, Spengler, & Erfanian, 1988; Matson & Taras, 1989).

DRO refers to the delivery of a reinforcer at the end of a predetermined interval during which the targeted maladaptive behavior did not occur. If a target behavior is emitted before the end of the predetermined interval, the therapist restarts the interval and reinforcement is withheld thus placing the target behavior under extinction. An important variable in the DRO intervention is the length of the interval during which the target behaviors must not be emitted to obtain the reinforcement (O'Brien & Repp, 1990). As O'Brien and Repp (1990) pointed out, the selected interval should be sufficiently short to "catch" the individual not emitting SIB. The length of initial intervals is especially difficult to gauge when the individual engages in high-frequency SIB. Conversely, if the selected interval is too short and the type of reinforcer is not varied, the individual may become satiated

(Mazaleski et al., 1993; O'Brien & Repp, 1990). A serious disadvantage of the DRO procedure is the possibility of inadvertently reinforcing other "inappropriate" behaviors (e.g., screaming, body rocking).

Recently, we have also seen an adapted form of DRO called *momentary DRO* being used in reduction of stereotypy (Barton, Brulle, & Repp, 1986; Derwas & Jones, 1993; Repp, Barton, & Brulle, 1983). The difference between these two DRO procedures is in the reinforcement criterion: In the whole interval DRO the target behavior must not occur at any time, whereas with momentary DRO the target behavior must not occur at the interval end.

Mazaleski et al. (1993) studied the relative contribution of the two main components of DRO, extinction of the target behavior and reinforcement of the absence of the target behavior. They found for socially mediated SIB that the effectiveness of DRO procedures was related largely to extinction, rather than to the reinforcement of other behavior.

DRO is the differential reinforcement procedure most frequently reported in the literature (Matson & Taras, 1989). According to O'Brien and Repp's (1990) review of 20 years of research literature, 36 and 45% of published studies using DRO did so to suppress SIB and stereotypy, respectively, whereas 66 and 20% of published studies using DRI did so to treat SIB and stereotypy, respectively.

DRI is the differential reinforcement of predetermined behaviors that are incompatible with the targeted maladaptive behavior (e.g., typing at a keyboard and head slapping). A distinct advantage of DRI over DRO is its differential reinforcement of a predetermined appropriate and topographically incompatible behavior, thus reducing the probability of an inadvertent reinforcement of other maladaptive behaviors. In a study of pica behavior (eating cigarette butts) in two adults with mental retardation, Donnelly and Olczak (1990) differentially reinforced gum chewing as an incompatible behavior to pica. A significant decrease in frequency of pica resulted and was accompanied by an increase in the frequency of the incompatible and more socially acceptable gum chewing. When comparing DRI and DRO, Tarpley and Schroeder (1979) observed a faster rate of suppression of SIB in three individuals with profound mental retardation when using DRI.

DRA is the differential reinforcement of predetermined appropriate behaviors that may not necessarily be topographically incompatible with the targeted SIB or stereotypy. In their review of reinforcement-based intervention literature published between 1968 and 1988, O'Brien and Repp (1990) reported only two published studies using DRA. A recent study by Sisson, Hersen, and Van Hasselt (1993) reported on a DRA plus overcorrection procedure used to suppress stereotypy in two individuals with sensory impairments and mental retardation. They differentially reinforced one individual for placing an envelope in a bin rather than engaging in hand flapping, rocking, and stereotypic manipulation of objects; for the second client, they identified on-task behavior as the alternative behavior to stereotypy. In both cases, DRA plus overcorrection resulted in significant reductions in stereotypy. Unfortunately, Sisson et al. (1993) did not counterbalance their intervention design and it is impossible to detect the contribution of DRA versus overcorrection on the suppression of stereotypy.

In an interesting variation of differential reinforcement procedures, researchers have begun to investigate the effectiveness of differential negative reinforcement schedules (DNR). This includes prohibition of successful escape contingent on the target behavior (escape extinction) and allows escape with some other behavior. Roberts, Mace, and Daggert (1995) compared differential negative reinforcement of other behavior (DNRO) with differential negative reinforcement of alternate behavior (DNRA) in the treatment of self-injurious tantrum behavior. DNRO permits escape after a time period in which the target behavior has not occurred. DNRA has a dual requirement: Only the omission of the target behavior and the display of a specific alternative behavior produce a reinforcer. In this preliminary study, DNRA was found to be more effective than DNRO.

Published studies report conflicting results of effectiveness for treatment interventions using differential reinforcement alone. More often than not, researchers use these techniques together with other approaches (e.g., extinction, response interruption, overcorrection). In fact, it is considered good clinical practice to incorporate differential reinforcement procedures into any treatment program to suppress SIB (Favell, McGimsey, & Schell, 1982).

Functional Communication Training

Functional communication training (FCT) is based on the assumption that SIB and stereotypy are a means to express needs or demands (Carr & Durand, 1985a,b; Carr et al., 1994; Cipani, 1990; Donnellan, Mirenda, Mesaros, & Fassbender, 1984; Evans & Meyer, 1985; Schroeder, Mulick, & Rojahn, 1980). FCT contains two essential elements: the accurate analysis of the social or communicative function of the target SIB or stereotypy and the careful selection of a functionally equivalent communication response that will replace the target SIB or stereotypy (Carr & Durand, 1985a). Functional analysis is an integral part of establishing whether the SIB or stereotypy serves a function of: (1) attention seeking/request for reinforcement or (2) escape/avoidance of an unpleasant situation. Carr and Durand (1985a) then prescribed the shaping and/or reinforcement of a functionally equivalent, but socially more appropriate alternative or replacement behavior. In many regards, FCT can be viewed as a more elaborate form of DRA.

Carr and Durand (1985b) tested functional communication training in a two-step process. In the first part of their study, they observed the frequency of maladaptive behaviors of four children during three typical educational situations: working on an easy academic task and receiving adult attention during either 33% (easy & 33%) or 100% (easy & 100%) of the session intervals; and working on a difficult academic task while receiving adult attention during 100% (difficult & 100%) of the session intervals. They randomly gave adult attention in the form of either a mand (e.g., "copy this drawing"), praise (e.g., "good job"), or a neutral comment (e.g., "it is cold outside"). Carr and Durand directed their experiment to study the effects of varying degrees of task difficulty on the frequency of aggression, tantrum behaviors, and SIB (escape/avoidance) and the effects of amounts of attention on the frequency of maladaptive behavior (attention seeking). The first part of their study revealed an increase in maladaptive behaviors: for two clients during the difficult & 100% (escape/avoid demand); for one client during the easy & 100% (seeking attention); and for the fourth client during both difficult & 100% (escape/avoidance) and easy & 33% (attention seeking).

In the second part of their study, Carr and Durand (1985b) used the observational information obtained from the first experiment to hypothesize the communicative function of the maladaptive behavior for each of the four participants. They then trained their clients with the appropriate replacement behavior/phrase (1) requesting help in cases of escape-mediated behaviors (e.g., "I don't understand") or (2) requesting some adult attention or social interaction (e.g, "Am I doing good work?"). During this second phase the adult provided attention only during the low-attention tasks or assistance only during the difficult tasks, and only after the clients' request using the appropriate replacement phrase. The more effective verbal request for attention replaced attention-seeking maladaptive behaviors. Similarly, the maladaptive behaviors that were functioning for escaping a difficult task, were replaced by the more functional requests for assistance. Others have successfully used sign language in FCT (Bird, Dores, Moniz, & Robinson, 1989; Duker, Jol, & Palmen, 1991; Wacker et al., 1990) or assistive technology (a micro switch that activated a prerecorded message [Wacker et al., 1990]). Moreover, generalization (Bird et al., 1989) and maintenance of acquired functional communication ability at a 2-year follow-up (Durand & Carr, 1991) have been shown.

Extinction and Time-Out

Extinction is a treatment procedure that consists of identifying the reinforcing agent of the SIB or stereotypy and withholding the reinforcer whenever the target maladaptive behavior is emitted. If a functional analysis suggests that the stereotypy is reinforced by parental attention, the treatment plan would consist of withholding parental attention (ignoring) whenever the target stereotypy is emitted. If it is difficult to clearly identify the reinforcer or when good control over the reinforcer is difficult to establish, it is preferable *not* to employ an extinction procedure (Favell, Azrin, et al., 1982). An obvious concern with extinction procedures of severe SIB is the danger of injury to the client especially during the increase in frequency and/or intensity expected during the typical extinction burst. Some authors have nonetheless used extinction with SIB. Duker and Seys (1983) used extinction procedures with six individuals with severe mental retardation and presenting a variety of SIB. Reductions in SIB were achieved for only two participants. In a meta-analysis of the scientific literature of interventions for stereotypy, Wehmeyer (1995) concurred with previous reviews that both extinction and time-out are ineffective treatment strategies for the reduction of stereotypy. It must be mentioned, however, that most of the published applied behavior analysis research studies prior to the mid-1980s did not report functional analysis data. It is possible that some of the interventions that were found ineffective were not based on a careful functional analysis and may have been inappropriate for the functional properties of the target behavior.

Time-out consists of a temporary removal of the individual's access to reinforcing activities or objects. Time-out can involve physically removing the client from the environment (*exclusionary time-out*) or permitting the individual to remain (*nonexclusionary time-out*) (Malcuit,

Pomerleau, & Maurice, 1995). Rose, Sloop, and Baker (1980) reported reducing head banging in a 19-year-old man with profound mental retardation by moving the individual to an isolation room when he engaged in head banging. Besides the time-out procedure, Rose et al. (1980) used terry-cloth restraints to prevent injury during the exclusionary time-out procedure. Of all decelerative treatment practices reviewed by Lennox et al. (1988), time-out was the least effective procedure (20 versus at least 55% for other procedures) in suppressing SIB. Again, we need to take into consideration that in earlier studies time-out may have been used in inappropriate circumstances.

Environmental Manipulation

Treatment may at times consist of modifying the environment in which the maladaptive behaviors are most frequent. An understimulating environment (Berkson, 1967; Edelson, 1984) may cause or maintain stereotypies and some forms of SIB (Lovaas, 1982). Loud and continuous noise may even increase stereotypy (Adams et al., 1980).

As previously mentioned, some individuals engage in self-stimulation in an attempt to regulate their levels of arousal. One form of treatment may therefore consist of increasing the access to toys, music or other objects that may heighten the environment's level of sensory stimulation (e.g., Mulick et al., 1878). Conversely, a treatment plan may equally consist of reducing noise levels, bright lights, or the temperature in the room to regulate the heightened level of sensory stimulation present in the environment.

Sensory Extinction

Sensory extinction is founded on the hypothesis that sensory consequences rather than social consequences maintain some forms of SIB and stereotypy (see also Table 1). Sensory extinction is a procedure by which the proprioceptive properties of stereotypies or SIB are reduced or eliminated (Rincover, 1978). Sensory extinction focuses on masking or dampening the tactile, vestibular, or sensory feedback produced by the maladaptive behavior. Rincover and Devany (1982) reported good results with three children who engaged in SIB. The authors used protective helmets to reduce the tactile sensations of hand-to-head contact of two children who engaged in head banging; they lined the floors and walls with gym mats to reduce the tactile feedback for one child who hit his head on the floor and walls; and they used rubber gloves to cover the hands of a child who self-injured by scratching herself. This procedure was used in combination with DRO. The frequency of SIB decreased rapidly in all three participants and the protective equipment was gradually faded with a maintenance of suppression of SIB at a 3-month follow-up. Luiselli (1991) used protective mittens with a visually impaired woman who engaged in high-frequency eye pressing, and Kennedy and Souza (1995) provided their participant, who also engaged in eye poking, protective goggles to counter the sensory stimulation produced by the maladaptive behavior. Both studies found suppression of SIB. Rincover, Cook, Peoples, and Packard (1979) used a sensory extinction treatment approach with four children with autism who engaged in stereotypy. Employing a standardized procedure, Rincover and colleagues assessed the sensory function of stereotypy for each client and planned individualized treatment strategies. They placed a vibrating device on the back of the hand of two children who engaged in stereotypic finger and hand movements, seemingly a proprioceptive reinforcement. The vibrator was used to mask the sensory feedback produced by finger and hand waving. Also used for a similar type of stereotypy was a blindfold or turning off the overhead lights to reduce visual stimulation. The authors also placed a carpet over a table surface to eliminate the sound produced by the plate spinning of a fourth participant. The authors reported durable suppression of the stereotypies. An important variable to observe is topographical substitution. Norton (1986) noted

that maladaptive behaviors placed under sensory extinction were suppressed but that there was an increase in equally maladaptive but topographically different SIB. Some authors have also been critical of sensory extinction because of the possibility that the protection equipment used may merely physically prevent the behavior or be perceived by the clients as an aversive and thus confound the extinction versus punishing components of this procedure (Lovaas, 1982).

In a rare example of sensory extinction of escape/avoidance motivated behavior (avoidance of internal stimuli such as chronic pain), Linn, Rojahn, Helsel, and Dixon (1988) explored the use of transcutaneous electric nerve stimulation (TENS) with two clients with multiple forms of SIB. TENS is a noninvasive treatment procedure often prescribed for chronic and acute pain. Unfortunately, the results of TENS on SIB were ambivalent.

Alternate Sensory Activities

Favell, McGimsey, and Schell (1982) were among the first to show clinically that a treatment program could effectively reduce SIB by providing alternate sensory activities that provided the same stimulation as that sought by the target SIB. Alternate sensory activities and sensory extinction are two treatment approaches based on the hypothesis that sensory reinforcement is mediating SIB or stereotypies (see Table 1). Favell, McGimsey, and Schell (1982) suppressed pica, hand mouthing, and eye poking by making available alternate objects and activities that were intended to produce sensory input similar to that provided by the target SIB. Giving toys to the subject reduced hand mouthing in a child who initially used the toys to provide gustatory stimulation by placing them in his mouth. Mouthing toys completely replaced SIB (hand mouthing). The authors then suppressed and replaced mouthing toys with more appropriate toy playing using a differential reinforcement procedure. Others have used different forms of alternate sensory activities such as access to a video game (Kennedy & Souza,

1995) and bright and colorful toys (Favell, McGimsey, & Schell, 1982) to replace eye poking; mouthing rubber toys to replace pica (Favell, McGimsey, & Schell, 1982). Steege, Wacker, Berg, Cigrand, and Cooper (1989) reported a decrease in SIB when they gave a client access to a switch that activated a radio or fan.

A distinct advantage of the alternate sensory activity treatment over sensory extinction treatment is its inclusion of shaping and reinforcing of alternative behaviors that can functionally replace (in terms of sensory feedback) SIB and stereotypy.

Punishment

Punishment refers to any response contingent procedure in which the presentation of an *aversive* stimulus or the removal of a pleasant stimulus results in the *suppression* of the frequency of the target behavior (Azrin & Holz, 1966; Matson & DiLorenzo, 1984; Repp & Singh, 1990). Several authors reviewed the punishment outcome literature in mental retardation and concluded that aversive stimuli have been generally highly effective in suppressing SIB (Cataldo, 1991; Favell, Azrin, et al., 1982; Lennox et al., 1988; Matson & Taras, 1989) and stereotypy (Gorman-Smith & Matson, 1985; LaGrow & Repp, 1984; Lennox et al., 1988). However, the propriety of using any form of punishment in individuals with mental retardation—no matter how dangerous the behavior at hand—was the focus of a long and bitter debate in the late 1980s, which split many professionals in this field into polarized groups of irreconcilable opinions. The book edited by Repp & Singh (1990) presents some of the ethical, political, and methodological considerations that were advanced during that divisive controversy.

Over the years many types of aversive stimuli have been investigated as treatment options for SIB and (less so) for stereotypy, including: electric shock (Corte, Wolf, & Locke, 1971; Linscheid, Iwata, Ricketts, Williams, & Griffin, 1990), Tabasco sauce (Altemeyer, Williams, & Sams, 1985), water mist (Rojahn, McGonigle,

Curcio, & Dixon, 1987), visual screening procedures (Rojahn & Marshburn, 1992; Watson, Singh, & Winton, 1986), ammonia vapors (Altman, Haavik, & Cook, 1978), lemon juice (Sajwaj, Libet, & Agras, 1974), slapping (Romanczyk, 1977), contingent application of a protective device (Luiselli, 1986), mechanical restraints (Hamad, Isley, & Lowry, 1983), physical restraint (Konarski & Johnson, 1989), movement suppression (Rolider & Van Houten, 1985), forced exercise (Baumeister & MacLean, 1984), and overcorrection (Ollendick, Matson, & Martin, 1978).

In a technical sense, not all stimuli that are generally regarded as unpleasant are *aversive* for everybody. For example, most would agree that being mechanically restrained is an unpleasant experience. However, several authors have demonstrated that restraints may possess reinforcing properties for some individuals (Favell, McGimsey, & Jones, 1978; Favell, McGimsey, Jones, & Cannon, 1981; Foxx, 1990). For instance, Foxx (1990) demonstrated that SIB of a man with mild mental retardation could be reduced by using arm splints as reinforcers in a nonexclusionary time-out paradigm. If the client engaged in SIB while wearing the arm splints, the restraints were temporarily removed. This procedure rapidly suppressed SIB.

Overcorrection is the treatment most frequently found in the SIB and stereotypy literature (Gorman-Smith & Matson, 1985; Matson & Taras, 1989). Foxx and Azrin (1973) presented the use of overcorrection in the treatment of stereotypy in four children. Overcorrection procedures can involve one or both of two treatment components: *positive practice* and *restitution*. Positive practice involves several repetitions of an appropriate or desired behavior that is topographically similar to the target behavior and that is performed in the environment where the SIB or stereotypy was emitted. Carey and Bucher (1986), for example, followed each instance of finger flicking or hand waving by a 2-minute positive practice procedure. This required the clients to pick up marbles and to place them in a hole on a pegboard. Another example of positive practice used by Azrin and Wesolowski (1975) involved a woman with severe mental retardation and self-induced vomiting. The procedure had the person walk to the bathroom and do the action of vomiting into the sink or toilet. This positive practice lasted approximately 20 to 30 minutes. Restitution also has an aspect of repetition and involves rectifying the consequences of the target behavior or correcting the environment. Azrin and Wesolowski (1975) also used a restitution procedure with the woman who self-induced vomiting. Restitution consisted of returning the environment to its previous condition before the maladaptive behavior. In this case, the individual had to mop the floor where she vomited and change her clothes or bedsheets. The cleaning of the floor and changing of clothes or bedsheets was repeated for 15 practice trials.

Although Foxx and Azrin (1973) described overcorrection as an educative procedure, Foxx and Bechtel (1982) later clarified that it was the punitive component of this procedure that made it an effective treatment approach. Overcorrection is an effective yet time-consuming, staff-intensive, and complex procedure to follow (MacKenzie-Keating & McDonald, 1990; Sisson, Van Hasselt, Hersen, & Aurand, 1988). Some of its limitations include a poor transfer of treatment effects across situations (Rojahn and Sisson, 1990); reports of negative collateral effects, such as an increase in nontargeted SIB (see LaGrow & Repp, 1984); and poor maintenance of the treatment effects at follow-up (Matson & Stephens, 1981).

The use of aversive stimuli has demonstrated strong and immediate suppressive effects on SIB and stereotypy. However, these effects are frequently situation-specific and generalize poorly to other settings. The use of punitive procedures has attracted much controversy and debate over the years.

In summary, behavioral techniques are generally very effective in reducing problem behaviors such as stereotypies and SIB, and they are the treatment of choice. Their main disadvantage is the financial cost and human effort in having highly trained and experienced staff to carry out the program on an ongoing basis, including programming for generalization and maintenance. Only if such staff is available are behavioral techniques successful.

Psychopharmacological Intervention

Medication has been used extensively to reduce maladaptive behaviors in people with mental retardation (Aman, 1993; Aman & Singh, 1991). Medication has frequently been used for general suppression of maladaptive behavior, without regard for the precipitating or maintaining factors (Gardner & Sovner, 1994). In a survey of their large service-delivery network, Altemeyer et al. (1987) reported that 39% of their SIB population was receiving psychotropic medications. Among the different types of medications used to suppress SIB and stereotypy reported in the literature, we find neuroleptics (Aman, White, & Field, 1984; Durand, 1982; Singh & Winton, 1984), antimanics (Singh & Winton, 1984), and antidepressants (Bodfish & Madison, 1993; Garber et al., 1992; Sovner et al., 1993). Neuroleptics are by far the most frequently used medication in controlling maladaptive behaviors. Several extensive reviews exist regarding the use of medication in controlling maladaptive behaviors; the interested reader should consult Aman (1993).

Naloxone/Naltrexone

Another type of medication frequently used to reduce SIB and stereotypy are the opioid antagonists naloxone and naltrexone. Naloxone must be given by injection and its half-life is short compared with that of naltrexone, which has the added advantage of being administered orally (see Werry & Aman, 1993). With the shorter half-life and the difficulties posed by having to inject naloxone while an individual may be engaging in high-frequency SIB or stereotypy, naltrexone is the preferred choice of the two.

The action of the opioid antagonists is two-fold. First, they lower the pain threshold increased by the high concentration of endorphin produced by SIB. Second, the opioid antagonists reduce the narcoticlike "high" resulting from the increased concentration of endogenous opiates generated by SIB. This reinforcement-based hypothesis of endogenous opiates seems confirmed by the observation of an extinction burst following the start of treatment of SIB with naltrexone (Benjamin, Seek, Tresise, & Price, 1995; Knabe, Schulz, & Richard, 1990). A recent review of the use of naloxone and naltrexone in the suppression of SIB seems to suggest a high rate of success, 78 and 89%, respectively (Ricketts, Ellis, Singh, & Singh, 1993).

Sandman, Barron, and Coleman (1990) attempted to determine the optimal dosage of naltrexone in suppressing SIB. Sandman and his collaborators, using a double-blind procedure and a Latin square design, gave four clients four fixed doses of 0, 25, 50, or 100 mg once a day, on Monday and Wednesday. The subjects were videotaped during two 10-minute segments each day over the entire week. The authors observed a significant suppression of SIB for all four clients with doses of 25 mg (ranging from 0.36 to 0.63 mg/kg) and 50 mg (ranging from 0.71 to 1.26 mg/kg). Naltrexone further suppressed SIB for three of the four clients when used at a fixed dosage of 100 mg (equivalent to 1.43, 2.11, and 2.27 mg/kg). SIB increased for one of the four clients at the 100 mg dosage. This client was the lightest of the four individuals, where the 100 mg dosage represented 2.53 mg/kg.

Although many studies using naltrexone have shown significant reductions in SIB and stereotypy, 4 of the 23 studies surveyed by Willemsen-Swinkels, Buitelaar, Nijhof, and van Engeland (1995) failed to obtain significant reductions in SIB. In their own study of naltrexone, Willemsen-Swinkels et al. (1995) actually observed a significant increase in the frequency of stereotypy. Others have also reported SIB topographical specificity in the suppressive effects of naltrexone (Thompson, Hackenberg, Cerutti, Baker, & Axtell, 1994). Thompson and his collaborators reported within-client differential effects of naltrexone for some SIB topographies of four clients. One client's self-injurious behavior of hand-to-head hitting and wrist biting was reduced with naltrexone, but the treatment had no effect on the frequency of throat poking. The authors also observed another client for whom naltrexone effectively suppressed hand-to-chin SIB, but did not suppress nose poking and actually worsened face slapping. It would seem plausible to conduct a functional analysis before administering an opiate blocker. This medication ought to be particularly useful if the behavior were maintained by positive internal stimuli (e.g., endorphin release) or negative internal stimuli (opiate blocker attenuates pain or discomfort).

Willemsen-Swinkels et al. (1995) employed a double-blind, placebo-controlled, crossover design to study the suppressive effects of naltrexone on the SIB and autistic behavior of 33 clients, who ranged in age from 18 to 46 and in level of severity of mental retardation from mild to profound. They were recruited based on a diagnosis of autism ($n = 24$) or presence of SIB ($n = 9$). The behavioral impact of naltrexone was assessed using behavioral questionnaires; direct observations were obtained for only 11 of the 33 clients. None of the clients showed a significant decrease in SIB while receiving single daily doses of 50 or 150 mg of naltrexone. This study, along with Campbell et al. (1993) and Zingarelli et al. (1992), is a large-sample naltrexone study with negative results regarding SIB and stereotypy. Clearly, more controlled studies with adequate sample sizes are needed to shed more light on the dose effects found in some reports and the overall efficacy of naltrexone on SIB and stereotypy.

CASE STUDY

Judy was a 31-year-old woman with Down's syndrome who had lived in a large state institution since early childhood. Intellectually, and in terms of her adaptive behavior, she functioned in the profound range of mental retardation. She attended a functional living skills program during the day, three times a week. Judy was visually impaired (blind in her left eye and myopic in her right eye). Scoliosis had seriously impaired her gross motor development and restricted her movement. She was able to move independently by pushing herself around the room on the floor. However, with assistance she was able to walk a few steps. Otherwise, Judy was in good physical health. As for her self-help skills, Judy was able to feed herself with a spoon, but needed much help getting dressed and for her hygiene. Interaction with other people in the day program was rare, although she seemed to enjoy being with certain staff members if they initiated the contact. Judy had no functional language and lacked other means of expressive communication as well. She seemed to understand only simple instructions when given in a context, such as "sit down" or "come eat." Her group home, where she lived with 10 other adults with severe to profound mental retardation, was clean and physically quite appealing, but socially and otherwise understimulating.

During the past year, Judy's SIB consisting of head banging, head butting, and face slapping had dramatically escalated in intensity and frequency. Although she had shown these behaviors for at least 10 years, the behavior had recently begun to cause lacerations from butting the back of her head against the wall and on her forehead from banging her head with her fist. Her cheeks were often reddened and swollen from slapping her face with the palm of her right hand. Her medical treatment for SIB and general agitation consisted of 300 mg of Mellaril per day, which the psychiatrist had increased from 200 mg 8 months earlier.

At that point, the day program treatment team requested a functional behavior analysis for her SIB, and the consulting psychologist began administering several diagnostic and assessment procedures. Beginning with interviews of direct care staff and review of the charts, the psychologist determined that there was no obvious traumatic or otherwise extraordinary event in Judy's life that could have explained the behavior deterioration. To screen for mental health problems, the Diagnostic Assessment for the Severely Handicapped (Matson, Gardner, Coe, & Sovner, 1990) was completed by the psychologist interviewing staff. No mental health problems were detected. The psychologist instructed residential and day program staff to conduct systematic behavior observations throughout Judy's waking hours. Each SIB incident was to be recorded by a detailed behavior description, along with its antecedents and consequences, the time of day it occurred, location, and activity. The data sheet used was similar to the functional observation form recommended by O'Neill et al. (1990). Staff submitted the completed data sheets to the psychologist on a daily basis, who monitored progress by plotting the data. When this information was presented by the psychologist to the interdisciplinary treatment team, it was soon revealed that SIB occurred predominately during times when staff members were particularly busy (e.g., preparing meals, setting or cleaning the tables, aiding residents taking baths), and when Judy was left unattended. The data further showed that only when Judy hit herself did a staff member pay attention to her during those times. Staff attention consisted of holding her arms and rubbing her back to calm her down. Judy usually stopped her SIB as soon as a staff member touched her. Further observations also showed that SIB was more frequent in "downtimes" at the residential unit, as compared with organized day activities or meal times. In other words, the hypothesis that staff attention motivated SIB seemed warranted. Therefore, no further corroborative information by a more involved experimental functional analysis seemed necessary. As a general guideline, staff was instructed to record the frequency of appropriate attention-getting behavior, such as making eye contact, or reaching for somebody's hand.

In accordance with the least restrictive, effective treatment alternative, the psychologist developed a nonaversive treatment package that consisted of a functional communication training component and an extinction procedure. Throughout the day, staff was instructed to provide systematic positive attention to Judy every 15 minutes. When SIB occurred, staff was to delay attention for at least 1 minute to avoid unintended reinforcement of SIB. The psychologist also instructed staff to respond to Judy whenever she was appropriately trying to initiate contact with them (i.e., reinforcing behavior that is functionally equivalent to SIB). During daily 30-minute sessions, the psychologist began communication training with Judy, shaping appropriate behavior to gain staff attention. Functional communication training started by reinforcing two behaviors that were already in Judy's repertoire, namely, making eye contact and reaching out to touch the therapist's hand. When Judy did either one, the therapist said "Yes, Judy, what do you want?" The therapist also attempted to shape rudimentary vocal behavior into a functional response signaling the desire for interaction.

After an initial increase of SIB in the residential unit, which was probably the result of the unaccustomed ignoring of her behavior (extinction burst), SIB quickly decreased in all settings and Judy's appropriate social behavior increased proportionally in frequency. Three weeks after the psychologist started the intervention, the attending psychiatrist reduced the dosage of Mellaril to 150 mg without any negative consequences. Several months later, it so happened that Judy had to transfer to a new day program where the staff was not informed about Judy's communication training. Within 2 days, her SIB started to reemerge. When the new day program staff brought this to the psychologist's attention, she set up staff training, and SIB quickly disappeared in the new environment as well.

SUMMARY

Stereotyped behavior and SIB in individuals with mental retardation refer to a group of conspicuous, idiosyncratic, recurring behaviors that are typically considered problematic. Particularly some forms of SIB can have devastating effects on the individual displaying the behavior, but also for the family and other caretakers. Both types of behavior are highly correlated with the level of cognitive functioning and adaptive behavior. DSM-IV (APA, 1994) classifies stereotypies and SIB in the category of Stereotypic Movement Disorders. Despite this diagnostic practice, we have only little evidence for the validity of classifying all of these different topographies in a single response class. Most stereotypic behaviors and SIB are caused by a combination of biological and environmental factors. It is plausible to assume that certain individuals have a neurobiological disposition for certain types of repetitive behaviors, and that a personal learning history shapes the behavioral manifestation. In most cases, both types of behaviors can be effectively treated and managed by behavioral forms of interventions, particularly if these interventions are carefully designed on the basis of a comprehensive functional behavior analysis. Although behavioral interventions are very effective, they are often very costly. They are time consuming and require highly skilled personnel for program development and implementation. Psychopharmacology so far has not proven to be very effective, particularly for SIB. However, there are promising developments. Recent advances in the design of new medications based on recent findings about neurobiological irregularities in individuals with stereotypy and SIB justify hope for a series of breakthroughs in the near future.

REFERENCES

Adams, G. L., Tallon, R. J., & Stangl, J. M. (1980). Environmental influences on self-stimulatory behavior. *American Journal of Mental Deficiency, 85,* 171–175.

Allen, J. J. (1980). Jogging can modify disruptive behaviors. *Teaching Exceptional Children, 12,* 66–70.

Altemeyer, B. K., Lock, B. J., Griffin, J. C., Ricketts, R. W., Williams, D. E., Mason, M., & Stark, M. T. (1987). Treatment strategies for self-injurious behavior in a large service-delivery network. *American Journal of Mental Deficiency, 91,* 333–340.

Altemeyer, B. K., Williams, D. E., & Sams, V. (1985). Treatment of severe self-injurious and aggressive biting. *Journal of Behavior Therapy and Experimental Psychiatry, 16,* 159–167.

Altman, K., Haavik, S., & Cook, W. J. (1978). Punishment of SIB in natural settings using contingent ammonia. *Behavioral Research and Therapy, 16,* 85–96.

Aman, M. G. (1993). Efficacy of psychotropic drugs for reducing self-injurious behavior in the developmental disabilities. *Annals of Clinical Psychiatry, 5,* 171–188.

Aman, M. G., Hammer, D., & Rojahn, J. (1993). Mental retardation. In T. H. Ollendick & M. Hersen (Eds.), *Handbook of child and adolescent assessment* (pp. 321–345). Boston: Allyn & Bacon.

Aman, M. G., & Singh, N. N. (1991). Pharmacological intervention. In J. L. Matson & J. A. Mulick (Eds.), *Handbook*

of mental retardation (2nd ed., pp. 347–372). Elmsford, NY: Pergamon Press.

Aman, M. G., Singh, N. N., Stewart, A. W., & Field, C. T. (1985). The Aberrant Behavior Checklist: A behavior rating scale for the assessment of treatment effects. *American Journal of Mental Deficiency, 89,* 485–491.

Aman, M. G., Tassé, M. J., Rojahn, J., & Hammer, D. (1996). The Nisonger CBRF: A child behavior rating form for children with developmental disabilities. *Research in Developmental Disabilities, 17,* 41–57.

Aman, M. G., White, A. J., & Field, C. (1984). Chlorpromazine on stereotypic and conditioned behavior of severely retarded patients: A pilot study. *Journal of Mental Deficiency Research, 28,* 253–260.

American Psychiatric Association. (1994). *Diagnostic and statistical manual of mental disorders* (4th ed.). Washington, DC: Author.

Azrin, N. H., & Holz, W. C. (1966). Punishment. In W. K. Honig (Ed.), *Operant behavior: Areas of research and application* (pp. 380–447). New York: Appleton Century Crofts.

Azrin, N. H., & Wesolowski, M. D. (1975). Eliminating habitual vomiting in a retarded adult by positive practice and self-correction. *Journal of Behavior Therapy and Experimental Psychiatry, 6,* 145–148.

Barton, L. E., Brulle, A. R., & Repp, A. C. (1986). Maintenance of therapeutic changes by momentary DRO. *Journal of Applied Behavior Analysis, 19,* 277–282.

Baumeister, A. A., & MacLean, W. E. (1984). Deceleration of SIB and stereotypic responding by exercise. *Applied Research in Mental Retardation, 5,* 385–394.

Baumeister, A. A., & Rollings, J. P. (1976). Self-injurious behavior. In N. R. Ellis (Ed.), *International review of research in mental retardation* (Vol. 9, pp. 55–96). New York: Academic Press.

Benjamin, S., Seek, A., Tresise, L., & Price, E. (1995). Case study: Paradoxical response to naltrexone treatment of self-injurious behavior. *Journal of the American Academy of Child and Adolescent Psychiatry, 34,* 238–242.

Berkson, G. (1967). Abnormal stereotyped motor acts. In J. Zubin & H. F. Hunt (Eds.), *Comparative psychopathology—animal and human* (pp. 76–94). New York: Grune & Stratton.

Berkson, G. (1983). Repetitive stereotyped behaviors. *American Journal of Mental Deficiency, 88,* 239–246.

Berkson, G., & Davenport, R. K. (1962). Stereotyped movements in mental defectives. *American Journal of Mental Deficiency, 66,* 849–852.

Berkson, G., Gutermuth, L., & Baranek, G. (1995). Relative prevalence and relations among stereotyped and similar behaviors. *American Journal on Mental Retardation, 100,* 137–145.

Berkson, G., & Mason, W. A. (1963). Stereotyped movements of mental defectives: III. Situational effects. *American Journal of Mental Deficiency, 68,* 409–412.

Berkson, G., & Mason, W. A. (1964). Stereotyped movements of mental defectives. IV. The effects of toys and the character of the acts. *American Journal of Mental Deficiency, 68,* 511–524.

Berkson, G., McQuiston, S., Jacobson, J. W., Eyman, R., & Borthwick, S. (1985). The relationship between age and stereotyped behavior. *Mental Retardation, 23,* 31–33.

Bird, F., Dores, P. A., Moniz, D., & Robinson, J. (1989). Reducing severe aggressive and self-injurious behavior with functional communication training. *American Journal of Mental Retardation, 94,* 37–48.

Bodfish, J. W., Crawford, T. W., Powell, S. B., Golden, R. N., & Lewis, M. H. (1995). Compulsions in adults with mental retardation: Prevalence, phenomenology, and comorbidity with stereotypy and self-injury. *American Journal on Mental Retardation, 100,* 183–192.

Bodfish, J. W., & Madison, J. T. (1993). Diagnosis and fluoxetine treatment of compulsive behavior disorder of adults with mental retardation. *American Journal on Mental Retardation, 98,* 360–367.

Borthwick, S. A., Meyers, C. E., & Eyman, R. K. (1981). Comparative adaptive and maladaptive behavior of mentally retarded clients of five residential settings in three western states. In R. H. Bruininks, C. E. Meyers, B. B. Sigford, & K. C. Lakin (Eds.), *Deinstitutionalization and community adjustment of mentally retarded people* (AAMD Monograph No. 4, pp. 351–359). Washington, DC: American Association on Mental Deficiency.

Campbell, M. (1985). Timed Stereotyped Behavior Scale. *Psychopharmacology Bulletin, 21,* 1082.

Campbell, M., Anderson, L. T., Small, A. M., Adams, P., Gonzalez, N. M., & Ernst, M. (1993). Naltrexone in autistic children: Behavioral symptoms and attentional learning. *Journal of the American Academy of Childhood and Adolescent Psychiatry, 32,* 1283–1291.

Carey, R. G., & Bucher, B. D. (1986). Positive practice overcorrection: Effects of reinforcing correct performance. *Behavior Modification, 10,* 73–92.

Carr, E. G. (1977). The motivation of self-injurious behavior: A review of some hypotheses. *Psychological Bulletin, 84,* 800–816.

Carr, E. G. (1994). Emerging themes in the functional analysis of problem behavior. *Journal of Applied Behavior Analysis, 27,* 393–399.

Carr, E. G., & Durand, V. M. (1985a). The social-communicative basis of severe behavior problems in children. In S. Reiss & R. Bootzin (Eds.), *Theoretical issues in behavior therapy* (pp. 221–245). New York: Academic Press.

Carr, E. G., & Durand, V. M. (1985b). Reducing behavior problems through functional communication training. *Journal of Applied Behavior Analysis, 18,* 111–126.

Carr, E. G., Levin, L., McConnachie, G., Carlson, J. I., Kemp, D. C., & Smith, C. E. (1994). *Communication-based intervention for problem behavior.* Baltimore: Paul H. Brookes.

Cataldo, M. F. (1991). The effects of punishment and other behavior reducing procedures on the destructive behaviors of persons with developmental disabilities. In National Institutes of Health (Ed.), *Treatment of destructive behaviors in persons with developmental disabilities* (pp. 231–343). (NIH Publication No. 91-2410). Washington, DC: U.S. Government Printing Office.

Christopher, R., & Lewis, B. (1984). The effects of auditory tempo changes on rates of stereotypic behavior in handicapped children. *The Mental Retardation and Disability Bulletin, 12,* 105–114.

Cipani, E. (1990). The communicative function hypothesis: An operant behavior perspective. *Journal of Behavior Therapy and Experimental Psychiatry, 21,* 239–247.

Corte, H. E., Wolf, M. M., & Locke, B. J. (1971). A comparison of procedures for eliminating self-injurious behavior of retarded adolescents. *Journal of Applied Behavior Analysis, 3,* 201–213.

Davenport, R. K., & Berkson, G. (1963). Stereotyped movements of mental defectives: II. Effects of novel objects. *American Journal of Mental Deficiency, 67,* 879–882.

Day, H. M., Horner, R. H., & O'Neill, R. E. (1994). Multiple functions of problem behaviors: Assessment and intervention. *Journal of Applied Behavior Analysis, 27,* 279–289.

DeLissevoy, V. (1963). Head banging in early childhood: A suggested cause. *Journal of Genetic Psychology, 102,* 109–114.

Derby, K. M., Wacker, D. P. Peck, S., Sasso, G., DeRaad, A., Berg, W., Asmus, J., & Ulrich, S. (1994). Functional analysis of separate topographies of aberrant behavior. *Journal of Applied Behavior Analysis, 27,* 267–278.

Derwas, H., & Jones, R. S. (1993). Reducing stereotyped behavior using momentary DRO: An experimental analysis. *Behavioral Residential Treatment, 8,* 45–53.

Donnellan, A. M., Mirenda, P. L., Mesaros, R. A., & Fassbender, L. L. (1984). Analyzing the communicative functions of aberrant behavior. *Journal of the Association for Persons with Severe Handicaps, 9,* 201–212.

Donnelly, D. R., & Olczak, P. V. (1990). The effects of differential reinforcement of incompatible behavior (DRI) on pica for cigarettes in persons with intellectual disability. *Behavior Modification, 14,* 81–96.

Duker, P. C., Jol, K., & Palmen, A. (1991). The collateral decrease of self-injurious behavior and teaching communicative gestures to individuals who are mentally retarded. *Behavioral Residential Treatment, 6,* 183–196.

Duker, P. C., & Seys, D. M. (1983). Long-term follow-up effects of extinction and overcorrection procedures with severely retarded individuals. *British Journal of Mental Subnormality, 29,* 74–80.

Dunlap, G., Dyer, K., & Koegel, R. L. (1983). Autistic self-stimulation and intertrial interval duration. *American Journal of Mental Deficiency, 88,* 194–202.

Dura, J. R., Mulick, J. A., & Rasnake, L. K. (1987). Prevalence of stereotypy among institutionalized non-ambulatory profoundly mentally retarded people. *American Journal of Mental Deficiency, 91,* 548–549.

Durand, V. M. (1982). A behavioral/pharmacological intervention for the treatment of severe self-injurious behavior. *Journal of Autism and Developmental Disorders, 12,* 243–251.

Durand, V. M., & Carr, E. G. (1987). Social influences on "self-stimulatory" behavior: Analysis and treatment application. *Journal of Applied Behavior Analysis, 20,* 119–132.

Durand, V. M., & Carr, E. G. (1991). Functional communication training to reduce challenging behavior: Maintenance and application in new settings. *Journal of Applied Behavior Analysis, 24,* 251–264.

Durand, V. M., & Crimmins, D. B. (1983, October). *The motivation assessment scale: A preliminary instrument which assesses the functional significance of children's deviant behavior.* Paper presented at the meeting of the Berkshire Association of Behavior Analysis and Therapy, Amherst, MA.

Durand, V. M., & Crimmins, D. B. (1988). Identifying the variables maintaining self-injurious behavior. *Journal of Autism and Developmental Disorders, 18,* 99–117.

Edelson, S. M. (1984). Implications of sensory stimulation in self-destructive behavior. *American Journal of Mental Deficiency, 89,* 140–145.

Evans, I. M., & Meyer, L. H. (1985). *An educative approach to behavior problems: A practical decision model for interventions with severely handicapped learners.* Baltimore: Paul H. Brookes.

Eyman, R. K., & Call, T. (1977). Maladaptive behavior and community placement. *American Journal of Mental Deficiency, 82,* 137–144.

Favell, J. E., Azrin, N. H., Baumeister, A. A., Carr, E. G., Dorsey, M. F., Forehand, R., Foxx, R. M., Rincover, A., Risley, T. R., Romanczyk, R. G., Russo, D. C., Schroeder, S. R., & Solnick, J. V. (1982). The treatment of self-injurious behavior. Task force report of the Association for the Advancement of Behavior Therapy. *Behavior Therapy, 13,* 529–554.

Favell, J. E., McGimsey, J. F., & Jones, M. L. (1978). The use of physical restraint in the treatment of self-injury and as positive reinforcement. *Journal of Applied Behavior Analysis, 11,* 225–241.

Favell, J. E., McGimsey, J. F., Jones, M. L., & Cannon, P. R. (1981). Physical restraint as positive reinforcement. *American Journal of Mental Deficiency, 86,* 425–432.

Favell, J. E., McGimsey, J. F., & Schell, R. M. (1982). Treatment of self-injury by providing alternate sensory activities. *Analysis and Intervention in Developmental Disabilities, 2,* 83–104.

Forehand, R., & Baumeister, A. A. (1970). Body rocking and activity level as a function of prior movement restraint. *American Journal of Mental Deficiency, 74,* 608–610.

Foxx, R. M. (1990). «Harry»: A ten year follow-up of the successful treatment of a self-injurious man. *Research in Developmental Disabilities, 11,* 67–76.

Foxx, R. M., & Azrin, N. H. (1973). The elimination of self-stimulatory behavior of autistic and retarded children by overcorrection. *Journal of Applied Behavior Analysis, 6,* 1–14.

Foxx, R. M., & Bechtel, D. R. (1982). Overcorrection. In M. Hersen, R. M. Eisler, & P. M. Miller (Eds.), *Progress in behavior modification* (pp. 227–288). New York: Academic Press.

Foxx, R. M., McMorrow, M. J., Fenlon, S., & Bittle, R. G. (1986). The reductive effects of reinforcement procedures on the genital stimulation and stereotypy of a mentally retarded adolescent male. *Analysis and Intervention in Developmental Disabilities, 6,* 239–248.

Frankel, F, Freeman, B. J., Ritvo, E., & Pardo, R. (1978). The effect of environmental stimulation upon the stereotyped behavior of autistic children. *Journal of Autism and Developmental Disorders, 8,* 389–394.

Fraser, W. I., Leudar, I., Gray, J., & Campbell, I. (1986). Psychiatric and behaviour disturbance in mental handicap. *Journal of Mental Deficiency Research, 30,* 49–57.

Garber, H. J., McGonigle, J. J., Slomka, G. T., & Monteverde, E. (1992). Clomipramine treatment of stereotypic behaviors and self-injury in patients with developmental disabilities. *Journal of the American Academy of Child and Adolescent Psychiatry, 31,* 1157–1160.

Gardner, W. I., & Sovner, R. (1994). *Self-injurious behaviors: Diagnosis and treatment.* Willow Street, PA: VIDA Publishing.

Gary, L. A., Tallon, R. J., & Stangl, J. M. (1980). Environmental influences on self-stimulatory behavior. *American Journal of Mental Deficiency, 85,* 171–175.

Goldberg, D. P., Cooper, B., Eastwood, M. R., Kedward, H. B., & Shephard, M. (1970). A standardized psychiatric interview for use in community surveys. *British Journal of Preventive and Social Medicine, 24,* 18–23.

Goodall, E., & Corbett, J. (1982). Relationships between sensory stimulation and stereotyped behavior in severely mentally retarded and autistic children. *Journal of Mental Deficiency Research, 26,* 163–175.

Gorman-Smith, D., & Matson, J. L. (1985). A review of treatment research for self-injurious and stereotyped responding. *Journal of Mental Deficiency Research, 29,* 295–308.

Greenberg, F., Guzzetta, V., De Oca-Luna, R. M., Magenis, R. E., Smith, A. C. M., Richter, S. F., Kondo, I., Dobyns, W. B., Patel, P. I., & Lupski, J. (1991). Molecular analysis of the Smith-Magenis syndrome: A possible contiguous-gene syndrome associated with del(17)(p 11.2). *American Journal of Human Genetics, 49,* 1207–1218.

Greer, R. D., Becker, B. J., Saxe, C. D., & Mirabella, R. F. (1985). Conditioning histories and setting stimuli controlling engagement in stereotypy or toy play. *Analysis and Intervention in Developmental Disabilities, 5,* 269–284.

Gualtieri, C. T., & Schroeder, S. R. (1989). Pharmacotherapy for self-injurious behavior: Preliminary tests of the D_1 hypothesis. *Psychopharmacology Bulletin, 25,* 364–371.

Guess, D., & Carr, E. (1991). Emergence and maintenance of stereotypy and self-injury. *American Journal on Mental Retardation, 96,* 299–319.

Hagberg, B. (1993). Clinical criteria, stages and natural history. In B. Hagberg (Ed.), *Rett Syndrome—Clinical and biological aspects* (pp. 4–20). London: Mac Keith Press.

Hamad, C. D., Isley, E., & Lowry, M. (1983). The use of mechanical restraint and response incompatibility to modify self-injurious behavior: A case study. *Mental Retardation, 21,* 213–217.

Hung, D. W. (1978). Using self-stimulation as reinforcement for autistic children. *Journal of Autism and Childhood Schizophrenia, 8,* 355–366.

Iwata, B. A., Dorsey, M. F., Slifer, K. J., Bauman, K. E., & Richman, G. S. (1982). Toward a functional analysis of self-injury. *Analysis and Intervention in Developmental Disabilities, 2,* 3–20.

Iwata, B. A., Pace, P. M., Dorsey, M. F., Zarcone, J. R., Vollmer, T. R., Smith, R. G., Rodgers, T. A., Lerman, D. C., Shore, B. A., Mazaleski, J. L., Goh, H. L., Cowdery, G. E., Kalsher, M. J., McCosh, K. C., & Willis, K. (1994). The functions of self-injurious behavior: An experimental–epidemiological analysis. *Journal of Applied Behavior Analysis, 27,* 215–240.

Iwata, B. A., Pace, G. M., Kissel, R. C., Nau, P. A., & Farber, J. M. (1990). The Self-Injury Trauma (SIT) Scale: A method for quantifying surface tissue damage caused by self-injurious behavior. *Journal of Applied Behavior Analysis, 23,* 99–110.

Iwata, B. A., Vollmer, T. R., & Zarcone, J. R. (1990). The experimental (functional) analysis of behavior disorders: Methodology, applications, and limitations. In A. C. Repp & N. N. Singh (Eds.), *Perspectives in the use of nonaversive and aversive interventions for persons with developmental disabilities* (pp. 301–330). Sycamore, IL: Sycamore Press.

Jacobson, J. W. (1982). Problem behavior and psychiatric impairment within a developmentally disabled population I: Behavior frequency. *Applied Research in Mental Retardation, 3,* 121–139.

Johnson, H. G., Ekman, P., Friesen, W., Nyhan, W. L., & Shear, C. (1976). A behavioral phenotype in the de Lange syndrome. *Pediatric Research, 10,* 843–850.

Kaufman, M. E., & Levitt, H. A. (1965). A study of three stereotyped behaviors in institutionalized mentally defectives. *American Journal of Mental Deficiency, 69,* 467–473.

Kennedy, C. H., & Souza, G. (1995). Functional analysis and treatment of eye poking. *Journal of Applied Behavior Analysis, 28,* 27–37.

Kern, L., Koegel, R. L., & Dunlap, G. (1984). The influence of vigorous versus mild exercise on autistic stereotyped behaviors. *Journal of Autism and Developmental Disorders, 14,* 57–67.

Kern, L., Koegel, R. L., Dyer, K., Blew, P. A., & Fenton, L. R. (1982). The effect of physical exercise on self-stimulation and appropriate responding in autistic children. *Journal of Autism and Developmental Disabilities, 12,* 399–419.

King, B. H. (1993). Self-injury in people with mental retardation: A compulsive behavior hypothesis. *American Journal on Mental Retardation, 98,* 93–112.

Knabe, R., Schulz, P., & Richard, J. (1990). Initial aggravation of self-injurious behavior in autistic patients receiving naltrexone treatment. *Journal of Autism and Developmental Disorders, 20,* 591–593.

Konarski, E. A., & Johnson, M. R. (1989). The use of brief restraint plus reinforcement to treat self-injurious behavior. *Behavioral Residential Treatment, 4,* 45–52.

Kraemer, G. W., Ebert, M. H., Schmidt, D. E., & McKinney, W. T. (1991). Strangers in a strange land: A psychobiological study of infant monkeys before and after separation from real or inanimate mothers. *Child Development, 62,* 548–566.

LaGrow, S. J., & Repp, A. C. (1984). Stereotypic responding: A review of intervention research. *American Journal of Mental Deficiency, 88,* 595–609.

Lennox, D. B., Miltenberger, R. G., Spengler, P., & Erfanian, N. (1988). Decelerative treatment practices with persons who have mental retardation: A review of five years of the literature. *American Journal on Mental Retardation, 92,* 492–501.

Lewis, M. H., & Baumeister, A. A. (1982). Stereotyped mannerisms in mentally retarded persons: Animal models and theoretical analyses. In N. R. Ellis (Ed.), *International review of research in mental retardation* (Vol. 11, pp. 123–161). New York: Academic Press.

Lewis, M. H., MacLean, W. E., Bryson-Brockman, W., Arendt, R., Beck, B., Fidler, P. S., & Baumeister, A. A. (1984). Time-series analysis of stereotyped movements: Relationship of body-rocking to cardiac activity. *American Journal of Mental Deficiency, 89,* 287–294.

Lewis, M. H., MacLean, W. E., Johnson, W. L., & Baumeister, A. A. (1981). Ultradian rhythms in stereotyped and self-injurious behavior. *American Journal of Mental Deficiency, 85,* 601–610.

Lewis, M. H., Silva, J. R., & Silva, S. G. (1995). Cyclicity of aggression and self-injurious behavior. *American Journal on Mental Retardation, 99,* 436–444.

Linn, D. M., Rojahn, J., Helsel, W. J., & Dixon, J. (1988). Acute effects of transcutaneous electric nerve stimulation on self-injurious behavior. *Journal of the Multihandicapped Person, 1,* 105–127.

Linscheid, T. R., Iwata, B. A., Ricketts, R. W., Williams, D. E., & Griffin, J. C. (1990). Clinical evaluation of the Self-Injurious Behavior Inhibiting System (SIBIS). *Journal of Applied Behavior Analysis, 23,* 53–78.

Lourie, R. (1949). The role of rhythmic patterns in childhood. *American Journal of Psychiatry, 105,* 653–660.

Lovaas, O. I. (1982). Comments on self-destructive behaviors. *Analysis and Intervention in Developmental Disabilities, 2,* 115–124.

Lovaas, O. I., Newsom, C., & Hickman, C. (1987). Self-stimulatory behavior and perceptual reinforcement. *Journal of Applied Behavior Analysis, 20,* 45–68.

Lovaas, O. I., & Simmons, J. Q. (1969). Manipulation of self-destruction in three retarded children. *Journal of Applied Behavior Analysis, 2,* 143–157.

Luckasson, R., Schalock, R. L., Coulter, D. L., Snell, M. E., Polloway, E. A., Spitalnik, D. M., Reiss, S., & Stark, J. A. (1992). *Mental retardation: Definition, classification, and systems of support* (9th ed.). Washington, DC: American Association on Mental Retardation.

Luiselli, J. K. (1986). Modification of self-injurious behavior: An analysis of the use of contingently applied protective equipment. *Behavior Modification, 10,* 191–204.

Luiselli, J. K. (1991). Functional assessment and treatment of self-injury in a pediatric, nursing-care resident. *Behavioral Residential Treatment, 6,* 311–319.

MacKenzie-Keating, S. E., & McDonald, L. (1990). Overcorrection: Reviewed, revisited and revised. *The Behavior Analyst, 13,* 39–48.

Malcuit, G., Pomerleau, A., & Maurice, P. (1995). *Psychologie de l'apprentissage: termes et concepts.* Paris: Edisem.

Matson, J. L. (1989). Self-injury and stereotypies. In T. H. Ollendick & M. Hersen (Eds.), *Handbook of child psychopathology* (2nd ed., pp. 265–275). New York: Plenum Press.

Matson, J. L., & DiLorenzo, T. M. (1984). *Punishment and its alternatives.* Berlin: Springer.

Matson, J. L., Gardner, W. I., Coe, D. A., & Sovner, R. (1990). *Diagnostic Assessment for the Severely Handicapped (DASH) scale (User manual).* Unpublished manuscript, Louisiana State University, Baton Rouge.

Matson, J. L., & Stephens, R. M. (1981). Overcorrection treatment of stereotyped behaviors. *Behavior Modification, 5,* 491–502.

Matson, J. L., & Taras, M. E. (1989). A 20 year review of punishment and alternative methods to treat problem behaviors in developmentally delayed persons. *Research in Developmental Disabilities, 10,* 84–104.

Maurice, P., & Trudel, G. (1982). Self-injurious behavior prevalence and relationships to environmental events. In J. H. Hollis & C. E. Meyer (Eds.), *Life-threatening behavior: Analysis and intervention* (Monograph No. 5, pp. 81–103). Washington, DC: American Association on Mental Retardation.

Mazaleski, J. L., Iwata, B. A., Vollmer, T. R., Zarcone, J. R., & Smith, R. G. (1993). Analysis of the reinforcement and extinction components in DRO contingencies with self-injury. *Journal of Applied Behavior Analysis, 26,* 143–156.

Morin, D. (1987). *Méta-analyse des facteurs contribuant au maintien à court et à long terme de la suppression des compotements d'automutilation* [Meta-analysis of the factors contributing to the short and long term maintenance of SIB suppression]. Unpublished master's thesis. Université du Quebéc à Montréal, Montreal.

Moseley, A., Faust, M., & Reardon, D. M. (1970). Effects of social and nonsocial stimuli on the stereotyped behav-

iors of retarded children. *American Journal of Mental Deficiency, 74,* 809–811.

Mulick, J. A., Hoyt, P., Rojahn, J., & Schroeder, S. R. (1978). Reduction of a "nervous" habit in a profoundly retarded youth by increasing toy play. *Journal of Behavior Therapy and Experimental Psychiatry, 9,* 381–385.

Murphy, G. H., Oliver, C., Corbett, C., Crayton, L., Hales, J., Head, D., & Hall, S. (1993). Epidemiology of self-injury, characteristics of people with severe self-injury and initial treatment outcome. In C. Kiernan (Ed.), *From Research to practice? Implications of research on the challenging behavior of people with learning disability* (pp. 1–35). Cleredon, Avon, UK: Bild Publications.

Newton, J. T., & Sturmey, P. (1991). The Motivation Assessment Scale: Interrater reliability and internal consistency in a British sample. *Journal of Mental Deficiency Research, 35,* 472–474.

Norton, R. S. (1986). Side effects of sensory extinction and an alternative procedure for high rates of self-injury [Letter to the editor]. *The Behavior Therapist, 8,* 86–87.

Nyhan, W. L. (1994). The Lesch-Nyhan disease. In T. Thompson & D. B. Gray (Eds.), *Destructive behavior in developmental disabilities: Diagnosis, measurement, and evaluating treatment outcome* (pp. 181–197). Beverly Hills: Sage.

O'Brien, S., & Repp, A. C. (1990). Reinforcement-based reductive procedures: A review of 20 years of their use with persons with severe or profound retardation. *Journal of the Association for Persons with Severe Handicaps, 15,* 148–159.

Oliver, C., Murphy, G. H., & Corbett, J. A. (1987). Self-injurious behavior in people with mental handicap: A total population study. *Journal of Mental Deficiency Research, 31,* 147–162.

Ollendick, T. H., Matson, J. L., & Martin, J. E. (1978). Effectiveness of hand overcorrection for topographically similar and dissimilar self-stimulatory behavior. *Journal of Experimental Child Psychology, 25,* 296–303.

O'Neill, R. E., Horner, R. H., Albin, R. W., Storey, K., & Sprague, J. R. (1990). *Functional analysis of problem behavior: A practical assessment guide.* Sycamore, IL: Sycamore Press.

Pohl, P. (1977). Tempo changes during body rocking. *Developmental Medicine and Child Neurology, 19,* 485–488.

Reid, A. H., Ballinger, B. R., & Heather, B. B. (1978). Behavioural syndromes identified by cluster analysis in a sample of 100 severely and profoundly retarded adults. *Psychological Medicine, 8,* 399–412.

Reiss, S. (1994). *Handbook of challenging behavior: Mental health aspects of mental retardation.* Worthington, OH: IDS Publishing Corporation.

Repp, A. C., Barton, L. E., & Brulle, A. R. (1983). A comparison of two procedures for programming the differential reinforcement of other behaviors. *Journal of Applied Behavior Analysis, 16,* 435–445.

Repp, A. C., Felce, D., & Barton, L. E. (1988). Basing the treatment of stereotypic and self-injurious behaviors on hypotheses of their causes. *Journal of Applied Behavior Analysis, 21,* 281–289.

Repp, A. C., & Singh, N. N. (Eds.). (1990). *Perspectives on the use of nonaversive and aversive interventions for persons with developmental disabilities.* Sycamore, IL: Sycamore Press.

Ricketts, R. W., Ellis, C. R., Singh, Y. N., & Singh, N. N. (1993). Opioid antagonists: II. Clinical effects in the treatment of self-injury in individuals with developmental disabilities. *Journal of Developmental and Physical Disabilities, 5,* 17–28.

Rincover, A. (1978). Sensory extinction: A procedure for eliminating self-stimulatory behavior in developmentally disabled children. *Journal of Abnormal Child Psychology, 6,* 299–310.

Rincover, A., Cook, R., Peoples, A., & Packard, D. (1979). Sensory extinction and sensory reinforcement principles for programming multiple adaptive behavior change. *Journal of Applied Behavior Analysis, 12,* 221–233.

Rincover, A., & Devany, J. (1982). Using sensory reinforcement and sensory extinction principles in the treatment of self-injury. *Analysis and Intervention of Developmental Disorders, 2,* 67–81.

Roberts, M. L., Mace, F. C., & Daggett, J. A. (1995). Preliminary comparison of two negative reinforcement schedules to reduce self-injury. *Applied Behavior Analysis, 28,* 579–580.

Rogers-Warren, A., & Warren, S. F. (Eds.). (1977). *Ecological perspectives in behavior analysis.* Baltimore: University Park Press.

Rojahn, J. (1986). Self-injurious behavior and stereotypic behavior in non-institutionalized mentally retarded people. *American Journal of Mental Deficiency, 91,* 268–276.

Rojahn, J. (1994). Epidemiology and topographic taxonomy of self-injurious behavior. In T. Thompson & D. B. Gray (Eds.), *Destructive behavior in developmental disabilities: Diagnosis and treatment* (pp. 49–67). Beverly Hills: Sage.

Rojahn, J., Borthwick-Duffy, S. A., & Jacobson, J. W. (1993). The association between psychiatric diagnoses and severe behavior problems in mental retardation. *Annals of Clinical Psychiatry, 5,* 163–170.

Rojahn, J., & Marshburn, E. (1992). Facial screening and visual occlusion. In J. K. Luiselli, J. L. Matson, & N. N. Singh (Eds.), *Self-injurious behavior: Analysis, assessment, and treatment* (pp. 200–234). Berlin: Springer.

Rojahn, J., McGonigle, J. J., Curcio, C., & Dixon, M. J. (1987). Suppression of pica by water mist and aromatic ammonia. *Behavior Modification, 11,* 65–74.

Rojahn, J. R., Polster, L. M., Mulick, J. A., & Wisniewski, J. J. (1989). Reliability of the Behavior Problem Inventory. *Journal of the Multihandicapped Person, 2,* 271–293.

Rojahn, J., & Schroeder, S. R. (1979). *Ecobehavioral assessment.* Unpublished manual available from the first author of this chapter.

Rojahn, J., & Schroeder, S. R. (1991). Behavioral assess-

ment. In J. L. Matson & J. A. Mulick (Eds.), *Handbook of mental retardation* (2nd ed., pp. 240–259). Elmsford, NY: Pergamon Press.

Rojahn, J., & Sisson, L. A. (1990). Stereotyped behavior. In J. L. Matson (Ed.), *Handbook of behavior modification with the mentally retarded* (2nd ed., pp. 181–223). New York: Plenum Press.

Rojahn, J., Tassé, M. J., & Sturmey, P. (1997). The Stereotyped Behavior Scale: Topographic classification of stereotyped behavior in mental retardation. *American Journal on Mental Retardation, 102,* 137–146.

Rolider, A., & Van Houten, R. (1985). Movement suppression time-out for undesirable behavior in psychotic and severely developmentally delayed children. *Journal of Applied Behavior Analysis, 18,* 275–288.

Romanczyk, R. G. (1977). Intermittent punishment of self-stimulation: Effectiveness during application and extinction. *Journal of Consulting and Clinical Psychology, 45,* 53–60.

Rose, V., Sloop, W., & Baker, P. (1980). Elimination of chronic self-injurious behavior by withdrawal of staff attention. *Psychological Reports, 46,* 327–330.

Runco, M. A., Charlop, M. J., & Schreibman, L. (1986). The occurrence of autistic children's self-stimulation as a function of familiar versus unfamiliar stimulus conditions. *Journal of Autism and Developmental Disorders, 16,* 31–44.

Rutter, M., Tizard, J., Yule, W., Graham, P., & Whitmore, K. (1976). Isle of Wight studies, 1964–1974. *Psychological Medicine, 6,* 313–332.

Sajwaj, T., Libet, J., & Agras, S. (1974). The control of life-threatening rumination in a six month old infant. *Journal of Applied Behavior Analysis, 7,* 557–563.

Sandman, C. A., Barron, J. L., & Coleman, H. (1990). An orally administered opiate blocker, naltrexone, attenuates self-injurious behavior. *American Journal on Mental Retardation, 95,* 93–102.

Schroeder, S. R., Hammock, R. G., Mulick, J. A., Rojahn, J., Walson, P., Fernald, W., Meinhold, P., & Sarphare, G. (1995). Clinical trials of D_1 and D_2 dopamine modulating drugs and self-injury. *Mental Retardation and Developmental Disabilities Research Reviews, 1,* 120–129.

Schroeder, S. R., Mulick, J. A., & Rojahn, J. (1980). The definition, taxonomy, epidemiology, and ecology of self-injurious behavior. *Journal of Autism and Developmental Disorders, 10,* 417–432.

Schroeder, S. R., Rojahn, J., & Mulick, J. A. (1978). Ecobehavioral organization of developmental day care for the chronically self-injurious. *Journal of Pediatric Psychology, 3,* 81–88.

Schroeder, S. R., Rojahn, J., & Reese, R. M. (1997). Reliability of instruments for assessing psychotropic medication effects on self-injurious behavior in mental retardation. *Journal of Autism and Developmental Disorders, 27,* 89–102.

Singh, N. N., & Winton, A. S. W. (1984). Behavioral monitoring of pharmacological intervention for self-injury. *Applied Research in Mental Retardation, 5,* 161–170.

Sisson, L. A., Hersen, M., & Van Hasselt, V. B. (1993). Improving the performance of youth with dual sensory impairment: Analyses and social validation of procedures to reduce maladaptive responding in vocational and leisure settings. *Behavior Therapy, 24,* 553–571.

Sisson, L. A., Van Hasselt, V. B., Hersen, M., & Aurand, J. C. (1988). Tripartite behavioral intervention to reduce stereotypic and disruptive behaviors in young multihandicapped children. *Behavior Therapy, 19,* 503–526.

Smith, R. G., Iwata, B. A., Vollmer, T. R., & Zarcone, J. R. (1993). Experimental analysis and treatment of multiply controlled self-injury. *Journal of Applied Behavior Analysis, 26,* 183–196.

Soraci, S., Deckner, C. W., McDaniel, C., & Blanton, R. L. (1982). The relationship between rate of rhythmicity and the stereotypic behaviors of abnormal children. *Journal of Music Therapy, 19,* 46–54.

Sovner, R., Foxx, C. J., Lowry, M. J., & Lowry, M. A. (1993). Fluoxetine treatment of depression and associated self-injury in two adults with mental retardation. *Journal of Intellectual Disability Research, 37,* 301–311.

Sparrow, S. S., Balla, D. A., & Cicchetti, D. V. (1984). *Interview edition. Expanded form manual. Vineland Adaptive Behavior Scales.* Circle Pines, MN: American Guidance Service.

Steege, M. W., Wacker, D. P., Berg, W. K., Cigrand, K. K., & Cooper, A. F. (1989). The use of behavioral assessment to prescribe and evaluate treatments for severely handicapped children. *Journal of Applied Behavior Analysis, 22,* 23–33.

Stevens, E. A. (1971). Some effects of tempo changes on stereotyped rocking movements of low-level mentally retarded subjects. *American Journal of Mental Deficiency, 76,* 76–81.

Strohmer, D. C., & Prout, H. T. (1989). *Strohmer-Prout Behavior Rating Scale manual.* Schenectady, NY: Genium Publishing Co.

Tarpley, H., & Schroeder, S. R. (1979). A comparison of DRO and DRI procedures in the treatment of self-injurious behavior. *American Journal of Mental Deficiency, 84,* 188–194.

Tassé, M. J., Aman, M. G., Hammer, D., & Rojahn, J. (1996). The Nisonger CBRF: Age and gender differences and norms. *Research in Developmental Disabilities, 17,* 59–75.

Tassé, M. J., Aman, M. G., Rojahn, J., & Kern, R. A. (in press). Developmental disabilities. In R. T. Ammerman & J. V. Campo (Eds.), *Handbook of pediatric psychology and psychiatry.* Boston: Allyn & Bacon.

Tate, B., & Barroff, G. (1966). Aversive control of self-injurious behavior in a psychotic boy. *Behavior Research and Therapy, 4,* 281–287.

Thelen, E. (1981). Rhythmical behavior in infancy: An ethological perspective. *Developmental Psychology, 17,* 237–257.

Thompson, T. J., & Berkson, G. (1985). Stereotyped behavior of severely disabled children in classroom and free-play settings. *American Journal of Mental Deficiency, 89,* 580–586.

Thompson, T., Hackenberg, T., Cerutti, D., Baker, D., & Axtell, S. (1994). Opioid antagonist effects on self-injury in adults with mental retardation: Response form and location as determinants of medication effects. *American Journal on Mental Retardation, 99,* 85–102.

Tierney, I. R., McGuire, R. J., & Walton, H. J. (1978). The effect of music on body-rocking manifested by severely mentally deficient patients in ward environments. *Journal of Mental Deficiency Research, 22,* 255–261.

Wacker, D. P., Steege, M. W., Northup, J., Sasso, G., Berg, W., Reimers, T., Cooper, L., Cigrand, K., & Donn, L. (1990). A component analysis of functional communication training across three topographies of severe behavior problems. *Journal of Applied Behavior Analysis, 23,* 417–429.

Watson, J., Singh, N. N., & Winton, A. S. W. (1986). Suppressive effects of visual and facial screening on self-injurious finger sucking. *American Journal of Mental Deficiency, 90,* 526–534.

Watters, R. W., & Watters, W. E. (1980). Decreasing self-stimulatory behavior with physical exercise in a group of autistic boys. *Journal of Autism and Developmental Disorders, 10,* 378–387.

Wehmeyer, M. L. (1995). Intra-individual factors influencing efficacy of interventions for stereotyped behaviours: A meta analysis. *Journal of Intellectual Disability Research, 39,* 205–214.

Werry, J. S., & Aman, M. G. (1993). Anxiolytics, sedatives, and miscellaneous drugs. In J. S. Werry & M. G. Aman (Eds.), *Practitioner's guide to psychoactive drugs for children and adolescents.* New York: Plenum Medical Book Company.

Wieseler, N. A., Hanson, R. H., Chamberlain, T. P., & Thompson, T. (1985). Functional taxonomy of stereotypic and self-injurious behavior. *Mental Retardation, 5,* 230–234.

Willemsen-Swinkels, S. H. N., Buitelaar, J. K., Nijhof, G. J., & van Engeland, H. (1995). Failure of naltrexone hydrochloride to reduce self-injurious and autistic behavior in mentally retarded adults. *Archives of General Psychiatry, 52,* 766–773.

Winnega, M., & Berkson, G. (1986). Analyzing the stimulus properties of objects used in stereotyped behavior. *American Journal of Mental Deficiency, 91,* 277–285.

Wolery, M., Kirk, K., & Gast, D. L. (1985). Stereotypic behavior as a reinforcer: Effects and side effects. *Journal of Autism and Developmental Disorders, 15,* 149–161.

Zarcone, J. R., Rodgers, T. A., Iwata, B. A., Rourke, D. A., & Dorsey, M. F. (1991). Reliability analysis of the Motivational Assessment Scale: A failure to replicate. *Research in Developmental Disabilities, 12,* 349–360.

Zingarelli, G., Ellman, G., Hom, A., Wymore, M., Heldorn, S., & Chicz-DeMet, A. (1992). Clinical effects of naltrexone on autistic behavior. *American Journal on Mental Retardation, 97,* 57–63.

13

Tics and Tourette's Disorder

FLOYD R. SALLEE AND EVE G. SPRATT

INTRODUCTION

Tics are the most common movement disorder of childhood. Although tics as such are common in the child population, it remains the task of the clinician to determine when tics are likely to be self-limited, as in transient tic disorder, or part of a more progressive and debilitating syndrome. The tic spectrum of disorders including Gilles de la Tourette syndrome (TS) and chronic motor tic disorder have been described in the pediatric, psychiatric, and neurological literature. TS represents a diversity of clinical presentations, with a wide range of associated symptoms of varying severity, as well as comorbid psychiatric conditions. New themes in the TS literature include the impact of comorbidity on prognosis and treatment as well as an increasing focus on the genetic aspects and heritability of the disorder.

The latest revision of the *Diagnostic and Statistical Manual of Mental Disorders* (DSM-IV; APA, 1994) contains new impairment criteria that will have considerable impact on the frequency of diagnosis within the tic spectrum. Tic phenomenon may often cause less impairment to the individual than a comorbid condition. Under DSM-IV, the absence of impairment caused by tics would exclude the diagnosis of a tic disorder because the individual would not meet full symptom criteria. In this chapter, an update of trends in assessment and treatment strategies will be highlighted.

PHENOMENOLOGY

Tic Phenomenology

The presence of tics is a key feature throughout the tic spectrum of which TS is the severest form. The distinction between "transient" and "chronic" tic is dependent on a history for less than versus more than 12 months. Frequently the signs and symptoms of tic disorder range from infrequent movements and sounds that are barely detectable or easily camouflaged to dramatic and disabling tic symptoms. Patients frequently consciously try to suppress their tic symptoms and can do so for a period of a few minutes to a few hours. Temporary suppress-

FLOYD R. SALLEE AND EVE G. SPRATT • Department of Psychiatry and Behavioral Science, Medical University of South Carolina, Charleston, South Carolina 29425-0742.

Handbook of Child Psychopathology, 3rd edition, edited by Ollendick & Hersen. Plenum Press, New York, 1998.

ibility distinguishes tic disorder from other hyperkinetic movement disorders. This contributes to making the assessment of tic symptoms in these patients a challenge (Kurlan, 1988).

Tics are sudden, repetitive, stereotyped movements, or vocal sounds that are brief and rapid and may involve multiple muscle groups. Tics occur at random intervals. Although tics can be voluntarily suppressed for periods of time, some patients describe premonitory sensory urges for which tics are voluntarily performed to relieve the urge. Tics in general tend to be exacerbated by several factors, including stress, fatigue, or underlying medical illness. Tics can also be triggered by environmental stimuli and over varying periods of time wax and wane in severity and change anatomical location.

Tics are categorized as "simple," and limited to individual muscle groups, or single nonsensical utterances, or "complex," such as coordinated patterns of movement (often looking purposeful), or word phrases and full sentences. Sudden onset of facial tics (eye blink, grimace, eye tic) is common at first presentation, with rostral–caudal progression over time. Many complex tics (e.g., touching, tapping, repetitive phrasing) can be difficult to differentiate from compulsions.

Clinical characteristics of Tourette's disorder described in patients from around the world have shown concurrence in age of onset, gender ratio, and tic symptom spectrum. Typical age of onset is 7 years, although onset of TS before 1 year of age has been reported (Burd & Kerbeshian, 1987). Eye tics are the most common first symptom (eye rolling, eye blinking, or wide eye opening) in 20 to 53% of patients (Bruun, 1988a,b; Nomura & Segawa, 1982), often prompting a referral to an ophthalmologist. Facial (grimacing, nose twitching, or licking movements) and vocal tics (sniffing, throat clearing, grunting, or coughing) are the next most common. Vocal tics often lead to investigations for allergy, upper respiratory infections, sinusitis, or other ENT abnormalities. Whole body tics such as body rocking, pelvic thrusting, shutters, or diaphragmatic tics may be encoun-

tered in a significant number of patients (Lees, Robertson, Trimble, & Murray, 1984). Coprolalia is the most dramatic of the vocal tics. It is the spontaneous interruption of speech flow with various obscenities with no obvious provoking cause. Coprolalia (2–4% incidence) is not necessary for the diagnosis of Tourette's disorder, nor is it pathognomonic, as it can be present in other neurological disorders. Other unusual symptoms of copropraxia, echolalia, or echopraxia are present in most patient series with varying frequency. Self-abusive tics such as hitting oneself or lip biting (significant enough to inflict damage) are present in 5 to 13% of patients (Bruun, 1988a,b; Comings & Comings, 1985). Complicated movements or unusual repetitive behaviors, such as touching or tapping of objects, can take on a compulsive quality as patients often report an internal drive to perform these behaviors.

Although natural history data are limited, Shapiro, Shapiro, Young, and Feinberg (1988a) reported that complete remissions in children are expected in 24–61% of patients, with improvement in the remainder and only a fraction showing no change or worsening of tics (3–24%). Symptoms tend to progress in TS as the patient enters adolescence, with amelioration of symptoms in late adolescence or adult life (Erenberg, Cruse, Rothner, & Rothner, 1987). The waxing and waning quality of symptoms tends to decrease with age and remission in adults is infrequent.

Associated Psychiatric Symptomatology

Psychiatric and learning disorders have been seen in association with Tourette's disorder, attention-deficit/hyperactivity disorder (ADHD), and obsessive-compulsive disorder (OCD) are most frequently encountered. Comings and Comings (1984, 1985) reported that in 250 cases of TS, ADHD is present in 54%. In the more severely disordered TS patients, the incidence of concurrent ADHD increases to 70–80%. Even in very mild cases of Tourette's disorder, the incidence of ADHD is seven- to eightfold greater than that in the general population. TS and ADHD may be etiologically related in some persons. However, a study by Pauls, Leckman, and Cohen (1993) of 338 first-degree relatives of 85 TS probands and 113 controls revealed that ADHD, learning problems, stuttering, and speech problems by themselves are not variant forms of TS. Learning disabilities have been suggested in a large proportion of patients, but it is undetermined whether these exist in the absence of ADHD. Hagin and Kugler (1988) reported that a series of Tourette-disordered patients have lower-than-expected school achievement in mathematics and reading comprehension.

Frankel et al. (1986) found an incidence of OCD in adult Tourette-disordered patients of 51%, using an inventory derived from the Leyton Obsessional Inventory (LOI) (Cooper, 1970). An epidemiological study of 431 patients diagnosed with Tourette's disorder commissioned by the Ohio Tourette's Syndrome Association found a point prevalence of 74% for OCD at some time during the illness (Stefl, 1983). Grad, Pelcovitz, Olson, Matthews, and Grad (1987) found that 7 of 25 patients with an average age of 11.1 years met criteria for OCD based on the child version of the LOI (Berg, Rapoport, & Flament, 1986). Stefl (1983) found a high incidence of aggression, hostility, and depression in a sample of Tourette's patients in addition to obsessive-compulsive behavior.

The phenomenology of OCD within the context of TS may be different than when OCD occurs alone. George, Trimble, Ring, Sallee, and Robertson (1993) found that subjects with comorbid TS and OCD had significantly more violent, sexual, and symmetrical obsessions and more touching, blinking, counting, and self-injurious compulsions. The group with OCD alone had more obsessions concerning dirt or germs or cleaning compulsions. However, in a study of 10 subjects with OCD and 15 subjects with OCD and comorbid TS, the latter subjects reported their compulsions arose spontaneously whereas the former subjects reported their compulsions were frequently preceded by

cognitions. Scales used included the Yale-Brown Obsessive Compulsive Scale (YBOCS; Goodman, Price, Rasmussen, Riddle, & Rapoport, 1991), the LOI, and a new questionnaire designed to emphasize the differences in symptoms between the two groups.

Social discomfort, shame, self-consciousness, irritability, and depressed mood frequently occur as secondary phenomena of TS. In severe cases of TS the tics may directly interfere with daily activities. Social, academic, and occupational functioning may be impaired because of rejection by others or anxiety about having tics in social situations (DSM-IV). Rare complications of TS include physical injury such as blindness resulting from retinal detachment associated with head banging or striking oneself, orthopedic problems from knee bending, neck jerking, or head turning, and skin problems from picking.

DIAGNOSIS

An accurate documented diagnosis of TS is often made 5–12 years after onset of symptoms (Golden & Hood, 1982). Tics are readily identifiable and rarely confused with other conditions, which suggests that clinicians may not readily recognize TS but attribute tic symptoms to psychological, ophthalmological, or ENT-related causes, or to incorrectly await the appearance of coprolalia for a diagnosis. There are several factors that contribute to failure of clinicians to diagnose TS. These include: (1) the assumption that coprolalia is necessary, (2) the belief that motor and vocal tics must be present simultaneously, and (3) misunderstanding that patients can suppress tics, suggesting that their tics must be volitional.

Key for DSM-IV criteria is the concept of "transient" and "chronic," now operationalized around symptoms being present for less than or greater than 1 year, respectively. To meet the criteria for the transient tic disorder, the symptoms must be present for at least 4 weeks but not longer than a year. A "Tic Disorder Not Otherwise Specified" category is included for tic disorders of atypical onset or duration, or with longer tic-free intervals than 3 months. New in DSM-IV are impairment criteria attributed to tics that significantly impact social, occupational, or other important functioning.

Transient tic disorder is a disorder of childhood in which stress is said to play a predominant role in the etiology. In some children, transient tics may recur over several years, but tics tend to be mild and not to persist for longer than a few weeks or months. Chronic motor or vocal tic disorder is stable in its symptomatology with tics that persist in the same anatomic location or with the same phenomenology. Patients display either vocal or motor tics, but not both, and limited motor tics are by far more common. Family studies suggest that this disorder is two to three times more prevalent than TS (Comings, Comings, Devor, & Cloninger, 1984). Family genetic studies support an etiological relationship between chronic motor tic disorder and TS (Pauls, Kruger, Leckman, Cohen, & Kidd, 1984; Pauls & Leckman, 1986).

A diagnosis of Tourette's disorder is clearly delineated in the DSM IV diagnostic criteria (Table 1), but assessment of the durational criteria is sometimes difficult. Both multiple motor and one or more vocal tics must be present for some time during the illness, although not necessarily concurrently. The anatomic location, number, frequency, and complexity of tics are noted to change over time, but the onset must be before age 18. Furthermore, the occurrence of tics should not be attributable to psychoactive substance intoxication or as a result of known central nervous system disease such as Huntington's chorea or postviral encephalitis. The differential diagnosis of TS must include exclusion of other idiopathic tic disorders and causes of secondary tics (see Table 2).

Differential diagnosis should include such movement disorders of childhood as chorea (dancing movements as in Sydenham's chorea), myoclonus (brief muscle contractions), athetosis (slow writhing of face, fingers, or toes), dystonia (slow twisting movements as in blepharospasm), hemiballismus, tremor, Huntington disease, neuroacanthocytosis, and tardive dyskinesia, as well as focal seizures. Simple tics may be difficult to distinguish from myoclonic or choreic jerks. Complex tics may be difficult to distinguish from repetitive stereotypes of mental retardation or psychosis, akathisia, restless legs syndrome, and the rituals of OCD.

ETIOLOGY

The concept of tic spectrum as advanced by Singer and Walkup (1991) is based on the lack of evidence that tics are environmentally based and may be principally dependent on variable expression of the same genetic diathesis (Kurlan, 1988). An explosion of research interest in the genetics of TS has been generated from exciting

---

Table 1. Diagnostic Criteria for 307.23 Tourette's Disorder

A. Both multiple motor and one or more vocal tics have been present at some time during the illness, although not necessarily concurrently. (A *tic* is a sudden, rapid, recurrent, nonrhythmic, stereotyped motor movement or vocalization.)
B. The tics occur many times a day (usually in bouts) nearly every day or intermittently throughout a period of more than 1 year, and during this period there was never a tic-free period of more than 3 consecutive months.
C. The disturbance causes marked distress or significant impairment in social, occupational, or other important areas of functioning.
D. The onset is before age 18 years.
E. The disturbance is not the result of the direct physiological effects of a substance (e.g., stimulants) or a general medical condition (e.g., Huntington's disease or postviral encephalitis).

Table 2. Etiology of Tics

Idiopathic
    Transient tic disorder
    Chronic motor or vocal tic disorder
    Tourette's disorder
    Tic disorder not otherwise specified
"Secondary" tics
    Postencephalitic
    Postrheumatic chorea
    Head injury
    Carbon monoxide poisoning
    Neuroancanthocytosis
    Drug-induced (stimulants, levodopa, neuroleptics
       ["tardive Tourette"], carbamazepine, phenytoin,
       phenobarbital)

evidence that it may be variably expressed as either TS or OCD (Pauls et al., 1986, 1990), and perhaps ADHD (Comings, Himes, & Comings, 1990; Pauls et al., 1993). The TS gene is believed to be an autosomal dominant pattern of inheritance with varying degrees of penetrance. At this time, 60% of the human genome has been studied, but no genetic linkage has been clearly established (Singer & Walkup, 1991). Though the dopamine system has been implicated in TS, linkage studies probing the D1 (Gerlenter et al., 1993) or D2 (Comings et al., 1992; Gerlenter et al., 1990) receptor locus with TS and/or tic spectrum disorders have been mixed, with uncertainty as to whether it even modifies TS severity (Gerlenter, Pauls, Leckman, Kidd, & Kurlan, 1994). Family and twin studies also support the genetic transmission of TS. In one large study, 53% of the monozygotic twins were concordant for TS compared with 8% of the dizygotic twins. When the data were analyzed using tic spectrum disorders including chronic motor tics, the concordance rate increases to 77% versus 23%, respectively (Price, 1985).

The roles of the environment and hormonal factors are viewed not as causative in TS, but as modifying either phenotypic expression or severity. Maternal life stress during pregnancy and nausea/vomiting during the first trimester may be associated with tic severity (Leckman et al., 1990). Environmental influence of sex hor-

mones at critical stages of development is implicated in phenotypic expression as males tend to exhibit tics and females tend to have OCD. The excessive trophic effect of sex hormones on later expression of a genetic predisposition for TS is expounded on by Kurlan (1992). This hypothesis is in part substantiated by reports of antiandrogen therapy improving tic symptoms, and clinical observation of altered tic symptoms at menarche, menopause, and during pregnancy. The greater frequency of TS in males suggests a possible role for testosterone or other sex hormones in development of the condition (Hyde & Weinberger, 1995).

Brain regions involved in TS include the basal ganglia, limbic system, and frontal cortex. Recent structural brain studies of basal ganglia volume in children with TS suggest that the left caudate, a part of the basal ganglia nucleus, is reduced in size (Singer, 1993). This finding has now been substantiated by an independent laboratory, showing reductions in regional basal ganglia volumes in TS versus normal controls, emphasizing the asymmetries found in the TS brain (Peterson et al., 1993). Positron emission tomography (PET) with ^{18}F-labeled fluoro-deoxy-D-glucose shows that glucose utilization in the basal ganglia averages 16% above control, with minor differences also apparent in frontal and temporal lobes bilaterally (Chase et al., 1984). The increase in glucose utilization indicates more metabolic activity in these areas.

The effectiveness of dopamine blockade in TS by the use of medications that are mixed D_1/D_2 antagonists (haloperidol, fluphenazine, pimozide) and sulpiride (D_2) (George et al., 1993) has led to a hypothesis of dopamine dysregulation, characterized by hypersensitive postsynaptic dopamine receptors (Singer, Butler, Tune, Seifert, & Coyle, 1982). This theory is supported by cerebrospinal fluid findings of lowered baseline and turnover levels of the dopamine metabolite homovanillic acid (Butler & Grace, 1979; Cohen, Shaywitz, Caparulo, Young, & Bowers, 1978) and is suggested by a PET study in TS using specially labeled ^{11}C-*N*-methylspiperone, which demonstrated elevated D_2 receptor density

(B_{max}) in basal ganglia (Wong et al., 1989). George et al. (1994), using the newly developed D_2/D_3 receptor SPECT ligand [123] I-6-methoxybenzamine, found no receptor occupancy differences between unmedicated TS patients and controls. In postmortem studies of TS, significant elevations of dopamine uptake carrier sites using [3H]mazindol binding have been identified in the basal ganglia (Singer & Walkup, 1991). This suggests that TS may involve increases in synaptically available dopamine.

Serotonin (5-HT) is also invoked as playing a role in TS pathophysiology, as furthered by recent clinical studies of synergistic effects between neuroleptics and selective serotonin reuptake inhibitors (SSRIs) for alleviating severe tics (McDougle et al., 1990), particularly in patients with comorbid TS and OCD (George et al., 1993). Cerebrospinal fluid studies in TS patients reveal low 5-hydroxyindoleacetic acid (5-HIAA), the principal serotonin metabolite (Butler & Grace, 1979; Cohen et al., 1978). Postmortem studies of TS patients demonstrate low levels of tryptophan (5-HT precursor) and low serotonin in basal ganglia (Anderson, Leckman, Riddle, Chappell, & Cohen, 1989). Plasma tryptophan is reduced in TS (Comings et al., 1990) as is whole blood serotonin (Comings et al., 1990). Dopamine transmission is modulated by serotonin through action at the 5-HT$_3$ receptor (George et al., 1993), as suggested by recent animal studies (Blandina, Goldfarb, Craddock-Royal, & Green, 1989). Weizman et al. (1992) studied platelets from patients with TS alone or comorbid with OCD (TS+OCD) and found reduced serotonin transporter protein sites via reduced [3H]imipramine binding capacity (B_{max}) in patients with TS+OCD.

Competing theories involving cholinergic (Sallee, Stiller, & Perel, 1992) and opioid systems (Haber, Kowall, Vonsattel, Bird, & Richardson, 1986; Leckman et al., 1988) also have been entertained. Four case studies have recently been described hypothesizing that an infection-triggered autoimmune response can cause or exacerbate cases of childhood OCD or tic disorder (Allen, Leonard, & Swedo, 1995).

EPIDEMIOLOGY

Although tic spectrum disorder may be more common among the school-age population than previously appreciated, the estimated prevalence of TS indicates that it remains a rare disorder. The point prevalence estimates of TS in schoolchildren range from 3.1–4.9/10,000 in teens (male–female, 16- to 17-year-old Israeli inductees) (Apter et al., 1993) to 105–13/10,000 (male–female) in children Grades K–8 (Caine et al., 1988; Comings et al., 1990). These estimates, based in differing methodologies, suggest that anywhere from 125,000 to over 1 million children in the United States may be suffering from TS. TS is more common in boys than in girls (5:1) (Witelson, 1993), and more frequent in Caucasians than African Americans or Hispanics. Typical mean age of onset is 6 years with the majority of patients being identified by age 13. Point prevalence estimates may appear to decrease in the future as a result of inclusion of impairment criteria in DSM-IV criteria.

ASSESSMENT

Tics are difficult to objectively quantify reliably because of their heterogeneous presentation (simple eye blinks and grunts must be measured along with copropraxia and coprolalia). Complicating assessment is the tendency for symptoms to wax and wane irrespective of treatments or interventions. Can the clinician be sure that this month's should shrug is equivalent to last week's grunt? Presence of partial volitional control and the tendency in most patients to suppress tics when observed, are additional obstacles to assessment of symptoms. For example, Goetz, Tanner, Wilson, and Shannon (1987) reported that motor tics recorded with the examiner present were 27% of that recorded in the absence of the examiner.

Clinical Interview

The anatomical location, number, frequency, intensity, complexity, and degree of disruption associated with minor and phonic tics should be documented by a clinician. The age of onset should be noted along with associated stressors and toxic insults such as stimulant medications. Clinicians should delineate the course of tics over the past year and over the past several months prior to presentation. Assessment should substantiate clinical waxing and waning of the disorder, duration of severe tic symptoms, and factors associated with exacerbation or improvement. Does the patient recognize sensory urges or mental phenomena associated with tics? Do external stimuli provoke or trigger tic symptoms? What impact on the individual's self-esteem, social adaptation, or academic performance do tic symptoms have? Finally, an assessment should be made of risk to self-injury as a result of the presence of tics. Such findings will serve as a record of tic symptom severity at the time of initial presentation and for documentation of impairment associated with motor and phonic tic phenomena. Associated behavioral phenomena should be assessed in addition to tics. These include the presence or absence of obsessive-compulsive symptoms and behaviors such as simple rituals, and full-fledged OCD. Does the patient have attentional problems, mood lability, or irritability, and is an affective disturbance also present? How does the patient get along with family or friends? What is his or her premorbid history and adjustment before tic onset? What are the life events associated with onset and exacerbation of tic symptoms? Are stability of family life, coping skills, and social support available to the patient?

A genetic family history should be taken about other relatives or family members who have unusual movement problems or obsessive-compulsive behaviors. The past medical or developmental history that may be relevant to the presence of tics, such as prenatal birth history, developmental delays, medication exposures, and injuries, must be included in a complete assessment. A neurological examination should be done with an assessment of soft neurological signs. If the results of the latter are abnormal, then further determination of presence or absence of electroencephalogram abnormalities or brain structural problems is warranted. If the patient has been on medication for tic symptoms, response to medication, adequate length of trials, and exacerbation resulting from medication treatment should be noted. In addition, assessment of school status, presence or absence of learning disabilities, and adequacy of school placement are essential to maximize academic functioning.

Neurological Examination

Results of the neurological examination of patients with primary TS are usually unremarkable with no focal or lateralizing signs. "Soft" signs such as coordination and fine motor performance problems are common particularly in TS with comorbid ADHD symptomatology. Motor tics are very characteristic and rarely confused with other forms of hyperkinetic movement disorders. Both clonic (e.g., rapid) and tonic (e.g., sustained) tics occur, but most often tics are brief and are of the clonic variety. Clonic tics can sometimes be confused with myoclonus and chorea. Tonic tics may be confused with dystonic movements. Buccal–lingual tics can be problematic in TS patients who have been exposed to neuroleptics, as it is difficult to readily distinguish these movements from neuroleptic-induced dyskinesias. Tics often involve ocular movements that are rare in other types of dyskinesias. Characteristics of abruptness, suppressibility, and the influence of stress or relaxation on movements should help the clinician make the determination that a tic is present. Most other dyskinesias are continuous and not abrupt and cannot be readily suppressed for long periods of time. Stress can exacerbate tics as well as other dyskinesias; however, tics are characteristically increased during periods of relaxation as well. A careful neurological workup should include screening for metabolic conditions or Wilson's disease, which may produce tremors that can be confused with tics.

On neurological examination, minor motor asymmetries (e.g., unilateral impairment of rapid alternating movements, increased tone on one side) are found in one-half of TS patients (Sweet, Solomon, Wayne, Shapiro, & Shapiro, 1973). In 12 to 38% of patients, EEG abnormalities exist but they are rarely epileptiform and are most often reported as nonspecific slowing (Bergen, Tanner, & Wilson, 1982). Neuroimaging of TS patients has been nonspecific with reports of asymmetrical lateral ventricles or prominent cortical sulci (Caparulo et al., 1981; Lees et al., 1984). At present, in the absence of localizing findings on neurological examination, an EEG and CT scan are not routinely performed in the evaluation of TS.

Assessment Instruments

Assessment tools are critical in the evaluation of TS, and recent developments in this area have bolstered the confidence of clinicians in their ability to quantify and track tic symptoms over time. In clinical practice, these instruments document the course of illness and monitor the waxing and waning of symptoms in treatment. These assessment tools were initially developed for research strategies to determine outcome in drug treatment studies (Goetz, Tanner, Wilson, Carroll, Como, & Shannon, 1987; Leckman, Walkup, Riddle, & Cohen, 1987) or to do epidemiological research (Stefl, 1983). The two strategies presently employed to quantitate tic symptoms in an objective fashion rely either on the microanalysis of a timed sample of tic behavior, as in the method of Tanner, Goetz, and Klawans (1982), or by the use of subjective clinical ratings after review of a patient's symptoms and history (Harcherick, Leckman, Detlor, & Cohen, 1984).

Parental and Self-Reports

Although patients and their parents may be unskilled at detecting tics, they have an advan-

tage over the clinician of frequent samplings across multiple settings. Structured parental and self-report instruments have often been used in epidemiological, genetic, and longitudinal studies. The Tourette's Syndrome Questionnaire (TSQ) (Jagger et al., 1982) systematically obtains historical information such as developmental history, course of tic behavior, and effect of TS on the individual. The Tourette's Syndrome Symptom Checklist (Cohen, Leckman, & Shaywitz, 1984) quantitates daily and weekly ratings of tic behaviors by asking the respondent to identify and estimate the frequency and disruption of tics and associated behavioral symptoms. In its present form as the Tourette Syndrome Symptom List (TSSL) (Walkup, Rosenberg, Brown, & Singer, 1992), this self-report is used to monitor the patient and family perception of improvement over treatment intervals.

Adjunctive symptoms of inattention, impulsivity, motoric hyperactivity, and internalizing symptoms are best delineated by relevant scales such as the Conners Parent Questionnaire (Goyette, Conners, & Ulrich, 1978) or Child Behavior Checklist and Profile (Achenbach & Edelbrock, 1983). Obsessive-compulsive symptoms can be quantitated on the Leyton Obsessional Inventory–Child Version (Berg et al., 1986), or the child version of the Yale-Brown Obsessive-Compulsive Rating Scale (Goodman et al., 1989).

Clinician Observer Assessment

Clinician observer methods employ the skill of the clinician to determine the nuances of tic symptoms and can, with varying degrees of success, provide a judgment concerning impairment as a result of the noted tics. Early attempts such as the Shapiro Tourette's Syndrome Severity Scale (STSSS) developed by Shapiro, Shapiro, Young, and Feinberg (1988b) and the Tourette's Syndrome Global Scale (TSGS) (Harcherick et al., 1984) are examples of this approach. The STSSS severity rating correlates well with tic counts obtained by trained clinicians ($r = .61$) and with global ratings of clinical improvement (.72). It also possesses good test–

retest reliability and internal consistency (Shapiro et al., 1988b). Most recently the STSSS has been used to evaluate potent pharmacological treatments such as pimozide and haloperidol (Shapiro et al., 1989).

The TSGS is a multidimensional scale not only of TS symptoms, but of behavioral symptoms as well, while incorporating a social functioning determination. The TSGS has a tic domain with four dimensions (simple motor tics, complex motor tics, simple phonic tics, complex phonic tics) and a social functioning domain with three dimensions (behavioral problems, motor restlessness, school or occupational dysfunctioning). Although the TSGS has been useful to quantitate the disorder, the social and behavioral scales can potentially weight adversely the total score (Harcherick et al., 1984). Using this scale, one can have the same score if tics are relatively mild but behavior and school functioning severely impaired (perhaps as a result of concomitant ADHD) as a patient with good school functioning and severe motor tics and coprolalia. Internal consistency in the tic symptom dimension is good (intraclass correlation = .71) and agreement of raters in the global score is excellent ($r = .89$) despite the wide diversity of symptom dimensions. Because of its compromised psychometric properties, the TSGS is somewhat out of favor as a rating instrument at this time.

Recently a new clinician-rated scale of tic severity, the Yale Global Tic Severity Scale (YGTSS), has been developed (Leckman et al., 1989). The YGTSS provides an evaluation of the number, frequency, intensity, complexity, and interference of motor and phonic symptoms. This semistructured interview gathers information on the specific character and anatomical location of tics during the course of a 1-week interval before assessment, then the clinician is asked to rate the severity of the tics along five separate dimensions. The YGTSS is a second-generation instrument derived from the earlier TSGS but focuses only on tic behaviors without attempting to assess a broader range of maladaptive behaviors or academic performance. The YGTSS has two subscale scores of motor and phonic tics, which are shown to be internally consistent. Moreover, factor analyses have shown that the items of the YGTSS can be recombined into categories that were identical to the a priori motor and phonic subscales. The scale has demonstrated good to excellent interrater reliability except for motor tic intensity measures. There is close agreement between the YGTSS and the TSGS and the TS-CGI and STSSS scales, but not with the ADHD-CGI. The scale has been validated with its reliability and psychometric properties well defined. It is used widely in drug trials in TS (Walkup et al., 1992).

Videotaped Assessment

Goetz, Tanner, Wilson, and Shannon (1987) developed a videotape rating scale that can be adapted clinically for routine assessment of tic symptoms. The advantage of such a method is that it obviates the subjective quantification of symptoms and can provide an objective measure of severity. Their method utilizes short, videotaped recordings and measures five tic variables including number of body areas affected, frequency of motor tics and vocalizations, and severity of motor tics and vocalizations. The videotaped ratings of Goetz, Tanner, Wilson, and Shannon (1987) accurately detected improvement in tic symptoms with neuroleptic treatment, suggesting that this method could be used to follow patients in therapy.

Chappell et al. (1994) demonstrated the short- and long-term stability of tic counts as reliable indexes of overall tic severity. Based on videotaped segments of at least 5 minutes' duration, they accurately measured motor and phonic tic frequency. Tic counts obtained in this manner were highly correlated with clinician ratings of frequency using the YGTSS scale. Videotaping using the shorter-duration format therefore becomes a feasible addition to self-rating and clinician-rated frequency. Drawbacks to videotaping include the need for expensive and cumbersome equipment and the time required to review tapes. The videotaped ratings seem least adaptable to a clinical setting where "blind" and unbiased review frequently cannot be obtained.

TREATMENT

Neuroleptic Pharmacotherapy

Although the onset of TS, and its aggressive management, usually begins during school age, few studies have specifically addressed neuroleptic efficacy and benefit/risk in TS children. Haloperidol has been the drug of choice for over 30 years. Pimozide, an alternative neuroleptic, has also shown efficacy in tic treatment. In direct comparison with each other, pimozide proved less favorable (i.e., less efficacious with no advantage in side effect spectrum) (Shapiro et al., 1989). However, neither haloperidol nor pimozide is ideal as both rely on dopamine blockade. Both have a risk of neurological sequelae such as withdrawal-emergent or tardive dyskinesia (TD), with recent reports of TD in children exposed to as little as 4 mg haloperidol daily for 4 years (Silva, Magee, & Friedhoff, 1993). The risk of extrapyramidal symptoms (EPS) is high in children exposed to neuroleptics for long treatment periods and EPS tends to go unrecognized (Richardson, Haugland, & Craig, 1991). In an institutionalized child sample, Richardson et al. (1991) found an incidence of EPS of 34% and risk of treatment-emergent TD to be 12%. In TS outpatients, our data (unpublished) suggest a similar incidence of EPS in neuroleptic-treated TS children (42%) even at low doses. As a result, alternatives to neuroleptic therapy continue to be appealing, despite the progressive lowering of neuroleptic therapeutic dose range over the last decade to the 1–4 mg/day range.

Alternative Pharmacological Treatments

Alternative nonneuroleptic treatments for TS (e.g., clonidine, tricyclic antidepressants, SSRI) (Kurlan, Como, Deeley, & McDermott, 1993; Leckman & Cohen, 1991; Sandyk & Bamford, 1988) have yielded mixed results in limited clinical trials. The most widely used of these, clonidine, has had many case reports and open-

label studies suggesting tic efficacy. Among four controlled clinical trials, two demonstrated tic efficacy (Borison, Arg, Hamilton, Diamond, & David, 1983; Leckman & Cohen, 1991) and two did not (Goetz, Tanner, Wilson, Carroll, et al., 1987; Singer et al., 1995), which may have been the result of dose and assessment differences. Even when clonidine dose is optimized (3–5 µg/kg), "in terms of clinical practice, there is little doubt that clonidine is not as effective as the D2-dopamine receptor-blocking agents, such as haloperidol and pimozide, in controlling tic behaviors" (Leckman & Cohen, 1991). Though clonidine is the treatment of first choice at many TS treatment centers, as few as 38% of clonidine-treated patients exhibit a potent response (>50% tic severity improvement; Leckman & Cohen, 1991). Neuroleptics ultimately are used because of greater tic potency (70–80% of patients exhibit >50% tic severity improvement). Retrospective open-label data for tricyclic antidepressants such as desipramine and nortriptyline suggest tic efficacy (Spencer, Biederman, Kerman, Steingard, & Wilens, 1993). A controlled study of desipramine in TS with ADHD comorbidity found superiority to placebo on only one analogue tic measure with more standardized scales not detecting a difference (Singer et al., 1995). Initial interest in SSRI treatment of tics in TS was generated by Kurlan et al. (1993) who found a trend for tic improvement with fluoxetine. George et al. (1993) did not find statistical evidence of tic efficacy of fluvoxamine in a controlled comparison with sulpiride, however. Though investigation of SSRI therapy for TS is still under way, it appears that equivalent tic efficacy to neuroleptics is unlikely and their most useful role may be in the treatment of OCD comorbidity.

Treatment of Comorbid TS and ADHD

Stimulants are first-line treatment in ADHD, and although use in TS+ADHD is problematic, the benefits frequently outweigh risks of tic exacerbation. Exacerbation in certain instances can be attributed to the natural waxing and waning course of the disorder (Shapiro et al., 1988a). Some authors advocate stimulants combined with neuroleptic therapy (Shapiro et al., 1988a), or careful monitoring for tic exacerbation when used alone (Erenberg, Cruse, & Rothner, 1985). Gadow, Sverd, and Nolan (1992) noted that whereas 20–30% of patients experience tic exacerbation, another 10–20% experience decreased tics with methylphenidate. Decreased tics with long-term stimulant treatment has been attributed to desensitizing of DA receptors (Price, Leckman, Pauls, Cohen, & Kidd, 1986). In a placebo-controlled trial of methylphenidate in prepubertal boys with TS+ADHD (DSM-III-R), Gadow et al. (1992) found significant decreases in vocal tics with methylphenidate versus placebo. In a separate double-blind, placebo-controlled study of low (0.2 mg/kg BID) and higher (0.4 mg/kg BID) dose methylphenidate in 11 children with TS+ADHD, Konkol, Fischer, and Newby (1990) found that ADHD improved in 9 of the 11 children and that tics worsened on the low dose for 1 child (9%) and on the higher-dose methylphenidate for 4 children (36%). Castellanos and Rapoport (1993), studying 10 boys with TS+ADHD, found decreased hyperactivity without significant tic worsening on moderate methylphenidate doses (0.45 mg/kg BID) and, although a higher dose (0.7 mg/kg BID) exacerbated tics with continuation of therapy, tics were desensitized and returned to placebo levels. The desensitization of stereotypic movements with continuation of stimulants has also been associated with pemoline treatment (Sallee, Stiller, Perel, & Everett, 1989).

Although tricyclic antidepressants have been advocated as treatments for TS+ADHD, they also can exacerbate tics (Riddle et al., 1988), have no established efficacy in controlling tics (Singer & Walkup, 1991; Spencer et al., 1993), and as a drug class have cardiovascular risks of sudden death. The potential benefits must be factored against the relative risks.

Clonidine is a centrally acting noradrenergic agent (alpha-2 agonist) whose mechanism of action (inhibition of locus ceruleus outflow and decreased norepinephrine turnover) should be compatible with both TS and ADHD pathophysiology. There have been 16 case reports and open-label studies of 416 patients, which suggest that clonidine is effective for tic therapy, and in 259 of 416 (62%) cases, behavioral improvement of comorbid ADHD was attributed to clonidine. Double-blind, placebo-controlled studies of clonidine's effectiveness in TS have not been as consistent, however (Goetz, Tanner, Wilson, Carroll, et al., 1987; Leckman & Cohen, 1991). At this point clonidine's efficacy in ADHD alone and in TS+ADHD has not been established. It is, however, considered the drug of first choice for TS+ADHD in many centers and is the first alternative to stimulants in the NIMH/USOE "Multisite Study for the Treatment of ADHD." The newer alpha-2 adrenergic agonist guanfacine may offer a less sedating alternative for ADHD with tics (Chappell, Leckman, & Riddle, 1995).

Pimozide as a neuroleptic is unique in also exhibiting stimulant pharmacology, and may be useful in TS+ADHD. We have advocated for pimozide monotherapy in TS+ADHD in low does (Sallee, Sethuraman, & Rock, 1994), where tics are severe or not treatable with clonidine. SSRI have been reported effective in open trials in ADHD (Barrickman, Noyes, Kuperman, Schumacher, & Verda, 1991), but their efficacy in TS is marginal for tics (Kurlan et al., 1993), making them of marginal utility in TS+ADHD. A potentially helpful alternative treatment is Deprenyl, a monoamine oxidase inhibitor (MAOI) that has been used in an open trial (at an average dose of 8.1 mg/day), with improvement noted in 26 of 29 children and adolescents with TS and disabling ADHD. Two patients in the series had exacerbation of their tics thought to be secondary to metabolization of Deprenyl to the L isomers of amphetamine and methamphetamine exacerbating or unmasking tics (Jankovic, 1993).

Treatment of Comorbid Depression and Anxiety

Studies of TS patients have noted the comorbidity of anxiety and depression which can exacerbate tics (Pittman et al., 1987). Tricyclic anti-depressant or SSRI therapy can be safely utilized if potential benefits outweigh the risks. Benzodiazepines have been used as treatment of TS patients with comorbid anxiety disorders. Clonazepam has been described as a useful adjunct to clonidine in seven children with tics and ADHD (Steingard et al., 1993).

Nonpharmacological Treatment

Self-monitoring is frequently used in TS studies as a method of gathering data on tic frequency in the child's natural environment. Motor and phonic tics are most likely to occur at home in an environment where the child feels comfortable and where he or she is least afraid of embarrassment or ridicule. Rarely have tic counts been employed in a natural setting, and so patients are asked to use wrist counters or notebooks or to fill out daily questionnaires for a specified period of time. This procedure alone seems to reduce tic frequency. Four case study reports document this effect of self-monitoring and have used it as a treatment (Billings, 1978; Hutzell, Platzek, & Logue, 1974; Ollendick, 1981; Thomas, Abrams, & Johnson, 1971). Furthermore, these improvements were shown to be maintained at 1-year follow-up (Hutzell et al., 1974; Ollendick, 1981). Therefore, careful assessment by the clinician focuses the patient's awareness and seemingly promotes an effort to diminish symptoms.

Behavioral treatments have capitalized on the very observable nature of tics and the ability of patients to control symptoms for various periods of time. Techniques of massed negative practice, contingency management, and relaxation training rely heavily on the accurate and ongoing assessment of treatment outcome documented on either direct observation or videotaping of sessions. Behavioral treatment research in this area has used within-subject designs exclusively, with no group studies to demonstrate generalizability (Azrin & Peterson, 1988). Although this research approach most closely approximates the clinical situation, it has contributed to the lack of enthusiasm for behavioral treatments in favor of pharmacotherapy. Behavioral treatment of OCD has shown greater promise (March, Mulle, & Herbel, 1994). Family, cognitive behavior, supportive, and other therapies may be needed to address the social–emotional difficulties that often accompany TS (Carter, Pauls, Leckman, & Cohen, 1994).

CASE STUDY

Ken is a 13-year-old white male seventh grader with a 1-year history of increasing irritability, temper tantrums, sad mood, and avoidance of personal hygiene. He exhibited compulsive tapping behaviors with a need to slide his foot or skip in a certain manner when walking and a need to trace letters over and over while writing. At 9 months from onset of the symptoms, Ken began taking over 1 hour to eat a meal or to shower.

A diagnosis of obsessive-compulsive disorder was made and the patient began treatment with an SSRI, fluoxetine. When after 8 weeks his symptoms of OCD continued unabated, he was subsequently treated with sertraline followed shortly thereafter with clomipramine monotherapy. Despite history of functioning as an honor student, he demonstrated academic deterioration with the start of a new school year. He began demonstrating a notable onset of facial grimacing, eye twitching, animal and birdlike sounds, and involuntary throat clearing sounds.

Clomipramine monotherapy was partially successful in decreasing compulsive behaviors but was followed by increased frustration and violent aggressive outbursts requiring psychiatric hospitalization. A review of the family history revealed a first cousin and uncle with similar symptoms. A diagnosis of TS was made. Combined haloperidol (2 mg/day) and fluvoxamine was started and OCD symptoms and irritability decreased greatly with return home from the hospital. On addition of haloperidol, the tic symptoms, both motor and vocal, decreased to rare occurrence.

Case Discussion

The co-occurrence of OCD and TS varies from 30 to 60% in TS populations. The appearance of tic symptoms is often in the context of life-stress, such as the start of school in this case. The severity of OCD symptomatology contributed to the worsening of symptoms. Clearly the OCD was initially the most disabling and impairing diagnosis with tics perhaps relegated to tic disorder NOS status. The lack of tic impairment may have led most clinicians to either exclude the diagnosis or to relegate it to nonimportance. Tic symptoms were, however, the precipitating reason for inclusion of haloperidol in the treatment regimen. Recent literature would suggest that severe cases of OCD may require dopaminergic augmentation with neuroleptics. The exacerbation of violent behavior and dyscontrol can be fueled by the frustration these patients feel and may be a frequent consequence of SSRI therapy in patients with comorbid OCD and tic disorders. The case illustrates the importance of considering comorbid conditions in therapy and the frequent association of tic symptoms with other disorders such as OCD although ADHD is the most common comorbid clinical presentation.

SUMMARY

TS, once thought to be of psychodynamic origin, is now recognized as a neuropsychiatric brain disorder influenced by genetic, environmental, developmental, hormonal, and other extragenetic factors (Hyde & Weinberger, 1995). It is a lifelong disorder frequently associated with significant comorbid psychiatric conditions. Although genetic aspects of the disorder are exciting, the identity of the defective gene for TS has proven elusive. Much progress has been made over the last 5 years in the assessment of TS, particularly because of second-generation measures such as the YGTSS. The emphasis in DSM-IV on impairment criteria will, to some extent, likely decrease the frequency of TS diagnosis. Specific treatments for TS have moved away from behavioral treatment in general in favor of pharmacological interventions. The neuroleptics as a class have been optimized by reducing overall dosing regimens to the 1–4 mg range for both haloperidol and pimozide. Alternative pharmacological therapies continue to be attractive with intense efforts directed at investigations of clonidine, guaneficine, tricyclic antidepressants, SSRI, and MAOI agents. Successful treatment must include comprehensive assessment and treatment of comorbid conditions in order to optimize potential functioning.

REFERENCES

Achenbach, T. M., & Edelbrock, C. S. (1983). *Manual for the Revised Child Behavior Checklist and Profile.* Burlington, VT: University Associates in Psychiatry.

Allen, A. J., Leonard, H. L., & Swedo, S. E. (1995). Case study: A new infection-triggered, autoimmune subtype of pediatric OCD and Tourette's syndrome. *Journal of the American Academy of Child and Adolescent Psychiatry, 34,* 307–311.

American Psychiatric Association. (1994). *Diagnostic and statistical manual of Mental Disorders* (ed. 4, pp. 78–105). Washington, DC: Author.

Anderson, G. M., Leckman, J. F., Riddle, M. A., Chappell, P. B., & Cohen, D. J. (1989). *Recent neurochemical research on Tourette's syndrome.* Paper presented at the Biological Aspects of Nonpsychotic Disorders Regional Congress. World Federation of Societies of Biological Psychiatry, Jerusalem.

Apter, A., Pauls, D. L., Bleich, A., Zohar, A. H., Kron, S., Ratzoni, G., Dycian, A., Kotler, M., Weizman, A., Gadot, N., & Cohen, D. J. (1993). An epidemiologic study of Gilles de la Tourette's syndrome in Israel. *Archives of General Psychiatry, 50,* 734–738.

Azrin, N. H., & Peterson, A. L. (1988). Behavior therapy for Tourette's syndrome and tic disorders. In D. J. Cohen, R. D. Bruun, & J. F. Leckman (Eds.), *Tourette's syndrome and tic disorders: Clinical understanding and treatment* (pp. 238–255). New York: Wiley.

Barrickman, L., Noyes, R., Kuperman, S., Schumacher, M. A., & Verda, M. (1991). Treatment of ADHD with fluoxetine: A preliminary trial. *Journal of the American Academy of Child and Adolescent Psychiatry, 30,* 762–767.

Berg, C. J., Rapoport, J. L., & Flament, M. F. (1986). The Leyton Obsessional Inventory–Child Version. *Journal of the American Academy of Child Psychiatry, 25,* 84–92.

Bergen, D., Tanner, C. M., & Wilson, R. (1982). The electroencephalogram in Tourette syndrome. *Annals of Neurology, 11,* 638–641.

Billings, A. (1978). Self-monitoring in the treatment of tics: A single-subject analysis. *Journal of Behavior Therapy and Experimental Psychiatry, 9,* 339–342.

Blandina, P., Goldfarb, J., Craddock-Royal, B., & Green, J. P. (1989). Release of endogenous dopamine by stimulation of 5-hydroxytryptamine receptors in rat striatum. *Journal of Pharmacology and Experimental Therapeutics, 251,* 803–809.

Borison, R. L., Arg, L., Hamilton, W. J., Diamond, B. I., & David, J. M. (1983). Treatment approaches in Gilles de la Tourette syndrome. *Brain Research Bulletin, 11,* 205–208.

Bruun, R. D. (1988a). The natural history of Tourette's syndrome. In D. J. Cohen, R. D. Bruun, & J. F. Leckman (Eds.), *Tourette's syndrome and tic disorders: Clinical understanding and treatment* (pp. 22–39). New York: Wiley.

Bruun, R. D. (1988b). Subtle and underrecognized side effects of neuroleptic treatment in children with Tourette's disorder. *American Journal of Psychiatry, 145,* 621–624.

Burd, L., & Kerbashian, J. (1987). Onset of Gilles de la Tourette's syndrome before 1 year of age. *American Journal of Psychiatry, 144,* 1066–1067.

Butler, B. S., & Grace, A. A. (1979). Acute and chronic haloperidol treatment: Comparison of effects on nigral dopaminergic cell activity. *Life Science, 23,* 1715–1728.

Caine, E. O, McBride, M. C., Chiverton, P., Bamford, K. A., Rediess, S., & Shiao, J. (1988). Tourette's syndrome in Monroe County school children. *Neurology, 38,* 472–475.

Caparulo, B. K., Cohen, D. J., Rothman, S. L., Young, D. G., Katz, J. D., Shaywitz, S. E., & Shaywitz, B. A. (1981). Computed tomographic brain scanning in children with developmental neuropsychiatric disorders. *Journal of the American Academy of Child Psychiatry, 20,* 338–357.

Carter, A. S., Pauls, D. L., Leckman, J. F., & Cohen, D. F. (1994). A prospective longitudinal study of Gilles de la Tourette's syndrome. *Journal of the American Academy of Child and Adolescent Psychiatry, 33,* 377–385.

Castellanos, F. X., & Rapoport, J. L. (1993). Stimulant treatment of ADHD and Tourette disorder. American Psychiatric Association Abstracts.

Chappell, P. B., Leckman, J. F., & Riddle, M. A. (1995). The pharmacologic treatment of tic disorders. *Pediatric Psychopharmacology, 4,* 197–216.

Chappell, P. B., McSwiggan-Hardin, M. T., Scahill, L., Rubenstein, M., Walker, D. E., Cohen, D. J., & Leckman, J. F. (1994). Videotape tic counts in the assessment of Tourette's syndrome: Stability, reliability, and validity. *Journal of the American Academy of Child and Adolescent Psychiatry, 33,* 386–393.

Chase, T. N., Foster, N. L., Fedro, P., Brooks, R., Mansi, L., Kessier, R., & DiChiro, G. (1984). Gilles de la Tourette syndrome: Studies with the fluorine-18-labeled fluorodeoxyglucose positron emission tomographic method. *Annals of Neurology, 15,* 175.

Cohen, D. J., Leckman, J. F., & Shaywitz, B. A. (1984). The Tourette syndrome and other tics. In D. Shaffer, A. A. Ehrhardt, & L. Greenhill (Eds.), *The clinical guide to child psychiatry.* New York: Free Press.

Cohen, D. J., Shaywitz, B. A., Caparulo, B., Young, J. G., & Bowers, M. B. (1978). Chronic multiple tics of Gilles de la Tourette's disease: CSF acid monoamine metabolites after probenecid administration. *Archives of General Psychiatry, 35,* 245–250.

Comings, D. E. (1990). Blood serotonin and tryptophan in Tourette syndrome. *American Journal of Medical Genetics, 36,* 418–430.

Comings, D. E., & Comings, B. G. (1984). Tourette's syndrome and attention deficit disorder with hyperactivity: Are they genetically related? *Journal of the American Academy of Child Psychiatry, 23,* 138–146.

Comings, D. E., & Comings, B. G. (1985). Tourette's syndrome: Clinical and psychological aspects of 250 cases. *American Journal of Human Genetics, 37,* 435–450.

Comings, D. E., Comings, B. G., Devor, E. J., & Cloninger, C. R. (1984). Detection of major gene for Gilles de la Tourette syndrome. *American Journal of Human Genetics, 36,* 586–600.

Comings, D. E., Comings, B. G., Muhleman, D., Dietz, G., Shahbahrami B., Tast, D., Knell, E., Kocsis, P., Baumgarten, R., Kovacs, B. W., Levy, D. L., Smith, M. A., Borison, R. L., Evans, D. D., Klein, D. N., MacMurry, J., Tosk, J. M., Sverd, J., Gysin, R., Flanagan, S. D. (1991). The dopamine D2 receptor locus as a modifying gene in neuropsychiatric disorders. *JAMA, 266,* 1793–1800.

Comings, D. E., Himes, J. A., & Comings, B. G. (1990). An epidemiologic study of Tourette's syndrome in a single school district. *Journal of Clinical Psychiatry, 51,* 463–469.

Cooper, J. (1970). The Leyton Obsessional Inventory. *Psychological Medicine, 1,* 48–64.

Erenberg, G., Cruse, R. P., & Rothner, A. D. (1985). Gilles de la Tourette's syndrome: Effects of stimulant drugs. *Neurology, 35,* 1346–1348.

Erenberg, G., Cruse, R. P., Rothner, D. O., & Rothner, A. D. (1987). The natural history of Tourette's syndrome: A follow-up study. *Annals of Neurology, 22,* 383–385.

Frankel, M., Cummings, J. L., Robertson, M. M., Trimble, M. R., Hill, M. A., & Benson, D. F. (1986). Obsessions and compulsions in Gilles de la Tourette's syndrome. *Neurology, 36,* 378–382.

Gadow, K. D., Sverd, J., & Nolan, E. E. (1992). Methylphenidate in hyperactive boys with comorbid tic disorder: II. Short-term behavioral effects in school settings. *Journal of the American Academy of Child and Adolescent Psychiatry, 31,* 462–471.

George, M. S., Robertson, M. M., Costa, D. C., Ell, P. J., Trimble, M. R., Pilowsky, L., & Verhoeff, N. P. L. G. (1994). Dopamine receptor availability in Tourette's syndrome. *Psychiatry Research: Neuroimaging, 55,* 193–203.

George, M. S., Trimble, M. R., Ring, H. A., Sallee, F. R., & Robertson, M. M. (1993). Obsessions in obsessive-compulsive disorder with and without Gilles de la Tourette's disorder. *American Journal of Psychiatry, 150,* 93–97.

Gerlenter, J., Kennedy, J. L., Grandy, D. K., Zhou, Q. Y., Civelli, O., Pauls, D. L., Pakstis, A., Kurlan, R., Sunahara, R. K., Niznik, H. B., et al. (1993). Exclusion of close linkage of Tourette's syndrome to D1 dopamine receptor. *American Journal of Psychiatry, 150,* 449–453.

Gerlenter, J., Pakstis, A. J., Pauls, D. L., Kurlan, R., Gancher, S. T., Civelli, O., Grandy, D., Kidd, K. K. (1990). Gilles de la Tourette syndrome is not linked to D2 dopamine receptor. *Archives of General Psychiatry, 47,* 1073–1077.

Gerlenter, J., Pauls, D. L., Leckman, J., Kidd, K. K., & Kurlan, R. (1994). D2 dopamine receptor alleles do not influence severity of Tourette syndrome. Results from four large kindreds. *Archives of Neurology, 51,* 397–400.

Goetz, C. G., Tanner, C. M., Wilson, R. S., Carroll, V. S., Como, P. G., & Shannon, K. M. (1987). Clonidine and Gilles de la Tourette's syndrome: Double-blind study using objective rating methods. *Annals of Neurology, 21,* 307–310.

Goetz, C. G., Tanner, C. M., Wilson, R. S., & Shannon, K. M. (1987). A rating scale for Gilles de la Tourette's syndrome: Description, reliability, and validity data. *Neurology, 37,* 1542–1544.

Golden, G. S., & Hood, O. J. (1982). Tics and tremors. *Pediatric Clinics of North America, 29,* 95–103.

Goodman, W. K., Price, L. H., Rasmussen, S. A., Riddle, M. A., & Rapoport, J. L. (1989). Children's Yale-Brown Obsessive Compulsive Scale: Validity. *Archives of General Psychiatry, 46,* 1012–1016.

Goyette, C. H., Conners, C. K., & Ulrich, R. F. (1978). Normative data on revised Conners Parent and Teacher Rating Scales. *Journal of Abnormal Child Psychology, 6,* 221–236.

Grad, L. R., Pelcovitz, D., Olson, M., Matthews, M., & Grad, G. (1987). Obsessive-compulsive symptomatology in children with Tourette's syndrome. *Journal of the American Academy of Child Psychiatry, 26,* 69–74.

Haber, S. N., Kowall, N. W., Vonsattel, J. P., Bird, E. D., & Richardson, E. P. (1986). Gilles de la Tourette's syndrome: A postmortem neuropathological and immunohistochemical study. *Journal of Neurological Sciences, 75,* 225–241.

Hagin, R. A., & Kugler, J. (1988). School problems associated with Tourette's syndrome. In D. J. Cohen, R. D. Bruun, & J. F. Leckman (Eds.), *Tourette's syndrome and tic disorders: Clinical understanding and treatment* (pp. 224–236). New York: Wiley.

Harcherick, D. F., Leckman, J. F., Detlor, J., & Cohen, D. J. (1984). A new instrument for clinical studies of Tourette's syndrome. *Journal of the American Academy of Child Psychiatry, 23,* 153–160.

Hutzell, R. R., Platzek, D., & Logue, P. E. (1974). Control of symptoms of Gilles de la Tourette's syndrome by self-monitoring. *Journal of Behavior Therapy and Experimental Psychiatry, 5,* 71–76.

Hyde, T. M., & Weinberger, D. R. (1995). Tourette's syndrome: A model neuropsychiatric disorder. *JAMA, 273,* 498–501.

Jagger, J., Prusoff, B. A., Cohen, D. J., Kidd, K. K., Carbonari, C. M., & John, K. (1982). The epidemiology of Tourette's syndrome. *Schizophrenia Bulletin, 8,* 267–278.

Jankovic, J. (1993). Deprenyl in attention deficit associated with Tourette's disorder. *Archives of Neurology, 50,* 286–288.

Konkol, R. J., Fischer, M., & Newby, R. F. (1990). Double-blind, placebo-controlled stimulant trial in children with Tourette's syndrome and attention deficit hyperactivity disorder. *Annals of Neurology, 28,* 424.

Kurlan, R. (1988). The spectrum of Tourette's syndrome. *Current Opinions in Neurology and Neurosurgery, 1,* 294–298.

Kurlan, R. (1992). The pathogenesis of Tourette's syndrome: A possible role for hormonal and excitatory neurotransmitter influences in brain development. *Archives of Neurology, 49,* 874–876.

Kurlan, R., Como, P., Deeley, C., & McDermott, M. P. (1993). A pilot controlled study of fluoxetine for obsessive-compulsive symptoms in children with Tourette's syndrome. *Clinical Neuropharmacology, 16,* 167–172.

Leckman, J. F., & Cohen, D. J. (1991). Clonidine treatment of Gilles de la Tourette's syndrome. *Archives of General Psychiatry, 48,* 324–328.

Leckman, J. F., Dolnansky, E. S., Hardin, M. T., Clubb, M., Walkup, J. T., Stevenson, J., & Pauls, D. L. (1990). Perinatal factors in the expression of Tourette's syndrome: An exploratory study. *Journal of the American Academy of Child and Adolescent Psychiatry, 29,* 220–226.

Leckman, J. F., Riddle, M. A., Berrettini, W. H., Anderson, G. M., Hardin, M., Chappel, P., Bissette, G., Nemeroff, C. B., Goodman, W. K., & Cohen, D. J. (1988). Elevated CSF dynorphan A [1-8] in Tourette's syndrome. *Life Science, 43,* 2015–2023.

Leckman, J. F., Riddle, M. A., Hardin, M. T., Ort, S. I., Swartz, K. L., Stevenson, J., & Cohen, D. (1989). The Yale Global Tic Severity Scale: Initial testing of a clinician-rated scale of tic severity. *Journal of the American Academy of Child and Adolescent Psychiatry, 28,* 566–573.

Leckman, J. F., Walkup, J. T., Riddle, M. A., & Cohen, D. J. (1987). Tic disorders. In H. Y. Meltzer, W. Bunney, J. Coyle, J. David, I. Kopin, C. Schuster, R. Shader, & G. Simpson (Eds.), *Psychopharmacology, the third generation of progress* (pp. 1239–1246). New York: Raven Press.

Lees, A. J., Robertson, M., Trimble, M. R., & Murray, N. M. F. (1984). A clinical study of Gilles de la Tourette's syndrome in the United Kingdom. *Journal of Neurology, Neurosurgery, and Psychiatry, 47,* 1–8.

March, J. S., Mulle, K., & Herbel, B. (1994). Behavioral psychotherapy for children and adolescents with obsessive-compulsive disorder: An open trial of a new protocol-driven treatment package. *Journal of the American Academy of Child and Adolescent Psychiatry, 33,* 333–341.

McDougle, C. J., Goodman, W. K., Price, L. H., Delgado, P. L., Krystal, J. H., Charney, D. S., & Heninger, G. R. (1990). Neuroleptic addition in fluvoxamine-refractory obsessive-compulsive disorder. *American Journal of Psychiatry, 147,* 652–654.

Ollendick, T. H. (1981). Self-monitoring and self-administered overcorrection: The modification of nervous tics in children. *Behavior Modification, 5,* 75–84.

Pauls, D. L., Kruger, S. D., Leckman, J. F., Cohen, D. J., & Kidd, K. K. (1984). The risk of Tourette syndrome and chronic multiple tics among relatives of Tourette syndrome patients obtained by direct interview. *Journal of the American Academy of Child Psychiatry, 23,* 134–137.

Pauls, D. L., & Leckman, J. F. (1986). The inheritance of Gilles de la Tourette's syndrome and associated behaviors: Evidence for an autosomal dominant transmission. *New England Journal of Medicine, 315,* 993–997.

Pauls, D. L., Leckman, J. F., & Cohen, D. J. (1993). Familial relationship between Gilles de la Tourette's syndrome, attention deficit disorder, learning disabilities, speech disorders, and stuttering. *Journal of the American Academy of Child and Adolescent Psychiatry, 32,* 1044–1050.

Pauls, D. L., Pakstis, A. J., Kurlan, R., Kidd, K. K., Leckman, J. F., Cohen, D. J., Kidd, J. R., Como, P., & Sparkes, R. (1990). Segregation and linkage analysis of Tourette's syndrome and related disorders. *Journal of the American Academy of Child and Adolescent Disorders, 29,* 195–203.

Pauls, D. L., Towbin, K. E., Leckman, J. F., Lahner, A. E., & Cohen, D. J. (1986). Gilles de la Tourette's syndrome and obsessive-compulsive disorder: Evidence supporting a genetic relationship. *Archives of General Psychiatry, 43,* 1180–1182.

Peterson, B., Riddle, M. A., Cohen, D. J., Katz, L. D., Smith, J. C., Harden, M. T., & Leckman, J. F. (1993). Reduced basal ganglia volumes in Tourette's syndrome using three-dimensional reconstruction techniques from magnetic resonance images. *Neurology, 43,* 941–949.

Pitman, R. K., Green, R. C., Jenike, M. A., & Mesulam, M. M. (1987). Clinical comparison of Tourette's disorder and obsessive-compulsive disorder. *American Journal of Psychiatry, 144,* 1166–1171.

Price, B. H. (1985). Gilles de la Tourette syndrome. *Neurology and Neurosurgery, 8,* 1–8.

Price, R. A., Leckman, J. F., Pauls, D. L., Cohen, D. J., & Kidd, K. K. (1986). Gilles de la Tourette's syndrome: Tics and central nervous system stimulants in turns and non-turns. *Neurology, 36*(2), 232–237.

Richardson, M. A., Haugland, G., & Craig, T. J. (1991). Neuroleptic use, parkinsonian symptoms, tardive dyskinesia, and associated factors in child and adolescent psychiatric patients. *American Journal of Psychiatry, 148,* 1322–1328.

Sallee, F. R., Sethuraman, G., & Rock, C. M. (1994). Effects of pimozide on cognition in children with Tourette syndrome: Interaction with comorbid attention deficit hyperactivity disorder. *Acta Psychiatrica Scandinavica, 90,* 4–9.

Sallee, F. R., Stiller, R. L., & Perel, J. M. (1992). Pharmacodynamics of pemoline in attention deficit disorder with hyperactivity. *Journal of the American Academy of Child and Adolescent Psychiatry, 31,* 244–251.

Sallee, F. R., Stiller, R. L., Perel, J. M., & Everett, G. (1989). Pemoline-induced abnormal involuntary movements. *Journal of Clinical Psychopharmacology, 9,* 125–129.

Sandyk, R., & Bamford, C. R. (1988). Beneficial effects of imipramine on Tourette's syndrome. *International Journal of Neuroscience, 39,* 27–29.

Shapiro, A. K., Shapiro, E., Young, J. G., & Feinberg, T. E. (1988a). *Gilles de la Tourette syndrome.* New York: Raven Press.

Shapiro, A. K., Shapiro, E. S., Young, J. G., & Feinberg, T. E. (1988b). Measurement in tic disorders. In A. K. Shapiro, E. S. Shapiro, J. G. Young, & T. E. Feinberg (Eds.), *Gilles de la Tourette syndrome* (pp. 127–193). New York: Raven Press.

Shapiro, E., Shapiro, A. K., Fulop, G., Hubbard, M., Mandeli, J., Nordlie, J., & Phillips, R. A. (1989). Controlled study of haloperidol, pimozide, and placebo for the treatment of Gilles de la Tourette's syndrome. *Archives of General Psychiatry, 46,* 722–730.

Silva, R., Magee, H., & Friedhoff, A. (1993). Persistent tardive dyskinesia and other neuroleptic-related dyskinesias in Tourette's disorder. *Journal of Child and Adolescent Psychopharmacology, 3,* 137–144.

Singer, H. S. (1993). Pathobiology. In R. Kurlan (Ed.), *Handbook of Tourette's syndrome and other related tic and behavioral disorders* (pp. 267–288). New York: Dekker.

Singer, H. S., Brown, J., Quaskey, S., Rosenberg, L. A., Mellits, E. D., & Denckla, M. B. (1995). The treatment of attention-deficit hyperactivity disorder in Tourette's syndrome: A double-blind placebo-controlled study with clonidine and desipramine. *Pediatrics, 95,* 74–81.

Singer, H. S., Butler, I. J., Tune, L. E., Seifert, W. E., & Coyle, J. T. (1982). Dopaminergic dysfunction in Tourette syndrome. *Annals of Neurology, 12,* 361–366.

Singer, H. S., & Walkup, J. T. (1991). Tourette syndrome and other tic disorders: Diagnosis, pathophysiology, and treatment. *Medicine, 70,* 15–32.

Spencer, T., Biederman, J., Kerman, K., Steingard, R., & Wilens, T. (1993). Desipramine treatment of children with attention-deficit hyperactivity disorder and tic disorder or Tourette's syndrome. *Journal of the American Academy of Child and Adolescent Psychiatry, 32,* 354–360.

Stefl, M. E. (1983). *The Ohio Tourette Study.* Cincinnati: University of Cincinnati School of Planning.

Steingard, R., Biederman, J., Spencer, T., Wilens, T., & Gonzalez, A. (1993). Comparison of clonidine response in the treatment of attention-deficit disorder with and without comorbid tic disorders. *Journal of the American Academy of Child and Adolescent Psychiatry, 32,* 350–353.

Sweet, R. D., Solomon, G. E., Wayne, H. L., Shapiro, E., & Shapiro, A. K. (1973). Neurological features of Gilles de la Tourette's syndrome. *Journal of Neurology, Neurosurgery, and Psychiatry, 36,* 1–9.

Tanner, C. M., Goetz, G. G., & Klawans, H. L. (1982). Cholinergic mechanisms in Tourette syndrome. *Neurology, 32,* 1315–1317.

Thomas, E. J., Abrams, K. S., & Johnson, J. B. (1971). Self-monitoring and reciprocal inhibition in the modification of multiple tics on Gilles de la Tourette's syndrome. *Journal of Behavior Therapy and Experimental Psychiatry, 2,* 159–171.

Walkup, J. T., Rosenberg, L. A., Brown, J., & Singer, H. S. (1992). The validity of instruments measuring tic severity in Tourette's syndrome. *Journal of the American Academy of Child and Adolescent Psychiatry, 30,* 472–477.

Weizman, A., Mandel, A., Barber, Y., Weitz, R., Cohen, A., Mester, R., & Rehavi, M. (1992). Decreased platelet imipramine binding in Tourette syndrome children with obsessive-compulsive disorder. *Society of Biological Psychiatry, 31,* 705–711.

Witelson, S. F. (1993). Clinical neurology as data for basic neuroscience: Tourette's syndrome and the human motor system. *Neurology, 43,* 859–861.

Wong, D. F., Pearlson, G. D., Young, L. T., Singer, H., Villemagne, V., Tune, L., Ross, C., Dannals, R. F., Links, J. M., Chan, B., Wilson, A. A., Ravert, H. T., Wagner, H. N., & Gjedde, A. (1989). D2 dopamine receptors are elevated in neuropsychiatric disorders other than schizophrenia. *Journal of Cerebral Blood Flow and Metabolism, 9*(Suppl. 1), 593.

14

Elimination Disorders

STEVEN J. ONDERSMA AND C. EUGENE WALKER

INTRODUCTION

The importance of toilet training in the lives of parents and children is difficult to overestimate. To parents, it is a major step in their child's progress toward independence, and has come to represent not only their own effectiveness as parents but also the intellectual and emotional health of their child. To children, toilet training is the first major developmental challenge they face that is more important to others than to them. Suddenly, they discover that their ability to control what were once involuntary processes is a matter of extreme social significance, and that failures in this regard merit the displeasure of parents and peers alike. When failures occur, then, the interactive consequences in terms of family functioning and the child's adjustment can be far-reaching (Walker, 1995).

Persistent failures in toilet training, or elimination disorders, have a wide range of causes. Enuresis and encopresis are elimination disorders that are not the direct result of a general

medical condition. Each will be discussed in turn.

ENURESIS

Phenomenology

Enuretic children typically come to the attention of mental health professionals after numerous home remedies and discipline strategies have been attempted. Frustration on the part of both parent and child is common (Foxman, Valdez, & Brook, 1986); many parents report bedwetting to be a significant problem for them and their child, and a significant proportion of these admit to blaming the child or dealing with it via punishment (Butler, Brewin, & Forsythe, 1986; Haque et al., 1981). Children who lack control over micturition are frequently embarrassed and fearful of the reaction of others to their difficulties, and are often frustrated by their inability to "grow up." These feelings only increase with age, as the child becomes more acutely aware of the social stigma of his or her difficulty. They typically believe that they are the only ones their age who still have such problems, a belief that only exacerbates their feelings of shame.

STEVEN J. ONDERSMA AND C. EUGENE WALKER • College of Medicine, University of Oklahoma Health Sciences Center, Oklahoma City, Oklahoma 73190.

Handbook of Child Psychopathology, 3rd edition, edited by Ollendick & Hersen. Plenum Press, New York, 1998.

Often, enuretic children avoid social activities such as staying overnight with friends, going on camping trips, or attending summer camp, for fear they will wet the bed.

Episodes of urinary incontinence are most often reported as occurring during the night only, although daytime enuresis either alone or in combination with nighttime enuresis will be reported as well.

Diagnosis

Enuresis is defined in the DSM-IV (American Psychiatric Association, 1994) as repeated voiding of urine in inappropriate places such as in clothes or in bed. Such voiding may be involuntary or intentional, and must: (1) be by a child with a chronological or developmental age of at least 5 years, (2) occur twice a week for at least 3 consecutive months (or cause clinically significant distress or impairment in social, academic, or other important areas of functioning), and (3) be functional, that is, not related to the direct effect of a general medical condition (APA, 1994). The DSM-IV further requires that the wetting be described as nocturnal, diurnal, or both.

Many investigators also categorize enuresis as either primary/continuous (existing from birth without any significant periods of continence) or secondary (appearing following a period of continence of at least 6 months in duration). Some research has suggested that secondary enuresis is more often associated with stressful life events (Fergusson, Horwood, & Shannon, 1990; Jarvelin, Moilanen, Vikevainen-Tervonen, & Huttunen, 1990), and many clinicians see secondary enuresis as reflecting acute onset of psychosocial stress. However, the clinical utility of this distinction is questionable, as other research comparing primary and secondary enuretics has shown them to be "more similar than different" (Scott, Barclay, & Houts, 1992, p. 94), and outcome studies have not found the distinction to predict treatment response (Houts, Berman, & Abramson, 1994).

Etiology

Etiological theories of enuresis fall into three general categories: biological, emotional, and learning. The evidence for and against each approach to the understanding of enuresis will be reviewed.

Biological Theories

Although enuresis by definition is inappropriate voiding not related to a general medical condition, some researchers have hypothesized that much wetting is the result of a distinct medical cause not yet widely recognized. Such biological theories of the pathogenesis of enuresis abound. They include broad implications of genetic factors, as well as suggestions of specific abnormalities in hormonal fluctuations, arousability, bladder capacity, and developmental maturity.

The evidence for a genetic component in enuresis is strong. Bakwin (1973) reported that, of children whose parents had no history of enuresis, 15% could be diagnosed as enuretic. In contrast, 44% of those with one parent with a history of enuresis and 77% of those with two parents with histories of enuresis met criteria for the disorder. Bakwin also reported a 68% concordance rate for monozygotic twins and a 36% concordance for dizygotic twins. A family predisposition for enuresis is clear, and it has emerged as the single best predictor of enuresis (Fergusson, Horwood, & Shannon, 1986).

Numerous specific physiological pathways (either environmental, genetic, or congenital in origin) leading to enuresis have also been proposed. The most recent of these has followed the discovery that enuretic children tend to respond well to administration of desamino-D-arginine vasopressin (DDAVP), an antidiuretic hormone analogue (see Moffat, Harlos, Kirshen, & Burd, 1993, for a review). Subsequent research showed a less marked nocturnal surge in vasopressin, or antidiuretic hormone (ADH), in enuretic than in nonenuretic children (Rittig, Knudsen, Norgaard, Pedersen, &

Djurhuus, 1989). ADH works by augmenting resorption of water via its effects on the epithelial cells of the tubules within the kidney that transport urine. Thus, a lack of a normal nocturnal increase in ADH may result in a higher nocturnal production of urine (polyuria) and less concentrated urine (low osmolality; Norgaard, Pedersen, & Djurhuus, 1985; Rittig et al., 1989).

However, more recent research has failed to find evidence of abnormal nocturnal polyuria in enuretic children (Evans & Meadow, 1992; Watanabe, Kawauchi, Kitamori, & Azuma, 1994). Further, not all children who produce high amounts of urine are incontinent. For example, virtually all children with sickle-cell anemia show polyuria as a result of their illness; yet, only 50% are enuretic (Readett, Morris, & Serjeant, 1990). Further, enuretic children are not thirsty in the morning and do not tend to wet the bed more often toward the end of a night's sleep, contrary to what would be expected if polyuria were indeed the cause of their bedwetting (Steele, 1993). There are also no population-based studies of the prevalence of relatively low levels of ADH in nonenuretic children. Finally, if low levels of ADH were the only or primary cause of enuresis, behavioral treatments would most likely be only minimally effective. This is clearly not the case (see the section entitled "Treatment").

Sleep abnormalities have also been implicated in the pathogenesis of enuresis. The fact that the majority of enuretic episodes are nocturnal and the report of many parents that their children are extremely difficult to awaken (Haque et al., 1981) has led to the suggestion that enuresis is a deficit in arousability in response to the sensations of a full bladder (e.g., Perlmutter, 1976). Numerous EEG studies of the relationship between bedwetting episodes and depth of sleep have found no significant correlation (Mikkelsen et al., 1980; Norgaard, Hansen, & Bugge, 1989). These studies, however, do not take into account the child's general arousability, or the rate at which they go from sleeping to alertness. Studies of general arousability are rare, and their results are inconsistent (Boyd, 1960; Braithwaite, 1956; Kaffman & Elizur, 1977). More careful research of arousability rather than sleep stages is needed. However, even positive findings in this area would be less than conclusive: these children may have learned to sleep through distracting stimuli as a result of their incontinence.

Much attention has also been given to the functional bladder capacity (FBC) of enuretic children. FBC is defined as the amount of urine voided after being asked to refrain from voiding for as long as possible, following the intake of 8 to 16 ounces of liquid. Some investigators have found a smaller FBC in enuretic than in continent children. They have speculated that this decreased capacity is the result of inadequate cortical inhibition, and the cause of nighttime wetting (Starfield, 1967; Zaleski, Gerrard, & Shokeir, 1973). However, there is considerable overlap in the FBCs of enuretic and nonenuretic children (Rutter, 1973), and increases in FBC have not been shown to correlate with improvement (Starfield & Mellits, 1968). Failure to withhold urine overnight likely results in inadequate stretching of the bladder, which in turn results in a smaller FBC in enuretic children (Rutter, 1973).

A final proposed biological pathway is developmental delay, specifically of the neurological mechanisms of bladder control. Although this hypothesis has intuitive appeal given the developmental aspects of the acquisition of continence, the research examining this issue is scant and inconsistent. Gross and Dornbusch (1983) referred to analyses of National Health Examination Survey data confirming that enuretic children were behind their nonenuretic peers in bone age and growth, and that they walked, talked, and became sexually mature later. Gross and Dornbusch also pointed out that males develop more slowly overall and are also more likely to be enuretic (this latter assertion, however, is suspect—see "Epidemiology," below). Whether or not enuretic children are delayed in these areas, however, is of little importance given the inevitability with which they do reach such milestones within a few months of their peers. Enuretic children are incontinent for up to 10 years or more past the point at which their peers have achieved dryness; if *specific* delays that can continue for a decade or more exist, they have yet to be identified.

Emotional Theories

As with many other disorders, psychoanalytic theory has assumed enuresis to be the expression of various neurotic conflicts (Fenichel, 1946; Imhof, 1956; Solomon & Patch, 1969). Such hypotheses cannot be tested, as random assignment to groups and experimental control over such intrapsychic phenomena is not possible. It *is* possible to study the effects of definable psychopathological features on the expression or severity of enuresis using prospective designs, but no such research has been conducted. Virtually all such research to date has been cross-sectional, comparing the prevalence of certain psychopathological variables (e.g., anxiety, depression) in enuretic children with that in nonenuretic children. The results of such research vary, but overall suggest slightly poorer adjustment (e.g., higher anxiety and lower self-esteem) in enuretic children (Shaffer, 1973). More recent research has found evidence for such an association even when studying a nonreferred community sample (Moilanen, Jarvelin, Vikevainen-Tervonen, & Huttunen, 1987).

However, the cross-sectional design of such research only affirms an association and does not show whether emotional distress is a cause or a result of enuresis. Further, the weak associations found do not support the notion that enuresis is strongly related to psychopathology of any kind. Finally, psychotherapeutic techniques based on the assumption of emotional causation have been ineffective (Houts et al., 1994; Walker, 1995). It appears that emotional difficulties in enuretic children are mild, and are as likely to be a result as a cause of their bedwetting.

Learning Theories

Enuresis is often conceptualized as the result of inadequate learning experiences and response contingencies. Whereas the majority of children learn to either awaken or contract the muscles of the pelvic floor in response to the sensations of a full bladder, enuretic children clearly do neither. Many investigators see this failure to respond appropriately as a failure in learning (e.g., Lovibond & Coote, 1970; Walker, 1995); enuretic children do not learn to attend to the sensations of a full bladder while they are asleep, and/or fail to respond appropriately on having done so. Others point out that biological factors such as developmental delay, low FBC, and deficient production of ADH, as well as psychosocial stress, can easily be seen as inhibiting acquisition or expression of the subtle skill of delaying the reflexive behavior of micturition (Scott et al., 1992; Walker, 1995). Numerous highly effective treatments are based on this etiological theory.

Epidemiology

Studies of the prevalence of nocturnal enuresis vary widely in their findings, primarily reflecting differences in populations, definitions of enuresis, and methods of data collection. The most commonly reported estimate is that approximately 15–20% of 5-year-old children are enuretic at least once per month (Fergusson et al., 1986; McGee, Makinson, Williams, Simpson, & Silva, 1984; Oppel, Harper, & Rider, 1968). By age 7, approximately 7–15% of children are enuretic at least once per month (Fergusson et al., 1986; McGee et al., 1984; Rutter, Yule, & Graham, 1973), and 7% of 7-year-old boys and 3% of 7-year-old girls are enuretic at least weekly (Rutter et al., 1973). Most studies of adolescents suggest that the prevalence of enuresis decreases to approximately 1% by the midteens (e.g., Martin, 1966; Rutter et al., 1973). The spontaneous annual remission rate for a clinic-referred sample has been estimated at approximately 15% (de Jonge, 1973; Forsythe & Redmond, 1974).

Most investigators assume that boys are much more frequently enuretic than girls (e.g., de Jonge, 1973). Although some studies of representative samples have supported this (Verhulst et al., 1985), the research suggesting such differences is often based on clinic-referred samples. Studies of representative population samples have at times found smaller differences between boys and girls. For example, McGee et al. (1984), studying children 5, 7, and 9 years old, found that 11% of boys were enuretic, as compared with 9.4% of girls. Similarly, in another study of a representative community sample, Fergusson et al. (1986) reported that boys were only slightly slower to attain bladder control than girls. The rate of enuresis does appear to decline more quickly in girls than in boys (Verhulst et al., 1985).

Diurnal enuresis is far less prevalent than nocturnal enuresis, occurring in approximately 1% of children between the ages of 7 and 12 (de Jonge, 1973). Diurnal enuresis, as opposed to nocturnal enuresis, appears to be more common in girls than in boys (de Jonge, 1973).

Assessment

The complex medical, social, and environmental issues associated with enuresis necessitate a multifaceted assessment. The first requirement of such an assessment is to ensure that a medical evaluation of the problem has been performed; this evaluation should include a screen for any urinary tract infections as well as a thorough history. If needed, more expensive and invasive procedures such as cystoscopy or excretory urograms may also be included. Although the possible medical causes of enuresis are many, the Committee on Radiology of the American Academy of Pediatrics (1980) has suggested that in the absence of signs such as current infection, daytime wetting, or a history of urological disease, the use of the more invasive procedures is not warranted.

A small proportion of enuretic children have urinary tract infections. Approximately 40% of these children will become dry following antibiotic treatment (Schmitt, 1982). A smaller proportion will be found to have more significant urological diseases that may or may not respond to medical intervention. In the majority of cases, however, no abnormalities will be found, allowing psychosocial evaluation to continue. Psychosocial assessment may also be needed in cases where successful medical treatment of underlying disorders or diseases is unsuccessful in ameliorating the enuresis (see Figure 1).

Following the exclusion of a general medical condition, an in-depth clinical interview is necessary. This interview should include all aspects of a typical clinical interview, including developmental history, family constellation, family mental health and medical history (especially history of enuresis), family environment, behavior problems, and recent stressors. Standardized checklists may be very useful in quickly screening for the presence of family and behavior problems. Additionally, the enuresis itself should be examined in detail: A full functional analysis including onset, frequency, and typical reactions of the child and caretakers to wetting should be made, as well as an examination of past attempts at treatment and the child's sleeping patterns (Walker & Shaw, 1988). It may also be important to determine the FBC of the child (the procedure is described in Starfield, 1967) and the arousability of the child. Finally, given the frequency with which parental disapproval and frustration can exacerbate the enuretic child's distress, thorough assessment of the quality of the parent–child relationship and parental reactions to wetting is suggested. Morgan and Young (1975) produced a scale designed to evaluate parental reactions to enuresis.

If the child is wetting during the day as well as or instead of at night, physiological causes are more likely to be primary. Regarding cases of diurnal enuresis that may respond to psychological/behavioral intervention, Schmitt (1982) suggested three categories: (1) urgency incontinence, or inadequate warning that the bladder is full; (2) stress-related incontinence, or urinating in response to specific crises or stressors;

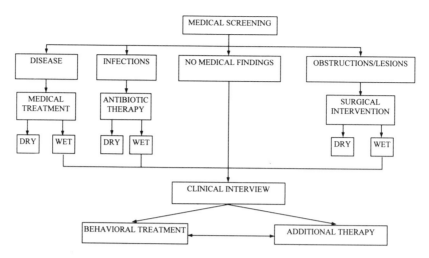

Figure 1. Flow chart of the steps in assessment of enuresis leading to a decision to use behavioral treatment. Complications include onset caused by trauma, family distress, and child behavior problems. Some complications such as poor motivation, negative parental attitudes, and previously treated failures may require more carefully monitored behavioral treatment than is normally required. (Adapted with permission from Scott, Barclay, & Houts, 1992.)

and (3) resistive incontinence, or refusal to toilet appropriately despite the ability to do so.

Treatment

The treatment of enuresis has a long and colorful history, having included such remedies as drinking tea made from the burnt crop of a cock and standing naked over a burning nest of the Phoebe bird (Glicklich, 1951). More recent behavioral and medical treatments, although less creative, have overall been quite successful in decreasing enuretic episodes. The treatment of nocturnal and diurnal enuresis will be discussed separately.

Nocturnal Enuresis

Medical Treatment. Medical treatment of nocturnal enuresis is the most common treatment modality used (Foxman et al., 1986; Gross & Dornbusch, 1983). Enuretic children are most often referred first to primary care physicians, who overwhelmingly use pharmacological inter-

ventions over behavioral interventions (Foxman et al., 1986). The most common medications used are tricyclic antidepressants and DDAVP.

Tricyclic antidepressants, especially imipramine (Tofranil), have until recently been the drug of choice by physicians treating nocturnal enuresis. Imipramine has two major actions, an anticholinergic effect (blocking parasympathetic nerves) and a noradrenergic effect (increasing norepinephrine), neither of which clearly account for its antienuretic properties (Gross & Dornbusch, 1983). However, it appears that a primary pathway for these effects may be the immediate increase in norepinephrine in the postsynaptic cleft that imipramine produces (through inhibiting norepinephrine reuptake), which in turn facilitates relaxation of muscles surrounding the bladder (Houts, 1991; Rapoport et al., 1980; Springer, Kropp, & Thor, 1994). The downregulation of beta receptors and its concomitant antidepressant effect, which takes approximately 3 weeks, does not appear to be related to the antienuretic actions of imipramine.

Regardless, imipramine typically results in a

decrease in enuretic episodes in 85% of cases within the first 2 weeks of treatment (Shaffer, 1977). However, only approximately one-half of all children will show a complete or nearly complete reduction in bedwetting episodes with imipramine (Gross & Dornbusch, 1983), and up to 95% relapse after medication is discontinued (Blackwell & Currah, 1973). Further, its negative side effects (e.g., sleep disturbance, tiredness, and gastrointestinal distress) can be significant (*Physicians' Desk Reference*, 1994). Cardiac irregularities can occur with doses higher than 3.5 mg/kg, requiring EKG monitoring. Overdoses of imipramine can be fatal.

Synthetic ADH, or DDAVP (desmopressin), has more recently emerged as the drug of choice for nocturnal enuresis. Available as an intranasally administered spray, it acts by concentrating urine, thereby reducing urine output from the kidney to the bladder. Its effects are immediate, and it has been shown to be reliably more effective than placebo. A review of 18 randomized, controlled trials of desmopressin found less wet nights as compared with placebo by proportions of 10 to 91% (Moffat et al., 1993). However, Moffat et al. also reported that, across studies, only 24.5% of subjects achieved short-term complete dryness. Moreover, in the three studies that reported long-term results, only 5.7% of subjects undergoing treatment with DDAVP achieved long-term dryness after discontinuing treatment. Although DDAVP is largely considered a remarkably safe medication, side effects such as headaches and abdominal pain have been noted (Moffat et al., 1993), as have rare instances of severe hyponatremia (sodium depletion in the blood) and hyponatremic seizures (Kallio, Rautava, Huupponen, & Korvenranta, 1993). Interestingly, some reports have suggested that DDAVP is far more effective for children with a family history of enuresis than for those without such a history (Hogg & Hussman, 1993; Miller, Goldberg, & Atkin, 1989).

Behavioral Treatment. Behavioral treatments for nocturnal enuresis have been in use since Mowrer and Mowrer popularized the bell-and-pad urine alarm in 1938. Since then a wide range of treatments have been investigated, including urine alarm treatment alone, urine alarm treatment plus a variety of added behavioral components, and behavioral treatment without a urine alarm.

Urine alarm systems have been extensively investigated. The typical system is made up of a pad that is placed underneath the sleeping child; wetness completes an electrical circuit, causing a loud alarm to go off. More recent devices do not use a pad, instead substituting a small absorbent strip that is placed in the child's pajamas or underwear. The mechanism by which such devices reduce enuresis is currently unclear. Original explanations were in terms of classical conditioning: Awakening and/or contraction of the muscles of the pelvic floor (the conditioned response) in response to a full bladder (the conditioned stimulus) resulted from pairing a full bladder with the unconditioned stimulus of a loud alarm. More recent investigators have suggested that mild punishment or aversion is the principle at work: Children may learn to retain urine until morning or to awaken and urinate so as to avoid the noxious stimulus of the alarm (Walker, Milling, & Bonner, 1988).

Rates of cessation of enuresis have typically been reported to be in the 70 to 90% range, with most estimates averaging approximately 75% (Doleys, 1977, 1979). However, Houts et al. (1994) reported the overall effectiveness rate (complete dryness) for urine alarms alone to be 59% in their meta-analysis. Regardless, the effectiveness of such treatment is clear.

Reported relapse rates for urine alarm treatments are as high as 41%. However, subsequent retreatments for subjects who relapse can result in successful reconditioning in 68% of cases (Doleys, 1977), typically much more quickly than during the initial treatment phase. Further, two simple methods have been developed that have greatly reduced the relapse rate following successful conditioning. First, intermittent reinforcement schedules have been used in place of continuous schedules. That is, rather than presenting the alarm on all wetting incidents, it is presented on a variable and intermittent schedule. Although it appears to take longer to reach dryness using such variable negative reinforcement schedules, relapse rates are significantly lower when using this method (Finley, Wansley, & Blenkarn, 1977; Turner, Young, & Rachman, 1970).

A second technique for reducing relapse rates is overlearning, which involves having the child increase his or her fluid intake before bedtime while the alarm is still being used. Possibly through helping the child learn to have control with greater levels of bladder distension, such techniques have been shown to be effective in reducing relapse (Morgan, 1978; Taylor & Turner, 1975).

Despite their effectiveness, urine alarms often take between 5 and 12 weeks to produce cessation of enuresis. This span, combined with the difficulty of using urine alarms appropriately, makes this treatment difficult for some families, especially if other stressors are present. In an effort to increase effectiveness, obtain results more quickly, and reduce relapse rates, numerous behavioral components have been added to urine alarm treatment. These include rewards for dry nights, retention control training (in which children are rewarded for retaining larger and larger amounts of urine), overlearning, positive training in rapid awakening and appropriate toileting, and self-correction of wetting accidents in which the child washes him- or herself and changes the bedsheets. Two multicomponent treatment packages, Dry Bed Training (Azrin, Sneed, & Foxx, 1974) and Full Spectrum Home Training (Houts & Liebert, 1984), have been researched.

Dry bed training (Azrin & Besalel, 1979; Azrin et al., 1974) is an intensive program consisting of a urine alarm, retention control training, positive reinforcement for appropriate toileting, training in rapid awakening, and cleanliness training. Parents are trained to wake their children hourly; rewards are given for dryness and for voiding appropriately. If the child has wet the bed, a mild reprimand is given and multiple positive practice sessions take place in which the child practices getting out of bed and going to the toilet. This program was reported by Azrin to achieve nearly 100% success (e.g., Azrin et al., 1974). Other researchers have found it effective, but not to the degree reported by Azrin (e.g., Bollard & Nettlebeck, 1982; Doleys, Ciminero, Tollison, Williams, & Wells, 1977). Investigation of the components of dry bed training have suggested that the urine alarm is an essential and not an optional component (as suggested by Azrin and colleagues), that the waking schedule is the most important addition to the urine alarm, and that the chief advantage of dry bed training over basic urine alarm treatment is the speed at which dryness is acquired (Scott et al., 1992). Relapse does not appear to be significantly different from that of standard urine alarm treatment (Scott et al., 1992).

Full spectrum home training includes the use of a urine alarm, retention control training, overlearning, and cleanliness training (Houts & Liebert, 1984). A chart in the child's bedroom includes instructions and a record of wet and dry nights. The child is instructed to change the bedding after every wetting episode, and is also rewarded for retaining urine during daily retention control training sessions. Overlearning was originally achieved using Young and Morgan's (1972) procedure of having the child drink large amounts of liquid each night. Later research, however, has suggested that a method of gradual increases in prebedtime liquid intake is more successful in reducing relapse (Scott et al., 1992). Success rates with full spectrum home training have been approximately 80%, at times with only one session of direct therapist contact in a group format (Houts, Liebert, & Padre, 1983). Relapse has been approximately 20%, a significant improvement over the 40% relapse rate of basic urine alarm treatment. Interestingly, it appears that the addition of overlearning decreases short-term effectiveness but also decreases relapse rates (Houts, Peterson, & Whelan, 1986). Some evidence has suggested that retention control training does add to treatment effectiveness, but only for children with small FBCs (Geffken, Bennett-Johnson, & Walker, 1986).

Numerous studies have investigated the success of behavioral interventions without the use of a urine alarm (e.g., dry bed training without an alarm, retention control training). Such methods have been found to be less effective than the same treatment with the urine alarm, both for dry bed training (Scott et al., 1992) and for retention control training (Walker, 1995). A meta-analysis of the enuresis outcome literature suggests that such methods alone have an effectiveness rate of approximately 36% (Houts et al., 1994). However, many clinicians experienced in treating enuresis prefer to begin treatment with the use of minimal behavioral reinforcers such as sticker charts, and add components such as urine alarms if the child does not respond.

Other Treatments. Hypnosis, individual psychotherapy, and family therapy have all been utilized in treating enuresis. Hypnosis as a primary intervention for enuresis is not frequently reported in the treatment literature, despite excellent results in the few published studies that exist. Olness (1975) reported that 31 of 40 children ceased bedwetting, most of them within the first month of treatment, using a self-hypnosis procedure. Similarly, Collison (1970) used hypnotic interventions and reported that 9 of 11 cases (most of them children) were dry at follow-up. Banerjee, Srivastav, and Palan (1993) reported hypnosis and imipramine to be equally effective for children over 7 years of age after 3 months of treatment; imipramine was more effective for children 7 or younger, whereas hypnosis was significantly more effective than imipramine at 9-month follow-up. More research is clearly needed to further explore this promising intervention.

In contrast, less specific psychotherapeutic interventions such as individual or family therapy have not proven effective. Such therapies have not been shown to be more effective than no-treatment control conditions (Lovibond,

1964; Novick, 1966) or other active forms of treatment (DeLeon & Mandell, 1966).

Nocturnal Enuresis Treatment Summary

Nocturnal enuresis is clearly a treatable disorder, although a significant proportion of treated cases either relapse or fail to respond at all. Comparisons of the various treatment techniques can be difficult; Houts et al. (1994) highlighted the fact that success in urine-alarm studies is typically reported as percentage of children reaching a criterion of 14 consecutive dry nights, whereas pharmacological studies most often report percentage reduction in enuretic episodes. In their meta-analysis, Houts et al. (1994) converted all studies to a common metric and controlled for investigator allegiance (measured via examinations of the introduction sections of the studies). They reported, overall, the highest success rates for psychological treatment using urine alarms, although the difference between such treatment and DDAVP was not significant at posttreatment. Urine alarm treatment did show a significantly higher efficacy rate than medical treatment (tricyclics or DDAVP) at follow-up (see Table 1).

In the only direct comparison of DDAVP and urine alarm treatment, similar results were found: DDAVP was found to be less effective at posttreatment, although the difference was not statistically significant (Wille, 1986). However, at follow-up, those in the urine alarm treatment condition remained dry at a significantly higher rate. Thus, it seems clear that urine alarm treatment may be superior in the long-term management of enuresis. Wille (1986) noted, however, that DDAVP is significantly faster in producing increased dryness than the urine alarm and is relatively free of side effects. For very short-term needs (e.g., a family vacation or summer camp), DDAVP may be a useful intervention.

Houts et al. (1994) also examined the various components of psychological therapy in their meta-analysis. Urine alarms emerged as the single most effective treatment component. Although adding additional components to urine

Table 1. Percentage of Children Who Ceased Bedwetting for Different Categories of Treatment

Treatment	N of groups	% of Ceased bedwetting		
		M	SD	Adjusted M[a]
Posttreatment				
Psychological				
With urine alarm	46	66	25	60$_a$
Without urine alarm	16	31	26	34$_b$
Tricyclics	28	40	14	39$_b$
Desmopressin	4	46	12	46$_a$
Other medications	9	23	25	25$_b$
Follow-up				
Psychological				
With urine alarm	30	51	21	44$_a$
Without urine alarm	11	21	26	26$_b$
Tricyclics	12	17	18	18$_b$
Desmopressin	3	22	17	21$_b$
Other medications	5	13	10	17$_b$

Note: Reprinted with permission from Houts, Berman, and Abramsom (1994).
[a]Means adjusted for investigator allegiance. Adjusted means with different subscripts at posttreatment and adjusted means with different subscripts at follow-up differ reliably ($p \leq .05$) from one another. Tests from the analysis of covariance were based on pooled $MS_e = 366.9$ ($df = 55$) at follow-up.

alarm treatment did result in greater efficacy, the difference between urine alarm treatment with and without other procedures was nonsignificant both at posttreatment and at follow-up (Houts et al., 1994). Nevertheless, the addition of various procedures (e.g., waking schedules, overlearning) to urine alarm treatment is relatively simple, and has been shown in some studies to speed acquisition of dryness and reduce relapse (e.g., Houts et al., 1983, 1986).

Diurnal Enuresis

The literature on treatment of functional diurnal enuresis is sparse. As previously noted, Schmitt (1982) suggested categorizing children based on whether their incontinence appears to be caused by inadequate perception of bladder distension, sudden urination in response to stressors, or simple unwillingness to toilet appropriately. For children with urgency incontinence, training in the recognition of and control over the need to urinate is crucial. For children who respond to stressors with urination, training in sphincter contraction rather than relaxation in response to feared stimuli may be very helpful. For children who are capa-

ble of withholding but choose not to, a simple system of rewards for appropriate voiding may be effective (Schmitt, 1982). Although such suggestions may appear intuitively valid, there is a dearth of appropriate outcome studies of children with diurnal enuresis.

CASE STUDY 1

Jay was a 7-year-old boy who had never achieved nighttime continence. He wet the bed an average of 4 days per week, but had been essentially continent in the daytime for several years. No other significant behavior problems were present, other than some mild academic difficulties. His developmental history was unremarkable except for mild hypoxia at birth and a delay in acquiring speech. His biological father reportedly had wet the bed until age 9.

During one of two evaluation sessions, Jay's mother and stepfather reported that they differ in how they regard his bedwetting; his mother felt he would simply grow out of it, whereas his stepfather saw the bedwetting as laziness and removed privileges following enuretic episodes. Both parents changed the sheets when they were wet and used fluid restriction prior to bedtime. Further assessment using Morgan and Young's (1975) scale of parental perceptions of enuresis revealed both that it had become a significant source of distress for the family, and that conflict in how to deal with it was exacerbating the situation.

A crucial first step in working with this family was to alleviate the distress and conflict surrounding Jay's enuresis. The involuntary nature, prevalence, and difficulties associated with enuresis were explained to the family in detail; they were helped to see that their situation was common and understandable, and that no one (especially Jay) needed to feel responsible for the bedwetting.

Second, the family was given a clear rationale for why urine alarm treatment worked: They were told that bladder control at night is a complex and difficult skill, and that it is a wonder more children do not have difficulty learning it. The urine alarm was framed as a device for helping children learn to wake up when their bladder is full (Morgan, 1974). They were told that treatment typically took up to 12 weeks and that temporary relapses were common. They were then asked to purchase a urine alarm (a version of which is available from Palco Laboratories, 8030 Soquel Ave., Santa Cruz, CA 95062) and to make a wall chart with which to record wet and dry nights. A system of rewards for dry nights was used to invest Jay in the treatment program. The parents were instructed to sleep nearby for the first week to ensure that Jay woke up in response to the alarm (children with poor arousability may need training in going from sleep to waking quickly, and/or additional measures such as shaking to help the alarm become a stimulus for waking). They were told to have him change his sheets and practice appropriate voiding following any wetting episodes. He was rewarded if he was able to at least partially void in the toilet during these exercises.

Jay began to show significant decreases in wet nights within 3 weeks of treatment. When he was down to approximately 1 wet night per week, overlearning was initiated. Based on the system described by Scott et al. (1992), he was asked to drink 4 ounces of water 15 minutes before bedtime. This amount was then increased by 2 ounces for every two consecutive dry nights, up to a maximum of 9 ounces (Berger, Maizels, Moran, Conway, & Firlit, 1983).

The family showed an almost immediate decrease in distress with the normalization of their situation and the promise of relief. Additionally, Jay reached the criterion of 14 consecutive dry nights within 6 weeks. He remained dry at 6-month follow-up.

ENCOPRESIS

Introduction

Encopresis, or fecal incontinence, accounts for approximately 3% of all pediatric medicine outpatient visits (Levine, 1975) and approximately 25% of all pediatric gastroenterology clinic visits (Taitz, Wales, Urwin, & Molnar, 1986). It occurs during the day more often than at night, and is thus markedly more socially evident than enuresis. However, research on encopresis lags behind that of enuresis in terms of both quantity and quality.

Phenomenology

Encopresis, carrying even more social stigma than enuresis, can be a significant source of distress for both parents and children (Becker, 1994; Fireman & Koplewicz, 1992; Walker et al., 1978). This distress is evident in terms of both self-esteem (Landman, Rappaport, Fenton, & Levine, 1986) and behavior/emotional problems (Buchanan & Clayden, 1992; Gabel, Hegedus, Wald, Chandra,& Chiponis, 1986). Parents may present as overwhelmed and frustrated, and often feel that their child could be continent if he or she wished; punishment for soiling episodes is commonly reported. In contrast, encopretic children may appear indifferent to their problem. They are often unaware of the foul odor they carry, and insist that they have no control over their bowel functions. However, a majority are in fact eager to be continent (Landman et al., 1986).

The social stigma of fecal soiling and the belief of parents that it is simply a problem of inadequate motivation combine to greatly reduce the willingness of parents to bring a child's encopresis to the attention of a health care provider. Direct questioning as part of a comprehensive intake is often necessary to elicit information about fecal soiling (Walker et al., 1988).

Fecal soiling is most often reported as occurring during the daytime, and can range in frequency from once per month to several times per day or more (Walker et al., 1988). The typical soiling episode involves relatively small amounts of a yellowish, pasty, and foul-smelling material, but occasionally involves huge amounts of very dark stool. In addition, encopretic children tend to have infrequent bowel movements that are hard, dark, and often bloody, and many show reluctance to use the toilet.

Diagnosis

The DSM-IV (APA, 1994) defines encopresis as the passage of feces in inappropriate places such as in clothing or on the floor. This elimination of feces may be involuntary or intentional, and must: (1) be by a child with a chronological or developmental age of at least 4 years; (2) occur at least once a month for a minimum of 3 months; and (3) be functional, or not related to the direct effect of a general medical condition. The DSM-IV further requires that the presence or absence of constipation with overflow incontinence be indicated.

Although not included in the DSM-IV, specification of subtypes of encopresis has proven to be crucial in making treatment decisions. Walker (1978) identified three general subtypes of encopresis: retentive (resulting from constipation and overflow incontinence), manipulative (intentional soiling for secondary gain), and stress-related (anxiety-induced and diarrhetic). In reference to the DSM-IV, manipulative and stress-related encopresis can be seen as subtypes of encopresis not related to constipation with overflow incontinence.

It has been estimated that 80–95% of encopretic children are chronically constipated, and are classified as having constipation with overflow incontinence (or retentive encopresis). Retentive encopresis will thus be discussed first, and in most detail.

Etiology of Retentive Encopresis

As with enuresis, etiological theories of retentive encopresis fall into three general categories: biological, emotional, and learning. Dietary and behavioral factors also appear to be involved. Following a description of the physiological process of elimination and how constipation can paradoxically result in fecal incontinence, the evidence for and against each approach to the understanding of retentive encopresis will be reviewed.

Physiology of Retentive Encopresis

Children become constipated for a number of reasons, including inadequate intake of dietary fiber, underhydration, a hereditary tendency toward constipation, neurological and/or endocrine abnormalities, and voluntary withholding of stools (see below for a more detailed discussion). Once constipation develops in children, it can quickly become chronic, as the child becomes progressively less responsive to internal cues. This process is facilitated by stretching of the bowel walls, which causes the muscles of the colon to become flaccid, weak, and unresponsive. Thus, the child becomes insensitive to cues, which gradually decrease in intensity (Meunier, Mollard, & Marechal, 1976); simultaneously, the colon loses the muscle tone necessary to expel stools. Chronic constipation can result in discomfort and lethargy, reducing the child's activity level and thus further exacerbating the condition (Christopherson & Rapoff, 1992).

In this manner, dry, hard fecal material can become firmly impacted or lodged in the colon. As a result, the colon becomes enlarged and the tissue stretched relatively thin, a condition known as *psychogenic megacolon*. The impaction prevents liquid wastes proximal to it from passing through the colon normally so that nutrients can be absorbed and solid waste formed into stools. Instead, this liquid collects in a pool above the impaction and seeps around it, causing a pasty stain in the clothing of the child. As this is an entirely passive process, children are in fact quite correct when they state that they were unaware of the need to defecate and that they had no control over the soiling. Occasionally, the impaction itself may suddenly become loosened and the child may have a spontaneous and extremely large bowel movement.

Such impactions are a significant health hazard warranting active and aggressive treatment (Walker, 1978). Fortunately, the colon can regain its muscle tone and sensitivity after the impaction has been removed and normal elimination has been reestablished. Dietary fiber and liquids are crucial in this process, and inadequate amounts of both of these are a clear contributor to constipation (Christopherson & Rapoff, 1992; Murray, 1994; Walker, 1995). Other possible etiological factors can be categorized as biological, emotional, and learning.

Biological Theories of Retentive Encopresis

Encopresis by definition excludes fecal incontinence related to the direct effect of a general medical condition. However, the possibility exists that "functional" soiling is actually the result of a medical condition not yet clearly recognized. Constipation can indeed be caused by a wide range of biological factors, including anatomical abnormalities, endocrine disorders, and neurological disorders. Whether or not most cases of encopresis are related to such factors is the issue of interest, along with whether or not the presence of physiological abnormalities necessitates the use of surgical or pharmacological interventions. Current estimates suggest that clear medical causes for fecal soiling can be found only in 2 to 15% of children with bowel problems (Liebman, 1979; Schmitt, 1984).

One theory is that chronic constipation and the resultant overflow incontinence primarily reflects a genetic predisposition to such difficulties. In one of the few studies in this area, Bakwin and Davidson (1971) found concordance rates for constipation in monozygotic twins to be six times greater than in dizygotic twins. Pettei and Davidson (1991) reported that a significant proportion of constipated children showed evidence of infrequent bowel movements in the first 6 months of life. Further, some investigators have noted poor health as an infant to be associated with later encopresis (Buchanan & Clayden, 1992), and that encopresis can be linked to developmental delays and neurological impairment (Bemporad, Pfeifer, Gibbs, Cortner, & Bloom, 1971). Difficulties for this theory include inconsistencies in the evidence that genetic predispositions are primary in the development of constipation (Doleys, 1981), and the lack of an agreed-upon mechanism by which such effects might occur (Houts & Abramson, 1990).

Recent research, however, has suggested that some encopretic children do show specific abnormalities in the physiological mechanisms of defecation. Anorectal manometry is a technique used to measure the point at which rectal distention is perceived, resting sphincter tone, and sphincter tone during defecation attempts. It is most often performed via an apparatus made up of three consecutive inflatable balloons that is inserted in the rectum. The most consistently supported specific abnormality found in encopretic children is a paradoxical tightening of the external sphincter during defecation. Numerous studies have shown that from 43 to 78% of constipated children contract rather than relax the external anal sphincter during defecation attempts (Keren, Wagner, Heldenberg, & Golan, 1988; Loening-Baucke & Cruikshank, 1986; Wald, Chandra, Chiponis, & Gabel, 1986). Although such contractions during defecation attempts undoubtedly contribute to retentive encopresis, it is unclear whether they represent neurological dysfunction or learned behavior (as the external sphincter is under voluntary control).

A second specific abnormality identified during manometric studies is an increased threshold of perceived distention in constipated and encopretic children (Loening-Baucke & Cruikshank, 1986; Meunier, Marechal, & de-Beaujeu, 1979; Molnar, Taitz, Urwin, & Wales, 1983). Such an increased threshold for the perception of distention could result in failure to adequately recognize the need for a bowel movement, thus leading to constipation and encopresis. However, some controlled studies have found no such abnormalities in the thresholds of encopretic children (Keren et al., 1988; Wald et al., 1986). Further, where such abnormalities exist, it is unclear whether they are the result of neurological abnormalities or simple adaptation.

Poor resting internal anal sphincter tone has also been reported in some constipated and encopretic children (Loening-Baucke, 1984; Loening-Baucke & Younoszai, 1984), which could result in failure to prevent fecal material from leaking inappropriately. In contrast to these findings, Wald et al. (1986) found no differences in resting sphincter tone between encopretic and continent children.

Emotional Theories of Retentive Encopresis

As with enuresis, many psychodynamically oriented theorists have suggested that encopresis is a symptom of underlying conflict

(Lifshitz & Chovers, 1972; Silber, 1969). Other authors have suggested that family conflict, coercive toilet training, or general psychopathology in the child may be the cause of soiling (Amsterdam, 1979; Bemporad, 1978; Ringdahl, 1980). It does appear that encopretic children exhibit more emotional and behavior problems than continent children (Abrahamian & Lloyd-Still, 1984; Gabel et al., 1986; Landman et al., 1986). However, these problems are less severe than those in children referred for mental health services, and are as likely to be a result as a cause of the encopresis (Abrahamian & Lloyd-Still, 1984; Gabel et al., 1986). Psychotherapy focusing on underlying conflict, emotional issues, and/or relationships has not been proven effective in treating retentive encopresis (Achenbach & Lewis, 1971; Berg & Jones, 1964; Doleys, Schwartz, & Ciminero, 1981). However, psychotherapeutic techniques may be more applicable to manipulative and stress-related encopresis, and may have an indirect role in retentive encopresis.

Learning Theories of Retentive Encopresis

Learning theorists suggest that retentive encopresis may be a result of one of two learning principles. First, pain during defecation, unsanitary or less than private school bathrooms, a lack of confidence in one's toileting skills, or simple unwillingness to stop a more pleasant activity can all result in learned avoidance of defecation. This avoidance is further strengthened by the large and painful nature of the infrequent bowel movements that follow prolonged withholding. Withholding stools eventually leads to constipation and soiling.

A second possible cause of retentive encopresis is a failure to acquire the discriminative and behavioral skills necessary for a successful bowel movement. Stated most simply, the cues of rectal distention simply may not have become discriminative for appropriate defecation in the toilet. This, coupled with the fact that the child may have difficulty with the mechanics of toileting (e.g., opening the bathroom door, undoing clothes, sitting on a toilet designed for adults,

and so on) may result in "accidental" soiling of clothes.

The many cases of encopresis for which no medical cause can be found can easily be understood in this way. Further, the consistent finding that encopretic children actually contract rather than relax external anal sphincter muscles during attempts at defecation supports this notion: They could be voluntarily withholding, or their sphincters could be contracting involuntarily as a classically conditioned response following the association of defecation with aversive stimuli.

Interestingly, either medical conditions (e.g., anal fissures) or emotional difficulties (e.g., anxiety or depression) can be seen as indirect contributors to retentive encopresis with learning as the mechanism. A child could learn to avoid defecation following painful experiences that were the direct result of medical conditions such as perianal fissures. Further, overly anxious children could be predisposed to withholding because of inordinate fears, and depressed children might be predisposed to constipation as a result of inactivity.

Epidemiology

Estimates of the prevalence of encopresis vary, in large part because of differences in populations studied and definitions of encopresis used. No current studies separate retentive from other forms of encopresis. Estimates of overall prevalence average approximately 2 to 3% for 7- to 8-year-olds (Bellman, 1966; Levine, 1975; Yates, 1970). Incidence drops to approximately 1.5% by age 10–12 (Rutter, Tizard, & Whitmore, 1970). Boys are four to five times more likely to be encopretic than girls at all ages (Bellman, 1966; Rutter et al., 1970).

Assessment of Encopresis

Medical

Medical evaluation is a crucial first step in the assessment of an encopretic child, given the possibility that a significant medical condition may exist. No agreed-upon guidelines exist as to what a standard encopresis evaluation should entail, nor is there agreement as to the value of the many possible procedures (Houts & Abramson, 1990). Most physicians will perform a thorough history and physical, including a rectal examination, palpation for fecal masses, testing for occult blood in the stool, and urinalysis in females, given the likelihood of concomitant urinary tract infections. More invasive procedures such as anorectal manometry, radiological studies, and rectal biopsies may or may not be performed, depending on the physician's approach and the presence of warning signs. Typical conditions to be ruled out via medical evaluation include Hirschsprung's disease (inadequate innervation of colonic segments), hypothyroidism (which may result in inadequate peristalsis), and anorectal abnormalities (e.g., anal stenosis or fissures).

Psychological

Psychological assessment should be broad and multifaceted (Walker & Shaw, 1988). A general clinical interview of the parent or parents is required to assess their level of frustration, their reactions to soiling episodes, the child's developmental history (especially with regard to toilet training), marital/relationship problems within the home, environmental stressors, family medical and psychiatric history, potential for compliance, and medication usage. Further, the parents may be asked to complete a detailed diary of toileting and elimination behavior, including number of self-initiated visits to the toilet, parental response to appropriate toileting behavior as well as to soiling episodes, the time of day of all such behavior, and diet. A primary goal of such an interview is to determine if the child's soiling is retentive, manipulative, or stress-related, and if the child has been incontinent all of his or her life, or if he or she suddenly became incontinent. An evaluation of other behavior problems is also necessary. The use of standardized behavior checklists may be helpful in this.

The child should be interviewed thoroughly as well. Of special interest is whether or not he or she is aware of the need to defecate, and whether or not fear of pain or phobias of public bathrooms or other stimuli are present. The child should also be asked for help in developing a list of potential rewards. The extent of the child's toileting skills can be determined via a direct interview, through the use of dolls or drawings, and/or by an interview with the parent(s).

Treatment

The treatment outcome research with encopresis is decades behind that of enuresis (Houts & Abramson, 1990). Greatly complicating the formation of conclusions based on this literature is the failure of most researchers to separate subtypes of encopretics or to use dismantling strategies to study treatment methods in isolation. There is a great need for research that examines the effectiveness of specific techniques with retentive, manipulative, and stress-related encopretics separately.

Three primary treatment methods have shown effectiveness with retentive encopresis; all have the goal of reducing fecal retention and increasing appropriate toileting. These methods have been studied both singly and in combination.

Medical Treatment

A commonly used form of treatment for retentive encopresis is laxative and purgative therapy, the goal of which is to remove any impaction and establish regular bowel movements (Berg & Jones, 1964; Murray, 1994; Parker & Whitehead, 1982). The establishment of regular bowel movements in this manner is meant to allow the colon to regain its normal size and muscle tone, increasing the child's ability to defecate on his or her own and decreasing the possibility of further impaction (Murray, 1994). The decreased size and increased softness of stools also serve to reduce pain and fear associated with having bowel movements (Walker, 1995). As oral laxatives are sometimes ineffective in removing impactions (instead simply causing pain and increased overflow incontinence), purgatives such as enemas and suppositories are frequently used when severe impactions are present. Once the impaction is removed, stool softeners and laxatives such as mineral oil and dietary fiber are used, sometimes for up to a year or longer before being gradually faded out (Abrahamian & Lloyd-Still, 1984; Behrman, Vaughan, & Nelson, 1987; Murray, 1994). As mineral oil tends to inhibit the absorption of fat-soluble vitamins, it should be taken 1–3 hours after meals, and vitamin supplements should be added to the diet. Although there has been some concern about laxative dependence following such treatment (Houts & Abramson, 1990; Schaefer, 1979), evidence seems to suggest that dependence does not typically occur (Murray, 1994). The nutritional safety of such programs has been documented (McClung et al., 1993).

The effectiveness of medical treatments alone with retentive encopresis has not been thoroughly studied. Investigations of medical management typically include a mixed group of encopretics, and also frequently include supportive counseling and scheduled toilet sittings. Of four studies of purgative/laxative treatment alone with retentive encopretics, initial success rates range from 38 to 84%, with most averaging approximately 70% (Abrahamian & Lloyd-Still, 1984; Berg & Jones, 1964; Loening-Baucke & Cruikshank, 1986). The only long-term follow-up done reported that 47% of the children treated in this manner remained symptom-free 5 years later; 36% had only minor symptoms, which were controlled with intermittent use of laxatives, and none were laxative dependent (Abrahamian & Lloyd-Still, 1984).

Biofeedback

Biofeedback has also been used successfully with retentive encopresis, although most studies using biofeedback are of children with fecal incontinence secondary to medical conditions (Cerulli, Nikoomanesh, & Schuster, 1979; Ker-

en et al., 1988; Whitehead, Parker, Masek, Cataldo, & Freeman, 1981). In an excellent study comparing biofeedback plus conventional treatment (purgatives, laxatives, scheduled toilet sittings, and supportive counseling) versus conventional treatment alone, Loening-Baucke (1990) found biofeedback to add significantly to conventional treatment. At 12-month follow-up, 16% of children treated with conventional treatment alone and 50% of children treated with conventional treatment plus biofeedback were symptom-free. Normal defecation dynamics (e.g., relaxing rather than contracting the external anal sphincter during defecation attempts) were correlated with treatment success (Loening-Baucke, 1990).

Behavioral Treatment

Some investigators have used behavioral treatments alone with retentive encopretics. Most protocols involve some combination of education, reinforcement for appropriate toileting, scheduled toilet sittings, and regular pants checks with positive reinforcement for clean pants and mild punishment for soiled pants. A number of single case studies have reported cessation of soiling using such techniques (Bach & Moyland, 1975; Conger, 1970; Neale, 1963; Rolider & Van Houten, 1985). The only group study in this area found that 36% of retentive encopretics treated with behavioral methods alone were symptom-free at 12 months (Nolan, Debelle, Oberklaid, & Coffey, 1991).

Combined Behavioral and Medical Treatment

A number of studies have utilized complex combinations of behavioral techniques and laxatives with retentive encopretics, most including an initial clean-out phase as well. For example, Fireman and Koplewicz (1992) evaluated a short-term treatment protocol using an initial cleanout phase (using purgatives or laxatives), education, scheduled toilet sittings, diet modifications, rewards for appropriate toileting and for no soiling, cleanliness training (the child being responsible for cleaning soiled clothes), penalties for soiling, and laxatives or suppositories if the child was unable to defecate. Of the 52 children studied, 44 were retentive. The authors found that 84.6% of children were symptom-free posttreatment, and that 78.8% were still symptom-free after a 7-week-phaseout period. Wright (1975) reported nearly 100% success using an initial cleanout phase, education, reinforcers for appropriate toileting, scheduled toilet sittings, suppositories and enemas, dietary changes, rewards for clean underpants, and mild punishments for soiling episodes. Stark and colleagues used a short-term therapy group for retentive encopretics; it included behavioral methods and a cleanout phase, and placed special emphasis on fiber intake in lieu of laxatives (Stark, Owens-Stively, Spirito, Lewis, & Guevremont, 1990). They reported that only 2 of 18 children were soiling by the end of a 6-week treatment phase, and that those 2 responded completely to additional therapy. Notably, this study included only children who had previously failed standard medical therapy.

Other studies have reported similar results with combined programs (Davidson, Kugler, & Bauer, 1963; Houts, Mellon, & Whelan, 1988; Houts & Peterson, 1986; Nolan et al., 1991). Several other large-scale investigations have found success rates of only approximately 50% (e.g., Levine & Bakow, 1976; Taitz et al., 1986), but these appear to have used mixed groups of retentive and nonretentive encopretics. Overall, such programs appear to be highly effective when used with retentive encopretics; further, children who initially fail to respond to other methods have been shown to frequently become continent when treatment using combined methods is employed (Walker, 1978).

Unfortunately, very little research has investigated which components of combined treatments are most important. In an excellent review of the encopresis treatment literature, Houts and Abramson (1990) suggested that positive reinforcement for appropriate toileting is an important component of most treatment packages. Research by Stark, Spirito, et al. (1990) and by

Houts and colleagues (Houts et al., 1988; Houts & Peterson, 1986) suggests that high fiber intake is an effective alternative to mineral oil or other laxatives. Berg, Forsythe, Holt, and Watts (1983) reported that laxative use did not add to the effectiveness of behavioral treatment. Similarly, Nolan et al. (1991) found that cleanout with purgatives and subsequent laxative use only added to treatment effectiveness with less compliant subjects; they did not add to effectiveness for more compliant subjects. However, most research and extensive clinical experience suggests that clearing of the colon (whether by diet or laxative), along with behavioral interventions, is necessary for effective treatment. Research on biofeedback with encopretic children suggests that it may be a valuable addition to treatment when abnormal defecation dynamics are present (Loening-Baucke, 1990).

Other Treatments

As with enuresis, a small number of investigators have reported successful treatment of encopresis using hypnosis. Olness (1976) used self-hypnosis with four preschoolers who had not responded to medical interventions; three of the four were able to achieve continence. Other researchers have reported similar results (e.g., Goldsmith, 1962; Tilton, 1980). Although these results are promising, more systematic and controlled research is needed.

Various individual and family therapies have also been explored as interventions for encopresis in children. Individual psychotherapy has not been shown to be more effective than no treatment (Achenbach & Lewis, 1971; Berg & Jones, 1964; Doleys et al., 1981). Family therapy, investigated more recently (e.g., Wells & Hinkle, 1990), has not been proven useful without the addition of behavioral, dietary, and/or medical components (Walker, 1995).

CASE STUDY 2

Susan was a 6-year-old girl who had been soiling at least once per day almost continually since birth; the frequency of soiling had not decreased, despite nearly constant attempts at convincing her to use the toilet appropriately. Manometric studies performed by a pediatric gastroenterologist showed that her sphincter strength was normal, and plain radiograph revealed a substantial amount of fecal material in her colon. In all respects, results of her physical examination were normal and her physician was confident that all possible medical causes of her current constipation and soiling had been ruled out.

During one of two evaluation sessions, Susan's mother reported that both she and her daughter were becoming very frustrated, especially as there appeared to be "no reason" for the soiling. It became clear that Susan was experiencing significant anxiety and pain with toileting, and that the soiling had begun to impact her social functioning and self-esteem. Her knowledge of toileting skills was adequate, and no significant behavior problems were evident.

It seemed clear that Susan had learned to retain stools and fear toileting because of early experiences with large and painful bowel movements, and that the withholding she developed as a result had prevented the extinction of that fear. This conceptualization was explained clearly to all parties involved, so as to decrease frustration and blame and to provide a framework for the amelioration of Susan's soiling. The physiology of retentive encopresis was explained to Susan and her mother, and a full behavioral and medical treatment plan was developed. It was strongly emphasized in a positive way to the patient's mother that there was every reason to believe that the problem could be eliminated, but that consistency was of utmost importance. She appeared to understand and was eager to continue.

With the help of her physician, Susan underwent a thorough cleanout via two consecutive daily enemas and a cup per night of Goletely (an oral cathartic that the physician felt could be effective even in the presence of impaction). High amounts of dietary fiber were worked into her diet, along with an increase in fluids (especially fruit juices) and a decrease in amount of dairy products (which can have a constipatory effect). Such dietary changes were framed for Susan and her parents as permanent and important changes in her eating habits.

The behavioral program developed for her followed that outlined in a previously tested protocol (Calkins, Walker, & Howe, 1994; Walker et al., 1988). Susan helped develop a list of reinforcers, which were wrapped and put in a basket in the bathroom. She earned a prize for producing stool at regularly scheduled toilet sittings four times per day.

At the end of each day, Susan's clothing was examined for soiling. If she had soiled (or if soiling at any other time of day occurred), she had to actively participate in cleaning herself and her clothes. If she had not soiled, she was given a reward. Her success at the regular toilet sittings and at the nightly soiling check was charted daily, with Susan's help. The therapist monitored Susan's progress via weekly return visits or phone contacts.

Susan showed significant improvement in 3 weeks. The program was maintained for a total of 14 weeks, at which point Susan had demonstrated 8 consecutive weeks of appropriate toileting without soiling. A graduation ceremony was held in which the reward system was officially discontinued, her success was celebrated and praised, and an activity of her choice (going to her favorite restaurant) took place. At 6-month follow-up, there had been no further episodes of soiling, and Susan's social functioning had improved dramatically.

MANIPULATIVE SOILING

Soiling used for manipulative purposes has not been studied in any depth, perhaps in part because of its relative rarity (Walker, 1995).

Following evaluation by a physician, a thorough functional analysis will typically reveal any manipulativeness in a child's soiling. Warning signs include initiation of soiling when angry or not receiving attention, threats by the child that he or she will soil, no evidence of constipation or diarrhea, and apparent secondary gain such as being taken home when a test is being given at school.

Treatment techniques for the child who uses soiling in a manipulative way have not been systematically evaluated. However, typical family counseling, emotional expression, and behavioral techniques appear to generalize well (Walker et al., 1988). The child should be encouraged to find more acceptable ways of expressing him or herself, and the parent should be helped to respond in an appropriate manner to soiling episodes. All possible sources of reinforcement for soiling behavior should be eliminated.

DIARRHEA-RELATED ENCOPRESIS

Physical examinations of children with chronic diarrhea who soil in response to stress may include anorectal manometry to rule out poor sphincter tone as a causative factor. Conditions causing chronic diarrhea, such as inflammatory bowel disease and infections, should also be ruled out.

In most cases it is clear that the child soils when directly confronted with a feared stimulus or when under increased general stress. Diarrhea is almost always present in such children, who insist that they are unable to control their soiling. They remain continent when not experiencing any significant or sudden anxiety.

Treatment techniques for children with chronic diarrhea who soil in response to stress have not been systematically evaluated. However, a combination of decreasing the diarrhea, increasing anal sphincter control, and reducing the effects of stress on the child appears indicated (Walker et al., 1988). Some studies have reported success using systematic desensitization in treating chronic diarrhea (Cohen & Reed, 1968; Hedberg, 1973). In vivo exposure to stressful situations, paired with relaxation of skeletal muscles and contraction of anal sphincters, may be a fruitful treatment technique for these children. Also helpful are standard treatment techniques such as stress inoculation training (Meichenbaum, 1977), relaxation training (Walker, Hedberg, Clement, & Wright, 1981), and assertiveness training (Walker et al., 1981). The specific treatment techniques selected should vary depending on the particular characteristics of the case (Walker et al., 1988).

SUMMARY

Elimination disorders are among the more common and treatable disorders that health care professionals are faced with. Despite this, a great deal of confusion surrounds enuresis and encopresis. This confusion is caused in large part by the use of the terms *enuresis* and *encopresis* to refer to incontinence related to medical conditions, a situation that is further exacerbated by the assertion that even "functional" elimination disorders are biogenic.

Although the etiology of enuresis and encopresis has yet to be clearly defined, it seems clear that a diathesis-stress model is highly applicable. Elimination disorders can be seen as the result of genetic predispositions toward polyuria, developmental delays, or constipation, in combination with stressors such as a poor diet, poor acquisition of toileting skills, or maladaptive contingencies.

Comprehensive behavioral treatments for both enuresis and encopresis have been shown to be safe and highly effective, *when* the presence of a general medical condition has been ruled out. However, primary care physicians are the providers most often sought out by parents with enuretic or encopretic children, and very few physicians are either trained in behavioral techniques or refer to behavioral practitioners. There is thus a clear need for a more active partnership between physicians and psychologists to ensure both a thorough consideration of all medical aspects involved, and the most effective treatment possible (Houts & Abramson, 1990).

An equally pressing need is outcome research, especially of encopresis, that clearly clarifies subtypes and that uses dismantling strategies to isolate which aspects of treatment are most effective, when, and for whom. Such research strategies will be crucial in the attempt to increase already high treatment effectiveness, reduce relapse, and decrease length of treatment.

ACKNOWLEDGEMENTS

The authors would like to thank James Allen, M.D., for his help with the pharmacological sections of this chapter.

REFERENCES

Abrahamian, F. P., & Lloyd-Still, J. D. (1984). Chronic constipation in childhood: A longitudinal study of 186 patients. *Journal of Pediatric Gastroenterology and Nutrition, 3*, 460–467.

Achenbach, T. M., & Lewis, M. (1971). A proposed model for clinical research and its application for encopresis and enuresis. *Journal of the American Academy of Child Psychiatry, 10*, 535–554.

American Academy of Pediatrics: Committee on Radiology. (1980). Excretory urography for evaluation of enuresis. *Pediatrics, 65*, 644–645.

American Psychiatric Association. (1994). *Diagnostic and statistical manual of mental disorders* (4th ed., rev.). Washington, DC: Author.

Amsterdam, B. (1979). Chronic encopresis: A system based psychodynamic approach. *Child Psychiatry and Human Development, 9*, 137–144.

Azrin, N. H., & Besalel, V. A. (1979). *Parent's guide to bedwetting control: A step-by-step method*. New York: Simon & Schuster.

Azrin, N. H., Sneed, T. J., & Foxx, R. M. (1974). Dry-bed training: Rapid elimination of childhood enuresis. *Behaviour Research and Therapy, 12*, 147–156.

Bach, R., & Moylan, J. J. (1975). Parents administer behavior therapy for inappropriate urination and encopresis: A case study. *Journal of Behavior Therapy and Experimental Psychiatry, 6*, 239–241.

Bakwin, H. (1973). The genetics of enuresis. *Clinics in Developmental Medicine, 48–49*, 73–77.

Bakwin, H., & Davidson, M. (1971). Constipation in twins. *American Journal of Diseases of Children, 121*, 179–181.

Banerjee, S., Srivastav, A., & Palan, B. M. (1993). Hypnosis and self-hypnosis in the management of nocturnal enuresis: A comparative study with imipramine therapy. *American Journal of Clinical Hypnosis, 36*, 113–119.

Becker, J. H. R. (1994). An approach to the treatment of encopresis. *Surgery Annual, 26*, 49–66.

Behrman, R. E., Vaughan, V. C., & Nelson, W. E. (1987). *Textbook of pediatrics* (13th ed.). Philadelphia: Saunders.

Bellman, M. (1966). Studies on encopresis. *Acta Paediatrica Scandinavica, 170*(Suppl.), 1–137.

Bemporad, J. R. (1978). Encopresis. In B. B. Wolman, J. Egan, & A. O. Ross (Eds.), *Handbook of treatment of mental disorders in childhood and adolescence* (pp. 161–178). Englewood Cliffs, NJ: Prentice–Hall.

Bemporad, J. R., Pfeifer, C. M., Gibbs, L., Cortner, R. H., & Bloom, W. (1971). Characteristics of encopretic patients and their families. *Journal of the American Academy of Child Psychiatry, 10*, 272–292.

Berg, I., Forsythe, I., Holt, P., & Watts, J. (1983). A controlled triad of Senokot in faecal soiling treated by behavioural methods. *Journal of Child Psychology and Psychiatry, 24*, 543–549.

Berg, I., & Jones, K. V. (1964). Functional faecal incontinence in children. *Archives of Disease in Childhood, 39*, 465–472.

Berger, R. M., Maizels, M., Moran, G. C., Conway, J. J., & Firlit, C. F. (1983). Bladder capacity (ounces) equals age (years) plus 2 predicts normal bladder capacity and aids in diagnosis of abnormal voiding patterns. *Journal of Urology, 129*, 347–349.

Blackwell, B., & Currah, J. (1973). The psychopharmacology of nocturnal enuresis. In I. Kolvin, R. C. MacKeith, & S. R. Meadow (Eds.), *Bladder control and enuresis* (pp. 231–257). Philadelphia: Lippincott.

Bollard, J., & Nettlebeck, T. (1982). A comparison analysis of dry-bed training for treatment of bedwetting. *Behaviour Research and Therapy, 20*, 383–390.

Boyd, M. M. (1960). The depth of sleep in enuretic school children and in non-enuretic controls. *Journal of Psychosomatic Research, 4*, 274–281.

Braithwaite, J. V. (1956). Some problems associated with enuresis. *Proceedings of the Royal Society of Medicine, 49*, 33–39.

Buchanan, A., & Clayden, G. (1992). *Children who soil: Assessment and treatment.* New York: Wiley.

Butler, R. J., Brewin, C. R., & Forsythe, W. I. (1986). Maternal attributions and tolerance for nocturnal enuresis. *Behaviour Research and Therapy, 24*, 307–312.

Calkins, D. L., Walker, C. E., & Howe, A. C. (1994). Elimination disorders: Psychological issues. In R. A. Olson, L. L. Mullins, J. B. Gillman, & J. M. Chaney (Eds.), *The sourcebook of pediatric psychology* (pp. 46–54). Boston: Allyn & Bacon.

Cerulli, M. A., Nikoomanesh, P., & Schuster, M. M. (1979). Progress in biofeedback conditioning for fecal incontinence. *Gastroenterology, 76*, 742–746.

Christopherson, E. R., & Rapoff, M. A. (1992). Toileting problems in children. In C. E. Walker & M. C. Roberts (Eds.), *Handbook of clinical child psychology* (2nd ed., pp. 399–411). New York: Wiley.

Cohen, S. I., & Reed, J. L. (1968). The treatment of nervous diarrhoea and other conditioned autonomic disorders by desensitization. *British Journal of Psychiatry, 114*, 1275–1280.

Collison, D. L. (1970). Hypnotherapy in the management of nocturnal enuresis. *Medical Journal of Australia, 1*, 52–54.

Conger, J. C. (1970). Treatment of encopresis by the management of social consequences. *Behavior Therapy, 1*, 386–309.

Davidson, M., Kugler, M. M., & Bauer, C. H. (1963). Diagnosis and management in children with severe and protracted constipation and obstipation. *Journal of Pediatrics, 62*, 261–275.

de Jonge, G. A. (1973). Epidemiology of enuresis: A survey of the literature. In I. Kolvin, R. C. MacKeith, & S. R. Meadow (Eds.), *Bladder control and enuresis* (pp. 39–46). Philadelphia: Lippincott.

DeLeon, G., & Mandell, W. (1966). A comparison of conditioning and psychotherapy in the treatment of functional enuresis. *Journal of Clinical Psychology, 22*, 326–330.

Doleys, D. M. (1977). Behavioral treatments for nocturnal enuresis in children: A review of the recent literature. *Psychological Bulletin, 84*, 30–54.

Doleys, D. M. (1979). Assessment and treatment of childhood encopresis. In A. J. Finch & P. C. Kendall (Eds.), *Treatment and research in child psychopathology* (pp. 185–205). New York: Spectrum.

Doleys, D. M. (1981). Encopresis. In J. M. Ferguson & C. B. Taylor (Eds.), *The comprehensive handbook of behavioral medicine* (Vol. 2, pp. 145–157). New York: Spectrum.

Doleys, D. M., Ciminero, A. R., Tollison, J. W., Williams, C. L., & Wells, K. C. (1977). Dry-bed training and retention control training: A comparison. *Behavior Therapy, 8*, 541–548.

Doleys, D. M., Schwartz, M. S., & Ciminero, A. R. (1981). Elimination problems: Enuresis and encopresis. In E. J. Mash & L. G. Terdal (Eds.), *Behavioral assessment of childhood disorders* (pp. 109–117). New York: Guilford Press.

Evans, J. H. C., & Meadow, S. R. (1992). Desmopressin for bed wetting: Length of treatment, vasopressin secretion, and response. *Archives of Disease in Childhood, 67*, 184–188.

Fenichel, O. (1946). *The psychoanalytic theory of neurosis.* London: Routledge & Kegan Paul.

Fergusson, D. M., Horwood, L. J., & Shannon, F. T. (1986). Factors related to the age of attainment of nocturnal bladder control: An 8-year longitudinal study. *Pediatrics, 78*, 884–890.

Fergusson, D. M., Horwood, L. J., & Shannon, F. T. (1990).

Secondary enuresis in a birth cohort of New Zealand children. *Paediatric and Perinatal Epidemiology, 4,* 53–63.

Finley, W. W., Wansley, R. A., & Blenkarn, M. M. (1977). Conditioning treatment of enuresis using a 70% intermittent reinforcement schedule. *Behaviour Research and Therapy, 15,* 419–427.

Fireman, G., & Koplewicz, H. S. (1992). Short-term treatment of children with encopresis. *Journal of Psychotherapy Practice and Research, 1,* 64–71.

Forsythe, W. I., & Redmond, A. (1974). Enuresis and spontaneous cure rate: Study of 1129 enuretics. *Archives of Disease in Childhood, 49,* 259–263.

Foxman, B., Valdez, R. B., & Brook, R. H. (1986). Childhood enuresis: Prevalence, perceived impact, and prescribed treatments. *Pediatrics, 77,* 482–487.

Gabel, S., Hegedus, A. M., Wald, A., Chandra, R., & Chiponis, D. (1986). Prevalence of behavior problems and mental health utilization among encopretic children: Implications for behavioral pediatrics. *Developmental and Behavioral Pediatrics, 7,* 293–297.

Geffken, G., Bennett-Johnson, S., & Walker, D. (1986). Behavioral interventions for childhood nocturnal enuresis: The differential effect of bladder capacity on treatment progress and outcome. *Health Psychology, 5,* 261–272.

Glicklich, L. B. (1951). An historical account of enuresis. *Pediatrics, 8,* 859–876.

Goldsmith, H. (1962). Chronic loss of bowel control in a nine year old child. *American Journal of Clinical Hypnosis, 4,* 191–192.

Gross, R. T., & Dornbusch, S. M. (1983). Disordered processes of elimination: Enuresis. In M. D. Levine, W. B. Carey, A. C. Crocker, & R. T. Gross (Eds.), *Developmental–behavioral pediatrics* (pp. 573–586). Philadelphia: Saunders.

Haque, M., Ellerstein, N. S., Gundy, J. H., Shelov, S. P., Weiss, J. C., McIntire, M. S., Olness, K. N., Jones, D. J., Heagarty, M. C., & Starfield, B. H. (1981). Parental perceptions of enuresis: A collaborative study. *American Journal of Diseases of Childhood, 135,* 809–811.

Hedberg, A. G. (1973). The treatment of chronic diarrhea by systematic desensitization: A case report. *Journal of Behavior Therapy and Experimental Psychiatry, 4,* 67–68.

Hogg, R. J., & Hussman, D. (1993). The role of family history in predicting response to desmopressin in nocturnal enuresis. *Journal of Urology, 150,* 444–445.

Houts, A. C. (1991). Nocturnal enuresis as a biobehavioral problem. *Behavior Therapy, 22,* 133–151.

Houts, A. C., & Abramson, H. (1990). Assessment and treatment for functional childhood enuresis and encopresis: Toward a partnership between health psychologists and physicians. In S. B. Morgan & T. M. Okwumabua (Eds.), *Child and adolescent disorders: Developmental and health psychology perspectives* (pp. 47–103). Hillsdale, NJ: Erlbaum.

Houts, A. C., Berman, J. S., & Abramson, H. (1994). Effectiveness of psychological and pharmacological treatments for nocturnal enuresis. *Journal of Consulting and Clinical Psychology, 62,* 737–745.

Houts, A. C., & Liebert, R. M. (1984). *Bedwetting: A guide for parents and children.* Springfield, IL: Thomas.

Houts, A. C., Liebert, R. M., & Padre, W. (1983). A delivery system for the treatment of primary enuresis. *Journal of Abnormal Psychology, 11,* 513–520.

Houts, A. C., Mellon, M. W., & Whelan, J. P. (1988). Use of dietary fiber and stimulus control to treat retentive encopresis: A multiple baseline investigation. *Journal of Pediatric Psychology, 13,* 435–445.

Houts, A. C., & Peterson, J. K. (1986). Treatment of a retentive encopretic child using contingency management and diet modification with stimulus control. *Journal of Pediatric Psychology, 11,* 375–383.

Houts, A. C., Peterson, J. K., & Whelan, J. P. (1986). Prevention of relapse in full-spectrum home training for primary enuresis: A components analysis. *Behavior Therapy, 17,* 462–469.

Imhof, B. (1956). Bettwasser in der erziehungsberatung. *Heilpaedagogische Werkblaetter, 25,* 122–127.

Jarvelin, M. R., Moilanen, I., Vikevainen-Tervonen, L., & Huttunen, N. P. (1990). Life changes and protective capacities in enuretic and non-enuretic children. *Journal of Child Psychology and Psychiatry, 31,* 763–774.

Kaffman, M., & Elizur, E. (1977). Infants who become enuretic: A longitudinal study of 161 kibbutz children. *Child Development Monographs,* No. 42.

Kallio, J., Rautava, P., Huupponen, R., & Korvenranta, H. (1993). Severe hyponatremia caused by intranasal desmopressin for nocturnal enuresis. *Acta Paediatrica, 82,* 881–882.

Keren, S., Wagner, Y., Heldenberg, D., & Golan, M. (1988). Studies of manometric abnormalities of the rectoanal region during defecation in constipated and soiling children: Modification through biofeedback therapy. *American Journal of Gastroenterology, 83,* 827–831.

Landman, G. B., Rappaport, L., Fenton, T., & Levine, M. D. (1986). Locus of control and self-esteem in children with encopresis. *Developmental and Behavioral Pediatrics, 7,* 111–113.

Levine, M. D. (1975). Children with encopresis: A descriptive analysis. *Pediatrics, 56,* 412–416.

Levine, M. D., & Bakow, H. (1976). Children with encopresis: A study of treatment outcome. *Pediatrics, 58,* 845–852.

Liebman, W. M. (1979). Disorders of defecation in children: Evaluation and management. *Postgraduate Medicine, 66,* 105–110.

Lifshitz, M., & Chovers, A. (1972). Encopresis among Israeli kibbutz children. *Israel Annals of Psychiatry and Related Disciplines, 10,* 326–340.

Loening-Baucke, V. (1984). Abnormal rectoanal function in children recovered from chronic constipation and encopresis. *Gastroenterology, 87,* 1299–1304.

Loening-Baucke, V. A. (1990). Modulation of abnormal defecation dynamics by biofeedback treatment in chronically constipated children with encopresis. *Journal of Pediatrics, 116,* 214–222.

Loening-Baucke, V. A., & Cruikshank, B. M. (1986). Abnormal defecation in chronically constipated children with encopresis. *Journal of Pediatrics, 108,* 562–566.

Loening-Baucke, V. A., & Younoszai, M. K. (1984). Abnormal and sphincter pressure in chronically constipated children. *Journal of Pediatrics, 100,* 213–218.

Lovibond, S. H. (1964). *Conditioning and enuresis.* New York: Macmillan Co.

Lovibond, S. H., & Coote, M. A. (1970). Enuresis. In C. G. Costello (Ed.), *Symptoms of psychopathology: A handbook* (pp. 373–396). New York: Wiley.

Martin, C. R. A. (1966). *A new approach to nocturnal enuresis.* London: H. K. Lewis.

McClung, H. J., Boyne, L. J., Linscheid, T., Heitlinger, L. A., Murray, R. D., Fyda, J., & Li, B. U. K. (1993). Is combination therapy for encopresis nutritionally safe? *Pediatrics, 91,* 591–594.

McGee, R., Makinson, T., Williams, S., Simpson, A., & Silva, P. A. (1984). A longitudinal study of enuresis from five to nine years. *Australian Paediatric Journal, 20,* 39–42.

Meichenbaum, D. (1977). *Cognitive behavior modification.* New York: Plenum Press.

Meunier, P., Marechal, J. M., & deBeaujeu, M. J. (1979). Rectoanal pressures and rectal sensitivity studies in chronic childhood constipation. *Gastroenterology, 77,* 330–336.

Meunier, P., Mollard, P., & Marechal, J. M. (1976). Physiopathology of megarectum: The association of megarectum with encopresis. *Gut, 17,* 224–227.

Mikkelsen, E. J., Rapoport, J. L., Nee, L., Gruenau, C., Mendelson, W., & Gillin, J. C. (1980). Childhood enuresis: I. Sleep patterns and psychopathology. *Archives of General Psychiatry, 37,* 1139–1144.

Miller, K., Goldberg, S., & Atkin, B. (1989). Nocturnal enuresis: Experience with long-term use of intranasally administered desmopressin. *Journal of Pediatrics, 114,* 723.

Moffat, M. E. K., Harlos, S., Kirshen, A. J., & Burd, L. (1993). Desmopressin acetate and nocturnal enuresis: How much do we know? *Pediatrics, 92,* 420–425.

Moilanen, I., Jarvelin, M. R., Vikevainen-Tervonen, L., & Huttunen, N. P. (1987). Personality and family characteristics of enuretic children. *Psychiatria Fennica, 18,* 53–61.

Molnar, D., Taitz, L. S., Urwin, O. M., & Wales, J. (1983). Anorectal manometry results in defecation disorders. *Archives of Disease in Childhood, 58,* 257–261.

Morgan, R. T. T. (1974). *Enuresis and the enuresis alarm: A clinical manual for the treatment of nocturnal enuresis.* Unpublished manuscript.

Morgan, R. T. T. (1978). Relapse and therapeutic response in the conditioning treatment of enuresis: A review of recent findings on intermittent reinforcement, over-

learning and stimulus intensity. *Behaviour Research and Therapy, 16,* 273–279.

Morgan, R. T. T., & Young, G. C. (1975). Case histories and shorter communications. *Behaviour Research and Therapy, 13,* 197–199.

Mowrer, O. H., & Mowrer, W. M. (1938). Enuresis: A method for its study and treatment. *American Journal of Orthopsychiatry, 8,* 436–459.

Murray, R. D. (1994). Elimination disorders: Medical issues. In R. A. Olson, L. L. Mullins, J. B. Gillman, & J. M. Chaney (Eds.), *The sourcebook of pediatric psychology* (pp. 42–45). Boston: Allyn & Bacon.

Neale, D. H. (1963). Behavior therapy and encopresis in children. *Behaviour Research and Therapy, 1,* 139–149.

Nolan, T., Debelle, G., Oberklaid, F., & Coffey, C. (1991). Randomised trial of laxatives in treatment of childhood encopresis. *Lancet, 338,* 523–527.

Norgaard, J. P., Hansen, J. H., & Bugge, N. J. (1989). Sleep patterns in enuretic children: A polygraphic study of EEG and bladder activity. *Scandinavian Journal of Urology and Nephrology* (Suppl. 125), 73–78.

Norgaard, J. P., Pedersen, E. B., & Djurhuus, J. C. (1985). Diurnal anti-diuretic-hormone levels in enuretics. *Journal of Urology, 134,* 1029–1031.

Novick, J. (1966). Symptomatic treatment of acquired and persistent enuresis. *Journal of Abnormal Psychology, 71,* 363–368.

Olness, K. (1975). The use of self-hypnosis in the treatment of childhood nocturnal enuresis. *Clinical Pediatrics, 14,* 273–279.

Olness, K. (1976). Autohypnosis in functional megacolon in children. *American Journal of Clinical Hypnosis, 19,* 28–32.

Oppel, W. C., Harper, P. A., & Rider, R. V. (1968). The age of attaining bladder control. *Pediatrics, 42,* 614–626.

Parker, L., & Whitehead, W. (1982). Treatment of urinary and fecal incontinence in children. In D. C. Russo & J. W. Varni (Eds.), *Behavioral pediatrics: Research and practice* (pp. 143–174). New York: Plenum Press.

Perlmutter, A. D. (1976). Enuresis. In T. P. Kelalis & L. R. King (Eds.), *Clinical pediatric urology* (pp. 166–181). Philadelphia: Saunders.

Pettei, M. J., & Davidson, M. (1991). Idiopathic constipation. In W. A. Walker, P. R. Durie, J. R. Hamilton, J. H. Walker-Smith, & J. B. Watkins (Eds.), *Pediatric gastrointestinal disease: Vol. 1. Pathophysiology, diagnosis, management* (pp. 818–829). Philadelphia: B. C. Decker.

Physicians' desk reference. (1994). Montvale, NJ: Medical Economics Data Production Company.

Rapoport, J. L., Mikkelsen, E. J., Zavadil, A., Nee, L., Gruenau, C., Mendelson, W., & Gillin, J. C. (1980). Childhood enuresis: II. Psychopathology, tricyclic concentration in plasma, and antienuretic effect. *Archives of General Psychiatry, 37,* 1146–1152.

Readett, D. R. J., Morris, J., & Serjeant, G. R. (1990). Nocturnal enuresis in sickle cell haemoglobinopathies. *Archives of Disease of Childhood, 65,* 290–293.

Ringdahl, I. C. (1980). Hospital treatment of the encopretic child. *Psychosomatics, 21,* 65–71.

Rittig, S., Knudsen, U. B., Norgaard, J. P., Pedersen, E. B., & Djurhuus, J. C. (1989). Abnormal diurnal rhythm of plasma vasopressin and urinary output in patients with enuresis. *American Journal of Physiology, 256,* F664–F671.

Rolider, A., & Van Houten, R. (1985). Treatment of constipation-caused encopresis by a negative reinforcement procedure. *Journal of Behavior Therapy and Experimental Psychiatry, 16,* 67–70.

Rutter, M. (1973). Indication for research. In I. Kolvin, R. C. MacKeith, & S. R. Meadow (Eds.), *Bladder control and enuresis* (pp. 137–147). Philadelphia: Lippincott.

Rutter, M., Tizard, J., & Whitmore, K. (1970). *Education, health, and behaviour.* London: Longmans & Green.

Rutter, M., Yule, W., & Graham, P. (1973). Enuresis and behavioral deviance: Some epidemiological considerations. In I. Kolvin, R. C. MacKeith, & S. R. Meadow (Eds.), *Bladder control and enuresis* (pp. 137–147). Philadelphia: Lippincott.

Schaefer, C. E. (1979). *Childhood encopresis and causes and therapy.* New York: Van Nostrand Reinhold.

Schmitt, B. D. (1982). Daytime wetting (diurnal enuresis). *Pediatric Clinics of North America, 29,* 9–20.

Schmitt, B. D. (1984). Encopresis. *Primary Care, 11,* 497–511.

Scott, M. A., Barclay, D. R., & Houts, A. C. (1992). Childhood enuresis: Etiology, assessment, and current behavioral treatment. In M. Hersen, R. M. Eisler, & P. M. Miller (Eds.), *Progress in behavior modification* (Vol. 28, pp. 83–117). Sycamore, IL: Sycamore Publishing Company.

Shaffer, D. (1973). The association between enuresis and emotional disorder: A review of the literature. In I. Kolvin, R. C. MacKeith, & S. R. Meadow (Eds.), *Bladder control and enuresis* (pp. 118–136). Philadelphia: Lippincott.

Shaffer, D. (1977). Enuresis. In M. Rutter and L. Hersov (Eds.), *Child psychiatry: Modern approaches* (pp. 581–612). Oxford: Blackwell.

Silber, D. L. (1969). Encopresis. Discussion of etiology and management. *Clinical Pediatrics, 8,* 225–231.

Solomon, P., & Patch, V. D. (1969). *Handbook of psychiatry.* Los Altos, CA: Lange Medical Publications.

Springer, J. P., Kropp, B. P., & Thor, K. B. (1994). Facilitatory and inhibitory effects of selective norepinephrine reuptake inhibitors on hypogastric nerve-evoked urethral contractions in the cat: A prominent role of urethral beta-adrenergic receptors. *Journal of Urology, 152,* 515–519.

Starfield, B. (1967). Functional bladder capacity in enuretic and nonenuretic children. *Journal of Pediatrics, 70,* 777–781.

Starfield, B., & Mellits, E. D. (1968). Increase in functional bladder capacity and improvements in enuresis. *Journal of Pediatrics, 72,* 483–487.

Stark, L. J., Owens-Stively, J., Spirito, A., Lewis, A., & Guevremont, D. (1990). Group behavioral treatment of retentive encopresis. *Journal of Pediatric Psychology, 15,* 659–671.

Stark, L. J., Spirito, A., Lewis, A. V., & Hart, K. J. (1990). Encopresis: Behavioral parameters associated with children who fail medical management. *Child Psychiatry and Human Development, 20,* 169–179.

Steele, B. T. (1993). Nocturnal enuresis: Treatment options. *Canadian Family Physician, 39,* 877–880.

Taitz, L. S., Wales, J. K. H., Urwin, O. M., & Molnar, D. (1986). Factors associated with outcome in management of defecation disorders. *Archives of Disease in Childhood, 61,* 472–477.

Taylor, P. D., & Turner, R. K. (1975). A clinical trial of continuous, intermittent, and overlearning "bell and pad" treatments of nocturnal enuresis. *Behaviour Research and Therapy, 13,* 281–293.

Tilton, P. (1980). Hypnotic treatment of a child with thumbsucking, enuresis, and encopresis. *American Journal of Clinical Hypnosis, 22,* 238–240.

Turner, R. K., Young, G. C., & Rachman, S. (1970). Treatment of nocturnal enuresis by conditioning techniques. *Behaviour Research and Therapy, 8,* 368–381.

Verhulst, F. C., Van Der Lee, J. H., Akkerhuis, G. W., Sanders-Woudstra, J. A. R., Timmer, F. C., & Donkhorst, I. D. (1985). The prevalence of nocturnal enuresis: Do DSM-III criteria need to be changed? *Journal of Child Psychology and Psychiatry, 26,* 989–993.

Wald, A., Chandra, R., Chiponis, D., & Gabel, S. (1986). Anorectal function and continence mechanisms in childhood encopresis. *Journal of Pediatric Gastroenterology and Nutrition, 5,* 346–351.

Walker, C. E. (1978). Toilet training, enuresis, and encopresis. In P. Magrab (Ed.), *Psychological management of pediatric problems* (Vol. 1, pp. 129–189). Baltimore: University Park Press.

Walker, C. E. (1995). Elimination disorders: Enuresis and encopresis. In M. C. Roberts (Ed.), *Handbook of pediatric psychology* (2nd ed.). New York: Guilford Press.

Walker, C. E., Hedberg, A. G., Clement, P. W., & Wright, L. (1981). *Clinical procedures for behavior therapy.* Englewood Cliffs, NJ: Prentice–Hall.

Walker, C. E., Milling, L. S., & Bonner, B. L. (1988). Incontinence disorders: Enuresis and encopresis. In D. K. Routh (Ed.), *Handbook of pediatric psychology* (pp. 363–397). New York: Guilford Press.

Walker, C. E., & Shaw, W. (1988). Assessment of eating and elimination disorders. In P. Karoly (Ed.), *Handbook of child health assessment* (pp. 434–469). New York: Wiley.

Watanabe, H., Kawauchi, A., Kitamori, T., & Azuma, Y. (1994). Treatment system for nocturnal enuresis according to an original classification system. *European Urology, 25,* 43–50.

Wells, M. E., & Hinkle, J. S. (1990). Elimination of childhood encopresis: A family systems approach. *Journal of Mental Health Counseling, 12,* 520–526.

Whitehead, W. E., Parker, L., Masek, B. J., Cataldo, M. F., & Freeman, J. M. (1981). Biofeedback treatment of fecal incontinence in patients with myelomeningocele. *Developmental Medicine and Child Neurology, 23,* 313–322.

Wille, S. (1986). Comparison of desmopressin and enuresis alarm for nocturnal enuresis. *Archives of Disease in Childhood, 61,* 30–33.

Wright, L. (1975). Outcome of a standardized program for treating psychogenic encopresis. *Professional Psychology, 6,* 453–456.

Yates, A. J. (1970). *Behavior therapy.* New York: Wiley.

Young, G. C., & Morgan, R. T. T. (1972). Overlearning in the conditioning treatment of enuresis. *Behaviour Research and Therapy, 10,* 147–151.

Zaleski, A., Gerrard, J. W., & Shokeir, M. H. K. (1973). Nocturnal enuresis: The importance of a small bladder capacity. In I. Kolvin, R. C. MacKeith, & S. R. Meadow (Eds.), *Bladder control and enuresis* (pp. 95–101). Philadelphia: Lippincott.

III

Psychological Aspects of Physical Conditions

15

Pediatric Headaches

ELISE E. LABBÉ

INTRODUCTION

It is surprising to many to discover that children have headaches and that these headaches can serve to significantly disrupt children's school and home lives. Parents' reactions vary from believing that their child is trying to get out of doing chores or homework to the possibility of their child having a brain tumor. Although headaches can be caused by brain tumors, other neurological disorders, postconcussive reactions, sinus, and a variety of diseases, the most common type of headache in children is migraine headache (Bush, 1987; Labbé, 1991). In adolescence, youngsters' reports of muscle-contraction (MCH) or tension headaches become a concern as well (Labbé, 1988). Thus, the focus of this chapter will be on migraine and MCH in children and adolescents. This focus was chosen because other types of headaches are usually part of other syndromes and are treated primarily with medication or surgery. In contrast, psychosocial factors have been shown to cause, maintain, or exacerbate migraine headaches or

MCHs (Andrasik et al., 1988; Labbé, 1991). And psychological and behavioral treatments have been demonstrated to be quite effective in reducing migraine and MCHs in youngsters (Duckro & Cantwell-Simmons, 1989; Hoelscher & Lichstein, 1984; Rapoff, Walsh, & Engel, 1988).

PHENOMENOLOGY

Description and Characteristics of Migraine

Migraine headaches involve several symptoms. The most common symptoms are throbbing or pulsating pain, unilateral location (usually in the frontal or temporal area), nausea, vomiting, and photophobia. In classic migraine, the child experiences symptoms of scotomata, parathesis of the face and head, and vertigo *prior* to the headache. These symptoms are *prodromes*, or premonitory symptoms. Scotomata is loss of vision in a part of the visual field. Headaches can last a few hours to most of the day. Head pain is often described by the child as moderate to severe. The headache is often relieved by sleep. Rest can reduce the head pain. Children report two to eight headaches per month, although the

ELISE E. LABBÉ • Department of Psychology, University of South Alabama, Mobile, Alabama 36688.

Handbook of Child Psychopathology, 3rd edition, edited by Ollendick & Hersen. Plenum Press, New York, 1998.

frequency can vary greatly between children, as well as for a given child over several years. Most studies on migraines only include those children who have at least two headaches per month. Children can experience a greater number of headaches during certain times of the year. Many children report fewer headaches in the summer, possibly reflecting less school-related stress. This can be a confounding variable when evaluating treatment effects. A family history of migraine has been reported for 66–98% of children in several studies (Prensky, 1976). Common migraine is more frequently diagnosed than classic migraine. In common migraine the symptoms may vary and the pain is usually bilateral. The distinguishing feature between classic and common migraine is that children experience prodromes in classic migraine but not in common migraine.

Developmental Features

There are reports that children as young as 2 years old may experience migraines. Children have a difficult time describing their pain and the characteristics of the headache. Techniques to increase the reliability and validity of children's reports will be addressed in the section on assessment. A subgroup of children, usually at the younger ages, may experience recurrent abdominal pains (Symon & Russell, 1986), with vascular changes, such as pallor or flushing, loss of appetite, and vomiting. These children tend to experience migraine symptoms or develop migraines later in life.

Description and Characteristics of MCH

Children with MCHs report more frequent, sometimes daily headaches that are not as severe as the migraine headaches. The pain is described as a tightness around the head. The pain is often in the back of the head and shoulders although frequently in the frontal region. Children do not experience nausea or vomiting. The head pain will increase during the day and often the child will awake with the headache. Massage and stretching can help reduce the pain.

DIAGNOSIS

Care should be taken that a complete health and neurological examination is made. It is important to rule out other causes of headaches that may be fatal or more responsive to medication. Prior to any form of psychological or behavioral treatment, the psychologist should require a medical consent from the child's physician with a statement of diagnosis.

Diagnosis can be difficult with younger children as they are not able to verbalize the pain in a way that can be easily understood and characterized. Increasing the reliability and validity of children's reports will be addressed in the section on assessment. In both research and clinical practice the most commonly used diagnostic criteria for pediatric migraine were suggested by Prensky and Sommer (1979) (see Table 1 for these criteria). The diagnostic criteria of the Ad Hoc Committee on Classification of Headaches (1962) are also used. In general, reliability of diagnosis may be low.

Diagnosis of migraine headache must be differentiated from that of MCH or mixed headache. See Table 1 for the criteria for MCH. Mixed headache is the occurrence in an individual of MCH and migraine headaches, either separately or at the same time. Joffe, Bakal, and Kaganov (1983) argued that reports of headaches from children make it difficult to classify migraine headache versus MCH. They proposed the severity model of headache, which is supported by data indicating that as the headache increases in severity so do the number of symptoms related to vascular as well as muscular systems. In the adult research literature this controversy also exists; however, there are several studies that report being able to differentiate migraine headache from MCH (Blanchard, 1992; Williamson, 1981).

Table 1. Diagnostic Criteria for Pediatric Migraine and Muscle-Contraction Headaches

Common migraine	Classic Migraine	Muscle-contraction headache
Throbbing, pulsating pain	Throbbing, pulsating pain	Bandlike, constant dull aching pain
Unilateral or bilateral pain in frontal or temporal area	Unilateral or bilateral pain in frontal or temporal area	Bilateral or back of head or neck
Relief after rest	Relief after rest	No relief after rest
Photophobia	Photophobia	Responds to massage
Nausea	Nausea	
Vomiting	Vomiting	
	Prodromes	
	Dizziness	
	Scotomata	
	Flashing lights	

ETIOLOGY

Migraine Headaches

To date, no definitive statement can be made on the pathophysiology of migraine. There is evidence for biochemical, neural, and vascular changes in response to psychological, environmental, or other physical factors. Most researchers support a headache model positing that a variety of triggering events cause intracranial and extracranial arteries in the brain to constrict. These triggering events may be environmental stimuli, as well as psychological and/or internal physical responses. In response to vasoconstriction, some extracranial arteries dilate, causing pressure in surrounding tissue, sterile inflammation, and biochemical changes. These responses are perceived as painful. Within the past 5 years, studies support the idea that changes in levels of endogenous opiate peptides are associated with reports of headache. Canitano, Guidetti, Piano, and Ippoliti (1994) reported that several neurotransmitter pathways and neuropeptides have been investigated in order to elucidate the basic mechanisms involved in the pathogenesis of migraine. Goads-

by (1994) suggested that since the finding that serotonin (5-HT) could alleviate an acute attack of migraine, the definition of a multiplicity of serotonin receptors has provided neurological patients with many new therapeutic options. There remains considerable disagreement as to the site at which these newer therapies may act. Research has been directed toward determining if the receptor involved in the alleviation of headaches could be dissociated from unwelcome effects, such as diarrhea and flushing. Initially, there were two clearly defined 5-HT receptor subtypes, D and M, together with an atypical group. Recent research supports the new classification system, with seven subclasses of the 5-HT_1 receptor being identified, of which the 5-HT_{1D} subtype has emerged as an effective target for migraine treatment.

Goadsby (1994) also argued that the trigemini–vascular system plays a role in the pain of migraine. The well-established vascular component of the headache has focused attention on the trigeminal innervation of pain-sensitive intracranial structures, such as the dura mater and large vessels. Goadsby pointed out that there is considerable animal research indicating that these structures are innervated by the ophthalmic branch of the trigeminal nerve. Innervation of the trigeminal nerve involves release of vasoactive peptides such as substance P2 and calcitonin gene-related peptide. Moskowitz (1992) hypothesized that migraine is the clinical manifestation of trigeminal activation leading to sterile inflammation in the dura mater. This hypothesis is supported by research indicating that plasma extravasation, resulting from trigeminal ganglion stimulation, is blocked by a variety of drugs that have positive effects on the head pain. Problems with this model are that serotonin does not block plasma extravasation following trigeminal ganglion stimulation, and plasma extravasation consequent to trigeminal ganglion stimulation can be blocked by pretreatment with sumatriptan, whereas pretreatment of headache in patients using sumatriptan during aura does not block headache. Plasma extravasation has not been observed in humans during migraine. Goadsby (1994) argued that finding the location of a central site of action may be the key to understanding the effects of 5-HT_1 agonists in reducing headaches.

The role of psychological and environmental factors can be elucidated by research into the impact of cognitive and social learning principles on the experience of pain. Modeling, environmental reinforcement, anxiety, depression, and cognitive responses have been hypothesized as factors that may cause, exacerbate, or maintain the headache.

Anxiety, depression, and/or psychological conflicts have been viewed as potential causes of chronic headache (Andrasik et al., 1988; Cunningham et al., 1986; Lanzi, Balottin, Borgatti, Guderzo, & Scarabello, 1988). Problems with these earlier conclusions are that the studies report only those children whose parents were seeking treatment for them, and thus are not representative of all child migraineurs. Also, although personality traits may be found to differentiate children headache sufferers from those without headache, a causal relationship cannot be inferred. Several investigators suggest the psychological difficulties found may be a consequence of living with the pain (Andrasik et al., 1988; Hoelscher & Lichstein, 1984). More re-

cent studies based on well-designed procedures report statistical differences on measures of anxiety, depression, and other psychological problems between the headache and control groups. However, in most instances the headache group scores are still within the normal range. A study that not only used a no-pain control group but also included a "pain" control group found no significant differences between scores on a variety of psychological tests between the migraine headache group and the "pain" control group (Cunningham et al., 1986). The latter group consisted of children suffering from chronic musculoskeletal pain, including juvenile rheumatoid arthritis and patella-femoral knee pain. The only difference found between the migraine group and the pain control group was on a somatic complaints score, which included items such as vomiting, nausea, and perceptual disturbances (all of which are migraine symptoms). Cunningham et al. (1986) did report significant differences between the no-pain control group and the migraine group, in that the children with headaches showed less social participation and scored higher on a measure of anxiety. Although there were significant differences, the headache group scores were not in the clinical range. In summary, children who experience chronic headaches, although not clinically depressed or anxious, may be at risk for developing emotional problems. Furthermore, research indicates that many children will continue to experience headache as adults; thus, they may continue to experience these higher levels of emotional difficulties.

Secondary gain and positive reinforcement for reporting pain has been suggested as a factor in maintaining headache activity in children. This in turn could foster development of a maladaptive coping pattern of responding to stress with reports of headaches. Ramsden, Friedman, and Williamson (1983) reported on a single case study using contingency management procedure to treat a young girl with migraine headache. Results indicated a significant reduction in the child's complaint of headache.

Although effects of behavioral conditioning have been studied in adults with chronic pain and have been found to be an important aspect to consider in understanding chronic pain, they have not been systematically studied in children who have headaches.

Modeling and ineffective coping skills may also contribute to development of chronic headaches in children. It is well known that there is a significant familial factor associated with headaches. Genetics and/or family functioning may contribute to this finding. Mikail and von Baeyer (1990) reported an intriguing study of parents who did versus did not have chronic headache. They also evaluated children of both groups. They found that children of the headache group were more likely to experience headache than those of pain-free parents. They also found that children had higher mean scores on the Personality Inventory for Children (PIC), and significant differences were found on the social skills, delinquency, and general adjustment scales. The mean scores, although significantly different, were within the normal range. Mikail and von Baeyer also found a significant correlation between headache parents' self-report of emotional difficulties and the child's scores on the PIC. This was not found for the headache-free parent group. This study provided some initial evidence for the possible interplay between parental response to chronic pain and the child's experience of head pain. The researchers suggested that children may lack effective coping skills as their parents are not effective models, and the child may also be experiencing greater degrees of stress in response to their parents' pain behavior.

Muscle-Contraction Headaches

Etiological models of MCHs often include not only muscular but vascular and biochemical factors as well. The general consensus is that various emotional or environmental events may trigger or cause scalp and neck muscles to contract for prolonged periods of time, resulting in such pain. Vasoconstriction in contracted muscles might also contribute to the pain experience by producing ischemia. Other proposed contributors to the headache are abnormal vascular reactivity in the muscles, with accumulation of pain-provoking substances in the muscle or a central deficiency of inhibiting neurotransmitter substances. These etiological explanations, although commonly articulated, have not been experimentally validated.

The literature on children with MCHs often describes these children as having experienced significant school or family stress or an inability to cope with stress. As with the physiological factors proposed, the assumption about the role stress plays in the development and maintenance of MCH has not been experimentally validated.

EPIDEMIOLOGY

Distribution of Disease

Migraine headaches are equally as common in males and females prior to puberty. After puberty, many more females report migraine headaches, and males report a reduction or complete cessation of headaches (Williamson, Baker, & Cubic, 1993). A similar pattern holds for MCH patients.

Prevalence

About 5% of children aged 7 to 15 seen in a pediatric practice may be diagnosed as having migraine headaches (Labbé, 1991). A family history of migraine has been reported for 66–90% of children in several studies.

Controversy exists on the prevalence of MCHs in children (Labbé, 1988). Part of the difficulty in determining prevalence of MCH in children is that most studies include a category for classic and common migraine and lump all other types of headaches together. Children are rarely diagnosed with MCH before puberty. However, adolescents are more likely to seek treatment for MCH.

ASSESSMENT

Prior to commencing any type of psychological treatment, the psychologist should obtain records of the medical examination of the child. If no medical evaluation has been made, the psychologist should require one before implementing any type of intervention. The assessment of headache typically involves an interview with the child and a significant other adult, usually the mother, followed by completion of questionnaires assessing the headache experience, as well as overall psychological functioning of the child. The interview should involve obtaining history of the headache activity, a complete description of the pain, and exploration of the antecedents and consequences of the pain behavior. Table 2 presents an example of an interview format that has been used by Labbé in research and clinical practice.

Most research and clinical protocols require the child to keep a pain diary or log for 4 weeks. The headache log should allow the child to record information on the frequency, intensity, duration of the headache, and medication used. Visual analog scales can be used for younger children. Table 3 provides an example of a headache diary that could be used for children over 8 years old. The child is often required to keep the headache log throughout assessment and treatment phases. The headache log is the usual tool for the researcher and clinician to determine if treatment is reducing headache activity, as well as to help the child identify patterns and/or triggers of headache activity. Once the child begins treatment, home exercises and results of practice can be recorded in the log.

The clinician may also want to have the child draw how the headache feels. This can be done while the child is experiencing the headache as he or she may have a difficult time remembering how the pain felt when questioned later. Children's reports on duration of headache activity and time between headaches may be unreliable. Labbé, Williamson, and Southard (1985) found insignificant correlations between parents' observation of headache duration and the child's report. Children over 12 often give a more reliable report of headache pain (Marcon & Labbé, 1990).

Psychophysiological assessment is sometimes used to determine the child's physiological response during stress and relaxation. However, there is little support in the literature for using psychophysiological assessment in making differential diagnosis of types and/or severity levels of headaches. More often the child's physiological responses, particularly frontalis muscle tension and fingertip skin temperature, are assessed prior to, during, and at the completion of treatment. The clinician can then determine if these responses were improved by comparing data from baseline to treatment phases. Reductions in muscle tension and increases in skin temperature indicate that greater degrees of relaxation and increased parasympathetic nervous system arousal were achieved by the child.

Overall psychological functioning of the child as well as family functioning should also be evaluated. These factors can be assessed during the interview and through the use of objective questionnaires. Family issues and the child's current psychological functioning should be addressed because if significant problems exist the clinician may have a difficult time carrying out treatment protocols focused only on headaches. A questionnaire that can be used to assess family functioning is the Family Environment Scales by Moos and Moos (1986) that can be completed by the child and parent; parents can also complete the Symptom Checklist-90 for themselves (Derogatis, 1992). To screen for significant clinical psychological problems that the child may be experiencing, the parent an also complete a behavior checklist such as the Child Behavior Checklist (Achenbach & Edelbrock, 1983) and the child can complete questionnaires such as

Table 2. Headache Interview

1. You have had headache problems since the age of _____.
2. You have approximately _____ headaches per month.
3. Headaches last about _____ hours.
4. Have you been to the doctor for care of headaches?
   Yes _____ No_____ If yes, the diagnosis was _____.
5. What medication was prescribed for you? _____
   Dosage _____ Frequency of use _____
6. Have you had any of the following?
   eye problems _____ ear problems _____
   dental problems _____ sinus problems _____
   head injury _____ seizures _____
   or other neurological problems _____
   If you have had any of the above, how have they been related to your headache?
7. Have your headaches changed in any way during menstruation (girls) or beginning puberty (boys)? increased
   _____ decreased _____
8. Have you been under stress which may be related to your headache? Yes _____ No _____
9. Do you have a parent who suffers from headaches? Yes _____ No _____
   If yes, which parent? _____
10. Does any other family member suffer from headaches? Yes _____ No_____
    If yes, which family member? _____
11. Is there a seasonal pattern to your headache? Yes _____ No _____
    If yes, when? _____
13. Do you have difficulty sleeping? Yes _____ No _____
    If yes, please describe your difficulty: _____.
14. Are you involved in extracurricular activities? Yes _____ No _____
    What are they? _____.
15. What kind of grades have you received? _____.
Use the scale shown to rate the following:
    1 = never   2 = rarely   3 = sometimes   4 = usually   5 = always
16. Does your headache interfere with school or homework? _____
17. Does vigorous physical exercise precede your headaches? _____
18. The headaches occur: in school _____ in home _____ other places _____
19. The headaches occur: during the morning _____ afternoon _____ sleep _____ all day _____
    weekdays _____ weekends _____ certain days _____
20. Do headaches occur when the following people are present? parents _____ siblings _____ friends
    _____ teachers _____ others _____
21. When at home what is the child doing before a headache? (include frequency) _____
    _____
22. What happens at home when a headache is reported?
    rest _____ medication _____ prefers to be alone _____ special requests _____ stays home from
    school _____ doesn't do homework _____ doesn't do housework _____ other _____
23. Are there certain classes the child reports headaches in? Yes _____ No _____
    If yes, indicate which classes and include frequency _____
    _____
24. What happens when the child reports a headache at school? rest _____ medication _____ goes home
    _____ doesn't do schoolwork _____

the Youth Self-report form (Achenbach & Edelbrock, 1983), State–Trait Anxiety Test (Speilberger, Edwards, Lushene, Montuori, & Platzek, 1973), or the Beck Depression Inventory for Children (Kovacs, 1981). If significant clinical problems are discovered, a more comprehensive and in-depth psychological evaluation may be recommended before preceding to or at least in combination with treatment of the child's headaches.

Table 3. Headache Log

Page 1   Rating Scale
0 = No headache (HA)
1 = Very mild HA, I'm aware of it only when thinking
    about it.
2 = Mild HA, I ignore it at times.
3 = Moderate HA, pain all the time.
4 = Severe HA, difficult to concentrate, but can do simple
    things.
5 = Extremely intense HA, I want to go to bed, can't do
    anything!

Page 2   Instructions
Rate your head pain four times daily. Record how long
you've had the headache. Record name and amount of
medication used. If between ratings, how long has pain
lasted?

Repeated on Pages 3–10 (one for each day)
DATE _____
TIME   RA   LONG   MEDS/AMT

Breakfast_____
Lunch_____
Dinner_____
Bedtime_____

TREATMENT

A review of the literature on the efficacy of
nonpharmacological treatments with children
indicates positive or equivocal outcomes. No
studies have been reported that found such
treatments to be harmful or having a negative effect on the child (Duckro & Cantwell-
Simmons, 1989). A problem in determining appropriateness of prescriptive treatment is that
many studies included a variety of headache
types—migraine, classic migraine, and mixed.
Most studies report using 8–10 sessions at a rate
of slightly more than one session per week. Frequency of headache is reported to be the most
consistently modified pain characteristic. Intensity of the head pain is often unchanged. Duckro and Cantwell-Simmons (1989) reported
finding a "floor effect," as patients with less severe headaches prior to treatment did not improve significantly with behavioral intervention.

Booster sessions may be used to maintain the effects of treatment. However, as few studies include long-term follow-up, efficacy of booster
sessions has not been determined.

Compliance to treatment has been a concern
with children as psychological and behavioral
treatments involve an investment of time and
money. Also with young children there may be
difficulties in having them cooperate during
treatment and carrying out home instructions.
There is also the question of how involved the
parents should become during treatment and
with home practice. In general, recommendations from the literature suggest that parents
should become less involved as the child gets
older. Younger children may need to be reminded and encouraged to carry out skills
learned. In a large study focusing on personality characteristics and compliance, 161 children who had migraine headaches participated
in a behavioral-oriented treatment program
(Guibert, Firestone, McGrath, Goodman, &
Cunningham, 1990). Guibert et al. studied factors that might predict adherence and compliance to treatment, including demographic factors, emotional status, and credibility ratings of
treatment. Results indicate that older children
were less likely to drop out during treatment,
children with fewer headaches were more likely
to adhere to the treatment regimen, and children who thought the treatment less credible
were more likely to drop out. Most of the demographic data and personality measures did not
distinguish between compliant children and
dropouts.

Children with migraine headaches are more
easily recruited and more likely to comply with
treatment than children with MCH because of
the greater disturbance migraine may cause in
their lives. Migraine headaches tend to be more
severe and periodic and include more alarming
symptoms, such as nausea, than MCHs. Parents
may not take MCHs as seriously as migraine
headaches, and the child may learn to live with
the daily less severe MCH. Parents of children
with MCH, as well as their children, may not
be as motivated to seek treatment or keep up

with treatment demands. Treatment compliance may be increased by providing intervention in a school setting. Larson and Melin (1986) were successful in conducting relaxation training and providing information and self-directed interventions in the school setting with children who had MCH and/or migraine headaches.

Children may respond better to nonpharmacological treatments than adults (Labbé & Williamson, 1984). Providing treatment to youngsters may prevent development of a lifelong chronic pain syndrome that can become resistant to treatment over time. Interventions to be described in this chapter have been used in the treatment of migraine as well as MCH, with the exception of skin-temperature biofeedback, which is primarily used for migraine headaches. Treatments discussed are skin-temperature biofeedback, progressive muscle relaxation, EMG biofeedback, self-hypnosis, cognitive coping strategies, and behavior modification. In most situations these treatments involve individual therapy sessions.

Skin-Temperature Biofeedback with Autogenic Training and Home Practice

Skin-temperature biofeedback with autogenic training and home practice is a popular approach and one that has been consistently evaluated over the past 10 years. Table 4 presents an example of a treatment protocol for biofeedback. The treatment session usually lasts for about 45 minutes. Skin-temperature biofeedback requires the child to increase her or his skin temperature assisted by continuous auditory and/or visual feedback. Most therapists will allow the child to adjust to the ambient temperature, which should be 76 ± 1 °F (Kelton & Belar, 1983). This may take 10 to 20 minutes. After the baseline period the therapist may include a self-control phase for about 5 minutes in which the child is asked to warm both hands without feedback. The rationale behind the self-control phase is to encourage independence from the biofeedback machine, which is one of

the goals of the therapy. After the self-control phase the child is asked to continue hand warming with the help of feedback. The autogenic component involves the therapist giving the child verbal phrases to think about. These phrases consist of statements that involve feelings and sensations of relaxation. The final component is the home practice. Children are instructed to practice once or twice a day for about 15 to 20 minute. Some therapists give the child a home biofeedback monitor to use or ask the child to practice hand warming using the autogenic phrases without feedback. Children are usually treated for 10–12 sessions over 7–8 weeks. The child may be seen twice a week for the first 2 weeks, then sessions are spaced out over the rest of the treatment phase. To date several studies ranging from case studies to controlled group studies have been reported and indicate that skin-temperature biofeedback with autogenic training and home practice is an effective approach in reducing pediatric headache activity. Labbé (1994) reported on a series of studies examining the potent components of this treatment package. Results indicated no statistically significant difference between the skin temperature plus autogenic component or autogenic component only. However, when evaluating the clinical significance between these components by examining those children who were symptom-free versus improved, the autogenic combined with the skin-temperature biofeedback fared better than the autogenic only. Labbé suggested that children may find the biofeedback more interesting and thus they were more eager to participate. Also, feedback is a more concrete form of encouragement that the child can more readily understand. Surprisingly, the home practice component was found not to be as critical and did not provide any additional benefits as compared with those children who were not given specific practice instructions or a home monitor device. Blanchard (1992) reported conflicting results of two studies evaluating effectiveness of the home practice component. Home practice and long-term maintenance are areas that need to be further studied with children. Use of booster sessions may be beneficial in maintaining treatment success although most of the studies have included adult subjects (Blanchard, 1992). Few studies have provided long-term follow-up data.

Progressive Muscle Relaxation (PMR) and EMG Biofeedback

PMR has been used to treat both migraine and MCH. A few studies, mostly case reports or small uncontrolled group designs, have been reported that have evaluated PMR for MCH (Labbé, 1988). Some of the studies also paired electromyographic (EMG) biofeedback with PMR. In general, results indicated significant improvement of headache pain over time. Most PMR treatment protocols used 10 sessions over an 8-week period. Children were also instructed to practice the relaxation exercise daily. Sessions generally lasted 45 minutes with a brief baseline period, instructions on PMR, and 20 minutes of EMG biofeedback. Because of the small number of studies evaluating these procedures with children and adolescents, it is premature to make firm conclusions about PMR or EMG biofeedback for MCH. This is an area in which larger-scale and more well-controlled treatment studies are desperately needed.

PMR has also been reported to be useful in treating migraine headache. Researchers have pointed out that similar results have been found for PMR alone and for biofeedback techniques. They argue that PMR does not involve expensive equipment and can be easily learned by children. Both clinical practice and research results indicate that children appear more eager to interact with the biofeedback equipment and appreciate the concrete nature of the feedback display (Labbé, Delaney, Olson, & Hickman, 1993). Further studies should look at the impact of the biofeedback equipment on increasing children's interest and ultimately their compliance and cooperation with the treatment.

Self-Hypnosis

Some researchers have evaluated self-hypnosis with children suffering from headaches (Olness, MacDonald, & Uden, 1987). The child is taught to use visual or other sensory stimuli to change the pain experience. Self-hypnosis is also used to increase relaxation and lower anxiety levels. More research exploring the relative effectiveness of self-hypnosis to other psychological techniques may help determine whether this approach should be used more frequently in the clinic.

Cognitive Coping Skills, Behavior Management, and Self-Directed Treatments

Recent reports have evaluated the combination of cognitive coping skills, behavior management, and self-directed techniques. Some studies have compared these treatments and medication therapy. In general, results of these studies indicate these approaches to be quite effective in treating pediatric migraine. Often, biofeedback and/or relaxation training are included in the treatment package. It is difficult to determine which components are effective because of the heterogeneous treatment components used.

An example of a recent study is that by Müller, Metsch, Pothmann, and Sartory (1994), who reported a comparison study between relaxation with stress inoculation training, cephalic vasomotor biofeedback with stress inoculation training, and medication therapy using Metoprolol. At 4-week follow-up, all three approaches had significantly reduced migraines, with the relaxation with stress inoculation group displaying a slightly better improvement than the other groups.

A current trend in the literature is to evaluate self-directed or home-based treatment. It is believed that home-based regimens may increase accessibility to treatment, reduce number of sessions with health professionals, and increase cost-effectiveness and generalization to the natural environment (Allen & McKeen, 1991). Allen and McKeen compared a home-based program for young migraineurs to a clinic-based program. They found that a home-based treatment program requiring only three clinic visits was successful in treating the children, with treatment effects maintained at 3- and 8-month follow-up. The home-based treatment included skin-temperature biofeedback and parent-implemented behavior management guidelines designed to encourage reliance on biofeedback rather than maladaptive pain behaviors. Parental compliance with behavior management guidelines was the best predictor of headache outcome. Thus, when using home-based interventions for the younger child, parental cooperation may be necessary.

There is now a wealth of treatment studies available; however, mechanisms for success are not clearly understood. Documentation of physiological changes has been rare but is needed to elucidate the biobehavioral mechanisms involved in treatment success. Plasma β-endorphin levels in young migraine patients were assessed before and after behavior therapy for children who had migraines and children who did not have a history of headaches (Helm-Hylkema, Orlebeke, Enting, Thussen, & van Ree, 1990). A first group of children, both migraine and controls, was assessed and treated in the winter; and the second group of children, both migraine and controls, in the summer. The controls did not receive therapy. Therapy consisted of four group sessions and four individual sessions. Sessions included information about pain, migraine, and pain-coping strategies, and various methods of physical relaxation were taught and the principles of rational emotive therapy were practiced to try to reduce tension. In individual sessions patients were taught skin-temperature biofeedback and given biodots to practice at home. Helm-Hylkema et al. (1990) found reduced plasma β-endorphin, whereas ACTH concentration was normal. These findings are similar to those for adult migraine sufferers. A disturbance in either the conversion of β-LPH to β-endorphin or the release of

β-endorphin from the hypophysis may occur. This lower level of β-endorphin may be one of the factors determining the sensation of pain during headaches. Helm-Hylkema et al. found lower levels of β-endorphin, cortisol, and prolactin in winter than summer, for the migraine children as well as the controls. Seasonal differences thus may influence hormone production, or the higher levels of environmental stress caused by school may play a part in increasing the headache activity. They also found that children in the winter group reported more headaches than those in the summer group. Other findings were that after behavior therapy, the β-endorphin level in plasma was significantly higher than before, but not for those who were in a waiting period. Control subjects demonstrated no significant changes. It is not known how behavior therapy affects the activity of the endorphin system. Genazzani et al. (1985) suggested that catecholamines play a part in the release of β-endorphin. Relaxation training reduces sympathetic activity, which in turn may influence the release of β-endorphin.

Medical Treatment

Medical intervention can generally be grouped in two categories: symptomatic or abortive therapy and prophylactic therapy. An ergot preparation or an analgesic plus sedative or antinausea agent is often used for an abortive or symptomatic approach. A prophylactic approach includes use of such medications as propranolol, anticonvulsant, antihistamines, antidepressants, or calcium channel blockers. Usually these medications will not rid the child of headaches but rather reduce headache activity to a more manageable level. The long-term side effects of most of these medications are unknown and the few studies comparing medication therapy to biofeedback or relaxation techniques have consistently demonstrated the relaxation techniques to have equal or superior effects (Olness et al., 1987; Müller et al., 1994).

MCH is rarely treated with medication. Over-the-counter pain relievers, such as acetamino-phen, are usually recommended. Massage and use of local heat or cold packs may also reduce pain. Antidepressants are often prescribed if the physician suspects the child to have emo-tional problems.

CASE STUDY

A case study will be presented that gives a description of how a child with pediatric migraine may be evaluated and given therapy. The case described is fictitious and characteristics of the child and her response to the procedures described are typical of the many youngsters seen in my clinic as well as research programs.

Calley is an 11-year-old Caucasian female. She was referred by her pediatrician as her parents did not want her to take medication for her headaches. An intake interview was conducted, a headache ques-tionnaire was filled out by Calley, and the Child Behavior Checklist was completed by her parents. She was instructed to keep a headache log over the next 4 weeks in order to determine more specifically the frequency, duration, and intensity of the headaches and medication usage.

Assessment indicated that Calley was not experiencing any signifi-cant emotional or behavior problems at home or school. She is in the fifth grade and is an above-average student. She takes dance and pi-ano lessons and is a safety patrol officer for her school. Calley's father is a financial planner and her mother is a real estate agent. She has a 16-year-old brother who is also a good student.

Calley reports having moderate to severe headaches about three times a month. These headaches occur at home and school and last 6 to 8 hours. The pain becomes so severe that she is unable to carry out her usual activities and requires a quiet place without lights on, to rest in. She makes up any work that she is unable to do during the headache. Calley reports feeling frustrated about the headaches and will feel upset when she "feels a headache coming on." She also expe-riences nausea and occasional vomiting during the headache. She has been reporting headaches since age 8, but these headaches have increased in frequency within the last 6 months. She experienced her first menstrual period 3 months ago. She takes acetaminophen when headaches begin.

The treatment protocol chosen for Calley was skin-temperature biofeedback, with autogenic training and home practice. Table 4 presents an outline of the treatment protocol. Calley's first session lasted about 45 minutes in which a baseline recording was made of her skin temperature during quiet sitting and then during a 15-min-ute period in which she was asked to warm her hands using her imag-ination. During this self-control period, she was not able to consis-tently raise her temperature. Her headache logs were collected and she was asked to continue recording her headaches. The next nine sessions were scheduled over a 12-week period. An explanation of the equipment was made during the first two sessions. Calley was asked to explain how it worked to her mother so as to demonstrate under-standing of the procedure. Sessions included a 15-minute baseline and adaptation phase, followed by 15 minutes of skin-temperature biofeedback. Continuous auditory and visual feedback was given. Calley was also instructed in autogenic phrases to help facilitate fo-cusing of images and sensations of warmth and relaxation. Feedback

Table 4. Treatment Protocol

• 9 sessions	15 minutes of baseline and adaption
	15 minutes of feedback
	5 minutes of self-control
• 10th session	15 minutes of baseline and adaption
	15 minutes of self-control
• Explanation of equipment used: visual and auditory feedback	
• Autogenic and imagery instructions	
• Verbal shaping	
• Home practice:	twice daily

was followed by 5 minutes of self-control with the instructions to con-tinue warming her hands without the feedback. The final and tenth session involved the adaptation phase with 15 minutes of self-control.

During the first two treatment sessions Calley had some difficulty relaxing and increasing her skin temperature. She appeared to be trying too hard. We discussed the importance of releasing any ten-sion and not forcing herself to relax. Calley complied and was able to increase her skin temperature about 2–3 °F during the following feedback sessions and she was able to maintain that increase during the self-control phase. Calley was asked to practice warming her hands twice daily for about 10 to 20 minutes. She was instructed to initially select a quiet place to practice in. She was encouraged to practice in more challenging environments as she improved her abil-ity to relax. She was also warned that once a headache began, relax-ation might help to reduce the pain but not completely remove it. Calley began reporting a decrease in headache activity at about the 6th week of treatment. This is typical, and parents and children are informed that it may take a few weeks before significant changes in headache activity occur. By the end of treatment Calley reported she had been headache free for the past 2 weeks. A follow-up booster ses-sion was scheduled for 4 weeks. She reported continued success with headache reduction. Another booster session was scheduled for 2 months, at which time Calley reported having had one headache. She was given 15 minutes of feedback and instructed to continue practicing at home. At 6- and 12-month follow-up, Calley reported that she had been headache free.

SUMMARY

Migraine and MCH headaches are frequently observed in children and adolescents. Differen-tial diagnosis should be made between migraine and MCH headaches, and the child's emotional and psychological status needs to be assessed so as to determine the best treatment approach. Within the past 10 years a variety of psychologi-cal and behavioral approaches have been stud-ied and found effective in reducing chronic head pain in children. Skin-temperature biofeedback with autogenic training has been the most well studied of the treatments for migraine headaches and the results indicate it is superior to no treatment. EMG biofeedback and PMR training have been the most well-studied treatments for MCH and appear to be more effective than no treatment. Medication is often prescribed, and a few studies have shown nonpharmacological approaches to be equal to or superior to pharmacological approaches.

Issues to address in treatment are compliance to the time-consuming techniques and how much the parents should be involved. Providing treatment may be more cost-effective than traditional individual, outpatient treatment sessions. Psychological and behavioral treatments appear to be safe alternatives for the treatment of chronic headache in children.

REFERENCES

Achenbach, T. M., & Edelbrock, C. (1983). *Manual for the Child Behavior Checklist and Revised Child Behavior Profile.* Burlington: University of Vermont Department of Psychiatry.

Ad Hoc Committee on Classification of Headaches. (1962). Classification of headaches. *Journal of the American Medical Association, 179,* 127–128.

Allen, K. D., & McKeen, L. R. (1991). Home-based multicomponent treatment of pediatric migraine. *Headache, 31,* 467–472.

Andrasik, F., Kabela, E., Quinn, S., Attanasio, V., Blanchard, E. B., & Rosenblum, E. L. (1988). Psychological functioning of children who have recurrent migraine. *Pain, 34,* 43–52.

Blanchard, E. B. (1992). Psychological treatment of benign headache disorders. *Journal of Consulting and Clinical Psychology, 60,* 537–551.

Bush, J. P. (1987). Pain in children: A review of the literature from a developmental perspective. *Psychology and Health, 1,* 215–236.

Canitano, R., Guidetti, V., Piano, G., & Ippoliti, F. (1994). Correlation between childhood migraine and the opiatergic system: A neuroimmunological approach. In F. C. Rose (Ed.), *New advances in headache research* (Vol. 3, pp. 77–80). London: Smith-Gordon.

Cunningham, S. J., McGrath, P. J., Ferguson, H. B., Humphreys, P., D'Astous, J., Latter, J., Goodman, J. T., & Firestone, P. (1986). Personality and behavioral characteristics in pediatric migraine. *Headache, 27,* 16–20.

Derogatis, L. R. (1992). *SCL-90-R: Administration, scoring and procedures manual-II.* Towson, MD: Clinical Psychometric Research.

Duckro, P. N., & Cantwell-Simmons, E. (1989). A review of studies evaluating biofeedback and relaxation training in the management of pediatric headache. *Headache, 29,* 428–433.

Genazzani, A. R., Petraglia, F., Facchinetti, F., Sances, G., Storchi, R., & Nappi, G. (1985). Central regulation of circulating β-endorphin: Possible implications in headache treatments. *Cephalalgia, 1,* 102–104.

Goadsby, P. J. (1994). New insights into the pathogenesis of migraine. In F. C. Rose (Ed.), *New advances in headache research* (Vol. 4, pp. 5–7). London: Smith-Gordon.

Guibert, M. B., Firestone, P., McGrath, P., Goodman, J., & Cunningham, J. S. (1990). Compliance factors in the behavioral treatment of headache in children and adolescents. *Canadian Journal of Behavioural Science, 22,* 37–44.

Helm-Hylkema, H. V. D., Orlebeke, J. F., Enting, L. A., Thussen, J. H. H., & van Ree, J. (1990). Effects of behaviour therapy on migraine and plasma β-endorphin in young migraine patients. *Psychoneuroendocrinology, 15,* 39–45.

Hoelscher, T. J., & Lichstein, K. L. (1984). Behavioral assessment and treatment of child migraine: Implications for clinical research and practice. *Headache, 24,* 94–103.

Joffe, R., Bakal, D. A., & Kaganov, J. (1983). A self-observation study of headache symptoms in children. *Headache, 23,* 20–25.

Kelton, A., & Belar, C. (1983). The relative efficacy of autogenic phrases and autogenic-feedback training in teaching hand warming to children. *Biofeedback and Self-regulation, 8,* 461–474.

Kovacs, M. (1981). Rating scales to assess depression in school aged children. *Acta Paedopsyciatrica, 46,* 305–315.

Labbé, E. (1988). Childhood muscle contraction headache: Current issues in assessment and treatment. *Headache, 28,* 430–434.

Labbé, E. (1991). Headache. In F. D. Burg, J. R. Ingelfinger, & E. R. Ward (Eds.), *Current pediatrics therapy* (Vol. 14, pp. 92–96). Philadelphia: Saunders.

Labbé, E. (1994). Treatment of childhood migraine with skin temperature biofeedback, autogenic training and home practice: A component analysis. In F. C. Rose (Ed.), *New advances in headache research* (Vol. 4, pp. 123–128). London: Smith-Gordon.

Labbé, E., Delaney, D., Olson, K., & Hickman, H. (1993). Skin-temperature biofeedback training: Cognitive and developmental factors in a nonclinical child population. *Perceptual and Motor Skills, 76,* 955–962.

Labbé, E. E., & Williamson, D. A. (1984). Treatment of childhood migraine using autogenic feedback training. *Journal of Consulting and Clinical Psychology, 52,* 968–976.

Labbé, E., Williamson, D., & Southard, D. (1985). Reliability and validity of children's reports of migraine headache symptoms. *Journal of Psychopathology and Behavioral Assessment, 7*, 375–383.

Lanzi, G., Balottin, U., Borgatti, R., Guderzo, M., & Scarabello, E. (1988). Different forms of migraine in childhood and adolescence: Notes on personality traits. *Headache, 28*, 618–622.

Larson, B., & Melin, L. (1986). Chronic headaches in adolescents: Treatment in a school setting with relaxation training as compared with information-contact and self-regulation. *Pain, 25*, 325–326.

Marcon, R. A., & Labbé, E. E. (1990). Assessment and treatment of children's headaches from a developmental perspective. *Headache, 30*, 586–592.

Mikail, S. F., & von Baeyer, C. L. (1990). Pain, somatic focus, and emotional adjustment in children of chronic headache sufferers and controls. *Social Science Medicine, 31*, 51–59.

Moos, R. H., & Moos, B. S. (1986). *Family Environment Scale manual* (2nd ed.). Palo Alto, CA: Consulting Psychologists Press.

Moskowitz, M. A. (1992). Neurogenic versus vascular mechanisms of sumatriptan and ergot alkaloids in migraine. *Trends in Pharmacological Science, 13*, 307–311.

Müller, B., Metsch, J., Pothmann, R., & Sartory, G. (1994). A comparison of psychological and pharmacological prophylaxis of childhood migraine. In F. C. Rose (Ed.), *New advances in headache research* (Vol. 4, p. 328). London: Smith-Gordon.

Olness, K., MacDonald, J. T., & Uden, D. L. (1987). Comparison of self-hypnosis and propranolol in the treatment of juvenile classic migraine. *Pediatrics, 79*, 593–597.

Prensky, A. L. (1976). Migraine and migrainous variants in pediatric patients. *Pediatric Clinics of North America, 23*, 461–471.

Prensky, A. L., & Sommer, D. (1979). Diagnosis and treatment of migraine in children. *Neurology, 29*, 506–510.

Ramsden, R., Friedman, B., & Williamson, D. A. (1983). Treatment of childhood headaches reports with contingency management procedures. *Journal of Clinical Child Psychology, 12*, 202–206.

Rapoff, M., Walsh, D., & Engel, J. M. (1988). Assessment and management of chronic pediatric headaches. *Issues in Comprehensive Pediatric Nursing, 11*, 159–178.

Speilberger, C. D., Edwards, C., Lushene, R., Montuori, J., & Platzek, D. (1973). *STAIC: Preliminary manual.* Palo Alto, CA: Consulting Psychologists Press.

Symon, D. N. K., & Russell, G. (1986). Abdominal migraine: A childhood syndrome defined. *Cephalalgia, 6*, 223–228.

Williamson, D. (1981). Behavioral treatment of migraine and muscle contraction headache: Outcome and theoretical explanation. In M. Hersen, R. M. Eisler, & P. M. Miller (Eds.), *Progress in behavior modification* (Vol. 11, pp. 163–201). New York: Academic Press.

Williamson, D. A., Baker, J. P., & Cubic, B. A. (1993). Assessment in pediatric headache research. In T. H. Ollendick & P. J. Prinz (Eds.), *Advances in clinical child psychology* (Vol. 15, pp. 275–304). New York: Plenum Press.

16

Childhood Asthma

THOMAS L. CREER

INTRODUCTION

Pediatric asthma is increasingly a problem for children, their families, and society. An estimated 20 to 30 million Americans—8 to 12% of the population—have asthma (Pope, Patterson, & Burge, 1993). Approximately half of the Americans with asthma are children; it is conservatively estimated that 10% of all children in the United States have the disorder (Gergen, Mullally, & Evans, 1988). Asthma is the major cause of school absenteeism related to chronic physical conditions and is the leading cause of child hospitalization. In 1990 alone, children between the ages of 5 and 17 missed more than 10 million days of school, had an estimated 160,000 hospitalizations, and made 860,000 emergency room visits (Weiss, Gergen, & Hodgson, 1992). Treatment of pediatric asthma is expensive; Marion, Creer, and Reynolds (1985) found that childhood asthma consumed up to one-third of a family's income. These findings were almost identical to those reported by Vance and Taylor (1971) a decade earlier. Darkening the bleak

THOMAS L. CREER • Department of Psychology, Ohio University, Athens, Ohio 45701.

Handbook of Child Psychopathology, 3rd edition, edited by Ollendick & Hersen. Plenum Press, New York, 1998.

picture created by these bits of data is the fact that there is no cure for asthma.

Despite the problems posed by the disorder, considerable progress has been made with respect to childhood asthma. These advances are critical to our understanding of the disorder and how it is controlled. The progress may, at times, seem subtle and unimportant. However, these advances offer considerable hope to those children and their families trapped by asthma.

PHENOMENOLOGY

Definition of Asthma

Asthma has been defined in many ways, usually in accordance with the needs of various groups working with the condition. Clinicians treating patients want a different definition than epidemiologists studying patient populations or immunologists investigating the pathogenesis of the disorder (Busse & Reed, 1988). The frames of reference are so diverse and the types of phenomena studied so different, it was thought that agreement on a single definition would be impossible. The difficulty in defining asthma is further increased, continued Busse and Reed (1988), because "of the complexity and heterogeneity of the genetic, environmental, psychosocial, physiologic, and molecular biologic factors in its pathogenesis, course, and manifestations" (p. 969). Defining asthma in terms of its cause is impossible as the cause of asthma is unknown (Creer & Bender, 1995a,b).

Despite difficulties inherent in the task, two major attempts were recently made to provide a working definition of asthma. First, a panel of U.S. experts was assembled by the National Heart, Lung, and Blood Institute to provide guidelines for the definition, diagnosis, and management of asthma. The panel proposed an operational definition they anticipated could be used by all scientists who work with asthma. The definition states:

> Asthma is a lung disease with the following characteristics: (1) airway obstruction (or airway narrowing) that is reversible (but not completely so in some patients) either spontaneously or with treatment; (2) airway inflammation; and (3) airway hyperresponsiveness to a variety of stimuli. (National Institutes of Health, 1991, p. 1)

Second, a panel of international experts on asthma, also assembled by the National Heart, Lung, and Blood Institute, arrived at a definition for asthma:

> Asthma is a chronic inflammatory disorder of the airways in which many cells play a role, including mast cells and eosinophils. In susceptible individuals, this inflammation causes symptoms which are usually associated with widespread but variable airway obstruction that is often reversible, either spontaneously or with treatment, and causes an associated increase in airway responsiveness to a variety of stimuli. (National Institutes of Health, 1992, p. 1)

Although there are differences between the two operational definitions of asthma, the descriptions are marked more by similarity than by dissimilarity. Both definitions, for example, present characteristics of asthma per se. Arriving at an operational definition of what is meant by an asthma attack, episode, or flareup involves a totally separate process that entails obtaining an agreement among medical personnel, behav-

ioral scientists, patients, and, in the case of children, their parents (Creer, 1992; Creer & Bender, 1993, 1995b).

The work of the expert panels on asthma, particularly the group of U.S. experts, has had several positive consequences. First, the guidelines were published in their entirety and widely circulated not only by the National Institutes of Health, but also by leading respiratory journals including *The Journal of Allergy and Clinical Immunology* and *Pediatric Allergy, Asthma, and Immunology* in 1991. Second, the guidelines achieved their goal in that they have served to direct the treatment and research of those involved with asthma. They are heavily cited both by clinicians and by researchers. Finally, realization that new innovations would require revised and updated guidelines led to the formation of a second panel of U.S. experts. Their report was recently published (National Institutes of Health, 1997). The aim is to update guidelines for the definition, diagnosis, and treatment of asthma every 5 years. Development of guidelines for asthma has been widely welcomed by all involved with the disorder, including children and their families. They should be read by anyone interested in childhood asthma.

Characteristics of Asthma

The definitions of asthma composed by the two expert panels identify the major characteristics of asthma. Three characteristics—its intermittent, variable, and reversible nature—have been used to describe asthma for centuries; they serve as the hallmark characteristics of asthma observed both by patients and by those who treat or investigate the disorder (Creer & Bender, 1995b). Two other characteristics—airway hyperresponsiveness and airway inflammation—are increasingly of interest to scientists and to patients.

Intermittency

Frequency of attacks vary from patient to patient and, for a given patient, from time to time.

A child may have a number of attacks during a period of a few days, and then be asymptomatic for several weeks, months, or even years. A second patient may experience perennial asthma and have attacks most days throughout the year. Intermittency of attacks experienced by patients is a function of several classes of variables, including the number of stimuli that precipitate episodes, hyperreactivity of airways, degree of control established over asthma, physical changes, health care variables such as access to appropriate medical care, and patient variables such as medication compliance. Any of these classes of variables is capable of producing dramatic changes in a patient's asthma (Creer & Bender, 1993, 1995b).

Intermittency of asthma presents three problems to scientists (Creer & Bender, 1995b). First, the unique sequence of each patient's asthma attacks makes it difficult, if not impossible, to recruit a homogeneous population of subjects. Recruiting only patients with perennial asthma does not control the problem because these patients may be differentially affected by factors unrelated to a study (e.g., an outbreak of flu or changes in their medical treatment) that independently alter their rates of attacks. Matching patients in asthma studies is difficult and can only occur when large populations of subjects are available. Second, intermittency of asthma makes it difficult to recruit and maintain subjects in a study. Patients with asthma readily volunteer for studies when they are experiencing attacks. However, once asthma remits, they lose interest. Their reaction makes it hard, if not impossible, to recruit and maintain patients in control conditions in studies that employ randomized control groups (Wigal, Creer, Kotses, & Lewis, 1990). Finally, the intermittent nature of asthma generates a wide range of expectancies in patients (Renne & Creer, 1985). Children with perennial asthma and their parents anticipate the youngsters will experience asthma throughout the year; consequently, they may be more compliant with treatment regimens and better prepared to manage episodes. Children with more intermittent patterns of asthma and their parents may view at-

tacks as a transitory phenomenon that will abate spontaneously without treatment. If long periods of time elapse between attacks, children and their parents often forget how to treat attacks and are unprepared to manage asthma (Creer, 1991a).

Variability

Variability refers to severity both of a patient's asthma and of discrete attacks. Use of the term is often unexplained, and it is not always clear whether severity is being used to refer to the general condition of a patient's asthma or to the specific attacks he or she experiences (Creer & Bender, 1993, 1995b). There is ambiguity to use of the term in the literature, although both the national (National Institutes of Health, 1991) and international (National Institutes of Health, 1992) guidelines for the diagnosis and management of asthma contain a general classification for asthma severity, and an outline for the treatment of mild, moderate, or severe asthma attacks.

Reversibility

Asthma is characterized by airway obstruction that remits either spontaneously or with treatment. This feature distinguishes the condition from other respiratory disorders, particularly emphysema, where reversibility does not occur. As with other characteristics of asthma, however, there are exceptions (Creer & Bender, 1995b). First, reversibility may be relative. Although most patients show complete reversibility of airway obstruction with appropriate treatment, others do not achieve total reversibility even with intensive therapy (Loren et al., 1978). Second, ability of attacks to remit spontaneously makes it impossible to prove a cause–effect relationship between changes in a child's asthma and a treatment for the condition (Creer, 1982). Although outcome data may support a particular intervention as producing change in a patient's asthma, there remains the possibility that a remission of symptoms could have occurred spontaneously and coincidental to treatment.

Airway Hyperresponsiveness

Airway hyperreactivity or hyperresponsiveness is an exaggerated airway response, commonly called *bronchoconstriction,* that occurs when the airways are exposed to a number of stimuli. Bronchoconstriction in asthma is a reduction in small-airway diameter because of muscle spasm, mucosal swelling or edema, mucosal inflammation, and increased mucus secretion. Stimuli that produce bronchoconstriction in children include: (1) viral respiratory infections; (2) allergens such as pollens, dust mites, molds, cat dander, and cockroach parts; (3) irritants such as tobacco smoke, air pollution, and strong odors; (4) drugs such as aspirin and chemicals such as food additives; (5) exercise; (6) weather changes; and (7) emotional responses, particularly laughing, shouting, and crying. Airway hyperreactivity is ubiquitous in asthma; in addition, the level of airway responsiveness correlates with the clinical severity of asthma (National Institutes of Health, 1991). Patients with the most reactive airways usually require more potent medications, including oral steroids, whereas patients with milder degrees of airway hyperreactivity require fewer and less potent medications (Kaliner & Lemanske, 1992).

Airway Inflammation

Precisely how inflammation occurs in the airways and how it interacts with bronchial hyperresponsiveness are unknown. It is believed that inflammation is not caused by a single cell or single inflammatory mediator; rather, inflammation is thought to result from a complex interaction among inflammatory cells, mediators, and the cells and tissues present in the airways (National Institutes of Health, 1991). Various stimuli, such as exposure to pollens, release inflammatory mediators from airways cells, including mast cells, macrophages, epithelial cells, and nerve cells. Some mediators, such as histamine, produce immediate bronchospasm by inducing contraction of smooth muscle cells in airways or by enhancing neurotransmitter re-

lease from cholinergic nerve terminals that innervate the muscle (Madison, 1991). Other mediators, such as platelet-activating factor, may or may not contribute to immediate bronchospasm, but attract additional mediators. These mediators promote vascular leakiness, increased mucosal production, and the development of bronchial hyperresponsiveness. Once bronchial hyperreactivity occurs, pointed out Madison (1991), "the airways become exquisitely sensitive to normally innocuous stimuli, such as cold air, low concentrations of inhaled histamine or methacholine, and exercise" (p. 177). The key words are "exquisitely sensitive." It explains why when exposed to a minute quantity of a stimulus that causes no harm in others—a peanut is a good example—some individuals may experience a severe respiratory response, anaphylaxis, that can lead to severe respiratory distress or even death.

Developmental Features

Ellis (1993) noted that signs and symptoms of asthma are present during the first year or two of life in most children later diagnosed as having the disorder. These are children who exhibit recurrent periods of coughing or wheezing. The major provocateur of coughing and wheezing, continued Ellis (1993), is viral respiratory infection. A male predominance in rate of asthma emerges and persists through childhood. A number of anatomical and physiological peculiarities predispose infants and young children to wheezing. The most important of these are a disproportionate narrowing of the peripheral airways and decreased static elastic recoil of the lungs. Decreased bronchodilator smooth muscle and mucous gland hyperphasia with increased secretion of mucus may also predispose children to airway obstruction. Physiological changes, particularly in midchildhood, often result in an improvement in a child's asthma (Ellis, 1993). Continuous interaction between maturational and environmental variables is apt to produce developmental changes throughout childhood. As the two types of variables are inextricably interrelated, it is often impossible to delineate which factors produce changes in pediatric asthma.

DIAGNOSIS

The diagnosis of asthma is based on the child's medical history, physician examination, X rays, pulmonary function testing, and laboratory testing. Ellis (1993) noted that the medical history is the most important component in the diagnostic evaluation of children suspected of having asthma. Asthma history guidelines were proposed by Ellis (1993) and by the U.S. expert panel on asthma (National Institutes of Health, 1991). The guidelines suggest topics of interest to both medical and behavioral scientists. A definitive diagnosis of asthma is often difficult to obtain early in a child's illness. Most children who wheeze in infancy do not go on to develop asthma. However, according to a longitudinal study conducted by Martinez et al. (1995), wheezing episodes in infants are probably related to a predisposition to asthma. Smith (1993) indicated that 40 to 50% of children with severe wheezing from viral infections in infancy have repeated episodes of wheezing throughout childhood, and many children have increased reactivity to exercise or histamine when tested at 8 or 9 years. A chronic cough lasting more than 6 weeks and persisting after a viral upper respiratory infection, Smith (1993) pointed out, is a major indicator of childhood asthma.

Whereas patient symptoms, particularly wheezing and coughing, are used to diagnose asthma, confirmation of asthma comes about through use of two procedures. A 15 to 20% or greater improvement in results of pulmonary function tests, particularly FEV-1 (forced expiratory volume in 1 second or the total amount of air that can be exhaled in 1 second), after use of a bronchodilator is a commonly used indicator of asthma. The patient must present airway obstruction for this procedure to be used, however. Smith (1993) suggested that response to

asthma treatment, either bronchodilators or anti-inflammatory drugs, is the best diagnostic indicator of cough-only asthma. When the patient is not experiencing airway obstruction, a procedure may be used where a child is challenged by exercise, inhalation of methacoline, or to other stimuli. A 20% fall in FEV-1 in response to such a challenge is indicative of asthma. These two procedures for establishing the diagnosis of asthma are invaluable to both medical and behavioral scientists. They confirm the diagnosis of the condition for both clinical and research purposes.

ETIOLOGY

Etiological factors are related both to onset of asthma and to onset of specific attacks.

Risk Factors for Asthma

Most research on etiology has been directed at what could initially provoke asthma. Several major factors have been reported.

Genetic and Familial Factors

There is ample evidence of a hereditary basis to asthma. Ellis (1993) suggested that the most compelling evidence of these factors comes from the study of twins. Studies indicate that there is a substantial concordance of asthma in monozygotic twins (15–20%) compared with dizygotic twins (5–9%). Familial factors are equally important. When one parent has asthma, there is a 25% risk of their child developing asthma; when two parents have asthma, the risk is doubled to 50%. Longitudinal studies indicate that parental asthma is one of the most powerful predictors of asthma.

Bronchial Reactivity

Ellis (1993) emphasized that increased bronchial reactivity or responsiveness is "a fundamental and intrinsic characteristic of all individuals with asthma, both children and adults" (p. 1228). Although a spectrum of bronchial reactivity emerges in various population samples, Ellis (1993) continued, virtually all children with asthma have an abnormal degree of responsiveness when challenged with methacholine or cold air. Exposure to environmental factors, including allergens, dust mite droppings, and cockroach parts, is likely to interact with bronchial reactivity and trigger the initial asthma attack in many children.

Atopy

Atopy is defined as an increased predisposition to synthesize specific antibodies against environmental allergens (Ellis, 1993). It tends to occur in families, and is often applied to a group of disorders, including asthma. Atopy is reflected by positive skin tests, positive skin tests plus asthma symptoms, or the presence of asthma symptoms only. Overall, 75 to 80% of children with asthma show positive skin tests to common allergies. However, the exact role played by atopy in producing the onset of asthma remains confusing (Smith, 1993).

Sex

Asthma is diagnosed more frequently in male children before the age of 10. The male/female ratio ranges from 1.4:1 to 2:1. Severity of asthma also tends to be more severe in young boys than young girls. After the age of 10, however, the male preponderance begins to lessen. Longitudinal studies that follow children into adulthood generally have found no sex difference in prevalence or rate of asthma (Smith, 1993).

Age

One-third of children with asthma experience the onset of their symptoms before the age of 2; 80% have symptoms before the age of 5 (Smith, 1993). It was once thought that more severe and persistent asthma occurred before the age of 1 year. However, Smith (1993) explained,

the frequency of asthma attacks and the need for continual medication during childhood are more important indicators for persistence of the condition than onset of asthma before 1 year.

Respiratory Tract Infection

The role of respiratory infections in provoking asthmatic symptoms was established in the past two decades. Viral agents, and not bacterial agents, have been found to be the principal factors in provoking asthma. Ellis (1993) pointed out that the two most common viral agents implicated in the onset of asthma are the respiratory syncytial virus (RSV) and the parainfluenza virus. RSV infection was particularly a risk factor in young children as its presence was almost always associated with wheezing.

Emotional Stressors

In a longitudinal investigation, Klinnert, Mrazek, and Mrazek (1994) followed 150 children at genetic risk for developing asthma. Early findings indicate the potential interactive effects of stressful life events and parenting difficulties at a critical point after the birth of the child. These factors could prove to be significant predictors of later asthma in children genetically predisposed to the disorder.

Risk Factors for Attacks

In the past two decades, increasing attention has been directed toward determining potential risk factors for given attacks. In most instances, the specific trigger of a given episode is unknown. However, once a class or classes of stimuli have been identified as precipitating a child's attacks, steps can be taken to eliminate many of the stimuli from the child's environment. The approach of avoiding triggers and other allergens, particularly in the indoor environment, is indicative of the shift toward preventing asthma attacks as much as is possible (National Institutes of Health, 1991, 1992).

Environmental stimuli, found both indoors and outdoors, can pose major risk factors to patients with asthma, including children. A study by Stoddard and Miller (1995), for example, examined exposure to parental smoking as a risk factor for asthma or wheezing in childhood. Based on a cross-sectional analysis of the National Medical Expenditure Survey of 7578 children below the age of 18, investigators estimated that maternal smoking was responsible for 380,000 cases of childhood asthma or wheezing, or 7.5% of such symptomatic children. It is estimated that most Americans spend 93% of their time indoors (Pope et al., 1993). Maternal smoke, dust mites, cockroach parts, and household odors are but a few of the indoor stimuli that may trigger attacks in children with asthma.

A number of studies have examined outdoor stimuli as potential triggers of asthma. For example, a recent study found that 28% more hospital emergency room visits were made by patients with asthma when higher ambient levels of ozone were present (Weisel, Cody, & Lioy, 1995). These findings demonstrated that ozone adversely affects patients with asthma at levels below the current U.S. standards for air pollution. Also illustrative of current research is a study by Targonski, Persky, and Ramekrishnan (1995). They found that the odds of death caused by asthma occurring on days with exposure to 1000 spores per cubic meter or greater were 2.16 higher than on days on which the mold spore counts were less than 1000 spores per cubic meter.

EPIDEMIOLOGY

Three types of epidemiological data, pertaining to prevalence, morbidity, and mortality, are of interest in childhood asthma.

Prevalence

Asthma is the most common chronic illness in children. Newacheck, Budetti, and Halfon (1986) reported that asthma, along with other respiratory diseases, accounted for approximately 25% of all limitation of activity in childhood. According to data gathered in the National Health Interview Survey, prevalence of asthma in children younger than 18 in the United States was 3.2% in 1981 and 4.3% in 1988 (Taylor & Newacheck, 1992). This is below the 10% prevalence rate of pediatric asthma reported by Gergen et al. (1988). However, the latter estimate may be the most accurate: A report from the Centers for Disease Control (CDC) recently indicated that for persons aged 5–34, considered the most stable population to study, the rate of asthma increased 52%, from 34.6 per 1000 to 52.6 per 1000 from 1982 to 1992. The rate for males increased by 29% (from 39.7 to 51.4 per 1000) and increased 82% for females (from 29.4 to 53.6 per 1000) (*Morbidity and Mortality Weekly Reports,* 1995).

The difficulty of determining which populations of U.S. children are apt to experience asthma was described by Creer and Bender (1993). Among children most at risk for childhood asthma are members of racial or ethnic minorities who are poor and who live in urban areas (Evans, 1992; Weiss, Gergen, & Crain, 1992). This is shown in several sets of data. Weitzman, Gortmaker, and Sobol (1990) described data from the National Health Interview Survey indicating that black children were more likely to have asthma than white children. Other data, also gathered in national health and nutritional surveys, found the highest prevalence of active asthma among Puerto Rican children (Carter-Pokras & Gergen, 1993). Risk factors thought to contribute to asthma in minority children, particularly black children who live in the inner city, include: (1) poverty; (2) environmental factors; (3) psychological factors; (4) familial factors, particularly family dysfunction, large family size, and smaller homes; and (5) physical factors, especially low birth rate and maternal age younger than 20 years at the child's birth (Evans, 1992; Weitzman et al., 1990).

The role of risk factors in affecting asthma is neither clear nor consistent across minority groups, in part because of the paucity of information about these factors (Creer & Bender, 1995b). This is best exemplified by data concerning passive smoke and pediatric asthma. In the National Health Interview Survey of 1988, passive smoke was considered a major health risk in the homes of black children (Weiss, Gergen, & Crain, 1992). These data led some experts, including Evans (1992), to conclude that black children are more likely to have been exposed to cigarette smoke. Carter-Pokras and Gergen (1993), however, suggested that Puerto Rican children may be at increased risk for asthma because of greater exposure to passive smoke. Differing conclusions, based on different sets of data, graphically illustrate the limitations of our knowledge regarding risk factors and childhood asthma. In addition, little is known about the extent of pediatric asthma in rural areas (Weiss, Gergen, & Crain, 1992), although the overall rate of chronic illness is reportedly higher in rural than in urban areas (Creer & Bender, 1995b).

Morbidity

Morbidity data reflect the quantitative or qualitative states or conditions affected by asthma. Until recently, the major focus was almost entirely on changes in morbidity of patients with asthma. There is a rich vein of available information (Creer and Bender, 1995b). Findings from the National Ambulatory Medical Care Survey indicated that physician visits for asthma as a first-listed diagnosis increased from 6.5 million in 1985 to 7.1 million in 1990 (*Morbidity and Mortality Weekly Reports,* 1992). Between 1979 and 1987, hospitalizations for asthma among children aged 0 to 17 years increased 4.5% per year, with the largest increase among children 0 to 4 years of age. Among children aged 0 to 4 years, blacks had approximately 1.8 times the increase of whites (Gergen & Weiss, 1990). Data from the CDC (*Morbidity and Mortality Weekly Reports,* 1995) suggested that the age-adjusted hospital discharge rate for asthma as the primary diagnosis for patients 5 to 34 years of age was constant in both 1982 and 1992. Rates of asthma

for females were consistently higher than for males, and rates for blacks were consistently higher than for whites. Increased rates of hospitalization suggest a disparity between medical care available to white and black children. Many white children are able to receive outpatient treatment and avoid most severe attacks. Black children, however, tend to receive less outpatient treatment and are often forced to resort to hospital visits, particularly those to hospital emergency rooms, for treatment of attacks.

Access to medical care is a variable in the level of treatment provided children with asthma. Halfon and Newacheck (1993) analyzed data from the National Health Interview Survey on Child Health, and reported that poor children were more likely than nonpoor children to have spent more than 7 days in bed a year because of asthma. Poor children also had 40% fewer doctor visits and 40% had more hospitalizations for their asthma than nonpoor children. These findings were thought to reflect a diminished accessibility to appropriate outpatient health services for poor children. The burden of childhood asthma was examined further in a study by Taylor and Newacheck (1992). Relative to children with asthma, those with asthma missed an additional 10.1 million days of school, and had 12.9 million more contacts with physicians in 1988.

The economic impact of asthma has been scrutinized in a number of studies. Weiss, Gergen, and Hodgson (1992) found that costs of the disorder were an estimated $6.2 billion in 1990. Direct costs for asthma, including expenditures for hospitalizations, approached $1.6 billion. This represented the largest single direct medical expenditure for the condition, and indicated an increase of $500,000 over comparable data reported for 1985. Costs of outpatient hospital care for asthma were reported to be approximately $190.3 million; expenditures for care for asthma provided in hospital emergency rooms were approximately $295 million. Experts consider asthma as a condition that can be treated on an outpatient basis (National Institutes of Health, 1991). Costs for outpatient services were approximately $537.3 million; costs for inpatient services, however, were estimated to be $2000.6 billion by Weiss and his colleagues (1992). Medication costs, including those for childhood asthma, added approximately $1009.7 million to the total bill; this constituted an increase over estimated medication costs in 1985 of $712.7 million. Indirect costs for asthma totaled $2568.4 million. The largest component of indirect costs ($726.1 million) was attributed to the loss of more than 10 million school days among children 5 to 17 years of age.

Weiss, Gergen, and Hodgson (1992) concluded their review by pointing out that although asthma is often a mild chronic illness that can be treated with ambulatory care, 43% of its economic impact was associated with emergency room use, hospitalization, and death. Recent data collected from 25,614 patients with asthma enrolled in a national HMO indicated that members aged 18 and under consumed 47% of direct medical expenses for asthma-related illness (Stempel, Sturm, Hedblom, & Durcanin-Robbins, 1995). If these expenses were extrapolated to the total U.S. population, suggested Stempel et al. (1995), the annual direct medical costs for asthma would exceed $5 billion. This is 40% higher, corrected for inflation, than what was projected from an estimate in 1990.

Mortality

Until recently, deaths from asthma were considered rare. Relative to deaths from other causes (e.g., cancer, accidents), mortality from asthma is still low. Nevertheless, an increasing rate of deaths from asthma has been of concern both to professionals who treat the disorder and to the lay public. The rising rate of deaths is striking: From 1982 through 1991, the CDC reported that the annual age-adjusted death rate for asthma increased 40% from 13.4 per million population (3154 deaths) to 18.8 per million (5106 deaths). During the period, the rate increased 59% for females (from 15.4 to 24.6) and 34% for males (from 11.7 to 15.7). The data showed that for people aged 5–34, the rate increased 42% from 3.4 (401) deaths to 4.9 (569)

deaths (*Morbidity and Mortality Weekly Reports*, 1995). The annual death rate, continued the CDC, was consistently higher for blacks than for whites. During the period, the rate increased 41% for females (from 3.6 to 4.6) and 43% for males (3.7 to 5.3). Deaths from asthma from 1968 through 1987 among patients aged 5 to 34 were examined by Weiss and Wagener (1990). They reported that during the 1970s, mortality attributable to the condition declined by 7.8% per year in the United States. During the 1980s, however, mortality attributable to asthma rose by 6.2% per year, increasing faster among those aged 5 to 14 than among those aged 15 to 34. These findings are probably conservative, in that asthma mortality rates, determined through death certificate information, may underestimate actual asthma-related mortality (Hunt et al., 1993).

The increased number of deaths caused by asthma is of concern for three reasons. First, newer and more effective medications for the disorder, as well as guidelines for their use (National Institutes of Health, 1991, 1992) should have produced a decline in the mortality. This has not occurred, although there has been a recent plateau in the upward trend of deaths linked to asthma (Sly, 1994). Second, despite data indicating that the guidelines have improved the medical care provided some patients with the condition, especially those seen in hospital emergency rooms (Lantner & Ros, 1995), other reports have tied the increase in deaths from asthma to physician ignorance (Altman, 1993). In short, despite detailed guidelines for treating asthma, many medical personnel fail to follow them. Finally, perhaps the cruelest aspect concerning deaths from asthma is that, as pointed out by Ellis (1988), any mortality is unacceptable with a potentially reversible disorder such as asthma.

ASSESSMENT

The assessment and treatment provided to children with asthma by behavioral scientists is, in part, a function of how individual scientists perceive the disorder. Asthma has traveled a road from being portrayed as a purely psychological disorder at one end of the spectrum to a purely immunological disease at the other end of the continuum. The prevailing view, however, is that described by a number of authors in discussing chronic illness in children (Creer & Christian, 1976; Desguin, Holt, & McCarthy, 1994; Perrin & MacLean, 1988; Russo & Varni, 1982). According to their conceptual framework, children with chronic illness including asthma are like healthy children. Basically, children with chronic diseases or disorders are perceived as normal children in abnormal situations. Like other children, they are influenced by a variety of developmental, cognitive, and environmental factors (Desguin et al., 1994).

Assessment of children with asthma by behavioral scientists is similar to that conducted on children without the condition. Asthmatic children are referred for evaluation because of typical childhood problems, ranging from inappropriate interactions with peers to problems in the classroom. There are situations, however, when asthma is a reason for assessment. Behavioral scientists may be called on to assess problems that may be related to asthma per se or to specific asthma-related problems.

Problems with Asthma

A history of asthma is invaluable to both medical and behavioral scientists. Physicians learn about the physical characteristics of asthma; the information, as noted earlier, serves as the basis for diagnosing the disorder. The history of asthma also provides considerable information to behavioral scientists. The National Institutes of Health (1991) suggested topics to be reviewed in obtaining a history from patients with the disorder. The suggested topics have been expanded into an asthma questionnaire and presented in Table 1. Responses to the questionnaire provide a profile of asthma that is useful to medical and behavioral scientists. The discussion here, however, focuses on the value of each of the topics to psychologists and other behavioral scientists.

Symptoms

It is important to determine what individual children perceive as symptoms of asthma. Some may give what is a thorough clinical description of the disorder, and others may claim they rarely experience any symptoms of asthma. There are youngsters who describe more symptoms than they actually experience, and other children who deny they have asthma. Comparing information obtained separately from children and their parents is useful because it often reveals marked discrepancies in the way the two sets of informants view asthma symptoms.

Pattern of Symptoms

It is useful to know the pattern of asthma symptoms experienced by a child. Knowing whether a youngster experiences perennial or seasonal asthma, the topography of symptoms, and anything about the events that constitute an attack yields invaluable information. It permits the development of an intervention program to help a child manage asthma, as well as teaching the youngster realistic expectations necessary to control the disorder. The pattern of symptoms provides information that is useful in determining the type of intervention that may be required if a family is to optimize its ability to cope with childhood asthma and their asthmatic child.

Precipitating and/or Aggravating Factors

Factors that serve as triggers or aggravants of asthma are of interest to medical scientists in diagnosing and planning a treatment regimen. The information is no less important to behavioral scientists. Factors such as emotional reactions or family dysfunction are of concern to anyone involved with childhood asthma. Less obvious, asthmatic children may be evaluated to

Table 1. Asthma Questionnaire

I. Symptoms
   A. Cough, wheezing, shortness of breath, chest tightness, and sputum production of a modest degree
   B. Conditions associated with asthma, such as rhinitis, sinusitis, nasal polyposis, or atopic dermatitis

II. Pattern of symptoms
   A. Perennial, seasonal, or perennial symptoms with seasonal exacerbations
   B. Continuous, episodic, or continuous symptoms with acute exacerbations
   C. Onset, duration, and frequency of symptoms (days per week or month)
   D. Diurnal variation with special reference to nocturnal symptoms

III. Precipitating and/or aggravating factors
   A. Viral respiratory infections
   B. Exposure to environmental allergens such as pollen, mold, house dust mite, cockroach, animal dander, or secretory products, e.g., saliva
   C. Environmental change, such as moving, going on vacation, etc.
   D. Exposure to irritants, including tobacco smoke, strong odors, and air pollution
   E. Emotional reactions, such as crying or laughing hard, shouting, etc.
   F. Family dysfunction, such as parent separation, divorce, alcoholism, etc.
   G. Drugs, such as aspirin
   H. Food additives, such as sulfites or yellow food coloring
   I. Changes in weather or exposure to cold air
   J. Exercise
   K. Endocrine factors, such as menses

IV. Development of disorder
   A. Age of onset and age at diagnosis
   B. Progress of disorder, e.g., whether asthma is better or worse
   C. Previous evaluation, treatment, and response
   D. Present management and response, including plans for managing acute episodes
      1. Preventative measures taken to avoid symptoms
         a. Degree of adherence to preventive measures
      2. Stepwise regimen taken to manage acute episodes
         a. Degree of adherence to management regimen

V. Profile of typical exacerbation
   A. Prodromal signs and symptoms (e.g., itching of skin on the anterior neck, nasal allergy symptoms)
   B. Temporal progression
      1. Typical sequence of events taken during an acute episode
   C. Usual management
      1. Usual strategies taken by child and family
      2. Degree of confidence in management strategies

VI. Living situation
   A. Home age, location, cooling and heating systems, such as central with oil, electric, and/or wood-burning stove or fireplace
   B. Carpeting over a concrete slab
   C. Humidifier
   D. Description of patient's room with special attention to pillow, bed, floor covering, and other items that collect dust
   E. Animals in home
   F. Exposure to cigarette smoke in home
   G. Day care, school, or work environment

VII. Impact of disorder
   A. Impact on patient
      1. Number of emergency room visits and hospitalizations
      2. History of life-threatening acute exacerbations, intubation, or oral steroid therapy
      3. Number of days absent and academic performance
      4. Limitation of activity, especially sports
      5. History of nocturnal awakening
      6. Effect on growth, development, behavior, peer relationships, school or work achievement, and lifestyle

(continued)

Table 1. (Continued)

B. Impact on family
  1. Disruption of family
  2. Effect on siblings
  3. Economic impact
VIII. Assessment of patient's and family's perception of illness
  A. Patient and parental knowledge of asthma and belief in the chronicity of asthma and in the efficacy of treatment
  B. Ability of patient and parents to cope with asthma
  C. Level of family support and patient's and parent's capacity to recognize severity of an exacerbation
  D. Economic resources
IX. Family history
  A. Allergy in close relatives
  B. Asthma in close relatives
X. Medical history
  A. General medical history and history of other allergic disorder, history of injury to the airways, viral bronchiolitis, recurrent croup, gastroesophagael reflux, or passive exposure to smoke
  B. Review of symptoms

determine if any of a range of potential problems exist, including whether children smoke, use illegal drugs such as marijuana (most adolescents with asthma know that marijuana, at least when used occasionally, is a bronchodilator), or experience psychological distress because of delayed menses. With the increasing trend toward preventing asthma by altering environmental variables, there is a stronger attempt to determine what and how environmental stimuli might be altered in a child's environment to reduce asthma.

Development of the Disorder

Medical scientists probe for certain information related to the development and onset of childhood asthma. Behavioral scientists probe the same topics, but for different information. If, for example, children have had asthma for a period but it has only been recently diagnosed, they will have a number of questions about what is going to happen to them. Referral is apt to be made to help youngsters cope with the disorder and to change unrealistic expectations ranging from ignoring attacks to perceiving asthma as totally disabling. The increased severity of asthma generates a variety of psychological reac-

tions in both children and their parents. These reactions range from denial to increased anxiety to depression. Finally, management and response to asthma treatment generates a number of questions: Does a child know how to prevent asthma attacks? Are appropriate strategies taken, including use of preventative medications? Does the child comply with medication instructions? Does the child follow a stepwise strategy to relieve symptoms? These are common questions raised regarding childhood asthma.

Profile of Typical Exacerbation

This is a significant topic: Exactly what does a child and his or her family do during an attack? It is imperative to know the prodromal signs and symptoms exhibited by a child. Responses such as scratching the neck or humping the shoulders may signal the onset of asthma before wheezing is observed. Some parents note that changes in their child's behaviors, ranging from hyperlike behaviors to a sudden silence, are sometimes indicative of an approaching episode. Early intervention in these cases may abort the episode before it becomes a full-fledged attack. The temporal sequence of an attack is important. Does an episode occur rapidly or does the sequence slowly unfold so as to allow early intervention? Strategies taken to manage attacks yield important data, particularly information that indicates patients are attempting to adhere to medical instructions for asthma management. Finally, it is important to determine how confident patients are with respect to their ability to perform whatever steps are required to manage asthma, as well as the anticipated outcomes of their efforts. Positive self-efficacy and outcome beliefs are required for the control of childhood asthma (Creer, 1991a).

Living Situation

Environmental factors that could affect asthma are of interest to anyone treating childhood asthma. In most instances, medical personnel will offer suggestions for altering the environment so as to reduce the frequency and severity of asthma attacks. Consultation with behavioral scientists often occurs with respect to issues that arise in school and with animals in the home. School issues cover a gamut of topics, including how to help a child make up missed schoolwork caused by a high absenteeism to overcoming the resistance of many physical education teachers to have asthmatic children in their classes (physical education teachers show the widest range of attitudes of educators toward asthma: some believe it is a psychosomatic disorder and the child with asthma can do anything children without asthma can do, whereas others think any kind of exercise will provoke attacks and, therefore, do not want a child with asthma in their classes). Consultation, sometimes including a brief education program on childhood asthma, can overcome these problems. Of greater concern is asking a family to rid a home of a pet. Many behavioral scientists are shocked to discover that many families seemingly prefer the company of a dog to that of their child with asthma.

Impact of the Disorder

The effect the condition has on children and their families is of interest to all who treat childhood asthma. This section of the questionnaire reflects the variety of topics that can be explored in an interview with children and their families. The answers to these questions alone will provide considerable information about the role asthma plays in the lives of children and their families.

Assessment of Perception of Illness

How children and their families perceive asthma can determine whether or not the condition is controlled. Medical personnel often have some interest in these topics, but it is the behavioral scientist who is apt to learn more about attitudes and beliefs regarding asthma.

Family History

Knowledge about a family history of allergy or asthma permits medical personnel to pinpoint factors that might influence the course of a child's asthma. Family history is important to behavioral scientists because it provides clues concerning family characteristics and dynamics where there is a child with asthma. If a youngster has a parent who had asthma as a child, that youngster is often treated in a different manner than is the case with families where there is no history of asthma.

Medical History

Reviewing past medical history can be skewed toward the needs of the interviewer. It provides the opportunity to fill in any areas where additional information would be useful for either medical or behavioral reasons.

Specific Asthma-Related Problems

Behavioral scientists have been called on to assess a number of behavior problems exhibited by children with asthma. The list would include such problems as panic during attacks, overuse of hospitals, lack of medication compliance, inappropriate use of medication dispensers, problems in symptom detection, as well as about every other behavior problem exhibited by children without asthma (Creer, 1979, 1982, 1991a). The tools of assessment range from psychometric testing to observational procedures (Creer, 1991b, 1992). There are specific asthma-related behaviors, however, that require assessment. An illustration of such a problem is provided by the research of Bender and his colleagues. They use a broad array of psychometric and behavioral techniques to examine behavioral and psychological effects that occurred as a result of the administration of asthma medications. The research they have conducted has had broad implications for how children with asthma are treated medically. A study by Mazer, Figueroa, and Bender (1990) found that oral β-agonists produced a fine motor tremor, but did not affect the completion of more complex motor tasks. β-Agonists are often used to treat acute episodes. Two studies (Bender, Lerner, & Poland, 1991; Milgrom & Bender, 1993) confirmed that changes occurred in the effect on children treated with corticosteroids. The children, particularly those with a preexisting history of emotional problems, were more anxious and depressed when receiving higher doses of corticosteroids. Finally, in two definitive studies, the psychological side effects of theophylline, a commonly prescribed medication for asthma, were evaluated. Both studies investigated asthmatic children in placebo-controlled, randomized protocols with identical parent questionnaires and tests measuring attention, impulsivity, activity level, hand steadiness, memory, and self-reported mood. In an open-label study by Bender, Lerner, Ikle, Comer, and Szefler (1991), children showed improved attention on laboratory measures, although their parents reported conduct problems and hyperactivity which they attributed to hyperactivity. In a blinded study by Bender and Milgrom (1992), the children again showed improved attention, along with slightly increased hand tremor and anxiety. However, the parents were unable to discriminate between placebo and theophylline treatment conditions, a striking finding as only children with a

history of theophylline-induced psychological side effects reported by their parents participated in the study.

TREATMENT

The National Institutes of Health (1991, 1992) emphasize that management of asthma relies on four integral components: (1) objective measures of lung function, (2) pharmacological therapy, (3) environmental manipulation, and (4) patient education. Effective asthma management has the following goals: (1) to maintain a patient's normal respiratory function, (2) to maintain normal activity levels, (3) to prevent chronic and troublesome asthma symptoms, (4) to prevent recurrent exacerbations of asthma, and (5) to avoid adverse side effects from asthma medications. Prevention of attacks and management of ongoing episodes are the two basic approaches to asthma management.

Prevention of Asthma

Two general approaches are taken to the prevention of asthma: the use of preventive or maintenance medications and environmental manipulation.

Preventive Medications

Preventive medications are anti-inflammatory drugs often prescribed for children with moderate to severe asthma. They interrupt the development of bronchial inflammation and have a prophylactic or preventive action. They may also modulate or terminate ongoing inflammatory reactions in the airways (National Institutes of Health, 1991). Commonly prescribed medications include corticosteroids, particularly inhaled corticosteroids, cromolyn sodium, and nedocromil sodium. If taken as directed, these medications should prevent most attacks. These are prophylactic medications only; they have no value when used in the treatment of acute asthma. If anything, in fact, taking preventive medications during an attack may exacerbate the episode.

Environmental Manipulation

Depending on the triggers of their asthma, children with asthma and their families may be asked to rid their homes of carpeting, feather pillows and mattresses, pets, and anything else that could precipitate a child's asthma. Increasingly, medical personnel visit a child's home to uncover potential environmental triggers for the child's asthma. In a move that would warm the heart of the most ardent radical behaviorist, families are often asked to make drastic environmental changes, such as removing carpeting, stuffed furniture, draperies, certain plants, and other items that may collect dust or permit mold formation. Air conditioning or special air filters may be requested. These changes entail an initial expense, but in the long run they are likely to prevent unnecessary asthma attacks.

An important component to the control of asthma is the stepwise management of attacks. With the stepwise approach, the number of medications and frequency of administration are increased as necessary. The aim is to use the optimum medication needed to establish or maintain control with minimal risk of drug side effects (National Institutes of Health, 1991, 1992).

Attack Management

Sometimes an attack may be controlled when a child escapes a precipitating stimulus. This usually only occurs in the incipient stage of an episode, however. In most instances, children are asked to use a bronchodilator. Bronchodilators act primarily to relax bronchial smooth muscle and dilate the airways. Two types of bronchodilators are β-adrenergic agonists and methylxanthines. β-Adrenergic agonists relax

airway smooth muscle and may modulate mediator release from mast cells or basophils. In particular, they act on β-adrenergic receptors in the airways. They are used not only to control ongoing attacks, but also to prevent exercise-induced asthma. Methylxanthines, principally theophylline, are also used to manage ongoing attacks. Theophylline serves as a bronchodilator, and is particularly useful in controlling nighttime asthma. As theophylline has the potential for adverse effects, it must be carefully prescribed and monitored. Anticholinergic agents are occasionally used to help control attacks, but rarely with children.

Contributions of behavioral scientists to treatment are threefold: First, behavioral scientists are called on to help change inappropriate behaviors that occur in any population of children. Most problems exhibited by children with asthma are identical to those that may be observed in children without the condition. Second, referrals may be made to help alter behavioral patterns that can occur across chronic illnesses. Typical problems include anxiety, depression, marital discord, and family dysfunction (Creer & Bender, 1995b). Any other psychological or problem behavior noted in children in an abnormal situation may prompt referral to a behavioral scientist. Finally, there are problems related to the management of asthma. Those relevant to the prevention of asthma and attack management will be described.

Preventive Medications

A major problem in childhood asthma is noncompliance or nonadherence to medication regimens. The problem cannot be covered in a few paragraphs or pages; a more detailed account of compliance in children (Krasnegor, Epstein, Johnson, & Yaffe, 1993) and childhood asthma is found elsewhere (Creer, 1993; Creer & Levstek, in press). The methodology for assessing noncompliance in asthma is quite sophisticated. Not only has every assessment procedure been used in measuring medication compliance, but techniques unique to the evaluation of adherence in asthmatic patients have been developed. The classic example is the chronolog. This instrument fits an inhaler like a glove. Each time an inhalation occurs, it is recorded on a disk; the disk can be inserted into a translator and output provided as to the time of each inhaler activation. Unfortunately, assessment of compliance in asthma is far ahead of our knowledge about both determinants of noncompliance and how to change patterns of nonadherence (Creek & Levstek, in press). Although we can determine with some accuracy those who are noncompliant, we are less apt to know why they are nonadherent or how to modify the pattern.

There are two caveats that must be issued before behavioral scientists attempt to increase medication compliance in children with asthma. First, medical personnel usually blame children and their families for being noncompliant, but in all likelihood the children have not been taught to properly take medications via inhalers, metered dose inhalers (MDI), nebulizers, spacers, and other equipment. The specialized equipment is designed to transfer the proper dose of inhaled medication directly to children's airways. When children perform the simple motor skills required to use inhalers and other equipment correctly, inhaled medication can quickly produce bronchodilation. However, an increasing number of investigations have studied the knowledge and skills of both medical personnel and patients regarding the proper use of the inhalers and similar equipment. Generally, results are similar to those reported by Goodman et al. (1994) who, in a study that investigated MDI use by patients, concluded, "Our findings confirm those of others [i.e., proper use of the MDI is rare]; 75% of the subjects did not perform an acceptable MDI maneuver as defined by standard criteria." Whereas any number of reasons may be generated as to why medical personnel and patients do not use inhalers and similar apparatus correctly, Chapman, Hanania, and Kesten (1995), three veteran investigators of the problem, offered as good a reason as any when they recently lamented: "It

is regrettable that patient care is often suboptimal for lack of simple instruction inhaler use. We believe that much of the blame lies with academic medicine, which regards such a prosaic skill as beneath its dignity" (p. 290).

The second caveat could be more important to behavioral scientists: Physicians do not always prescribe the correct dose or appropriate medications for children with asthma. The problem was noted by Sublett, Pollard, Kadlec, and Karibo (1979) in studying compliance to theophylline regimens in children with asthma. They found that only 1 of 50 patients tested had theophylline levels within the therapeutic range. This indicated a 2% rate of compliance. However, the one patient thought to be adherent was not totally compliant: had the child been totally compliant, the dose of theophylline would have been so high (about 20 μg/ml) it could have easily resulted in seizures and possibly death. These warnings should alert the behavioral scientist to evaluate not only whether children take medications as directions, but also that an appropriate treatment regimen has been prescribed.

Environmental Manipulation

Behavioral scientists are often called on to help families change their environments to benefit children with asthma. Skills in developing checklists and other reminders for children are useful. The task of persuading families to rid the home of pets is often left to behavioral scientists. In most cases, families can be induced to find a new home for the dog and other furry members of the household. If all attempts at persuasion fail, the only recourse may be to turn in the parents for child abuse. By keeping the pet and ignoring their child's asthma, they are endangering the youngster's health to a degree that is no less harmful than if the child were subject to some other form of child abuse.

Attack Management

Both expert panels on asthma recommended the inclusion of patient education in any treatment program for the disorder (National Institutes of Health, 1991, 1992). Indeed, asthma has been at the forefront of the development of educational and self-management programs. The result has been the development and evaluation of a number of educational and self-management programs for childhood asthma. Wigal et al. (1990) reviewed 19 such programs. Despite some methodological shortcomings typical of first-generation programs, overall the programs did make a contribution to: (1) preventing and managing attacks, (2) reducing asthma-related health-care costs, (3) reducing the impact asthma had on the quality of life of children and their families, and (4) teaching patients to accept responsibility for the management of asthma. Several second-generation programs are currently being developed. These not only use more technologically advanced teaching methods (e.g., use of interactive television and personalized audiotapes) but also tailor programs for the needs of individual children. These programs offer considerable hope for improving the management of asthma in that they will synthesize the skills of medical and behavioral scientists with those of children and their families to optimize control over asthma. All children with asthma are entitled not only to appropriate medical treatment, but also to learning how they can help control their condition. Children and their families must learn the basic skills of self-management; programs that teach these skills are becoming more available every year. If self-management does nothing more, children are bound to learn the skills necessary to correct inhaler use.

CASE STUDY

Loren is a 12-year-old boy with moderate to severe asthma. For the fourth time in a year he was hospitalized because of asthma. At morning rounds in the hospital, Loren's asthma was reviewed by medical personnel and behavioral scientists. His physician pointed out that the boy's asthma could be controlled if he avoided triggers of his asthma, including exercise-induced attacks, and if he complied with his medication regimen. It was pointed out by a member of the nursing staff that Loren did not use a nebulizer properly. Instead of alleviating his respiratory distress, most of the medication was wasted because of inappropriate inhaler use. Lack of quick relief frustrated Loren. As a result, he tended to become angry, a behavior that only

exacerbated his asthma. Based on these discussions, it was decided to: (1) teach Loren to identify and avoid triggers of his asthma, (2) review his medications and adjust the regimen if possible, (3) improve his compliance to his medication treatment regimen, (4) teach him how to use a nebulizer correctly, and (5) teach him skills to control his frustration. The treatment team agreed to work together to attain these five goals.

Identify and Avoid Triggers

Loren was interviewed separately by both his physician and a staff psychologist using the asthma questionnaire. This provided enough information to warrant a visit to his home and school. At home, it was noted that he slept in a room with carpeting, drapes, and a number of stuffed animals. His parents were asked to remove these stimuli; they did so. The family had a pet cat. It was suggested that the cat be given a bath once a week—a common procedure to remove cat saliva and dander. The parents thought it would be easier to give the cat to a neighbor, and to set up an aquarium that could be enjoyed by the entire family. At school, it was noted that a hamster was kept in the classroom. When the teacher was informed that the hamster could be precipitating asthma in Loren, it was removed. All other potential triggers of his asthma were reviewed with Loren and his family. Loren did not realize that certain stimuli precipitated his asthma, and vowed to avoid or escape from these triggers whenever possible.

Review Medications

His physician reviewed Loren's medications with him and his parents. Several changes were made: First, the number of medications was reduced. This was achieved by increasing the dose of one drug and cutting another entirely out of the treatment regimen. Second, Loren was placed on longer-lasting medication. This avoided his having to take a dose late at night or very early in the morning. Third, all medications were prescribed to be taken with meals. This meant that the dose he formerly took at school was eliminated. Finally, the purpose of each medication was described, and Loren was taught to take them in a stepwise manner. Loren had been taking a preventive medication during attacks. It was explained that this only exacerbated the severity of his attacks. The physician stressed the importance of taking a preventive medication before Loren engaged in sports. It was explained to Loren that taking medications would allow him to enjoy athletic games, and that 67 of 596 (11%) U.S. athletes in the 1984 Olympics had asthma. Forty-one of the 67 won medals. Loren seemed elated to hear that he was no different from many excellent athletes because he has asthma.

Medication Compliance

The psychologist tailored a procedure to improve Loren's compliance to medication regimens. It was noted that his parents controlled the drugs, a situation that led to constant disagreements between Loren and his parents. "They bug me," Loren asserted. The psychologist negotiated an agreement with Loren, his parents, and his physician. It was decided that control of medications should be shifted to Loren and the control exercised by his parents faded out of the process. Periodic reviews of Loren's progress were made by his physician. In return for his compliance, Loren was receive an increase in his allowance for each week he was compliant. A contract was drawn up and signed by Loren, his parents, his physician, and the psychologist. Loren was also taught to record basic information each day on a diary. Only information related to his asthma and medication use was recorded; completed diary forms were mailed every 2 weeks to Loren's physician.

Use of Nebulizer

The psychologist asked Loren to demonstrate how he used a nebulizer to take medications. It was observed that Loren did not coordinate the responses necessary to activate the equipment, and to inhale or exhale properly. Using a shaping procedure described by Renne and Creer (1976), Loren was quickly taught to use the devise properly. He was given a checklist to use as a reminder of the behaviors he had to coordinate when he used a nebulizer or inhaler at home.

Management of Frustration

As part of a self-management training provided Loren by the psychologist and health educator, Loren was taught to identify and control the frustration that often interfered with treatment and exacerbated his asthma. In particular, he was taught progressive relaxation exercises. Loren was told that if he could relax, he might promote bronchodilation. More importantly, it was stressed that if he could relax using self-instructions, Loren could perform whatever steps were required to control his asthma, and prevent an episode from increasing in severity.

Loren's progress was periodically monitored by his treatment team. His treatment team soon found that Loren's asthma was under excellent control. Loren not only reported he had fewer attacks, but he required no further hospitalizations for his asthma. Loren's parents described a family where asthma was no longer at the center of their activities. They noted that asthma was rarely the cause of any disputes between them and Loren. Members of the nursing staff reported that Loren used the nebulizer correctly when he visited his physician. Finally, by taking a preventive medication before he exercised, Loren increased his participation in sports. He was elated when he made the seventh-grade basketball team.

SUMMARY

Pediatric asthma is of concern not only to children and their families, but also to medical and behavioral scientists. Epidemiological data concerning the disorder indicate a sharp increase in almost every category from the number of children with asthma to skyrocketing economic costs. The further deterioration of our environment portends more and more children will experience a condition, childhood asthma, that has no cure. Prevalence of the disorder could reach epidemic proportions by the end of the century. There are no signs from biological, medical, or behavioral research that we can totally reverse what can only be untold suffering and misery caused by asthma.

There are three potential trends that do offer a glimmer of hope not only for patients and their families, but also for those who treat the disorder. First, the creation of expert panels on asthma by the National Institutes of Health (1991, 1992) has generated guidelines that can be used both by clinicians and by investigators. They serve as a gold standard for everyone who works with the disorder. For patients, the guidelines have already produced better treatment; for scientists, it provides a framework helpful to designing and conducting research. Nothing is comparable in other areas of pediatrics as information that is provided on the definition, diagnosis, and treatment of asthma. As the guidelines will be updated every 5 years, they offer a foundation for both experts and novices in the area of asthma management and research.

The second trend is the view that success of any treatment protocol for childhood asthma is a function of the contribution made by children and their families. Almost two decades ago, the National Heart, Lung, and Blood Institute made patient education and self-management a high priority in asthma control. The initial result was the development and evaluation of a large number of programs aimed at childhood asthma. The first-generation programs, most of which were designed by behavioral scientists, have been widely accepted by patients and the medical community. More sophisticated programs are on the horizon. They not only incorporate components with proven value from the first-generation educational and self-management programs, but also utilize newer and more effective ways to teach patients about their disorder. The trend toward teaching asthmatic patients to become partners with medical and behavioral personnel in the management of asthma will become stronger as the prevalence and costs of the condition escalate.

The final trend is of interest to behavioral scientists: They can play a large role in childhood asthma if they desire. Most of the strategies developed to teach patients to be allies with their physicians in the management of asthma were developed by behavioral scientists. Their input has generally been welcomed by pediatric allergists, pulmonary physicians, and other medical personnel who treat the disorder. Unlike other specialists, pediatricians and other physicians do not see such help as an intrusion on their territory, but welcome any assistance they can obtain. The potential is great: There is a widespread belief that a drug will eventually be developed to cure asthma, but that patients won't take it as directed. Behavioral scientists will be called on to teach and maintain medication compliance. There are downsides to this rosy scenario, however. First, fewer and fewer psychologists and psychiatrists are electing to specialize in research and clinical work with asthmatic patients. The trend has become far more sharp than was the case when the author started working with childhood asthma three decades ago. Health educators, respiratory therapists, and nurses have moved into the vacuum, but their skills, although considerable, are not the same skills as those possessed by psychologists and psychiatrists. Consequently, the band of behavioral skills needed to help control asthma is not as broad as it must be; the specialized skills of all behavioral scientists, respiratory therapists, and nurses are required to help control childhood asthma. Second, it is impossible to make a contribution in asthma without a basic understanding of the physical nature of asthma and how the condition is treated. Without this background, any contribution by behavioral scientists is apt to be insignificant. In addition, as was pointed out earlier in describing medication compliance, the lack of knowledge about asthma increases our potential to do grave harm to children and their families. The solution is to become well versed in both the psychological and medical literature. Many chil-dren with asthma and their parents will applaud your efforts.

ACKNOWLEDGMENTS

The author is indebted to Kathleen Steiner and Deirdre Levstek for their invaluable comments and assistance.

REFERENCES

Altman, J. K. (1993, May 4). Rise in asthma deaths is tied to ignorance of many physicians. *The New York Times*, p. B8.

Bender, B. G., Lerner, J. A., Ikle, D., Comer, C., & Szefler, S. (1991). Psychological change associated with theophylline treatment of asthmatic children: A six-month study. *Pediatric Pulmonology, 11,* 233–242.

Bender, B. G., Lerner, J. A., & Poland, J. E. (1991). Association between corticosteroids and psychological change in hospitalized asthmatic children. *Annals of Allergy, 66,* 410–419.

Bender, B. G., & Milgrom, H. (1992). Theophylline-induced behavior change in children: An objective evaluation of parent's perceptions. *Journal of the American Medical Association, 267,* 2621–2624.

Busse, W. W., & Reed, C. E. (1988). Asthma: Definitions and pathogenesis. In E. Middleton, Jr., C. E. Reed, E. F. Ellis, N. F. Adkinson, Jr., & J. W. Yunginger (Eds.), *Allergy: Principles and practice* (3rd ed., pp. 969–998). St. Louis: Mosby.

Cater-Pokras, O. D., & Gergen, P. J. (1993). Reported asthma among Puerto Rican, Mexican-American, and Cuban children, 1982–1984. *American Journal of Public Health, 83,* 580–582.

Chapman, K. R., Hanania, N. A., & Kesten, S. (1995). Medical personnel's knowledge of the ability to use inhaling devices. *Chest, 107,* 290.

Creer, T. L. (1979). *Asthma therapy: A behavioral health care system for respiratory disorders.* New York: Springer Publishing.

Creer, T. L. (1982). Asthma. *Journal of Consulting and Clinical Psychology, 50,* 912–921.

Creer, T. L. (1991a). The application of behavioral procedures to childhood asthma: Current and future perspectives. *Patient Education and Counseling, 17,* 9–22.

Creer, T. L. (1991b). Psychologic and behavioral assessment of childhood asthma. Part I: Psychologic instruments. *Pediatric Asthma, Allergy, and Immunology, 5,* 317–328.

Creer, T. L. (1992). Psychological and behavioral assessment of childhood asthma. Part II. Behavioral approaches. *Pediatric Asthma, Allergy, and Immunology, 6,* 21–34.

Creer, T. L. (1993). Medication compliance and childhood asthma. In N. A. Krasnegor, L. Epstein, S. B. Johnson, & S. J. Yaffe (Eds.), *Developmental aspects of health compliance behavior* (pp. 303–333). Hillsdale, NJ: Erlbaum.

Creer, T. L., & Bender, B. G. (1993). Asthma. In R. J. Gatchel & E. B. Blanchard (Eds.), *Psychophysiological disorders* (pp. 151–208). Washington, DC: American Psychological Association.

Creer, T. L., & Bender, B. G. (1995a). Recent trends in asthma research. In A. J. Goreczyny (Ed.), *Handbook of health and rehabilitation psychology* (pp. 31–53). New York: Plenum Press.

Creer, T. L., & Bender, B. G. (1995b). Pediatric asthma. In M. C. Roberts (Ed.), *Handbook of pediatric psychology* (2nd ed., pp. 219–240). New York: Guilford Press.

Creer, T. L., & Christian, W. P. (1976). *Chronically-ill and handicapped children: Their management and rehabilitation.* Champaign, IL: Research Press.

Creer, T. L., & Levstek, D. (in press). Adherence to asthma regimens. In D. S. Gochman (Ed.), *Handbook of health behavior research.* New York: Plenum Press.

Desguin, B. W., Holt, I. J., & McCarthy, S. M. (1994). Comprehensive care of the child with a chronic condition. Part 1. Understanding chronic conditions in childhood. *Current Problems in Pediatrics, 24,* 199–218.

Ellis, E. F. (1988). Asthma in infancy and childhood. In E. Middleton, Jr., C. E. Reed, E. F. Ellis, N. F. Adkinson, Jr., & Y. W. Yunginger (Eds.), *Allergy: Principles and practice* (3rd ed., pp. 969–998). St. Louis: Mosby.

Ellis, E. F. (1993). Asthma in infancy and childhood. In E. Middleton, Jr., C. E. Reed, E. F. Ellis, N. F. Adkinson, Jr., J. W. Yunginger, & W. W. Busse (Eds.), *Allergy: Principles and practice* (4th ed., pp. 1225–1262). St. Louis: Mosby.

Evans, R., III. (1992). Asthma among minority children: A growing problem. *Chest, 101,* 368S–371S.

Gergen, P. J., Mullally, D. I., & Evans, R. (1988). National survey of prevalence of asthma among children in the United States, 1976–1980. *Pediatrics, 81,* 1–7.

Gergen, P. J., & Weiss, K. B. (1990). Changing patterns of asthma hospitalization among children: 1979 to 1987. *Journal of the American Medical Association, 264,* 1688–1692.

Goodman, D. E., Israel, E., Rosenberg, M., Johnston, R., Weiss, S. T., & Drazen, J. M. (1994). The influence of age, diagnosis, and gender on proper use of metered-dose inhalers. *American Journal of Respiratory and Critical Care Medicine, 150,* 1256–1261.

Halfon, N., & Newacheck, P. W. (1993). Childhood asthma and poverty: Differential impacts and utilization of health services. *Pediatrics, 91,* 56–61.

Hunt, L. W., Jr., Silverstein, M. D., Reed, C. E., O'Connell, E. J., O'Fallon, W. M., & Yunginger, J. W. (1993). Accuracy of the death certificate in a population-based study of asthmatic patients. *Journal of the American Medical Association, 269,* 1947–1952.

Kaliner, M., & Lemanske, R. (1992). Rhinitis and asthma.

Journal of the American Medical Association, 268, 2807–2829.

Klinnert, M. D., Mrazek, P. J., & Mrazek, D. A. (1994). Early asthma onset: The interaction between family stressors and adaptive parenting. *Psychiatry, 57,* 51–61.

Krasnegor, N. A., Epstein, L., Johnson, S. B., & Yaffe, S. J. (Eds.). (1993). *Developmental aspects of health compliance behavior.* Hillsdale, NJ: Erlbaum.

Lantner, R. R., & Ros, S. P. (1995). Emergency management of asthma in children: Impact of NIH guidelines. *Annals of Allergy, Asthma, and Immunology, 74,* 188–190.

Loren, M. L., Leung, P. K., Cooley, R. L., Chai, H., Bell, T. D., & Buck, V. M. (1978). Irreversibility of obstructive changes in severe asthma in children. *Chest, 74,* 126–129.

Madison, J. M. (1991). Chronic asthma in the adult: Pathogenesis and pharmacotherapy. *Seminars in Respiratory Medicine, 12,* 175–184.

Marion, R. J., Creer, T. L., & Reynolds, R. V. C. (1985). Direct and indirect costs associated with the management of childhood asthma. *Annals of Allergy, 54,* 31–34.

Martinez, F. D., Wright, A. L., Taussig, L. M., Holberg, C. J., Halonen, M., Morgan, W. J., & the Group Health Medical Associates. (1995). Asthma and wheezing in the first six years of life. *New England Journal of Medicine, 332,* 133–138.

Mazer, B., Figueroa, R. W., & Bender, B. (1990). The effect of albuterol aerosol on fine-motor performance in hospitalized asthmatic children. *Journal of Allergy and Clinical Immunology, 86,* 243–248.

Milgrom, H., & Bender, B. G. (1993). Current issues in the use of theophylline. *American Review of Respiratory Disease, 147,* S33–S39.

Morbidity and Mortality Weekly Reports. (1992). Asthma—United States, 1980–1990.

Morbidity and Mortality Weekly Reports. (1995). Asthma—United States, 1982–1992.

National Institutes of Health. (1991). *Executive summary: Guidelines for the diagnosis and management of asthma* (NIH Publication No. 91-3024A). Washington, DC: U.S. Government Printing Office.

National Institutes of Health. (1992). *International consensus report on diagnosis and management of asthma* (DHHS Publication No. 92-3091). Washington, DC: U.S. Government Printing Office.

National Institutes of Health. (1997). *Highlights of the Expert panel Report 2: Guidelines for the diagnosis and management of asthma* (NIH Publication No. 97-4051A). Washington, DC: U.S. Department of Health and Human Services.

Newacheck, P. W., Budetti, P. P., & Halfon, N. (1986). Trends in activity-limiting chronic conditions among children. *American Journal of Public Health, 76,* 178–184.

Perrin, J. M., & MacLean, W. E. (1988). Children with chronic illness. *Pediatric Clinics of North America, 35,* 1325–1337.

Pope, A. M., Patterson, R., & Burge, H. (Eds.). (1993). *Indoor allergens: Assessing and controlling adverse health effects.* Washington, DC: National Academy Press.

Renne, C. M., & Creer, T. L. (1976). Training children with asthma to use inhalation therapy equipment. *Journal of Applied Behavioral Analysis, 9,* 1–11.

Renne, C. M., & Creer, T. L. (1985). Asthmatic children and their families. In M. L. Walraich & D. K. Routh (Eds.), *Advances in developmental and behavioral pediatrics* (Vol. 6, pp. 41–81). Greenwich, CN: JAI Press.

Russo, D. C., & Varni, J. W. (1982). Behavioral pediatrics. In D. C. Russo & J. W. Varni (Eds.), *Behavioral pediatrics* (pp. 3–24). New York: Plenum Press.

Sly, R. M. (1994). Changing asthma mortality and sales of inhaled bronchodilators and antiasthmatic drugs. *Annals of Allergy, 73,* 439–443.

Smith, L. (1993). Childhood asthma: Diagnosis and treatment. *Current Problems in Pediatrics, 23,* 271–305.

Stempel, D. A., Sturm, L. L., Hedblom, E. C., & Durcanin-Robbins, J. F. (1995). Total costs of asthma care. *Journal of Allergy and Clinical Immunology, 95,* 217.

Stoddard, J. J., & Miller, T. (1995). Impact of parental smoking on the prevalence of wheezing respiratory illness in children. *American Journal of Epidemiology, 141,* 96–102.

Sublett, J. L., Pollard, S. J., Kadlec, G. J., & Karibo, J. M. (1979). Noncompliance in asthmatic children: A study of theophylline levels in pediatric emergency room population. *Annals of Allergy, 43,* 95–97.

Targonski, P. V., Persky, V. W., & Ramekrishnan, V. (1995). Effect of environmental molds on risk of death from asthma during pollen season. *Journal of Allergy and Clinical Immunology, 95,* 955–961.

Taylor, W. R., & Newacheck, P. W. (1992). Impact of childhood asthma on health. *Pediatrics, 90,* 657–662.

Vance, V. J., & Taylor, W. F. (1971). Status and trends in residential asthma homes in the United States. *Annals of Allergy, 29,* 428–437.

Weisel, C. P., Cody, R. P., & Lioy, P. J. (1995). Relationship between summertime ambient ozone levels and emergency department visits for asthma in central New Jersey. *Environmental Health Perspectives, 103,* 97–102.

Weiss, K. B., Gergen, P. J., & Crain, E. F. (1992). Inner-city asthma: The epidemiology of an emerging U.S. public health concern. *Chest, 101,* 362S–367S.

Weiss, K. B., Gergen, P. J., & Hodgson, T. A. (1992). An economic evaluation of asthma in the United States. *New England Journal of Medicine, 326,* 862–866.

Weiss, K. B., & Wagener, D. K. (1990). Changing patterns of asthma mortality: Identifying target populations at high risk. *Journal of the American Medical Association, 264,* 1683–1687.

Weitzman, M., Gortmaker, S., & Sobol, A. (1990). Racial, social and environmental risks for childhood asthma. *American Journal of Diseases of Children, 144,* 1189–1194.

Wigal, J. K., Creer, T. L., Kotses, H., & Lewis, P. D. (1990). A critique of 19 self-management programs for childhood asthma. Part I. The development and evaluation of the programs. *Pediatric Asthma, Allergy, and Immunology, 4,* 17–39.

17

Juvenile Diabetes

Suzanne Bennett Johnson

INTRODUCTION

Pancreatic beta cell destruction and the resultant inability of the pancreas to produce insulin is the pathological process underlying insulin-dependent diabetes mellitus (IDDM). This form of diabetes, also known as *type I diabetes,* is typically diagnosed in childhood or adolescence. Hence, it is commonly referred to as *juvenile* or *childhood diabetes.* Juvenile diabetes is a chronic disease for which there is no cure. Consequently, the child or adolescent is faced with lifelong demands associated with the disease and its management.

As early as the seventeenth century, psychological factors have been associated with diabetes. Thomas Willis (1684) suggested that it was a disease resulting from "prolonged sorrow." Two centuries later, Maudsley (1899) pointed to anxiety as a correlate of diabetes onset. However, as insulin was not discovered until 1922, children with diabetes had little time to

live, and psychological factors were generally ignored in view of the physical realities.

In the twentieth century, juvenile diabetes changed from a relatively short-term mortal illness to a chronic disorder associated with reasonable life expectancies (although even today, life expectancy remains only 75% of normal; Travis, Brouchard, & Shiner, 1987). Improved medical management of IDDM came at a time of widespread interest in psychosomatic medicine. Heavily influenced by psychoanalytic theory, psychological research initially focused on the elucidation of a "diabetic personality," which would predispose the individual to this disease. Dunbar's (1954) work is illustrative of this view. Patients with diabetes were presumed to have certain personality characteristics that differentiated them from healthy individuals and from other illness groups. Most of these characteristics were certainly unflattering and suggested substantial psychopathology: dependence–independence conflicts, poor sexual adjustment, anxiety, depression, paranoid suspicion. Empirical evidence suggests that there is, in fact, no specific diabetic personality, although individuals in poor health do report more adjustment problems than those in good diabetes control (Dunn & Turtle, 1981; Johnson, 1980).

Although the search for the "diabetic person-

SUZANNE BENNETT JOHNSON • Center for Pediatric Psychology and Family Studies, University of Florida Health Science Center, Gainesville, Florida 32610-0165.

Handbook of Child Psychopathology, 3rd edition, edited by Ollendick & Hersen. Plenum Press, New York, 1998.

ality" no longer dominates psychological research on diabetes, an interest in behavioral, social, cognitive, and emotional factors remains. However, the focus of current psychological research has changed. Earlier studies emphasized the study of variables within the individual (e.g., personality) and the comparison of patients, conceptualized as a homogeneous group, with healthy controls. More recent research seeks to elucidate psychological variables relevant to health and functioning within the diabetes population. This approach presumes great heterogeneity in how people respond to and manage this disease. With good diabetes control now known to delay, diminish, or prevent complications of diabetes (DCCT Research Group, 1993), there is a greater emphasis on improving patient adherence to medical management programs. Adherence behaviors and their modification are clearly psychological phenomena. As a consequence, the medical community is increasingly seeking psychological expertise to assist them and their patients.

This chapter focuses on the phenomenology, diagnosis, medical management, etiology, and epidemiology of juvenile diabetes as well as psychological assessment considerations and treatment options available to psychologists working with this population.

PHENOMENOLOGY

The classic onset symptoms of juvenile diabetes include fatigue, thirst, hunger, frequent urination, and weight loss despite excessive eating. Because insulin is necessary for utilization of available blood sugar, the child with diabetes is literally "starving" despite eating large quantities of food. Without insulin, high levels of circulating blood glucose cannot be utilized. The body responds as if it is in a state of starvation, breaking down body fats into fatty acids, and the child may exhibit marked breath odor. The liver converts the fatty acids to ketone bodies to be used by peripheral tissues. However, because insulin also plays a critical role in the inhibition of

fat breakdown, fatty acids and ketones soon begin to accumulate in excessive amounts. The body's attempt to eliminate such excessive glucose and ketone buildup results in frequent urination. The child exhibits thirst and repeated trips to the bathroom; dehydration can easily result. In untreated juvenile diabetes, when the kidney cannot effectively eliminate the high levels of ketones entering the bloodstream, ketosis or ketoacidosis occurs. This is a very serious condition that, if left untreated, produces coma and ultimately death (Davidson, 1991).

The child with diabetes is managed by exogenous insulin replacement by one or more daily injections. However, current treatment methods only approximate normal pancreatic function. Consequently, both hyperglycemia (excessively high blood glucose levels) and hypoglycemia (excessively low blood glucose levels) can and do occur. Hypoglycemia (also called insulin shock), in particular, can lead to relatively rapid cognitive disorientation, convulsions, and coma.

Diabetes is also associated with a number of serious complications that typically occur 15–20 years after disease onset. It is the leading cause of new cases of blindness in persons aged 20–74 (Klein & Klein, 1985). It accounts for approximately one-quarter of all new cases of end-stage renal disease in the United States (Herman & Teutsch, 1985). Forty to forty-five percent of all nontraumatic amputations in this country are done on patients with diabetes whose peripheral vascular disease has diminished arterial perfusion to the legs and feet to such an extent that ulcers and gangrene have resulted (Palumbo & Melton, 1985). However, atherosclerotic heart disease is the single most common cause of mortality in this population, accounting for one-third of all deaths in patients over 40 years of age (Barrett-Conner & Orchard, 1985).

DIAGNOSIS AND MEDICAL MANAGEMENT

Presence of the classic symptoms of diabetes, polyuria (frequent urination), polydipsia (excessive thirst), ketonuria (ketones in the urine), and rapid weight loss, with a random blood glucose level >200 mg/dl is considered diagnostic. The disease may also be diagnosed in asymptomatic youngsters with an oral glucose tolerance test. The child arrives for the test in the fasting state. Blood glucose is measured and then the youngster is given by mouth a glucose dose of 1.75 g/kg ideal weight (up to a maximum of 75 g). Subsequent blood glucose tests are conducted for 2 hours after glucose ingestion. IDDM is diagnosed if: (1) the fasting plasma glucose level is ≥ 140 mg/dl and (2) on at least one occasion after the glucose is ingested and at 2 hours postingestion, the plasma glucose level is ≥ 200 mg/dl (Davidson, 1991).

Recently, it has become possible to identify persons at high risk for diabetes using samples from a single blood draw (Riley et al., 1990; Schatz et al., 1994). Large-scale screening programs are now under way for a multisite Diabetes Prevention Trial (DPT-1), funded by the National Institutes of Health. Individuals selected for participation are offered experimental interventions to assess whether disease onset can be delayed or prevented.

Because insulin insufficiency is the underlying cause of juvenile diabetes, treatment of diagnosed patients involves insulin replacement by injection at least once and usually two or more times per day. Two types of insulin are commonly used: short-acting (Regular or Semilente) and intermediate-acting (NPH or Lente). They vary in absorption rate, time of maximal action, and duration of action. Comparing the two types, short-acting insulin has an earlier onset of action (30–60 minutes versus 3–4 hours after injection), an earlier time of maximal action (2–6 versus 10–16 hours after injection), and a shorter total duration of action (4–12 versus 20–24 hours after injection). Intermediate-acting insulin, either alone or in combination with short-acting insulin, is usually prescribed (Davidson, 1991). Combining insulins may be helpful as short-acting insulin injected before breakfast will handle the glucose produced by the breakfast meal, minimizing the rise in blood glucose

that would have occurred if only intermediate-acting insulin had been used.

The goal of therapy is to maintain the patient's blood glucose within the normal range. However, even combining types of insulin will not guarantee normoglycemia. In the healthy person without diabetes, the pancreas produces insulin in response to blood glucose (e.g., after eating), maintaining blood glucose within a constant and relatively narrow range (80–120 mg/dl). Insulin replacement by injection once or twice a day does not permit rapid changes in insulin availability in response to increases or decreases in blood glucose. If the patient eats too much, given the available supply of insulin, hyperglycemia will result. If the patient eats too little, given the available supply of insulin, hypoglycemia will occur. Consequently, the patient is told to eat small amounts frequently throughout the day. Three small meals and three snacks are recommended.

Other factors, in addition to diet, can affect or induce blood glucose excursions. Exercise, considered beneficial because it improves insulin action, may also result in hypoglycemia if insufficient calories are consumed. Illness and stress may impair insulin action, leading to hyperglycemia. Because of the interacting influences of diet, exercise, illness, emotional state, and insulin action, blood glucose variability is to be expected. As a consequence, blood glucose levels must be monitored on a daily basis so as to appropriately manage hypo- or hyperglycemic episodes, should they occur. Home blood glucose monitoring is accomplished by obtaining a small sample of blood from a finger stick and placing it on a reagent strip. The strip changes color depending on the available glucose in the sample. The color change is compared to a color chart that specifies for the patient the blood glucose level associated with that particular color. Alternatively, the patient may use one of a number of available computerized blood glucose meters in which the reagent strip is simply inserted, the meter "reads" the strip, and the result appears on the screen. Home blood glucose monitoring, although now widely accepted in the United States, is a relatively new phenomenon. It is the product of technological advances that permit reliable and accurate blood glucose measurement in the home environment. Prior to these developments, urine glucose tests were the usual method of monitoring blood glucose. However, because urine glucose tests are an indirect measure of blood glucose, they are far less satisfactory.

Recently published results of the Diabetes Complications and Control Trial (DCCT) are expected to significantly impact diabetes care. The DCCT was launched in 1982 by the NIH to test whether intensive therapy (IT), consisting of a rigorous regimen of increased insulin injection frequency ($\geq$ three shots per day), increased blood glucose testing frequency ($\geq$ four tests per day), frequent insulin adjustment, and increased provider contact (monthly clinic visits plus weekly phone contact) could result in near-normal blood glucose levels and a reduction in risk for the complications of diabetes. IT was compared with conventional therapy, which represented usual care of patients with diabetes, in a 29-site trial involving over 1400 patients. The trial was terminated a year early when the marked advantage of IT over conventional therapy became apparent; IT was associated with lower mean blood glucose and a significant delay in onset and a slower progression of eye disease (retinopathy), kidney disease (nephropathy), and nerve disease (neuropathy) (DCCT Research Group, 1993). However, associated costs of IT included increased weight gain and increased frequency of severe hypoglycemia. Nevertheless, the DCCT Research Group recommended that most patients with IDDM, including adolescent patients, should be treated with IT.

Because the DCCT was conducted with a carefully selected group of highly motivated, predominantly adult, IDDM patients, its impact on everyday clinical practice remains to be seen. Although IDDM is typically diagnosed in childhood, adolescents were underrepresented in the DCCT and no children were included in the trial. Nevertheless, the DCCT Research Group and the National Diabetes Information Clearing House (NDICH) recommend IT use with youngsters aged 13 and older (DCCT Research Group, 1993; NDIC, 1994). We have yet to elucidate which adolescents are most likely to succeed and fail when offered IT, and what specific risks may be associated with IT in this particular age group. Neither the DCCT Research Group nor the NDICH formally recommended IT use with children.

ETIOLOGY

Etiology of IDDM remains unclear, although genetic factors are clearly implicated. Relatives of IDDM patients are at greatly increased risk for developing the disease themselves. Nevertheless, only about 1 child in 50 who is a brother or sister of an IDDM patient will actually develop diabetes before 20 (LaPorte & Cruickshanks, 1985). Barnett, Eff, Leslie, and Pyke (1981) studied 81 identical twin pairs in which one twin had developed IDDM before the age of 20. Over 40% of these co-twin pairs were discordant for diabetes. Other factors, in addition to some type of genetic predisposition, appear to be involved in the development of this disease.

Currently, there is good evidence to suggest that IDDM is an autoimmune disease in which the body attacks and destroys its own insulin-producing islet cells within the pancreas. Overt diabetes occurs only when sufficient numbers of islet cells have been destroyed. However, the mechanism that triggers this autoimmune process is unknown (Thai & Eisenbarth, 1993). Nevertheless, islet cell antibodies appear to predate the onset of the disease by months or even years and are currently being used in large-scale screening programs as a predictive marker of who will develop this disease in the future (Riley et al., 1990; Schatz et al., 1994).

EPIDEMIOLOGY

There are two types of diabetes mellitus: (1) juvenile or type I or IDDM, which is the focus of this chapter, and (2) adult or type II or non-insulin-dependent diabetes (NIDDM). When discussing the prevalence of IDDM, it is common to compare it with the prevalence of NIDDM. This comparison makes the problem of diabetes in children appear small because only 5% of all diabetics in the United States have IDDM or the juvenile form. However, when comparing IDDM with other chronic diseases of childhood, a different picture emerges. In the United States, about 1 child in 600 has IDDM, or approximately 120,000 youngsters (LaPorte & Tajima, 1985). Risk for developing IDDM is higher than that for most other chronic diseases of childhood. It is equal to that for all childhood cancers combined and is much greater than that for other well-known diseases such as cystic fibrosis, muscular dystrophy, and rheumatoid arthritis (LaPorte & Cruickshanks, 1985). Although international comparisons are difficult because of lack of accurate prevalence data, it appears that the IDDM rate in the United States is comparable to the rate in non-Scandinavian European countries, lower than that of Scandinavian countries, and higher than that of Asian countries. There appear to be true geographic–racial differences in the risk for developing IDDM. For example, in the United States, males and females are at equal risk for IDDM but whites are 1.5 times more likely to develop IDDM than blacks. Disease onset can occur at any age, although peak incidence appears to be around puberty (LaPorte & Cruickshanks, 1985; Zimmet, 1983).

ASSESSMENT

There are multiple assessment issues relevant to the treatment of children with diabetes. Although chronic disease does place youngsters at increased risk for psychological disorders (Lavigne & Faier-Routman, 1992), most children with diabetes appear similar to healthy peers on measures of general psychological adjustment (see Johnson, 1995a, for a review). However, both children and parents may experience mild anxiety and depression at the time of diagnosis, but this typically dissipates within 6 months (Kovacs, Brent, Steinberg, Paulauskas, & Reid, 1986; Kovacs et al., 1985). Clinically significant levels of anxiety have also been documented in persons identified through screening programs as high risk for diabetes as well as in their family members; much initial anxiety usually returns to normal levels within 3–4 months (Johnson, Riley, Hansen, & Nurick, 1990; Johnson & Tercyak, 1995). Nevertheless, mothers often reported considerable parenting stress attempting to cope with the multiple, complex demands of managing diabetes in a growing child (Hauenstein, Marvin, Snyder, & Clarke, 1989; Wysocki, Huxtable, Linscheid, & Wayne, 1989).

Youngsters with diabetes usually function adequately in the classroom, with IQ scores in the normal range. However, hypoglycemia is clearly associated with cognitive and motor impairments. Even when the child is not hypoglycemic, there is increasing evidence of subtle neuropsychological effects that may interfere with some children's cognitive functioning. Risk factors for poor neuropsychological performance include disease diagnosis before age 5 and a history of poor glucose control. However, frequent school absences related to illness may also contribute to the problem (see Ryan, 1990, for a review).

Rather than focusing on more general issues of psychological adjustment and school performance, this chapter will emphasize disease-specific assessment (i.e., how the patient and family manage the youngster's illness). This type of information is typically less well known to psychologists and is particularly relevant to difficult-to-manage cases referred by the medical community. For the interested reader, the available literature relevant to these children's general adjustment, cognitive functioning, and school performance has been reviewed elsewhere (Johnson, 1995a).

Knowledge about Diabetes

Chronic illnesses, like diabetes, require the patient to manage the disease on a daily basis.

Clinic visits occur only intermittently with the physician serving in a consultant role. The physician may make specific recommendations but it is up to the patient to deal with the variable and often complex management issues presented by the disease on a daily basis. Consequently, to effectively manage diabetes, the patient must be highly knowledgeable. Unfortunately, one of the most consistent findings noted in this literature is the inadequacy of patient knowledge whether the patients are children or adults (Johnson et al., 1982; Lorenz, Christensen, & Pichert, 1985; Page, Verstraete, Robb, & Etzwiler, 1981; Watkins, Roberts, Williams, Martin, & Coyle, 1967).

Because children exhibit significant cognitive changes as they mature, it is not surprising that children with diabetes demonstrate age-related variability in their disease knowledge. As expected, adolescents generally exhibit more sophisticated knowledge than their younger counterparts; some of the diabetes management skills are sufficiently complex that very young children exhibit considerable difficulty. For example, most youngsters are able to accurately self-inject insulin by age 9 (Gilbert et al., 1982; Johnson et al., 1982; Kohler, Hurwitz, & Milan, 1982; Naughten, Smith, & Baum, 1982). Encouraging youngsters to take total responsibility for this component of their care before age 9 may be detrimental to their health as most young children will not be cognitively or socially mature to successfully accept the responsibility. However, just because a child may not yet be capable of carrying out some or all diabetes management tasks does not mean the child should be excluded from the process. Parents may need to take primary responsibility but most children are capable of significant participation, albeit with parental supervision.

With the recent realization that knowledge about diabetes is as complex as the disease itself, there is increasing recognition that diabetes knowledge cannot be accurately assessed by brief questionnaire or by taking the patient's word that he or she knows how to accurately inject insulin or test blood glucose. Fortunately,

alternative, more extensive assessment methodologies are now available. The Test of Diabetes Knowledge, given in a multiple-choice format, tests the patient's or parent's level of basic knowledge about diabetes (general information) as well as the respondent's ability to choose appropriate treatment options when presented with varying situations (problem-solving). The instrument has proved to be reliable and sensitive to children's acquisition of new knowledge (Harkavy et al., 1983; Johnson, 1995b; Johnson et al., 1982). Behavioral observation methods have been particularly useful for the assessment of diabetes management skills, such as insulin injection and glucose testing; excellent interobserver agreement is usually obtained (e.g., Gilbert et al., 1982; Harkavy et al., 1983; Johnson et al., 1982).

Although adequate knowledge about diabetes may be a necessary condition for good diabetes care, it is not a sufficient condition. Understanding diabetes and acquiring the necessary disease management skills does not guarantee that a patient and family will consistently adhere to provider recommendations.

Adherence to Treatment Recommendations

Patient nonadherence to prescribed treatment regimens is a problem faced by the medical community at large. As might be expected, diabetes, which is characterized by both chronicity and complexity, presents numerous problems in this regard (see Johnson, 1992, for a review). Longitudinal studies of newly diagnosed youngsters suggest that adherence is best at the time of diagnosis and deteriorates thereafter (Jacobson et al., 1990).

Adolescent patients appear to be particularly vulnerable to adherence difficulties (Christensen, Terry, Wyatt, Pichert, & Lorenz, 1983; Johnson, 1995b; Johnson, Silverstein, Rosenbloom, Carter, & Cunningham, 1986). Tattersall and Lowe (1981) eloquently described how diabetes often interferes with most of the goals of normal adolescence. During this developmental period when it seems so important to conform to peer standards, youngsters with diabetes may feel "different" because of disease-associated delayed sexual maturation as well as numerous unusual behaviors (e.g., injections, glucose testing) associated with their daily management regimen. Dietary demands require frequent meals and snacks and the avoidance of food high in fat and concentrated sweets. The adolescent with diabetes is faced with the paradox of needing to eat foods when no one else is eating and needing to avoid foods everyone else consumes! Perhaps it is not surprising that these adolescents find it more and more difficult to refuse "junk" food and to eat when others are not eating.

As mentioned above, adolescents are often very knowledgeable about diabetes management, but at the same time can be extremely nonadherent, illustrating the discordant association that can occur between disease knowledge and adherence behaviors. Nevertheless, it is important to be sensitive to inadvertent noncompliance in both adolescent and childhood populations, although this is probably more common in the latter. In such cases, the patient believes he or she is adherent with the treatment regimen and may report good to excellent compliance but, because of ignorance or lack of skill, the patient is making one or more serious diabetes management errors. The patient is described as inadvertently noncompliant because the patient is unaware of the compliance problem and, in fact, believes there is none. Inadvertent noncompliance can occur with patients of any age. However, it may be particularly common in younger children who are given much responsibility for their own care but who may have not yet developed the cognitive sophistication to accurately carry out certain management tasks. Johnson et al. (1982) found that 40% of the youngsters they studied were making insulin injection errors; errors were more common in younger patients.

Because younger patients are not always (or even usually) capable of managing this complex illness alone, parental responsibility or involvement in these children's care seems necessary for adequate adherence. Johnson (1995b) published one of the few studies examining the link between parental supervision and diabetes regimen adherence. Parental supervision was a significant predictor of five of the six diabetes adherence behaviors studied: insulin injection, exercise, type of diet consumed, calories consumed, and concentrated sweet consumption. Only glucose testing was not significantly predicted by the amount of parental supervision.

Adolescents are frequently encouraged to manage this disease on their own. However, in view of the poor adherence associated with this developmental period, some authors are now suggesting that parents should become or remain more involved with their older children's daily care. Ingersoll, Orr, Herrold, and Golden (1986) studied patient–parent participation in insulin management in youngsters aged 12–21. As might be expected, parental participation decreased with increasing patient age. By the time the child was 15, parental participation had virtually ceased. The authors argued that for some adolescents, who are not yet sufficiently mature to handle the social demands of this developmental phase, parental withdrawal from the treatment process may be premature with resultant deterioration in the youngster's adherence and diabetes control.

When assessing patient adherence, most health providers rely on patients' or parents' answers to general inquiries about daily care procedures. Unfortunately, what patients or parents say they usually do may bear little resemblance to their actual behavior.

Empirical investigations have often used health provider estimates of patient adherence. This assessment strategy is problematic because health providers are usually very much aware of their patient's health status, making it difficult to obtain the necessary independence between physician ratings of patient adherence and their knowledge of their patients' diabetes control. Because providers may rate patients' adherence as a function of their health status rather than as a function of their actual behaviors, such ratings tell us more about physician beliefs concerning adherence–health status linkages than they do about actual patient or parent disease-related behaviors.

This problem of conceptual confounding between compliance and diabetes control is further highlighted by a survey of pediatric diabetologists in the United States; over 89% reported using glycosylated hemoglobin (a biological assay that is an index of average blood glucose levels over the past 2–3 months; Ziel & Davidson, 1987) to assess patient compliance (Clarke, Snyder, & Nowacek, 1985). Most health care providers appear to view patients with persistent hyperglycemia (indexed by high glycosylated hemoglobin levels) as noncompliant, whereas those with blood glucose levels nearer to the normal range (as indexed by low glycosylated hemoglobin levels) are presumed to be compliant. As glycemic control in diabetes is a function of more than adherence (including the appropriateness of the medical management program prescribed; see Johnson, 1994, for an extensive discussion of these issues), confounding these terms in this way can easily lead to faulty conclusions concerning patients' actual diabetes management behaviors. Measures of health status offer no information as to what the patient is or is not doing. Perhaps more importantly, the physician is inclined to blame patients for their poor diabetes control (i.e., it is their refusal to follow the prescribed regimen) rather than carefully assessing all possible etiologies for each patient's condition, only one of which is noncompliance.

Psychologists are often referred children in poor diabetes control because physicians have been unsuccessful in managing the children's illness and, as a consequence, psychological–behavioral factors are presumed to be involved. In such cases, a careful assessment of the child's and parents' adherence behaviors is required. Physician ratings and health status measures may provide important clues that something is wrong but they do not tell us what is wrong. In such cases, there is simply no substitute for a good behavioral assessment.

A behavioral assessment of adherence behaviors can be conducted in a number of ways. Observational methods can be used when the problem behavior is readily apparent and there is patient–parent willingness to carefully monitor and record the behaviors targeted. Lowe and Lutzker (1979), for example, had a mother observe her daughter's foot care, glucose testing, and dietary behavior. However, observational methods are clearly labor intensive, often requiring extensive training to ensure that the observer reliably records the behaviors of interest. Issues of measurement reactivity also need to be considered. If the patient knows diabetes-related behaviors are being observed, she or he may seek ways to deceive the observer by making observation exceeding difficult or by attempting to appear more adherent than is actually the case.

Patients are sometimes asked to keep daily written records of their diabetes-management behaviors. Although self-monitoring has long been of interest to behavioral psychologists, this method of measuring adherence behaviors in chronically ill childhood populations has not been extensively tested. In our experience, such data are reliable if patients keep complete records, but only 50% of patients are compliant with this request. Diabetes is an extremely complex disease. Adding detailed recordkeeping to an already demanding schedule seems more than many patients are willing to accept. Another alternative is to ask patients to keep written records on only a limited subset of all possible adherence behaviors. Schafer, Glasgow, and McCaul (1982), for example, asked three 16 to 18-year-olds to self-monitor three behaviors: wearing diabetic identification, exercise frequency, and glucose testing frequency. Only two of the three youngsters were able to provide reliable self-monitoring data, illustrating the importance of patient cooperation even when the number of behaviors to be recorded is limited.

In many cases, however, we do not know which of a myriad of possible adherence behaviors we should ask even cooperative patients to monitor. Often we want some overview of all of the patient's diabetes-relevant behaviors to help us target one or two for further assessment and intervention. In such cases, 24-hour recall interviews with patient and parent can prove very useful. Although 24-hour recall interviews are commonly used in the nutrition field, Johnson and her colleagues have modified this method to assess multiple adherence behaviors in diabetes patients. The patient is asked to recall yesterday's events from the time of awakening until retiring to bed. All diabetes-related behaviors are recorded by the interviewer. The parent is also interviewed (independently) about the youngster's behavior. By combining data from both the parent and patient interviews, errors resulting from forgetting or lack of knowledge (e.g., the parent is probably ignorant of many of the child's activities at school) are minimized. Multiple interviews of this type permit a more representative sample of the patient's behavior. In a series of studies, the reliability and validity of this technique have been examined and documented (Freund, Johnson, Silverstein, & Thomas, 1991; Johnson, 1995b; Johnson et al., 1986, 1992; Johnson, Freund, Silverstein, Hansen, & Malone, 1990; Johnson, Tomer, Cunningham, & Henretta, 1990; Reynolds, Johnson, & Silverstein, 1990; Spevack, Johnson, Riley, & Silverstein, 1991). Special consideration should be given when interviewing young children about behaviors involving time (e.g., time of insulin administration, time of meals, duration of exercise). However, with brief practice, children as young as 6 can provide reliable information about the multiple components of their daily diabetes care (Freund et al., 1991). This assessment strategy has a number of advantages: reliable information can be obtained about the multiple components of diabetes care, interviews can be conducted by telephone, and little is demanded of the patient other than the time (approximately 20 minutes) to conduct the interview. However, trained interviewers are required and when multiple interviews are conducted with multiple informants, the process becomes labor intensive.

Also available are self-report questionnaires that ask patients to rate their adherence to specific behaviors relevant to diabetes management such as medication administration, diet, exercise, glucose testing, and foot care; from these ratings a total compliance score is obtained (Brownlee-Duffeck et al., 1987; Cerkoney & Hart, 1980; Hanson, Henggeler, & Burghen, 1987). Few studies have examined the reliability of this approach (Brownlee-Duffeck et al., 1987; Hanson et al., 1988). Further, convincing evidence is now available indicating that diabetes adherence is a multivariate construct; multiple behaviors are involved and they are not highly related to one another (Glasgow, McCaul, & Schafer, 1987; Johnson et al., 1986; Johnson, Tomer, et al., 1990; Orne & Binik, 1989). Questionnaires that yield single compliance scores will be insensitive to this underlying complexity. If certain adherence behaviors (e.g., timing of insulin administration) are related to glycemic control while others (e.g., foot care) are not, then measures yielding single compliance scores will fail to identify which behaviors are most important for good health.

Stress

The impact of physical stress, such as an illness, on diabetes control is well documented (Craig, 1981). Theoretically, psychological stress could play a similarly disruptive role. Stress hormones, like epinephrine and norepinephrine, when produced in sufficient amounts, could antagonize the peripheral metabolic effects of insulin as well as stimulate glycogenolysis and gluconeogenesis by the liver resulting in hyperglycemia. These catecholamines also encourage mobilization of free fatty acids and thereby their conversion to ketone bodies by the liver. As mentioned previously, excessive ketone production can lead to diabetic ketoacidosis.

One of the earliest demonstrations of psychological stress effects on metabolic control is provided in a case report by Hinkle and Wolfe (1949). A 15-year-old girl with a history of repeated diabetic ketoacidotic episodes kept a diary of daily stressful events and her urine ketone test results, demonstrating a striking relationship between the two.

Early attempts to study the relationships of psychological stress and metabolism in a controlled laboratory environment reported stress-related increases in free fatty acids and urine volume, but inconsistent effects on blood glucose (Hinkle & Wolf, 1952; Vandenbergh, Sussman, & Titus, 1966; Vandenbergh, Sussman, & Vaughan, 1967). Methodological problems including lack of statistical analyses, failure to completely characterize and differentiate between patients (i.e., IDDM versus NIDDM; adolescents versus adults; those in good versus poor diabetes control prior to the stress induction), and failure to obtain quantitative data from the patients themselves as to the level of stress experienced, make interpretation of these initial studies difficult. More recent and more methodologically sophisticated studies of adults and adolescents with IDDM have failed to demonstrate metabolic derangements in response to laboratory stressors (Delamater et al., 1988; Gilbert, Johnson, Silverstein, & Malone, 1989; Kemmer et al., 1986). The authors of these studies concluded that for most IDDM patients, acute metabolic derangement is probably not a common consequence of the ordinary stresses of daily life. Major life events may have a stronger impact on glycemic control (Goldston, Kovacs, Obrosky, & Iyengar, 1995), but for ethical reasons cannot be manipulated within the context of a carefully controlled laboratory experiment. Furthermore, survey data suggest that patients believe that stress influences their glycemic control (Cox, Taylor, Nowack, Holley-Wilcox, & Pohl, 1984); it is possible that there are subgroups of patients for whom there is a consistent association between daily stress and hyperglycemia (Gonder-Frederick, Carter, Cox, & Clarke, 1990; Halford, Cuddihy, & Mortimer, 1990). Some authors have suggested that patient coping style may influence stress–glycemic control relationships, with less adaptive coping styles resulting in poorer glycemic control (Aiken, Wallander, Bell, & Cole, 1992; Brand,

Johnson, & Johnson, 1986; Delamater, Kurtz, Bubb, White, & Santiago, 1987; Hanson et al., 1987; Kager & Holden, 1992; Peyrot & McMurry, 1992; Stabler et al., 1987). However, there appears to be little consensus as to what constitutes adaptive coping.

Although it is generally assumed that stress causes poor diabetes control, poor diabetes control could easily make a patient feel more stressed. Stress is also presumed to influence diabetes control through the metabolic effects of the stress hormones. An alternative hypothesis views stress as a disruptive influence on regimen adherence. Stressed individuals may change their eating or sleeping habits, which, in turn, could negatively impact their metabolic status. Very few studies have attempted to simultaneously assess the direct effect of stress on glycemic control and its indirect effect through adherence, and results of this limited literature are inconclusive. Hanson and Pichert (1986) found that stress disrupted adherence and had a direct, negative effect on glycemic control. Balfour, White, Schiffrin, Dougherty, and Dufresne (1993) reported stress effects that were primarily indirect, through dietary disinhibition. In contrast, Hanson et al. (1987) and Aiken et al. (1992) found evidence for a direct effect of stress but no indirect effects through adherence.

Although psychological stress–glycemic linkages remain an intriguing area of inquiry, the nature and clinical significance of such associations remain to be clarified.

Family Context

Family context is of obvious importance to the acquisition of diabetes knowledge and adherence to the daily demands of disease management. Family context can be a source of stress for the child or a source of support, encouraging successful adaptation to the disease. Family conflict, particularly unresolved conflict, played a central role in Minuchin and colleagues' conceptualization of the "psychosomatic family," which became a popular explanation for cases of repeated hospitalizations for keto-acidotic episodes (Baker, Minuchin, Milman, Liebman, & Todd, 1975; Minuchin et al., 1975; Minuchin, Rosman, & Baker, 1978). More recently, the "psychosomatic family" has come under considerable scientific scrutiny, as more sophisticated models of family functioning within the context of childhood illnesses have been developed (Anderson & Coyne, 1993; Coyne & Anderson, 1988, 1989).

Although the early literature consistently pointed to less-than-ideal family circumstances as a determinant of poorer health in children with diabetes (see Johnson, 1980, for a review), only recently have investigators begun to identify the specific family components critical to good health or adjustment in this population. Some studies have identified low conflict and high organization as important for medical regimen compliance (Bobrow, AvRuskin, & Siller, 1985; Hauser et al., 1990; Schafer, Glasgow, McCaul, & Dreher, 1983), whereas others have emphasized the role of family flexibility and diabetes-specific supportive behaviors (Hanson, DeGuire, Schinkel, & Henggeler, 1992; Hanson, Henggeler, et al., 1992; Schafer et al., 1983; Schafer, McCaul, & Glasgow, 1986; Wysocki et al., 1989). As was true of the stress–diabetes literature, the family context literature would benefit from clear testable hypotheses in which the behavioral linkages between specific family context variables and patient health or adjustment are specified and studied in the same investigation.

Thus far, we have focused on the importance of family context to the patient's adjustment and health. We have selected this approach because psychologists are often referred patients who are in trouble, and it is the psychologist's task to assess the possible causes of the patient's predicament. Family context variables are certainly important from this perspective. However, it is also the case that the child's illness may impact on the family. There is an interesting literature addressing the effect of a child's chronic illness or disability on parental and marital adjustment, family interaction patterns, sibling adjustment, and the family's economic status. In the interest of space, this literature will not be discussed in detail here, and the interested reader is referred to reviews available elsewhere (e.g., Johnson, 1995a).

TREATMENT

Psychological treatments for children with diabetes include education, behavioral or social-learning interventions, and relaxation/biofeedback training.

Education

Although education is a standard component of diabetes care, controlled studies of the effects of an education program on children with this disease are rare. In an extensive review, Padgett, Mumford, Hynes, and Carter (1988) located 14 controlled studies of the use of an education program (didactic or multicomponent programs that included self-monitoring) with IDDM patients. Of these, only 5 focused on children and adolescents. In 3 of the 5 studies, knowledge was used as an outcome variable, and in all 3 there was evidence of better knowledge in the education group compared with the control group (although effect sizes varied considerably). This small literature is consistent with a much larger literature examining the effects of educational instruction with adults who have diabetes (Brown, 1990; Padgett et al., 1988); although knowledge frequently improves subsequent to an education program, this does not always translate into improved adherence or better glycemic control. Glasgow and Osteen (1992) argued that education programs need to be evaluated from a broader perspective, including short and long-term health outcomes as well as assessments of the intervening variables that are presumed to translate the education program (e.g., improved knowledge, improved adherence) into improved health.

Behavioral or Social-Learning Interventions

Because improved knowledge does not always translate into improved diabetes care, several behavioral and social-learning interventions have been used in an effort to improve patient adherence and glycemic control. In fact, a meta-analysis of the education and psychosocial intervention literature suggested that behavioral/social-learning programs produce some of the largest effect sizes seen in the literature (Padgett et al., 1988). However, there have been few controlled studies documenting the effects of behavioral or social-learning programs with children or adolescents who have diabetes. Only five such studies were identified in the 1988 review by Padgett and colleagues. Since that time, several additional controlled intervention studies have been published. Satin, LaGreca, Zigo, and Skyler (1989) documented positive effects of a family-oriented group intervention program, and Anderson, Wolf, Burkhart, Cornell, and Bacon (1989) successfully employed a peer-group problem-solving intervention for adolescents with diabetes. Delamater et al. (1990) focused their self-management training program on newly diagnosed cases, documenting positive health status effects 2 years postdiagnosis. Although this literature would also benefit from increased attention to the issues raised by Glasgow and Osteen (1992) in their critique of the education literature, the preponderance of the evidence clearly suggests that the behavioral or social-learning strategies can be successfully employed to assist patients and their families.

Relaxation/Biofeedback Training

As stress is presumed to induce hyperglycemia, stress reduction techniques might be expected to improve glycemic control. Relaxation training has been the most commonly used intervention strategy, with inconsistent effects. Padgett and colleagues' (1988) meta-analysis found that relaxation training exhibited the weakest of all educational and psychosocial intervention effects. However, there is some evidence that this approach may be more effective in NIDDM than IDDM populations (Feinglos, Hastedt, & Surwit, 1987; Surwit & Feinglos, 1983). Most studies of relaxation training with IDDM patients have been limited to case reports. In a rare, controlled treatment outcome study, McGrady, Bailey, and Good (1991) improved IDDM adults' self-reported blood glucose test results subsequent to a 10-session treatment program of biofeedback-assisted relaxation plus stress management; treatment effects were later replicated with the control group. Boardway, Delamater, Tomakowsky, and Gutai (1993) also used a control group design to test the effect of stress management training with IDDM adolescents. Their intervention emphasized methods of identifying and appropriately coping with stress, rather than relaxation techniques. The intervention significantly reduced diabetes-specific stress experienced by these youngsters, but had no effect on adherence or glycemic control. As discussed previously, individual differences may underlie the inconsistencies found in the stress and diabetes literature. Certain patients may be particularly stress sensitive whereas others are not. A better understanding of stress–glycemic control linkages in this population may be necessary before successful stress intervention programs, which yield consistently positive effects, can be designed and implemented.

CASE REPORT: A PSYCHOLOGICAL ASSESSMENT OF AN IDDM ADOLESCENT WITH A HISTORY OF REPEATED EPISODES OF KETOACIDOSIS

Lisa L. is a 14-year-old white female with a 4-year history of IDDM. Her mother reports problems with her diabetes management since diagnosis, but these have escalated during the last year. Lisa has been hospitalized 10 times in the past 12 months. Her insulin dose has been raised from 0.7 to 1.5 units/kg, but her glucose levels have failed to stabilize. She was referred by her pediatrician.

Lisa is the only adopted child in a family of four youngsters. She has three brothers, aged 20 years, 2 years, and 1 month. The oldest sibling is out of the home, attending college. Lisa spends a great deal of time assisting her mother with the two youngest boys. The 2-year-old was born seriously ill, and required several operations, although his health is good now. Mr. L. has worked for 17 years as a mechanic. Mrs. L. worked for an insurance company for 7 years, but has not worked since the birth of her two youngest sons.

The assessment interview indicated that Lisa has multiple problems in addition to her diabetes management. During the past year, she began junior high school, but missed 48 days because of diabetes-related illness. Her grades slipped from A's and B's to C's and D's. She has few friends, is emotionally volatile, and behaviorally noncompliant with parental requests. On the Behavior Problem Checklist, both parents rated Lisa high on the Conduct and Personality Problem dimensions.

On the Test of Diabetes Knowledge-R, Lisa performed exceptionally well, scoring 90% on the General Information component and 83% on the Problem Solving component. Lisa's mother exhibited a similarly high level of knowledge (General Information 90%, Problem Solving 80%), whereas her father showed deficits in all areas (General Information 72%, Problem Solving 69%). On the Skills Tests, Lisa proved to be very knowledgeable and more proficient than both of her parents. Lisa obtained an 81% accuracy score on the Glucose Testing Skills Test and 96% on the Insulin Injection Skills Test. In contrast, her parents' scores on these same tests ranged from 59% to 74%.

On the Diabetes Opinion Survey, developed by Johnson and colleagues to measure youngsters' attitudes toward the disease, Lisa indicated that she felt very stigmatized by her diabetes. Her Lie Scale score also indicated that she was attempting to present herself in a favorable light and that she was unlikely to be completely truthful about her own problems and difficulties.

On the Parent Diabetes Opinion Survey, also developed by Johnson to measure parental attitudes toward diabetes, both Mr. and Mrs. L. indicated that Lisa's diabetes is highly disruptive to the family. They feel that they are stigmatized (i.e., they view other people as treating them and their family differently because of Lisa's diabetes). Both parents see Lisa as using her diabetes to manipulate people around her and both are extremely rule-oriented about how Lisa's diabetes should be managed. For example, both believe that Lisa should never be permitted any sweets, even on special occasions.

Lisa claims to be adherent with her daily diabetes management requirements but her reports are suspect. For example, she states that she tests her urine for glucose and ketones three times per day and her blood twice per day. However, she keeps no records of these test results and when asked what the results were, she reported unusually "good" results. Lisa's descriptions are highly inconsistent with her history of poor glucose control. Moreover, she reports always following her diet, although she admits she *used* to "cheat a lot" (but insists she does not do so now). Both Lisa and her mother attribute her repeated keto-acidotic episodes to "emotional upset." For example, when Lisa was caught stealing $25 from a neighbor and her mother confronted her, Lisa became "upset" and was hospitalized within 48 hours.

The family interaction patterns observed during the assessment interview are particularly worthy of note. Mrs. L. did all the talking; Mr. L. responded only to direct questions. Mrs. L. openly expressed her hostility toward Lisa. Privately she expressed dissatisfaction with her husband because of his lack of assistance with her child care demands. Lisa is viewed by both parents as openly hostile toward her father. She is always involving herself in family arguments (even those that do not concern her), during which she sides with her mother. The oldest son is seen as near perfect (if not perfect), in contrast to

Lisa. Mrs. L.'s exceptionally nurturant behavior toward her youngest sons was obvious in the first assessment interview; she refused to let other available persons care for her children. Mr. and Mrs. L. have never left the two youngest boys with a sitter, and consequently have not had an evening together without the children in several years.

In summary, this 14-year-old adolescent presents with a variety of behavior and health status problems. Her difficulties have escalated in the past year, probably as a result of changed interaction patterns within the family. Mrs. L. has had two sons in the past 2 years, one of whom was born with serious health problems. Both of these sons clearly changed Lisa's role within the family from youngest child to sibling caretaker. Whereas Mrs. L. may have previously exhibited her nurturant behavior toward Lisa, she is now directing this toward her young sons. Her decision to quit work to care for her boys may have further highlighted for Lisa the changed focus of her mother's caretaking behaviors. Mrs. L. is feeling stressed with the increased demands of these young children coupled with Lisa's difficulty adjusting to this new situation. She is angry at her husband for his passive stance. The decision of her oldest son to leave home for college leaves her without any male support, further exacerbating her unexpressed hostility toward her husband. Lisa becomes the target of Mrs. L.'s anger. Lisa is adopted, has diabetes, and engages in numerous behaviors that would annoy or anger any parent.

Lisa is angry too. She is angry at her two youngest siblings but can never express this. Instead, she is very nurturant toward them as this is approved of by her mother. The primary target of Lisa's anger is her father. In this manner, she speaks indirectly for her mother. It is possible that she may be receiving some subtle encouragement from her mother for this response. At the same time, Lisa's difficulties pull her parents together. Although Mr. L. did not say much, he did come to the assessment session and, no doubt, often listens to Mrs. L.'s complaints about Lisa. In this manner, Mrs. L. may feel some minimal, although certainly not sufficient, support from her husband. Lisa's behavior and repeated hospitalizations also change the family's focus of attention toward her and away from her "perfect" older brother and her two younger siblings. Lisa is highly knowledgeable about diabetes, and is capable of using her illness to manipulate the focus of attention within the family.

Successful treatment will require an improved parenting bond between Mr. and Mrs. L., who will need to clearly specify what is acceptable and unacceptable behavior for Lisa and to respond consistently to Lisa's behavior. Mr. and Mrs. L. will need to become knowledgeable about all aspects of Lisa's diabetes management and supervise injections and glucose testing rigorously so as to prevent Lisa's manipulative use of her diabetes. Lisa needs to develop a caring relationship with someone with whom she can feel sufficiently safe to begin to examine her own behavior less defensively. Given her parents' anger at her, this could best be done in the context of a therapeutic relationship. However, the goal of treatment should be to reduce parental hostility toward Lisa by inducing sufficient improvement in Lisa's behavior. Lisa's parents should then be able to reestablish the emotional capability of expressing toward her some of the same warmth and positive regard they exhibit toward their sons.

SUMMARY

At the beginning of this century, the leading causes of death were influenza, pneumonia, diphtheria, tuberculosis, and gastrointestinal infections. Today, few people die of these disorders. In the early 1900s, children with diabetes lived less than 1 year. Today they have a life expectancy approximately 75% of normal. The remarkable medical advances of this century have changed the health care problems faced by industrialized societies. Chronically ill children are now comprising an ever larger portion of pediatric practice. It is estimated that 10–20% of all children in the United States have a chronic condition (Gortmaker & Sappenfield, 1984). These children require approximately 10 times more health care services than their more physically normal peers (Smyth-Staruch, Breslau, Weitzman, & Gortmaker, 1984). Chronic conditions, like diabetes, place lifelong, daily demands on the patient and family. Often these demands are multiple and complex. The patient must learn to live and manage diabetes with only occasional consultation from the physician. However, successful disease management requires more than an appropriate medical prescription. The patient must understand the prescription, adhere to it, and in some cases even make prescription modifications in the face of the vicissitudes of daily life.

By definition, chronic illnesses have no cure. Although medical management of these disorders has improved, in most cases it remains imperfect. Consequently, the patient must struggle not only with the daily demands of a disease management regimen, but also with the knowledge that even perfect adherence will not guarantee completely normal function either now or in the future. Although chronic illnesses always come under the purview of physicians, there is increasing recognition of the inherently psychological processes required for their successful management. Physician–patient communication, patient education, patient knowledge about the disease, patient adherence, and patient adjustment to a disease that has no cure and that can be imperfectly medically managed at best, are all psychological phenomena. We psychologists are faced with an opportunity and a responsibility. We must diligently learn about the medical–physical aspects of the chronically ill children we treat. We must educate and increase the sensibilities of the medical community to the behavioral and emotional aspects of managing chronically ill children. And we must rigorously apply our own scientific expertise to the study of behavior–health status relationships so as to advance the field.

ACKNOWLEDGMENT

Preparation of this chapter was supported by grant RO1 HD13820 from the National Institute of Child Health and Human Development.

REFERENCES

Aiken, J., Wallander, J., Bell, D., & Cole, J. (1992). Daily stress variability, learned resourcefulness, regimen adherence, and metabolic control in type 1 diabetes mellitus: Evaluation of a path model. *Journal of Consulting and Clinical Psychology, 60*, 113–118.

Anderson, B., & Coyne, J. (1993). Family context and compliance behavior in chronically ill children. In N. Krasnegor, L. Epstein, S. B. Johnson, & S. Yaffe (Eds.), *Developmental aspects of health compliance behavior* (pp. 77–89). Hillsdale, NJ: Erlbaum.

Anderson, B., Wolf, F., Burkhart, M., Cornell, R., & Bacon, G. (1989). Effects of peer-group intervention on metabolic control of adolescents with IDDM: Randomized outpatient study. *Diabetes Care, 12*, 179–183.

Baker, L., Minuchin, S., Milman, L., Liebman, R., & Todd, T. (1975). Psychosomatic aspects of juvenile diabetes mellitus: A progress report. In Z. Laron (Ed.), *Diabetes in juveniles: Medical and rehabilitation aspects* (pp. 332–343). Basel: Karger.

Balfour, L., White, D., Schiffrin, A., Dougherty, G., & Dufresne, J. (1993). Dietary disinhibition, perceived stress and glucose control in young type I diabetic women. *Health Psychology, 12*, 33–38.

Barnett, A., Eff, C., Leslie, R., & Pyke, D. (1981). Diabetes in identical twins. *Diabetologia, 20*, 87–93.

Barrett-Connor, E., & Orchard, T. (1985). Diabetes and heart disease. In M. Harris & R. Hamman (Eds.), *Diabetes in America* (NIH Publication No. 85–1468, pp. XVI–XVI–41). Bethesda: U.S. Department of Health and Health and Human Services, National Institutes of Health.

Boardway, R., Delamater, A., Tomakowsky, J., & Gutai, J. (1993). Stress management training for adolescents with diabetes. *Journal of Pediatric Psychology, 18*, 29–45.

Bobrow, E., AvRuskin, R., & Siller, J. (1985). Mother–daughter interaction and adherence to diabetes regimens. *Diabetes Care, 8,* 146–151.

Brand, A., Johnson, J., & Johnson, S. (1986). Life stress and diabetic control in children and adolescents with insulin-dependent diabetes. *Journal of Pediatric Psychology, 11,* 481–496.

Brown, S. (1990). Studies of educational interventions and outcomes in diabetic adults: A meta-analysis revisited. *Patient Education and Counseling, 16,* 189–215.

Brownlee-Duffeck, M., Peterson, L. Simonds, J., Goldstein, D., Kilo, C., & Hoette, S. (1987). The role of health beliefs in the regimen adherence and metabolic control of adolescents and adults with diabetes mellitus. *Journal of Consulting and Clinical Psychology, 55,* 139–144.

Cerkoney, K., & Hart, L. (1980). The relationship between the health belief model and compliance of persons with diabetes mellitus. *Diabetes Care, 3,* 594–598.

Christensen, N. K., Terry, R. D., Wyatt, S., Pichert, J. W., & Lorenz, R. A. (1983). Quantitative assessment of dietary adherence in patients with insulin-dependent diabetes mellitus. *Diabetes Care, 6,* 245–250.

Clarke, W. L., Snyder, A. L., & Nowacek, G. (1985). Outpatient pediatric diabetes—I. Current practices. *Journal of Chronic Diseases, 38,* 85–90.

Cox, D., Taylor, A., Nowacek, G., Holley-Wilcox, P., & Pohl, S. (1984). The relationship between psychological stress and insulin-dependent diabetic control: Preliminary investigations. *Health Psychology, 3,* 63–75.

Coyne, J., & Anderson, B. (1988). The "psychosomatic family" reconsidered: Diabetes in context. *Journal of Marital and Family Therapy, 14,* 113–123.

Coyne, J., & Anderson, B. (1989). The "psychosomatic family" reconsidered II: Recalling a defective model and looking ahead. *Journal of Marital and Family Therapy, 15,* 139–148.

Craig, O. (1981). *Childhood diabetes and its management* (2nd ed.). London: Butterworths.

Davidson, M. B. (Ed.). (1991). *Clinical diabetes mellitus: A problem-oriented approach.* New York: Thieme Medical.

DCCT Research Group. (1993). The effect of intensive treatment of diabetes on the development and progression of long-term complications in insulin-dependent diabetes mellitus. *New England Journal of Medicine, 329,* 977–986.

Delamater, A., Bubb, J., Davis, S., Smith, J., Schmidt, L., White, N., & Santiago, J. (1990). Randomized prospective study of self-management training with newly diagnosed diabetic children. *Diabetes Care, 13,* 492–498.

Delamater, A., Bubb, J., Kurtz, S., Kuntze, J., Smith, J., White, N., & Santiago, J. (1988). Physiologic responses to acute psychological stress in adolescents with type I diabetes mellitus. *Journal of Pediatric Psychology, 13,* 69–86.

Delamater, A., Kurtz, S., Bubb, J., White, N., & Santiago, J. (1987). Stress and coping in relation to metabolic control of adolescents with type 1 diabetes. *Developmental and Behavioral Pediatrics, 8,* 136–140.

Dunbar, F. (1954). *Emotions and bodily changes.* New York: Columbia University Press.

Dunn, S., & Turtle, J. (1981). The myth of the diabetic personality. *Diabetes Care, 4,* 640–646.

Feinglos, M., Hastedt, P., & Surwit, R. (1987). Effects of relaxation therapy on patients with type I diabetes mellitus. *Diabetes Care, 10,* 72–75.

Freund, A., Johnson, S. B., Silverstein, J., & Thomas, J. (1991). Assessing daily management of childhood diabetes using 24-hour recall interviews: Reliability and stability. *Health Psychology, 10,* 200–208.

Gilbert, B., Johnson, S. B., Silverstein, J., & Malone, J. (1989). Psychological and physiological responses to acute laboratory stressors in insulin-dependent diabetes mellitus adolescents and nondiabetic controls. *Journal of Pediatric Psychology, 14,* 577–591.

Gilbert, B. O., Johnson, S. B., Spillar, R., McCallum, M., Silverstein, J. H., & Rosenbloom, A. (1982). The effects of a peer-modeling film on children learning to self-inject insulin. *Behavior Therapy, 13,* 186–193.

Glasgow, R., McCaul, K., & Schafer, L. (1984). Barriers to regimen adherence among persons with insulin-dependent diabetes. *Journal of Behavioral Medicine, 9,* 65–77.

Glasgow, R., & Osteen, V. (1992). Evaluating diabetes education: Are we measuring the most important outcomes? *Diabetes Care, 15,* 1423–1432.

Goldston, D., Kovacs, M., Obrosky, D., & Iyengar, S. (1995). A longitudinal study of life events and metabolic control among youths with insulin-dependent diabetes mellitus. *Health Psychology, 14,* 409–414.

Gonder-Frederick, L. Carter, W., Cox, D., & Clarke, W. (1990). Environmental stress and blood glucose change in insulin-dependent diabetes mellitus. *Health Psychology, 9,* 503–515.

Gortmaker, S. L., & Sappenfield, W. (1984). Chronic childhood disorders: Prevalence and impact. *Pediatric Clinics of North America, 13,* 186–193.

Halford, W., Cuddihy, S., & Mortimer, R. (1990). Psychological stress and blood glucose regulation in type I diabetic patients. *Health Psychology, 9,* 516–528.

Hanson, C., DeGuire, M., Schinkel, A., & Henggeler, S. (1992). Comparing social learning and family systems correlates of adaptation in youths with IDDM. *Journal of Pediatric Psychology, 17,* 555–572.

Hanson, C., Henggeler, S., & Burghen, G. (1987). Model of associations between psychosocial variables and health-outcome measures in adolescents with IDDM. *Diabetes Care, 10,* 752–758.

Hanson, C., Henggeler, S., Harris, M., Cigrang, J., Schinkel, A., Rodrigue, J., & Klesges, R. (1992). Contributions of sibling relations to the adaptation of youths with insulin-dependent diabetes mellitus. *Journal of Consulting and Clinical Psychology, 60,* 104–112.

Hanson, C., Henggeler, S., Harris, M., Mitchell, K., Carle, D., & Burghen, G. (1988). Associations between family members' perceptions of the health care system and the health of youths with insulin-dependent diabetes mellitus. *Journal of Pediatric Psychology, 13*, 543–554.

Hanson, S., & Pichert, J. (1986). Perceived stress and diabetes control in adolescents. *Health Psychology, 5*, 439–452.

Harkavy, J., Johnson, S. B., Silverstein, J., Spillar, R., McCallum, M., & Rosenbloom, A. (1983). Who learns what at diabetes summer camp. *Journal of Pediatric Psychology, 8*, 143–153.

Hauenstein, E., Marvin, R., Snyder, A., & Clarke, W. (1989). Stress in parents of children with diabetes mellitus. *Diabetes Care, 12*, 18–19.

Hauser, S., Jacobson, A., Lavori, P., Wolfsdorf, J., Herskowitz, R., Milley, J., & Bliss, R. (1990). Adherence among children and adolescents with insulin-dependent diabetes mellitus over a four-year longitudinal follow-up: II. Immediate and long-term linkages to family milieu. *Journal of Pediatric Psychology, 15*, 527–542.

Herman, W. H., & Teutsch, S. M. (1985). Kidney diseases associated with diabetes. In M. Harris & R. Hamman (Eds.), *Diabetes in America* (NIH Publication No. 85-1468, pp. XIV-1–XIV-31). Bethesda: U.S. Department of Health and Human Services, National Institutes of Health.

Hinkle, L. E., & Wolf, S. (1949). Experimental study of life situations, emotions, and the occurrence of acidosis in a juvenile diabetic. *American Journal of the Medical Sciences, 217*, 130–135.

Hinkle, L., & Wolf, S. (1952). Importance of life stress in course and management of diabetes mellitus. *Journal of the American Medical Association, 148*, 513–520.

Ingersoll, G. M., Orr, D. P., Herrold, A. J., & Golden, M. P. (1986). Cognitive maturity and self-management among adolescents with insulin-dependent diabetes mellitus. *Journal of Pediatrics, 108*, 620–623

Jacobson, A., Hauser, S., Lavori, P., Wolfsdorf, J., Herskowitz, R., Milley, J., Bliss, R., Gelfand, E., Wertlieb, D., & Stein, J. (1990). Adherence among children and adolescents with insulin dependent diabetes mellitus over a four year longitudinal follow-up: I. The influence of patient coping and adjustment. *Journal of Pediatric Psychology, 15*, 511–526.

Johnson, S. B. (1990). Psychosocial factors in juvenile diabetes: A review. *Journal of Behavioral Medicine, 3*, 95–115.

Johnson, S. B. (1992). Methodological issues in diabetes research: Measuring adherence. *Diabetes Care, 15*, 1658–1667.

Johnson, S. B. (1994). Health behavior and health status: Concepts, methods, and applications. *Journal of Pediatric Psychology, 19*, 129–141.

Johnson, S. B. (1995a). Insulin-dependent diabetes mellitus in childhood. In M. Roberts (Ed.), *Handbook of pediatric psychology* (2nd ed., pp. 263–285). New York: Guilford Press.

Johnson, S. B. (1995b). Managing insulin-dependent diabetes mellitus in adolescence: A developmental perspective. In J. Wallander & L. Siegel (Eds.), *Adolescent health problems: Behavioral perspectives* (pp. 265–288). New York: Guilford Press.

Johnson, S., Freund, A., Silverstein, J., Hansen, C., & Malone, J. (1990). Adherence–health status relationships in childhood diabetes. *Health Psychology, 9*, 606–631.

Johnson, S., Kelly, M., Henretta, J., Cunningham, W., Tomer, A., & Silverstein, J. (1992). A longitudinal analysis of adherence and health status in childhood diabetes. *Journal of Pediatric Psychology, 17*, 537–553.

Johnson, S. B., Pollack, T., Silverstein, J., Rosenbloom, A., Spillar, R., McCallum, M., & Harkavy, J. (1982). Cognitive and behavioral knowledge about insulin diabetes among children and parents. *Pediatrics, 69*, 708–713.

Johnson, S. B., Riley, W., Hansen, C., & Nurick, M. (1990). Psychological impact of islet cell-antibody screening: Preliminary results. *Diabetes Care, 13*, 93–97.

Johnson, S. B., Silverstein, J., Rosenbloom, A., Carter, R., & Cunningham, W. (1986). Assessing daily management in childhood diabetes. *Health Psychology, 5*, 545–564.

Johnson, S. B., & Tercyak, K. (1995). Psychological impact of islet cell antibody screening for IDDM on children, adults, and their family members. *Diabetes Care, 18*, 1370–1372.

Johnson, S., Tomer, A., Cunningham, W., & Henretta, J. (1990). Adherence in childhood diabetes: Results of a confirmatory factor analysis. *Health Psychology, 9*, 493–501.

Kager, V., & Holden, E. (1992). Preliminary investigation of the direct and moderating effects of family and individual variables on adjustment of children and adolescents with diabetes. *Journal of Pediatric Psychology, 17*, 491–502.

Kemmer, F., Bisping, R., Steingruber, H., Baar, H., Hardtmann, R., Schlaghecke, R., & Berger, M. (1986). Psychological stress and metabolic control in patients with type I diabetes mellitus. *New England Journal of Medicine, 314*, 1078–1084.

Klein, R., & Klein, B. E. K. (1985). Vision disorders in diabetes. In M. Harris & R. Hamman (Eds.), *Diabetes in America* (NIH Publication No. 85–1468, pp. XII-1–XII-36). Bethesda: U.S. Department of Health and Human Services, National Institutes of Health.

Kohler, E., Hurwitz, L. S., & Milan, D. (1982). A developmentally staged curriculum for teaching self-care to the child with insulin dependent diabetes mellitus. *Diabetes Care, 5*, 300–304.

Kovacs, M., Brent, D., Steinberg, T., Paulauskas, S., & Reid, J. (1986). Children's self-reports of psychological adjustment and coping strategies during first year of insulin dependent diabetes mellitus. *Diabetes Care, 9*, 472–479.

Kovacs, M., Finkelstein, R., Feinberg, R., Crouse-Novak, M., Paulauskas, S., & Pollack, M. (1985). Initial psychological responses of parents to the diagnosis of insulin-dependent diabetes mellitus in their children. *Diabetes Care, 8,* 568–575.

LaPorte, R. E., & Cruickshanks, K. J. (1985). Incidence and risk factors for insulin-dependent diabetes. In M. Harris & R. Hamman (Eds.), *Diabetes in America* (NIH Publication No. 85-1468), pp. III-1–III-11). Bethesda: U.S. Department of Health and Human Services, National Institutes of Health.

LaPorte, R. E., & Tajima, N. (1985). Prevalence of insulin-dependent diabetes. In M. Harris & R. Hamman (Eds.), *Diabetes in America* (NIH Publication No. 85-1468, pp. V-1–V-8). Bethesda: U.S. Department of Health and Human Services, National Institutes of Health.

Lavigne, J., & Faier-Routman, J. (1992). Psychological adjustment to pediatric physical disorders: A meta-analytic review. *Journal of Pedatric Psychology, 17,* 133–157.

Lorenz, R., Christensen, N., & Pichert, J. (1985). Diet-related knowledge, skill, and adherence among children with insulin-dependent diabetes mellitus. *Pediatrics, 75,* 872–876.

Lowe, K., & Lutzker, J. R. (1979). Increasing compliance to a medical regimen with a juvenile diabetic. *Behavior Therapy, 10,* 57–64.

Maudsley, H. (1899). *The pathology of mind* (3rd ed.). New York: Appleton.

McGrady, A., Bailey, B., & Good, M. (1991). Controlled study of biofeedback-assisted relaxation in type 1 diabetes. *Diabetes Care, 14,* 360–365.

Minuchin, S., Baker, L., Rosman, B. L., Liebman, R., Milman, L., & Todd, T. C. (1975). A conceptual model of psychosomatic illness in children. *Archives of General Psychiatry, 32,* 1031–1038.

Minuchin, S., Rosman, B., & Baker, L. (1978). *Psychosomatic families.* Cambridge, MA: Harvard University Press.

Naughten, E., Smith, M. A., & Baum, J. D. (1982). At what age do diabetic children give their own injections? *American Journal of Diseases of Children, 136,* 690–692.

NDIC. (1994). *Diabetes control and complications trial (DCCT)* (NIH Publication No. 94-3874). Bethesda: U.S. Department of Health and Human Services, National Institutes of Health.

Orne, C., & Binik, Y. (1989). Consistency of adherence across regimen demands. *Health Psychology, 8,* 27–43.

Padgett, D., Mumford, E. Hynes, M., & Carter, R. (1988). Meta-analysis of the effects of educational and psychosocial interventions on management of diabetes mellitus. *Journal of Clinical Epidemiology, 41,* 1007–1030.

Page, P., Verstraete, D., Robb, J., & Etzwiler, D. (1981). Patient recall of self-care recommendations in diabetes. *Diabetes Care, 4,* 96–98.

Palumbo, P. J., & Melton, L. J., III. (1985). Peripheral vascular disease and diabetes. In M. Harris & R. Hamman (Eds.), *Diabetes in America* (NIH Publication No. 85-1468, pp. XV-1–XV-21). U.S. Department of Health and Human Services, National Institutes of Health.

Peyrot, M., & McMurry, J. (1992). Stress buffering and glycemic control: The role of cooping styles. *Diabetes Care, 15,* 842–846.

Reynolds, L., Johnson, S. B., & Silverstein, J. (1990). Assessing daily diabetes management by 24-hr recall interview: The validity of children's reports. *Journal of Pediatric Psychology, 15,* 493–509.

Riley, W., Maclaren, N., Krischer, J., Spillar, R., Silverstein, J., Schatz, D., Schwartz, S., Malone, J., Shah, S., Vadheim, C., & Rotter, J. (1990). A prospective study of the development of diabetes in relatives of patients with insulin-dependent diabetes. *New England Journal of Medicine, 323,* 1167–1172.

Ryan, C. (1990). Neuropsychological consequences and correlates of diabetes in childhood. In C. Holmes (Ed.), *Neuropsychological and behavioral aspects of diabetes* (pp. 58–84). Berlin: Springer-Verlag.

Satin, W., La Greca, A., Zigo, M., & Skyler, J. (1989). Diabetes in adolescents: Effects of multifamily group intervention and parent simulation of diabetes. *Journal of Pediatric Psychology, 14,* 259–275.

Schafer, L., Glasgow, R., & McCaul, K. (1982). Increasing adherence of diabetic adolescents. *Journal of Behavioral Medicine, 5,* 353–363.

Schafer, L., Glasgow, R., McCaul, K., & Dreher, M. (1983). Adherence to IDDM regimens: Relationship to psychosocial variables and metabolic control. *Diabetes Care, 6,* 493–498.

Schafer, L., McCaul, K., & Glasgow, R. (1986). Supportive and nonsupportive family behaviors: Relationships to adherence and metabolic control in persons with type 1 diabetes. *Diabetes Care, 9,* 179–185.

Smyth-Staruch, K., Breslau, N., Weitzman, M., & Gortmaker, S. (1984). Use of health services by chronically ill and disabled children. *Medical Care, 22,* 310–328.

Spevack, M., Johnson, S. B., Riley, W., & Silverstein, J. (1991). The effect of diabetes summer camp on adherence behaviors and glycemic control. In J. Johnson & S. B. Johnson (Eds.), *Advances in child health psychology* (pp. 285–292). Gainesville: University Presses of Florida.

Stabler, B., Surwit, R., Lane, J., Morris, M., Litton, J., & Feinglos, M. (1981). Type A behavior pattern and blood glucose control in diabetes children. *Psychosomatic Medicine, 49,* 313–316.

Surwit, R., & Feinglos, M. (1983). The effects of relaxation on glucose tolerance in non-insulin-dependent diabetes. *Diabetes Care, 6,* 176–179.

Tattersall, R. B., & Lowe, J. (1981). Diabetes in adolescence. *Diabetologia, 20,* 517–523.

Thai, A., & Eisenbarth, G. (1993). Natural history of IDDM. *Diabetes Reviews, 1,* 1–14.

Travis, L., Brouchard, B., & Shiner, B. (1987). *Diabetes mellitus in children and adolescents.* Philadelphia: Saunders.

Vandenbergh, R., Sussman, K., & Titus, C. (1966). Effects of

hypnotically induced acute emotional stress on carbohydrate and lipid metabolism in patients with diabetes mellitus. *Psychosomatic Medicine, 28,* 382–390.

Vandenbergh, R., Sussman, K., & Vaughan, G. (1967). Effects of combined physical–anticipatory stress on carbohydrate–lipid metabolism in patients with diabetes
mellitus. *Psychosomatics, 8,* 16–19.

Watkins, J. D., Roberts, D. E., Williams, T. F., Martin, D. A., &
Coyle, V. (1967). Observations of medication errors
made by diabetic patients in the home. *Diabetes, 16,*
882–885.

Willis, T. (1684). Pharmaceutice rationalis. In *The works of
Thomas Willis.* London: Dring, Harper & Leigh.

Wysocki, T., Huxtable, K., Linscheid, T., & Wayne, W.
(1989). Adjustment to diabetes mellitus in preschoolers and their mothers. *Diabetes Care, 12,* 524–
529.

Ziel, R., & Davidson, M. (1987). The role of glycosylated serum albumin in monitoring glycemic control in stable
insulin-requiring diabetic out-patients. *Journal of Clinical Endocrinology and Metabolism, 64,* 269–273.

Zimmet, P. (1983). Epidemiology of diabetes mellitus. In M.
Ellenberg & H. Rifkin (Eds.), *Diabetes mellitus: Theory
and practice* (3rd ed., pp. 451–468). New York: Medical
Examination Publishing.

18

Childhood Cancer

ALICE G. FRIEDMAN, SUSAN A. LATHAM,
AND LYNNDA M. DAHLQUIST

INTRODUCTION

During the past decade there has been remarkable progress in understanding the psychological impact of chronic disease on children. This is particularly true in pediatric oncology settings where close collaboration between behavioral researchers and their medical colleagues has resulted in improved medical outcomes and quality of life for children undergoing treatment and among the increasing number of survivors of childhood cancer.

In an earlier edition of this volume, Dolgin and Jay (1989) noted that links between the biomedical and behavioral aspects of research and clinical practice within pediatric oncology serve as a model for the fields of pediatric psychology and behavioral medicine. This has proven to be a visionary remark. Over the past decade the zeitgeist in the medical community has changed considerably. There now tends to be more attention to the full range of domains relevant to positive outcomes for individuals experiencing a range of medical problems. Although improved technologies have often resulted in prolonged life for children, there is growing concern about the quality of this added time. There is now a movement calling for a broader definition of outcome extending beyond an exclusive focus on biomedical outcomes to include the psychological factors that are highly pertinent to good outcome and higher quality of life for children with chronic illnesses (Chesler 1993; Kazak & Nachman, 1991; Van Eys, 1991).

In this chapter we focus on the *psychological* aspects of childhood cancer. To fully understand the challenges imposed by the disease and its treatment, we present a brief overview of medical aspects of the disease and their implications for psychosocial functioning. This is followed by a discussion of the most common etiology of psychological distress and issues related to assessment and treatment of these challenges. The final section presents a case illustrating some of the major principles discussed throughout the chapter. One of our primary objectives is to illustrate the range of demands confronting children and their families after receiving a di-

ALICE G. FRIEDMAN AND SUSAN A. LATHAM • Department of Psychology, Binghamton University, Binghamton, New York 13905. LYNNDA M. DAHLQUIST • Department of Psychology, University of Maryland Baltimore County, Baltimore, Maryland 21228.

Handbook of Child Psychopathology, 3rd edition, edited by Ollendick & Hersen. Plenum Press, New York, 1998.

agnosis of cancer and to demonstrate how behavioral research has contributed to improved care and overall adjustment.

A thorough discussion of concerns related to all types of childhood cancer is beyond the scope of this chapter. We have chosen to highlight the most critical issues relevant to children diagnosed before age 15 with the most common forms of childhood cancer, namely, leukemia (specifically acute lymphoblastic leukemia) and brain tumors. However, many of these issues are pertinent to children undergoing treatment for other types of cancer as well. Likewise, these issues may also generalize to other chronic diseases of childhood. However, for a more thorough review of the full scope of biomedical and psychosocial aspects of childhood cancer, readers are referred to the scholarly and comprehensive edited volume by Bearison and Mulhern (1994). For an overview of issues related to other pediatric conditions, readers are referred to the comprehensive handbook edited by Roberts (1995).

Prior to proceeding with a discussion of the medical aspects of cancer, brief discussion of two issues is warranted. The first is related to the placement of this topic in a volume on child psychopathology. In contrast to many of the chapters in this book, the majority of children diagnosed with cancer are typical children who are exposed to unusual and demanding circumstances (Armstrong, 1992; Russo & Varni, 1982). Understanding the factors that contribute to the resiliency demonstrated by the vast majority of diagnosed children and their families may provide useful information for others faced with multiple challenges. Second, it is increasingly apparent that the family is a critical mediator to child coping. It is therefore important to consider the child within the context of his or her family and the extraordinary circumstances associated with pediatric cancer.

Medical Aspects and Implications

Approximately 10,000 children and adolescents in the United States are diagnosed with cancer each year. Of those, approximately two-thirds will survive the disease (Lampkin, 1993). This represents a marked improvement in prognosis over a relatively short period of time. Three decades ago, most forms of childhood cancer were invariably fatal and survival was measured by days or months. Today, most children are cured and those who are not live longer than ever before. Improved prognosis is mainly attributable to aggressive treatments that may last for years. Medical advances in cancer treatment have been accompanied by a shift in focus from conceptualizing pediatric cancer as an acute disease to considering it as a chronic illness with implications across the life span (Kazak, 1993).

The term *cancer* refers to a heterogeneous group of disorders, each involving the proliferation of abnormal cells, but otherwise being quite different. Type and length of treatment, prognosis, prevalence, etiology, symptoms, and ramifications for the child and his or her family differ greatly depending on the type and stage (extent) of the cancer and the age of the child (Anderson, 1992; Boman, 1992). Although the disease can involve any organ system, certain forms of cancer are more common in childhood. Children under age 15 are most likely to be diagnosed with leukemia or brain and nervous system tumors. Together these account for roughly half of the cases. Children may also be diagnosed with lymphomas (involving the lymph nodes), neuroblastoma (sympathetic nervous tissue), Wilms' tumor (involving the kidney), and a variety of other forms, although these are quite rare (Mulvihill, 1989). The causes of childhood cancer remain poorly understood. In rare instances cancer can be traced directly to genetic or environmental factors, but most commonly the reasons a particular child has cancer are unknown. For most children, cancer is undoubtedly the unfortunate result of a complex interaction of environmental, genetic, and viral factors (Mulvihill, 1989).

The diagnosis of cancer is often made after a child has experienced persistence of symptoms that mimic those associated with mild childhood illnesses. In the case of leukemia, fatigue, flulike symptoms, leg pain, or fever may linger or recur prompting parents to seek medical attention. For brain tumors, initial symptoms may include headache, nausea and vomiting, and unsteadiness. If cancer is suspected, confirmation of the diagnosis generally follows a series of diagnostic tests (Nesbit, 1989). The specific tests conducted are dependent on the type of suspected cancer but typically include tests that are invasive and painful. In the case of leukemia, for example, diagnostic studies normally include a bone marrow aspiration (and biopsy) and a lumbar puncture. These tests, used to evaluate the presence of cancer cells in the central nervous system, are among the most painful and dreaded of all invasive medical procedures (Rape & Bush, 1994). A needle is inserted into a bone, typically the back or hip, for withdrawal of bone marrow and spinal fluid for evaluation. Although the procedures last just a few minutes, the pain has been described as excruciating. In the case of brain tumor or other solid tumors, diagnostic procedures may involve various forms of imaging studies such as X rays, magnetic resonance imaging (MRI) or computed tomography (CT) scans; although not painful, these tests require a high level of cooperation by the child.

Most local hospitals and pediatricians are not equipped to provide treatment for pediatric cancer. Therefore, the majority of children are referred to a specialized pediatric oncology center for treatment. The major advances in survival have been accomplished through the use of multimodal treatments designed to obliterate cancer cells at each phase of cell reproduction and involve some combination of surgery, chemotherapy, radiation therapy, and bone marrow transplantation. Regardless of the type of cancer, the treatment goal is to achieve and maintain remission, or disease-free state. Surgery is generally used, if possible, to remove solid tumors. Chemotherapy, administered orally, through intravenous, intramuscular, or direct injections into the CNS, is a systemic approach aimed at preventing abnormal cell growth and division. Chemotherapy is the primary treatment for leukemia but may be used for solid tu-

mors, in conjunction with surgery, to obliterate remaining cells. Multiple drugs are generally given in specific sequences over courses that may last a few days and may be repeated for years. Radiation therapy, used to eliminate remaining abnormal cells or, in the case of leukemia, used as a prophylactic measure to eliminate occult cells remaining in the CNS, may be administered daily over the course of a few weeks. Bone marrow transplantation (BMT), the newest form of treatment, involves destroying the patient's own marrow via chemotherapy and radiation and replacing it with marrow donated by a matched donor. BMT results in temporary loss of immune functioning rendering children highly susceptible to infection. To limit exposure to infection, children are usually kept in isolation for a few weeks following the procedure.

Unfortunately, each of these forms of treatment affects healthy cells in addition to abnormal cells. Resulting toxicities cause short- and long-term side effects. Short-term effects of chemotherapy may include nausea and vomiting, loss of appetite, lowered immune functioning, and hair loss. Long-term consequences result from damage to vital organs and can include impaired growth, cardiac complications, and second cancers, among others. Radiation therapy also causes undesirable side effects including gastrointestinal difficulties, fatigue, and damage to tissue proximal to the irradiated site, and possible later malignancies. Patients undergoing BMT typically experience symptoms related to rejection of the new marrow (graft-versus-host disease). Acute symptoms may include mouth sores, nausea, and vomiting and longer-term difficulties may include hearing loss, growth and endocrine abnormalities, cataracts, and second malignancies (Ramsay, 1989). The isolation imposed by BMT is often accompanied by increased feelings of depression (Ramsay 1989).

Late Effects

Many early papers touting medical advances were quite optimistic about eventual cures.

However, as the number of survivors increases, and as assessments become more systematic, the initial optimism is tempered by concerns about late effects. Long-term medical effects resulting from delayed toxic effects of treatment may include difficulties in any organ system, recurrence, and a second malignancy (Neglia & Nesbit, 1993). In addition, survivors have shown an increased incidence of developmental, academic, cognitive, and social sequelae (Buckley, 1993; Kazak, 1993; Meadows et al., 1993). There is now greater attention to evaluating the health status, quality of life, and functional status of cancer survivors (Eiser, 1994; Jenney, Kane, & Lurie, 1995). Many oncology centers offer specialized clinics to provide surveillance and intervention for patients after they have completed treatment. Patients regularly return to the clinics where their physical and psychological well-being are monitored.

It is estimated that there are now approximately 50,000 survivors of childhood cancer in the United States, corresponding to approximately 1 of every 1000 individuals reaching age 20 (Raymond, 1988). As this is really the first generation of survivors, their future is still uncertain (van Eys, 1991). Compared with their healthy peers, survivors who are now in their 20s are less likely to graduate from college and have health insurance coverage. Survivors are also more likely to experience work-related limitations and receive public assistance (Hayes, 1993).

Collaborative Treatment Approaches

As childhood cancer is a rare disease, no one institution could accrue a sufficient number of patients to provide reliable information about treatment efficacy. Advances in care and improved psychological and medical outcome have been accomplished through cooperative multisite, multidisciplinary, collaborative study groups. The two major groups are the Children's Cancer Group (CCG) and the Pediatric Oncology Group (POG). Most children now receive treatment at institutions participating in CCG or POG collaborative studies. Children who have diagnoses under study are typically enrolled in treatment protocols with the goal of improving cure rates and reducing negative side effects (Hammond et al., 1993; Meadows et al., 1993).

Role of Psychology in Pediatric Oncology Settings

The relationship between psychology and medicine within medical settings can be characterized as ambivalent. It is often marred by misunderstanding between the disciplines about their roles and responsibilities, and by differences in patterns of communication, charting, professional etiquette, and approaches toward conceptualizing patient difficulties (Wright & Friedman, 1991). Although these difficulties can exist in pediatric oncology settings, they tend to be less pervasive than in many other disciplines. Here, successful collaboration between medicine and psychology has fostered integration of mental health services and medical care resulting in coordinated patient care as well as in important cooperative studies that have provided information to guide medical treatment.

Psychologists also typically work closely with their social work and other mental health colleagues. Although there can be confusion about which discipline is responsible for certain aspects of care, most centers have formal mechanisms in place to facilitate ongoing communication between the two disciplines. One method is through mental health rounds conducted weekly to review patient information. Typically social workers provide routine psychosocial care consisting of assisting families during diagnosis, securing tangible resources, monitoring adjustment, and following families throughout their contact with the oncology center. The psychology service may be contacted when a family is experiencing problems beyond those that typically accompany the diagnosis. In larger oncology centers employing a range of mental health professionals, mental health services may be provided by child life workers, social workers, neuropsychologists, and developmental, child clinical, and pediatric psychologists. In all cases, the goal is close collaboration to ensure the most cost-effective means for providing appropriate support and timely interventions to all families.

ETIOLOGY OF PSYCHOLOGICAL DISTRESS

The diagnosis of cancer is accompanied by extraordinary stressors for the child and family that place them at risk for psychological difficulties associated with the disease and may increase their vulnerability to non-disease-related stressors (Baum & Baum, 1989; Eiser, 1994). During and following treatment, children continue to have the same developmental demands as healthy children, along with those associated with cancer. Bull and Drotar (1991) asked children and adolescents in remission to identify personal situations they found stressful. They found that children generated far more non-cancer-related stressors than cancer-related ones. Most common were concerns related to school, siblings, and parents—issues similar to their healthy peers. Nevertheless, cancer-related concerns were also expressed.

The majority of children undergoing treatment for cancer appear to fare remarkably well (Kupst & Schulman, 1988; Kupst et al., 1983, 1984), although there is evidence that a subgroup of children do experience cognitive, behavioral, and emotional difficulties during and following treatment (Mulhern, Wasserman, Friedman, & Fairclough, 1989; Overholser & Fritz, 1990; Sanger, Copeland, & Davidson, 1991). In this section we outline potential sources of general distress and associated risk factors followed by a discussion of more specific treatment-related issues.

Psychological Adjustment to Cancer-Related Stressors

Treatment for cancer progresses across predictable stages and the nature and intensity of the associated stressors change as the child proceeds through these stages.

Diagnosis

The initial impact of the diagnosis comes at a time when rapid changes are taking place. Families are presented with complicated information regarding the specific diagnosis, prognosis, treatment plans, side effects, and available resources. Often, concrete arrangements must be made for transportation, lodging close to a hospital, leave from jobs, and child care of other children. At the same time, treatment decisions must be made and emotional resources are typically depleted (Lansky, List, & Ritter-Sterr, 1989). Children and families who have to travel long distances for treatment are apt to have higher levels of distress and more financial hardships than those who live closer to the hospital (Aitken & Hathaway, 1993).

Families report that the initial diagnosis is the most stressful period during the course of the illness (Barnhart et al., 1994; Brown, 1989). Feelings of anxiety, sadness, and need to gather information are common (Kupst, 1993; et al., 1983) as are feelings of guilt related to speculation about potential causes of the disease (Lansky et al., 1989). This is a particularly vulnerable time for parents, and a significant proportion experience marital discord (Dahlquist et al., 1993). Families who are more resilient are those with more emotional and economic resources, higher levels of social support, and higher levels of premorbid functioning. These families are also better equipped to deal with the multiple emotional and concrete challenges of the new diagnosis (Kozak & Meadows, 1989; Kupst et al., 1983, 1995; Speechley & Noh, 1992). Studies have documented elevated levels of distress and behavioral difficulties for the child and anxiety and depression for parents at the time of diagnosis with improvement noted over time (Kupst et al., 1983; Mulhern, Fairclough, Smith, & Douglas, 1992; Sawyer, Antoniou, Nguyen, Rice, & Baghurst, 1995).

Certain aspects of the oncology setting and the relationship between the family and oncology staff at this stage may play a critical role in later adjustment. In one of the few prospective longitudinal studies of a cohort of children undergoing treatment for leukemia and their families, Kupst (1993) reported that families feel they benefit most from interventions geared toward: (1) providing concrete information and direction, (2) providing support and someone to act as a liaison, and (3) providing assistance with mobilizing their own coping strategies to deal with stress (Kupst, 1993).

Active Treatment

Treatment typically involves an initial induction period characterized by intensive treatment with the goal of attaining an initial remission, followed by a less rigorous course of maintenance therapy. During this period the child is generally exposed to numerous aversive medical procedures, toxic therapies, and disruption of age-appropriate activities (including absences from school). Factors associated with positive adjustment during this period include the age of the child (older age at diagnosis leads to better coping on the part of the mother), previous coping abilities, coping abilities of other family members, a good support system, and lack of additional stressors (Kupst et al., 1983).

Parents and children are generally advised to resume their usual activities and to maintain as normal an environment as possible. However, there are numerous impediments to this goal, including constraints imposed by medical complications, increased levels of general distress within the family, and changes in how families interact. In a recent study, Claflin and Barbarin (1991) interviewed adolescents about their experiences during cancer treatment. A substantial proportion of the children reported that their families treated them differently after their diagnosis. A primary complaint of the adolescents was that their families "babied" them.

Parents are often unsure about how much information to give their child about the diagnosis and its ramifications and there are no clear guidelines for health professionals (Chesler, Allswede, & Barbarin, 1991). Positive long-term adaptation of the child is associated with early knowledge of the diagnosis (Slavin, O'Malley, Koocher, & Foster, 1982). Withholding information from children does not alleviate anxiety and is therefore not endorsed (Claflin & Barbarin, 1991). Age-appropriate discussion about illness within families and with the oncology staff can prevent the child from arriving at erroneous conclusions (Claflin & Barbarin, 1991).

Treatment Completion

The completion of active treatment represents a major milestone for most families but can be accompanied by additional stressors and ambivalence. By the time a child completes treatment, the family has often established a strong support system within the medical setting. For many families being treated some distance from their homes, the end of treatment can mean loss of support and reduction in contact with medical staff and other families undergoing similar experiences. Further, because the cancer is no longer being actively treated, some families experience increased anxiety related to loss of protection and fears of recurrence (Cincotta, 1993; Eiser, 1994).

Treatment can leave many children with a range of physical impairments from cosmetic to functional. Functional impairment and physical disability are associated with increases in depressive symptomatology (Fritz, Williams, & Amylon, 1988; Greenberg, Kazak, & Meadows, 1989) and social problems, and decreases in academic achievement (Carpentieri, Mulhern, Douglas, Hanna, & Fairclough, 1993; Fritz et al., 1988; Mulhern et al., 1989). To help ameliorate these difficulties, a variety of interventions may be warranted including aggressive physical rehabilitation, modifications in the children's environment to accommodate their disabilities, counseling to accept their limitations and retain good self-concept, and close monitoring of their academic progress (Carpentieri et al., 1993).

As the time since diagnosis increases, the number and severity of problems decrease and adjustment usually improves significantly (Kupst & Schulman, 1988; Wasserman, Thompson, Wilimas, & Fairclough, 1987). Many children and adolescents in remission look remarkably like their peers on measures of popularity, school adjustment, and social competence (Fritz et al., 1988; Noll, Bukowski, Davies, Koontz, & Kulkarni, 1993; Spirito et al., 1990). These children are more apt to report general life stressors as being problematic than cancer-related stressors (Bull & Drotar, 1991). Positive adjustment is associated with open communication, current school functioning, social/peer interaction, and lack of concurrent stressors (Fritz et al., 1988; Kupst & Schulman, 1988).

Relapse

If relapse occurs, therapy becomes more intense and hospital admissions for fever and infections can be as frequent as those during therapy (Rochester, 1989). Recurrence is reported by some patients and their families as being more stressful and fear provoking than the initial diagnosis (Cincotta, 1993; Rolland, 1990; Wasserman et al., 1987). Relapse for most forms of cancer does represent a serious threat to survival. Children with leukemia who undergo treatment following relapse have a lower rate of survival and a higher incidence of late effects of treatment (Mulhern et al., 1987).

Death

Despite improved treatments, one-third of the children diagnosed do not survive. The increased expectancies for survival of childhood cancer patients can make the death of a child even harder to bear (Eiser, 1994). There has been far less systematic research on how to best assist children and families during this difficult time. Recommendations are generally based more on general psychological principles than on empirical findings. Unambiguous communication of the child's condition from the medical team is recommended to assist the family deal with the impending death. The focus of medical and behavioral intervention shifts from being future-oriented to being present-oriented. Families typically take a more active role in the daily care of the child (Martinson & Papadatou, 1994). Adequate support and pain management are critical during this period (Chesler, 1993; Rolland, 1990; Whittam, 1993). Parents are generally informed of all medical options so that they may make informed decisions concerning their child's care (Rochester, 1989; Whittam, 1993). It is recommended that questions concerning their child's condition be addressed honestly and openly. Open communication can allow the family to attend to unresolved relationship issues and make the most of their remaining time together (Rolland, 1990; Whittam, 1993).

Options for care in terms of setting are typically discussed with the family. There are now a number of hospice and home-care programs designed especially for children (Martinson & Papadatou, 1994). Home care is appropriate for some families, whereas others feel safer and better cared for in the hospital (Rochester, 1989; Whittam, 1993). Most home-care programs are structured to allow the families to be the primary caregivers, with nurses facilitating care and doctors serving as consultants. The goal is to enable the child to live in the customary setting of the home, cared for by those closest to the child. Home care can lessen the guilt felt by parents after the death of their child and improve the adjustment of well siblings (Lauer, Mulhern, Wallskog, & Camitta, 1983; Mulhern, Lauer, & Hoffmann, 1983). It can also allow for greater family communication and can decrease the child's sense of isolation (Whittam, 1993).

Home care is not desired by nor is it feasible for all families. Single parents or those of low SES may not have the resources to provide such intensive care. Insurance may not provide for home care and some doctors are not comfortable with this option. In some cases the child's condition may make this course unfeasible. Clear communication concerning the family's wishes and the realities of the patient's medical condition is necessary for the family to make an informed decision concerning palliative care (Whittam, 1993).

Bereavement care is important for the family's adjustment after the child dies. A postmortem conference with the medical team to review the course of the child's illness and key decisions made along with the proximate causes of death can help reassure the family that their child received the best care possible (Chesler, 1993; Whittam, 1993).

Parental Adjustment

Having a child diagnosed with cancer challenges the coping resources of the entire family. Parents must meet the physical and emotional needs of their ill child while attempting to juggle the demands of work and normal family household responsibilities. Despite the many trials faced by these families, research has demonstrated that their adjustment can be similar to that of families without a chronically ill child (Davies, Noll, DeStefano, Bukowski, & Kulkarni, 1991; Kazak & Meadows, 1989; Kupst et al., 1995).

A number of factors appear to be associated with positive parental (usually maternal) adjustment. The importance of social support as a buffer for parents coping with the stressors associated with cancer has been demonstrated in numerous studies (Barbarin, 1987; Dahlquist et al., 1993; Mulhern, Fairclough, Smith, & Douglas, 1992; Overholser & Fritz, 1990; Speechley & Noh, 1992; Varni, Katz, Colegrove, & Dolgin, 1994). Barrera (1986) identified three major dimensions of social support: perceived social support, social embeddedness, and enacted social support. Perceived social support is defined as the satisfaction with the perceived availability

and adequacy of social support. Social embeddedness refers to the size of the social network. Enacted social support is the frequency of helping behaviors from others. Perceived social support is the most frequently assessed dimension of this construct and it has been consistently found to be negatively correlated with psychological distress.

Whereas adequate levels of perceived social support are associated with positive adjustment, low levels are predictive of increased depressive symptomatology in both mothers and fathers (Mulhern, Fairclough, et al., 1992; Speechley & Noh, 1992). This has implications for the ill child as well in that the quality of parental coping and adjustment is associated with the quality of the child's coping and adjustment (Mulhern, Fairclough, et al., 1992; Overholser & Fritz, 1990).

The quality of the marital relationship is also correlated with adjustment (Kupst et al., 1984; Kupst & Schulman, 1988; Speechley & Noh, 1992). Whereas social support is important for fathers of a child with cancer, marital satisfaction is a greater buffer for them. In other words, the support offered by marriage is particularly important for the well-being of fathers in this situation (Speechley & Noh, 1992). Factors that have been found to be predictive of marital distress early in the course of the disease include discrepancy between the couple's state anxiety levels and use of stimulus approach coping (Dahlquist et al., 1993). The greater the difference in the parents' anxiety levels surrounding the stressors associated with the diagnosis, the greater is the reported marital distress. Stimulus approach coping implies a belief that something can be done about the situation and efforts are made to somehow alter it. During the early months of the cancer diagnosis, treatment for the child is placed in the hands of the cancer treatment team, and in reality, parents can only await the outcome. Avoidant coping strategies may be more adaptive at this time because the situation is uncontrollable. Avoidant coping strategies may even help to maintain marital satisfaction (Dahlquist et al., 1993).

Low SES is also associated with poor adjustment (Kupst et al., 1995). Financial concerns are a major stressor for all families caring for a child with cancer (Barnhart et al., 1994; Overholser & Fritz, 1990). Costs not only include treatment, hospitalization, and medication, but travel and lodging expenses, and time away from work. For parents with few resources, additional economic hardships may seem insurmountable.

Sibling Adjustment

When a child in the family is diagnosed with a catastrophic disease, available family resources may be targeted toward the affected child and away from other children in the family. Siblings may be left to contend with mixed feelings of fear and sadness along with guilt and jealousy toward the afflicted child while parents are unavailable both physically and emotionally. Research on the impact of having a sibling with cancer has been somewhat contradictory. There is some evidence that, on global measures of long-term adjustment, siblings fare adequately. For example, studies have found siblings' levels of adjustment to be similar to established norms and to those of children who don't have a chronically ill sibling (Evans, Stevens, Cushway, & Houghton, 1992; Horowitz & Kazak, 1990; Madam-Swain, Sexson, Brown, & Ragab, 1993). Yet there is no doubt that these children are affected by their sibling's illness and are at elevated risk for difficulties in adjusting during the time of crisis. Scores within the normal range on various measures of adjustment suggest that the siblings' distress may be interpreted by them and by their parents as a normal response to an abnormal situation. Further, problems may be transient and not sufficiently severe to categorize them as maladjusted. Some studies do confirm an elevated incidence of distress and related adjustment problems (Sahler & Carpenter, 1988; Sargent et al., 1995).

Healthy siblings report experiencing distress over disruptions in family routines in terms of separations, role changes, and alterations in normal family activities. Some children express difficulties in school in terms of concentrating on schoolwork and in dealing with difficult comments from peers regarding their sibling's condition. Siblings report feeling jealous of the extra attention received by the ill child. At the same time, many report fearing the possible death of their ill sibling (Adams-Greenly, Shiminski-Maher, McGowan, & Meyers, 1986; Evans et al., 1992; Sargent et al., 1995).

In a recent review of studies about siblings, Carpenter and LeVant (1994) identified three major sources of distress for siblings: (1) lack of adequate parental communication about the afflicted sibling and inadequate involvement in treatment, (2) isolation from parents, and (3) insufficient emotional and social resources including insufficient peer support. They estimated that approximately 50% of siblings experience adjustment problems at some point following the cancer diagnosis (Carpenter & LeVant, 1994).

Several buffering factors for the positive adjustment of healthy siblings have been identified. Better adaptation has been found in larger families. This may be because there is more emotional support available; older siblings may be able to take greater responsibility for household chores and care for younger siblings (Madam-Swain et al., 1993). Sibling knowledge of their ill brother or sister's cancer is positively associated with social competence. This in turn is related to better psychological adjustment (Evans et al., 1992). The directionality of this association is unclear. It may be that more socially competent children are able to elicit the information they need. Or it may be that socially competent children have better coping skills overall.

Age and gender also have an effect on healthy siblings' adjustment. Sargent et al. (1995) found that boys aged 6–11 were at highest risk for developing problems. Young children in general were found to have a more difficult time in adjusting to the disruptions imposed by the cancer diagnosis. This may be a developmental issue in that young children are more dependent on their families than are older children and, therefore, are more vulnerable to changes in the family's functioning. They may also suffer more from withdrawal of parental attention and have fewer coping resources available to them to deal with changes. The reason boys were differentially affected remains unclear although young boys may be more apt to express problems overtly.

On a final note, some researchers have found that there may be some positive results of having to cope with the illness of a sibling. Horowitz and Kazak (1990) found higher rates of some prosocial behaviors in a sample of preschool siblings of children with cancer. Sargent et al. (1995) found that older siblings were more likely to report that they had become more compassionate and caring, felt that family members were closer to each other, that they had experiences they might not otherwise have had, and that they felt they had been helpful to the ill child and their family.

Procedure-Related Distress

Treatment almost invariably involves repeated exposure to aversive medical procedures. Some children undergo daily finger-sticks and as many as 300 venipunctures for purposes of drawing blood and administering chemotherapy, anesthesia, or hydration (Jacobsen et al., 1990). Bone marrow aspirations (BMAs) and lumbar punctures (LPs) are routine for many treatment protocols. Children are generally awake and restrained by a nurse and/or parent during these procedures (Katz, Kellerman, & Siegel, 1980). Postsurgical pain related to removal of sutures and wound cleansing are common causes of pain.

Children vary in the amount of distress they exhibit during procedures and their ability to cope with it. During BMAs and LPs, young children typically exhibit more distress-related behaviors such as crying, screaming, and clinging. Older children (age 7 and up) are more apt to express their distress verbally (Katz et al., 1980).

A clear relationship between a child's naturally preferred coping style and his or her level of distress during the procedures has yet to be established (Manne, Bakeman, Jacobsen, & Redd, 1993). In contrast to other fear-provoking situations where anxiety dissipates with repeated exposure, distress toward these procedures appears to increase each time (Katz et al., 1980). Further, previous experiences with procedure-related distress may increase anticipatory anxiety toward subsequent events.

Children's expressions of pain and distress during medical procedures are highly related to specific behaviors exhibited by parents (Blount, Sturges, & Powers, 1990; Manne, Bakemann, Jacobsen, Gorfinkle, & Redd, 1994) and staff (Dahlquist, Pendley, Power, Landthrip, & Jones, 1994; Dahlquist, Pendley, Power, Landthrip, Jones, & Steuber, 1995; Dahlquist, Power, & Carlson, 1995). When adults use strategies geared toward directing attention away from the medical procedure, children appear to show fewer behavioral signs of distress (such as crying) and more behaviors geared toward coping (Manne, Bakemann, et al., 1992). In contrast, parental behaviors, presumably emitted with the goal of comforting their child, can result in increased distress-related behaviors. For example, parental use of reassuring comments or apologies can serve to increase rather than decrease distress. Directives, on the other hand, appear to lower distress. A recent study by Dahlquist and colleagues (Dahlquist, Power, Cox, & Fernbach, 1994) provides evidence for the hypothesis that parents' own anxiety and attitude may be conveyed to the child through their overt behaviors during the procedure. In a study of 66 children undergoing BMA, child anxiety and distress were related to parental anxiety and rewarding of dependency. Studies of healthy children undergoing inoculation, which experimentally manipulated parental presence, have also found that children cry more when their mothers are present versus remain in the waiting room (Gonzales et al., 1989; Gross, Stern, Levin, Dale, & Wojnilower, 1983; Shaw & Routh, 1982).

Children may respond differently to medical practitioners than to their parents. In a study involving observations of children during medical procedures, Dahlquist and colleagues (Dahlquist, Power, & Carlson, 1995) found a relationship between reassuring comments by practitioners and lower levels of child distress. It may be that practitioners provide more reassurance to those children who are exhibiting less behavioral distress. Alternatively, children may respond differently to practitioner and parental reassurance. If the later is correct, children may benefit from distraction and coaching offered by parents along with reassurance from the medical staff.

Academic and Neuropsychological Impact

While children are undergoing treatment, academic concerns generally focus on helping the child maintain his or her developmental level. For younger children this means facilitating exposure to opportunities to try new tasks and to strive to achieve developmental milestones. For older children this means keeping up with peers on academic subjects. With normalization being the goal, efforts are made to ensure that the children return to school as soon after diagnosis as possible and to attend whenever medically feasible. Most children do miss a substantial portion of the school year during the first few years following diagnosis. Although Copeland (1992) noted that studies have failed to document an association between amount of school missed and educational and academic performance, sustained absences can impede social adjustment and make future school reintegration more difficult (Varni, Katz, Colegrove, & Dolgin, 1993).

A second and perhaps more critical educational concern focuses on the long-term impact of cancer and its treatment on the child's intellectual, cognitive, and academic abilities. Most studies on academic and neuropsychological impact of cancer and its treatment have focused on children with leukemia and brain tumors as

these constitute the largest group and appear at greatest risk. For children with leukemia, most of the concern focuses on the long-term negative effects of CNS prophylactic treatments. The latter involves injection of chemotherapy directly into the CNS and/or cranial irradiation to obliterate any cancerous cells present in the CNS. Use of prophylactic treatment has greatly reduced the incidence of recurrence but there is mounting concern about whether these children experience subtle or significant neuropsychological deficits (Butler & Copeland, 1993; Copeland, 1992; Cousens, Ungerer, Crawford, & Stevens, 1991; Mulhern, Ochs, & Fairclough, 1992).

Research examining the impact of prophylactic treatments is fraught with methodological difficulties related to problems in measurement (such as the use of global measures that may be insensitive to subtle difficulties), experimental designs that lack appropriate controls, small sample sizes limiting power to detect differences, and lack of consideration of potential confounds such as the impact of SES, illness severity, and school absence (for review see Butler & Copeland, 1993; Mulhern, 1994). These limitations are related to difficulties inherent to studying this population rather than to lack of rigor on the part of the investigators.

However, the emerging consensus is that CNS prophylactic treatment can result in significant declines in IQ (Copeland, 1992; Cousens, Waters, Said, & Stevens, 1988; Stehbens et al., 1991) and deficits in specific abilities such as memory, attention and concentration, visual processing speed, and sequencing abilities (Cousens et al., 1991). Children treated before the age of 3 appear to be particularly vulnerable to the effects of cranial irradiation. Deficits may not be apparent for 3 or more years following treatment (Mulhern, Ochs, & Fairclough, 1992). According to Cousens et al. (1991), CNS prophylaxis appears to cause multiple deficits rather than a specific one.

In contrast to the contradictory findings about CNS prophylaxis, there is consistent evidence that children who relapse requiring a second course of CNS treatment experience significant declines in intellectual and academic functioning. In a retrospective study of survivors of CNS relapse, Mulhern et al. (1987) found a marked (10-fold) increase in incidence of mental retardation.

Children with brain tumors constitute another group at sharply elevated risk for long-term deficits in intellect and academic achievement. The type and extent of deficits are highly dependent on aspects of the tumor (type, location, and size), type of treatment, side effects, and complications. Study findings have consistently documented significant declines in IQ following treatment. Children younger than 7 at the time of cranial irradiation averaged a 25-point decline in IQ (Packer et al., 1989). Studies have also documented deficits across numerous specific sensory and motor abilities (for a comprehensive review see Mulhern, 1994).

ASSESSMENT

Global Strategy

Assessment of the child and family is an ongoing process that begins at diagnosis and continues for years after treatment is completed. Just as the range of stressors changes across different phases of treatment, so does the focus and scope of assessment. Assessment early in treatment typically focuses on evaluating the family's adjustment, determining their level of understanding of the medical condition and its treatment, and assessing the child's level of adjustment. A formal evaluation of the child's cognitive development and academic achievement may be undertaken to provide a baseline for later comparison. During treatment more focused assessments targeting specific areas of concern may be conducted. This is particularly likely in cases where children are exhibiting behavior problems, extreme anxiety or distress during medical procedures, or appear withdrawn. For many years following completion of treatment, routine

assessments may be scheduled for the purpose of long-term surveillance.

Psychological Adjustment to Cancer-Related Stressors

Evaluating adjustment of children and parents early in the course of treatment is complicated by lack of information about what constitutes dysfunction and what specific behaviors correlate with positive long-term outcome (Barbarin, 1987). Comparing children with control samples or with a standardization sample on standardized measures of psychological adjustment has limited utility because behaviors indicative of dysfunction among healthy children may be appropriate and adaptive expressions of distress among sick children. The Child Behavior Checklist (CBCL; Achenbach, 1991), for example, is frequently used to evaluate adjustment in healthy and medically ill populations. However, instrument development and item selection was based on relationships among specific behaviors and mental health problems in healthy children. Even efforts to develop new norms for cancer patients do not solve the problem, as different behaviors may be predictive of problems for this population (Perrin, Stein, & Drotar, 1991).

Researchers have generally used a number of tactics to circumvent the measurement problems. One strategy is to use broadband instruments, such as the CBCL (Achenbach, 1991), Personality Inventory for Children (PIC), Wirt, Lachar, Klinedinst, & Seat, 1990), or others as general screening instruments. Children who appear to be experiencing problems may be interviewed or otherwise further assessed. Other investigators have used a number of more targeted assessment tools to evaluate specific dimensions of emotion such as depression (Mulhern, Fairclough, Smith, & Douglas, 1992), self-esteem (Greenberg et al., 1989), and self-competency (Varni et al., 1993). These measures may introduce similar measurement problems. They may not provide valid measures of the intended construct when used with medically ill populations. In the case of depression, for example, items may not distinguish symptoms related to medical problems from those related to depression (Mulhern et al., 1992). An alternative approach is the use of new instruments designed expressly for this population. Recent efforts have focused on developing measures to assess overall quality of life (Bradlyn, Harris, Warner, Ritchey, & Zaboy, 1993; Jenney et al., 1995; Mulhern, Fairclough, Friedman, & Leigh, 1990) and coping (Spirito, Stark, & Williams, 1988). These instruments have the advantage of facilitating comparisons with other children with similar difficulties. Being relatively new, however, they have not been well validated.

A few investigators have combined a number of measurement approaches. In a comprehensive study of family coping, Kupst and colleagues (Kupst et al., 1983, 1984; Kupst, Natta, Richardson, Schulman, Lavigne, & Das, 1995) included measures designed to assess an entire family's well-being such as adequacy of child coping, parental report of child adjustment, symptom checklists, assessment of disease/disability variables (such as medical status), and inventories to determine the parents' level of functioning (parental coping, parental personality). Information derived from different sources may provide very different perspectives about the same child (Mulhern, Fairclough, et al., 1992), thereby providing a more complete understanding of the child's behavior across situations and toward different people.

Although there are no specific assessment tools that have known utility for this population, a number of principles of assessment have emerged. The first is that child assessment must be conducted within the context of the family setting and with a full appreciation of the demands of the medical illness. Fluctuations in the behavior of the child and family may be viewed as responses to changes in cancer-related challenges and are not necessarily indicative of pathological processes. Testing while children are experiencing temporary treatment-related side effects is avoided as this could depress the child's scores resulting in an inaccurate measure of level of functioning. The evaluation should include identification of strengths and available concrete and emotional coping resources rather than exclusively focusing on deficits. Further, assessment should encompass the full scope of domains relevant to child and family adjustment and the focus of assessment should change over time to reflect changes in the child's developmental level (and related developmental milestones) and changes in the phase of treatment. Peer status, for example, may not be a priority during diagnosis but will become a more important issue as the child is reintegrated into school and social activities. Last, because of lack of appropriately standardized measures, interpretation of assessment findings must be guided by clinical judgments rather than strict adherence to available, but perhaps inappropriate, norms.

Parental Adjustment

Assessment of parental adjustment is generally conducted within the context of the child's treatment. This may occur informally during the early phases of the child's treatment with psychosocial staff assessing parental understanding of disease-related issues, availability of resources and social support, general adequacy of parenting, and presence of concurrent stressors or preexisting emotional problems. Unless parents are participating in a particular project, their level of adjustment may not be formally assessed in the absence of indications of difficulties.

A variety of strategies have been used in research focused on family and parental adjustment. These include using semistructured interviews with parents to assess specific coping strategies (Barbarin & Chesler, 1986), questionnaires designed to evaluate aspects of family functioning, such as the Family Adaptability and Cohesion Evaluation Scales (Olson, Portner, & Bell, 1982, as in Kazak & Meadows, 1989) or the Family Environment Scales (Moos & Moos,

1981, as in Greenberg et al., 1989), or evaluation of specific emotions of interest, such as depression and anxiety (Dahlquist et al., 1993). Interpretation of assessment results is complicated by the same issues relevant to assessing the patients. The discriminative validity of these instruments has typically not been established with parents of chronically ill children. However, these measures may be useful to examine relationships among variables of interest. Used with caution, they may also help to identify families in particular distress.

Sibling Adjustment

Siblings are often the neglected members of the family. Parents are generally involved in most aspects of treatment making them accessible to informal surveillance by medical and mental health practitioners. In contrast, during the period of diagnosis and early treatment, care of siblings is often relegated to relatives. Information about the medically ill child's diagnosis, aspects of treatment, and the day-to-day activities of parents and the ill child may be conveyed to siblings third- or fourthhand. Likewise, there may be little communication to parents about the behaviors of siblings. As a result, siblings may experience significant disturbances that are not apparent until problems are seen in school or with peers. Although some pediatric oncology centers routinely evaluate families at specific intervals, siblings who live a distance from the treatment setting may not be included.

Most studies on sibling adjustment have used instruments validated on typical children. When assessments are conducted during a time of turmoil in the family, expressed distress by siblings may reflect adaptive responses rather than connote psychopathology. Nevertheless, if clinical judgment is used to carefully consider expressed behavioral distress within the medical context, these instruments can be helpful for generating hypotheses about how a child is doing.

Targets for assessment include the child's understanding of his or her sibling's medical condition, presence of adjustment problems with particular emphasis on recent changes in behavior corresponding to the sibling's diagnosis, availability of social and peer support, and availability of opportunities for the sibling to discuss feeling about changes occurring in the family.

Procedure-Related Distress

The major goal of assessing a child's response to painful medical procedures is to identify potentially modifiable resources of distress and to develop strategies to alleviate distress related to those not modifiable. Modifiable sources of distress often include inadequate pharmacological pain management or aspects of the clinic setting that are less than ideal for some children. Pressure to hurry the procedure, fueled by the need to treat large numbers of children, may not give the child adequate preparation time. Small changes in how the early parts of the procedure are handled may alleviate considerable distress. Children's misconceptions about the procedures are another common source of distress. One child who was particularly upset about receiving a bone marrow aspiration thought that the practitioner was going to stick a "bow and arrow" into his back. Information about the nature of the procedure helped reduce the child's distress.

Evaluating pain in children is complicated by aspects of pain itself. Pain is a subjective experience that is determined by a complex interaction of affective, cognitive, behavioral, developmental, and situational factors (McGrath & Unruh, 1987). There is therefore little relationship between the extent of tissue damage and perceptions of pain. The association between subjective experiences of pain and observable behavior differs depending on a host of factors such as the child's age and temperament, demand characteristics of the setting, parental expectations, and practitioner behaviors.

An additional complication is that many of the most common forms of cancer are most prevalent in very early childhood, a time when most children lack the verbal ability to communicate their subjective experiences. As a result, the extent or severity of the child's pain is generally inferred by observations of the child's behavior and comparing them to the child's responses toward other situations. This approach is complicated by the fact that different observers of the same child provide significantly different assessments of the child's level of pain and distress. In a recent study, Manne, Jacobsen, and Redd (1992) found ratings of children's pain completed by nurses, parents, and the child to differ considerably, with ratings apparently based on different variables. Nurses' ratings were related to the child's overt distress during the procedure, whereas parents' ratings appeared to be influenced by how much pain they anticipated their child would experience and by their own level of anxiety. Children's ratings were related more to their age, with younger children reporting higher ratings of pain and distress than older ones.

Different observers have access to different information about the child, which influences their interpretation of the child's behavior. Parents have the advantage of knowing the characteristic behavior of their child. On the other hand, their perceptions of their child's distress may be influenced by their own emotions. Practitioners who have observed numerous children undergoing the same procedures have an informal standardization sample to use as a yardstick for comparison. They, however, may not know the child sufficiently well to judge the child's level of distress on the basis of overt behavior alone.

In light of these complexities, assessment of the child's distress is generally accomplished by combining the results of a few different assessment approaches: self-report, parental and practitioner ratings, and direct observations. Asking the child about his or her fears and anxiety is the most direct way to assess distress. This may be accomplished by using one of the available self-report instruments designed for this purpose. These visual analogue scales are picto-rial representations of familiar items, such as a yardstick or thermometer or faces varying from happy to sad. Children are asked to convert their subjective level of distress into ratings by pointing to a picture corresponding to how much distress they are experiencing. A potential problem with this approach is that young children may lack the verbal ability to understand and respond to the task.

Medical practitioners (usually nurses) and parents are also asked to rate the child's pain on a similar scale. There are a number of observational procedures designed to measure the child's distress-related behaviors during specific procedures. Typically, independent raters record the incidence and duration of the child's distress and coping-related behaviors in specific situations. Observations are generally divided into three procedural phases (anticipatory, insertion of the needle, completion/recovery) as children may display significantly different behaviors across these three periods. For some children, for example, the anticipation phase may be the most difficult. Others may cope well initially but have difficulty complying to practitioner demands during the procedure itself. New observation strategies also enable recording of triadic (among child, parent, medical practitioner) behavior—acknowledging the interactive and reciprocal nature of behavior among all individuals in the setting (Dahlquist et al., 1995).

There is no standard way to combine information obtained from these various sources to derive a global measure of distress. Therefore, clinicians typically obtain information from these multiple sources and use their clinical experience to make interpretations on which to base their interventions.

Academic and Neuropsychological Impact

Research on the negative late effects of cancer suggests that children may be vulnerable to a range of deficits with the potential for interfering with learning. There are currently no established standards for the timing or content of cognitive and academic assessment for children with cancer. Children at high risk for late neurological effects related to the nature of their cancer or to its treatment may be routinely evaluated in the oncology center at regularly scheduled intervals. Testing may be part of their treatment protocol or may be advised for clinical purposes. Mulhern (1994) recommends that the timing and scope of the assessments be guided by current knowledge of the amount of risk associated with the child's history. For example, a child treated as an infant for a brain tumor should be evaluated every 6 months for several years and then yearly. A survivor of leukemia who did not receive cranial irradiation is at lower risk and could be evaluated at the end of treatment and 3 to 5 years later (Mulhern, 1994).

No tools or approaches have been developed specifically to evaluate cognitive abilities and academic achievement in children with cancer. Because of the potential for subtle deficits, however, the most useful evaluations include broadband instruments to evaluate a range of abilities and more specific tests to assess the presence of subtle difficulties that may impede learning. Butler and Copeland (1993) pointed out that selection of assessment tools should be guided by a logical and coherent rationale. Choice of specific measures is based on information about the child's disease (such as extent or site of the tumor) and the empirical findings about resultant difficulties related to the disease and its treatment. With research supporting an elevated incidence of a range of problems, assessments usually include evaluation of information processing abilities, memory, attention, math skills, ability to plan and learn new material, and perceptual-motor coordination (Butler & Copeland, 1993). The timing of the evaluation, particularly during baseline assessment, should be arranged to avoid the introduction of measurement error related to transient treatment-related side effects. Findings are conveyed to school personnel in the child's school district to ensure that the child is receiving appropriate services and that evaluations and interventions are well coordinated.

TREATMENT

Global Strategy

The psychological demands of cancer treatment are well appreciated by practitioners in pediatric oncology settings although the extent to which these settings provide formal mechanisms to enhance adjustment and prevent future problems differs widely. Interestingly, most centers do not have well-delineated psychosocial programs. Psychological interventions are most likely to be targeted to specific problems when they arise rather than provided for prevention. Only 26% of pediatric oncology programs routinely offer psychological consultation (Kaufman, Harbeck, Olson, & Nitschke, 1992). There has clearly been more research on delineating stressors and their impact than on developing validated methods of prevention and treatment. The exceptions to this are in the area of pain control, where there has been considerable work.

Psychological Adjustment to Cancer-Related Stressors

Kupst et al. (1983) described one of the earliest and most clearly delineated psychosocial interventions designed to facilitate adjustment for families with cancer across the many phases of treatment. Newly diagnosed children with leukemia and their families were assigned randomly to receive one of three levels of intervention: total, moderate, and no-project intervention (control group). For families in the total and moderate intervention conditions, assistance was provided at well-designated periods during the child's course of treatment. Early intervention focused on helping families understand the medical aspects of the disease and its treatment and assisting families develop support systems. Team members also functioned as liaisons between parents and medical staff and were available to discuss any difficulties that arose. Families provided with total intervention were seen during every clinic visit whereas those in the moderate intervention group were seen less often. The control group was provided with the level of care they would normally have received had they not participated in the study.

Families appeared to cope well regardless of the group to which they were assigned. Mothers who received the total or moderate intervention were rated by physicians as coping better than those in the control group at 6 months following diagnosis. However, differences were not apparent 6 months later (Kupst et al., 1983). In fact, only 6 of 64 families were characterized by low levels of coping. Children returned to school quickly, and discipline reverted back to normal within the family. Ten years following treatment, the families continued to fare well. Mothers' coping abilities and overall adequacy of adjustment were the strongest predictors of the child's coping and adjustment (Kupst et al., 1995).

Social opportunities and peer relations constitute another important influence on adjustment. A major goal is to help children return to their usual activities and lifestyle as quickly as possible; particularly to school which serves as the child's major opportunity for social interaction. Cancer and its treatment present numerous obstacles to school reintegration and some families thus opt for homebound instructions. Children may be absent for an extended period immediately following diagnosis and intermittently during treatment. Inconsistent attendance may challenge the school system particularly in districts that strictly adhere to an attendance-based criterion for passing. Children may experience anxiety about how peers will respond to treatment-related changes in appearance. School systems may be reluctant to have the child in the classroom and may actually encourage homebound instruction. Homebound instruction may be helpful if school attendance is impossible but it is typically overused and can impede school reentry.

Interventions designed to facilitate school reentry can be an effective strategy to assist children, parents, school personnel and peers cope with the multiple challenges associated with return to school. Katz and colleagues (Katz, Rubenstein, Hubert, & Blew, 1988; Katz, Varni, Rubenstein, Blew, & Hubert, 1992; Varni et al., 1993) developed a multicomponent treatment package that has been validated and has served as a model school reintegration program. The program includes several different strategies including: (1) *prevention education* geared toward establishing a collaboration among school personnel; (2) *a hospital-based liaison* to enhance communication between the medical professionals and the school personnel; (3) *preparation* of the child, parents, and school personnel to help anticipate and cope with predictable problems and potential needs of the child; (4) *conferences and presentations* designed to educate peers and school personnel about cancer and its treatment; (5) *social skills training* for the child to provide explicit training in problem-solving of cancer-related interpersonal difficulties, assertiveness training, and instruction about how to cope with verbal and physical teasing about appearance changes from peers; and (6) *follow-up* contacts with teachers, children, and parents to assess ongoing needs.

Children and parents appeared to benefit from participating in the project. Children experienced fewer behavioral and emotional difficulties, greater self-perceived social cognitive and physical competence, and higher levels of school behavior (Katz et al., 1988). Children, parents and teachers rated the program highly (Katz et al., 1992). Social skills training appears to be an important aspect of the program. Compared with children who did not receive social skills training, those who did were rated by parents as having fewer behavior problems. They also viewed themselves as more scholastically competent and felt that their classmates and teachers were more supportive. These difficulties were apparent 9 months after the intervention.

Summer camps provide another opportunity for children to develop social competence and to participate in age-appropriate recreational activities. Children with cancer may be excluded from typical camps that lack available medical support to accommodate them. In contrast, special camps designed for children with cancer enable attendance during any phase of treatment. These camps are designed to provide education and the opportunity to socialize with peers. They also encourage independence, particularly from parents who may tend to be overprotective (Spirito, Forman, Ladd, Wold, & Fitz, 1992). There have been few evaluations of the impact of the camps on adjustment, however. Smith, Aotlieb, Aururtch, & Blotcky (1987) did find that children who attended camp continued to be more involved in social and physical activities for weeks following the end of camp. This study did not use a comparison group, however. Future research may help delineate the types of experiences that are particularly effective for encouraging socialization.

Parental Adjustment

Historically, parents have been discounted as potential resources for helping their child adjust. However, there is mounting evidence that parents may be *the* critical ingredient in determining long-term outcome. Psychosocial interventions in the form of providing medical information, teaching coping skills, and recommending membership in support groups have been found to be effective ways of increasing parents' perceived social support and helping them to cope with stressors associated with taking care of a child with cancer (Kupst et al., in press; Speechley & Noh, 1992). Social support continues to be of importance long after the initial diagnosis. Kupst et al. found that 6 years postdiagnosis, the benefits of social support were still evident; however, by 10 years the effect was no longer as important.

Close cooperation is necessary between husband and wife to meet the many demands of caring for their ill child while attending to their normal family duties. Helping couples to communicate openly, develop common goals, and support each other can reduce friction between partners and lead to greater marital satisfaction while coping with these difficult circumstances. There has not been any study of the efficacy of marital or family therapy on parental adjustment of children with cancer. It may be that early identification of distressed families and timely interventions would have a positive impact on marital stability and child adjustment.

Other targets for intervention with parents include helping them deal with pragmatic issues. Parents need to have a clear understanding of their insurance coverage and hospital and doctor billing policies. The hospital social worker can make appropriate referrals to Medicaid, financial assistance, and Supplemental Security Income. Families may be referred to the Leukemia Society and the American Cancer Society for assistance and information. The Ronald McDonald House provides housing for families who live more than 50 miles from the hospital (Brown, 1989). Social work services are automatically provided in 80% of cancer centers and are either offered or available on request in another 17% of these facilities (Kaufman et al., 1992). Parents are encouraged to be active consumers of health care and to serve as advocates for their children.

Parents are taking a more active role in their child's care than ever before. In a study of parental involvement in their child's medical care, Lozowski, Chesler, and Chesney (1993) reported a high level of parental intervention. Over half of the parents surveyed reported that they had intervened to prevent or correct a medical mistake. Parents with high levels of income and education and who were active in local self-help groups were more likely to intervene.

Sibling Adjustment

The number of siblings of childhood cancer patients is far greater than the number of children with cancer, yet there has been far less attention paid to them. There has been little research on psychosocial programs for siblings and even descriptive papers are scarce. In one of the few available papers, Adams-Greenly et al. (1986) described a workshop conducted by an interdisciplinary team for siblings at Memorial Sloan-Kettering Cancer Center in New York. Their program included: (1) *education* about cancer and its treatment, (2) *social support* geared toward validating the children's feelings, and (3) *recreation time* during which children were encouraged to get to know each other. Social workers also meet with parents to discuss the themes of the workshop and show them a videotape. Evaluation of the program is purely descriptive. Nearly all of the 124 children who completed the program rated it highly.

Summer camps are another vehicle for helping siblings adjust to cancer-related stressors. Like those designed for children with cancer, these camps are designed to provide peer support, education, and a fun environment away from the family crisis. Some camps include the child with cancer and siblings whereas others are exclusively for siblings.

There is a need for increased attention to the well-being of siblings, particularly during the most intense phases of cancer treatment. Siblings should be provided with age-appropriate information regarding the ill sibling's condition and they should be encouraged to discuss their feelings openly. Healthy siblings may also benefit from the type of social skills programs sometimes offered to children with cancer with the goal of helping them deal with questions from their peers. Given the importance of perceived social support discussed earlier, it is surprising that little research has addressed this construct with this population. Evans et al. (1992) found that approximately one-third of their sample of siblings reported that they had no one to talk to about their fears and concerns. Support groups for healthy siblings are rarely offered in oncology centers (Kaufman et al., 1992). It seems reasonable to expect that increased social support would be beneficial for these children as well.

Procedure-Related Distress

There has been much discussion about the relative merits of pharmacological and cognitive-behavioral interventions for children during brief painful medical procedures (Ellis & Spanos, 1994). Until recently many children were restrained without any intervention during invasive procedures for which adults were routinely premedicated (Friedman et al., 1991; Hockenberry & Bologna-Vaughn, 1985). Historically, arguments against using premedication included increased risk associated with sedation, difficulty titrating dosage in children, and the probability that it would increase "downtime" during which children cannot participate in age-appropriate activities. The current recommendations are that children receive the optimal combination of behavioral and pharmacological interventions (Jay, Elliott, Woody, & Siegel, 1991).

The most commonly employed interventions designed to alleviate distress in children are multicomponent treatments that include combinations of preparatory information, attentional distraction, hypnosis, relaxation training and related strategies, preparatory information and modeling, and reinforcement for cooperation and completing the procedure. Parents and practitioners may also be trained as coaches to help children implement the strategies they have learned while undergoing the procedures (Blount, Powers, Cotter, Swan, & Free, 1994). The most well-controlled studies have been those examining the efficacy of cognitive-behavioral treatments for distress reduction during BMAs and LPs and venipuncture (Ellis & Spanos, 1994). Emphasis has shifted from establishing that these approaches reduce distress to delineating the specific mechanisms underlying their efficacy.

Most of the validated interventions designed to reduce distress are based on principles of social, operant, and classical learning theory. Children are given preparatory information, exposure to films modeling children undergoing similar procedures, and opportunities to rehearse the desired behavior. These approaches are predicated on the principle that children can learn coping strategies by observing others and that practicing the desired responses increases self-efficacy about abilities to successfully cope during the procedure. Children are also taught some form of relaxation or breathing exercises and positive self-talk, behaviors that are incompatible with fear responses. Lastly, children are rewarded for completing the procedure (Dahlquist, Gil, Armstrong, Ginsberg, & Jones, 1985; Jay, Elliott, Katz, & Siegel, 1987; Jay, Elliott, Ozolins, Olson, & Pruitt, 1985; Jay, Elliott, Woody, & Siegel, 1991).

These programs appear to be very effective. Jay and colleagues noted that some children showed a 50% reduction in behavioral distress following intervention (Jay et al., 1985, 1987). Unfortunately, the programs are expensive and time intensive, making them prohibitive for most centers. Children do not appear to be able to use the strategies independently even after intense training, necessitating the presence of a coach during each procedure. Further, children who receive training for one medical procedure do not appear to benefit during subsequent ones (Jay et al., 1987). It remains unclear what aspects of coaching are important, and which components of the treatment program are essential. However, one of the most effective aspects of the various treatment programs may be their value as distractors for the child. The coach may serve as a potent distractor during the procedures. Support for this hypothesis comes from evidence that when adults in the setting use distraction strategies, children exhibit lower levels of distress and increased coping (Manne, Bakeman, Jacobsen, Gorfinkle, Bernstein, & Redd, 1992).

Selection of appropriate interventions must be guided by the child's age and level of cognitive development. There has been very little research on interventions designed to alleviate pain in infants and very young children. Soothing stroking, rocking, massage, soothing talk, and use of pacifiers or other nonnutritive sucking may be helpful, although formal research in this area is lacking. Most interventions that have been evaluated are more suitable for preschool-aged or older children. They generally require children to attend to instructions and respond to simple commands. As

children get older, their ability to respond to requests and use coping strategies improves. Helping very young children cope with procedures can be a challenge. Recently some oncology settings have used party blowers to distract children during the procedure (Manne et al., 1994; Manne, Redd, Jacobsen, Gorfinkle, Schorr, & Rapkin, 1990). Although this represents an effort to match skill requirements of the intervention with the child's abilities, over half of the children refused to use the blower during the procedures (Manne et al., 1994) and many children are too young to use blowers.

Children treated in settings without resources to provide elaborate interventions may still benefit from some simple interventions. In a study of healthy children undergoing routine inoculations, Blount et al. (1990) found that when adults simply used directive commands (such as asking the child to "breathe"), children were more likely to use deep breathing strategies. These children also exhibited fewer distress-related behaviors during procedures.

Not all children require or even benefit from behavioral interventions. Manne, Bakeman, et al. (1992) suggested that adults should be responsive to the child's initial levels of distress. Children who are initially upset seem to benefit from directives to use coping strategies. In contrast, children who are not upset may become more distressed if given directives.

A further consideration is parental level of anxiety, which has repeatedly been shown to be related to children's level of behavioral distress. The most effective interventions for all children may be those designed to lower parental anxiety, teach parents methods to inhibit expression of their distress, and to increase their use of behaviors known to help children cope.

Academic and Neuropsychological Impact

Most of the research to date has focused on documenting deficits rather than on remediation. It is unknown, for example, whether children who experience deficits related to cancer benefit differentially from interventions compared with healthy children with similar performance levels and learning difficulties. A potentially important difference between children with congenital deficits and those with deficits secondary to cancer is their level of premorbid functioning. Children who acquire deficits are often aware of decrements in their own performance relative to previous levels. Parents and the child may be acutely aware of and frustrated by the emerging difficulties. Some may be reluctant to acknowledge deficits or approve special services for their child.

Although formal studies are lacking, many of the recent advances in understanding how to treat children with learning disabilities are probably relevant to this population. It remains to be determined whether there may be groups of children who fit a particular subtype of learning disability who may benefit from a particular approach to remediation.

The school system has a responsibility to ensure that all children receive appropriate instruction. Public Law 94-142.47,59–62 ensures the rights of all handicapped children to an appropriate free education. Parents whose children had been typical prior to the diagnosis may be unaware of this law or the range of available educational services. Even those who are aware of these rights may be reluctant to "pressure" the school system to accommodate their child. Some parents benefit from a liaison serving as their child's advocate.

Children at risk for cognitive late effects need close monitoring. Parents and school personnel should be informed about the potential for subtle and more global difficulties. Emerging cognitive and emotional difficulties can be an added source of frustration and further impair school adjustment. Timely provision of psychological and academic interventions may prevent children from developing feelings of inadequacy related to their emerging disabilities.

CASE STUDY

Children diagnosed with cancer, and particularly those with leukemia, may spend a major portion of their childhood dealing with the challenges imposed by the disease and its treatment. The following case illustrates how these demands can interfere with the usual developmental milestones and accomplishments of childhood.

Penny was first diagnosed with leukemia at age 10. She underwent 3 years of chemotherapy and had been off treatment for 2 years when she relapsed at 15. She was started on reinduction therapy and then underwent an allogeneic bone marrow transplant. Her 18-year-old brother served as bone marrow donor. Penny and her parents were referred for routine psychological screening at diagnosis and again prior to bone marrow transplant. Mr. and Mrs. Jones had been married for 24 years. They reported that they had tried for several years to conceive prior to the births of their two children. At the time of the initial diagnosis both parents were successful attorneys in a small town. The family moved to a city to be closer to a major cancer center. Mrs. Jones quit her job to take Penny to treatments.

Penny was described as a sweet girl who presented no behavior problems at home or school. She was an A or B student prior to her illness and had maintained good grades since diagnosis. However, her school attendance had been variable as a result of side effects of treatment. She had been on homebound instruction the first year of her illness and again since her relapse. She was anticipating another year of homebound schooling at the completion of the bone marrow transplant.

Penny's parents denied any psychological difficulties personally or in the family. In fact, Penny's mother reported an almost unbelievably low level of state anxiety on the State-Trait Anxiety Inventory (T score of 37) and accompanied her test answer sheet with a note stating that they were a "good Christian family that had no problems." In contrast, Mr. Jones reported high levels of anxiety and depression. Both parents reported significant martial dissatisfaction on the Dyadic Adjustment Scale (DAS), scoring well below the 100 point cutoff for marital distress mentioned in the literature (Mrs. Jones's total DAS score was 82 and Mr. Jones's 52). At the time of evaluation, both parents appeared very unhappy in their marriage and very concerned about their daughter's illness. However, their ability to communicate their feelings and support each other was extremely impaired.

Penny also denied any emotional distress. Her State-Trait Anxiety Inventory T scores ranged from 33 to 41 and she denied any symptoms of depression. She remained cheerful in most settings and said she had no worries about her transplant. She did not volunteer any concerns about her own mortality.

Because Mrs. Jones was so guarded, the initial role played by psychology involved support and assistance communicating with the medical staff. During her prolonged hospital stay, it quickly became apparent that Mrs. Jones was extremely worried about her daughter but dealt with her concerns by attempting to control all aspects of her medical care to ensure that no mistakes were made. This resulted in many conflicts with staff. As Penny's condition worsened as a result of side effects, Mrs. Jones began to lose sleep and became increasingly irritable. She often swore at staff and lashed out abusively. At one point none of the nurses wanted to care for Penny.

Through the process of helping Mrs. Jones communicate more effectively with staff, it was possible to establish a moderate level of trust in the therapeutic relationship. She began to discuss her feelings of anger at the injustice of her daughter's illness, anger at her husband for their bad marriage, anger at her son who was acting up while they were going through the stress of Penny's treatment, and anger at parents of healthy children in general. However, she remained quite guarded and usually retreated into a superficial cheerfulness after a session of self-disclosure.

Penny remained pleasant and friendly in general throughout the hospitalization for her bone marrow transplant. However, she appeared to regress in her style of coping with pain and discomfort. She became increasingly tearful and dependent on her mother to do things for her when she was not feeling well. She she was feeling the worst, she refused to speak with the medical staff for herself. Her mother talked for her and handled all communication with the staff. Penny said she did not want to talk about her progress or her prognosis and did not want to be present during any meetings with the medical staff.

After successful engraftment, Penny was discharged with precautions to maintain social isolation for the first few months until her ability to fight infection was totally recovered. Approximately 4 months after discharge her mother called and requested an outpatient appointment to help Penny get back to school. In her mother's opinion, Penny was self-conscious about her hair and was embarrassed to return to school.

An interview with Penny revealed much more pervasive anxiety than mere cosmetic concerns. She acknowledged being self-conscious about her hair and fears that peers would tease her. However, she had a long blond wig valued at several hundred dollars that was stylishly cut and indistinguishable from real hair. Thus, her fears of obviously standing out from peers appeared exaggerated. Penny acknowledged feeling afraid to be with other teens her age in a variety of social situations as well as in school, citing primarily her fears that others would stare at her. She had no peer contact over the past 2 years and thus had no opportunities for these fears to extinguish.

Over time, Penny had grown increasingly dependent on her mother to handle things for her (at a time when she would normally have been developing greater autonomy and confidence in her ability to manage for herself). She had been living in the same room with her mother in the hospital for over 6 months. Her mother had handled nearly every detail of her care, many of which Penny would not have been able to handle herself. The social isolation at discharge served to further this somewhat developmentally inappropriately close contact with her mother at home. As a result, her confidence waned and her fears seemed to generalize. She now felt too afraid to walk anywhere in the hospital by herself or to drive the car to the corner market (she had a learner's permit). At the time of evaluation, she was even unable to ride the elevator to the very familiar oncology clinic without her mother.

Many of Penny's concerns appeared initially to be developmentally appropriate worries that would have extinguished under normal conditions had she simply faced her peers and allowed the natural consequences to follow. However, her illness created an artificial situation in which most opportunities to face her fears or gain confidence were avoided, thus negatively reinforcing her fear/avoidance behaviors. The forced isolation allowed this situation to generalize extensively.

Penny expressed a strong desire to begin driving again and to visit her friends from school. She recognized that she relied on her mother too much and was embarrassed that she could not go anywhere without her. As she appeared ready to change, she was offered short-term anxiety management treatment. An individualized hierarchy of anxiety-provoking situations was constructed. Penny was taught two competing responses to use in these situations: progressive muscle relaxation and cognitive reframing. She then participated in an in vivo desensitization program. For example, her initial item on her hierarchy was riding the elevator with an adult other than her mother. We gradually worked up to more difficult hierarchy items such as riding the elevator in the clinic building alone. These behaviors were developmentally appropriate for most children her age. Penny made excellent progress, and in about 2 months was able to drive to the local fast-food market alone (during daylight hours), and walk down a crowded street and past groups of people.

Penny's experiences illustrate how the medical treatment of cancer can interfere with the normal developmental process. Classically conditioned fears, maintained by operant contingencies, are both common and understandable. They can also be successfully treated. Penny's family difficulties, however, were more longstanding and resistant to change. Her mother never remained forthright enough in therapy on a regular basis

to make any progress in dealing with her own grief and anger. Neither parent wanted marital or family therapy. By separating Penny from her mother in the individual therapy session, it was possible to provide her some initial success experiences with autonomy in a very nonthreatening atmosphere. The extinction of many of her fears followed relatively rapidly.

SUMMARY

Children with cancer and their families are faced with multiple challenges. Most cope extraordinarily well despite the rigors of treatment, disruption of normal routines, resulting disabilities, cosmetic impairments, and uncertainty about the future. The medical and psychological advances seen in the past few decades are largely attributable to bold efforts by practitioners and researchers to collaborate closely and to strive for medical cures and positive psychosocial outcomes. The overall approach embraced by pediatric oncology has served as a template for other disciplines faced with similar issues.

As we approach the new millennium the focus of pediatric health care is apt to change considerably. Childhood cancer was once a somewhat esoteric disorder, garnering considerable resources relative to the number of children afflicted. Today this distinction has been replaced by HIV where medical technology has been less successful. Most major oncology settings are now focusing on developing new strategies to deal with the growing number of children afflicted with AIDS. The collaborative multidisciplinary efforts of the major study groups (POG and CCG) have demonstrated how cooperation rather than competition across institutions can speed the search for cures. Hopefully this will serve as a model in the search for solutions to the AIDS epidemic.

Psychology and pediatric oncology have worked together to ensure the best possible outcome for children under treatment and their families. This union has been so successful, in fact, that Bearison and Mulhern (1994) coined the term pediatric psychooncology to connote the psychological perspective of pediatric oncology. One limitation of this union has been the predominance of research focused on medically relevant questions rather than on psychological questions. As childhood cancer becomes more similar to other chronic childhood diseases, its commonalities may encourage more theoretically driven research on more general questions of vulnerability and resiliency in childhood.

ACKNOWLEDGMENT

Preparation of this chapter was supported in part by a grant from the Prospect Group awarded to the first author. We greatly appreciate their generosity and support.

REFERENCES

Achenbach, T. M. (1991). *Manual for the Revised Child Behavior Checklist.* Burlington: University of Vermont, Department of Psychiatry.

Adams-Greenly, M., Shiminski-Maher, T., McGowan, N., & Meyers, P. A. (1986). A group program for helping siblings of children with cancer. *Journal of Psychosocial Oncology, 4,* 55–67.

Aitken, T. J., & Hathaway, G. (1993). Long distance related stressors and coping behaviors in parents of children with cancer. *Journal of Pediatric Oncology Nursing, 10,* 3–12.

Anderson, B. L. (1992). Psychological interventions for cancer patients to enhance the quality of life. *Journal of Consulting and Clinical Psychology, 60,* 552–568.

Armstrong, F. D. (1992). Psychosocial intervention in pediatric cancer: A strategy for prevention of long-term problems. In T. M. Field, P. M. McCabe, & N. Schneiderman (Eds.), *Stress and coping in infancy and childhood* (pp. 197–218). Hillsdale, NJ: Erlbaum.

Barbarin, O. A. (1987). Psychosocial risks and invulnerability: A review of the theoretical and empirical bases of preventive family-focused services for survivors of childhood cancer. *Journal of Psychosocial Oncology, 5,* 25–41.

Barbarin, O. A., & Chesler, M. (1986). The medical context of parental coping with childhood cancer. *American Journal of Community Psychology, 14,* 221–235.

Barnhart, L. L., Fitzpatrick, V. D., Sidell, N. L., Adams, M. J., Shields, G. S., & Gomez, S. J. (1994). Perception of family need in pediatric oncology. *Child and Adolescent Social Work Journal, 11,* 137–148.

Barrera, M. (1986). Distinctions between social support concepts, measures, and models. *American Journal of Community Psychology, 14,* 413–445.

Baum, B. J., & Baum, E. S. (1989). Psychosocial challenges of childhood cancer. *Journal of Psychosocial Oncology, 7,* 119–129.

Bearison, D. J., & Mulhern, R. M. (Eds.). (1994). *Pediatric psychooncology: Psychological perspectives on children with cancer.* London: Oxford University Press.Benner, A. E., & Marlow, L. S. (1991). The effect of a workshop on childhood cancer on students' knowledge, concerns, and desire to interact with a classmate with cancer. *Children's Health Care, 20,* 101–107.

Blount, R. L., Powers, S. W., Cotter, M. W., Swan, S., et al. (1994). Making the system work: Training pediatric oncology patients to cope and their parents to coach them during BMA/LP procedures. *Behavior Modification, 18,* 6–31.

Blount, R. L., Sturges, J. W., & Powers, S. W. (1990). Analysis of child and adult behavioral variations by phase of medical procedure. *Behavior Therapy, 21,* 33–48.

Boman, K. (1992). Influence of factors related to illness, treatment, and demographic background on psychological coping in childhood cancer survivors. *Reports from the Department of Psychology, University of Stockholm, 757,* 1–12.

Bradlyn, A. S., Harris, C. V., Warner, J. E., Ritchey, A. K., Zaboy, K. (1993). An investigation of the validity of the quality of well-being scale with pediatric oncology patients. *Health Psychology, 12,* 246–250.

Brown, P. G. (1989). Families who have a child diagnosed with cancer: What the medical caregiver can do to help them and themselves. *Issues in Comprehensive Pediatric Nursing, 12,* 247–260.

Buckley, J. (1993). Infrastructure for pediatric intervention trials. *Cancer, 71,* 3241–3243.

Bull, B. A., & Drotar, D. (1991). Coping with cancer in remission: Stressors and strategies reported by children and adolescents. *Journal of Pediatric Psychology, 16,* 767–782.

Butler, R. W., & Copeland, D. R. (1993). Neuropsychological effects of central nervous system prophylactic treatment in childhood leukemia: Methodological considerations. *Journal of Pediatric Psychology, 18,* 319–338.

Carpenter, P. J., & LeVant, C. S. (1994). Sibling adaptation to the family crisis of childhood cancer. In D. J. Bearison & R. K. Mulhern (Eds.), *Pediatric psychooncology: Psychological perspectives on children with cancer* (pp. 122–142). London: Oxford University Press.

Carpentieri, S. C., Mulhern, R. K., Douglas, S., Hanna, S., & Fairclough, D. L. (1993). Behavioral resiliency among children surviving brain tumors: A longitudinal study. *Journal of Clinical Child Psychology, 22,* 236–246.

Chesler, M. A. (1993). Introduction to psychosocial issues. *Cancer, 71,* 3245–3250.

Chesler, M. A., Allswede, J., & Barbarin, O. A. (1991). Voices from the margin of the family: Siblings of children with cancer. *Journal of Psychosocial Oncology, 9,* 19–41.

Chesler, M. A., Heiney, S. P., Perrin, R., Monaco, G. P., Kupst, M. J., Cincotta, N. F., Katz, E. R., Deasy-Spinetta, P. D., Whittam, E. H., & Foley, G. V. (1993). Principles of psychosocial programming for children and cancer. *Cancer, 71,* 3210–3212.

Cincotta, N. (1993). Psychosocial issues in the world of children with cancer. *Cancer, 71,* 3251–3260.

Claflin, C. J., & Barbarin, O. A. (1991). Does "telling" less protect more? Relationships among age, information disclosure, and what children with cancer see and feel. *Journal of Pediatric Psychology, 16,* 169–191.

Copeland, D. R. (1992). Neuropsychological and psychosocial effects of childhood leukemia and its treatment. *CA-A Cancer Journal for Clinicians, 42,* 283–295.

Cousens, P., Ungerer, J. A., Crawford, J. A., & Stevens, M. M. (1991). Cognitive effects of childhood leukemia therapy: A case for four specific deficits. *Journal of Pediatric Psychology, 16,* 475–488.

Cousens, P., Waters, B., Said, J., & Stevens, M. (1988). Cognitive effects of cranial irradiation in leukemia: A survey and meta-analysis. *Journal of Child Psychology and Psychiatry, 29,* 839–852.

Dahlquist, L. M., Czyzewski, D. I., Copeland, K. G., Jones, C. L., Taub, E., & Vaughan, J. K. (1993). Parents of children newly diagnosed with cancer: Anxiety, coping, and marital distress. *Journal of Pediatric Psychology, 18,* 365–376.

Dahlquist, L., Pendley, J., Power, T., Landthrip, D., & Jones, C. (1994). Manual for the Pediatric Medical Interaction Scale (PMIS). Unpublished manuscript, Baylor College of Medicine.

Dahlquist, L., Pendley, J., Power, T., Landthrip, D., Jones, C., & Steuber, P. (1995). Adult command structure and child distress during invasive medical procedures. Unpublished manuscript, Baylor College of Medicine.

Dahlquist, L., Power, T., & Carlson, L. (1995). Physician and parent behavior during invasive cancer procedures: Relationships to child behavioral distress. *Journal of Pediatric Psychology, 20,* 477–490.

Dahlquist, L., Power, T. G., Cox, C. N., & Fernbach, D. J. (1994). Parenting and child distress during cancer procedures: A multidimensional assessment. *Children's Health Care, 23,* 149–166.

Davies, W. H., Noll, R. B., DeStefano, L., Bukowski, W. M., & Kulkarni, R. (1991). Differences in the child-rearing practices of parents of children with cancer and controls: The perspectives of parents and professionals. *Journal of Pediatric Psychology, 16,* 295–306.

Dolgin, M. J., & Jay, S. M. (1989). Childhood cancer. In T. H. Ollendick & M. Hersen (Eds.), *Handbook of child psychopathology* (2nd ed., pp. 327–340). New York: Plenum Press.

Eiser, C. (1994). Making sense of chronic disease: The Eleventh Jack Tizard Memorial Lecture. *Journal of Child Psychology and Psychiatry, 35,* 1373–1389.

Ellis, J. A., & Spanos, N. P. (1994). Cognitive-behavioral interventions for children's distress during bone marrow aspirations and lumbar punctures: A critical review. *Journal of Pain and Symptom Management, 9,* 96–108.

Evans, C. A., Stevens, M., Cushway, D., & Houghton, J. (1992). Sibling response to childhood cancer: A new approach. *Child: Care, Health and Development, 18,* 229–244.

Friedman, A. G., Mulhern, R. K., Fairclough, D., Ward, P., Baker, D., Mirro, J., & Rivera, G. K. (1991). Midazolam premedication for pediatric bone marrow aspiration and lumbar puncture. *Medical and Pediatric Oncology, 19,* 499–504.

Fritz, G. K., Williams, J. R., & Amylon, M. (1988). After treatment ends: Psychosocial sequelae in pediatric cancer survivors. *American Journal of Orthopsychiatry, 58,* 552–561.

Gonzales, J., Routh, D., Saab, P., Armstrong, D., Shifman, L., Guerra, E., & Fawcett, N. (1989). Effects of parent presence on children's reactions to injections: Behavioral, physiological, and subjective aspects. *Journal of Pediatric Psychology, 14,* 449–462.

Greenberg, H. S., Kazak, A. E., & Meadows, A. T. (1989). Psychologic functioning in 8-to 16-year old cancer survivors and their parents. *The Journal of Pediatrics, 114,* 488–493.

Gross, A. M., Stern, R. M., Levin, R. B., Dale, J., & Wojnilower, D. A. (1983). The effect of mother–child separation on the behavior of children experiencing a diagnostic medical procedure. *Journal of Consulting and Clinical Psychology, 51,* 783–785.

Hammond, G. D., Haase, G. M., Krawiec, V., Bleyer, W. A., Severson, R. K., Bernstein, L., Krisher, J. P., Smith, M. A., Brady, A. M., & Menck, H. (1993). Patterns of care. *Cancer, 71,* 3202–3205.

Hays, D. M. (1993). Adult survivors of childhood cancer: Employment and insurance issues in different age groups. *Cancer, 71,* 3306–3309.

Hockenberry, M. J., & Bologna-Vaughan, S. B. (1985). Preparation for intrusive procedures using noninvasive techniques in children with cancer: State of the art vs. new trends. *Cancer Nursing, 8,* 97–102.

Horowitz, W. A., & Kazak, A. E. (1990). Family adaptation to childhood cancer: Sibling and family systems variables. *Journal of Clinical Child Psychology, 19,* 221–228.

Jacobsen, P., Manne, S., Gorfinkle, K., Schorr, O., Rapkin, B., & Redd, W. (1990). Analysis of child and parent behavior during painful medical procedures. *Health Psychology, 9,* 559–576.

Jay, S. M., Elliott, C. H., Katz, E., & Siegel, S. E. (1987). Cognitive-behavioral and pharmacologic interventions for children's distress during painful medical procedures. *Journal of Consulting and Clinical Psychology, 55,* 860–865.

Jay, S. M., Elliott, C. H., Ozolins, M., Olson, R., & Pruitt, S. (1985). Behavioral management of children's distress during painful medical procedures. *Behaviour Research and Therapy, 23,* 513–520.

Jay, S. M., Elliott, C. H., Woody, P. D., & Siegel, S. (1991). An investigation of cognitive-behavior therapy combined with oral valium for children undergoing painful medical procedures. *Health Psychology, 10,* 317–322.

Jenney, M. E. M., Kane, R. L., & Lurie, N. (1995). Developing a measure of health outcomes in survivors of childhood cancer: A review of the issues. *Medical and Pediatric Outcome, 24,* 145–153.

Katz, E. R., Kellerman, J., & Siegel, S. E. (1980). Behavioral distress in children undergoing medical procedures: Developmental considerations. *Journal of Consulting and Clinical Psychology, 48,* 356–365.

Katz, E. R., Rubinstein, C. L., Hubert, W. C., & Blew, A. (1988). School and social reintegration of children with cancer. *Journal of Psychosocial Oncology, 6,* 123–140.

Katz, E. R., Varni, J. W., Rubenstein, C. L., Blew, A., & Hubert, N. (1992). Teacher, parent, and child evaluative ratings of a school reintegration intervention for children with newly diagnosed cancer. *Children's Health Care, 21,* 69–75.

Kaufman, K. L., Harbeck, C., Olson, R., & Nitschke, R. (1992). The availability of psychosocial interventions to children with cancer and their families. *Children's Health Care, 21,* 21–25.

Kazak, A. E. (1993). Editorial: Psychological research in pediatric psychology. *Journal of Pediatric Psychology, 18,* 313–318.

Kazak, A. E., & Meadows, A. T. (1989). Families of young adolescents who have survived cancer: Social-emotional adjustment, adaptability, and social support. *Journal of Pediatric Psychology, 14,* 175–191.

Kazak, A. E., & Nachman, G. S. (1991). Family research on childhood chronic illness: Pediatric oncology as an example. *Journal of Family Psychology, 4,* 462–483.

Kupst, M. J. (1993). Family coping supportive and obstructive factors. *Cancer, 71,* 3337–3341.

Kupst, M. J., Natta, M. B., Richardson, C. C., Schulman, J. L., Lavigne, J. V., & Das, L. (1995). Family coping with pediatric leukemia: Ten years after treatment. *Journal of Pediatric Psychology, 20,* 601–617.

Kupst, M. J., & Schulman, J. L. (1988). Long-term coping with pediatric leukemia: A six-year follow-up study. *Journal of Pediatric Psychology, 13,* 7–22.

Kupst, M. J., Schulman, J. L., Maurer, H., Honig, G., Morgan, E., & Fochtman, D. (1983). Family coping with leukemia: The first six months. *Medical Pediatric Oncology, 11,* 269–278.

Kupst, M. J., Schulman, J. L., Maurer, H., Honig, G., Morgan, E., & Fochtman, D. (1984). Coping with pediatric leukemia: A two-year follow-up. *Journal of Pediatric Psychology, 9,* 149–163.

Kupst, M. J., Schulman, J. L., Maurer, H., Morgan, E., Honig, G., & Fochtman, D. (1983). Psychosocial aspects of pediatric leukemia: From diagnosis through the first six months of treatment. *Medical and Pediatric Oncology, 11,* 269–278.

Lampkin, B. C. (1993). Introduction and executive summary. *Cancer, 71,* 3199–3201.

Lansky, S. B., List, M. A., & Ritter-Sterr, C. (1989). Psychiatric and psychological support of the child and adolescent with cancer. In P. A. Pizzo & D. G. Poplack (Eds.), *Principles and practice of pediatric oncology* (pp. 885–897). Philadelphia: Lippincott.

Lauer, M. E., Mulhern, R. K., Wallskog, J. M., & Camitta, B. M. (1983). A comparison study of parental adaptation following a child's death at home or in the hospital. *Pediatrics, 1,* 107–112.

Lozowski, S., Chesler, M. A., & Chesney, B. K. (1993). Parental intervention in the medical care of children with cancer. *Journal of Psychosocial Oncology, 11,* 63–88.

Madam-Swain, A., Sexson, S. B., Brown, R. T., & Ragab, A. (1993). Family adaptation and coping among siblings of cancer patients, their brothers and sisters, and nonclinical controls. *The American Journal of Family Therapy, 21,* 60–70.

Manne, S. L., Bakeman, R., Jacobsen, P. B., Gorfinkle, K., Bernstein, D., & Redd, W. H. (1992). Adult–child interaction during invasive medical procedures. *Health Psychology, 11,* 241–249.

Manne, S. L., Bakeman, R., Jacobsen, P. B., Gorfinkle, K., & Redd, W. H. (1994). An analysis of a behavioral intervention for children undergoing venipuncture. *Health Psychology, 13,* 556–566.

Manne, S. L., Bakeman, R., Jacobsen, P., & Redd, W. H. (1993). Children's coping during invasive medical procedures. *Behavior Therapy, 24,* 143–158.

Manne, S. L., Jacobsen, P. B., & Redd, W. H. (1992). Assessment of acute pediatric pain: Do child self-report, parent ratings, and nurse ratings measure the same phenomenon? *Pain, 48,* 45–52.

Manne, S. L., Redd, W. H., Jacobsen, P. B., Gorfinkle, K., et al. (1990). Behavioral intervention to reduce child and parent distress during venipuncture. *Journal of Consulting and Clinical Psychology, 58,* 565–572.

Martinson, I. M., & Papadatou, D. (1994). Care of the dying child and the bereaved. In D. J. Bearison & R. K. Mulhern (Eds.), *Pediatric psychooncology: Psychological perspectives on children with cancer* (pp. 193–221). London: Oxford University Press.

Meadows, A. T., Black, B., Nesbit, M. E., Strong, L. C., Nicholson, H. S., Green, D. M., Hays, D. M., & Lozowski, S. L. (1993). Long-term survival: Clinical care, research, and education. *Cancer, 71,* 3213–3215.

Mulhern, R. K. (1994). Neuropsychological late effects. In D. J. Bearison & R. K. Mulhern (Eds.), *Pediatric psychooncology: Psychological perspectives on children with cancer* (pp. 99–121). London: Oxford University Press.

Mulhern, R. K., Fairclough, D., Friedman, A. G., & Leigh, (1990). Play performance scale as an index of quality of life in children with cancer. *Psychological Assessment: A Journal of JCCP, 2,* 149–155.

Mulhern, R. K., Fairclough, D. L., Smith, B., & Douglas, S. M. (1992). Maternal depression, assessment methods, and physical symptoms affect estimates of depressive symptomatology among children with cancer. *Journal of Pediatric Psychology, 17,* 313–326.

Mulhern, R. K., Lauer, M. E., & Hoffmann, R. G. (1983). Death of a child at home or in the hospital: Subsequent psychological adjustment of the family. *Pediatrics, 71,* 743–747.

Mulhern, R. K., Ochs, J., & Fairclough, D. (1992). Deterioration of intellect among children surviving leukemia: IQ test changes modify estimates of treatment toxicity. *Journal of Consulting and Clinical Psychology, 60,* 477–480.

Mulhern, R. K., Ochs, J., Fairclough, D., Wasserman, A., Davis, K., & Williams, J. M. (1987). Intellectual and academic achievement status after CNS relapse: A retrospective analysis of 40 children treated for ALL. *Journal of Clinical Oncology, 5,* 933–940.

Mulhern, R. K., Wasserman, A. L., Friedman, A. G., & Fair-clough, D. (1989). Social competence and behavioral adjustment of children who are long-term survivors of cancer. *Pediatrics, 83,* 18–25.

Mulvihill, J. J. (1989). Clinical genetics of pediatric cancer. In P. A. Pizzo & D. G. Poplack (Eds.), *Principles and practices of pediatric oncology* (pp. 19–38). Philadelphia: Lippincott.

Neglia, J. P., & Nesbit, M. E. (1993). Care and treatment of long-term survivors of childhood cancer. *Cancer, 71,* 3386–3391.

Nesbit, M. D. (1989). Clinical assessment and differential diagnosis of the child with suspected cancer. In P. A. Pizzo & D. G. Poplack (Eds.), *Principles and practice of pediatric oncology* (pp. 83–92). Philadelphia: Lippincott.

Noll, R. B., Bukowski, W. M., Davies, W. H., Koontz, K., & Kulkarni, R. (1993). Adjustment in the peer system of adolescents with cancer: A two-year study. *Journal of Pediatric Psychology, 18,* 351–364.

Overholser, J. C., & Fritz, G. K. (1990). The impact of childhood cancer on the family. *Journal of Psychosocial Oncology, 8,* 71–85.

Packer, R. J., Sutton, L. N., Atkins, T. E., Radcliffe, J., Bunnin, G. R., D'Angio, G., Siegel, K. R., & Schut, L. (1989). A prospective study of cognitive function in children receiving whole brain radiotherapy and chemotherapy: Two year results. *Journal of Neurosurgery, 70,* 707–713.

Perrin, E. C., Stein, R. E. K., & Drotar, D. (1991). Cautions in using the child behavior checklist: Observations based on research about children with a chronic illness. *Journal of Pediatric Psychology, 16,* 411–421.

Ramsay, N. K. (1989). Bone marrow transplantation in pediatric oncology. In P. A. Pizzo & D. G. Poplack (Eds.), *Principles and practice of pediatric oncology* (pp. 971–990). Philadelphia: Lippincott.

Rape, R. N., & Bush, J. P. (1994). Psychological preparation for pediatric oncology patients undergoing painful procedures: A methodological critique of the research. *Children's Health Care, 23,* 51–67.

Raymond, C. A. (1988). Fate of childhood cancer survivors comes under scrutiny. *Journal of the American Medical Association, 260,* 3246–3247.

Roberts, M. C. (Ed.). (1995). *Handbook of pediatric psychology* (2nd ed.). New York: Guilford Press.

Rochester, C. (1989). The child and family facing death. *Issues in Comprehensive Pediatric Nursing, 12,* 261–267.

Rolland, J. S. (1990). Anticipatory loss: A family systems developmental framework. *Family Process, 29,* 229–244.

Russo, D. C., & Varni, J. W. (1982). Behavioral pediatrics. In D. C. Russo & J. W. Varni (Eds.), *Behavioral pediatrics: Research and practice* (pp. 3–24). New York: Plenum Press.

Sahler, O. J., & Carpenter, P. J. (1988). Relationship between family functioning and sibling adaptation to the pediatric cancer experience. *Journal of Developmental and Behavioral Pediatrics, 9,* 106–107.

Sanger, M. S., Copeland, D. R., & Davidson, E. R. (1991). Psychosocial adjustment among pediatric cancer patients: A multidimensional assessment. *Journal of Pediatric Psychology, 16,* 463–474.

Sargent, J. R., Sahler, O. J. Z., Roghmann, K. J., Mulhern, R. K., Barbarin, O. A., Carpenter, P. J., Copeland, D. R., Dolgin, M. J., & Zelter, L. K. (1995). Sibling adaptation to childhood cancer collaborative study: Siblings' perceptions of the cancer experience. *Journal of Pediatric Psychology, 20,* 151–164.

Sawyer, M. G., Antoniou, G., Nguyen, A.-M. T., Rice, M., & Baghurst, P. (1995). A prospective study of the psychological adjustment of children with cancer. *American Journal of Pediatric Hematology/Oncology, 17,* 39–45.

Shaw, E. G., & Routh, D. K. (1982). Effect of mother presence on children's reaction to aversive procedures. *Journal of Pediatric Psychology, 7,* 33–42.

Slavin, L. A., O'Malley, J. E., Koocher, G. P., & Foster, D. J. (1982). Communication of the cancer diagnosis to pediatric patients: Impact on long-term adjustment. *American Journal of Psychiatry, 139,* 179–183.

Smith, K. E., Gotlieb, S., Gurwitch, R. H., & Blotchky, A. D. (1987). Impact of a summer camp on daily activity and family interactions among children with cancer. *Journal of Pediatric Psychology, 12,* 533–542.

Speechley, K. N., & Noh, S. (1992). Surviving childhood cancer, social support, and parents' psychological adjustment. *Journal of Pediatric Psychology, 17,* 15–31.

Spirito, A., Forman, E., Ladd, R., Wold, E., & Fitz, X. (1992). Remembrance programs at camps for children with cancer. *Journal of Psychosocial Oncology, 10,* 103–113.

Spirito, A., Stark, L. J., Cobiella, C., Drigan, R., Androkites, A., & Hewett, K. (1990). Social adjustment of children successfully treated for cancer. *Journal of Pediatric Psychology, 15,* 359–371.

Spirito, A., Stark, L. J., & Williams, C. (1988). Development of a brief checklist to assess coping in pediatric patients. *Journal of Pediatric Psychology, 13,* 555–574.

Stehbens, J. A., Kaleita, T. A., Noll, R. B., MacLean, W. E., O'Brien, R. T., Waskerwitz, M. J., & Hammond, D. G. (1991) CNS prophylaxis of childhood leukemia: What are the long-term neurological, neuropsychological, and behavioral effects: *Neuropsychological Review* 147–177.

Van Eys, J. (1991). The truly cured child? *Pediatrician, 18,* 90–95.

Varni, J. W., Katz, E. R., Colegrove, R., Jr., & Dolgin, M. (1993). The impact of social skills training on the adjustment of children with newly diagnosed cancer. *Journal of Pediatric Psychology, 18,* 751–767.

Varni, J. W., Katz, E. R., Colegrove, R., Jr., & Dolgin, M. (1994). Perceived social support and adjustment of children with newly diagnosed cancer. *Developmental and Behavioral Pediatrics, 15,* 20–26.

Wasserman, A. L., Thompson, E. I., Wilimas, D. L., & Fairclough, D. L. (1987). The psychological status of survivors of childhood/adolescent Hodgkins's disease. *American Journal of Diseases of Children, 141,* 626–631.

Whittam, E. H. (1993). Terminal care of the dying child. *Cancer, 71,* 3450–3462.

Wirt, R. D., Lachar, D., Klinedinst, J. K., & Seat, P. D. (1990). *Multidimensional description of child personality. A manual for the Personality Inventory for Children. 1990 edition.* Los Angeles: Western Psychological Services.

Wright, L., & Friedman, A. G. (1991). Challenge of the future: Psychologists in medical settings. In J. J. Sweet, R. H. Rozensky, & S. M. Tovian (Eds.), *Handbook of clinical psychology in medical settings* (pp. 603–614). New York: Plenum Press.

19

Pediatric AIDS

LISA ARMISTEAD, REX FOREHAND, RIC STEELE, AND BETH KOTCHICK

INTRODUCTION

Pediatric acquired immune deficiency syndrome (AIDS) currently is, and most likely will continue for some time to be, one of the biggest challenges faced by psychologists, physicians, and other health care workers. It is such a monumental challenge, at least in part, because of the vast array of difficulties that accompany the diagnosis. For instance, in all cases of vertically transmitted (i.e., transmitted from mother to child) pediatric AIDS (the most common mode of transmission), the child's mother is infected with the virus responsible for AIDS (human immunodeficiencyvirus [HIV]); thus, she probably will be ill or even dead before her child reaches adulthood (Lewis, Haiken, & Hoyt, 1994). Over the past several years, it has become clear that children with AIDS are at incredibly high risk for psychosocial difficulties (Jansen & Ammann, 1994). The myriad of issues that make pediatric AIDS

uniquely challenging will be addressed in this chapter, including a discussion of the course and etiology of the illness, as well as an overview of assessment, prevention, and treatment issues.

As is consistent with many of the related articles and surveillance statistics (e.g., CDC, 1994a; Taylor-Brown & Kumetat, 1994a), this chapter will discuss pediatric AIDS cases in children up to and including 12-year-olds. Many issues often differ for infected adolescents (e.g., mode of transmission), and a chapter on AIDS that encompasses the age range from birth to late adolescence could not begin to be thorough without becoming a book.

With regard to the biomedical aspects of pediatric AIDS, significant progress has been made in terms of diagnosis, prevention, and treatment of this illness since it was first described in 1982 (Jansen & Ammann, 1994). Despite progress, the incidence of HIV in children continues to increase and brings with it a myriad of physical, psychological, social, and school-related problems. Furthermore, with improved medical care, infected children are living longer than before, often into school age and adolescence. With longer life expectancies come additional psychosocial issues requiring the attention of health care professionals and society as a whole (Lewis et al., 1994).

LISA ARMISTEAD • Department of Psychology, Georgia State University, Atlanta, Georgia 30302-5010. REX FOREHAND, RIC STEELE, AND BETH KOTCHICK • Psychology Department, University of Georgia, Athens, Georgia 30602.

Handbook of Child Psychopathology, 3rd edition, edited by Ollendick & Hersen. Plenum Press, New York, 1998.

Despite the need for research to address the multitude of AIDS-related psychosocial issues, the current literature is in its infancy and research involving families affected by pediatric AIDS is very meager (Cohen, 1994). Furthermore, most of the published studies that address psychosocial issues are not data-based in nature. The few empirical psychosocial studies that have been done mostly address hemophilic children who are HIV seropositive as a result of their reliance on blood products, which were contaminated with HIV until 1985. Currently, children with hemophilia represent a tiny minority of pediatric HIV/AIDS cases (< 1%), and their psychosocial issues usually are quite different from those of the majority of children with HIV and/or AIDS (Taylor-Brown & Kumetat, 1994a). Although there is a paucity of available articles, this chapter discusses the relevant literature and attempts to expound on it by way of offering suggestions and guidelines for assessment and treatment.

To facilitate an understanding of the issues related to pediatric AIDS, the environment from which most children with AIDS hail must be addressed. Most of these children are members of ethnic minorities, are from families that are economically disadvantaged (CDC, 1993), and are more likely to reside in inner-city areas (Hoff et al., 1988). These families often find themselves rejected by a society that discriminates against their ethnic background and/or socioeconomic status (Armistead & Forehand, 1995; Herek & Glunt, 1988). As a result, these families have limited access to or use of medical and social services, and experience poor housing and inner-city violence (Mellins & Ehrhardt, 1994). Furthermore, given that most seropositive women are infected via injection drug use or via sexual contact with a man who is injecting drugs, the families from which these children originate are likely to encounter numerous drug-related difficulties (Mellins & Ehrhardt, 1994).

Another important issue that is unique to this population is that, in addition to the infected child, other family members are likely to be HIV infected (Indacochea & Scott, 1992). For instance, there may be more than one infected child in a family. Thus, parent(s) or alternative caregiver for the infected child is likely to be overtaxed in terms of caregiving responsibilities (Armistead & Forehand, 1995). Additionally, in almost all cases of pediatric AIDS, the mother and perhaps her partner also are infected with HIV. Frequently, neither parent survives to care for the infected child. Mellins and Ehrhardt (1994) found that the most stressful experience for infected children was the AIDS-related death of a sibling and/or parent. Furthermore, as a result of parental death, abandonment, or substance abuse, many ill children are forced to cope with the already overburdened foster care system (Mellins & Ehrhardt, 1994).

The stigma surrounding AIDS cannot be overlooked in terms of its relevance for the child living with AIDS. Unlike most other childhood illnesses, a substantial social stigma is associated with AIDS (Mason & Olson, 1989). For example, the media has reported several stories involving children living with AIDS who have not been allowed to attend school or families that have been "run out of town" because of the child's HIV status. Researchers (e.g., Armistead & Forehand, 1995; Mellins & Ehrhardt, 1994) also have noted the negative impact that the secrecy and ostracism of AIDS-related stigma may have on pediatric AIDS patients and their families. Clearly, many families that have a child infected with HIV are already stretched to the limit in terms of their ability to cope with their living environment, the infection of multiple family members, and the social stigma associated with AIDS. These issues and others will be addressed in the remaining sections of this chapter. In each section we will first discuss the medical issues and then address the relevant psychosocial issues.

PHENOMENOLOGY

Having briefly outlined the social environment of most children living with AIDS, we now present an overview of the typical medical course of AIDS. Following this overview, we discuss the phenomenology of the psychosocial aspects of HIV/AIDS.

HIV, once considered an acute disease, is now described as a chronic disease that involves multiple systems of the body (Indacochea & Scott, 1992). Currently, AIDS is understood as the severe end of the spectrum of the medical sequelae of HIV infection. More simply, AIDS is a fatal disorder that is caused by HIV, a virus that attacks and weakens the immune system (Jaret, 1986). Specifically, HIV infects T4 or "helper T cells," which, in a normally functioning immune system, are responsible for activating the "killer T cells" that destroy viruses entering the body. Once HIV has infected the T4 cells, it may remain "latent" for up to 8 years or it may rapidly reproduce, destroying T4 cells and resulting in clinical symptoms much earlier (Beckford & Dossett, 1992). As HIV destroys an increasing number of T4 cells, the individual's immune system becomes unable to defend against other infections, which eventually results in death (Olson, Huszti, Mason, & Seibert, 1989).

The first case of pediatric AIDS was described in 1982, before the discovery of HIV in 1983 (Ammann, 1994). It should be noted that the course of HIV, described above, is usually accelerated in pediatric cases compared with adults. Specifically, after infection with the virus, over 80% of untreated children will evidence some symptoms by 18–24 months of age, whereas the average adult will not display HIV-related symptoms until 8–10 years after infection (Pizzo et al., 1995).

Beckford and Dossett (1992) reported a number of clinical signs of pediatric HIV infection. These include, but are not limited to, failure to thrive, recurrent or intermittent fevers, lymphadenopathy (swollen lymph nodes), recurrent pulmonary disease (such as pneumonia), recurrent diarrhea, hepatitis, and skin rashes. Neurological signs (e.g., paresis, delayed neurological development) are present in up to 90% of children with HIV infection. Behavioral signs include change in gait, loss of acquired motor or

language skills, and deterioration of play (Belman, 1990). Children who are infected with HIV also suffer from recurrent or multiple bacterial and/or viral infections, which they have difficulty warding off because of their decreased immune response. In particular, *Pneumocystis carinii* pneumonia (PCP), a very serious opportunistic infection in children with AIDS, is a typical presenting illness, bringing with it a high morbidity and mortality (CDC, 1991). Clearly, HIV/AIDS extracts a substantial toll from its young victims in terms of the physical symptoms accompanying HIV infection.

The prognosis of HIV infection can vary substantially across children and across developmental levels. Studies have shown that, on average, 80% of infected children will live to at least 3 years of age with 50 to 65% living to at least 5 years of age (Blanche et al., 1994; European Collaborative Study, 1991; Scott et al., 1989).

Researchers (e.g., Blanche et al., 1994; Oxtoby, 1990) have described two patterns of disease course in vertically infected children. These vary as to when symptoms first appear. The first pattern includes those children who present with symptomatic disease before 1 year of age, and the second pattern relates to children who have vertically acquired infection but do not develop AIDS-related symptoms until after the first few years of life (Pizzo et al., 1995).

The first pattern occurs in about 20% of vertically infected infants and typically results in medical difficulties, such as severe failure to thrive, PCP, and/or encephalopathy. These children tend to have a rapid progression of disease and early death. The second pattern describes children who present with symptoms after the first year of life, often with lymphadenopathy and/or pneumonitis, and have a slower disease course (Pizzo et al., 1995). Children following the second pattern may survive into their late school-age, or even adolescent, years, evidencing a *median* survival age of 6 to 8 years (Rogers et al., 1987; Wilfert, 1993).

Of those children who are not infected vertically, a small group are infected via contaminated blood or blood products (e.g., those with hemophilia). These children generally have a slower progression of disease than those who are vertically infected (Krasinski, Borkowsky, & Holzman, 1989).

Neurological complications caused by HIV infection most often occur during development of the central nervous system (CNS) and can have a particularly negative impact on child development. There is evidence that HIV affects CNS structures responsible for motor and spatial memory development (Boivin et al., 1995), as well as those involved in affective and behavioral regulation (Price et al., 1988). Behaviorally, this may result in cognitive and motor delays, dementia, loss of developmental milestones, ataxia, and seizures (Schmitt, Seeger, Kreuz, Enenkel, & Jacobi, 1991). Even asymptomatic or mildly ill children may show subtle neurodevelopmental deficits (Cohen et al., 1991).

In addition to, or perhaps as a result of, the numerous medical difficulties associated with this disease, most of the available literature indicates that pediatric AIDS usually has a considerable impact on child development and psychosocial functioning. For example, Boivin et al. (1995) found that HIV-seropositive children scored significantly lower on a test of intelligence than did two control groups. When psychosocial functioning has been examined, vertically acquired HIV is seen to be particularly detrimental. Mellins and Ehrhardt (1994) reported that more than 50% of their sample of children living with AIDS evidenced behavior problems (e.g., hyperactivity, temper tantrums), developmental delays, and/or learning disabilities. A second study found that over 79% of their sample of infected children met criteria for one or more psychiatric diagnoses, the most common being attention-deficit/hyperactivity disorder, oppositional defiant disorder, and separation anxiety disorder (Havens, Whitaker, Feldman, & Ehrhardt, 1994). By contrast, a third study found that children's self-report scores on standardized measures of depression, anxiety, and self-esteem fell within the normal range (Bose, Moss, Brouwers, Pizzo, & Lorion, 1994).

The discrepancy between the Bose et al. study and the first two studies might be explained by the socioeconomic status (SES) of the families and the mode of infection. Specifically, the Bose et al. sample consisted mainly of children from middle-class families who were infected via contaminated blood products. In contrast, the samples in the other two studies were primarily from families of much lower SES and involved children who were vertically infected. Thus, environments of the children in the Bose et al. study differed in a number of ways from those the children in the Mellins and Ehrhardt and Havens et al. studies, including number of available parents (i.e., single- versus dual-parent households) and other family members being infected with the virus (Bose et al., 1994). Furthermore, as noted earlier, children infected via contaminated blood products typically have a slower progression of disease than those vertically infected, and this may account for differences across studies. Again, it is important to note that the vast majority of pediatric AIDS cases involve vertical infection and lower SES.

Other psychosocial considerations in children living with AIDS are that many experience peer-related difficulties or low self-esteem due to differences in their appearance, resulting from their smaller stature, wasting, dermatologic conditions, and/or distended abdomens (Lewis et al., 1994). In summary, children living with AIDS or who are infected with HIV appear to be at high risk for adjustment problems across a variety of areas, including the domains of psychological, social, and academic functioning.

DIAGNOSIS

Typically, the first clinical warning signs of the presence of HIV infection are recurrent bacterial and viral infections, which range in severity from mild ear infections to the more serious meningitis. Recurrent infections, in conjunction with specific historical features (e.g., sexual abuse, a mother who uses intravenous drugs or has a partner who uses), indicate the need for HIV testing in children. Another indicator of the need for testing is birth to a mother who is known to be seropositive (Arpadi & Caspe, 1992).

Currently, there are three means by which an individual can be diagnosed as having HIV: antibody detection, virus detection, or meeting the CDC's diagnostic criteria for AIDS. Initially, HIV testing in infants and children, as with adults, involved detecting the presence of antibodies to HIV within an individual's bloodstream (Arpadi & Caspe, 1992). However, such testing procedures are complicated regarding their use in very young populations where perinatal transmission is suspected. The complication is caused by presence of the mother's antibodies to HIV in the infant's system whether or not the infant is infected. These antibodies cross the placental barrier and, when using the most common tests (enzyme-linked immunosorbant assay [ELISA] and Western blot), their presence in the infant indicates a positive serostatus whether the infant is seropositive or not (Arpadi & Caspe, 1992). Thus, when relying on the ELISA and Western blot procedures, medical personnel and families have to wait up to 18 months (the point at which a mother's antibodies are no longer present in an infant's bloodstream) to know for certain if an infant is infected. This waiting period is a crucial time for early medical treatment for those infants who are infected; however, the negative side effects of current medical therapies prohibit treatment of infants who may not be infected (NIAID, 1994).

More recently, an alternative antibody detection assay has been used to detect infant-specific antibodies (e.g., IgA antibodies). These antibodies cannot have come from the mother as they are too large to have crossed the placental barrier and, thus, when present in the infant's bloodstream, indicate HIV infection (Arpadi & Caspe, 1992). This assay is simple, quick, inexpensive, and can detect the presence of HIV as early as 3–6 months of age (with excellent sensitivity achieved by 6 months; Indacochea & Scott, 1992). The drawback of this procedure is that it

may not be accurate at less than 6 months of age as the infant's system may not have yet developed its own antibodies to the virus (NIAID, 1994).

The second category of laboratory tests is viral detection. Three methods of viral detection have been used, and all have their strengths and weaknesses. HIV culture detects presence of the virus in the bloodstream or cells and, as opposed to common antibody screens, can be very accurate for infants less than 15 months old (Connor et al., 1994). However, it has many drawbacks, especially in children, including the fact that it requires large quantities of blood. Furthermore, it is expensive and labor intensive and the ability to detect the virus in the blood varies with disease stage (Arpadi & Caspe, 1992).

A second type of viral detection, which is less expensive than HIV culture, is viral antigen detection. This method involves detection of p24 core antigens in the blood. The disadvantage of this method is that levels of p24 also vary by disease stage such that not all infected children will have detectable antigenemia; thus, a negative test does not always exclude infection (Arpadi & Caspe, 1992). Viral antigen (p24) detection seems to be most accurate early and late in the disease course (Beckford & Dossett, 1992).

A third type of viral detection is polymerase chain reaction (PCR), which identifies specific HIV DNA sequences. In adults, this test has been demonstrated to detect the presence of HIV as much as 6 months before antibodies can be detected (Arpadi & Caspe, 1992). Because of its ability to detect the virus earlier than in antibody testing, PCR is particularly useful in young infants suspected of being infected (Beckford & Dossett, 1992). Furthermore, unlike HIV culture and p24 detection, the test is capable of detecting very small amounts of the virus and, thus, does not require large amounts of blood and is less dependent on disease stage (Beckford & Dossett, 1992). However, PCR is relatively new and, therefore, more expensive than ELISA, Western blot, and p24 antigen detection (NIAID, 1994).

In summary, with regard to laboratory tests and children, it appears that the common ELISA and Western blot methods are most useful for children older than 15 months of age or as screening devices for young infants (<15 months). One or more of the alternative methods discussed above typically are necessary for definitive results in infants under age 15 months (Indacochea & Scott, 1992).

Finally, a child can be diagnosed with HIV if she or he meets the CDC's diagnostic criteria for AIDS. (See CDC, 1990, for an update on the complete definition of pediatric AIDS).

Given the unique issues surrounding HIV, it is important that HIV diagnostic testing in children be conducted in a sensitive and confidential manner. Arpadi and Caspe (1991) recommended counseling for the child's parent or guardian that includes: (1) a description of the virus, (2) the "nature and purpose of the HIV test," (3) information regarding confidentiality and disclosure-related issues, (4) information about risk reduction, (5) the implications of a positive result, and (6) the benefits of early medical intervention. Furthermore, they recommend that results only be given in person and that appropriate referrals for treatment are provided.

ETIOLOGY

The vast majority of children with AIDS acquired their infection via vertical transmission from the mother. The CDC reported in 1994 that 89% of the cumulative total of pediatric AIDS cases were the result of vertical transmission, and 10% of the cumulative total were acquired via contaminated blood products prior to regular screening of the blood supply in 1985. In 1% of the cases, the source was not reported or could not be identified (CDC, 1994a). It is important to note that these percentages are cumulative and, thus, include children who are no longer living. When only current cases are considered, percentage for transmission via contaminated blood products is even lower than 10% (CDC, 1994a).

HIV may be passed from mother to child in utero via transplacental transmission, during labor and delivery via contact with infected maternal blood, or through breastfeeding. However, when an HIV-infected woman becomes pregnant, it is often found that the virus is not transmitted to the child. In the United States, vertical transmission is reported to occur between 15 and 30% of the time (CDC, 1993). One factor influencing such transmission is the mother's health status during her pregnancy. Likelihood of transmission appears to increase with the clinical severity of the mother's infection and is inversely related to her CD4+ cell count (Blanche et al., 1994). Additionally, if a woman has AIDS (versus only HIV infection) during pregnancy or up to 1 year after delivery, her child appears more likely to be vertically infected (Hague, Mok, MacCallum, Burns, & Yap, 1991).

Another route of transmission for pediatric AIDS is via contaminated blood products. As already noted, this is much less common than vertical transmission. Nevertheless, at least 10% of all child cases were infected through contaminated blood products. Six percent of these children were infected subsequent to blood transfusions and the remaining 4% suffered from a coagulation disorder (hemophilia) and were infected through blood products contaminated with HIV (CDC, 1994a). Hemophilia is transmitted genetically from mother to son and results in very low amounts of one of two factors in the blood that are responsible for the clotting mechanism serving to prevent excessive bleeding (Bussing & Johnson 1992). In the 1960s, it was discovered that the missing clotting factor could be separated from large quantities of blood and stored at home as a concentrate, resulting in fewer hospital visits for children with hemophilia and an overall improvement in quality of life (Mason, Olson, Myers, Huszti, & Kenning, 1989). Unfortunately, for many people with hemophilia, this improvement in quality of life was only temporary, as the blood supply became contaminated with HIV in the late 1970s and was not screened out of the supply until 1985. Consequently, 60% of individuals with hemophilia became infected with HIV (Dew, Ragini, & Nimorwicz, 1990). Thus, many children were afflicted with two chronic illnesses, hemophilia and HIV/AIDS.

Finally, we should note that child sexual abuse is another vehicle for HIV transmission (Hutto, 1994). However, statistics for percentage of children acquiring HIV through such abuse could not be located. We assume that relatively few children are infected by this route.

In summary, the vast majority of children acquire HIV through vertical transmission from the mother, and a much smaller percentage acquire the virus through contact with contaminated blood products. The latter method of acquisition no longer occurs, having been ended by screening and treatment of donated blood. Finally, a minute proportion of infected children may have been infected through sexual abuse; however, data have not been reported for this group (Hutto, 1994).

Because of the high risk of emotional, academic, and/or behavior problems in children with HIV/AIDS, the etiology of these difficulties will be explored. Four areas have been examined in an attempt to understand their causes: (1) illness-related issues, (2) gestational conditions, (3) family environment issues, and (4) societal issues.

Regarding illness-related issues, evidence that HIV itself has a direct impact on child psychosocial functioning is accumulating. Autopsies indicate that the virus causes calcification of portions of the basal ganglia, a subcortical brain structure that is involved in the modulation of behavior and affect (Price et al., 1988). Behavior is directly affected by such calcification. Other researchers have found "widespread myelin damage" (p. 319) in the central nervous system of patients with AIDS (Brouwers, Belman, & Epstein, 1990). Furthermore, the improved cognitive ability and social development observed on treatment with AZT indicate that the virus has direct physiological effects on child functioning (Pizzo et al., 1988).

Illness-related issues also may have secondary effects on child adjustment. These secondary issues include school absences and frequent hospitalizations (Melvin & Sherr, 1993). School absences typically are associated with lower academic achievement and increased social isolation (e.g., Markova, McDonald, & Forbes, 1980). Additionally, many infected children are frequently hospitalized and must undergo invasive medical procedures that may influence psychosocial functioning (Blount, Smith, & Frank, in press). Thus, beyond its direct effects on the body, HIV has secondary effects, such as school absences, which influence child adjustment.

Some gestational conditions occur at high rates within the pediatric AIDS population and can influence child functioning. These conditions compound the negative impact that the virus has on child psychosocial functioning. Intravenous drug use is the most common risk factor for HIV infection in women, as 41% of the current AIDS cases in women have been attributed to this behavior (CDC, 1994a). Maternal drug use during pregnancy, independent of HIV status, has been associated with a variety of behavior problems in offspring (Chasnoff, Griffith, MacGregor, Dirkes, & Burns, 1989; Naeye, Blanc, Leblanc, & Khatamee, 1973).

Havens et al. (1994) examined the psychosocial effects of HIV in the context of maternal drug use during pregnancy. Using a diagnostic interview, as well as standardized instruments, they studied three groups of children, all of whom were believed to have been exposed to maternal drug use in utero. The three groups were an HIV seropositive group, an HIV seroreverted group (i.e., children who initially tested positive for HIV but reverted to a negative status probably as a result of clearing of the mother's antibodies) and a non-HIV-exposed group. High rates (over 70%) of behavior disorders were found in all of the children in their sample, with the HIV seropositive group differing only by evidencing higher rates of subjective distress (i.e., anxiety) than either of the other two groups. This study provides evidence that difficulties in psychosocial functioning can result not only from HIV infection, but also from prenatal exposure to the most common maternal risk factor for HIV, drug use.

An additional gestational condition reflects the fact that many women living with HIV have a marginalized status in society. As a result, they do not receive adequate nutrition or adequate access to health care (Mellins & Ehrhardt, 1994). Poor nutrition and lack of prenatal care are other gestational factors that may negatively influence child functioning (Cohen, 1994).

With respect to family factors, research focusing on chronic illness in children has shown that a secure, supportive, and open family environment with adequate external support can have a positive impact on adjustment and the course of illness in children (Eiser, 1985; Lask & Fosson, 1989). Unfortunately, mothers of most HIV-infected children are themselves infected with the virus and often are dealing with financial problems, depression, and lack of social support, as well being the only available parent for the child (Armistead & Forehand, 1995; Mellins & Ehrhardt, 1994). As a consequence, many children living with AIDS do not have benefits of a secure and supportive family environment (Kurth, 1993). As would be expected, data, though limited, indicate that health of the mother and the subsequent home environment can negatively influence the psychosocial functioning of HIV-infected children (e.g., cognitive performance; Boivin et al., 1995).

One mechanism by which the family environment may negatively influence child adjustment is through the impact of the mother's HIV infection on her parenting abilities (Melvin & Sherr, 1993). There is an existing literature supporting the relationship between disrupted parenting and poorer child outcomes (Forehand & McMahon, 1981; Wierson & Forehand, 1994). In the case of mothers infected with HIV, they are likely to experience physical and/or emotional distress, as well as recurrent hospitalizations, which can interfere with effective parenting (Armistead & Forehand, 1995; Armistead, Klein, & Forehand, 1995). Many of these mothers also experience overwhelming guilt and a sense of responsibility for infecting their child, which may further compromise parenting (Weiner, Theut, Steinberg, Riekert, & Pizzo, 1994). Furthermore, the child's illness can negatively impact parenting as caring for an ill child places considerable stress and greater challenges on caregivers compared with caring for a nonill child (Burke & Dawson, 1987; Kohrman, 1991).

Uncertainties inherent in HIV infection also may negatively influence child and family functioning. Initially, there may be uncertainty regarding whether the child is actually infected. Such uncertainty is likely to increase or create anxiety for the child and/or parent(s), which may further contribute to the child's development of emotional difficulties (Melvin & Sherr, 1993).

A third family-related factor is that multiple losses may occur in a family or kinship network. Approximately 38% of women are infected via heterosexual contact (CDC, 1994a), indicating that the partner, who is possibly the father of the infected child, also is infected. Additionally, siblings or extended family members may be infected, leading to the parent(s) and child potentially having to cope with the loss of multiple family members. Related literature supports the notion that parent and/or child emotional or behavior disorders may develop as a result of experiencing these multiple losses (Bor, Miller, & Goldman, 1993; Garmezy, 1991).

Another subset of children may be affected in a different way by family factors. For this subgroup, care and nurturing are no longer provided by the family of origin. These children are left to cope with the already overburdened foster care system or are residing in the homes of relatives because their mothers are deceased, too ill to care for them, or unwilling to care for them, typically as a result of continued substance abuse (American Academy of Pediatrics, 1992). Although some of these alternative family environments are supportive and stable, others are far from ideal (Cohon & Cooper, 1993). These children may find themselves passed from one caregiver to another or, in the worst-case scenario, abandoned in hospitals where they live as "boarder babies" until caregivers can be found (Mellins & Ehrhardt, 1994).

In summary, mothers of HIV-infected children must invest substantial energy in caring for these children. Unfortunately, at least some of these women will be lacking in resources and energy that they can apply to parenting because of the toll exacted by their own illness (Armistead & Forehand, 1995). Still other mothers will be unable to care for their infected children at all, relying instead on the foster care system or extended family network. These factors, combined with the emotional strain associated with uncertainties surrounding HIV-related issues and the experience of multiple losses to HIV-related illness, may serve to stretch mothers (most of whom are also immunocompromised) beyond their capacity for adequate parenting.

The society in which children with AIDS reside also may have negative repercussions for their psychosocial functioning. Hailing primarily from economically disadvantaged communities of color, these children and their families are likely to face not only rejection and discrimination from mainstream society, but also limited access to and use of medical and social services (Mellins & Ehrhardt, 1994). Additionally, because of the social stigma associated with AIDS, some families will face rejection on the basis of their illness, as there are members of society who blame the infection on the behavior of the ill individual or who consider infection a punishment for immoral or illegal behavior (Blendon & Donelan, 1988). Furthermore, myths and ignorance regarding the transmission of HIV persist, which also may result in social ostracism of the infected family (Weiner et al., 1994). Lastly, given their often impoverished socioeconomic status, families with children infected with AIDS often are residing in extremely violent and crime-ridden areas of the United States. In addition to anxiety and/or stress response syndrome related to witnessing violence on a routine basis, this may result in additional loss of family members to death or imprisonment (Mellins & Ehrhardt, 1994).

EPIDEMIOLOGY

Worldwide, an estimated 1 million children have been infected with HIV and, by the year 2000, an estimated 10 million children will have been infected since the start of the epidemic (WHO/Global Programme on AIDS, 1993). Within the United States, there are 5891 pediatric AIDS cases (CDC, 1994b) and an estimated additional 10,000 children are infected with HIV (NIAID, 1994). There are about 7000 infants born each year to women who are HIV seropositive. Of these 7000, approximately 1000 to 2000 are infected (CDC, 1994b). To date, cases of pediatric AIDS have been reported in every state within the United States (Hutto, 1994). Furthermore, the proportion of cases among women, which is closely tied to the epidemic in children, has risen steadily to 18% of all AIDS cases (CDC, 1994a). If the rate of HIV infection in women continues to increase, the incidence of infection in children is likely to also increase (Ammann, 1994).

Rates of pediatric AIDS are disproportionately high among children of color. More than 50% of children with pediatric AIDS are African American and 25% are Latino (Oxtoby, 1991). In fact, within some U.S. cities, AIDS is the first or second leading cause of death among Latino and African American children (Weiner et al., 1994). Given the current trends, it is essential that the unique needs of the pediatric AIDS population be addressed.

ASSESSMENT

Assessment of the medical condition and psychosocial functioning of HIV-infected children needs to occur on a regular basis (Mendez, 1992). Medical assessment of disease progression and effects is performed in a variety of ways. In addition to a complete history and physical examination, laboratory studies provide important information regarding the child's condition. For example, CD4 counts and CD4/CD8 ratios are common and relatively reliable indicators of disease progression (Mendez, 1992). Brain imaging techniques (e.g., computed tomographic examination, magnetic resonance scans) are employed to assess for abnormalities in brain structure, such as cerebral atrophy, calcification of the basal ganglia, and/or decreased attenuation of white matter. Further, brain imaging techniques are useful not only to monitor disease progression, but also to demonstrate reversals in disease progression as a result of antiretroviral therapy (Brouwers et al., 1990).

Given that the data, though limited, appear to indicate that many children with AIDS experience a range of psychosocial problems and because some children are surviving to school age and adolescence (Lewis et al., 1994), it is important to assess for the myriad of psychosocial difficulties that these children are at risk for experiencing. Lack of a guiding literature to inform treatment of mental health problems in this population makes a thorough assessment even more crucial (Havens et al., 1994).

It is critical to incorporate the family and community systems into assessment and treatment whenever possible (Indacochea & Scott, 1992). Because of their significant impact on child development in general, parents or alternative caregivers of infected children simply cannot be ignored if an assessment is to be thorough. This is especially true because previous research has shown that parents of children with other serious illnesses experience psychosocial distress related to providing care for the ill child (Frank et al., 1991). Parental distress can, in turn, impact child adjustment (Armistead et al., 1995; Forehand, 1993).

This section initially focuses on the assessment of psychosocial difficulties in the child. Subsequently, assessment of the family unit is considered.

Child Psychosocial Assessment

When assessing the child, a psychoeducational battery should be given regularly, as progres-sion of disease results in cognitive decline and additional neuropsychological symptoms (Brouwers et al., 1990). Pizzo et al. (1995) recommend that batteries be administered as often as every 12 weeks except for those tests that are more susceptible to practice effects (e.g., intelligence tests). They recommend that the latter tests be given no more frequently than every 24 weeks.

The battery should include an intelligence test (e.g., Kaufman Assessment Battery for Children) and a measure of language development (e.g., Peabody Picture Vocabulary Test-Revised) for younger children or an achievement test (e.g., Peabody individual Achievement Test-Revised) for school children. Memory, attention, and motor functioning also should be assessed as the literature indicates that many infected children experience deficits in these domains (Brouwers et al., 1990). Additionally, neuropsychological functions not measured in the basic test battery should be evaluated (Brouwers et al., 1990).

For the purposes of treatment planning or educational interventions, it is important that test reports include the child's strengths and weaknesses. Scores on tests can provide information about disease progression as "maintenance of normal scores provides reassurance that CNS progression is not occurring" (Pizzo et al., 1995, p. 37). The positive impact of antiretroviral therapy also can be measured by improvements in functioning evidenced in test outcome (Pizzo et al., 1995).

Ideally, standard test instruments can be utilized according to the specific test guidelines. However, it is not always possible to administer tests in the standardized way. For instance, difficulty may arise in assessing young and sometimes developmentally delayed HIV seropositive children because of "floor" effects. This occurs when a child is functioning well below her or his chronological age and, thus, is unable to obtain any score on an age-appropriate test. In these cases, it may be necessary to utilize tests intended for younger children so that a "mental age or age equivalent" can be obtained (Brouwers et al., 1990).

It is important that optimal testing conditions be maintained. Children should not be tested immediately following painful medical procedures, after administration of sedating medications, when they are ill with another infection, or when they have a fever (Brouwers et al., 1990). Lastly, motoric or sensory impairment related to HIV may require the use of alternative test instruments in order to improve validity.

Behavioral functioning in the home can be examined by the Vineland Adaptive Behavior Scales (Wolters, Brouwers, Moss, & Pizzo, 1994). Results from this instrument can inform the medical and psychosocial treatments that are geared toward increasing the child's independent daily living skills. For example, Wolters et al. (1994) found that antiretroviral therapy resulted in an improvement in adaptive behavior that would not have been detected by a standard batter of cognitive tests. Assessment of adaptive behavior also may serve to facilitate planning for educational interventions for these children in the classroom.

Assessment of socioemotional difficulties is a necessity when evaluating HIV-infected children. Such an evaluation should include assessment for disorders within the broadband categories of internalizing problems (e.g., anxiety, depression) and externalizing problems (e.g., oppositional defiant disorder). Social competence and peer-related problems should be evaluated, particularly with school children or those in day-care settings (Cohen, 1994). Structured and unstructured interviews, as well as pencil-and-paper measures with older children, may be used for this portion of the assessment. Furthermore, this part of the assessment should involve, whenever feasible multiple reporters (e.g., child report, parent or caregiver report, teacher or day-care worker report), as well as behavioral observation. The latter can occur under conditions similar to those specified by Forehand and McMahon (1981) for children with other problems.

In addition to assessment of the aforementioned domains, an attempt to identify risks and resource factors that serve to modulate the impact of HIV on child functioning should be completed. Relevant risk factors include, but are not limited to, severity of physical symptoms, inadequate coping skills, and negative life events (Bose et al., 1994). Assessment of negative life events is particularly relevant for this population as many HIV-infected children live in crime-ridden, inner-city environments.

Some children experience significant stress and, yet, continue to function quite well. Research with populations other than HIV has identified a number of factors that appear to contribute to "normal" child adjustment in the face of exceptional stress (e.g., Emery & Forehand, 1994). These resiliency factors include social support from family and peers and an adequate coping skills repertoire.

An additional resource factor that should be assessed is self-worth. Given "our society's largely negative view of HIV positive individuals" (p. 196), children living with HIV are at increased risk for low self-worth and, in turn, a variety of psychosocial problems (Andrews, Williams, & Neil, 1993). Alternatively, adequate self-worth can serve as a protective factor against many types of problems (Neighbors, Forehand, & McVicar, 1993). Assessment for risk and resource factors can be completed in a manner similar to assessment for socioemotional difficulties.

Family Psychosocial Assessment

Events occurring in the family environment contribute to a child's psychological health (Rutter, 1985). Children living with AIDS are at high risk for being in less than ideal family situations because of the low socioeconomic status and drug use of many infected women (Gayetal, 1995). Thus, safety of the home environment, as well as the ability of the parent(s) to meet the child's physical needs (e.g., food and clothing), should be evaluated through parent report and, when possible, home visits and/or behavioral observation. Evaluation of these conditions is important in order to facilitate access to needed social and medical resources (Lewis et al., 1994).

Given the interplay between family stress and child adjustment (Forehand, 1993), the family members, especially the parent(s), should be assessed across a variety of areas. Weiner et al. (1994) elucidated some of the relevant areas when they found high rates of depression and anxiety in parents of children with HIV infection. Additional areas to assess, based on related literature, include marital distress (in dual-parent families), parenting stress, parental coping, parent social support, and parent–child attachment or interaction (Cohen, 1994). Again, these areas should be assessed using multiple reporters and multiple methods where possible.

With verbal children and with all caregivers, an assessment of the individual's concepts of AIDS should be undertaken (Siegel, 1993). Walsh and Bibace (1991) developed an open-ended questionnaire that can be useful in identifying HIV/AIDS myths and misconceptions held by the child and family. This assessment can inform educational needs, as well as interventions addressing disclosure of HIV status to the child.

Culturally Sensitive Assessment

Given that most children living with AIDS and their families are members of minorities, mental health workers conducting assessments need to utilize instruments that are suitable for and culturally sensitive to these populations. Unfortunately, because minority groups have been virtually excluded from research (Sherwen & Boland, 1994), valid standardized measures for assessing the majority of children living with AIDS and their families are rare (Jansen & Ammann, 1994). For instance, many pencil-and-paper questionnaires designed to assess psychological symptoms were developed with white middle-class individuals and may not be appropriate for use with other populations (Melvin & Sherr, 1993). One must attempt to use measures with established reliability and validity for the target population (Bose et al., 1994). Along this line, differences in sociocultural expectations should

be considered in the interpretation of assessment measures. Finally, in cases where English is not the first language, appropriate modifications in instrumentation should occur if reliable interpreters are unavailable (Melvin & Sherr, 1993).

PREVENTION AND TREATMENT

Interventions for children living with HIV and/or AIDS must involve medical and psychosocial components and are best implemented by a multidisciplinary team of professionals (Hutto, 1994). Although there is no medical cure for HIV and the disease is assumed to be 100% fatal, advances have been made in terms of preventing infection, as well as improving the quality of life for infected children.

Prevention

As just noted, because there is no cure for AIDS, prevention is the key to decreasing the spread of the disease. With regard to medical prevention of HIV in children, one of the most recent and exciting findings is that an antiretroviral drug, zidovudine, reduces the rate of mother-to-child transmission of the virus by as much as 67% (Connor et al., 1994) when administered pre-, peri-, and postnatally. However, as significant as this discovery is, there remains a need for additional prevention strategies. Specifically, it is important to continue to attempt to alter the sexual and drug-related behavior of women in their childbearing years, as well as the behavior of their sexual partners. Possible methods for efforts in this regard include, but are not limited to, the use of community education, media campaigns, family planning clinics, and condom distribution programs (Armistead & Forehand, 1995). However, it is critical that prevention efforts take into consideration "the existing social structure of the risk group that reinforces or maintains participation in risk behaviors" (Olson et al., 1989, p. 4).

Treatment

In terms of medical treatment, zidovudine administered to infected children results in improved immunological response with minimal side effects (Indacochea & Scott, 1992), as well as improvement across a variety of behavioral domains, including daily living, communication, and socialization skills (Wolters et al., 1994). Other antiretroviral medications (e.g., didanosine) show similar results in infected children (Hutto, 1994). In addition to treatment with antiretrovirals, HIV-infected children should be closely monitored for infection and can be given antibiotic prophylaxis in an attempt to prevent infections such as life-threatening PCP (Hutto, 1994).

In addition to medical treatment, studies (e.g., Havens et al., 1994) indicate that most children living with AIDS and their families can benefit from a variety of psychosocial interventions. Unfortunately, very little research has explored factors that might lead to improved psychosocial adjustment. Furthermore, treatment studies involving children with other chronic illnesses have minimal applicability to the pediatric AIDS population because of the unique aspects of the disease (e.g., stigma, multiple infected family members). Furthermore, research with other chronic illnesses has been conducted primarily with white middle-class families that differ in many ways from the majority of families afflicted with AIDS (Mellins & Ehrhardt, 1994). Nevertheless, we will present several target areas and suggest interventions for remediation of the psychosocial difficulties associated with HIV/AIDS.

Child-Based Psychosocial Treatments

Psychological treatment may serve to prevent development of some emotional difficulties related to frequent hospitalizations and painful procedures that many infected children undergo. Specifically, Melvin and Sherr (1993) recommended minimizing separation and isolation from family members during hospitalizations.

Additionally, Eiser (1985) called for "demystifying the hospital environment" (p. 40) by familiarizing children with the setting and preparing them for medical procedures. Along similar lines, pain management, such as relaxation or distraction techniques, may decrease trauma caused by painful medical procedures (Sherwen & Boland, 1994). Lastly, as children age and become more independent from adults, treatment may need to focus on compliance with medical protocols and dietary recommendations (Swales, 1994).

Given that many infected children are surviving to school age, educational needs cannot be ignored. Like all other children, those with HIV are entitled to appropriate educational services (Sherwen & Boland, 1994). Psychologists can serve as advocates for the child in the school system, facilitating special education placement when necessary.

Some infected children will evidence a need for treatment for internalizing and/or externalizing problems. Treatment focusing on alleviating depression or anxiety may include individual therapy, family therapy, or social support groups that provide opportunities for expression of grief and discussion of health status (Lewis et al., 1994). Behavior management programs implemented by parents and teachers are needed when a child has attention/deficit/hyperactivity disorder (which is not uncommon among this population) (Swales, 1994) or other externalizing problems.

Children with AIDS will sometimes suffer from dementia and/or delirium related to their medical condition. In these cases, they would benefit from environmental interventions, such as decreasing stimulation, increasing the safety of the environment, and providing diversional activities (Swales, 1994).

Coping with death and dying should be a focus of treatment as the child becomes increasingly ill. In accomplishing this, the therapist must first understand the family's philosophy and religious beliefs related to death. Subsequently, children who are aware that they are close to death may be told the following in order to allay fear: (1) they will not be alone at the time of death, (2) death itself is not painful, (3) it is okay to cry and feel sad, (4) they will have a chance to say goodbye if they so desire, and (5) they will always be remembered (Spinetta, Swarner, & Sheposh, 1981).

Family-Based Psychosocial Treatments

Almost without exception, researchers investigating the effects of pediatric AIDS have elucidated the need for treatment to be "family centered." As Cohen (1994) stated, it is clear that chronic and terminal illnesses, such as HIV, have "profound and long lasting effects on families" (p. 34). Thus, in addition to those issues directly related to the child's illness, a number of psychosocial problems may be present in families with an HIV seropositive child.

Initially, the non-disease-related challenges faced by some of these families (e.g., poverty, parental drug abuse) may overshadow the impact of the virus (Condrini et al., 1989). For instance, these families may require the efforts of social service workers to facilitate the resolution of financial and housing problems (Melvin & Sherr, 1993). Additionally, treatment for substance abuse may be necessary for the parent(s) as many have acquired HIV through injection drug use. Unfortunately, the safety and welfare of the child cannot be maintained in the face of persistent drug use; thus, social service agencies may need to arrange for alternative placement in these situations (Swales, 1994).

In the case where families are able to provide adequate care for infected children, it may be necessary to focus on parenting in order to prevent or remediate serious psychological symptoms in the infected child (Weiner et al., 1994). Parents will need to be educated about transmission prevention and the disruptions that HIV incurs on child development. In some instances, they may require instruction in general parenting skills, which they can apply to the child's emotional and behavior problems possibly resulting from HIV. These parenting skills, which are readily available in other sources (e.g., Fore-

hand & McMahon, 1981), include reinforcing appropriate behavior and utilizing procedures such as time-out for disruptive behavior.

Families may benefit from efforts designed to find a balance between denial of the child's illness versus excessive attention to the illness. They may need assistance with maintaining normal routines in the context of illness demands (Bor et al., 1993). Psychological support for the parents, which targets anxiety and depression, may further help to minimize disruptions in parenting (Weiner et al., 1994). This can be provided through the venues of individual therapy or support groups where individuals can share their disease-related experiences (Mellins & Ehrhardt, 1994).

Often families with HIV are fearful of ostracism and rejection and choose to keep their HIV experience a secret. As a consequence, they may not have access to the individuals who would typically provide important support in the case of chronic illness. Treatments designed to increase social support through either facilitating disclosure to support networks or introducing individuals to support groups may remediate support-related issues. Related to limited support is the lack of available respite care for parents of children with AIDS. Respite care was one of the two most common psychosocial needs reported by Mellins and Ehrhardt's (1994) sample of families with an infected child.

There are two other major issues facing most families with an HIV-infected child: disclosure of HIV status to the child and future planning for the child in cases where the parent also is infected. With regard to these decisions, the role of the psychologist or other mental health professional is to be informed about the issues concerning HIV in order to be a viable source of information for parents. In addition to providing information, the professional can offer support during and after the decision-making process. It clearly is never the mental health professional's role to make decisions for families (Armistead & Forehand, 1995).

Parents must decide whether to reveal the child's illness status to him or her. For pediatric cancer patients, professionals recommend providing the children with their diagnosis regardless of age (Stehbens, 1988). However, again, there are many differences between the diagnosis of AIDS and cancer. According to Swales (1994), most parents have not told their seropositive child of the diagnosis for fear of a negative impact on medical and psychological functioning. Unfortunately, there are no data available to guide parents or professionals about the positive and negative consequences of informing children about their HIV status. Thus, we are left with only "hunches" to guide parents in the decision-making process.

There are a number of reasons why a parent would choose not to reveal the diagnosis. Parents may be concerned about the young child's ability to understand or cope with this life-taking illness, especially given the large number of stressors these children already face. Additionally, the parent may have concerns about the child's ability to "keep the secret" of HIV in the family, which may be necessary to avoid ostracism and stigmatization (Armistead & Forehand, 1995).

In contrast, there also are a number of ways in which revealing HIV status may benefit the child and family. Havens et al. (1994) found that "exploration with HIV positive children of their understanding and concerns about their illness can be helpful in relieving anxiety and reducing isolation" (p. 24). Disclosure may be particularly useful in cases where children already are aware that they are ill but have not been informed of the cause. As illness-related uncertainty can be detrimental (Mischel, 1981), these children may function better when they know the truth (Armistead & Forehand, 1995). This may be particularly true as they age and begin to ask their caregivers questions about their illness (Swales, 1994).

In summary, a variety of issues must be considered in making the decision whether to disclose HIV status. These include the child's developmental level, health status, coping skills repertoire, and current knowledge about the illness (Armistead & Forehand, 1995). If a parent does

decide to disclose, whether it is best to inform the child using the term *AIDS* or *HIV* remains in debate. However, it has been proposed that, at a minimum, the child should have the following information: (1) his or her illness is serious, (2) treatment is necessary, (3) physicians have no cure but will continue to look for one, and (4) the child will be updated about his or her health status (Swales, 1994).

The second major decision for many parents of infected children is care for the child when the parent (or parents) becomes too ill to provide adequate care or, in the worst-case scenario, dies. This decision is complicated by a number of factors, such as a lack of alternative caregivers within the kinship network and a lack of flexible public policy to facilitate the transfer from biological parent to alternative caregiver (Armistead & Forehand, 1995). With regard to the latter, innovative policies, such as New York's recently established Standby Guardianship Law and Early Permanency Planning Program, will be important (Armistead & Forehand, 1995).

In conclusion, a wide range of medical and psychosocial problems face the victims of pediatric AIDS and their families. In attempting to address these issues, mental health professionals must remain nonjudgmental, culturally sensitive, and flexible (Mendez, 1992). Furthermore, education and treatment should be commensurate with developmental level and cognitive abilities. Lastly, the importance of family and community care cannot be overstressed (Indacochea & Scott, 1992) and is best accommodated by "one-stop" care centers where all family members can be treated across both medical and psychosocial domains (Ammann, 1994).

CASE STUDY

As is evident from the content of the present chapter, HIV/AIDS can have a dramatic impact on child adjustment across all domains of functioning. The psychosocial impact of HIV/AIDS on child adjustment varies depending on the child's developmental stage, as well as the severity of the disease. Here, we present the case study of Rochelle, a 7-year-old girl vertically infected with HIV and whose disease course is more typical of the second pattern discussed above, as she presented with symptoms after her second birthday.

Rochelle's father was an IV drug user who infected Rochelle's mother, Maggie, with HIV approximately 8 years ago. Maggie, who has a second daughter 1½ years younger than Rochelle, was unaware of her own infection until Rochelle was diagnosed with HIV at age 2. The younger daughter, Alicia, is not HIV infected. Maggie was diagnosed with AIDS when Rochelle was 5 years old and has been living in failing health ever since. The father, with whom Rochelle had only sporadic contact after age 2, was shot outside of his home when she was 6 years old.

In terms of social support, Maggie relies only on her family of origin, consisting of her mother and older brother. Maggie's mother, Dionne, learned of her daughter's and granddaughter's HIV diagnoses from Rochelle's father, who informed Dionne subsequent to an argument with Maggie. Maggie's brother was not informed of the dyad's positive serostatus but was told instead that Rochelle has cancer. Maggie also attempts to hide her own illness from her brother, which has become increasingly difficult given the deterioration of her health.

Beginning at age 1½, Rochelle started having recurrent fevers and diarrhea for which the emergency room physicians could offer no explanation. Subsequent to the fourth such episode and because of some developmental delay (e.g., onset of walking at 17 months), the physicians recommended HIV testing for Rochelle.

On learning of her daughter's diagnosis, as well as her own, Maggie suffered an episode of schizoaffective disorder, during which time Rochelle and Alicia resided with Dionne. Rochelle's health and emotional status declined significantly during this 1-year period. She lost weight and had two episodes of severe sinusitis. Additionally, Rochelle was very withdrawn and did not engage in play behavior. Maggie was able to resume care for her children on Rochelle's third birthday.

The next 2 years of Rochelle's life were relatively crisis-free. Her health remained fairly stable and she enjoyed typical childhood activities. During this time, Maggie struggled with whether to inform Rochelle of her illness. Maggie feared that disclosing her daughter's health status would lead to a decline in her physical health and fragile emotional well-being, as well as promote social alienation should Rochelle reveal the family's secret of AIDS. However, the medical staff encouraged Maggie to tell Rochelle of both her own and her daughter's illnesses, primarily because they suspected that Rochelle was already aware that something was wrong with her. Indeed, Rochelle had begun to question why she had to visit the doctor so often and why other children were so much bigger than she was. Ultimately, Maggie decided against disclosing to Rochelle until she felt her daughter could "handle it better." In this context, Maggie worked hard to hide her own failing health from the children and called Rochelle's various medications "vitamins."

At age 5, Maggie enrolled Rochelle and Alicia in a local Head Start program. During the school year, Rochelle experienced frequent sinusitis and ear infections. Although her illness resulted in frequent school absences, Rochelle enjoyed "going to school" with her sister. During this time, Rochelle's health continued to deteriorate and she was diagnosed with AIDS after two episodes of pneumonia.

By age 6, Rochelle had become quite frail; however, despite her failing health, she had a strong desire to continue with her sister in the Head Start program. Because of her age, the school district that ran the program recommended that Rochelle enter kindergarten rather than remain in Head Start. Rochelle's mother, her pediatrician, and the family's social worker all expressed concern that Rochelle would be too traumatized by the separation from her sister if she were to attend a different school. Cognitively, Rochelle demonstrated sufficient skills and development to advance in school; however, emotionally, as well as physically, Rochelle was very vulnerable. She would continue to miss much of school and, because her prognosis was very poor, her educational development was less of a concern than her physical and emotional well-being. A decision was made to keep Rochelle in the Head Start program for the coming year.

Currently, at age 7, Rochelle's health has deteriorated considerably. She is treated via home infusion several times daily and has a permanent GT tube through which nutrients are infused because she cannot tolerate normal foods. She is no longer able to attend school. Her prognosis is poor, with a life expectancy of 6 months to a year. Furthermore, Rochelle is socially withdrawn and cries easily. She still has not been told the name of her disease. Instead, both Alicia and Rochelle have been told that Rochelle has a sickness that makes her tired and weak and that doctors are working very hard to make it go away.

Maggie is having serious health complications of her own and is unable to care for her children independently. Currently, her mother is assisting her in caring for the children but this arrangement is not permanent as Dionne is willing to take custody of Alicia but not Rochelle. Social workers are assisting the family in finding alternative care arrangements for Alicia and Rochelle, whom Maggie wants to keep together as long as possible. However, it is unclear whether this option will be possible because of the paucity of available foster placements.

SUMMARY

Despite progress in preventing HIV in children, mainly through the positive impact of zidovudine in reducing vertical transmission, there is no cure or vaccine for this tragic disease. Thus, pediatric AIDS will continue to be a major challenge for medical and mental health workers beyond the twentieth century. Mental health professionals are increasingly called on to respond to the psychosocial issues inherent in pediatric AIDS. Unfortunately, there has not been a corresponding increase in empirical research to guide their efforts. Psychosocial research in this area must be a priority if the needs of the afflicted children and their families are to be met (Taylor-Brown & Kumetat, 1994b). In our attempts to meet the needs of these individuals, we cannot neglect their sociopolitical environment. This environment influences the whole range of issues associated with pediatric AIDS, from access to medical care, to disclosure of disease status, to future planning for the child's care. It is critical that the interventions targeted to these issues be informed by the sociopolitical environment of the children and their families.

ACKNOWLEDGMENTS

The support of the Centers for Disease Control and Prevention and the Institute for Behavioral Research at the University of Georgia is gratefully acknowledged.

REFERENCES

American Academy of Pediatrics: Task Force on Pediatric AIDS. (1992). Guidelines for human immunodeficiency virus-infected children and their foster families. *Pediatrics, 89,* 681–683.

Ammann, A. J. (1994). Human immunodeficiency virus infection/AIDS in children: The next decade. *Pediatrics, 93,* 930–935.

Andrews, S., Williams, A. B., & Neil, K. (1993). The mother–child relationship in the Hiv-1 positive family. *Image: Journal of Nursing Scholarship, 25,* 193–198.

Armistead, L., & Forehand, R. (1995). For whom the bell tolls: Parenting decisions and challenges faced by mothers who are HIV seropositive. *Clinical Psychology: Science and Practice, 2,* 239–250.

Armistead, L., Klein, K., & Forehand, R. (1995). Parental physical illness and child functioning. *Clinical Psychology Review, 15,* 1–15.

Arpadi, S., & Caspe, W. B. (1992). HIV testing. *Journal of Pediatrics, 119,* 8–13.

Beckford, A. P., & Dossett, J. H. (1992). Acquired immunodeficiency syndrome (AIDS) and human immunodeficiency virus (HIV) infection. In R. A. Hoekelman (Ed.), *Primary pediatric care* (pp. 115–125). St. Louis: Mosby Year Book.

Belman, A. L. (1990, August). AIDS and pediatric neurology. *Pediatric Neurology, 8,* 571–603.

Blanche, S., Mayaux, M., Rouzioux, C., Teglas, J., Firtion, G., Monpoux, F., Ciraur-Vigneron, N., Meier, F., Tricoire, J., Courpotin, C., Vilmer, E., Griscelli, C., Delfraissy, J., & the French Pediatric HIV Infection Study Group.

(1994). Relation of the course of HIV infection in children to the severity of the disease in their mothers at delivery. *New England Journal of Medicine, 330,* 308–312.

Blendon, R., & Donelan, K. (1988). Discrimination against people with AIDS: The public's perspective. *New England Journal of Medicine, 319,* 1022–1026.

Blount, R., Smith, A., & Frank, N. (in press). Preparation to undergo medical procedures. In A. J. Goreczny & M. Hersen (Eds.), *Handbook of pediatric and adolescent health psychology.* Boston: Allyn & Bacon.

Boivin, M. J., Davies, A. G., Mokili, J. K. L., Green, S. D. R., Giordani, B., & Cutting, W. A. M. (1995). A preliminary evaluation of the cognitive and motor effects of pediatric HIV infection in Zairian children. *Health Psychology, 14,* 13–21.

Bor, R., Miller, R., & Goldman, E. (1993). HIV/AIDS and the family: A review of research in the first decade. *Journal of Family Therapy, 15,* 187–204.

Bose, S., Moss, H. A., Brouwers, P., Pizzo, P., & Lorion, R. (1994). Psychologic adjustment of human immunodeficiency virus-infected school-age children. *Developmental and Behavioral Pediatrics, 15,* 26–33.

Brouwers, P., Belman, A. L., & Epstein, L. G. (1990). Central nervous system involvement: Manifestations and evaluation. In P. A. Pizzo & K. M. Wilfert (Eds.), *Pediatric AIDS: The challenge of HIV infection in infants, children, and adolescents* (pp. 318–335). Baltimore: Williams & Wilkins.

Burke, M., & Dawson, T. A. (1987). Temporary care foster parents: Motives and issues of separation and loss. *Child and Adolescent Social Work, 4,* 178–186.

Bussing, R., & Johnson, S. B. (1992). Psychosocial issues in hemophilia before and after the HIV crisis: A review of current research. *General Hospital Psychiatry, 14,* 387–403.

CDC. (1990). Update: Acquired immunodeficiency syndrome—United States. *MMWR, 39,* 81.

CDC. (1991). Working Group on PCP Prophylaxis in Children: Guidelines for prophylaxis against *Pneumocystis carinii* pneumonia for children infected with human immunodeficiency virus. *MMWR, 40,* 1–13.

CDC. (1993). HIV/AIDS Surveillance Report. U.S. Department of Health and Human Services, Atlanta.

CDC. (1994a). HIV/AIDS Surveillance Report. U.S. Department of Health and Human Services, Atlanta.

CDC. (1994b). Zidovudine for the prevention of HIV transmission from mother to infant. *MMWR, 43,* 285–287.

Chasnoff, I. J., Griffith, D. R., MacGregor, S., Dirkes, K., & Burns, K. A. (1989). Temporal patterns of cocaine use during pregnancy. *Journal of the American Medical Association, 261,* 1741–1744.

Cohen, F. L. (1994). Research on families and pediatric human immunodeficiency virus disease: A review and needed directions. *Developmental and Behavioral Pediatrics, 15,* 34–42.

Cohen, S. E., Mundy, T., Karassik, B., Lieb, L., Ludwig, D. D.,

& Ward, J. (1991). Neuropsychological functioning in human immunodeficiency virus type 1 seropositive children infected through neonatal blood transfusion. *Pediatrics, 88,* 58–68.

Cohon, J. D., & Cooper, B. A. B. (1993). A first look: Foster parents of medically complex, drug-exposed, and HIV+ infants. *Children and Youth Services Review, 15,* 105–130.

Condrini, A., Cattalan, C., Viero, F., Casella, S., Zampiron, M., & Laverda, A. M. (1989). Psychic development of children born to HIV infected Italian mothers. Fifth International Conference on AIDS. *Abstracts, 5,* 316.

Connor, E. M., Sperling, R. S., Gelber, R., Kiselev, P., Scott, W., O'Sullivan, M. J., VanDyke, R., Bey, M., Shearer, W., Jacobson, R. L., Jimenez, E., O'Neill, I. E., Bazin, B., elfraissy, J., Culnane, M., Coombs, R., Elkins, M., Moye, J., Stratton, P., & Balsley, J. (1994). Reduction of maternal–infant transmission of human immunodeficiency virus type 1 with zidovudine treatment. *New England Journal of Medicine, 331,* 1173–1180.

Dew, M. A., Ragini, M. V., & Nimorwicz, P. (1990). Infection with human immunodeficiency virus and vulnerability to psychiatric distress. *Archives of General Psychiatry, 47,* 737–744.

Eiser, C. (1985). *The psychology of childhood illness.* New York: Wiley.

Emery, R., & Forehand, R. (1994). Parental divorce and children's well-being: A focus on resiliency. In R. J. Haggerty, N. Garmezy, M. Rutter, & L. R. Sherrod (Eds.), *Stress, coping and development: Risk and resilience in children.* (pp. 64–99). London: Cambridge University Press.

European Collaborative Study. (1991). Children born to women with HIV-1 infection: Natural history and risk of transmission. *The Lancet, 337,* 253–260.

Forehand, R. (1993). Twenty years of research: Does it have practical implications for clinicians working with parents and children? *Clinical Psychologist, 46,* 169–176.

Forehand, R., & McMahon, R. (1981). *Helping the noncompliant child: A clinician's guide to parent training.* New York: Guilford Press.

Frank, S. J., Olmstead, C. L., Wagner, A. E., Laub, C. C., Freeark, K., Breitzer, G. M., & Peters, J. M. (1991). Child illness, the parenting alliance, and parenting stress. *Journal of Pediatric Psychology, 16,* 361–371.

Garmezy, N. (1991). Resiliency in children's adaptation to negative life events and stressed environments. *Pediatrics Annual, 20,* 459–466.

Gay, C. L., Armstrong, F. D., Cohen, D., Lai, S., Hardy, M. D., Swales, T. P., Morrow, C. J., & Scott, G. B. (1995). The effects of HIV or cognitive and motor development in children born to HIV− seropositive women with no reported drug use: Birth to 24 months. *Pediatrics, 96,* 1078–1082.

Hague, R. A., Mok, J. Y. Q., MacCallum, L., Burns, S., & Yap, P. L. (1991). *Do maternal factors influence the risk of vertical transmission of HIV?* VII International Conference on AIDS, Florence, Italy.

Havens, J. F., Whitaker, A. H., Feldman, J. F., & Ehrhardt, A. A. (1994). Psychiatric morbidity in school-age children with congenital human immunodeficiency virus infection: A pilot study. *Developmental and Behavioral Pediatrics, 15,* 18–25.

Herek, G. M., & Glunt, E. K. (1988). An epidemic of stigma: Public reactions to AIDS. *American Psychologist, 43,* 886–891.

Hoff, R., Berardi, V. P., Weiblen, B. J., Mahoney-Trout, L., Mitchell, M. L., & Grady, G. F. (1988). Seroprevalence of human immunodeficiency virus among childbearing women. *New England Journal of Medicine, 318,* 525–530.

Hutto, S. C. (1994). Pediatric HIV infection and AIDS: Medical issues. In R. A. Olson, L. L. Mullins, J. B. Gillman, & J. M. Chaney (Eds.), *Sourcebook of pediatric psychology* (pp. 218–236). Boston: Allyn & Bacon.

Indacochea, F. J., & Scott, G. B. (1992). HIV-1 infection and the acquired immunodeficiency syndrome in children. *Current Problems in Pediatrics, 3,* 166–204.

Jansen, J. K., & Ammann, A. J. (1994). Priorities in psychosocial research in pediatric human immunodeficiency virus infection. *Developmental and Behavioral Pediatrics, 15,* 3–4.

Jaret, P. (1986). Our immune system: The wars within. *National Geographic, 169,* 701–735.

Kohrman, A. F. (1991). Medical technology: Implications for health and social service providers. In N. J. Hochstadt & D. M. Yost (Eds.). *The medically complex child: The transition to home care* (pp. 3–13). New York: Harwood.

Krasinski, K., Borkowsky, W., & Holzman, R. S. (1989). Prognosis of human immunodeficiency virus infection in children and adolescents. *Pediatric Infectious Diseases Journal, 8,* 216–220.

Kurth, A. (1993). Reproductive issues, pregnancy and childbearing in HIV-infected women. In F. Cohen & J. Durhan (Eds.), *Women, children and HIV/AIDS* (pp. 115–123). Berlin: Springer.

Lask, B., & Fosson, A. (1989). *Childhood illness. The psychosomatic approach.* New York: Wiley.

Lewis, S. Y., Haiken, H. J., & Hoyt, L. G. (1994). Living beyond the odds: A psychosocial perspective on long-term survivors of pediatric human immunodeficiency virus infection. *Developmental and Behavioral Pediatrics, 15,* 12–17.

Markova, I., McDonald, K., & Forbes, C. (1980). Impact of hemophilia on child rearing practices and parental cooperation. *Journal of Child Psychology and Psychiatry and Allied Disciplines, 21,* 153–162.

Mason, P. J., & Olson, R. A. (1989). Psychosocial aspects of AIDS and HIV infection in pediatric hemophilia patients. In J. Seibert & R. Olson (Eds.), *Children, adolescents, and AIDS* (pp. 61–91). Lincoln: University of Nebraska Press.

Mason, P. J., Olson, R. A., Myers, J. G., Huszti, H. C., & Kenning, M. (1989). AIDS and hemophilia: Implications for families. *Journal of Pediatric Psychology, 14,* 341–355.

Mellins, C. A., & Ehrhardt, A. A. (1994). Families affected by pediatric acquired immunodeficiency syndrome: Sources of stress and coping. *Developmental and Behavioral Pediatrics, 15,* 54–60.

Melvin, D., & Sherr, L. (1993). The child in the family responding to AIDS and HIV. *AIDS Care, 5,* 35–42.

Mendez, H. (1992). Ambulatory care of HIV-seropositive infants and children. *Journal of Pediatrics, 119,* 14–17.

Mischel, M. H. (1981). The measurement of uncertainty in illness. *Nursing Research, 30,* 258–263.

Naeye, R. L., Blanc, W., Leblanc, W., & Khatamee, M. A. (1973). Fetal complications of maternal heroin addiction: Abnormal growth, infections, and episodes of stress. *Journal of Pediatrics, 83,* 1055–1061.

National Institute of Allergy and Infectious Diseases. (1994). *An overview: NIAID research on pediatric AIDS.* U.S. Department of Health and Human Services, Bethesda.

Neighbors, B., Forehand, R., & McVicar, D. (1993). Adolescents who are resilient to interparental conflict: What makes them different? *American Journal of Orthopsychiatry, 63,* 462–471.

Olson, R. A., Huszti, H. C., Mason, P. J., & Seibert, J. M. (1989). Pediatric AIDS/HIV infection: An emerging challenge to pediatric psychology. *Journal of Pediatric Psychology, 14,* 1–21.

Oxtoby, M. J. (1990). Perinatally acquired human immunodeficiency virus infection. *Pediatric Infectious Diseases Journal, 9,* 609–619.

Oxtoby, M. J. (1991). Perinatally acquired HIV infection. In P. A. Pizzo & C. Wilfert (Eds.), *Pediatric AIDS* (pp. 3–21). Baltimore: Williams & Wilkins.

Pizzo, P. A., Eddy, J., Falloon, J., Balsi, F. M., Murphy, R. F., Moss, H., Wolters, P., Brouwers, P., Jarosinski, P., Rubin, M., Broder, S., Yarchoan, R., Brunetti, M. M., Nusinoff-Lehrman, S., & Poplack, D. G. (1988). Effects of continuous intravenous infusion of zidovudine (AZT) in children with symptomatic HIV infection. *New England Journal of Medicine, 319,* 889–896.

Pizzo, P. A., Wilfert, C. M., & the Pediatric AIDS Siena Workshop II. (1995). Report of a Consensus Workshop, Siena, Italy, June 4–6, 1993: Markers and determinants of disease progression in children with HIV infection. *Journal of Acquired Immune Deficiency Syndromes and Human Retrovirology, 8,* 30–44.

Price, D. B., Inglese, C. M., Jacobs, J., Haller, J. O., Kramer, J., Hotson, G. C., Loh, J. P., Schlusselberg, D., Menez-Bautista, R., Rose, A. L., & Fikrig, S. (1988). Pediatric AIDS: Neuroradiologic and neurodevelopmental findings. *Pediatric Radiology, 18,* 445–448.

Rogers, M. F., Thomas, P. A., Starcher, E. T., Noa, M. C., Bush, T. J., & Jaffe, H. W. (1987). Acquired immunodeficiency syndrome in children: Report of the Centers for Disease Control National Surveillance, 1982 to 1985. *Pediatrics, 79,* 1008–1014.

Rutter, M. (1985). Resiliency in the face of adversity: Protective factors and resistance to psychiatric disorder. *British Journal of Psychiatry, 147,* 598–611.

Schmitt, B., Seeger, J., Kreuz, W., Enenkel, S., & Jacobi, G. (1991). Central nervous system involvement of children with HIV infection. *Developmental Medicine and Child Neurology, 33,* 535–540.

Scott, G. B., Hutto, C., Makuch, R. W., Mastrucci, M. T., O'Connor, T., Mitchell, C. D., Trapido, E. J., & Parks, W. P. (1989). Survival in children with perinatally acquired human immunodeficiency virus type 1 infection. *New England Journal of Medicine, 321,* 1791–1796.

Sherwen, L. N., & Boland, M. (1994). Overview of psychosocial research concerning pediatric human immunodeficiency virus infection. *Developmental and Behavioral Pediatrics, 15,* 5–11.

Siegel, L. J. (1993). Editorial: Children's understanding of AIDS: Implications for preventive interventions. *Journal of Pediatric Psychology, 18,* 173–176.

Stehbens, J. A. (1988). Childhood cancer. In D. K. Routh (Ed.), *Handbook of pediatric psychology* (pp. 135–161). New York: Guilford Press.

Taylor-Brown, S., & Kumetat, S. H. (1994a). Psychosocial aspects of pediatric human immunodeficiency virus and acquired immunodeficiency syndrome: Annotated literature review and call for research. *Developmental and Behavioral Pediatrics, 15,* 71–76.

Taylor-Brown, S., & Kumetat, S. H. (1994b). What we don't know: Children and human immunodeficiency virus. *Developmental and Behavioral Pediatrics, 15,* 77.

Walsh, M. E., & Bibace, R. (1991). Children's conceptions of AIDS: A developmental analysis. *Journal of Pediatric Psychology, 16,* 273–285.

WHO/Global Programme on AIDS. The HIV/AIDS pandemic: 1993 overview.

Weiner, L., Theut, S., Steinberg, S. M., Riekert, K. A., & Pizzo, P. A. (1994). The HIV-infected child: Parental responses and psychosocial implications. *American Journal of Orthopsychiatry, 64,* 485–492.

Wierson, M., & Forehand, R. (1994). Parent behavioral training for child noncompliance: Rationale, concepts and effectiveness. *Current Directions in Psychological Science, 3,* 146–150.

Wilfert, C. (1993). Pediatric AIDS: Part III: The natural history of HIV infection in children. *AIDS Clinical Care, 5,* 48, 50.

Wolters, P. L., Brouwers, P., Moss, H. A., & Pizzo, P. A. (1994). Adaptive behavior of children with symptomatic HIV infection before and after zidovudine therapy. *Journal of Pediatric Psychology, 19,* 47–61.

20

Intrafamilial Child Maltreatment

SANDRA T. AZAR, MONICA H. FERRARO, AND SUSAN J. BRETON

INTRODUCTION

Unlike the other disorders in this volume that are ostensibly nested within *individual children,* intrafamilial child maltreatment is considered a disorder nested in a *relationship.* To understand its impact, one must, therefore, examine it using a broader lens than is typical within other childhood disorders. It needs to be considered as occurring in the context of a more general breakdown in caregiver behavior that negatively influences both children's self system and the ecological context in which they develop. Developmental research has told us that children's outcomes evolve out of the multiple transactions between their characteristics and both caregiver adequacy and environmental factors that occur over time (Sameroff & Chandler, 1975). Child psychopathology as a result of maltreatment is more likely to occur when some continuous factor or set of factors is present that results in children "organizing" their world in a manner that is maladaptive. Thus, child abuse

and neglect can be viewed as heterogeneous events (e.g., in content, severity, chronicity, psychological meaning) whose impact encompass a continuum of responses. This fact makes both assessment and intervention more complex. Cognitive, behavioral, developmental, and family systems perspectives will be used to frame our discussion.

PHENOMENOLOGY

Consensus does not exist as to how maltreatment should be defined. Initial attempts at definition were legal and medical ones that were aimed at identification and prosecution. These focused narrowly on the intent of the perpetrator or the extent of physical consequences (e.g., broken bones). Such definitions, however, were not useful for treatment planning. As the emphasis shifted to intervention, maltreatment came to be seen as specific acts of omission or commission by perpetrators that are judged by a mixture of community values and professional expertise to be inappropriate or damaging (Garbarino & Giliam, 1980). Although such a definition is "socially mediated," it allows for a narrow versus a broad continuum in thinking

SANDRA T. AZAR, MONICA H. FERRARO, AND SUSAN J. BRETON • Frances L. Hiatt School of Psychology, Clark University, Worcester, Massachusetts 01610.

Handbook of Child Psychopathology, 3rd edition, edited by Ollendick & Hersen. Plenum Press, New York, 1998.

about impact (e.g., demonstrable harm versus endangerment) and encompasses a broad continuum of actions (e.g., from failure to supervise appropriately, to use of a gun or knife against). With more focus on child outcome, even broader definitions have emerged, including seeing maltreatment as part of a more general breakdown in caregiver capacities (Azar, Barnes, & Twentyman, 1988) or as part of a larger category of events labeled as *trauma* (Terr, 1991).

Four main types of maltreatment have emerged in the literature: physical abuse, sexual abuse, neglect, and emotional maltreatment. *Physical abuse* involves the use of aversive or inappropriate control strategies with a child (e.g., beatings, consistent use of coercive responses). *Neglect* is an act of omission of actions that leads to harm or endangerment of children's health or well-being, including a failure to provide minimal caregiving in the areas of medical care, education, nutrition, supervision, emotional contact, and safety, as well as providing inadequate environmental stimulation and structure (Wolfe, 1987). *Sexual abuse* has been defined in many ways, but definitions typically focus on the element of sexual exploitation (based on an inequality of power) involving anal, oral, genital, or breast contact between a child and another person (Cohen & Mannarino, 1993). As a high percentage of perpetrators tend to be people known to children, we will focus on intrafamilial abusers (e.g., fathers, stepfathers, other relatives). The hardest to define is *emotional abuse,* which has been seen as both central to all types of maltreatment and as occurring as a distinct entity. Such acts are ones that are psychologically damaging to the behavioral, cognitive, affective, or physical functioning of a child (Brassard, Germain, & Hart, 1987) (Table 1).

These four types often co-occur, and their interactive effect is not well understood. Clinically, other dimensions may also be important to consider. These include: severity and frequency/chronicity, the developmental period of a child's life in which maltreatment occurs, the

Table 1. Examples of Emotional Maltreatment

Rejection	A particular child in the family is scapegoated and is continually given feedback regarding his orher lack of worth.
Terrorizing	In sexual abuse, children are often threatened with harm if they tell anyone.
Isolating	Children are locked in closets for long periods or in basements for days.
Degrading	A child is continually called names and belittled even when he or she is doing well.
Missocializing	Adolescents may be encouraged to drink and smoke with parents or to shoplift items from stores to support the family.

number of perpetrators and their relationship to the child, and the nature of societal responses (e.g., foster care placements; a child's testifying in court against a parent) (Cicchetti & Barnett, 1991; Zuravin, 1991). One last factor discussed only recently is the meaning that the child takes from his or her experience (Azar & Bober, in press). Children may incorporate into schema regarding the self, others, and the world, elements of their maltreatment that are distorted and that influence their later functioning. Indeed, their view of the abuse may be the best predictor of outcome (McGee, Wolfe, Yuen, & Wilson, 1995).

Finally, maltreatment is also typically associated with a series of events, any one of which might "derail" development (e.g., poverty, domestic violence) or act in a compensatory way (e.g., nonperpetrator parent's supportive reaction to disclosure of sexual abuse).

DIAGNOSIS

Maltreatment may leave physical, social, and/or emotional "scars" that, for some children, have little in the way of observable consequences and for others, severely affect functioning. This continuum of impact and multidetermined outcomes needs to be considered carefully when making clinical decisions. Clinicians may be too ready to see such children as troubled and overlook their strengths, especially in sexual abuse (Vitulano, Lewis, Doran, Nordhaus, & Adnopoz, 1986).

Abusive parents and abused children exhibit a variety of disturbances that may not always reach the level of a diagnosis. A more useful way to think about "diagnosis" is to consider domains of functioning that might be *causal* to maltreatment in the parent, and might be *outcomes* in the child. Table 2 illustrates disturbances that have been observed.

There are five areas that may be considered high-probability candidates for intervention across types of abuse: interpersonal and emotional disturbances, cognitive disturbances, impulse control, stress coping, and anger control problems (Azar & Twentyman, 1986). In some cases, specific diagnostic difficulties may also need to be targeted as they may act as *setting events* or as *triggers* for abuse (e.g., parental drug abuse, child oppositional defiant disorder). Each of these areas will be discussed first for the parent and then for abused and neglected children. Finally, a systemic framework will be outlined for viewing cases during each era of childhood.

Disturbances in Abusive Parents

The most pervasive disturbance seen in abusive parents is a variety of *parenting skill deficits.* Abusive parents engage in fewer positive interactions with their children and less overall interaction. They also tend to use more negative, coercive, and rigid control tactics (Bousha & Twentyman, 1984; Burgess & Conger, 1978; Oldershaw, Walters, & Hall, 1986). Mothers who are at risk for physically abusing and/or neglecting their children also use explanation less when disciplining (Barnes & Azar, 1990; Trick-

ett & Kuczynski, 1986). Explanation is crucial for social development (e.g., empathy, perspective-taking).

Social cognitive problems have also been found (Azar, 1989; Milner, 1993). Physically abusive and neglectful parents have been shown to have poorer problem-solving ability in childrearing situations, to make more negative attributions to children, and to judge child misbehavior more harshly in some domains (Azar, Robinson, Hekimian, & Twentyman, 1984; Chilamkurti & Milner, 1993; Hansen, Pallotta, Tishelman, & Conaway, 1989; Larrance & Twentyman, 1983). They also appear to have more unrealistic expectations regarding what is appropriate child behavior (Azar et al., 1984; Azar & Rohrbeck, 1986) and may have subtle interpersonal discrimination problems that may cause them to be poor trackers of child behavior (Wahler & Dumas, 1989). These difficulties have been linked to more coercive and ineffective parenting responses (Barnes & Azar, 1990; Dix, Ruble, & Zambarano, 1989).

Although less work has been done with sexual abusers, they too appear to show cognitive distortions about children (e.g., seeing them as "wanting" the sexual contact; seeing themselves as "educating" children; Abel et al., 1989; Stermac & Segal, 1989) and problem-solving deficits (Hoagwood, 1990).

Contributing further to a negative developmental environment are parental skill deficits that prohibit regulating behavior both within and outside the family. Maltreaters appear to have *difficulties managing stress* and experience some events as more stressful than do nonabusive parents. For example, they show greater physiological arousal in response to both child-related stimuli (Frodi & Lamb, 1980; Hall & Hirschman, 1992; Wolfe, Fairbanks, Kelly, & Bradlyn, 1983) and non-child-related events (Casanova, Domanic, McCanne, & Milner, 1992). Physical abusers also appear to show *poorer ability to inhibit impulsive behavior* (Rohrbeck & Twentyman, 1986), and as a result, they may respond aggressively to behaviors that would not provoke

Table 2. Skill Deficits in Parents that May Increase the Risk of Abuse at Different Points in Children's Development and the Outcomes Observed among Abused Children and Adolescents

	Parent problem area	Child problem area
Infancy and toddlerhood	Insensitive and noncontingent responsiveness Poor ability to tolerate stresses such as prolonged crying, sleep problems, and feeding difficulties Failures to engage in behaviors that foster language, social, and emotional development Lack of attention to safety issues and health needs/knowledge deficit Expectancies that infants and toddlers are able to perspective take, are capable of intentional provoking behavior, and can provide the parent comfort Deficits in skills to comfort/soothe child, utilize distraction, redirection, and environmental management as a means to reduce aversive child behavior and manage child behavior	Attachment problems Health-related difficulties, such as undernourishment, low birth weight, prematurity, and physical trauma (e.g., shaken baby syndrome) Lags in toilet training, motor skills, speech, and language development, and socialization Anxiety Inappropriate sexual behavior Nightmares
Early and middle childhood	Inconsistent and indiscriminant use of discipline Overuse of physical stategies to manage behavior Lack of use of optimal socialization strategies (such as explanation) General lack of interaction A negative bias in overlabeling child behavior as evidence of misbehavior (even developmentally appropriate behavior) Poor ability to deal with stress of self-regulation problems in children (e.g., noncompliance) Unrealistic expectations of children's perspective-taking abilities, self-regulation skill, ability to place parental needs ahead of their own, to engage in self-care, and other household duties	High levels of noncompliance Developmental and academic problems Social cognitive difficulties (e.g., expression and recognition of affect; perspective-taking; empathy, social problem-solving) Heightened aggression Poor social skills Conduct problems; firesetting Social withdrawal Cognitive delays such as greater distractibility Inconsistent school attendance Fatigue Low self-esteem Difficulty trusting others Trauma/stress-related symptoms (regressed behavior) Poor conflict resolution skills
Adolescence	Failure to use age-appropriate child management strategies Excessive attempts to control Decreased ability to tolerate teenagers' moves toward autonomy Poor ability to deal with emerging sexuality Unrealistic expectations of taking on adult responsibilities	Overrepresented among runaways, delinquents, and truants Poor academic performance Poor stress/anger management skills Social skill and peer interaction problems Conduct problems Depression, suicidal, or self-injurious behavior

such responses in others. Similarly, sexual abusers tend to display a greater impulsivity within the sexual realm (e.g., dependence on pornography, compulsive masturbation; Kafka & Prentky, 1993).

A final area of disturbance is seen in the area of social support, and suggests *social skills deficits*. Social support provides parents with important buffers against stress (e.g., instrumental help, information, feedback). Physical abusers have smaller social support networks (Salzinger, Kaplan, & Artemyeff, 1983), tend to view themselves as more isolated (Newberger, Hampton, Marx, & White, 1986), and tend to overattribute responsibility for aversive behavior to others (Miller & Azar, 1996). Similarly, Kafka and Prentky (1993) found an elevated level of social phobia among sexual abusers. Thus, interpersonal difficulties may characterize all of these parents' social transactions.

Other problems, such as substance abuse (Famularo, Stone, Barnum, & Wharton, 1986), neurological problems (Elliot, 1988), and low intellectual functioning (Schilling & Schinke, 1984), have been cited as characterizing abusive and neglectful parents, but to date, the data supporting each are limited. Heightened stress has also been noted (e.g., divorce, domestic violence; Deblinger, Hathaway, Lippman, & Steer, 1993; MacFarlane, 1986), although all stressed parents do not engage in child abuse.

An intergenerational transmission of abuse has also been posited, although this link has been questioned (Widom, 1989). Recent estimates suggest that between 25 and 35% of maltreated children grow up to abuse their children (Kaufman & Zigler, 1987). Some reviews suggest that this is an overestimate or that it may vary by type of maltreatment (e.g., lower rates for neglect [Starr, MacLean, & Keating, 1991], higher rates for sexual abuse [Williams & Finkelhor, 1990]). Because abuse varies with other forms of family dysfunction, it may be that such histories are a "marker" variable, rather than causal. However, having such experiences may foster disturbed relationship patterns (e.g., "scripts"

for parenting; Azar, 1991a; Zeanah & Zeanah, 1989), placing the next generation at risk.

Disturbances among Abused and Neglected Children

Predicting outcomes seen in abused children and adolescents is very complex and no single pattern has been identified. A bidirectional interaction of several factors determines child outcome with both parent and child contributing to transactions that shape it (Azar et al., 1988; Cicchetti & Carlson, 1989; Parke & Collmer, 1975). Furthermore, outcome may relate not only to the maltreatment experience(s), but also to contextual factors associated with it (e.g., domestic violence, violent neighborhoods) and/or society's responses to it (e.g., foster care). For example, in one study, children with abuse histories reacted more strongly to adult interpersonal conflict (Hennessy, Rabideau, Cicchetti, & Cummings, 1994), suggesting these factors may combine to increase overall vulnerability. Finally, debate in the field varies between those trying to link specific outcomes to specific forms of maltreatment, to those arguing for the global impact of the stress produced, irrespective of type.

We will not resolve this question, but provide examples of both global problems observed among maltreated children and ones that may be more specific to particular types of abuse. Although each of the domains is discussed separately, they are intrinsically linked. For example, health issues may lead to attentional problems in school, resulting in lower academic performance.

Health-related difficulties found among maltreated children are often neglected in psychology reviews (Dubowitz, 1991). Consequences of physical abuse can include trauma, such as bruises, burns, and skeletal, head, and internal injuries (Pagelow, 1984). In sexual abuse, physical trauma may also occur (e.g., vaginal abrasions), as well as exposure to sexually transmitted disease (e.g., as many as 13% of sexually abused children evidence STDs; White, Loda, Ingram, & Pearson, 1983). Hormonal activity may also be affected, triggering premature onset of puberty (Trickett & Putnam, 1993).

Physical abuse can leave lasting effects (e.g., neuropsychological deficits, disabilities), resulting in need for further coping on the child's part (e.g., ongoing medical care, adjusting to a disability). These can also influence social interaction (e.g., dealing with the awkwardness of having burns stared at by peers). Although such extreme outcomes are more common in younger children, teenagers' health should not be ignored.

Neglected children may suffer the most physical consequences (e.g., resulting from undernourishment, lack of medical and dental care, as well as failures to monitor and supervise). Indeed, the majority of fatalities may be from neglect (e.g., mostly lack of supervision resulting in deaths from house fires or accidental poisoning) (Dubowitz, 1991). Failure to thrive can also result from neglect and can have long-term developmental outcomes. Finally, although causality is not clear, emotional abuse can produce physical complaints through chronic anxiety (e.g., stomachaches, headaches).

Developmental effects of maltreatment are numerous. Children must direct energy typically used for developmental growth into protection from abusive parents and for basic survival, resulting in multiple *lags in development* (e.g., language, motor skills; Azar & Twentyman, 1986; Martin, 1976).

Such children show *cognitive delays* and *academic difficulties* (Eckenrode, Laird, & Doris, 1993; Trickett, McBride-Chang, & Putnam, 1994) and *problems in emotional development,* including lower self-esteem, disturbances in healthy conceptions of self, mood, trust in others, and in basic emotional skills (e.g., recognition and expression of emotion) (Azar et al., 1988; Kendall-Tackett, Williams, & Finkelhor, 1993; Wolfe, 1987). In the extreme, some children, especially emotionally and sexually abused ones, show evidence of *posttraumatic stress disorder* (e.g., sleep problems, exaggerated startle re-

sponse, panic, hypervigilance, and developmental regressions [e.g., clinging behavior]; Terr, 1991).

Maltreated children experience a significant amount of stress, which may be chronic and have an impact on the *development of stress management skills and anger control.* Not only may such children fail to learn adaptive coping skills from their parents, they may also develop coping strategies that work in their maladaptive home environments (e.g., dissociation), but that do not serve them well outside the family.

Numerous *behavioral self-regulation difficulties,* such as overly compliant or aggressive, demanding, and rageful behaviors, are shown by maltreated children (Fantuzzo, 1990; Widom, 1989). Overly compliant behavior may help physically abused children avoid confrontations with parents. On the other hand, the aggressive behavior may be caused by continual frustration of their needs and the modeling of an aggressive response to frustration. Sexually abused children also exhibit inappropriate sexual and regressed behavior which may be specific to their experience (Kendall-Tackett et al., 1993). Clearly, these regulation difficulties confuse others (e.g., teachers, peers) and lead to adjustment problems.

Social development problems have also been prominent. Types of social problems may vary with development. Attachment difficulties and heightened unresponsiveness have been observed in infants and toddlers (Bee, Disbrow, Johnson-Crowley, & Barnard; 1981; Carlson, Cicchetti, Barnett, & Braunwald, 1989; Crittenden, 1985), whereas poor social skills (e.g., empathy, perspective-taking, poor problem-solving) have been found among older children (Barahal, Waterman, & Martin, 1981; George & Main, 1980; Haskett, 1990).

A study by Salzinger, Kaplan, Pelcovitz, Samit, and Krieger (1984) suggests that physically abused children may evidence cognitive distortions around interpersonal relationships. Maltreated 8- to 12-year-olds they studied identified peers who did not even like them as being "friends." Noteworthy, however, in this study was the fact that 13 of the 87 abused children were rated as popular with peers, reinforcing the idea that some children appear to have resilience. Farber and Egeland (1987) suggested that such resiliency may stem from having alternative social support during development or from an early period of competency that acts as a foundation for later adjustment.

Systemic Disturbances in the Maltreating Family across Childhood and Adolescence

Maltreatment develops against the backdrop of the tasks all families face across children's development and this needs to be taken into consideration clinically (Azar & Siegel, 1990). For example, maltreatment that emerges in adolescence may be related to unique cues that emerge during this period (e.g., developing sexuality, independence), whereas physical abuse that occurs in the late preschool years and re-emerges in adolescence may be related to the tensions of increasing autonomy demands made by the children during both of these periods. In our discussion of a systemic view, it must be pointed out that less is known about transactions in sexually abusive families and our discussion here will be more speculative.

In the *parenting of infants and toddlers,* the transition to parenthood becomes a relevant issue. The demands of infants are great and the birth of children may uncover preexisting interpersonal inadequacies. Parents at risk for maltreatment appear to begin their parenting earlier (National Research Council, 1993). Many disturbances in family interaction have been documented in abusive families in this age period (e.g., insensitive caregiving) that may set the stage for later difficulties. Social isolation during this highly stressful period of parenting may also contribute further to risk.

Prematurity, poor nutrition, and inadequate prenatal care may increase children's caretaking needs during this period. As they become more mobile, environmental risks and lack of supervision may result in injuries. Triggers for physical abuse may include: prolonged crying, feeding and sleeping problems, and soiling (Herrenkohl, Herrenkohl, & Egolf, 1983).

Parents may mistakenly believe that babies need discipline and that shaking them is better than striking them. This can result in shaken baby syndrome, where infants suffer from intracranial bleeding, brain swelling, or damage to the blood vessels of the eyes.

Social relationship disturbances found in some abused children may have their roots in this early period (i.e., attachment problems) (Azar et al., 1988; Cicchetti, 1989). Infants and toddlers may come to experience their world as one in which they cannot depend on much (e.g., food, safety, nurturance), affecting their basic trust of others.

Increases in children's abilities to operate autonomously, which occur during the *preschool and school-age years,* may result in behaviors that could be perceived by all parents as oppositional. To provide for development of children's autonomy and self-regulation that begin to develop in this period, parents need child management and social cognitive skills, both of which are areas of deficit for maltreaters. Parents who have low frustration tolerance or attribute this behavior as intended to annoy them may be particularly vulnerable to physical abuse during this period.

Heightened autonomy seen during middle childhood may also mislead the neglectful parent to expect the child to engage in more self-care and parental need fulfillment (e.g., being left home alone, caring for siblings). Injuries caused by house fires where children are unsupervised may occur during this period (Dubowitz, 1991). Poor nutrition and fatigue related to a lack of a structured routine may influence school performance and social behavior.

Sexual abuse of girls is usually initiated during this period. Ages 4 to 9 are especially high-risk years. It has been suggested that such increased risk to young girls may be the result of perpetrators' exploitation of the desire to please adults present during this period (Gelinas, 1983).

The adolescent years have not received much attention in the abuse literature, except for sexual abuse. Rates of *identified* maltreatment appear lower during this period, but in reality may be just as high. Maltreated children may exhibit behavior that fosters labeling them during this period (e.g., as runaways, truant, delinquent, or oppositional defiant).

Triggers for physical abuse during adolescence may have to do with teenagers shifting some of their allegiance to peers and the need for parents to adjust to emerging sexuality. The socially isolated parent may be particularly at risk during this period. Adolescents' focus on identity formation may make them particularly susceptible to the effects of emotional maltreatment (e.g., name calling and belittling). Neglect may take different forms during adolescence. Educational neglect (truancy), poor nutrition, and lack of supervision may be especially prominent and may influence long-term health and adjustment. Also, lack of supervision may make teenagers more vulnerable to sexual abuse. It has been suggested that perpetrators may be more likely to use force during this period (Gelinas, 1983), which may result in more trauma symptoms.

In summary, it is crucial to take a systemic/developmental view of families in case formulation. Intervention targets are highly dependent not only on the parent's stage of adult development and mastery of the parenting tasks here, but also on the stage-salient tasks the child must accomplish.

ETIOLOGY

Theories of maltreatment have varied on a number of different dimensions (Azar, 1991b). First, each has defined it differently (e.g., from a narrow focus on abuse as aggression, to viewing it as part of a larger category of social relational problems). Second, some models have attempted to explain all types of maltreatment, whereas others have addressed only one type. For example, incest has been seen as separate from other forms of abuse or other sexual offenses (e.g., rape) or combined with these other disturbances. Placement of causality has also varied, stemming from a defect within the perpetrator to the result of larger societal values (e.g., condoning of violence). It should be noted that little attention has been paid to theories explaining neglect.

Theories of maltreatment have shifted from single-cause models (e.g., stress) to more complex, multiple-cause frameworks (e.g., lists of possible causes) to more recent integrated perspectives (e.g., social ecological models of abuse). These integrated approaches hold the most promise for intervention development. A sampling of early theories and more recent ones is given in the hope of providing potential clinical frameworks.

Early models focused on single causes in perpetrators (e.g., personality problems, psychopathology; Johnson & Morse, 1968; Lanyon, 1986; Melnick & Hurley, 1969); the child (e.g., heightened care needs); the parent–child relationship (e.g., bonding failure; Klaus & Kennell, 1982); or the sociological/sociocultural context (e.g., stress [Garbarino, 1976], society's validation of use of violence [Gil, 1970], male dominance [Herman, 1981]). Single factors, however, have proved to be inadequate explanations.

Social-situational models began to be posited, but these were still not specified enough to foster targeted interventions. These approaches argue that individual and social contextual factors combine to produce abuse. The most comprehensive framework is Belsky's (1980) social ecological model. He posited four levels of influence that may affect the probability of abuse's occurrence. These levels are: individual characteristics (e.g., parental IQ), aspects of the family (e.g., marital satisfaction), forces within the community (e.g., poverty), and cultural factors (e.g., attitudes toward corporal punishment). Cicchetti and Rizley (1981) further argued that whether these factors are enduring or more transient would affect children's outcome.

As social learning theorists entered the field,

models that focused on skill deficits in perpetrators appeared. Numerous deficits have been posited in maltreating parents (Azar & Twentyman, 1986; Williams & Finkelhor, 1990). For example, sexual abusers have been seen as socially inept, having difficulties in empathy and cognitive distortions regarding children and sexual behavior (Williams & Finkelhor, 1990).

Integrated models have recently emerged that are more specified and hold promise for developing more focused interventions. These models, with some exceptions, have focused on one type of maltreatment and have either had a developmental or social learning theory foundation.

One such model is that of Wolfe (Wolfe, 1987; Wolfe, Kaufman, Aragona, & Sandler, 1981), which focuses on development of aggressive behavior. His view posits that abuse results from parental overreliance on coercive processes of child management that over time must escalate in order to produce the same level of child compliance. This framework also posits stages in the development of abusive patterns, contextual factors that hasten the process, and interventions that might reduce risk.

Taking a broader focus, Azar (1986, 1989) posited that physically and emotionally abusive and neglectful parents tend to exhibit skill deficits and cognitive disturbances in areas necessary for optimal parenting, with abuse or neglect merely the most visible evidence of dysfunction. These factors include cognitive disturbances, such as unrealistic expectations regarding age-appropriate responses (e.g., children should care for their parents' needs) and poor problem-solving (e.g., inflexibility, a limited childrearing repertoire). When children inevitably violate parents' expectations, these parents may develop a negative attributional bias toward them (e.g., thinking the child is intentionally misbehaving). Over time this would lead to increased frustration in parents. These same disturbances also have implications for development of children more generally. Disparity between parents' expectancies as to their children's capacities and the true abilities of their children, could lead to responses that would not

support children's developmental needs. Other deficits (e.g., poor impulse control, stress and anger management difficulties, poor social skills) may combine to increase further the risk of abuse, as well as foster a context where development is hampered (e.g., poor social supports to the family, financial problems). Similar skill deficits and cognitive disturbances appear to characterize sexual abusers (Abel et al., 1989), but have not yet been incorporated into this model.

Recent models have also emerged focusing exclusively on specific disturbances seen in children. Attachment theory has been invoked as an explanation of the social problems of abused children (i.e., abuse leading to insecure or disorganized attachment style; Crittenden & Ainsworth, 1989). Attempting to explain PTSD symptoms, abuse has been seen as a type of trauma, in which symptoms occur when children's typical coping capacities are exceeded and coping responses are employed that will not serve them well over time (e.g., dissociation) (Terr, 1991).

Finally, recent descriptions of abuse view it as a heterogeneous event, associated with multiple stressors that may in some cases overshadow its impact (e.g., separations and losses related to foster placement) or combine to produce negative child outcomes (Azar & Bober, in press). This may foster the growth of more complex theories. For example, Spaccarelli (1994) proposed a framework to explain the impact of sexual abuse that focuses on the children's cognitive response (e.g., their appraisal of the self as damaged), as well as responses within the parent–child dyad and the community.

Each of the models described has a different goal and might be applied in different clinical situations. Single-factor models that focus attention on parental deficits have utility in individual therapy with parents, whereas ones focusing on the context of maltreatment and on the multiple contributory factors may direct clinicians toward the use of specific external resources to help the family change (e.g., financial support to reduce economic stress, vocational help). The integrative models provide frameworks for working with the parent–child dyad and the family as a whole.

EPIDEMIOLOGY

Because the pattern of abuse varies depending on the definition used and on the observer, discussing epidemiology with any certainty is difficult. Official records (i.e., Child Protective Service [CPS] data) typically provide lower figures than community surveys. Moreover, both are subject to bias. Abuse is often a private event and, as such, true incidence may remain unknown.

Based on a survey of the 50 states, almost 2.9 million reports of child maltreatment were investigated by CPS agencies in 1993 (NCCAN, 1993), suggesting that 43 per 1000 children are affected. Primary reporters are professionals (educators, law enforcement, medical professionals, social service staff). Of the reports, approximately 38% are substantiated after being investigated, translating to 1,018,692 children in 1993 as victims. The largest number of these cases (49%) were substantiated for neglect, with 24% physically abused, 14% sexually abused, 7% medical neglect and emotional abuse, and about 15% victims of other forms of maltreatment (e.g., congenital drug addiction, abandonment). Many victims encounter more than one form.

Although maltreatment occurs at all ages, younger children are more likely to appear in the CPS caseloads. In community surveys, however, teens are more equally represented (Berkowitz & Sedlak, 1993; Wauchope & Straus, 1989). Although children's gender does not relate to reported neglect in state survey data, rates appear to decrease generally with age, regardless of sex. For sexual abuse, however, females are twice as likely as males to be victims in identified samples. It may be that males are just less likely to report sexual abuse because of the social stigma attached. For physical abuse, gender and age interact. Under the age of 12, males are more likely than females to be physically abused, whereas for victims 12 and older, the reverse is true.

Although subject to reporting biases (Azar & Benjet, 1994; Hampton & Newberger, 1985), maltreatment appears to vary by socioeconomic status (Pelton, 1978), ethnicity (Lauderdale, Valiunas, & Anderson, 1980; Long, 1986), and race (Long, 1986). Effects of abuse may be exacerbated for those who also experience racial and ethnic discrimination.

Some research suggests that family structure and size may also be important factors. Presence of a stepfather, for example, may double a girl's vulnerability for sexual abuse (Finkelhor & Baron, 1986).

Once maltreatment is identified, recidivism appears to be high (e.g., 20 to 70%; Hansen, Steffy, & Gauthier, 1993; Williams, 1983). As most estimates are based on treated samples, actual rates may be much higher.

ASSESSMENT

Given heterogeneity of parental deficits and child outcomes, providing a single assessment strategy is difficult. Our discussion above, however, suggests areas that commonly require attention. Because evaluations often involve the courts, unique assessment issues occur. Detailing these special problems is beyond the scope of this chapter, but will be outlined briefly below (for further information see Azar, 1992; Melton, Petrila, Poythress, & Slobogin, 1987).

There is little empirical guidance for deciding on assessment strategies. A multidisciplinary approach is useful (Azar & Wolfe, 1989; Hansen & Warner, 1992), including medical, behavioral, neurological, educational, and speech evaluations with children, as well as determinations of parents' behavioral strengths and weaknesses. For children out of parental custody, the resources of foster placements should also be examined.

Four assessment goals have been highlighted (Azar & Wolfe, 1989). First, immediate child risk must be determined. In cases where children are still in parental custody, their removal or that of the perpetrator may be necessary to provide safety and allow therapy to proceed. Although violence prediction is controversial, evaluating level of risk may have some utility (Grisso & Appelbaum, 1992). Some instruments exist for examining physical abuse potential (e.g., Child Abuse Potential Inventory; Milner, 1986, 1989), although they must be used cautiously as their validity is limited. Records from the school and social services involved with the family may provide invaluable information for beginning intervention and determining risk. For example, abuse that occurs at the end of each month may indicate economic triggers for the maltreatment, whereas abuse at the beginning of months, when AFDC payments are made, may reflect alcohol or drug problems.

Second, both functioning of individual family members and the family as a system in a larger community should be examined. Traditional cognitive, academic, and personality evaluations of the parent and child (e.g., the Minnesota Multiphasic Personality Inventory-2; Butcher, Dahlstrom, Graham, Tellegen, & Kaemmer, 1989) may help to rule out psychiatric disturbances, as well as obstacles to treatment. Screening for substance abuse might also be done (e.g., Michigan Alcohol Screening Test; Selzer, Vinokur, & vanRooijen, 1975). Physical and neurological examinations might also be helpful as head injuries and neurological disturbances have been linked with aggression (Elliot, 1988).

The McMaster model of family functioning may serve as a useful framework for structuring the systems assessment (Epstein, Bishop, & Baldwin, 1982). This model argues there are three levels of tasks that families must accomplish: (1) basic tasks, which involve the fundamental needs of survival (e.g., food, shelter); (2) developmental tasks, which involve adjusting to the shifting development needs of the family members and engaging in actions that foster developmental progress; and (3) emergency tasks, which involve the family's capacity

to handle emergency situations. Unlike most families, for whom mastery of the basic tasks is a given, maltreating families, especially neglectful ones, often have difficulties in all three areas. Six domains of family functioning are required to master these tasks: problem-solving, behavioral control, affective responsiveness, affective involvement, communication, and adequate distribution of family roles. Again, maltreating families may have disturbances in all of these areas. Measures of the family context both factually and as perceived by the parent are also crucial. Assessments of environmental stress and social support should include both quantity and quality.

The third goal of the assessment is to assess parental responses to childrearing needs (Azar & Wolfe, 1989). With physical abuse, in addition to the influence of *parental psychological functioning,* and *situational stressors,* there is a strong link between the abuse and events that, in some manner, involve the child (e.g., discipline situations; Wolfe, 1985). Assessment of parent–child interaction should include both self-report and observations. Structured observational assessments (e.g., situations where children must comply with parental commands, such as picking up toys, doing homework) that place stress on the parent–child interaction are most useful (Mash, 1991). Particular attention should be paid to affect expression. Detailed parental family background information may help provide ideas regarding past obstacles to learning new parenting strategies and potential resistances to intervention. Children's developmental history may uncover antecedents to maltreatment. For example, triggers for abuse that occur in developmental periods of children's increasing autonomy may differ for incidents occurring around the emergence of illnesses or parental concurrent trauma (e.g., sexual abuse has been linked to domestic violence; Deblinger et al., 1993).

Cognitive and behavioral skills assessments should be conducted with both the parent and child(ren). For the parent, the skill areas outlined earlier may be assessed through struc-

Table 3. Sample Items from the Parent Opinion Questionnaire

Domain	Sample item
Self-Care	Most of the time a 4-year-old can choose the right clothing for the weather and get him- or herself off to school.
Family Responsibility & Care of Siblings	An older daughter, 12 years old, could reasonably be expected to discipline younger brothers and sisters.
Leaving Children Alone	It's OK to leave a 3-year-old, who is soundly sleeping in a bed, alone in a house or apartment while the parent walks a friend to the corner bus stop.
Help & Affection to Parents	Parents can expect infants to always show them love and affection.
Proper Behavior and Feelings	Most often a 3-year-old will know how to play quietly for longer periods of time when his or her mother is not feeling well.
Punishment	It's good for a parent to set a 4-year-old on the toilet for an hour after the child messed up his pants.

tured interviews or paper-and-pencil measures. Although well-validated paper-and-pencil measures of parenting competency have not been developed (Grisso, 1986), some measures exist for selected skill areas (e.g., parent problem-solving skills [Hansen et al., 1989; Wasik, Bryant, & Fishbein, 1981], anger inventories [Novaco, 1975]). Cognitively based problems have also begun to receive some attention. For example, to assess parental unrealistic expectations regarding appropriate behavior in children, the Parent Opinion Questionnaire has been found to distinguish abusive and neglectful mothers from controls (Table 3; Azar et al., 1984; Azar & Rohrbeck, 1986). The Adult/Adolescent Parenting Inventory (Bavolek, 1984) has been used to measure parenting attitudes in four areas: parental expectations of the child, empathy toward children's needs, belief in the value of physical punishment, and parent–child role reversal. Thought listing strategies can also be helpful to solicit cognitions (Interpersonal Process Recall; Elliott, 1986). Table 4 lists common narratives suggesting cognitive problems.

Neglect issues deserve special consideration, although fewer scales are available. Family resource scales have begun to emerge (Dunst, 1986; Magura & Moses, 1986), as well as rating scales of home cleanliness (Rosenfield-Schlicter et al., 1983; Watson-Perczel, Lutzker, Greene, & McGimpsey, 1988), safety (e.g., Home Accident Prevention Inventory; Tertinger, Greene, & Lutzker, 1984), and health (Magura & Moses, 1986).

In conducting all evaluations, consideration needs to be given to variation in cultural practices (Azar & Benjet, 1994). For example, high levels of parental control may be seen negatively in one culture, but be seen as a sign of caring and stability in another. Knowledge of the culture may also influence the interpretation of social cues. For example, a child's turning his or her eyes downward when speaking to an adult family member may be mistakenly seen as fear, when it may in fact be a sign of respect.

A final goal should be an assessment of children's special needs. Children's skills and specific contextual stresses might be examined both directly and through parents' and others' reports (e.g., teachers). Instruments such as the Child Behavioral Checklist (CBCL; Achenbach & Edelbrock, 1983) or the Eyberg Child Behavioral Inventory (Eyberg & Ross, 1978) can provide insight into the parenting difficulties and how, if at all, these child behaviors are manifested in the school setting. Abusive parents may negatively distort when assessing their children, making independent raters crucial. For older children, self-report instruments of symptoms may also be administered (see other chapters in this volume).

Nonperpetrator parental reports of child PTSD symptoms in sexual abuse cases can also

Table 4. Phrases in Parents' Narratives that May Signal the Need for Cognitive Work

Phrase	Example statements	Distorted underlying assumption/expectation/cognitive problem
"He/she knows"	He knew I was tired. He knows his father had a bad day. She knows I don't let her do that.	Assumption of mindreading
A string of personality-based comments	He's a sneak. She's a sneak.	Stable negative internal attributions
Evidence of a power struggle	She thinks she's boss! I can't let her get away with this! He thinks he can put one over on me!	Low self-efficacy
Overly personalized explanations of causality with strong language	He knew it would get to me. He knew people were watching and he did it anyway. She was trying to destroy me.	Misattributions
Self-deprecatory statements	He must think I'm stupid. She must really think I'm dumb!	Negative self-schema
Explanations that are similar to descriptions of others in the parent's life	He's just like his father—no good! She looks at me just like my mother did when I did something wrong. When she does that, she reminds me of me.	Discrimination failure

be solicited using items from the CBCL (CBCL-PTSD; Wolfe, Gentile, & Wolfe, 1989) or instruments such as the Impact of Event PTSD Symptom Questionnaire (Horowitz, 1986), PTSD Reaction Index (Pynoos et al., 1987), or Child Dissociative Checklist (Bernstein & Putnam, 1986). Some measures can also be given to older children (e.g., the PTSD Reaction Index; Pynoos et al., 1987).

Finally, conducting evaluations useful to legal proceedings requires special skills and should not be undertaken lightly (see Azar, 1992; Azar & Benjet, 1994). Expert testimony is often solicited in such cases (especially sexual abuse) and requires a knowledge of both legal criteria and measurement. Special techniques and knowledge may be needed (e.g., use of anatomically correct dolls). The literature is just beginning to develop in this area.

TREATMENT

In discussing treatment, our primary focus will be on perpetrators. No amount of child treatment may be entirely effective unless parental behaviors change. Although the literature is very limited, special issues in treating victims of abuse will be highlighted and promising approaches discussed.

Empirically based treatment guidelines cannot be made. Large-scale clinical trials have yet to be conducted in this field. Based on the small literature presently available, however, social learning theory-based interventions and lay self-help groups have shown the most promise (Berkeley Planning Associates, 1978; Daro, 1988). Traditional psychotherapy appears to be less useful. The former will, therefore, be emphasized in our review.

Treatment of Parents

Given the immediate risks involved to children, interventions with maltreating families may initially target improving parenting skills and decreasing aggressive responses (e.g., increasing responsiveness, use of positive management strategies, communication), stress management, anger control capacities, and cognitively based strategies (e.g., problem-solving, more positively or neutrally toned interpretations of children's behavior).

Outcome work with physically abusive parents of preschoolers and school-age children has typically included some sort of package approach targeting multiple areas. For example, Wolfe, Sandler, and Kaufman (1981) found group treatment that targeted child management skills, stress coping strategies, anger control, and developmental knowledge to be effective. In another effort of this sort, Egan (1983) found that stress management training produced changes in parents' feelings, whereas child management training resulted in positive changes in parental skills. A final comparative study with physically abusive and neglectful parents of preschoolers compared insight-oriented group therapy (with supportive home visiting adjunct work) to cognitive-behavioral group treatment. The latter included cognitive-behavioral home visiting adjuncts and employed a package similar to that of Wolfe, Sandler, and Kaufman (1981) described above, with the addition of problem-solving training and cognitive restructuring of maladaptive parenting expectations. Both forms of treatment produced positive changes in parental behavior in the home and in caseworker reports of parenting problems compared with wait listed controls, but only the cognitive-behavioral condition had no recidivism at 1-year follow-up (Azar, 1989; Azar & Twentyman, 1984).

Single case design studies have dealt with specific triggers for abuse (e.g., migraines, marital distress, low recreation time, low tolerance for infant crying; Campbell, O'Brien, Bickett, & Lutzker, 1983; Lutzker & Rice, 1984) and have shown effectiveness for cognitive and behavioral strategies.

Some efforts at larger-scale community-based interventions have been attempted using social learning theory principles with mixed results. Szykula and Fleischman (1985) found that individual parent training reduced out-of-home placements, but failed to be effective with more difficult families.

Less formal work with abusers has occurred in self-help settings, such as Parents Anonymous. Such groups appear to be helpful, are low cost, and build natural support systems for parents (National Research Council, 1993).

Preventive interventions with at-risk parents and with cases involving low-level physical abuse and/or neglect may target a broader array of problem areas and be more comprehensive. Areas that may act to support parenting can be addressed (e.g., health, vocational help, marital work). The work of Olds and his colleagues is notable here (Olds, 1989; Olds, Henderson, Chamberlin, & Tatelbaum, 1986).

Less work has been done in neglect. Single case design studies have included work aimed at improving nutrition using tokens and reinforcement strategies (e.g., meal planning, budgeting; Sarber, Halasz, Messmer, Bickett, & Lutzker, 1983), responding to children's medical illnesses (Delgado & Lutzker, 1985), and improving home safety (Tertinger et al., 1984).

Treatment work with sexual abusers has been less successful. Cognitive-behavioral skills training with sexually abusive men has been suggested (e.g., altering sexual preferences, modifying social incompetence, and changing distorted cognitions). Relapse prevention procedures may also be crucial. Such strategies have produced reductions in rates of recidivism from 64% to 25% for periods of up to 4 years (Marshall, Laws, & Barbaree, 1990). Although promising, findings are limited and need to be viewed cautiously. Nonperpetrator parents and their abused children's PTSD symptoms have also been targeted for treatment (e.g., increasing parental support of children and decreasing behaviors that may maintain symptoms; increasing child stress coping, education, prevention skills training, and gradual exposure) (Deblinger, McLeer, & Henry, 1990).

Regardless of strategy or type of maltreatment, it has been argued that given their social isolation, group work may be especially useful for maltreating parents. Some risks, however, may occur in such work (e.g., interpersonal skills deficits negatively affecting group process, modeling of inappropriate responses of other group members). To monitor child safety, it is crucial that some individual work with children and/or the family as a whole occur concurrently with group treatment (e.g., adjunct home visiting, careful child protective agency monitoring). The sequencing of material presented in cases of physical abuse is also important, selecting as the first areas of concern content that will improve parents' mood state and decrease stress level and introducing more demanding material only after parents feel they have mastery over these skills.

A final note of caution is offered regarding treatment with maltreating parents. Work is often very slow and can be very taxing. Resistance to advice, compliance issues, and attendance may need to be addressed (e.g., use of incentives, through problem-solving). As with parents, therapists need to set achievable goals for themselves and to monitor their own stress levels carefully.

Treatment with Children

Because of individual differences in victims' symptoms, a single treatment approach is difficult to describe. Treatment studies are almost nonexistent. Our discussion will, therefore, focus primarily on the special issues and adaptations required in work with this population.

The initial kinds of "treatments" that have been used with abuse and neglect victims include: therapeutic day care and foster care to provide safety and fostering of developmental skills (Ayoub, 1991; Culp, Heide, & Richardson, 1987). Recently, there have also been a few published studies on behavioral skills training (e.g., social skills; Fantuzzo et al., 1988) and interventions dealing with PTSD symptoms (Deblinger et al., 1990). Fantuzzo and colleagues (1988), for example, carried out studies focusing on the use of peer and teacher prompting techniques to improve the social skills of abused preschoolers. Interestingly, perhaps because of victims' relationship history with adults, peer treat-

ment agents have been found to be superior to teachers. In work with children evidencing PTSD, Lipovsky (1991) emphasized education, facilitation of emotional expression, anxiety control, and controlled exposure to memories. Stress management, anger control training, and work on their academic performance may also be useful. Specific work with children experiencing neglect has not occurred.

A number of issues must be considered in doing child treatment. First, safety should be foremost in therapists' minds. Therapy will be of little use if the child must continue to devote energy to concerns regarding harm. If the child remains in parental custody, concurrent work with parents should be required. Concurrent work with foster or adoptive parents may also be useful to help them cope with the children's response to their past maltreatment.

Second, although heterogeneity of child problems seen makes it difficult to suggest high-priority treatment targets, reduction of aversive child behaviors (e.g., being oppositional, aggression, wetting the bed) that may act as triggers for maltreatment might be the first order of business. Efforts should then be directed to increasing adaptive behaviors (e.g., social skills). High valence trauma symptoms (e.g., dissociation) may also be a high priority, as these may interfere most with overall functioning.

The psychological maltreatment (e.g., exploitation, humiliation) that often accompanies abuse gives rise to a number of common themes in therapy to which therapists need to be sensitive. These would include issues of trust, anticipation of rejection, feelings of loss, and fear of adults.

Some *primary prevention* efforts have been directed at children. These have been of two types: ones teaching children how to avoid sexual abuse by others (see Miller-Perrin & Wurtele, 1988, for a review) and ones directed at decreasing violence (Hammond & Yung, 1991). The former is mainly aimed at preventing sexual abuse, but the skills taught have implications for prevention of physical abuse as well (e.g., assertiveness, problem-solving).

CASE STUDY[1]

Dottie was a 32-year-old single welfare mother of three children: Sara (age 15), Jennifer (age 11) and Jeffrey (age 5). Frank, the father of Jennifer, died of a heart attack 10 years ago. Gene, Dottie's current boyfriend, is Jeffrey's father and an alcoholic. The family had multiple past reports of physical abuse and neglect, including: (1) Frank's beating the girls with a belt, (2) both parents' neglect as a result of alcohol abuse, exemplified by leaving the girls home alone while they went to bars, and (3) Dottie's failure to get Jeffrey to school on a regular basis and her hitting Sara with a ruler, leaving visible welts on her legs.

At the time Dottie came in for treatment, she and Gene were still occasionally seeing each other, but they argued frequently. At times, their disputes became physical and involved the children. Dottie often took her frustration out on them, blaming them for "getting her into trouble" with Gene. Although her drinking had abated somewhat after Frank's death, her parenting difficulties remained. Related in part to an increasing financial burden, social isolation, and mounting interpersonal stress, Dottie often became irritable with the children. She believed they were more capable of caring for themselves than they actually were. Dottie was also alienated from her relatives, who frequently found fault with her parenting and housekeeping, often blaming Dottie for the children's misbehavior. She frequently became inappropriate and coercive in her parenting, especially under stress, and received little support from Gene.

Family and Parent Assessment

Jeffrey's kindergarten teacher filed a child neglect report in response to his frequent absences and aggressive behavior. An assessment was conducted by child protective services in two home visits for observations of the family, and more formal evaluations were done by a clinical psychologist.

A systems-based evaluation indicated that Dottie was generally able to meet the basic needs of the family, as she managed housing, food, and clothing for her children on her welfare check. Assessment, however, showed evidence that the family had difficulties with developmental tasks. Dottie failed to attend to her children's age-appropriate needs for supervision. She was inconsistent in her discipline, often threatening punishment and not following through, and at times resorting to physical strategies. Dottie also failed to acknowledge (or praise) her children's social and academic accomplishments. Other elements of the family life were chaotic. Mealtimes were unpredictable and often lacked nutrition. She did not enforce bedtimes (e.g., the children stayed up very late watching television and went to school tired). Also, fearful of the urban neighborhood, Dottie would forbid her children from going out of the house, resulting in their frustration tolerance being taxed (e.g., frequent fights over a Nintendo game, the only source of entertainment). Yet, when necessity called very late at night, Dottie would sent her 5-year-old to the neighborhood store blocks away. Although behavioral control and problem-solving seemed poor, the family was affectively involved and responsive to each other. However, social resources were limited outside the immediate family.

Traditional psychological assessments of Dottie (MMPI-2) did not

[1]This case was created for purposes of illustration.

indicate major psychiatric or personality difficulties, although her intellectual level on the WAIS-R was low average and she appeared to have some continued difficulties with alcohol. Her responses on the Beck Depression Inventory indicated presence of some depressive symptoms.

Dottie's behavioral assessment showed her to possess poor stress coping ability, poor parenting skills, limited social skills, poor impulse control (anger outbursts were common), and cognitive problems such as unrealistic expectations regarding the children's abilities and their meeting her needs for affection and attention. She also showed a narrow repertoire of interpersonal problem-solving skills. Because Dottie's children inevitably violated her high expectations, she often made misattributions of negative intent to her children or blamed her own limited skill as a parent. This led to very low self-efficacy, depressed affect, and use of alcohol. Her limited anger management, combined with her narrow repertoire of parenting strategies and poor problem-solving, increased the probability of her overreacting to her children's behavior. She found little reward in her role as a parent and did not provide much cognitive stimulation to the children.

Assessment of the Children

Dottie's three children manifested a variety of outcomes associated with maltreatment. For example, Jeffrey, now age 5, had been abused by his mother as an infant and exhibited an insecure attachment style with her, being both overly clinging and rejecting. Sara, the eldest child (age 15), showed disturbances in her autonomy and seemed to regress at times, also being overly clingy to her mother. Jennifer, age 11, had great difficulty establishing peer relationships and remained a loner at school.

Medically, Jeffrey, who suffered the earliest abuse, manifested some CNS damage and had an unusual gait as a result of fractures he sustained to his left leg. Peers made fun of this. Sara had scars across the backs of her legs, which also caused her some social discomfort. All three children showed low intellectual functioning and were reported to be behind academically. Jeffrey had language delays and, based on both his mother's and the teacher's reports (CBCL), showed aggressive behavior and poor impulse control. Jennifer also showed clinically significant problems with externalized behaviors on the CBCL, particularly aggression. Her mother and teacher also described her as noncompliant and having conduct problems. Sara had a history of delinquency, running away, and truancy. As treatment progressed, it was divulged that she had been molested by a former boyfriend of her mother. Because of this abuse, she showed PTSD symptoms (e.g., sleep problems, hypervigilance, dissociation).

Assessment of the children found dysfunctional social behavior, aggressive and destructive behavior, poor frustration tolerance, deficits in being able to identify feelings and notice affective changes in context, as well as limited perspective-taking skills.

Family/Parent Treatment

As mother had demonstrated problems with alcohol abuse, the first priority was to involve her in AA. She was willing to contract to do this. It was decided that the family issues were of two types. The first involved mother needing some limited help with basic life tasks to reduce some of the burdens of single parenting (e.g., education on budgeting, nutrition, appropriate child supervision, bedtimes). With the help of CPS, a home visitor was provided to help with these issues. The second set of problems had to do with the family's social isolation and mother's parenting problems. It was decided that a group parenting program aimed at providing stress and anger management skills and increasing mother's repertoire of parenting responses would be most useful in dealing with both problems simultaneously. Special cognitive work was directed at unrealistic expectations of children and use of them as a social support network. An active component of the group sessions was to build social relationships among the parents who, once the training portion of the program was over, would then move to working in a self-help format using the Parents Anonymous model. The home visitor helped structure tasks with the children after school and coached Dottie through interactions, engaging the family in role plays designed for her to master new parenting strategies. Work also involved Dottie in dealing with Sara's PTSD symptoms (see below). Mother responded to this two-pronged treatment (group and home parent training) and began to develop a wider social network, which became a source of both emotional and physical support (e.g., babysitting). Dottie also began to attend more closely to the daily routine of the family, providing more structure, consistency, and cognitive stimulation. Her depressed affect decreased, as did her anger outbursts.

Child Treatment

The children's treatment involved a mixture of modalities. The focus of Jeffrey's therapy was on decreasing his aggressive behavior through anger control, frustration tolerance, and problem-solving skills training, which encouraged him to expand his verbal communication and social skills. Jennifer's treatment was similar, with the addition of role plays to address perspective-taking. Sara was enrolled in a group for abused adolescent girls. Group sessions involved teaching normal reactions to sexual abuse, to be better able to identify feelings, stress coping skills and prevention skills, facilitating emotional expression, and gradual exposure to material from their sexual abuse experiences. The group was also involved in social skills training. Concurrently, Dottie attended periodic mothers' sessions, which addressed stress management, increasing support to Sara, education as to symptoms typically experienced by sexual abuse victims, and how to decrease her own responses that may inadvertently serve to maintain them.

Dottie, with the help of the home visitor and fine tuning in parent group sessions, instituted a point system at home, where the children's time spent working on school assignments was reinforced with rewards designed for each child's developmental needs (e.g., game playing for Jeffrey, phone time for Sara). The children's symptoms improved significantly and they began to perform better in school. They also formed some friendships, although Sara, in particular, still struggled with interpersonal trust issues.

Continued work was needed with this multiproblem family given that any additional stressor might upset the family's newfound balance, propelling them back into old patterns (e.g., the children being drawn on for support).

SUMMARY

Research work is still limited in child abuse and neglect. Newer models that address relational aspects of maltreatment hold great promise for providing foundations for developing new interventions. Social learning theory and systemic perspectives appear particularly useful, and interventions are slowly beginning to emerge to combat intrafamilial maltreatment.

REFERENCES

Abel, G. G., Gore, D. K., Holland, C. L., Camp, N., Becker, J. V., & Rathner, J. (1989). The measurement of the cognitive distortions of child molesters. *Annals of Sex Research, 2,* 135–152.

Achenbach, T., & Edelbrock, C. S. (1983). *Manual for the Child Behavior Checklist and Revised Child Behavior Profile.* Burlington, VT: University Associates in Psychiatry.

Ayoub, C. (1991). Physical violence and preschoolers: The use of therapeutic day care in the treatment of physically abused children and children from violent families. *The Advisor, 4,* 1–18.

Azar, S. T. (1986). A framework for understanding child maltreatment: An integration of cognitive behavioral and developmental perspectives. *Canadian Journal of Behavioral Science, 18,* 340–355.

Azar, S. T. (1989). Training parents of abused children. In C. E. Shaefer & J. M. Briesmeister (Eds.), *Handbook of parent training* (pp. 414–441). New York: Wiley.

Azar, S. T. (1991a, April). *Concern about the physical abuse of adolescents: A case of neglect.* Paper presented at the annual meeting of the Eastern Psychological Association, New York.

Azar, S. T. (1991b). Models of physical child abuse: A metatheoretical analysis. *Criminal Justice and Behavior, 18,* 30–46.

Azar, S. T. (1992). Legal issues in the assessment of family violence involving children. In R. T. Ammerman & M. Hersen (Eds.), *Assessment of family violence* (pp. 47–70). New York: Wiley.

Azar, S. T., Barnes, K. T., & Twentyman, C. T. (1988). Developmental outcomes in physically abused children: Consequences of parental abuse or the effects of a more general breakdown in caregiving behaviors? *Behavior Therapist, 11,* 27–32.

Azar, S. T., & Benjet, C. L. (1994). A cognitive perspective on ethnicity, race, and termination of parental rights. *Law and Human Behavior, 18,* 249–268.

Azar, S. T., & Bober, S. L. (in press). Developmental outcomes in abused children: The result of a breakdown in socialization environment. In W. Silverman & T. Ollendick (Eds.), *Group intervention in the school and the community.* Boston: Allyn & Bacon.

Azar, S. T., Robinson, D. R., Hekimian, E., & Twentyman, C. T. (1984). Unrealistic expectations and problem solving ability in maltreating and comparison mothers. *Journal of Consulting and Clinical Psychology, 52,* 687–691.

Azar, S. T., & Rohrbeck, C. A. (1986). Child abuse and unrealistic expectations: Further validation of the Parent Opinion Questionnaire. *Journal of Consulting and Clinical Psychology, 54,* 867–868.

Azar, S. T., & Siegel, B. (1990). Behavioral treatment of child abuse: A developmental perspective. *Behavior Modification, 14,* 279–300.

Azar, S. T., & Twentyman, C. T. (1984, November). *An evaluation of the effectiveness of behaviorally versus insight oriented group treatments with maltreating mothers.* Paper presented at the annual meeting of the Association for Advancement of Behavior Therapy, Philadelphia.

Azar, S. T., & Twentyman, C. T. (1986). Cognitive-behavioral perspectives on the assessment and treatment of child abuse. In P. C. Kendall (Ed.), *Advances in cognitive-behavioral research and therapy* (Vol. 5, pp. 237–267). New York: Academic Press.

Azar, S. T., & Wolfe, D. (1989). Child abuse and neglect. In F. J. Mash & R. A. Barkley (Eds.), *Treatment of childhood disorders* (pp. 451–489). New York: Guilford Press.

Barahal, R. M., Waterman, J., & Martin, H. P. (1981). The social cognitive development of abused children. *Journal of Consulting and Clinical Psychology, 49,* 508–516.

Barnes, K. T., & Azar, S. T. (1990, August). *Maternal expectations and attributions in discipline situations: A test of a cognitive model of parenting.* Paper presented at the annual meeting of the American Psychological Association, Boston.

Bavolek, S. J. (1984). *Handbook of the Adolescent-Parenting Inventory.* Park City, UT: Family Development Resources, Inc.

Bee, H. L., Disbrow, M. A., Johnson-Crowley, N., & Barnard, K. (1981, April). *Parent–child interactions during teaching in abusing and non-abusing families.* Paper presented at the biannual convention of the Society for Research in Child Development, Boston.

Belsky, J. (1980). Child maltreatment. An ecological integration. *American Psychologist, 35,* 320–335.

Berkeley Planning Associates. (1978). *Evaluation of child abuse demonstration projects 1974–1977.* Washington, DC: U.S. Department of Health, Education and Welfare.

Berkowitz, S., & Sedlak, A. J. (1993). *Study of high risk: Child abuse and neglect groups. State survey report.* Washington, DC: NCCAN.

Bernstein, E. M., & Putnam, F. W. (1986). Development, reliability, and validity of a dissociation scale. *Journal of Nervous and Mental Disorders, 174,* 725–735.

Bousha, D., & Twentyman, C. T. (1984). Abusing, neglectful and comparison mother–child interactional style. *Journal of Abnormal Psychology, 93,* 106–114.

Brassard, M. R., Germain, R., & Hart, S. N. (1987). *Psychological maltreatment of children and youth.* Elmsford, NY: Pergamon Press.

Burgess, R. L., & Conger, R. D. (1978). Family interaction in abusive, neglectful and normal families. *Child Development, 49,* 1163–1173.

Butcher, J. N., Dahlstrom, W. G., Graham, J. R., Tellegen, A., & Kaemmer, B. (1989). *Minnesota Multiphasic Personality Inventory-2 (MMPI-2): Manual for administration and scoring.* Minneapolis: University of Minnesota Press.

Campbell, R. V., O'Brien, S., Bickett, A. D., & Lutzker, J. R. (1983). In-home parent training of migraine headaches and marital counseling as an ecobehavioral approach to prevent child abuse. *Journal of Behavior Therapy and Experimental Psychiatry, 14,* 147–154.

Carlson, V., Cicchetti, D., Barnett, D., & Braunwald, K. G. (1989). Finding order in disorganization: Lessons from research on maltreated infants' attachments to their caregivers. In D. Cicchetti & V. Carlson (Eds.), *Child maltreatment* (pp. 494–528). London: Cambridge University Press.

Casanova, G. M., Domanic, J., McCanne, T. R., & Milner, J. S. (1992). Physiological responses to non-child-related stressors in mothers at risk for child abuse. *Child Abuse and Neglect, 16,* 31–44.

Chilamkurti, C., & Milner, J. S. (1993). Perceptions and evaluations of child transgressions and disciplinary techniques in high- and low-risk mothers and their children. *Child Development, 64,* 31–44.

Cicchetti, D. (1989). How research on child maltreatment has informed the study of child development: Perspectives from developmental psychopathology. In D. Cicchetti & V. Carlson (Eds.), *Child maltreatment* (pp. 377–431). London: Cambridge University Press.

Cicchetti, D., & Barnett, D. (1991). Toward the development of a scientific nosology of child maltreatment. In D. Cicchetti & W. Grove (Eds.), *Thinking clearly about psychology* (pp. 346–377). Minneapolis: University of Minnesota Press.

Cicchetti, D., & Carlson, V. (Eds.). (1989). *Child maltreatment: Theory and research on the causes and consequences of child abuse and neglect.* London: Cambridge University Press.

Cicchetti, D., & Rizley, R. (1981). Developmental perspectives on the etiology, intergenerational transmission, and sequelae of child maltreatment. *New Directions for Child Development, 11,* 31–56.

Cohen, J. A., & Mannarino, A. P. (1993). A treatment model for sexually abused preschoolers. *Journal of Interpersonal Violence, 3,* 115–131.

Crittenden, P. M. (1985). Maltreated infants: Vulnerability and resilience. *Journal of Child Psychology and Psychiatry, 26,* 85–96.

Crittenden, P. M., & Ainsworth, M. D. S. (1989). Child maltreatment and attachment theory. In D. Cicchetti & V. Carlson (Eds.), *Child maltreatment* (pp. 432–463). London: Cambridge University Press.

Culp, E., Heide, J. S., & Richardson, M. T. (1987). Maltreated children's developmental scores: Treatment versus nontreatment. *Child Abuse and Neglect, 11,* 29–34.

Daro, D. (1988). *Confronting child abuse: Research for effective program design.* New York: Free Press.

Deblinger, E., Hathaway, C. R., Lippman, J., & Steer, R. (1993). Psychosocial characteristics and correlates of symptom distress in non-offending mothers of sexually abused children. *Journal of Interpersonal Violence, 8*, 155–168.

Deblinger, E., McLeer, S. V., & Henry, D. (1990). Cognitive behavioral treatment for sexually abused children suffering from post traumatic stress: Preliminary findings. *American Academy of Child and Adolescent Psychiatry, 29*, 747–752.

Delgado, A. E., & Lutzker, J. R. (1985, November). *Training parents to identify and report their children's illness.* Paper presented at the annual convention of the Association for Advancement of Behavior Therapy, Houston.

Dix, T. H., Ruble, D. N., & Zambarano, R. J. (1989). Mothers' implicit theories of discipline: Child effects, parent effects, and the attribution process. *Child Development, 60*, 1373–1391.

Dubowitz, H. (1991). The impact of child maltreatment on health. In R. H. Starr & D. A. Wolfe (Eds.), *The effects of child abuse and neglect* (pp. 278–294). New York: Guilford Press.

Dunst, C. H. (1986). *Family resources, personal well-being, and early intervention.* Unpublished manuscript. Family Infant and Preschool Program, Western Carolina Center, Morganton, NC.

Eckenrode, J., Laird, M., & Doris, J. (1993). School performance and disciplinary problems among abused and neglected children. *Developmental Psychology, 29*, 53–62.

Egan, K. (1983). Stress management and child management with abusive parents. *Journal of Clinical Child Psychology, 12*, 292–299.

Elliot, F. A. (1988). Neurological factors. In V. B. VanHasselt, R. L. Morison, A. S. Bellack, & M. Hersen (Eds.), *Handbook of family violence* (pp. 359–382). New York: Plenum Press.

Elliott, R. (1986). Interpersonal Process Recall (IPR) as a psychotherapy process research method. In L. S. Greenberg & W. M. Pinsof (Eds.), *The psychotherapeutic process: A research handbook* (pp. 503–527). New York: Guilford Press.

Epstein, N. B., Bishop, D. S., & Baldwin, L. M. (1982). McMaster model of family functioning. In F. Walsh (Ed.), *Normal family processes* (pp. 115–141). New York: Guilford Press.

Eyberg, S. M., & Ross, A. W. (1978). Assessment of child behavior problems: The validation of a new inventory. *Journal of Clinical Child Psychology, 7*, 113–116.

Famularo, R., Stone, I., Barnum, R., & Wharton, R. (1986). Alcoholism and severe child maltreatment. *American Journal of Orthopsychiatry, 56*, 481–485.

Fantuzzo, J. (1990). Behavioral treatment of the victims of child abuse and neglect. *Behavior Modification, 14*, 316–339.

Fantuzzo, J. W., Jurecic, L., Stovall, A., Hightower, A. D., Goins, C., & Schachtel, D. (1988). Effects of adult and peer social initiations on the social behavior of withdrawn, maltreated preschool children. *Journal of Consulting and Clinical Psychology, 56*, 34–39.

Farber, E. A., & Egeland, B. (1987). Invulnerability among abused and neglected children. In E. J. Anthony & B. J. Cohler (Eds.), *The invulnerable child* (pp. 253–288). New York: Guilford Press.

Finkelhor, D., & Baron, L. (1986). High-risk children. In D. Finkelhor, S. Araji, L. Baron, L. Browne, S. D. Peters, & G. E. Wyatt (Eds.), *Sourcebook on child sexual abuse* (pp. 60–88). Beverly Hills, CA: Sage.

Frodi, A. M., & Lamb, M. E. (1980). Child abusers' responses to infant smiles and cries. *Child Development, 51*, 238–241.

Garbarino, J. (1976). A preliminary study of some ecological correlates of child abuse: The impact of socioeconomic stress on mothers. *Child Development, 47*, 178–185.

Garbarino, J., & Giliam, G. (1980). *Understanding abusive families.* Lexington, MA: Lexington Books.

Gelinas, D. J. (1983). The persisting negative effects of incest. *Psychiatry, 46*, 312–332.

George, C., & Main, M. (1980). Social interactions of young abused children: Approach, avoidance and aggression. *Child Development, 50*, 306–318.

Gil, D. (1970). *Violence against children: Physical child abuse in the United States.* Cambridge, MA: Harvard University Press.

Grisso, T. (1986). *Evaluating competencies.* New York: Plenum Press.

Grisso, T., & Appelbaum, P. S. (1992). Is it unethical to offer predictions of future violence? *Law and Human Behavior, 16*, 621–633.

Hall, G. C. N., & Hirschman, R. (1992). Sexual aggression against children: A conceptual perspective of etiology. *Criminal Justice and Behavior, 19*, 8–23.

Hammond, W. R., & Yung, B. R. (1991). Preventing violence in at-risk African-American youth. *Journal of Health Care for Poor and Underserved, 2*(3), 359–373.

Hampton, R., & Newberger, E. (1985). Child abuse incidence and reporting in hospitals: Significance of severity, class, and race. *American Journal of Public Health, 751*, 56–60.

Hansen, D. J., Pallotta, G. M., Tishelman, A. C., & Conaway, L. P. (1989). Parental problem-solving skills and child behavior problems: A comparison of physically abusive, neglectful, clinic, and community families. *Journal of Family Violence, 4*, 353–368.

Hansen, D. J., & Warner, J. E. (1992). Child physical abuse and neglect. In R. T. Ammerman & M. Hersen (Eds.), *Assessment of family violence: A clinical and legal sourcebook* (pp. 123–147). New York: Wiley.

Hansen, R. K., Steffy, R. A., & Gauthier, R. (1993). Long-term recidivism of child molesters. *Journal of Consulting and Clinical Psychology, 61*, 646–652.

Haskett, M. E. (1990). Social problem-solving skills of young physically abused children. *Child Psychiatry and Human Development, 21,* 109–118.

Hennessy, K., Rabideau, G., Cicchetti, D., & Cummings, E. M. (1994). Responses of physically abused and non-abused children to different forms of interadult anger. *Child Development, 65,* 815–828.

Herman, H. (1981). *Father–daughter incest.* Cambridge, MA: Harvard University Press.

Herrenkohl, R. C., Herrenkohl, E. C., & Egolf, B. P. (1983). Circumstances surrounding the occurrence of child maltreatment. *Journal of Consulting and Clinical Psychology, 51,* 424–431.

Hoagwood, K. (1990). Parental functioning and child sexual abuse. *Child and Adolescent Social Work, 7,* 377–387.

Horowitz, M. (1986). *Stress response syndromes* (2nd ed.). Northvale, NJ: Jason Aronson.

Johnson, B., & Morse, H. A. (1968). Injured children and their parents. *Children, 15,* 147–152.

Kafka, M. P., & Prentky, R. (1992). A comparative study of nonparaphilic sexual addictions and paraphilias in men. *Journal of Clinical Psychiatry, 53*(10), 345–350.

Kaufman, J., & Zigler, E. (1987). Do abused children become abusive parents? *American Journal of Orthopsychiatry, 57,* 186–192.

Kendall-Tackett, K. A., Williams, L. M., & Finkelhor, D. (1993). Impact of sexual abuse on children: A review and synthesis of recent empirical studies. *Psychological Bulletin, 113,* 164–180.

Klaus, M. H., & Kennell, J. H. (1982). *Maternal–infant bonding* (2nd ed.). London: Cambridge University Press.

Lanyon, R. I. (1986). Theory and treatment in child molestation. *Journal of Consulting and Clinical Psychology, 54,* 176–182.

Larrance, D. T., & Twentyman, C. T. (1983). Maternal attributions in child abuse. *Journal of Abnormal Psychology, 92,* 449–457.

Lauderdale, M., Valiunas, A., & Anderson, R. (1980). Race, ethnicity, and child maltreatment: An empirical analysis. *Child Abuse and Neglect, 4,* 163–169.

Lipovsky, J. A. (1991). Posttraumatic stress disorder in children. *Family and Community Health, 14,* 42–51.

Long, K. (1986). Cultural consideration in the assessment and treatment of intrafamilial abuse. *American Journal of Orthopsychiatry, 56,* 131–136.

Lutzker, J. R., & Rice, J. M. (1984). Project 12-Ways: Treating child abuse and neglect from an ecobehavioral perspective. In R. F. Dangel & R. A. Polster (Eds.), *Parent training: Foundations of research and practice* (pp. 260–293). New York: Guilford Press.

MacFarlane, K. (1986). Child sexual abuse allegations in divorce proceedings. In K. MacFarlane & L. Richardson (Eds.), *Sexual abuse of young children* (pp. 121–148). New York: Guilford Press.

Magura, S., & Moses, B. S. (1986). *The Parent Outcome Interview.* Washington, DC: Child Welfare League.

Marshall, W. L., Laws, D. R., & Barbaree, H. E. (Eds.).

(1990). *The handbook of sexual assault: Issues, theories and treatment of the offender.* New York: Plenum Press.

Martin, H. P. (1976). *The abused child: A multidisciplinary approach to developmental issues and treatment.* Cambridge, MA: Ballinger.

Mash, E. H. (1991). Measurement of parent–child interaction in studies of maltreatment. In R. Starr & D. A. Wolfe (Eds.), *The effects of child abuse and neglect* (pp. 203–255). New York: Guilford Press.

McGee, R. A., Wolfe, D. A., Yuen, S. A., & Wilson, S. K. (1995). The measurement of maltreatment: A comparison of approaches. *Child Abuse and neglect, 19,* 233–249.

Melnick, B., & Hurley, J. R. (1969). Distinctive personality attributes of child-abusing mothers. *Journal of Consulting and Clinical Psychology, 33,* 746–749.

Melton, G. B., Petrila, J., Poythress, N. G., & Slobogin, C. (1987). *Psychological evaluations for the courts: A handbook for mental health professionals.* New York: Guilford Press.

Miller, L. R., & Azar, S. T. (1996). The pervasiveness of maladaptive attributions in mothers at-risk for child abuse. *Family Violence & Sexual Assault Bulletin, 12,* 31–37.

Miller-Perrin, C. L., & Wurtele, S. K. (1988). The child sexual abuse prevention movement: A critical analysis of primary and secondary approaches. *Clinical Psychology Review, 8,* 313–329.

Milner, J. S. (1986). *The Child Abuse Potential Inventory: Manual (revised).* Webster, NC: Psytec Corporation.

Milner, J. S. (1989). Additional cross-validation of the Child Abuse Potential Inventory. *Psychological Assessment, 1,* 219–223.

Milner, J. S. (1993). Social information processing and physical child abuse. *Clinical Psychology Review, 13,* 275–294.

National Center on Child Abuse and Neglect. (1993). *Child maltreatment 1993. Reports from the states to the National Center on Child Abuse and Neglect.* Washington, DC: U.S. Department of Health and Human Services.

National Research Council. (1993). *Understanding child abuse and neglect.* Washington, DC: National Academy Press.

Newberger, E. H., Hampton, R. L., Marx, T. J., & White, K. M. (1986). Child abuse and pediatric social illness. *American Journal of Orthopsychiatry, 56,* 589–601.

Novaco, R. W. (1975). *Anger control: The development and evaluation of an experimental treatment.* Lexington, MA: Lexington Books.

Oldershaw, L., Walters, G. C., & Hall, D. K. (1986). Control strategies and noncompliance in abusive mother–child dyads: An observational study. *Child Development, 57,* 722–732.

Olds, D. L. (1989). The prenatal/early infancy project: A strategy for responding to the needs of high-risk mothers and their children. *Prevention in Human Services, 7,* 59–87.

Olds, D. L., Henderson, C. R., Chamberlin, R., & Tatelbaum, R. (1986). Preventing child abuse and neglect: A randomized trial of nurse home visitation. *Pediatrics, 78,* 65–78.

Pagelow, M. D. (1984). *Family violence.* New York: Praeger Scientific.

Parke, R. D., & Collmer, C. W. (1975). Child abuse: An interdisciplinary analysis. In E. M. Hetherington (Ed.), *Review of child development research* (Vol. 5, pp. 509–590). Chicago: University of Chicago Press.

Pelton, H. (1978). Child abuse and neglect: The myth of classlessness. *American Journal of Orthopsychiatry, 48,* 608–617.

Pynoos, R. S., Frederick, C., Nader, K., Arroyo, W., Steingberg, A., Eth, S., Nunez, F., & Fairbanks, L. (1987). Life threat and posttraumatic stress in school-age children. *Archives of General Psychiatry, 44,* 1057–1063.

Rohrbeck, C. A., & Twentyman, C. T. (1986). A multimodal assessment of impulsiveness in abusing, neglectful, and nonmaltreating mothers and their preschool children. *Journal of Consulting and Clinical Psychology, 54,* 231–236.

Rosenfield-Schlicter, M. D., Sarber, R. E., Bueno, G., Greene, B. F., & Lutzker, J. R. (1983). Maintaining accountability for an ecobehavioral treatment of one aspect of child neglect: Personal cleanliness. *Education and Treatment of Children, 6,* 153–164.

Salzinger, S., Kaplan, S., & Artemyeff, C. (1983). Mothers' personal social networks and child maltreatment. *Journal of Abnormal Psychology, 92,* 68–76.

Salzinger, S., Kaplan, S., Pelcovitz, D., Samit, C., & Krieger, R. (1984). Parent and teacher assessment of children's behavior in child maltreating families. *Journal of the American Academy of Child Psychiatry, 23,* 458–464.

Sameroff, A. J., & Chandler, M. J. (1975). Reproductive risk and the continuum of caretaking casualty. In F. D. Horowitz (Ed.), *Review of child development research* (Vol. 4, pp. 187–243). Chicago: University of Chicago Press.

Sarber, R. E., Halasz, M. M., Messmer, M. C., Bickett, A. D., & Lutzker, J. R. (1983). Teaching menu planning and grocery shopping skills to a mentally retarded mother. *Mental Retardation, 21,* 101–106.

Schilling, R. F., & Schinke, S. P. (1984). Maltreatment and mental retardation. *Perspectives and Progress in Mental Retardation, 1,* 11–22.

Selzer, M. L., Vinokur, A., & vanRooijen, L. (1975). A self-administered Short Michigan Screening Test. *Journal of Studies of Alcohol, 36,* 117–126.

Spaccarelli, S. (1994). Stress, appraisal, and coping in child sexual abuse: A theoretical and empirical review. *Psychological Bulletin, 116,* 340–362.

Starr, R. H., MacLean, D. J., & Keating, D. P. (1991). Life span developmental outcomes of child maltreatment. In R. Starr & D. A. Wolfe (Eds.), *The effects of child abuse and neglect* (pp. 1–32). New York: Guilford Press.

Stermac, L. E., & Segal, Z. V. (1989). Adult sexual contact

with children: An examination of cognitive factors. *Behavior Therapy, 20,* 573–584.

Szykula, S. A., & Fleischman, M. J. (1985). Reducing out-of-home-placements of abused children: Two controlled studies. *Child Abuse and Neglect, 9,* 277–284.

Terr, L. (1991). Childhood traumas: An outline and overview. *American Journal of Psychiatry, 148,* 10–20.

Tertinger, D. A., Greene, B. F., & Lutzker, J. R. (1984). Home safety: Development and validation of one component of an ecobehavioral treatment program for abused and neglected children. *Journal of Applied Behavior Analysis, 17,* 150–174.

Trickett, P. K., & Kuczynski, L. (1986). Children's misbehaviors and parental discipline strategies in abusive and nonabusive families. *Developmental Psychology, 22,* 115–123.

Trickett, P. K., McBride-Chang, C., & Putnam, F. W. (1994). The classroom performance and behavior of sexually abused females. *Development and Psychopathology, 6,* 183–194.

Trickett, P. K., & Putnam, F. W. (1993). Impact of child sexual abuse on females. Toward a developmental psychobiological integration. *Psychological Science, 4,* 81–87.

Vitulano, L. A., Lewis, M., Doran, L. D., Nordhaus, B., & Adnopoz, J. (1986). Treatment recommendations, implementation, and follow-up in child abuse. *American Journal of Orthopsychiatry, 56,* 478–480.

Wahler, R. G., & Dumas, J. E. (1989). Attentional problems in dysfunctional mother–child interactions: An interbehavioral model. *Psychological Bulletin, 105,* 116–130.

Wasik, B. H., Bryant, D. M., & Fishbein, J. (1981, November). *Assessment of parent problem solving skills.* Paper presented at the Annual Meeting of the Association for the Advancement of Behavior Therapy, Toronto.

Watson-Perczel, M., Lutzker, J. R., Greene, B. F., & McGimpsey, B. J. (1988). Assessment and modification of home cleanliness among families adjudicated for child neglect. *Behavior Modification, 12,* 57–87.

Wauchope, B. A., & Straus, M. A. (1989). Physical punishment and physical abuse of American children: Incidence rates by age, gender, and occupational class. In M. A. Straus & R. J. Gelles (Eds.), *Physical violence in American families: Risk factors and adaptations to violence in 8,145 families* (pp. 1–15). New Brunswick, NJ: Transaction.

White, S. T., Loda, F. A., Ingram, D. C., & Pearson, A. (1983). Sexually transmitted diseases in sexually abused children. *Pediatrics, 72,* 16–21.

Widom, C. S. (1989). Does violence beget violence? A critical examination of the literature. *Psychological Bulletin, 106,* 3–28.

Williams, G. (1983). The urgency of authentic prevention. *Journal of Clinical Child Psychology, 12,* 312–319.

Williams, L. M., & Finkelhor, D. (1990). The characteristics of incestuous fathers: A review of recent studies. In W. L. Marshall, D. R. Laws, & H. E. Barbaree (Eds.), *The handbook of sexual assault: Issues, theories and treatment of the offender* (pp. 231–255). New York: Plenum Press.

Wolfe, D. A. (1985). Child-abusive parents: An empirical review and analysis. *Psychological Bulletin, 97,* 462–482.

Wolfe, D. A. (1987). *Child abuse: Implications for child development and psychopathology.* Beverly Hills, CA: Sage.

Wolfe, D. A., Fairbanks, J. A., Kelly, J. A., & Bradlyn, A. S. (1983). Child abusive parents' physiological responses to stressful and non-stressful behavior in children. *Behavioral Assessment, 5,* 363–371.

Wolfe, D. A., Kaufman, K., Aragona, J., & Sandler, J. (1981). *The child management program for abusive parents.* Winter Park, FL: Anna Publishing.

Wolfe, D. A., Sandler, J., & Kaufman, K. (1981). A competen-cy-based parent training program for abusive parents. *Journal of Consulting and Clinical Psychology, 49,* 633–640.

Wolfe, V. V., Gentile, C., & Wolfe, D. A. (1989). The impact of sexual abuse on children: A PTSD formulation. *Behavior Therapy, 20,* 215–228.

Zeanah, C. J., & Zeanah, P. D. (1989). Intergenerational transmission of maltreatment: Insights from attachment theory and research. *Psychiatry, 52,* 177–196.

Zuravin, S. J. (1991). Research definitions of child physical abuse and neglect: Current problems. In R. H. Starr & D. A. Wolfe (Eds.), *The effects of child abuse and neglect: Issues and research* (pp. 100–128). New York: Guilford Press.

21

Children under Stress

NORMAN A. MILGRAM

INTRODUCTION

This chapter deals with a form of reactive psychopathology in children, namely, disorders that arise as a consequence of exposure to stressful life events. Issues of diagnosis, incidence, etiology, and treatment are more difficult to resolve in stress-related disorders than in the traditional, established diagnostic categories presented elsewhere in this handbook, reflecting the problematic nature of the stress concept.

First, the term *stress* means different things to different people. For example, the term is frequently defined as a source of psychopathology, and just as frequently as the form that psychopathology takes or its consequences. One may conclude, therefore, that stress is a major factor to be considered in all forms of psychopathology. Or one may conclude the opposite, that indiscriminate use of the term is justification for eliminating it from professional parlance.

The lack of clarity about the term *stress* made it necessary to adopt an unusual format in presenting this topic. In Part One, the major concepts in the field of stress and coping that are related to the assessment and treatment of psychopathology are discussed. In Part Two, four stress-related disorders—Adjustment Disorder, Acute Stress Disorder, Post-traumatic Stress Disorder, and Disorder of Extreme Stress—are compared, four kinds of traumatic events that produce stress-related disorders in children are summarized (natural disaster, war, physical violence, and sexual abuse in the home and community), and a case study is presented.

A second problematic feature of the stress concept is its departure from the etiological model of the historically prior psychiatric disorders. The traditional psychiatric orientation states that afflicted individuals respond "abnormally" to stimuli that ordinarily elicit normal behavior in most people, because of their personal predispositions and longstanding adverse experiences. The detrimental character of these adverse experiences may not appear to the casual observer to be a sufficient cause for the resulting psychopathology, and is so regarded only by the trained professional worker.

The stress-related orientation, by contrast, focuses on intense, stressful life events regarded as detrimental by any observer. It states that most people exposed to these stressful life events exhibit adverse stress reactions and recover under

NORMAN A. MILGRAM • Department of Psychology, Tel Aviv University, Ramat Aviv 69978, Israel.

Handbook of Child Psychopathology, 3rd edition, edited by Ollendick & Hersen. Plenum Press, New York, 1998.

favorable postexposure circumstances. Some suffer the persisting effects of the initial exposure long after the upsetting experience has ended, because of preexposure personal vulnerabilities and/or the highly adverse properties of these stressful events. The two orientations are not mutually exclusive, some disorders fall in an overlap category, and people with established psychiatric disorders may also become exposed to stressful life circumstances. Nevertheless, many adherents of the one orientation find it difficult to appreciate the nuances and legitimate contributions of the other.

For these reasons the topic of stress-related disorders did not appear at all in the first edition of this handbook (Ollendick & Hersen, 1983) or in other child psychopathology texts designed for advanced mental health students and practitioners (e.g., Knopf, 1979; Quay & Werry, 1979; Schwartz & Johnson, 1981). This is not to suggest that texts dealing with children under stress did not exist. On the contrary, many texts have that very title or variations on it (e.g., Brenner, 1985; Humphrey, 1982; McNamee, 1982). These latter texts were written without regard for the systematic diagnostic categories of the DSM-III-R or the DSM-IV (American Psychiatric Association, 1987 and 1994, respectively), and the range of stress-related topics within these texts is broad and unselective (e.g., doing poorly in school, living in a home without a father, poverty and cultural deprivation, undergoing hospitalization for serious illness or surgery).

There have been some promising exceptions. Recent psychiatric texts (Ammerman, Last, & Hersen, 1993; King & Noshpitz, 1991) devote a few chapters to stress-related topics such as physical abuse, sexual abuse, divorce, and chronic illness. Unfortunately, they do not compare and contrast the assumptions and criteria that inform conventional psychiatric disorders versus those that inform stress-related disorders. Texts with the title *crisis intervention* (Auerbach & Stolberg, 1986; Dattilio & Freeman, 1994) deal with a wide variety of stress-related disorders, but they also include conventional psychiatric disorders in which crisis situations arise, and thereby dim the distinction between the two orientations.

PART ONE: BASIC CONCEPTS IN THE FIELD OF STRESS AND COPING

Conceptualization of Stress

The term *stress* has become one of the most popular terms in mental health research and practice. Its popularity is in large measure related to the wide variety of phenomena subsumed under that heading and to its convenient, if indiscriminate, usage with reference to stimulus events, subject responses, or both (Levine & Scotch, 1970). These different usages are discussed below in serial fashion, and a resolution of the difficulties is proposed.

Stress as a Stimulus Event

One way of defining stress is in terms of stimulus events that lead to changes in the organism (Dohrenwend & Dohrenwend, 1974). In this approach, a life event is stressful to the extent that it requires the individual to change or adapt in coping with the frustrations, conflicts, and/or pressures brought about by the event (Coleman, Butcher, & Carson, 1984). The degree of stressfulness is objectively defined by the normative ratings of social readjustment provided by adult judges across a broad range of stressful life events, first for adults (Holmes & Rahe, 1967) and subsequently for children and adolescents (Coddington, 1972). This approach conceptualizes the cumulative stressfulness of events as an objective, independent variable affecting the adjustment and physical and mental health of those exposed to these events. This conceptualization of event stressfulness is a major research strategy in examining stress–health relationships in epidemiological research (Dohrenwend & Dohrenwend, 1974).

When applied to the diagnosis and treatment of psychopathological disorders, this approach creates a number of problems. First, it assumes that all stressful events have adverse health consequences, when, in fact, only undesirable events are potentially detrimental (Johnson, 1986). Second, it presumes an authoritative classification and ordinal scaling of stressful life events, when none exists.

The list proposed below is an effort in this direction. It first cites ordinary, common stress situations and experiences to which most children and adolescents are exposed and then increasingly extraordinary, unusual ones.

1. Routine tasks of daily living that arouse minor emotional tension, upset, or distress (e.g., doing household chores, attending school)

2. Normal developmental tasks or transitions, generally long term in duration, of the kind that are associated with Erikson's psychosocial stages (e.g., separation from home, the challenge of academic achievement from middle childhood on, and resolving the identity conflicts of adolescence)

3. Conventional events, generally of brief duration, that are typically regarded as desirable, but may, nevertheless, be adversely stressful (e.g., the birth of a sibling, change of residence or school)

4. Upsetting events that happen to children from time to time (e.g., breaking an arm or leg, being beaten up by a bully, undergoing surgery)

5. Family disruptions (e.g., parental separation, divorce, long-term unemployment)

6. Misfortune within the family circle (e.g., death through illness, accident, suicide, or homicide of family members, serious illness of family members)

7. Personal misfortune experienced by children (e.g., physical or sexual abuse or assault at the hands of family members or strangers, witnessing acts of violence committed against others, life-threatening illness or permanent injury and their consequences)

8. Catastrophic group misfortune associated with natural disasters (e.g., floods, fires, and hurricanes)

9. Catastrophic man-made disasters (e.g., war, terrorist attack on civilian populations, incarceration, torture) with temporary and/or permanent consequences (e.g., death, physical and economic deprivation, uprooting and relocation elsewhere)

All of these hassling routines, transitions, unpleasant events, disasters, and catastrophes are objective events. Events that appear farther down the list are more intense and more likely to contribute to psychopathological behavior than those that appear earlier. On the other hand, to consider all of these events as sources of psychopathological behavior leads to confusion. Even if the term *stress* is restricted to statistically infrequent stimulus events that are commonly regarded as unmitigated disasters, the definition remains problematic because some children do not experience or evince a stressful reaction to these stressful events. It is difficult, if not unconvincing, to speak of stress when there is no experienced distress.

Stress as a Response to an Event

Many research and professional health workers prefer to define stressful phenomena in terms of stress reactions, i.e., disruption in perception, emotion, motivation, and/or problem-solving behavior (Mechanic & Volkart, 1962). Definition by stress reaction is open, however, to the same objections as definition by stressful event. The definition encompasses all of human behavior, apart from simple reflexes—from mild adjustment reactions to severe psychopathology. A well-known definition of stress formulated by Janis and Leventhal (1968) illustrates this difficulty: "*Any* [italics added] change in one's environment that elicits a high degree of emotional tension (e.g., anxiety, depression), interferes with normal patterns of response, and requires new behavioral adaptation is an instance of stress." This definition brings under one roof the efforts of Job to cope with the slings and arrows of outrageous fortune and the temporary embarrassment of a sensitive child in response to a casual slight from a stranger. In so doing, it overgeneralizes the unifying concept of stress in these diverse behavioral phenomena to the point where it becomes trivialized.

Second, if we restrict the definition to the more severe end of the response continuum, we find, as expected, that some children exhibit extreme behaviors in appropriately threatening situations, whereas others are equally distressed when exposed to relatively conventional life situations. It is confusing to regard routine life situations as stressful because some vulnerable children become disorganized and disturbed when exposed to them.

Stress as an Imbalance between Stimulus Demand and Response Supply

A practical resolution of this impasse is (1) to employ the word as an adjective or a prefix, but never as a self-sufficient term, (2) to define stress in terms of both stimulus events and subject responses, (3) to restrict its use to instances where an imbalance between event demands and one's personal resources and available interpersonal supports leads to a temporary or permanent failure in adaptive behavior, and (4) to make the further restriction that the demand characteristics of the stressful life event be such as to bring about this imbalance in many, if not most, normally functioning people. In this approach, we refer to stressors (aspects of the stimulus situation perceived as threatening and taxing one's adaptive capacities), stressor mediating variables (aspects of the situation, the child, and their interaction that affect the stressor–stress reaction relationship), stress reactions (transient, adaptive and maladaptive behaviors), and stress disorders (crystallized clinical syndromes that follow from maladaptive efforts to rectify this imbalance and that may undergo spontaneous remission, respond to treatment, or become chronic).

Stress and the Conservation of Resources

A new interactional model was formulated by Hobfoll (1989). His Conservation of Resources theory proposes that people strive to obtain, retain, and protect those things, possessions, or resources that they value. The term *stress* is applicable only when valued resources are threatened or lost or when an anticipated increase in certain resources following the investment of other resources does not occur. Resources may be material or immaterial and are loosely classified as objects, conditions, characteristics, and energies. Illustrative examples of each category for children follow: objects (e.g., one's home, prized personal possessions), conditions (e.g., living with happily married parents, enjoying the friendship and respect of age peers), personal characteristics (e.g., high self-esteem, moral integrity), and energies (e.g., having the time to do what one has to do and what one wants to do, possessing the knowledge and information necessary to pursue one's goals). People expend energy resources so as to conserve or increase the preceding three resource categories.

This theory has several advantages over previous imbalance, transition, or change formulations, especially when applied to children and youth. It distinguishes between desired imbalances or changes sought after by adventuresome, curious, growing organisms and unwelcomed, aversive intrusions that contribute to psychopathological behavior. It lends itself to developmental considerations, as resources and the values attached to them change in the course of maturation and socialization. The theory provides structure for effective definition of the problem (diagnosis), for planning, and for implementing solutions to the problem (therapeutic intervention).

This structure is provided by the kinds of questions raised in stress-related situations and the answers provided: What resources are threatened? What resources must be invested to avert the threatened loss or to reduce the extent of the anticipated loss? Alternately, what resources have been lost? How important were they to the child? What resources may replace them, who decides which ones, and who obtains them? How rapidly did the loss occur or the threat of loss materialize? How rapidly must one mobilize resources to eliminate the threat, to reduce further loss, to restore depleted resources, or to acquire new resources? Because resource concepts are less familiar than imbalance concepts to professional workers, this chapter will rely chiefly on the latter with judicious use of the former.

Parameters of Stressful Life Events

Stressful events may be classified and scaled for their potentially deleterious effect by recourse to imbalance theories, resource theories, or both. With the family being the source of major resources for the child, threats or losses that originate within the family circle are more upsetting (e.g., father murdered mother) than threats or losses that originated outside the family (e.g., mother died in an automobile accident). Stressors that constitute threat and resource loss to the child alone are less upsetting than stressors that affect the entire family, and jeopardize family resources that the child might have tapped *in extremis*. Primary victimization (e.g., suffering repeated beatings) is more disruptive than secondary victimization (e.g., watching a loved one being beaten repeatedly).

Other parameters of stressful life events include: the time dimension (how long one was exposed to the stressor and to its immediate consequences), controllability versus uncontrollability of what is happening and what may happen; external versus internal responsibility for what has happened and for what must be done to prevent further damage and to restore what has been damaged; reversibility versus irreversibility of what may have happened or has already happened; and natural versus man-made source of the destructive stressor. Some extraordinary, complex stressors encompass all of these parameters in their most disruptive forms. Wars that involve civilian populations cause enormous loss of life and property, disrupt or possibly destroy the social fabric, directly victimize children and their families for an extended period, and bring about severe, irreversible consequences for all survivors (Frederick, 1985; Garmezy, 1983; Macksoud, Dyregov, & Raundalen, 1993).

Cognitive Appraisal and Coping

Although some classes of environmental stressors produce more severe stress reactions than others, individual and group differences are evident within each class of stressors or in relation to a particular stressor. These differences are explained in part by cognitive processes that characterize all encounters between people and stressors and affect their reactions to the encounter. Two kinds of cognitive processes or appraisals have been identified (Lazarus & Folkman, 1984):

1. Primary cognitive appraisal looks outward to the stressor and assesses the extent of harm/loss that has already occurred and the threat of future harm/loss.

2. Secondary cognitive appraisal looks inward and outward and assesses the coping options that are available, the likelihood that a given option will accomplish what it is supposed to, and the likelihood that one will be able to apply the option effectively. Secondary appraisals are affected by the assessment of the available personal resources and interpersonal supports at any given point in a stress situation.

Tertiary cognitive appraisal (proposed by the author) refers to the ongoing assessment of one's self-efficacy in coping with the exigencies of an extended stressful situation: What answer does one give to the question, "How well am I doing?" A favorable reply elicits a euphoric mood and motivates one to persevere and prevail despite internal and external obstacles; an unfavorable reply has the opposite effect. Adults and children alike, when caught up in an extended crisis, ask themselves whether their behavior is a source of pride or shame, to them or to significant others (Taylor & Loebel, 1989).

Tertiary appraisals depend on the frame of reference applied by the appraiser:

a. Normative external reference: "Am I conducting myself the way I am supposed to in this kind of situation?"

b. Comparative situational reference: "Am I conducting myself as well as others (upward and downward reference groups) in this situation?"

c. Internal reference: "Am I conducting myself well by my own standards?"

These cognitive appraisals—primary, secondary, and tertiary—affect current functioning and future adjustment in extended stressful situations. They determine how one copes with the task demands of the stressful situation. Several major coping strategies have been identified:

1. Problem-focused coping refers to cognitive and behavioral efforts to meet the demands of the external situation that precipitated the imbalance or resource threat/loss in the first place.

2. Emotional-focused coping refers to corresponding efforts to maintain the emotional control necessary for sustained problem-focused coping.

3. Coping by problem reformulation entails reexamination of the problem in terms that permit its practical resolution, provided that corresponding emotion-focused efforts are made to make this reformulation tolerable, if not desirable. These coping behaviors affect the intensity and duration of adverse stress reactions. The more effective the strategies, the more mild and short-lived are the resulting stress reactions.

Children's Stress Reactions

Children's stress reactions are manifested in different ways and assessed in different ways by different people. Children tell us they are highly anxious or depressed (verbal report). Family members, friends, classmates, or teachers comment on children's behavior (naturalistic obser-

vations) or make systematic ratings of their behavior (ratings scales). Psychologists assess performance decrements systematically in different areas of children's lives (tests, interviews, and observations). Physiologists measure elevation of autonomic and corticotropic responses. Medical internists and psychiatrists ascertain the presence and extent of physical illness, disease, behavioral disturbance, or psychiatric disorder that follow from extended exposure to stressful situations (physical examinations, laboratory tests, and psychiatric interviews). These different indices of stress reaction are analyzed in relation to one another both in conducting basic stressor-outcome research in general and in diagnosing and treating stress-related disorders in particular.

Intrapersonal Resources

The recurrent finding that children differ widely in their stress reactions to a given stressful event (interindividual differences) and that the same child differs widely in his or her reactions to different stressful events (intraindividual differences) leads to an analysis of some of the sources of these differences in response to stressful life events. One source is intrapersonal resources. High self-esteem (Pearlin & Schooler, 1978), psychological hardiness (Kobassa, 1979), cognitive and behavioral coping strategies and skills (Lazarus & Folkman, 1984), self-regulatory competencies (Rosenbaum, 1983), and self-efficacy based on success expectancies (Bandura, 1977) are examples of intrapersonal resources that facilitate coping with stressful life events. These and other personal characteristics contribute to person–stressful environment interactions in the following ways (Atkinson, Atkinson, Smith, & Bem, 1990):

1. Proactive interaction: A child chooses situations and shapes them differently than other children do.

2. Reactive interaction: A child interprets, experiences, and reacts to situations in different ways than other children.

3. Evocative interaction: A child evokes different responses from significant people (e.g., potential sources of support) than other children.

Strelau (1991) emphasized the importance of temperament risk factors in the development of behavior disorders. These factors must be considered, precisely because they are less susceptible to modification than environmental factors and are, therefore, likely to be overlooked. When we identify these temperamental characteristics, we are better able to understand the development of the presenting symptoms and to plan environmental modifications that will produce a better person–environment fit. Strelau showed, for example, that children with a highly reactive temperament maintain optimal activation with a low level of environmental stimulation; conversely, children with a low reactive temperament do better with a high level of environmental stimulation. He also argued that specific temperamental characteristics are not inherently helpful or harmful, independent of the stressful circumstance in which children find themselves. One investigator (de Vries, 1987) noted that there may be stressful circumstances in which negative temperamental traits (e.g., hyperactivity, low frustration tolerance) are advantageous. Some Masai infants were fed more than their age peers during conditions of marginal nutrition because they were more irritable and irritating. We conclude (1) that children may exhibit or adopt unusual, "apparently maladaptive" coping behaviors in stressful situations, that on careful analysis are found to be highly adaptive, and (2) that practitioners should exercise humility and caution before attempting to eliminate these behaviors in a comprehensive treatment program.

Interpersonal Supports

Another source of variability is interpersonal support. This support may take any of the following forms:

1. Stable social networks—e.g., a cohesive, extended family or clan, collective settlement (kibbutz), neighborhood, or an entire ethnic group within society—set and maintain standards governing the behavior of group members in routine and in extraordinary situations that adversely affect individuals, families, or entire communities.

2. Naturally occurring support systems— e.g., members of the nuclear family, school or neighborhood friends, members of one's church or youth group, or unfamiliar members of the community—may assume informal support functions.

3. Some groups are formally organized to serve certain stress-related needs in the community, e.g., a home visiting program run by volunteers in the community to serve children recuperating from serious illness or handicapped children confined to their homes, or a telephone answering service for adolescents in crisis situations (e.g., unplanned pregnancy, suicidal intentions, drug overdose). These programs are run by lay and/or professional organizations and are designed for different levels of therapeutic intervention as discussed below.

Social support has been conceptualized as providing the following functions during stressful situations (derived from Thoits, 1986; Weiss, 1974):

1. Helping people to define, understand, and cope with stressful life events (guidance, wise counsel)

2. Communicating to people during trying times that they are valued for their own personal worth, despite circumstances that may lead them to think otherwise (reassurance of worth)

3. Spending time with others during difficult situations (providing companionship and sense of reliable alliance)

4. Providing material assistance to people in resolving the problem at hand (instrumental support)

5. Providing harassed people with opportunities for relaxation or other pursuits (respite)

Conceptualizations of social support have changed over time (Milgram, 1989). Early research in the field was characterized by adherence to the *availability imperative,* the notion that mere availability of social support was a guarantee of its efficacy. This naive notion was replaced by a more sophisticated notion, the *time lock-and-key imperative.* For every child or adolescent caught up in a stressful situation there is an appropriate kind of support that will be optimally effective if provided at a particular point in the coping process (much like a bank lock that can only be opened by a specific key and only at a specific time). The implicit assumption common to both conceptualizations is that social support is like manna from heaven that falls on the needy.

Recently, the emphasis has shifted from what others do for afflicted children to what these children do to attract, recruit, and conserve the particular kinds of support they desire at any point in the coping process. This third conceptualization may be termed *sequential search and selection.* It assumes that children in need of support exercise some control over the support they receive—soliciting support on their own, rejecting some kinds of support, and accepting others (Milgram & Toubiana, 1996). It further assumes that some people in need receive more social support than others because of their superior support-seeking and support-attracting characteristics (Sarason, Sarason, & Pierce, 1994). The concept does not imply that all children or adults are necessarily wise in the support they seek or accept, merely that many, if not most, initiate activity and exercise choice.

Research (summarized in Milgram & Palti, 1993) suggests that one reason some children growing up in impoverished families and communities make impressive achievements is that they are able to seek, attract, and maintain social support from peers and adults in and outside that environment. Children who lack these skills or who reject the well-meaning efforts of support providers require active intervention by professional workers to guarantee that they receive appropriate support.

Conventional definitions of social support have tended to exclude professional support—psychotherapy or counseling—and refer only to indigenous, lay support providers, such as strangers who volunteer to help others or intact family members who help other family members in distress (Caplan, 1976). This exclusion is inappropriate. Professional workers provide informational and emotional support as defined above, and their availability and utilization reduce the risk of stress-related psychopathology.

Levels of Mental Health Intervention

The help provided by the various social support agencies to people in need is classified according to level. Three levels are described in the crisis intervention literature, namely, primary, secondary, and tertiary intervention (Slaikeu, 1984):

1. Primary intervention refers to educational efforts directed at the entire community or high-risk groups within it. These endeavors provide police, teachers, and other social agents, as well as parents and children, with knowledge and skills in advance of a given crisis so that they can deal with it more effectively if and when it arises.

2. Secondary intervention is directed to high-risk groups within the community who are currently coping with or have recently been exposed to aversive stressors (e.g., rape, physical battering, homes destroyed by raging waters or winds). The intervention is designed to provide help during the active crisis situation so that exposed individuals are able to resolve the situation rapidly at the earliest stages of maladjustment and with minimal sequelae. Some of the support systems at the primary and secondary levels are mobilized by professional workers and operate under their direction or in consultation with them, whereas others arise spontaneously in the lay community and operate entirely on their own.

3. Tertiary intervention refers to formal treatment programs provided by professional

and paraprofessional organizations and workers to individuals or families unable to resolve the initial crisis successfully. These clients have developed definitive stress-related psychopathological symptoms, and there is concern that their current symptom picture will deteriorate further. Intervention is designed to minimize residual effects, prevent exacerbation and chronicity of symptoms, prevent relapse, and thereby facilitate partial or complete recovery. At this level professional people work directly with afflicted persons.

The mental health field has become increasingly aware of its responsibility in identifying in advance groups at risk for stress-related disorders and in providing primary and secondary intervention programs (e.g., crisis walk-in clinics, crisis telephone services, public education programs). It may occasionally fail to do so in the case of high-risk groups whose political allegiance, ethnic membership, or controversial stance places them beyond the pale of professional concern. For example, U.S. veterans returning from Vietnam in the late 1960s and early 1970s did not receive proper treatment from the mental health professions because of the antiwar attitudes of members of these professions (Milgram & Hobfoll, 1986). Similarly, Israeli settlers living in sections of Sinai that were to be returned to Egypt as part of a peace settlement received hostile treatment in the media and little professional understanding from the mental health professions, despite the fact that they were obviously at high risk for stress-related reactions and disorders (Toubiana, Milgram, & Falach, 1986). Examples of ideologically stigmatized children are legion, such as children suffering from AIDS, children victimized by chronic sexual abuse, children born of an incestuous union, Palestinian children whose fathers were killed as "collaborators with Israel" by other Palestinians. Such children are at high risk for stress-related disturbances and should receive prompt, appropriate treatment, notwithstanding bias or prejudice held against them by members of their own communities (Milgram & Toubiana, 1988).

Developmental and Social Considerations

A major consideration in dealing with children and adolescents under stress is developmental. When we compare a child of 3 with a child of 6, or a 6 with a 9, we observe enormous differences in cognitive appraisal, perceptual efficiency, emotional control, motivation for personal control, opportunity for personal control, coping strategies, and other intrapersonal variables affecting one's coping with stress. Children are less aware than adults of the realistic threat and harm in a particular stressful situation and of the realistic coping options available to them. As a result, they may be more traumatized by a given episode, or conversely, less traumatized, depending on the complex character of the stressor and its direct impact on them and on the significant others in their lives. No one age is more vulnerable than another for all forms of deprivation and brutalization, but we can identify characteristic vulnerabilities at different ages and specific classes of stress-related symptoms that are more prevalent at one age versus another. For example, somatic symptoms, compulsive restorative play, separation anxiety, and regression are more common in preschool children, whereas guilt feelings, belligerent behavior, and fantasy production are more common in older children (Mowbray, 1988).

Developmental maturation and change are not the sole consideration, however, in evaluating real and potential differences between children and adults exposed to stressful situations. There are equally important social considerations. These refer to the child's privileges and responsibilities within the context of the child's family, peer group, other adults, and the society at large. What is the child allowed to do, forbidden to do, or required to do when stressful events occur in these various contexts? Each family, community, ethnic, and national group promulgates age and gender norms for what is expected of and given to children. These determinations in turn affect children's appraisals of what is going on, who will come to their aid, and so on. Social codes in turn govern the community's attitude and response when parents physically punish their children, determine how child victims are perceived and what redress of grievances is available to them and their parents, and affect how aggressive children are perceived and treated by the community and the legal system. The answers to these questions are relevant to the psychological treatment of children who are the victims of adult or peer aggression or are the perpetrators of aggression against others.

PART TWO: STRESS-RELATED DISORDERS IN CHILDREN

Three stress-related disorders are cited in the DSM-IV (1994): Adjustment Disorder, Acute Stress Disorder, and Post-traumatic Stress Disorder (PTSD). A fourth disorder, identified in the DSM-IV Field Trials but not included in the DSM-IV, Disorder of Extreme Stress, will also be discussed (Blank, 1994). The diagnosis, etiology, epidemiology, incidence, and treatment of these disorders may be understood with reference to the stress and coping concepts discussed thus far. The essential feature common to all is a maladaptive stress reaction to identifiable psychosocial stressors. The differences are instructive, and all four disorders are described in some detail, with PTSD receiving far more attention than the others for reasons discussed below.

Adjustment Disorder

An essential feature of this common disorder is the development of clinically significant emotional or behavioral symptoms within 3 months following the onset of an identifiable psychosocial stressor (or multiple stressors). The stressor is usually an unpleasant event of mild to moderate severity that occurs with moderate frequency. DSM-IV examples of these events appear in the first four or five categories of the stressor list presented in Part One—developmental diffi-

culties or crises; discrete events (e.g., minor illness or injury in family members); recurrent events (e.g., parent out of work, family in financial difficulty); continuous events (e.g., residing in a deteriorating neighborhood or living with a family member with a chronic illness).

The various subtypes of Adjustment Disorder are determined by associated affective or behavioral features: depressed mood, anxiety, conduct disturbance, or combinations of the above. Symptoms of this disorder reflect emotional distress in excess of what would be expected from exposure to the stressor and/or signify significant impairment in social or occupational (academic for children and youth) functioning. The assessment of functional impairment is based on a comparison of presumed prestressor level and observed poststressor level of functioning. This assessment is first made by parents and teachers, and then by professional workers who interview and test the child.

The disturbance in Adjustment Disorder begins shortly after the onset of the stressor, and generally persists for less than 6 months after the stressor or its consequences have ceased. If the stressor is an acute event (e.g., suffering an injury before a major school athletic competition), the onset of the disturbance is usually immediate or within a few days and the duration relatively brief. If the stressor or its consequences persist beyond 6 months, the Adjustment Disorder may also persist and is then termed a Chronic Adjustment Disorder. When the disturbance persists beyond 6 months, in the absence of the further stressors or its consequences, other diagnoses are considered (e.g., PTSD).

Differential diagnosis does not pose a difficult problem. Adjustment Disorders may resemble certain Mood Disorders (e.g., Major Depressive Episode), Anxiety Disorders (e.g., Panic, Generalized Anxiety), and Personality Disorders (e.g., Schizoid or Histrionic), but there are several differentiating features: Mood Disorders, Anxiety Disorders, and Personality Disorders are characterized by persistent maladaptive patterns of behavior that are relatively intractable to brief treatment and do not undergo spontaneous remission or reduction in intensity. By contrast, Adjustment Disorders are seen as situation-specific forms of maladjustment that will disappear when the situation ceases, generally within a few months, or with the passage of time as one succeeds in adapting to a continuous stressor. Preexisting conditions, e.g., Mental Retardation or Attention-Deficit and Disruptive Behavior Disorder, may increase one's vulnerability to stress and to the development of Adjustment Disorder.

PTSD

In an ascending hierarchy of stressful life events, Acute Stress Disorder, a new diagnostic category appearing for the first time in the DSM-IV (1994), should follow. Because it is a more mild form of PTSD, a well-established disorder that appeared in earlier editions of the DSM (1980, 1987), the major features of the latter are presented first in considerable detail.

There are six defining features of PTSD: instigating circumstances and initial response, various reexperience phenomena, avoidant behaviors, increased autonomic arousal, persistent distress and/or impairment in important areas of functioning, and duration of the disturbance.

Traumatic Event and Initial Response

PTSD is defined by the exposure of a child to a traumatic event that is outside the range of usual human experience and is markedly distressing to almost anyone, and in fact elicits intense fear, helplessness, or horror in the particular child being diagnosed. The recognizable traumatic stressor may be well known to all, as in the case of a natural or man-made disaster. It may be reported by the victim, as in rape or physical assault. It may be reported by observers (e.g., parent, teacher, innocent bystander) when the victim is unable to report what transpired. Examples are a young child who cannot

effectively communicate to others, an uncommunicative older child with a severe avoidant or depressive reaction, or a child with an amnestic condition following exposure to a psychologically intolerable stressor (e.g., witnessing the parent's murder).

When we encounter a child with symptoms resembling those of PTSD as described below, but are unaware of a proximal, identifiable stressor that preceded these symptoms, we must obtain a comprehensive case history, and carefully examine the child in structured and unstructured natural life and testing situations. If our efforts do not uncover stressors of intensity sufficient to account for the presenting symptoms, we must consider other diagnoses.

The following three criteria refer to the nature of the reactions to the traumatic event.

Intrusive Replay of the Traumatic Event

The traumatic event is persistently reexperienced in at least one (or more) of the following ways in order to qualify for the PTSD diagnosis:

1. Recurrent and intrusive distressing recollections of the event—in young children, repetitive play in which themes or aspects of the trauma are expressed
2. Recurrent distressing dreams of the event
3. Acting or feeling as if the traumatic event were happening again, including a sense of reliving the experience, illusions, hallucinations, and dissociative (flashback) episodes
4. Intense psychological distress (or 5— physiological reactivity) when exposed to internal or external events that symbolize or resemble aspects of the traumatic event

These involuntary intrusions of features of the original upsetting event, occurring long after the event happened and in physical settings far removed from the scene of the original event, have some of the features of obsessional thinking. The definition of obsessions in the

DSM-IV (1994) could apply equally to intrusions, "persistent ideas, thoughts, impulses, or images that are experienced as intrusive and inappropriate and that cause marked anxiety or distress" (p. 418).

Intrusions differ from obsessions in content, variety, and comorbidity:

1. The content of intrusions refers to stimulus characteristics of the stressor and response characteristics of the child during exposure to the traumatic event and thereafter. We are often able to reconstruct the stressor and the stress reactions experienced at the time by attending to the content of the intrusions. By contrast, the content of obsessions is perceived by the person to be senseless or repugnant without any recognized connection to a particular precipitating external event.

2. The variety of intrusions is almost unlimited, whereas there are a relatively small number of obsessions. The most common examples of the latter are repetitive thoughts of violence (e.g., killing a loved one), contamination (e.g., becoming infected by shaking hands), and doubt (e.g., repeatedly wondering whether one locked all of the doors and windows in the house before retiring for the evening).

3. Obsessions typically occur in juxtaposition with compulsions, i.e., repetitive and apparently senseless behaviors that complete a cycle of anxiety arousal and discharge. For example, if the obsessional thought implies a repugnant act, the compulsion prevents it from happening or offers restitution for its having occurred. Intrusions, by contrast, are not accompanied or followed by compulsive acts.

Intrusions may take the form of recurrent dreams about the event, but differ from Sleep Terror Disorder in that the details of the dream are better recalled than in the latter. Moreover, the latter diagnosis is restricted to children in which a particular form of sleep disturbance is noted and the other waking state criteria of PTSD are absent.

Three instances of traumatic event replay—ideational intrusions, dreams, and suddenly acting or feeling as if the traumatic event were recurring—are regarded by psychoanalysts as evidence of a repetition compulsion. Freud (1914/1953) attributed this phenomenon to a regulatory feedback loop generated by a direct relationship between stressor intensity and anxiety level and an inverse relationship between the latter and permeability of a "stimulus barrier" that controls the perceptual processing of the stressor. The persistence of stressor-related intrusions may also be explained in terms of learning principles associated with classical and operant conditioning (see Janis, 1971, pp. 41–62). The replay phenomenon and intense conditioned reactions are elicited by relatively neutral environmental stimuli or ideational cues that became associated with the traumatic event because of contiguity in time or place and/or physical or symbolic similarity between aspects of the original traumatic event and current events.

Researchers and practitioners welcome intrusions because they point to those aspects of the stressor and one's stress reactions that represent unfinished business. The traumatic content of intrusions and intense emotional reactions associated with it are a major focus for therapeutic intervention.

Persistent Avoidance and Numbing of General Responsiveness

The child must exhibit three or more of the following:

1. Efforts to avoid thoughts, feelings, or conversations associated with the trauma

2. Efforts to avoid activities or situations that arouse recollections of the trauma

3. Inability to recall an important aspect of the trauma (psychogenic amnesia)

4. Markedly diminished interest and participation in significant activities (in young children, loss of recently acquired developmental skills such as toilet training or language skills)

5. Feeling of detachment or estrangement from others

6. Restricted range of affect, e.g., unable to have loving feelings

7. Sense of foreshortened future, e.g., does not expect to grow up, have a career, get married and have children, or enjoy a long life

Avoidant phobic behavior, including amnesia for an important aspect of the trauma, reduces the probability that stimulus cued intrusions will occur. On the other hand, it also guarantees that the acquired sensitivity to a given phobic stimulus will persist and may recur in exacerbated form over time.

The numbing or lack of responsiveness may be expressed in a variety of ways. The child may show little interest and not engage in activities that were important and frequently engaged in before the stressful event occurred. The child may not appear interested in maintaining prized relationships. Differential diagnosis from the various mood disorders is based on a number of considerations: the cyclical nature of depressive episodes, and the prominence and pervasive quality of the depression itself, as compared with the flatness of affect in PTSD. Sometimes the child's condition merits more than one diagnosis. A given child may merit a primary diagnosis of PTSD and a secondary one of depressive episode, or the reverse, depending on the relative severity of the two disorders. Both disorders may arise from the traumatic event or the mood disorder may precede or follow it.

Psychological numbing has been interpreted as a massive form of denial that permits the individual to maintain a modicum of appropriate functioning in other life routines, before gradually engaging oneself in confronting and working through the various aspects of the traumatic event (Lazarus, 1983; Lifton, 1964). Although denial may be beneficial for the short haul, persistent denial becomes a self-perpetuating feature of chronic PTSD.

Why psychological numbing alternates with intrusions in many children and adolescents with PTSD merits explanation. The two phenomena would appear to be at opposite poles of stressor–stress reaction relationship with reference to reactivity. An intrusion is equivalent to behaving as if the original traumatic event were still taking place, and is an instance of hyper-reactivity. Numbing is behaving as if neither the traumatic event, nor anything else important to the child was happening, and is an instance of underreactivity. Both phenomena are exercises in extremes and, as such, lend themselves to a single explanation. Horowitz (1976, 1983) argued that a major aspect of all cognitive information processing is a completion tendency. This concept is similar to Piaget's concept of cognitive adaptation to stimulus events (Piaget, 1954). In Piaget's terms, the occurrence of a familiar event is likely to be quickly and automatically assimilated to existing cognitive schemata. By contrast, an unfamiliar event cannot be assimilated until existing schemata are accommodated (changed) so as to reduce the discrepancy between the prior concept and the present percept.

In the Horowitz formulation, all events are initially incorporated into active or short-term memory storage where they are compared against existing memory schemata. If the incongruity between the prior schemata and those mandated by the new event is small, then a minimum of cognitive processing is required, the event is quickly removed from active memory and conscious awareness, and stored in inactive or long-term memory. Once an event becomes inactive, it will not appear spontaneously in conscious awareness. By contrast, a highly threatening stressful event is incongruous with prestress schemata, and this incongruity is not resolved in one sitting. Memories of a stressful event remain in active memory storage and are more easily elicited by environmental cues than is material in inactive storage. These upsetting memories will recur until continued cognitive processing reduces their incongruity.

Denial is posited by Horowitz as a control mechanism to protect oneself against intolerable levels of emotional upset associated with stressful stimuli. It takes place as an aspect of the initial clinical reaction to the stressful event and recurs periodically when intrusions occur and upset one's equilibrium. It may also take place before intrusions occur in order to ward them off. Denial as an exaggerated form of control turns off reactions to all emotionally arousing experiences, bringing about psychological numbness. Oscillations in control behavior and variations in the intensity of environmental cues that elicit intrusions account for the recurrence in the same child of the two complementary phenomena.

Persistent Symptoms of Increased Arousal

The child must exhibit two or more of the following symptoms (not present before the trauma): difficulty falling or staying asleep, irritability or outbursts of anger, difficulty concentrating, hypervigilance, and exaggerated startle response. The etiological basis for these increased arousal symptoms is derived from qualitative features of the stress and coping paradigm. The symptoms are exaggerated coping maneuvers or their consequences. Hyperalertness and exaggerated startle response are maladaptive carry-overs of the heightened autonomic arousal and perceptual vigilance required to detect and react effectively to a life-threatening event well in advance. Sleep disturbance follows from any or all of the following factors: a high arousal state, the intrusion of upsetting thoughts that prevent one from relaxing and falling asleep, and upsetting dreams that disturb healthy sleep patterns and establish aversive reactions to falling asleep. Attention and concentration difficulties are explained by heightened arousal-increasing response competition between situation-relevant and -irrelevant responses, lack of interest in external events (numbing and disinterest), lack of sleep, and so forth.

Irritability and outbursts of anger arise for many, diverse reasons. First, irritability may occur because of heightened fears of losing control, especially if loss of control occurred during the traumatic episode. Second, irritability and anger may occur as part of one's reaction to the frustrating consequences of the traumatic episode. Third, verbal and physical aggression are

more likely to occur if the child behaved aggressively during the traumatic episode, especially under reduced capacity for control over impulses. Fourth, children may blame others for what happened to them. Chief targets are their parents or other adult caretakers who failed to protect them against harm. Other targets for their anger are those who directly harmed them, with children entertaining retaliation fantasies against their attackers. Fifth, children may be angry at themselves because of their guilt feelings. Typically guilt feelings are associated with depression rather than anger, but the depressive reaction may take the form of agitation and irritability (Milgram et al., 1988).

The basis for these guilt feelings has been termed *survivor guilt*. Guilt about surviving when others did not, or about behavior required for survival is cited as an associated feature of PTSD in the DSM-IV (1994, p. 425). In many crisis situations the different outcomes of the original victims (unharmed, injured, deceased) and the different behaviors of those involved become an object of moral appraisal. Victims who were spared may experience guilt feelings for not having intervened to help primary victims who were not spared. Survivors may question their belief system and the value of their continued existence when they find that people more worthy than they did not survive, or when they escape a situation without injury, while others suffer crippling disabilities for life. This symptom is determined in part by the character of the traumatic event and in part by developmental considerations. Older children and adolescents may well regard themselves as responsible for traumatic events or their consequences and become depressed, whereas very young children may experience shame or other negative affects.

Duration and Consequences of the Symptom Disturbance

The symptoms must persist for at least 1 month, to meet this criterion for a diagnosis of PTSD. The disturbance must cause clinically significant distress or impairment in important areas of functioning—social and scholastic for children. If duration of symptoms is less than 3 months, it is diagnosed as an acute disorder, and if more than 3 months, a chronic disorder. If onset of symptoms is at least 6 months after the stressor, the disorder is classified as delayed onset.

To qualify for a diagnosis of PTSD, all six criteria must be fulfilled. These quantitative cutoff scores (e.g., at least one of the five reexperiencing symptoms, at least three of the seven avoidant responses, and two of the five arousal symptoms) reflect a trade-off between stringent criterion requirements that reduce the number of people who qualify for the diagnosis, and less stringent requirements that increase the number.

Closing Comments on Differential Diagnosis

In the absence of a clear and definitive stressor, we infer that the current symptom picture is the consequence of breakdown in an individual with particular vulnerabilities and we assign the psychopathological reactions observed to other diagnostic categories—Generalized Anxiety Disorder, Obsessive Compulsive Disorder, Panic Disorder, and Mood Disorders (especially Depression). This inference follows from an adaptation to the field of stress and coping of the familiar behavior–person–situation relationship: $S = V \times PE$, in which symptoms (S) are the product of premorbid vulnerabilities (V) times precipitating event (PE). With symptoms held constant, as PE goes down, V goes up, and vice versa.

These preexisting vulnerabilities are conceptualized in psychodynamic terms as inadequate defenses to handle the intrusion of unconscious, unacceptable wishes and fears; and in learning terms as maladaptive expectancies or response hierarchies based on classical and operant conditioned responses acquired in prior life experience. Vulnerable individuals develop symptoms similar in some respects to those found in PTSD, after exposure to mild stressors that in and of themselves do not bring about these symptoms in most people. In these cir-

cumstances, premorbid vulnerabilities and predispositions to breakdown are emphasized over situational factors, and the type and goals of treatment are different. Traumatic events may occur, however, in children with preexisting crystallized anxiety or personality disorders. In this case, both disorders are diagnosed, and treatment for PTSD takes into consideration the adjustment problems associated with the preexisting disorder.

Acute Stress Disorder

The DSM-IV introduced a new diagnostic category for what was called *posttraumatic stress reaction* in the earlier edition of this chapter in Ollendick and Hersen (1989, p. 409). The precipitating event and the symptom picture of Acute Stress Disorder are identical to those of PTSD. They differ from PTSD in earlier onset of symptoms, shorter duration and lower intensity and frequency of reexperiencing, avoidant, and increased arousal symptoms. It is also characterized by at least three of the following symptoms experienced during or shortly after the distressing event: absence of emotional responsiveness, reduced awareness of the surroundings, derealization (estrangement from reality), depersonalization (estrangement from oneself or one's body), and dissociative amnesia (inability to remember important aspects of the trauma).

This disorder occurs within 1 month of the traumatic experience, and lasts for a minimum of 2 days and a maximum of 4 weeks. Those who do not recover in 1 month or less and/or whose symptoms persist or increase in intensity and frequency over time qualify, first for a diagnosis of the acute form of PTSD, and second for a diagnosis of the chronic form.

Disorder of Extreme Stress

If Acute Stress Disorder is a mild form of PTSD, Disorder of Extreme Stress is a more complex, severe, and recalcitrant variation

(Blank, 1994). It occurs in survivors of prolonged and repeated trauma, including concentration and slave labor camps, coercive religious cults, brothels, abusive hostage situations, and homes characterized by physical battering and sexual abuse. The formal diagnosis requires six symptoms among the following: chronic disturbance in regulating affect and impulse, difficulty in controlling anger, self-destructive behavior and suicidal preoccupations, difficulty in managing one's sexual involvements (adults), impulsive and risk-taking behavior, seeing self as ineffective and permanently damaged, chronic guilt and shame, minimizing the importance of the traumatic event, unrealistic (idealizing) perceptions of the perpetrator, inability to maintain relationships based on trust, tendency to be victimized, tendency to victimize others, loss of previously sustaining beliefs and values, despair and hopelessness, amnesia and dissociation from the traumatic event, and somatization. This disorder represents a severe type of stress-related disorder that results from prolonged exposure to extraordinary stressors.

Treatment of Stress-Related Disorders in Children

The clinical literature on treatment of PTSD in adults is extensive, especially with reference to former combat veterans (Figley, 1978; Williams, 1980), but less extensive with reference to children. Some of the treatment principles are derived from work with combat veterans in World War I (Salmon, 1919) and in more recent wars (Solomon, 1993; Toubiana, Milgram, & Noy, 1986). Soldiers who were unable to continue functioning and displayed the symptoms associated with incipient PTSD were treated as soon as the symptoms appeared (*immediacy*), as close as possible to the site of victimization (*proximity*), and were told that they would recover very soon and be able to resume their prior activities (*expectancy*). These expectations were conveyed both in words and in the behaviors required of them in the days that followed. A

fourth treatment principle has also been emphasized when PTSD occurs in a group context (*community*). This principle states that the resources of the group whose members were exposed to the stressor are mobilized to help exposed members recover by capitalizing on the desire to regain or maintain identification with the group (Milgram et al. 1988).

A recent publication (March & Amaya-Jackson, 1993) stated succinctly, "Central to almost all treatment strategies is an emphasis on reexposing the individual to traumatic cues under safe conditions and incorporating reparative and mastery elements in a structured, supportive manner" (p. 2). There are many different treatment orientations toward specific PTSD features such as intrusions and psychic numbing, with most emphasizing the importance of systematic reminiscence and reexperiencing the original traumatic event. Depending on their therapeutic orientation, professional workers speak of abreaction, release, working through, systematic desensitization, and extinction through implosion (Craighead, Kazdin, & Mahoney, 1981; Frederick, 1985). Many approaches deal with the long- as well as the short-term consequences of the original traumatic event.

Some recent publications deal extensively with diagnosis and treatment of PTSD in children and are highly recommended: a special section of the *Journal of the American Academy of Child Psychiatry* (1986) entitled Children's Reactions to Severe Stress; a book entitled *Post-Traumatic Stress Disorder in Children* (Eth & Pynoos, 1985); two chapters by Pynoos and Nader (1991, 1993); and a series of child treatment chapters in the *International Handbook of Traumatic Stress Syndromes* (Wilson & Raphael, 1993).

Special Kinds of Stressor-Related Psychopathology

Many kinds of stressors may contribute to the stress-related disorders discussed above. To summarize and analyze them is to go well beyond the space allotment of this chapter. Four are briefly discussed here: natural disasters, war, physical violence in the home and community, and sexual abuse in the home and community, in that order. Each kind of stressor has unique diagnostic and treatment features as well as features common to the other kinds of stressors. The first two share a community emphasis, i.e., these disasters affect entire communities, adults and children. Accordingly, there is a necessary focus on the community in assessing the stressors, their consequences, and the requisite interventions. The third and fourth kinds of stressors affect many children, but only as individuals and not as a collective sharing a common experience, and the assessment and intervention are individualized.

Children in Natural Disasters

Until recently there was little work on the responses of children to natural disaster (e.g., earthquakes, hurricanes, floods, bushfires) as compared with the intensive efforts to diagnose, intervene, and follow-up the posttraumatic reactions and disorders of adults. This neglect was based, in part, on the commonly held myth that children and youth are more resilient and flexible, and, therefore, more likely to make a quick recovery, without professional intervention (Gordon & Wraith, 1993). This myth has been detrimental to providing appropriate intervention on behalf of children in need, and, fortunately, has been abandoned by researchers and practitioners alike.

This myth has been replaced by a balanced view that the number of children upset or traumatized by natural disasters and in need of some level of intervention ranges from 10 to 90%, depending on the intensity, duration, extent of injury, and loss of life and property of the particular disaster. Children may, for example, experience on their persons the threats and losses associated with a tidal wave that nearly inundates their community (Belter, Dunn, & Jeney, 1991). They may also observe the maladaptive responses and emotional distress of their parents and other responsible adults and suffer the loss of adult support when they need it most (Green et al., 1991). If the dislocation is extensive and enduring, as was the earthquake in Armenia in 1988, posttraumatic reactions in children may reach epidemic proportions, jeopardize the well-being of the child population of a large region, and threaten to alter the individual and social character of the people of the affected region (Pynoos et al., 1993).

When the earthquake was of lesser magnitude, as was the Loma Prieta earthquake in the San Francisco Bay Area (Bradburn, 1991), children resumed their regular routines 6 to 8 months later. Some children were still troubled and displayed a heightened startle pattern to cues that reminded them of the disaster (e.g., noises, crossing a bridge). Similarly, children directly exposed to extended life-threatening circumstances and the subsequent loss of their homes in Hurricane Hugo (Belter et al., 1991) were far more upset 5 months later than children farther inland whose lives were never in danger and whose property damage was less extensive (Sullivan, Saylor, & Foster, 1991). An extensive study 3 months after this hurricane confirmed the relationship between degree of perceived or actual victimization and the frequency of PTSD symptoms, and also showed the effect of predisaster predisposing factors: Children with a high premorbid level of manifest anxiety were more likely to exhibit and retain PTSD symptoms months later (Lonigan, Shannon, Finch, Daugherty, & Taylor, 1991) than children with a low premorbid level.

The behavior of parents and of other significant adults during and after the disaster—especially, the mothers—was found to be more critical to children's subsequent adjustment than their direct exposure to the disaster itself (Green et al., 1991). McFarlane (1987) found that three parental variables strongly contributed to long-term PTSD symptoms in exposed children: separation from the parents immediately after the disaster, continuing maternal (not paternal) preoccupation with the disaster, and deterioration in family functioning. Green et al. (1991) also confirmed the adverse effects of the mother's traumatic stress reaction level, and of a disturbed (irritable and/or depressed) family atmosphere.

Parental influence on children's symptom formation and on subsequent adjustment is, in turn, moderated by developmental factors. For example, a 2-year follow-up study on children exposed to the Buffalo Creek dam collapse showed that the youngest and the oldest children were most affected by their parents' reactions, for different reasons. Young children were unable to evaluate the implications of what had happened and took their cues from the parents; they showed, overall, fewer PTSD symptoms than older children. Adolescents understood full well the implications of what happened, experienced survivor guilt, identified with their parents' plight, and felt the burden of shared responsibility for rectifying the situation (Green et al., 1991). Adolescent survivors of a cruise ship sinking attributed to themselves responsibility for the loss of life of their age peers—a tragedy for which no one else held them responsible—and as a consequence experienced greater PTSD a year later (Joseph, Brewin, Yule, & Williams, 1993).

The emphasis on emotional ventilation following a disaster would suggest that the children who displayed many, acute, intense stress reactions would be less upset on follow-up than those who had exhibited few stress reactions. In fact, the opposite was found: Children with high anxiety and behavior disturbance levels at school at the 2- and 8-month follow-ups were more likely to manifest PTSD symptoms 26 months after a bushfire with enormous loss of property and livestock than the others (McFarlane, 1987).

Several studies highlighted the importance of emphasizing the ability to maintain normal routines after a disaster (e.g., Belter et al., 1991), as well as the importance of identifying pathological indicators so as to intervene with groups at risk for PTSD (e.g., Belter et al., 1991; Green et al., 1991; Milgram & Toubiana, 1988). The two

emphases—on indices of normal, healthy functioning as well as on the frequency and intensity of stress-related symptoms—complement one another and provide a proper sense of proportion to the general public and to professional workers. These foci have been termed the *salutogenic* and the *pathogenic orientation*, respectively (Antonovsky, 1979), and should be taken into account in assessing the effects of natural disasters and other stressors on children.

Single-minded focus on the immediate consequences of the disaster—e.g., the terrifying images of injury, death, and destruction to which children were exposed, the actual scope of loss of life and property—may lead interventionists to ignore the many secondary adversities that affect the mental health of survivors, parents, and children alike—e.g., unemployment and economic hardship, the problems of relocation, exacerbation of predisaster traumatic experiences, and family difficulties. Hence, the importance is seen of comprehensive screening for the presence of indicators that place some communities and families within communities at high risk for chronic, severe stress reactions and disorders. As the intervention principles in natural disasters are applicable to other kinds of disasters, they are presented in the next section.

Children in War

The clinical literature on the effects of war on children has grown considerably in recent years. The earliest work dates back to World War II and the classical work of Anna Freud and Dorothy Burlingham with English children during and after the London blitz (1943). Contrary to lay expectation at the time, they found that English children as a group did not exhibit traumatic and posttraumatic stress reactions to bombing incidents when they were in the care of their parents or familiar surrogates. In fact, children living with their parents during the blitz had fewer posttraumatic stress reactions than children separated from their parents and evacuated to tranquil, rural settings (Garmezy, 1983, pp. 67–68).

Major reviews on children in war have appeared in recent years: Israeli children (Milgram, 1982; Raviv & Klingman, 1981; Spielberger, Sarason, & Milgram, 1982), children in Northern Ireland (Fields, 1977), and children in a number of countries and conflicts (Dyregov & Raundalen, 1987; Garmezy, 1983; Leavitt & Fox, 1993; Macksoud et al., 1993).

It is difficult to generalize across the different wars and, equally important, across the different postwar experiences.

Consider the following groups of children:

1. U.S. children residing in diplomatic communities in Afghanistan and Pakistan following the assassination of the U.S. ambassador in the former and the razing of the U.S. embassy in the latter (Rigamer, 1986)

2. Jewish orphans who spent formative years in the traumatizing and depriving atmosphere of Nazi concentration camps in Europe in the early 1940s before emigrating to the United States or Israel (Langmeier & Matejcek, 1975)

3. Central American children, in the 1980s, who grew up malnourished and repeatedly traumatized by physical violence, death, and separation from parents before emigrating to the United States (Arroyo & Eth, 1985)

4. Cambodian children who were exposed to traumatic experiences (1975–1979) in their own homeland before emigrating to the United States (Kinzie, Sack, Angell, Manson, & Rath, 1986; Sack, Angell, Kinzie, & Rath, 1986)

5. Northern Ireland children, Protestant and Catholic alike, who have lived since birth in intact families on their own home grounds, but are constantly exposed to brutalizing, life-threatening stressors (Fields, 1977; Fraser, 1974)

6. Kuwaiti children who witnessed the rape, torture, and murder of others during the Gulf War (Nader & Pynoos, 1993)

The children's subsequent adjustment was a function of the intensity and duration of the traumatic stressors and the stressful features of the setting in which they recovered. The U.S. diplomatic children experienced temporary stress reactions, and only a few suffered from severe disorders before returning to the safety of their country. The Jewish orphans built new lives in receptive, adopting societies and were encouraged to regard their survival and success as evidence of their triumph over adversity. The Central American and Cambodian children had to overcome enormous cultural differences between the countries and cultures of origin and those of an indifferent or unfriendly adoptive country. The children of Northern Ireland live in a society torn by ethnic–religious animosities, mistrust, and guerrilla warfare, with recurrent acts of violence alternating with periods of quiet and anticipation of the next violent act and function normally in many contexts, but pay a psychic price in adapting to unpredictable, recurrent stressors. The Kuwaiti children were exposed to multiple atrocities and exhibited a very high frequency and intensity of posttraumatic stress reactions.

Several conclusions were reached from surveying the literature on the effects of natural and man-made disasters including war, on children (Pynoos, Goenjian, & Steinberg, 1994):

1. *The stressor–victimization relationship.* The greater the degree of victimization—multiplicity and intensity of stressors, duration of exposure, extent and irreversibility of adverse consequences—the greater are the frequency, severity, and chronicity of resulting symptomatology. The sheer number of stressors impinging on the child or the family or community in which one lives at a particular point in time is especially important because their effect is a geometric rather than an arithmetic function of their number (Rutter, 1979).

2. *The overriding importance of effective adult support systems.* Because children are less familiar with the world around them than are adults, they rely on adult appraisals of threat and imminent danger. When adults communicate to them that the situation is under control and is

not an occasion for emotional distress, they respond in kind. When bereft of adult presence, support, and reassuring appraisals, they become demoralized and traumatized (Hobfoll et al., 1991).

3. *The balance between frightening knowledge and anxious ignorance.* Children need accurate information about what may happen or has happened and why, and what kinds of behaviors are expected of them. One should never assume that children do not know what is going on, but rather that they have received numerous anxiety-provoking cues, that they are unable to connect to objective, manageable reality. It is necessary to help children and adolescents understand and work through the threats and losses in the stressful situation.

4. *The balance between responsibility and burden.* Children should not be sheltered from family or community difficulties, nor should they be burdened by their parents' fears or demands. They should be actively recruited to do useful things during any family or community crisis, but they should not be asked to shoulder responsibilities beyond their developmental capability.

5. *The personal allocation of responsibility.* Children, like adults, ask themselves: (1) Who is responsible for their being in the current predicament? (2) Who is responsible for extricating them from it? It makes a great deal of difference if children attribute responsibility to themselves (internal) or to other people or forces beyond their control (external) in answering these questions. Attributions affect cognitive appraisals, stress reactions, motivation to take action, planning, and coping behavior. As children are not able or permitted to assume complete responsibility for their actions, it is important to ascertain that they share the same attributions as their adult guardians and professional workers for their current difficulties and the solutions for them. If they do not, it is imperative to make the necessary clarifications and attribution corrections (Milgram, 1986).

6. *The overriding importance and the modest contribution of developmental status to postdisaster outcomes in children.* Children's immediate response to stressors and their subsequent functioning and psychiatric status are a function of their developmental stage-dependent perceptual, cognitive, emotional, motivational, and behavioral repertoires. This conclusion does not contradict a second conclusion, that these outcomes are also affected by countless situational variables. By way of clarification, birth order makes a lifetime difference in one's personal and social development, but one would be hard pressed to separate out a consistent effect of birth order across the myriad of other variables that affect personal and social development in first- versus later-born children.

7. *Roles during and after disaster.* How well children function during a natural or manmade disaster and recover thereafter is a function of the roles they undertake during and after the disaster. Any treatment plan for traumatized children and adolescents must delve into the actual behavior of these children. For example, children who were mobilized by warring factions to inform on others or to perform acts of violence against others must deal with different issues than children who were at the mercy of others during the same conflict (Macksoud et al., 1993).

Several intervention principles emerge from work with children in natural disasters and war (Cohen, 1988; Gordon & Wraith, 1993; Hobfoll et al., 1991; Milgram, Sarason, Schonplug, Jackson, & Schwarzer, 1995; Raphael, 1986). All are directed to professional workers and some are also directed to parents and significant adults in the community:

1. Assess the strengths and weakness of the parents and other significant adults in the child's community and offer them the support that will enable them to function in a responsible fashion until the crisis is over.

2. Encourage adults to provide warmth and reassurance to children without minimizing children's concerns.

3. Encourage adults to discover what is specifically upsetting to children exposed to a par-

ticular kind of disaster and to direct their efforts to deal with these concerns.

4. Admonish adults not to impose their own fears or burdens on children, and not to project adult concerns or stereotypes onto children.

5. Help children to replace fantasy with reality in a gradual, sensitive manner. The latter is usually far less threatening.

6. Foster mutual support networks of children for children.

7. Encourage a return to normal routines and relationships.

8. Plan community activities using disaster-relevant symbols and rituals to help restore shared meanings and cherished assumptions shattered by the disaster.

One source of difficulty in assessing psychopathology and treatment needs is the vested interest of the political leaders of the society or country in presenting a picture that furthers their own agenda. If incidence of pathology is low, difficult decisions do not have to be made. If high, then someone must be held accountable for letting this lamentable situation happen, and someone else is responsible for fixing it (Milgram et al., 1995). Distortion can also take place at the local level where parents encourage their children to exaggerate their symptoms to gain sympathy at one point in time and to minimize it at another time in order to demonstrate the fortitude of the civilian population, including the children, in the ideological struggle (Milgram, 1990).

Physical Violence in the Home or Community

According to Finkelhor and Dziuba-Leatherman (1994), victimization of children and adolescents, broadly defined, is very common and in some categories (physical assault by nonfamily members, corporal punishment by parents or parent surrogates, and sibling assault) pandemic. Several reasons are cited for this widespread phenomenon: Children are small in stature and weak in muscle, and cannot, there-fore, deter victimization or retaliate against it. They cannot choose with whom to associate or to place distance between themselves and potential or actual victimizers. Third, society tolerates many forms of child victimization (e.g., by parents, siblings, age peers). The present section and the following one document two kinds of child victimization, namely, physical violence and sexual abuse.

There is a high level of physical violence in the home and in the community, and much of it affects children directly or indirectly. According to Finkelhor and Dziuba-Leatherman (1994), the rate per 1000 children for physical abuse is 23; for physical assault, 311; for corporal punishment, 499; and for sibling assault, 800. In addition, many children witness physical violence against another person. There is a wide range of witnessing encounters—from seeing a schoolmate killed in the schoolyard by a deranged sniper (Pynoos & Eth, 1985) to seeing one's teacher or one's mother killed (Malmquist, 1986). Life-threatening direct victim encounters range from being kidnapped and buried alive in a school bus for many hours before being able to escape (Terr, 1983) to being terrorized or physically attacked by psychotic parents (Anthony, 1986). Pedersen (1994) found that 82% of sixth graders in low-income Los Angeles neighborhoods reported exposure to physical violence and 29% reported PTSD symptoms; and that there was a strong relationship between direct exposure to violence and severity of symptomatology.

Longitudinal follow-up of child victims of physical violence has documented the recalcitrant nature of posttraumatic stress reactions and disorders. Many children exposed to a fatal sniper attack on their elementary school playground were found to be suffering from PTSD 14 months later. The best predictor of their mental health status was the degree of exposure to violence during the sniper attack, but greater interpersonal involvement (i.e., knowing the child who was killed) and experiencing guilt feelings were also strongly associated with a greater number of symptoms (Nader, Pynoos,

Fairbanks, & Frederick, 1990). A 4-year follow-up of school-bus kidnap victims revealed that all exhibited posttraumatic effects, despite brief treatment 5–13 months after the kidnapping (Terr, 1983). Symptom severity was related to the child's prior vulnerabilities, family pathology, and weak community bonding. Other researchers have confirmed that children with precrisis vulnerabilities—personal, familial, and cultural—are more likely to develop extensive, chronic psychopathology than resilient children capable of recruiting on their own the support that they need or mobilizing personal resources to deal with the crisis (Garmezy, 1983; Pynoos & Eth, 1985; Terr, 1983).

In dealing with child victims of direct and indirect violence, it is necessary to assess three levels of stressor or press (the term used by Murray, 1938/1962):

1. Alpha press or what actually happened
2. Beta press or what the child reportedly perceived
3. Gamma press (this author's term) or the content of the child's fantasies about what happened

Attention to the child's fantasied recollection of what took place will clarify the child's subsequent fantasied reactions. The latter include retaliation against the aggressor, protective measures to ensure that the violent act will never again be directed against the child, denial that the violent act ever took place, miraculous undoing of the act, and restoration of the loved one or healing of the injury incurred.

Given a highly specific traumatizing stressor (e.g., a violent act against oneself or a loved one), it is necessary to offer incident-specific treatment. In evaluating the psychopathological implications of these phenomena in children, it is important to follow several guidelines:

1. Obtain baseline data from other traumatized and nontraumatized groups of children comparable in age and other demographic variables, in order not to exaggerate or minimize the severity of temporary or permanent psychic disability in the target group of children.

2. Analyze ghosts, unusual bereavement rituals, and bizarre behaviors displayed by children in terms of their adaptive as well as their defensive value.

3. Make flexible, concerted efforts to return the child to the scene of the crime to reconstruct and reinterpret what happened literally and/or through imagery.

4. Register empathy and not horror when confronting children who have been exposed to extraordinary stigmatizing stressors (e.g., rape, incest, witness to murder).

5. Distinguish in assessment and intervention between stress reactions to a threat to life or limb and grief reactions to the actual loss of life or limb. The two phenomena are conceptually independent, and the particular circumstances of the violent event(s) may elicit the one and not the other, or both. The former refers to a condition in which aversive events of the past continue to haunt us. The latter refers to the opposite: Many pleasurable experiences with a loved one or with one's intact body are no longer available and we grieve their loss. These two kinds of events lead to different psychological reactions and sequelae, have different timetables for spontaneous extinction, and require different kinds of intervention.

6. Formulate or adopt a structured psychological first aid and treatment approach both for children exposed as a group and for children exposed as individuals to a violent act. Apply this approach at the level of the child, the group, the classroom, the family, and the larger community (Pynoos & Nader, 1988).

Sexual Abuse in Children in the Home and Community

The phenomenon of sexual abuse in children is far more widespread than was assumed in the past, according to a recent major review of child victimization (Finkelhor & Dziuba-Leatherman,

1994; see also Chapter 20). The prevalence of sexual abuse based on agency reports has been placed at 6 per 1000 children, but it is thought to be substantially higher. Some clinical researchers (Herman, Russell, & Trocki, 1986) have estimated the risk of victimization to be as high as 1:10 for boys and 1:3 for girls. Whatever the true figures, the number of child victims of sexual abuse including rape is sufficiently dismaying to bring it to the attention of many researchers and professional workers. The concern has become so great that the first systematic review of the impact of child sexual abuse (Browne & Finkelhor, 1986) was followed by a second review with 45 new studies only 7 years later (Kendall-Tackett, Williams, & Finkelhor, 1993).

The review (Kendall-Tackett et al., 1993) concluded that the majority of child victims experience chronic suffering from their experiences, the most common being PTSD (53% of the cases), behavior problems (37%), fears (33%), sexualized behaviors (defined as sexualized doll play, placing objects in anuses or vaginas, excessive or public masturbation, seductive behavior, and so forth) (28–38%), and poor self-esteem (35%). Adult women who experienced childhood sexual abuse reported more dissociation (disruption of consciousness, memory, and/or identity), sexual problems, alcoholism and drug addiction, suicide attempts, and self-mutilation than nonabused outpatient psychiatric controls, and were more likely to have been raped or sexually assaulted as adults as well (Briere, 1988).

Child victims of sexual abuse are predominantly female. Some estimates place females at eight times the risk of males for rape and two times as much for sexual abuse. This overrepresentation of females is constant from early childhood through adolescence, indicating that male children also remain at substantial risk over the developmental period (Finkelhor & Dziuba-Leatherman, 1994).

A major review on male children and adolescents (Watkins & Bentovim, 1992) suggests that there is greater underreporting for boys than for girls for several reasons: Most boys have an intense fear of homosexuality, may conclude they were selected for abuse because they are latent homosexuals, and suppress or repress the experience. Boys tend to react to sexual abuse by remaining silent, and show great reluctance to talk about it even after discovery. They tend to "act out," and elicit far less sympathy and concern than girls who "act in" and show distress. Boys, unlike girls, are not seen as physically weak and in need of protection, and are more likely to be blamed if they are abused.

There are three other classes of underreporting of which clinicians should be aware: sexual abuse perpetrated by women, by fathers with their sons, and by children and adolescents with one another. It is inconceivable to most professional workers and to the lay public that some women sexually abuse their children or other people's children, but some do. Moreover, when women initiate sexual activity with a male child other than their own, it is often regarded as a normative sexualization experience rather than an abusive one for the young male. Society also turns a blind eye to father–son abuse, although fathers or stepfathers are the most frequent abusers of boys; and to child–child and adolescent–child abuse that are highly frequent in boarding schools and other single-sex day and residential settings.

The fallout of child sexual abuse is highly pathogenic throughout life, but it would be incorrect to conclude that all victims develop persistent symptoms or serious psychiatric disorders. A significant proportion of sexually abused children (between 21 and 49%) have been found to be asymptomatic (Kendall-Tackett et al., 1993). There are several possible explanations for this consistent, counterintuitive finding. First, asymptomatic children may, in fact, be symptomatic, but the relevant dimensions on which their symptoms are manifest were not assessed, or the measuring instruments were not sufficiently sensitive. Second, some asymptomatic children may have been successful in suppressing their symptoms, but may manifest them at some vulnerable period later in their lives; other asymptomatic children may have been too immature to process cognitively the dire implications of sexual abuse when first examined, and become symptomatic as they mature and come to understand what was done to them. Third, asymptomatic children may be genuinely less affected than symptomatic counterparts, because they were exposed to less damaging parameters of child abuse or because they were more resilient. Professional workers who are unaware of the large number of asymptomatic children may diagnose these children as psychiatrically disturbed precisely because they are asymptomatic, and urge their clients to ventilate suppressed feelings and to uncover exhaustively their memories of the traumatic events.

Terr's distinction between Type I and Type II trauma appears useful in planning treatment (Terr, 1991). Type I trauma is a sudden, unpredictable single incident that may recur (e.g., stranger rapes or otherwise molests the child). Type II is a chronic, predictable, expected, and repeated trauma (e.g., father sexually abuses his daughter repeatedly, over a period of years). Both kinds of sexual abuse are traumatic, but the latter is likely to be more damaging because it is associated with more pathogenic features (Briere, 1988; Kendall-Tackett et al., 1993). These features include:

1. Sexual penetration (oral, anal, or genital)
2. Duration and frequency of the abusive acts
3. Incestuous relationship between child and perpetrator
4. Tacit cooperation by mother in the abuse, or absence of maternal support to terminate it
5. Use of physical force during the abusive act
6. Bizarreness of the sexual abuse (bestiality, pseudoreligious rites, insertion of foreign objects, and torture)
7. Number of perpetrators (gang rape, "orgies")

The age and sex of the victim are not included among risk factors contributing to psychopathology, because any abusive act has different meanings, behavioral implications, and consequences for boys versus girls and for different ages.

Most of the treatment literature has focused on adults who suffered sexual abuse as adults or on adults who suffered sexual abuse as children. There have been few empirical evaluations of the efficacy of treatment of sexually abused children. The Browne and Finkelhor (1986) multifaceted model of abuse impact proposes that sexual abuse traumatizes children through four distinct mechanisms: traumatic and inappropriate sexualization, betrayal of basic trust, stigmatization (devaluation by self and others), and pervading sense of powerlessness (e.g., learned helplessness). Comprehensive, individualized treatment would address each of these mechanisms. A short-term individualized cognitive behavior modification treatment program of 12 sessions with children ages 3 to 16 and their parents yielded significant improvement in anxiety, depression, and behavioral measures (Deblinger, McLeer, & Henry, 1990). This treatment is based on the two-factor model of learning theory, classical and instrumental, in dealing with inappropriate affective and behavioral responses and on cognitive reformulation of what transpired during and after the abusive experiences. Group therapy has also been used with older children, especially abused boys, using conjoint male and female therapists (Watkins & Bentovim, 1992).

CASE STUDY

The following case of an incipient Acute Stress Disorder is taken from a report on crisis intervention following a school bus disaster (Toubiana, Milgram, Strich, & Edelstein, 1988). Without rapid and appropriate intervention, it is highly probable that the adolescent's condition would have become chronic over time and qualified for a formal diagnosis of PTSD.

Zack, a 12-year-old seventh grader, was a passenger on a school bus during an end-of-the year outing in which one bus was demolished at a railroad crossing by a passing train. Nineteen schoolchildren and three accompanying adults were killed, and the remaining 14 children were critically injured. In the days that followed the communal burial of the victims, all children in the junior high were exposed to crisis interventions at all levels: consulting with teachers in conducting their classes and handling disturbed children; encouraging children to visit their injured schoolmates in the hospital, and to visit the parents of deceased children during the week of mourning; engaging the children in classroom discussions of the tragedy, and in classroom art and literature exercises dedicated to the memory of their former classmates. Children who did not come to school were strongly encouraged to come, and told that they could receive help only on school premises.

Zack was truant for several days following the accident because he was afraid to leave the house. At the same time he acknowledged that images of the terrible accident haunted him when he was alone at home. He was contacted by a psychologist (Toubiana) and told that he must come to school if he wished help in coping, and was given an appointment. When he arrived, it was evident that he was emotionally blank and numb. Zack was asked to relate the events of the fateful day. He recalled that he had gone on the outing against his wishes. He doesn't like single-day bus trips, but was pressured into going by his father. He felt better as he traveled and began talking with some of his friends when the bus in front was struck by a train. He heard a terrible noise and saw smoke, and children in his bus began to cry.

He was unable to cry even though he wanted to. Afterwards he saw the injured children and felt guilty that he still did not cry. He hoped that his good friend who had been on the bus was only injured, but he made no effort to verify this. When he awoke in the morning and learned that his friend had died, he was shocked. From then on, he had difficulty sleeping, was fearful and confused, and could not enter into casual conversation or play sports he especially liked. His parents tried to console him by buying him expensive presents, but these gifts merely increased his anguish.

Zack said that he was ashamed that he did not attend his friend's funeral or visit the home of the bereaved parents during the mourning period. This avoidant behavior on his part made him feel helpless. In reviewing the names and pictures of all of the children who died, he discovered that two were boys who had insulted him several days earlier. His anger toward them changed to the feeling that he must have been responsible for the altercation. Nevertheless, he continued to express anger toward his friend and the other boys because they had not reacted fast enough to escape from the bus in time.

The psychologist asked him to imagine once again the circumstances of the trip and to conjure up the images of the three boys. Zack complied with this difficult request and spoke aloud to the boys with whom he had argued. He now resolved the argument and said good-bye to them and to his friend. The psychologist suggested that, perhaps, they had something to say to him. They told him to resume his regular activities as they would have done if they were still living. After this emotionally moving experience, he went at the psychologist's suggestion to the memorial erected in the memory of the children on the school premises, stood silent in respect for several minutes, and then returned to his classes. He subsequently visited his friend's bereaved parents.

These interactions took place during several individual sessions with the psychologist. Zack displayed the classical symptoms associated with PTSD: intrusions and psychic numbing in response to the sudden death of schoolmates and friends, sleep disturbance, inability to concentrate, avoidance of activities and settings that aroused recollection of the traumatic event, and guilt feelings. Treatment consisted of reducing his sense of helplessness by requiring him to come against his stated wishes to school and by encouraging him to engage in commemorative behaviors honoring his dead friend and schoolmates. Abreaction was encouraged, and Zack relived the course of events in the accident, and went on to role-play emotionally moving restitutive behaviors. When he resumed normal classroom activities, treatment ceased. Follow-up over the next year and a half did not show any indication of relapse or PTSD sequelae.

SUMMARY

This chapter deals with a form of psychopathology in children that arises as a consequence of exposure to stressful life events. In Part One, major concepts in the field of stress and coping were defined: stress, stressor, stress reaction, stress disorder, personal resources, interpersonal supports, cognitive appraisal, coping, and levels of crisis intervention. In Part Two, the major categories of reactive psychopathology were presented: Adjustment Disorder, Acute Stress Disorder, Post-traumatic Stress Disorder, and Disorder of Extreme Stress. They were compared with one another and with other disorders. The intensity and chronicity of the various stress-related disorders were related to parameters of the stress situation, pre- and postcrisis personal resources and vulnerabilities, availability of adult support systems, developmental considerations, threat and loss experienced, and assumed responsibility for what happened and what to do about it. Different kinds of treatment were discussed. Four classes of extraordinary stressors—natural disasters, war-related stressors, violence in the home or community, and sexual abuse in the home or community—were described and treatment implications were discussed.

A case was presented of a seventh grader with a severe stress reaction following a tragic school-bus accident (at which he was present) in which 19 of his schoolmates died and 14 were injured. He showed many defining characteristics of the disorder and his short-term treatment was based on the principles of immediacy, proximity, expectancy, and community that were formulated in the treatment of PTSD in adult contexts (combat soldiers).

REFERENCES

American Psychiatric Association. (1980). *Diagnostic and statistical manual of mental disorders* (3rd ed.). Washington, DC: Author.

American Psychiatric Association. (1987). *Diagnostic and statistical manual of mental disorders* (3rd ed. rev.). Washington, DC: Author.

American Psychiatric Association. (1994). *Diagnostic and statistical manual of mental disorders* (4th ed.). Washington, DC: Author.

Ammerman, R. T., Last, C. G., & Hersen, M. (Eds.). (1993). *Handbook of prescriptive treatment for children and adolescents.* Boston: Allyn & Bacon.

Anthony, E. J. (1986). Terrorizing attacks on children by psychotic parents. *Journal of the American Academy of Child Psychiatry, 25,* 326–335.

Antonovsky, A. (1979). *Health, stress, and coping.* San Francisco: Jossey–Bass.

Arroyo, W., & Eth, S. (1985). Children traumatized by Central American warfare. In S. Eth & R. S. Pynoos (Eds.), *Post-traumatic stress disorder in children* (pp. 101–120). Washington, DC: American Psychiatric Association.

Atkinson, R. L., Atkinson, R. C., Smith, E. E., & Bem, D. J. (1990). *Introduction to psychology* (10th ed.). New York: Harcourt Brace Jovanovich.

Auerbach, S. M., & Stolberg, A. L. (Eds.). (1986). *Crisis intervention with children and families.* Washington, DC: Hemisphere.

Bandura, A. (1977). Self-efficacy: Toward a unifying theory of behavioral change. *Psychological Review, 84,* 191–215.

Belter, R. W., Dunn, S. E., & Jeney, P. (1991). The psychological impact of Hurricane Hugo on children: A needs assessment. *Advances in Behavioral Research and Therapy, 13,* 155–161.

Blank, A. S., Jr. (1994). Clinical detection, diagnosis, and differential diagnosis of post-traumatic stress disorder. *Psychiatric Clinics of North America, 17,* 351–383.

Bradburn, I. S. (1991). After the earth shook: Children's stress symptoms 6–8 months after a disaster. *Advances in Behavioral Research and Therapy, 13,* 173–179.

Brenner, A. (1985). *Helping children cope with stress.* Lexington, MA: Lexington Books.

Briere, J. (1988). The long-term clinical correlates of childhood sexual victimization. *Annals of the New York Academy of Sciences, 528,* 327–334.

Browne, A., & Finkelhor, D. (1986). The impact of child sexual abuse: A review of the research. *Psychological Bulletin, 99,* 66–77.

Caplan, G. (1976). *Support systems and community mental health.* New York: Behavioral Publications.

Coddington, R. D. (1972). The significance of life events as etiological factors in the diseases of children: I. A survey of professional workers. *Journal of Psychosomatic Research, 16,* 7–18.

Cohen, R. (1988). Intervention programs for children. In M. Lystad (Ed.), *Mental health response to mass emergencies* (pp. 262–283). New York: Brunner/Mazel.

Coleman, J. C., Butcher, J. N., & Carson, R. C. (1984). *Abnormal psychology and modern life.* Glenview, IL: Scott, Foresman.

Craighead, W. E., Kazdin, A. E., & Mahoney, M. J. (1981). *Behavior modification: Principles, issues, and applications.* Boston: Houghton Mifflin.

Dattilio, F. M., & Freeman, A. (Eds.). (1994). *Cognitive-behavioral strategies in crisis intervention.* New York: Guilford Press.

Deblinger, E., McLeer, S. V., & Henry, D. (1990). Cognitive behavioral treatment for sexually abused children suffering post-traumatic stress: Preliminary findings. *Journal of the American Academy of Child and Adolescent Psychiatry, 29,* 747–752.

de Vries, M. W. (1987). Cry babies, culture, and catastrophe: Infant temperament among the Masai. In N. Scheper-Hughes (Ed.), *Child survival: Anthropological perspectives on the treatment and mistreatment of children* (pp. 165–185). Dordrecht: Reidel.

Dohrenwend, B. S., & Dohrenwend, B. P. (Eds.). (1974). *Stressful life events: Their nature and effects.* New York: Wiley.

Dyregov, A., & Raundalen, M. (1987). Children and the stresses of war: A review of the literature. In C. P. Dodge & M. Raundalen (Eds.), *War, violence, and children in Uganda* (pp. 109–132). Oslo: Norwegian University Press.

Eth, S., & Pynoos, R. S. (Eds.). (1985). *Post-traumatic stress disorder in children.* Washington, DC: American Psychiatric Association.

Fields, R. M. (1977). *Society under siege: A psychology of Northern Ireland.* Philadelphia: Temple University Press.

Figley, C. R. (Ed.). (1978). *Stress disorders among Vietnam veterans.* New York: Brunner/Mazel.

Finkelhor, D., & Dziuba-Leatherman, J. (1994). Victimization of children. *American Psychologist, 49,* 173–183.

Fraser, M. (1974). *Children in conflict.* Hammondsworth, Middlesex: Penguin Books.

Frederick, C. J. (1985). Children traumatized by catastrophic situations. In S. Eth & R. S. Pynoos (Eds.), *Post-traumatic stress disorder in children* (pp. 71–99). Washington, DC: American Psychiatric Association.

Freud, A., & Burlingham, D. T. (1943). *War and children.* London: Medical War books.

Freud, S. (1953). Remembering, repeating, and working-through. *Standard edition* (Vol. 12, pp. 145–150). London: Hogarth Press. (Original work published 1914)

Garmezy, N. (1983). Stressors of childhood. In N. Garmezy & M. Rutter (Eds.), *Stress, coping, and development in children* (pp. 43–84). New York: McGraw–Hill.

Gordon, R., & Wraith, R. (1993). Responses of children and adolescents to disaster. In J. P. Wilson & B. Raphael (Eds.), *International handbook of traumatic stress syndromes* (pp. 561–575). New York: Plenum Press.

Green, L. B., Korol, M., Grace, M. C., Vary, M. G., Leonard, A. C., Gleser, G. C., & Smitson-Cohen, S. (1991). Children and disaster: Age, gender, and parental effects on PTSD symptoms. *Journal of the American Academy of Child and Adolescent Psychiatry, 30*, 945–951.

Herman, J. L., Russell, D., & Trocki, K. (1986). Long-term effects of incestuous abuse in childhood. *American Journal of Psychiatry, 143*, 1293–1296.

Hobfoll, S. E. (1989). Conservation of resources: A new attempt at conceptualizing stress. *American Psychologist, 44*, 513–524.

Hobfoll, S. E., Spielberger, C. D., Breznitz, S., Figley, C., Folkman, S., Lepper-Green, B., Meichenbaum, D., Milgram, N. A., Sarason, I. G., & van der Kolk, B. (1991). War-related stress: Addressing the stress of war and traumatic events. *American Psychologist, 46*, 848–855.

Holmes, T. H., & Rahe, R. H. (1967). The social readjustment rating scale. *Journal of Psychosomatic Research, 11*, 213–218.

Horowitz, M. J. (1976). *Stress response syndromes.* New York: Jason Aronson.

Horowitz, M. J. (1983). Psychological response to serious life events. In S. Breznitz (Ed.), *The denial of stress* (pp. 129–159). New York: International Universities Press.

Humphrey, J. H. (Ed.). (1982). *Stress in childhood.* New York: AMS Press.

Janis, I. L. (1971). *Stress and frustration.* New York: Harcourt Brace Jovanovich.

Janis, I. L., & Leventhal, H. (1968). Human reactions to stress. In E. Borgatta & W. Lambert (Eds.), *Handbook of personality theory and research.* Chicago: Rand McNally.

Johnson, J. H. (1986). *Life events as stressors in childhood and adolescence.* London: Sage.

Joseph, S. A., Brewin, C. R., Yule, W., & Williams, R. (1993). Causal attributions and post-traumatic stress in adolescents. *Journal of Child Psychology and Psychiatry, 34*, 247–253.

Kendall-Tackett, K. A., Williams, L. M., & Finkelhor, D. (1993). Impact of sexual abuse on children: A review and synthesis of recent empirical studies. *Psychological Bulletin, 113*, 164–180.

King, R. A., & Noshpitz, J. D. (1991). *Pathways of growth: Essentials of child psychiatry: Vol. 2. Psychopathology.* New York: Wiley.

Kinzie, J. D., Sack, W. H., Angell, R. H., Manson, S., & Rath, B. (1986). The psychiatric effects of massive trauma on Cambodian children: I. The children. *Journal of the American Academy of Child Psychiatry, 25*, 370–376.

Knopf, I. J. (1979). *Childhood psychopathology: A developmental approach.* Englewood Cliffs, NJ: Prentice–Hall.

Kobassa, S. C. (1979). Stressful life events, personality, and health: An inquiry into hardiness. *Journal of Personality and Social Psychology, 37*, 1–11.

Langmeier, J., & Matejcek, Z. (1975). *Psychological deprivation in childhood.* New York: Halsted Press.

Lazarus, R. S. (1983). The costs and benefits of denial. In S. Breznitz (Ed.), *The denial of stress* (pp. 1–30). New York: International Universities Press.

Lazarus, R. S., & Folkman, S. (1984). *Stress, appraisal, and coping.* Berlin: Springer.

Leavitt, L. A., & Fox, N. A. (Eds.). (1993). *The psychological effects of war and violence on children.* Hillsdale, NJ: Erlbaum.

Levine, S., & Scotch, N. A. (1970). Social stress. In S. Levine & N. A. Scotch (Eds.), *Social stress* (pp. 1–18). Chicago: Aldine.

Lifton, R. J. (1964). On death and death symbolism: The Hiroshima disaster. *Psychiatry, 27*, 191–210.

Lonigan, C., Shannon, M. P., Finch, A. J., Jr., Daughterty, T. K., & Taylor, C. M. (1991). Children's reactions to a natural disaster: Symptom severity and degree of exposure. *Advances in Behavioral Research and Therapy, 13*, 135–154.

Macksoud, M. S., Dyregov, A., & Raundalen, M. (1993). Traumatic war experiences and their effect on children. In J. P. Wilson & B. Raphael (Eds.), *International handbook of traumatic stress syndromes* (pp. 625–633). New York: Plenum Press.

Malmquist, C. P. (1986). Children who witness parental murder: Posttraumatic aspects. *Journal of the American Academy of Child Psychiatry, 25*, 320–325.

March, J. S., & Amaya-Jackson, L. (1993). Post-traumatic stress disorder in children and adolescents. *PTSD Research Quarterly, 4*, 1–3. (White River Junction, VT: The National Center for Post-Traumatic Stress Disorder)

McFarlane, A. C. (1987). Posttraumatic phenomena in a longitudinal study of children following a natural disaster. *Journal of the American Academy of Child and Adolescent Psychiatry, 26*, 764–769.

McNamee, A. S. (Ed.). (1982). *Children and stress: Helping children cope.* Washington, DC: Association of Childhood Education International.

Mechanic, D., & Volkart, E. (1962). Stress, illness behavior, and the sick role. *American Sociological Review, 26*, 51–58.

Milgram, N. A. (1982). War related stress in Israeli children. In L. Goldberg & S. Breznitz (Eds.), *Handbook of stress: Theoretical and clinical aspects* (pp. 656–676). New York: Free Press.

Milgram, N. A. (1986). An attributional analysis of war-related stress: Modes of coping and helping. In N. A. Milgram (Ed.), *Stress and coping in time of war: Generalizations from the Israeli experience* (pp. 9–25). New York: Brunner/Mazel.

Milgram, N. A. (1989). Social support versus self sufficiency in traumatic and post-traumatic stress reactions. In B.

Lerer & S. Gershon (Eds.), *New directions in affective disorders* (pp. 455–458). Berlin: Springer-Verlag.

Milgram, N. A. (1990, August). *Childhood PTSD in Israel: A cross cultural frame of reference.* Paper presented at the annual meeting of the American Psychological Association, Boston.

Milgram, N. A., & Hobfoll, S. (1986). Generalizations from theory and practice to war-related stress. In N. A. Milgram (Ed.), *Stress and coping in time of war: Generalizations from the Israeli experience* (pp. 316–352). New York: Brunner/Mazel.

Milgram, N. A., & Palti, G. (1993). Psychosocial characteristics of resilient children. *Journal of Research in Personality, 27,* 207–221.

Milgram, N. A., Sarason, B., Schonplug, U., Jackson, A., & Schwarzer, C. (1995). Catalyzing community support. In S. E. Hobfoll & M. W. de Vries (Eds.), *Extreme stress and communities: Impact and intervention* (pp. 473–497). Dordrecht, The Netherlands: Kluwer.

Milgram, N. A., & Toubiana, Y. H. (1988). Bias in identifying and treating high risk client groups. *Professional Psychology: Research and Practice, 19,* 21–25.

Milgram, N. A., & Toubiana, Y. H. (1996). Children's selective coping after a bus disaster: Confronting behavior and perceived support. *Journal of Traumatic Stress, 9,* 701–716.

Milgram, N. A., Toubiana, Y. H., Klingman, A., Raviv, A., & Goldstein, I. (1988). Situational exposure and personal loss in children's acute and chronic stress reactions to a school disaster. *Journal of Traumatic Stress, 1,* 339–351.

Mowbray, C. T. (1988). Post-traumatic therapy for children who are victims of violence. In F. Ochsberg (Ed.), *Posttraumatic therapy and victims of violence* (pp. 196–212). New York: Brunner/Mazel.

Murray, H. A. (1962). *Explorations in personality.* New York: Science Editions. (Original work published 1938)

Nader, K., & Pynoos, R. S. (1993). The children of Kuwait following the Gulf crisis. In L. A. Leavitt & N. A. Fox (Eds.), *The psychological effects of war and violence on children* (pp. 181–198). Hillsdale, NJ: Erlbaum.

Nader, K., Pynoos, R. S., Fairbanks, L., & Frederick, C. J. (1990). Children's PTSD reactions one year after a sniper attack at their school. *American Journal of Psychiatry, 147,* 1526–1530.

Ollendick, T. H., & Hersen, M. (Eds.). (1983). *Handbook of child psychopathology.* New York: Plenum Press.

Pearlin, L. I., & Schooler, C. (1978). The structure of coping. *Journal of Health and Social Behavior, 19,* 2–21.

Pedersen, L. N. (1994, November). *Posttraumatic stress disorder and children exposed to community violence.* Paper presented at the annual meeting of the International Society for Traumatic Stress Studies, Los Angeles.

Piaget, J. (1954). *The construction of reality in the child.* New York: Basic books.

Pynoos, R. S., & Eth, S. (1985). Children traumatized by witnessing acts of personal violence: Homicide, rape, or suicide behavior. In S. Eth & R. S. Pynoos (Eds.), *Posttraumatic stress disorder in children* (pp. 17–44). Washington, DC: American Psychiatric Association.

Pynoos, R. S., Goenjian, A., & Steinberg, A. M. (1994, June). *Strategies of disaster intervention for children and adolescents.* Paper presented at the NATO Workshop on Stress and Communities, Chateau de Bonas, France.

Pynoos, R. S., Goenjian, A., Tashjian, M., Karakashian, M., Manjikian, R., Manoukian, G., Steinberg, A. M., & Fairbanks, L. A. (1993). Post-traumatic stress reactions in children after the 1988 Armenian earthquake. *British Journal of Psychiatry, 163,* 239–247.

Pynoos, R. S., & Nader, K. (1988). Psychological first aid and treatment approach to children exposed to community violence: Research implications. *Journal of Traumatic Stress, 1,* 445–473.

Pynoos, R. S., & Nader, K. (1991). Childhood post-traumatic stress disorder. In J. Weiner (Ed.), *The textbook of child and adolescent psychiatry* (pp. 955–984). Washington DC: American Psychiatric Press.

Pynoos, R. S., & Nader, K. (1993). Issues in the treatment of posttraumatic stress in children and adolescents. In J. P. Wilson & B. Raphael (Eds.), *International handbook of traumatic stress syndromes* (pp. 535–550). New York: Plenum Press.

Quay, H. C., & Werry, J. S. (1979). *Psychopathological disorders of childhood.* New York: Wiley.

Raphael, B. (1986). *When disaster strikes: How individuals and communities cope with catastrophe.* New York: Basic Books.

Raviv, A., & Klingman, A. (1981). Children under stress. In S. Breznitz (Ed.), *Stress in Israel* (pp. 138–162). New York: Van Nostrand.

Rigamer, E. F. (1986). Psychological management of children in a national crisis. *Journal of the American Academy of Child Psychiatry, 25,* 364–369.

Rosenbaum, M. (1983). Learned resourcefulness as a behavioral repertoire for the self-regulation of internal events: Issues and speculations. In M. Rosenbaum, C. M. Franks, & Y. Jaffe (Eds.), *Perspectives on behavior therapy in the eighties* (pp. 54–76). Berlin: Springer.

Rutter, M. (1979). Protective factors in children's responses to stress and disadvantage. In M. W. Kent & J. E. Rolf (Eds.), *Primary prevention of psychopathology: Social competence in children* (Vol. 3, pp. 49–74). Hanover, NH: University Press of New England.

Sack, W. M., Angell, R. H., Kinzie, J. D., & Rath, B. (1986). The psychiatric effects of massive trauma on Cambodian children: II. The family, the home, and the school. *Journal of the American Academy of Child Psychiatry, 25,* 377–383.

Salmon, T. (1919). The war neuroses and their lesson. *New York State Journal of Medicine, 59,* 933–944.

Sarason, I. G., Sarason, B. R., & Pierce, G. R. (1994). Social support: Global and relationship-based level of analysis. *Journal of Social and Personal Relationships, 11,* 295–312.

Schwartz, S., & Johnson, J. H. (1981). *Psychopathology of childhood*. New York: Plenum Press.

Slaikeu, K. (1984). *Crisis intervention: A handbook for practice and research*. Boston: Allyn & Bacon.

Solomon, Z. (1993). *Combat stress reaction: The enduring toll of war*. New York: Plenum Press.

Spielberger, C. D., Sarason, I. G. (Eds.), & Milgram, N. A. (Guest Ed.). (1982). *Stress and anxiety* (Vol. 8). Washington, DC: Hemisphere.

Strelau, J. (1991). Temperament risk factors in children and adolescents as studied in eastern Europe. In W. B. Carey & S. C. McDevitt (Eds.), *Clinical and educational applications of temperament research* (pp. 65–77). Amsterdam: Swets & Zeitlinger.

Sullivan, M. A., Saylor, C. F., & Foster, K. Y. (1991). Post-hurricane adjustment of preschoolers and their families. *Advances in Behavioral Research and Therapy, 13*, 163–171.

Taylor, S. E., & Lobel, H. (1989). Social comparison activity under threat: Downward evaluation and upward contacts. *Psychological Review, 96*, 569–575.

Terr, L. C. (1983). Chowchilla revisited: The effects of psychic trauma four years after a school-bus kidnapping. *American Journal of Psychiatry, 140*, 1543–1550.

Terr, L. C. (1991). Childhood traumas: An outline and overview. *American Journal of Psychiatry, 148*, 10–20.

Thoits, P. A. (1986). Social support as coping assistance. *Journal of Consulting and Clinical Psychology, 54*, 416–423.

Toubiana, Y. H., Milgram, N. A., & Falach, H. (1986). The stress and coping of uprooted settlers. In N. A. Milgram (Ed.), *Stress and coping in time of war: Generalizations from the Israeli experience* (pp. 275–293). New York: Brunner/Mazel.

Toubiana, Y. H., Milgram, N. A., & Noy, S. (1986). A therapeutic community in a forward army field hospital: Treatment, education, and expectancy. In N. A. Milgram (Ed.), *Stress and coping in time of war: Generalizations from the Israeli experience* (pp. 117–128). New York: Brunner/Mazel.

Toubiana, Y. H., Milgram, N. A., Strich, Y., & Edelstein, A. (1988). Crisis intervention in a school community disaster: Principles and practices. *Journal of Community Psychology, 16*, 228–240.

Watkins, B., & Bentovim, A. (1992). The sexual abuse of male children and adolescents: A review of current research. *Journal of Child Psychology and Psychiatry, 33*, 197–248.

Weiss, R. S. (1974). The provisions of social relationships. In Z. Rubin (Ed.), *Doing unto others* (pp. 17–26). Englewood Cliffs, NJ: Prentice–Hall.

Williams, T. (Ed.). (1980). *Post-traumatic stress disorders of the Vietnam veteran*. Cincinnati, OH: Disabled American Veterans.

Wilson, J. P., & Raphael, B. (Eds.). (1993). *International handbook of traumatic stress syndromes*. New York: Plenum Press.

IV

Prevention and Treatment

22

Psychodynamically Based Therapies

Sandra W. Russ

INTRODUCTION

The therapies described in this chapter use a variety of mechanisms of change and intervention techniques that are guided by psychodynamic conceptualizations. Psychodynamic approaches focus on underlying cognitive, affective, and interpersonal processes from a developmental perspective (Shirk & Russell, 1996). The level of development of these processes and the interaction among them partially determines the child's behavior, relationships, and internal state. The psychodynamic framework is applied in order to understand these internal processes and childhood disorders. The specific intervention approach is based on this understanding of the child's internal world.

The present chapter will discuss the continuum of psychoanalytic and psychodynamic therapies, types of psychodynamic therapies, use of play in psychodynamic psychotherapy, psychotherapy outcome research with psychodynamic approaches, and current trends and future directions.

SANDRA W. RUSS • Psychology Department, Case Western Reserve University, Cleveland, Ohio 44106-7123.

Handbook of Child Psychopathology, 3rd edition, edited by Ollendick & Hersen. Plenum Press, New York, 1998.

PSYCHOANALYTIC–PSYCHODYNAMIC CONTINUUM

Psychodynamic approaches have evolved from psychoanalytic theory and psychoanalytic therapy. As Fonagy and Moran (1990) pointed out, many forms of psychodynamic therapies are based on the psychoanalytic conceptualization of child development. Although similar conceptualizations guide psychoanalytic and psychodynamic therapies, there are a number of differences between these two broad approaches. First, psychodynamic therapies have less ambitious goals than psychoanalytic therapy (Fonagy & Moran, 1990; Tuma & Russ, 1993). Whereas psychoanalysis works to achieve major structural changes in the personality, psychodynamic approaches have more immediate goals and tend to be focused on a few underlying issues and processes. Both approaches strive to return the child to normal developmental pathways—psychoanalysis in a global way and psychodynamic in a more focused way in a few areas. The idea that psychotherapy should help the child get back on track developmentally is one overarching goal of psychoanalytic–psychodynamic approaches (A. Freud, 1965; Palmer, 1970; Shirk & Russell, 1996). Second, psychoanalytic therapy is more intense than psychodynamic therapies (Fonagy & Moran, 1990; Tuma & Russ, 1993). Psychoanalytic treatment tends to be carried out five times per week and long term, lasting an average of 2 years (Fonagy & Moran, 1990). Training of therapists is lengthy (4–6 years beyond training for an adult analyst). Thus, the number of trained child analysts is low. Psychodynamic therapies are less intensive, usually involve weekly sessions with the child, and may be short term (6–12 sessions) or long term. The less frequent and shorter-term nature of psychodynamic therapies require different goals, mechanisms of change, and intervention techniques than psychoanalysis. Tuma (1989) stated that psychoanalysis and psychodynamic approaches differ in degree rather than in the kind of psychotherapy. In psychodynamic approaches the therapist is more active in pointing out feelings and defenses in order to understand and change behavior. In psychoanalysis, with a longer time frame, there is more of a focus on understanding the origins of the feelings, especially anxiety (Tuma, 1989).

A third difference not often discussed in the literature is that of flexibility. Psychoanalysis involves a very standardized approach over a long period of time. Psychodynamic approaches are more flexible in terms of the types of intervention techniques used and the integration of other theoretical perspectives and techniques. For example, the therapist might include modeling techniques, role-playing, or family sessions with a particular child, but always within an overall psychodynamic conceptualization of the case.

History of Psychoanalytic–Psychodynamic Approaches

Psychoanalysis with children evolved from psychoanalytic theory and treatment of adults. Sigmund Freud was the first to apply psychoanalytic theory to work with children. In the "Little Hans" case, he supervised the treatment of a 5-year-old boy by his father (Freud, 1909/1955). Tyson and Tyson (1990) described

this treatment as a developmental study of childhood experiences based on actual observation of a child.

Chused (1988), Tuma and Russ (1993), and Tyson and Tyson (1990) reviewed the history of the development of child psychoanalysis. In essence, the techniques of adult psychoanalysis were applied to children. Hug-Hellmuth (1921, 1924), A. Freud (1927), and Burlingham (1932) are credited with adapting psychoanalytic techniques to children. Children's play was used as a vehicle for communication and the therapist was more responsive and gratifying to the child than to the adult. The therapist actively worked to develop a positive relationship with the child (A. Freud, 1927). Anna Freud made significant contributions to psychoanalytic theory by developing her work on the ego and mechanisms of defense (1936/1966). Melanie Klein, in a different approach, developed early concepts in object relations theory and discussed the process of interpersonal relations (Tyson & Tyson, 1990). Klein also utilized active interpretation of children's play.

Kessler (1966, 1988) discussed the major influence of psychoanalytic approaches in the utilization of play in child treatment. Both Klein and A. Freud, to varying degrees, stressed the value of play in communication and in understanding internal conflicts and fantasies (Gerard, 1952). Today, play is utilized in many forms of child psychotherapy. Koocher and D'Angelo (1992) stated that "play-oriented therapy remains the dominant and most enduring approach to child treatment . . . practiced by clinicians" (p. 458).

TYPES OF PSYCHODYNAMIC THERAPIES

In most forms of psychodynamic psychotherapies, the child and therapist meet individually once a week for a session of 45–50 minutes. The mutual agreement between the child and the therapist is that the therapist is there to help the child express feelings and thoughts, understand causes of behavior, and form a relationship with the therapist (Freedheim & Russ, 1992). Play is a major tool in therapy. Traditionally, the child structures the therapeutic hour by choosing the topics, forms of play, and, in general, determines the pace of the therapy. In most cases, individual work with the child is only one part of the treatment program. Parent guidance and education, family sessions, and work with the school usually occur simultaneously with individual child therapy. For reviews of the practical issues that arise in therapy such as setting limits, choosing toys, dealing with vacations and terminations, see Kessler (1966, 1988) and Chethik (1989) for good discussions.

Different types of psychodynamic psychotherapies have different treatment goals and utilize different intervention techniques and mechanisms of change. The psychodynamic conceptualization of the underlying factors involved in child psychopathology fits the psychodynamic conceptualization of the intervention (Tuma & Russ, 1993). The psychodynamic framework views childhood disturbance within a developmental context. Through the assessment process, one identifies which underlying processes have developed problems or deficits and need to be addressed in therapy.

Mechanisms of Change

How change occurs in any form of therapy is a fundamental question. Freedheim and Russ (1983, 1992) identified six major mechanisms of change that occur in individual psychodynamic child psychotherapy. These mechanisms are based on those identified by Applebaum (1978) and Garfield (1980) in the adult literature. Different mechanisms of change are utilized in different types of psychodynamic psychotherapy with different types of childhood disorders. However, there is rarely a

pure type of psychotherapy and frequently all of these mechanisms may occur in one case.

Catharses and Labeling of Feelings

Through talk and play, children express feelings and release emotion. Such release of emotion has long been thought to be therapeutic (Axline, 1947; A. Freud, 1965; Moustakas, 1953). By labeling affect, the therapist helps to make the feeling less overwhelming and more understandable. Often, the labeling of affect occurs during pretend play.

Corrective Emotional Experience

The therapist accepts the child's feeling and thoughts. Often, the child's learned expectations are not met and a corrective emotional experience occurs (Kessler, 1966). For example, the automatic connection between the child's angry feelings toward father and anxiety should gradually decrease as the therapist helps the child accept the feeling and understand the reasons for the anger. The therapist is not punitive, and often normalizes the experience of having angry feelings.

Insight and Working Through

The emotional resolution of conflict or trauma is a major mechanism of change in psychodynamic psychotherapy. One goal of the therapist when utilizing such mechanisms of change is to help the child reexperience major developmental conflicts or situational traumas in therapy. Cognitive insight into origins of feelings and conflicts, causes of symptoms, links between thoughts, feelings, and actions is a goal of psychotherapy when underlying conflicts are a major issue (Sandler, Kennedy, & Tyson, 1980; Shirk & Russell, 1996). Verbal labeling of unconscious impulses, conflicts, and causes of behavior helps lend higher-order reasoning skills to understanding problems. However, in many cases, especially with young children, cognitive insight does not occur. Rather, emotional reexperiencing, emotional working through, and mastery do occur and result in symptom reduction and healthy adjustment. This is an important point and is an often overlooked mechanism of change in child treatment. Messer and Warren (1995) also stated that the goal of making the unconscious conscious needs to be modified in child play therapy with many children. In Erikson's (1963) concept of mastery, the child uses play to gain mastery over traumatic events and everyday conflicts. Resolving conflicts through play is part of normal child development. Waelder (1933) described the play process as one in which the child repeats an unpleasant experience over and over until it becomes manageable. As he put it, the child "digests" the event. Freedheim and Russ (1992) described the slow process of gaining access to conflict-laden material and playing it out until the conflict is resolved. The therapist helps guide the play, labels thoughts, feelings, and events, and makes interpretations to facilitate conflict resolution and the working through process.

Learning Alternative Problem-Solving Techniques and Coping Strategies

The therapist, in a directive approach, helps the child think about alternative ways of viewing a situation and generate problem-solving strategies. Role-playing and modeling of coping strategies are used. For example, Singer (1993) gave examples of modeling techniques during therapy. Although this mechanism of change is not often associated with psychodynamic therapy, it is frequently part of an intervention within a psychodynamic conceptualization of the case.

Development of Internal Structure

Many children have structural deficits that result in problems with self/object differentiation, interpersonal functioning, self-esteem regulation, impulse control, object constancy, and separation of fantasy from reality. In these children, there are major deficits in underlying cognitive, affective, and interpersonal processes. Structure-building approaches are based on conceptualizations by Mahler (1968) and Kohut (1977). The therapist is viewed as being a stable, predictable, caring, and empathic figure. Development of good object relations is a major goal of therapy with these children. Gilpin (1976) stressed that the role of the therapist is to become an internalized object. The relationship between the therapist and child is probably the most important aspect of therapy in helping this process to occur. Genuine understanding and expression of empathy by the therapist is a major technique that enables the child to develop.

A Variety of Nonspecific Variables

Nonspecific variables function in child therapy as they do in adult therapy. Expectation of change, hope, awareness of parental concern, no longer feeling so alone, are all factors that contribute to change in therapy.

Treatment Approaches with Specific Populations

Three major types of psychodynamic therapies emerge in the current child psychotherapy literature (Chethik, 1989; Freedheim & Russ, 1983, 1992). The different types of therapy differ in their emphasis on insight and working through versus development of internal structure and object relations versus structured problem-solving and coping strategies. Different mechanisms of change are emphasized in each type. Catharsis and corrective emotional experience usually occur in all three types of therapy.

Insight-Oriented Therapy

As Tuma and Russ (1993) pointed out, the form of therapy most associated with the psychodynamic approach is insight-oriented therapy, and it is most appropriate for the child with anxiety and internalized conflicts. This approach is appropriate for children who have age-appropriate ego development, show evidence of internal conflicts, have the ability to trust adults, have some degree of psychological-mindedness, and can use play effectively. Insight-oriented therapy is most often recommended for internalizing disorders. Many of the anxiety disorders and depressive disorders are appropriate for insight-oriented therapy. Children with internalizing disorders often experience internal conflicts and have good ego development and good object relations. Anxiety disorders, depressive disorders, and intense reactions to traumas are examples of children with internalizing disorders. An insight-oriented approach with a focus on conflict resolution is most appropriate for internalizing disorders.

Goals of insight-oriented therapy are to help the child resolve internal conflicts and master developmental tasks. The major mechanism of change is insight and working through. Through the use of play and interpretation from the therapist, the child "calls forth forbidden fantasy and feelings, works through and masters developmental problems, and resolves conflicts" (Freedheim & Russ, 1983, p. 983). Active interpretation of the child's play, expressions, and resistances is a major technique.

Insight and working through can also be helpful for a child with good inner resources who has experienced a specific trauma (such as the loss of a parent). Altschul (1988) described the use of psychoanalytic approaches in helping children to mourn the loss of a parent. In this application, Webber (1988) stressed that the therapist must first address the question of whether the child can do his or her own psychological work. If not, therapy can be a major aid in the mourning process.

Structure-Building Approaches

A second major form of psychotherapy is the structure-building approach, which is used with children with structural deficits and major problems in developing good object relations. For children with impaired object relations, self/

other boundary disturbances, and difficulty distinguishing fantasy from reality, the therapist uses techniques that foster the development of object permanence, self/other differentiation, and modulation of affect. The major mechanism of change is the building of internal structure, such as object relations. Anna Freud (1965) described the development of object relations through a continual process of separation from the significant adult, usually the mother. Mahler (1975) elaborated on the separation-individuation process and described the development of object constancy and object representations. As Blank and Blank (1986) stressed, Mahler's concept of separation-individuation represented a new organizing principle to development. Object relations is not just another ego function, but plays a major role in the organization of intrapsychic processes.

The growing theory on the development of object relations reflects a new phase in psychoanalytic theory construction (Tuma & Russ, 1993). Good object relations involves well-developed object representations. The child must invest in the mental representation of the loved external object. Blank and Blank (1986) listed seven major functions served by object representations: Object representations provide a feeling of safety, establish internal regulatory functions, promote ego autonomy, serve as a model for character formation, promote superego development, provide an ego ideal, and enforce resolution of Oedipal wishes. Children who have inadequately developed object relations have structural deficits that impair a variety of functions. This impairment is evident in children with psychotic and characterological disorders. Children with severely impaired object relations, such as borderline children, have early developmental problems with a mix of severe dysfunction in the family and, in the case of borderline children, perhaps a genetic predisposition. These children require a structure-building psychotherapeutic approach.

In this approach, empathy on the part of the therapist (a general relationship factor) (Kohut & Wolfe, 1978) is a much more important intervention than is interpretation. Chethik (1989) provided an excellent discussion of psychotherapy with borderline children and narcissistically disturbed children. He pointed out that many of the therapeutic techniques are supportive in that they "shore up" defenses. The problems characteristic of borderline and narcissistic children are early developmental problems usually stemming from severe disturbance in the parent–child interaction. Kohut and Wolfe (1978) discussed the failure of empathy from the parent that is a major issue in the faulty parent–child interaction. Because of the frequency of this defect in parent–child relations, empathy from the therapist around the history of empathic failure becomes an important part of therapy. Frequently, help with problem-solving and coping is also used with these children. Therapy with these children is usually long term (1 to 2 years) to be effective.

Supportive Approaches

A third form of psychodynamic therapy is supportive psychotherapy, most appropriate for children with externalizing disorders. These children frequently act out, have antisocial tendencies, and are impulse-ridden. As Baum (1989) stated, several different labels have been used for these children. The broad syndrome of externalizing disorders includes labels of acting out, antisocial, character disorders, attention-deficit disorders, and conduct disorders. Theoretically, psychodynamic theory views these children as having major developmental problems. These children have not yet adequately developed the processes necessary for delay of gratification. In addition, these children are frequently egocentric, demonstrate an absence of shame and guilt, and their ability to empathize with others is impaired. Kessler (1988) recommended that structured, supportive therapy is more helpful to these children than any other kind of psychodynamic therapy. Therapy focuses on the here and now and on the development of problem-solving skills and coping resources. For example, the therapist might role-play with the child about how to handle teasing at school or how to be assertive with parents.

At this point, given the effectiveness of behavioral and cognitive-behavioral approaches in working with externalizing disorders, my own view is that supportive psychodynamic psychotherapy is not the treatment of choice. It should only be used as a supplement to other treatment approaches in order to work on a specific issue.

PLAY IN PSYCHODYNAMIC PSYCHOTHERAPIES

Play serves two major functions in psychotherapy (Russ, 1995). First, it is a major form of communication between the child and the therapist. It helps the therapist build a therapeutic alliance with the child. Chethik (1989) stressed that it is important that the therapist understand the "language of play." Because empathy on the part of the therapist is so important in developing a relationship, understanding and empathizing with play content and process is crucial. The second function of play is as a vehicle for change in psychotherapy. Many of the mechanisms of change just reviewed occur in play. Children use play to express feelings and to work through and master conflicts and traumas. The therapist labels, empathizes, interprets, and as Chethik (1989) stated, helps "the child work towards meaningful play" (p. 53). As reviewed by Tuma and Russ (1993), Chethik described four stages of play development (the reader is referred to Chethik, 1989, pp. 48–66 for a more detailed description):

1. *Initial period of nonengagement.* Setting the stage-setting expectations, structure, and limits. The therapist first defines how play will be used for communication, and how the child's internal life combined with play materials will express and replay the child's internal life for them both. "Meaningful play" must be developed, sometimes by varying the structure. This means that the overinstinctualized child (e.g.,

impulsive, fast to react) may require more structure, whereas the underinstinctualized child (e.g., obsessive, slow to react) may need to be encouraged to express instinctual life in play.

2. *Early phase of affective engagement.* As play develops, the therapist begins to share metaphors that emerge, and the child becomes attached to both the process and the therapist. When this happens, the therapist can then permit regressions by becoming a player in the play (by doing what the child asks him or her to do). The child can then express his or her instinctual life more freely because he or she identifies with the therapist and the therapist's sanctions. The safety the child feels in expressions are further ensured by imposing boundaries (e.g., by keeping forbidden expression in the room or having cleanup time). The unstructured quality, the accepting attitudes, and the boundaries all foster early "regression in the service of the ego." As the child feels more comfortable and masters anxiety, his or her play becomes more open. Those expressions at first defensively avoided are now displayed in full view of the therapist.

3. *Emergence of central fantasies.* As the process intensifies, the child elaborates highly invested fantasies in play. Repetitive play (characterized by the "compulsion to repeat") begins to deal with past traumatic and difficult situations. In the therapy process, however, the past has a changed outcome: Acceptance of the play and interpretations by the therapist permit new solutions, either verbally or through play. Now the situation is in the control of the child.

4. *Period of working through.* Specific symptoms or behaviors often have more than one meaning. A working through period is necessary where a series and variety of interpretations are made to bring about change in a symptom. Symptoms are discussed in different contexts until all of the meanings are worked out.

Play and Child Development

Another reason why play is helpful in therapy is that play is related to a number of important cognitive and affective processes and facilitates cognitive and emotional development (Russ, 1993, 1995; Singer & Singer, 1990). Thus, the therapist is helping the child to utilize play, which, in turn, is influencing cognitive and affective processes.

Singer and Singer (1990) suggested areas of cognitive development that are facilitated by pretend play. Play helps the child to expand vocabulary and link objects with actions, develop object constancy, form event schemas and scripts, learn strategies for problem-solving, develop divergent thinking ability, and develop flexibility in shifting between different types of thoughts. In a review of the literature in 1976, Singer and Singer concluded that the capacity for pretend play is positively related to verbal fluency, divergent thinking, and general cognitive functioning.

Play is related to and facilitates creative processes in children. Play has been found to facilitate divergent thinking in preschool children (Dansky, 1980; Dansky & Silverman, 1973). Divergent thinking is thinking that "goes in different directions" and has been found to be an important component of the creative process (Guilford, 1959). A typical question on a divergent thinking test would be "How many uses for a newspaper can you think of?" A good divergent thinker can generate a variety of solutions to a problem or associations to a word.

In the Dansky and Silverman (1973) study, children who had opportunities to play with a variety of objects gave significantly more uses for those objects than did control subjects. In a more refined study in 1980, Dansky found that make-believe play was the mediator of the relationship between play and divergent thinking. Free play enhanced divergent thinking, but only for children who engaged in make-believe play.

A number of correlational studies have found relationships between play and divergent thinking. Singer and Rummo (1973) found a relationship between playfulness and creativity in kindergarten boys. Lieberman (1977) found a relationship between "playfulness" and divergent thinking. She was looking at affective dimensions of spontaneity and joy in play. Russ and Grossman-McKee (1990) found a significant relationship between the amount of affect in play and the quality of fantasy in play and divergent thinking in first- and second-grade children, independent of intelligence. This finding was replicated in a different sample of children by Russ and Peterson (1990) and Russ (1993).

For the most part, the play and creativity research has focused on cognitive processes. Dansky's hypothesis that make-believe play would facilitate divergent thinking was based on the concept that the free combination of objects and symbolic transformations involved in make-believe play helped to loosen old associations. Sutton-Smith (1966) also speculated that play provides an opportunity to develop new combinations off ideas and new associations for old objects. Kogan (1983) suggested that in play the child searches for alternate uses for objects in divergent thinking tasks.

There has been little attention given to affective processes that may account for the play–creativity link. One of the main reasons for this lack of attention has been the lack of valid, standardized measures of affective expression in children's play. To investigate the area of affect in play and creativity, the author developed the Affect in Play Scale (Russ, 1987, 1993), which measures various dimensions of affect in play in a standardized puppet-play situation. In two studies, children who expressed more affect in play and a greater variety of affect categories were more creative on divergent thinking tasks, independent of IQ (Russ & Grossman-McKee, 1990; Russ & Peterson, 1990; see Russ, 1993). These results are consistent with those of Lieberman (1977), who found that "playfulness" which included affective components of spontaneity and joy was related to divergent thinking in children. In Russ's (1993) research, the psychodynamic theoretical basis for expecting a relationship between affect and creativity was that access to a wide range of affect and affect-laden thoughts should increase the associative network and broaden the range of associations. Psychodynamic theory postulates that individuals who do not repress and are open to affect and affect-laden thoughts, should be more open to memories and ideas in general and should have a broader range of associations than those who repress and are uncomfortable with affect-laden thoughts and fantasies. Experimental studies with adults by Isen, Daubman, and Nowicki (1987) found that inducing positive affect states in adults facilitated creative problem solving. Greene and Noice (1988) found similar results with eighth-grade children. Play may be one real-life example of self-induced affective states. Russ (1993) proposed that expression of affect states in play and expression of affect-laden thoughts in play are the two major affective dimensions that account for the relationship between play and creativity. These affective dimensions facilitate a broad associative network and the recombination of old ideas in new forms. Affective processes and cognitive processes interact in play and creativity.

Russ (1993, p. 59) reached the following conclusions from the play, affect, and creativity literature about how play aids in the development of creative thinking ability. Play helps the child to achieve the following:

1. Express affect and develop the ability to experience and express emotions as they arise.

2. Express and think about affect themes. Affect-laden content is permitted to surface and be expressed through play. Over time, the child develops access to a variety of memories, associations, and affective and nonaffective cognition. This broad repertoire of associations helps in creative problem-solving.

3. Resolve conflicts and master the many traumas of daily life. The child is freer to have access to a variety of affect states. Affective content does not get repressed and become unavailable.

4. Develop cognitive structure that enables the child to contain and modulate affect. Future stressors can then be more easily handled.

5. Experience positive affect, which is part of the play experience. Positive affect is important in creativity.

6. Practice with the free flow of associations that is part of divergent thinking.

Although there is much theory and clinical observation that play and adjustment are related, there is little empirical work to support this contention. There is some evidence that play is related to adjustment, however. Singer and Singer (1976), for example, found that children who are less imaginative in play are more aggressive. Singer and Singer (1990) concluded that imaginative play in children is related to academic adjustment and flexibility of thought. They also found that toddlers and preschoolers who engage in make-believe play are better adjusted across different situations. Burstein and Meichenbaum (1979) found that children who voluntarily played with stress-related toys prior to surgery demonstrated less distress and anxiety following surgery than children who avoided the toys. One might speculate that those children were accustomed to using play to deal with stress and problems. In a study of 4- to 11-year-olds, Kenealy (1989) investigated strategies that children use when they are feeling depressed and found that 50% of the children's responses included play strategies. Also, indirectly, if play facilitates flexible problem-solving, there is evidence that flexible problem-solving, in turn, aids the coping process (Follick & Turk, 1978).

In a study of urban children aged 4 and 5, Rosenberg (1984) found that the quality of fantasy play for children playing dyads was positively related to measures of social competence and ego resilience (Block-Q sort). Frequency of positive themes and relationship themes in the play was also related to ego resilience and social competence. In general, children with behavior problems and attachment problems had fewer positive and negative themes in play, with the exception of diffuse hostility.

Grossman-McKee (1990) found, using the Affect in Play Scale with first- and second-grade boys, that boys who expressed more affect in play had fewer pain complaints than boys with less affect in play. Good players were also less anxious on the State-Trait Anxiety Inventory for Children (Spielberger, 1973).

In a study of 7- to 9-year-olds, Christiano and Russ (1996) found a positive relationship between play and coping, and a negative relationship between play and distress. Children who were "good" players on the Affect in Play Scale implemented a greater number and variety of cognitive coping strategies (correlations ranged from .52 to .55) during an invasive dental procedure. In addition, good players reported less distress during the procedure than children who expressed less affect and fantasy in their play. Niec and Russ (1996) found that good players were more interpersonally oriented on a storytelling task. D'Angelo (1995) found that resilient children had better fantasy and more affect in their play than did internalizing and externalizing children on the Affect in Play Scale.

The research programs on children's play and the development of cognitive and affective processes have not had a direct impact on the use of play in psychotherapy. Many of these play and cognitive-affective links are probably at work in child psychotherapy, although not in a systematic fashion. Research that investigates the effect of specific play interventions on specific cognitive and affective processes is a crucial next step in play research. Only then will we be able to move from global play interventions that work in a hit-or-miss fashion to specific play interventions with a clear goal for a specific process.

RESEARCH WITH PSYCHODYNAMIC APPROACHES

There is little empirical support for the effectiveness of broad-based psychodynamic approaches with specific populations. The main reason for this lack of research is that the rather global approach and broad goals of psychodynamic approaches do not lend themselves easily to carefully controlled outcome studies (Fonagy & Moran, 1990). However, some studies do exist, and progress is being made in setting the stage for systematic research in the future.

In general, the early reviews of child therapy outcome studies concluded that there was little or no support for any type of child therapy. More recent work has concluded that there is support for the effectiveness of child psychotherapy if the research is well designed. For complete reviews, see Kazdin (1990), Russ (1995), and Weisz and Weiss (1993).

Tuma and Russ (1993) stated that psychodynamic treatment begins with a global assessment of the child's developmental level on a variety of dimensions. Based on this conceptualization, an individualized treatment plan is developed that outlines a basic therapeutic approach (e.g., insight or structure building), emphasizing different techniques and mechanisms of change. Because therapy is so individualized and the therapist is making decisions about intervention on a moment-to-moment basis, specific treatment guidelines based on research findings are few. The research needs to catch up with the seasoned therapist. Psychodynamic psychotherapy is still more of an art than a science and remains untested. This reality puts it at a disadvantage when compared with other treatment approaches such as behavior therapy. However, the richness of the psychodynamic treatment approach, its wealth of knowledge about child development, and its application to an individual child make it essential that we carry out sophisticated research studies that will answer specific questions about what interventions affect which specific processes.

In general, current reviews of child psychotherapy conclude that psychotherapy of all orientations is more effective than no treatment, and the size of the effect is similar to that found with adults (Casey & Berman, 1985; Kazdin, 1990; Tuma, 1989). Tuma (1986, 1989) reviewed 31 studies of traditional individual psychotherapies with children. In two-thirds of the studies, treated children showed greater improvement than untreated children. Tuma (1989) agreed with Casey and Berman's (1985) conclusion that no treatment modality has been shown to be more effective than any other. However, Weisz and Weiss (1993), in their recent review of major meta-analytic studies, concluded that in some meta-analyses behavioral approaches were superior to nonbehavioral approaches, including the psychodynamic. Behavior therapies yielded stronger effects than nonbehavioral approaches, but this finding was not consistent across meta-analyses. Weisz and Weiss also referred to the low number of psychodynamic therapy outcome studies in the literature.

Weisz and Weiss (1989, 1993) pointed out that most of the research studies in the meta-analyses involved controlled laboratory interventions. In many of these studies, children were recruited for treatment and were not clinic-referred; samples were homogeneous; there was a focal problem; therapy focused on the target problem; therapists were trained in the specific treatment approaches to be used; and the therapy relied primarily on those techniques. In essence, this was good research that followed many of the methodological guidelines for adequate research design. On the other hand, Weisz and Weiss (1993) cautioned that the evidence for the effectiveness of psychotherapy is based on studies that are not typical of conventional clinical practice. Thus, findings may not be generalizable to real clinical work. However, Weisz and Weiss (1989) made the important point that the control and precision of therapy for research purposes may be needed in clinical practice. Freedheim and Russ (1992) recommended that we need to begin to build bridges between research efforts and everyday treatment approaches.

The results of the meta-analyses also point to the need for specificity. Weisz (1993) concluded that studies showing positive results tend to be those that "zoom in" on a specific problem with careful planning of the intervention. Freedheim and Russ stated in 1983, and again in 1992, that we need to become very specific and ask: "Which specific interventions affect which specific cognitive, personality, and affective processes? How are these processes related to behavior and practical clinical criteria?" (1983, p. 988). It is only by asking these specific questions that we will be able to identify which interventions facilitate the development of specific cognitive and affective processes and which do not. Only then will we be able to "zoom in" in an optimal fashion.

Shirk and Russell (1996) developed a framework for conceptualizing intervention research that ties specific treatment processes to underlying cognitive, affective, and interpersonal processes, within a developmental framework. Psychodynamic conceptualizations of the effect of conflict and of deficits in developing processes should be testable within their framework. They stress the importance of specific investigation of specific processes and change mechanisms.

An important question is: How do we develop the kind of specificity that is called for in psychodynamic psychotherapy research? Bergin and Strupp (1972) and Barrett, Hampe, and Miller (1978) stressed the need for specificity. The problem was well phrased by Doleys (1989) in a review of enuresis and encopresis. When verbal psychotherapy was found to be effective with these children, it was unclear which specific features of the therapy were effective. He concluded, "Experimental approaches focusing on a component analysis are badly needed to determine which of the factors is most closely associated with success" (p. 304). Russ (1991) concluded that if psychodynamic approaches are to continue to be used, clinical researchers will need to become as specific as behavioral approaches in their research efforts. This need gains increasing impetus given the increasing need for "effectiveness and efficiency" demanded by third-party payers (Koocher & D'Angelo, 1992).

New forms for outcome studies must also be developed. Persons (1991) recently concluded that "contemporary outcome studies are incompatible with psychotherapy models because the outcome studies treat patients with standardized treatments that are assigned on the basis of psychiatric diagnosis rather than with individualized treatments based on theory-driven psychological assessment of the individual's difficulties" (p. 99). Individualized treatment based on theory-driven assessment is especially true of psychodynamic psychotherapy. Persons suggested ideographic outcome studies using a case formulation approach.

Kazdin (1993b) discussed numerous research issues in carrying out systematic assessment and evaluation in clinical practice. He concluded that we need to integrate systematic assessment and evaluation and single-case design wherever possible in clinical practice. Even though single-case designs have been used most frequently to evaluate behavioral intervention, Kazdin suggested that this approach is appropriate for other intervention approaches.

Fonagy and Moran (1990) applied many of the current guidelines for psychotherapy outcome research to evaluating the effectiveness of child psychoanalyses. Their studies are models for how to go about investigating the efficacy of psychodynamic approaches. They have carried out different types of studies that are well suited to the psychoanalytic or psychodynamic approach. In one study (Moran & Fonagy, 1987), they used a time series analysis to study the 184 weeks of treatment of a diabetic teenager. Time series analysis investigates whether or not there is a time-bound relationship between events. A relationship was found between major themes in analysis and diabetic control. Moran and Fonagy concluded that the interpretation of conflicts in the treatment brought about an improvement in diabetic control. The improved control led to temporary increases in anxiety and guilt. The improved diabetic control appeared to increase the likelihood of manifest psychological symptomatology. This pattern fit the psychodynamic understanding of this form of brittle diabetes.

In a second study, an inpatient program for

diabetes was evaluated (Fonagy & Moran, 1990). Eleven patients received psychotherapy and medical supervision, while the comparison group received medical treatment with no psychotherapy. The analytic treatment was well defined and based on the psychoanalytic understanding of brittle diabetes as being caused by the investment with unconscious emotional significance of the disease or its treatment regimen. This leads to a disregard for normal diabetic care. The goal of therapy was to make conscious the conflicts and anxieties that were interwoven with the regimen and to free the management of diabetes from the maladaptive effects of the symptom. The treated group showed significant improvement in diabetic control. None of the untreated group showed such an improvement. Improvement was maintained at 1-year follow-up. Fonagy and Moran (1990) stressed the importance and feasibility of systematic and specific intervention research that investigates changes in psychic structure such as affect regulation and empathy as a result of psychoanalysis. They reported that Wallerstein (1988) and his colleagues developed rating scales for these dimensions. Pauline Kernberg (1995) also developed a coding system for dimensions relevant to psychodynamic treatment. Shirk and Russell (1996) reviewed a number of research programs and measures relevant to assessing change in psychodynamic psychotherapy.

Another area where progress is being made in evaluating psychodynamic concepts is in play intervention research (Russ, 1995). Some studies have investigated the effect of play on specific types of problems or in specific populations. These studies are a good bridge between empirical laboratory studies of play and specific processes, like creativity, and more global clinical practice outcome studies. Russ (1995) labeled these as play intervention studies rather than play therapy because the focus is highly specific. Usually, they involve only a few sessions with no emphasis on forming "a relationship" with a therapist. On the other hand, these studies differ from specific process research in child development in that they are problem focused and are not as fine-tuned as they would be in laboratory research. Such play intervention studies seem to fit some of Weisz and Weiss's (1993) criteria by including children who were not clinic-referred, by having homogeneous samples, and by having a focal problem that the therapy focused on. Phillips (1985) reviewed two studies that would fall into this play intervention research category. Johnson and Stockdale (1975) and Cassell (1965) found that puppet play reduced anxiety in children undergoing surgery. (These studies are described in more detail in a later section.) In an excellent example of a well-designed play intervention study, Milos and Reiss (1982) used play therapy for preschoolers who were dealing with separation anxiety. They identified 64 children who were rated as high-separation-anxiety children by their teachers. The children were randomly assigned to one of four groups. Three play groups were theme related: the free-play group had appropriate toys; the directed-play group had the scene set with a mother doll bringing the child to school; the modeling group had the experimenter playing out a separation scene. A control group also used play with toys irrelevant to separation themes (blocks, puzzles, crayons). All children received three individual 10-minute play sessions on different days. Quality of play was rated. Results showed that all three thematic play conditions were effective in reducing anxiety around separation themes relative to the control group. An interesting finding was that when the free-play and directed-play groups were combined, quality of play ratings were significantly negatively related ($r = -.37$) to a posttest anxiety measure. High-quality play was defined as play that showed more separation themes and attempts to resolve conflicts. One might speculate that the children who were already good players used the intervention to master their separation anxiety. Milos and Reiss concluded that their results support the underlying assumption of play therapy, that play can reduce anxiety associated with psychological problems. The finding that quality of play was related to effectiveness of the intervention is consistent with the finding of Dansky (1980) that free play facilitated creativity only for those children who used make-believe well.

A well-designed study by Barnett (1984) also looked at separation anxiety and expanded on work by Barnett and Storm (1981) in which free play was found to reduce distress in children following a conflict situation. In the 1984 study, a natural stressor (the first day of school) was used. Seventy-four preschool children were observed separating from their mothers and were rated as anxious or nonanxious. These two groups were further divided into play or no-play conditions. The play condition was a free-play condition. The no-play condition was a story-listening condition. For half of the play condition, such play was solitary. For the other half, peers were present. The story condition was also split into solitary and peers-present segments. Play was rated by observers and categorized in terms of types of play. Play significantly reduced anxiety in the high-anxious group. Anxiety was measured by the Palmer Sweat Index. There was no effect for low-anxious children. For the anxious children, solitary play was best in reducing anxiety. High-anxious children spent more time in fantasy play than did low-anxious children, who showed more functional and manipulative play. They engaged more in fantasy play when no other children were present. Barnett interpreted these results to mean that play is used to cope with a distressing situation. The findings support the idea that it is not social play that is essential to conflict resolution, but rather imaginative play qualities that the child introduces into playful behavior. Actually, presence of peers increased anxiety in the high-anxious group.

These play intervention studies are a few examples of the kind of studies that tell us about how play can be helpful in dealing with specific problems. Results of these studies suggest that play helps children deal with fears and reduce anxiety and that something about play itself is important and serves as a vehicle for change. The play experience is separate from the experi-

ence of a supportive and empathic adult. Results also suggest that children who are already good players are more able to use play opportunities to resolve problems when these opportunities arise. Teaching children good play skills would provide children with a resource for future coping.

CURRENT TRENDS IN PSYCHODYNAMIC THERAPIES

Short-Term Therapy and Integrated Approaches

Conceptual frameworks exist for adult forms of brief psychodynamic intervention (Budman & Gurman, 1988; Mann & Goldman, 1982), but not for child forms of brief intervention. However, as Messer and Warren (1995) pointed out, short-term therapy (6–12 sessions) is a frequent form of psychodynamic intervention. The practical realities of HMOs and of clinical practice in general have led to briefer forms of treatment. Often, the time-limited nature of the therapy is by default, not by plan (Messer & Warren, 1995). The average number of sessions for children in outpatient therapy is six or less in private and clinic settings (Dulcan & Piercy, 1985).

There is little research or clinical theory about short-term psychotherapy with children (Clark, 1993; Messer & Warren, 1995). A few research studies have shown that explicit time limits reduced the likelihood of premature termination (Parad & Parad, 1968) and that children in time-limited psychotherapy showed as much improvement as those in long-term psychotherapy (Smyrnios & Kirby, 1993). The time is right for development of theoretically based short-term psychodynamic interventions for children with systematic research studies. Messer and Warren (1995) suggested that the developmental approach utilized by psychodynamic theory provides a useful framework for short-term therapy. One can identify the developmental problems and obstacles involved in a particular case. They also stressed the use of play as a vehicle of change and, as Winnicott (1970) has said, of development. They suggested that active interpretation of the meaning of the play can help the child feel understood, which in turn can result in lifelong changes in self-perception and experience. In other words, the understanding of the metaphors in the child's play could give the child insight, or an experience of empathy, or both.

Chethik (1989) discussed "focal therapy" as therapy that deals with "focal stress events" (p. 194) in the child's life. Chethik listed events such as death in the family, divorce, hospitalization, illness in the family or of the child as examples of specific stresses. Focal therapy focuses on the problem and is usually of short duration. The basic principles of psychodynamic therapy and play therapy are applied. The basic mechanism of change is insight and working through. Chethik viewed this approach as working best with children who have accomplished normal developmental tasks before the occurrence of the stressful event.

In general, brief forms of psychodynamic intervention are seen as more appropriate for the child who has accomplished the major developmental milestones. Lester (1968) viewed problems such as transient regressions, mild exaggerations of age-appropriate behaviors, and acute phobias as most appropriate for brief intervention. Proskauser (1969, 1971) stressed the child's ability to quickly develop a relationship with the therapist, good trusting ability, the existence of a focal dynamic issue, and flexible and adaptive defenses as criteria for short-term intervention. Messer and Warren (1995) concluded that children with less severe psychopathology are more responsive to brief intervention than children with chronic developmental problems. My own view is that the internalizing disorders are most appropriate for brief psychodynamic intervention. The therapist is active, at times directive, and uses all mechanisms of change in the therapy. Insight and working through are essential, but modeling, rehearsal, discussing coping strategies are also part of the

therapy. Children with major deficits in object relations and with early developmental problems need longer-term structure-building approaches.

Messer and Warren (1995) also stressed the importance of the family and social environment in maximizing the effectiveness of brief intervention. A supportive environment and, often, active engagement of the parents and school are essential for brief intervention to work.

The need for short-term intervention pushes therapists to search for optimal interventions. What will work most quickly and efficiently with a particular child? Conceptualizing in this way often leads to an integration of treatment approaches and techniques. The therapist decides to use both insight and problem-solving approaches. Kazdin (1990) pointed out that the field of child psychotherapy needs to combine treatment approaches for optimal results. Many children have multiple disorders, with a host of etiological factors involved, which require a combination of intervention techniques. Wachtel's (1977) sophisticated approach to integrating psychodynamic and behavioral techniques in a complementary way should apply to the child area as well as the adult. For example, Knell's (1993) cognitive-behavioral play therapy utilized behavioral interventions within a psychodynamic understanding of the meanings of play. She understands and interprets the play metaphors but also uses play to model problem-solving and reinforce desirable behaviors. The therapist might actively direct the play and act out scenes that express how the child feels and good problem-solving. The directed action speeds up the therapy process for many children.

Types of Settings and Populations

Psychodynamic conceptualizations and intervention techniques have been applied in modified forms in a variety of settings and to a variety of patient populations. One major advantage of working within settings other than a private office or clinic, such as the school or hospital, is that the therapist has access to significant others in the child's life (Schaefer & O'Connor, 1983).

Landreth (1983) discussed issues involved in carrying out play therapy in the schools. The therapist needs to have sessions at the least disruptive times, have 30-minute sessions rather than 50-minute sessions, and be sensitive to issues of confidentiality. Consultants to school settings have long used the psychodynamic conceptualization of problems during the consultation process. In the role of an educator, the consultant can help the teacher gain a better understanding of the reasons behind disruptive classroom behavior, underachievement, or general anxiety. The teacher can then develop techniques for working more effectively with the child in the classroom (Russ, 1978).

Psychodynamic principles and techniques have also been used in the hospital setting. Emma Plank established Child Life Programs in hospitals with the first in the hospitals of Case Western Reserve University in the 1950s. She used play techniques with hospitalized children to help them work through the fears and anxieties that are a natural part of illness and hospitalization (Plank, 1962). Contemporary Child Life Programs continue to use play to help prepare children for medical procedures. Children express fears and anxieties in the play and also receive information about medical procedures through play techniques. Golden (1983) viewed play sessions as helping children to deal with separation issues, fear of equipment and procedures; develop some sense of mastery and competence; and build trust with the hospital. Research with play intervention in hospital settings has supported play as a means of reducing anxiety. Johnson and Stockdale (1975) found that children who played with puppets before surgery showed less anxiety before and after surgery (as measured by the Palmer Sweat Index) than children who did not play with puppets. The one exception in their study was immediately before the surgery when anxiety was

elevated. Cassell (1965) used puppets with children undergoing cardiac catheterization and found that anxiety was reduced before surgery for the puppet-play group compared with the no-treatment control. There were no differences after surgery. The treatment group was less disturbed during the cardiac catheterization and expressed more willingness to return to the hospital for further treatment. Although results are encouraging, there are several methodological limitations in this study. First, the control group received no intervention or contact whatsoever, so that a number of variables, such as contact with a friendly adult, were not controlled. Second, the play intervention included a great deal of information-giving about the procedure. The play setting consisted of situation-appropriate puppets and equipment (doctors, parents, stethoscope) with an active therapist who played the cardiologist and demonstrated the procedure. Thus, it is impossible to tease out which aspect of the intervention— play, verbal support, or information-giving—accounted for the results.

In a study that did attempt to separate out play from verbal support, Rae, Worchel, Upchurch, Sanner, and Daniel (1989) investigated the effects of play on the adjustment of 46 children hospitalized for acute illness. Children were randomly assigned to one of four experimental groups:

• A therapeutic play condition in which the child was encouraged to play with medical and nonmedical materials. Verbal support, reflection, and interpretation of feelings were expressed by the research assistant.

• A diversionary play condition in which children were allowed to play with toys but fantasy play was discouraged. The toys provided did not facilitate fantasy, nor did the research assistant.

• A verbally oriented support condition in which children were encouraged to talk about feelings and anxieties. The research assistant was directive in bringing up related topics and would ask about procedures.

•   A control condition in which the research assistant had no contact with the child.

All treatment conditions consisted of two 30-minute sessions. The main result of this study was that children in the therapeutic play group showed significantly more reduction in self-reported hospital-related fears than children in the other three groups. There were no differences among the groups for parent ratings.

Modifications of basic psychodynamic play therapy techniques have been used with seriously developmentally delayed children. The therapist must assess the overall developmental level of the child and be flexible in altering the traditional approach. Mann and McDermott (1983) discussed play therapy with abused and neglected children. Frequently, these children must be guided and taught how to play. Therapists sometimes used food to help build the relationship with the child and attempt to address the severe unmet dependency needs. Irwin (1983) stressed the importance of teaching poor players how to play, so that they can have play experiences available to them.

FUTURE DIRECTIONS

The most urgent need in the area of psychodynamic psychotherapy is for systematic and focused outcome research. There are many types of studies that can be carried out, as I have reviewed. The field needs to overcome the myth that the psychodynamic approach is not "testable" and the inertia that has kept psychodynamic therapists from developing research studies. Shirk and Russell (1996) provided a framework for combining research and psychotherapy that fits psychodynamic approaches, as well as other approaches. Russ (1995) outlined the types of research programs in the field of play psychotherapy that are most likely to advance the field. These recommendations apply to psychodynamic therapies as well.

1.   *Specific-processes research on play and cognitive/affective processes.* Continuing the more tra-

ditional play in child development research is essential. Concurrent, longitudinal, and experimental studies on specific dimensions of play and specific cognitive, affective, and personality processes need to be carried out in a systematic fashion. Research at the micro level is necessary for investigating these processes. In addition, the results of these studies should inform child therapy. Shirk and Russell (1996) stressed the importance of integrating the extensive literature on the development of all psychological processes into child psychotherapy.

2.   *Focused-play intervention research.* We need to develop a body of studies that focus on different aspects of play intervention. There could be different types of play-intervention research.

a.   *Specific play interventions with specific populations and specific situations.* The Barnett (1984) study with children who were experiencing the first day of school is a good example of this type of study. There are a variety of natural stressors that could be used to investigate play intervention. Divorce, natural disasters, dental visits, presurgery, and loss of a parent are all situations in which play therapy is used. We need to develop an empirical base for play intervention in these situations.

b.   *Refining specific play techniques.* The general question of what kinds of intervention by the therapist best facilitate play needs to be studied empirically. There are many guidelines in the clinical literature about how to facilitate play, but few are based on empirical work. How do we best encourage affect in play? When is modeling more effective than a less directive approach? When is it less effective? For example, Gil (1991) pointed out that it is frequently important with sexually abused children to be nondirective, so that the child does not feel intruded on. What kinds of intervention most enhance the working-through process and conflict resolution? These kinds of research questions can be posed in well-controlled experimental studies and in psychotherapy-process research. Measures such as the Affect in Play Scale (Russ, 1993) are available to assess changes in play patterns as a result of play interventions.

c. *Research with play-intervention modules.* Kazdin (1993a) discussed the possibility of having different modules of intervention for different problems. Children with multiple problems might have different modules of intervention at different times. This concept is an intriguing one for the play area. We could develop 6- to 12-week play modules with different foci for different types of problems. Constricted children might benefit from play directed at increasing affective expression. Children who recently experienced trauma might benefit from the opportunity to play out the issues in a focused approach. Impulse-ridden children might benefit from a play module focused on helping them to regulate affect.

3. *Quasiexperimental studies in clinical practice.* Kazdin (1993b) recommended integrating assessment, evaluation, and single-case design wherever possible in clinical practice, despite the fact that controlled laboratory conditions cannot be achieved. Fonagy and Moran (1990) offered good models of how to accomplish this with psychodynamic therapies.

4. *Systematic integration of all types of research and clinical practice.* On a policy level, we need to find ways to support research programs and integrate them with clinical practice. These studies are possible to carry out, the concepts are measurable, and we need to find the policies and mechanisms that foster these research programs. Integrating these research programs is a long-term strategy. It is one that we will have to do, given the increasing need for "effectiveness and efficiency" demanded by third-party payers (Koocher & D'Angelo, 1992). This is consistent with Ross's (1981) call for the need to develop a programmatic series of "interrelated consecutive and simultaneous" studies that are both methodologically rigorous and clinically relevant. He stressed the importance of having a closer relationship between the clinic case study and the laboratory, with a reciprocal relationship between the clinic case study and the experiment. It is important to incorporate evolving research-based techniques into clinical practice.

As the field moves toward more short-term and integrated therapies, we need research-based guidelines about how and what to integrate. Which components of the psychodynamic approach can be utilized in short-term work and which cannot?

Psychodynamic theory is in the midst of a transition period. Some concepts referring to psychic structure as id, ego, and superego have not been found to be useful in a research framework. Current conceptualizations of cognitive, affective, and interpersonal processes such as object relations and affect regulation are able to be measured and evaluated. Research findings should guide us as to which concepts to keep and which to discard. The richness of psychodynamic theory captures the richness of the child. Subsequent research efforts will have to determine how much of this comprehensive theory will influence therapies of the future.

REFERENCES

Altschul, S. (1988). *Childhood bereavement and its aftermath.* New York: International Universities Press.

Applebaum, S. (1978). Pathways to change in psychoanalytic therapy. *Bulletin of the Menninger Clinic, 42,* 239–251.

Axline, V. M. (1947). *Play therapy.* Boston: Houghton–Mifflin.

Barnett, I. (1984). Research note: Young children's resolution of distress through play. *Journal of Child Psychology and Psychiatry, 25,* 477–483.

Barnett, I., & Storm, B. (1981). Play, pleasure and pain: The reduction of anxiety through play. *Leisure Science, 4,* 161–175.

Barrett, C., Hampe, T. E., & Miller, L. (1978). Research on child psychotherapy. In S. Garfield & A. Bergin (Eds.), *Handbook of psychotherapy and behavior change* (pp. 411–435). New York: Wiley.

Baum, C. G. (1989). Conduct disorders. In T. H. Ollendick & M. Hersen (Eds.), *Handbook of child psychopathology* (2nd ed., pp. 171–196). New York: Plenum Press.

Bergin, A. & Strupp, H. (1972). *Changing frontiers in science of psychotherapy.* Chicago: Aldine-Atherton.

Blank, R., & Blank, G. (1986). *Beyond ego psychology: Developmental object relations theory.* New York: Columbia University Press.

Budman, S. H., & Gurman, A. S. (1988). *Theory and practice of brief therapy.* New York: Guilford Press.

Burlingham, D. (1932). Child analysis and the mother. *Psychoanalytic Quarterly, 4,* 69–92.

Burstein, S., & Meichenbaum, D. (1979). The work of worrying in children undergoing surgery. *Journal of Abnormal Child Psychology, 7,* 121–132.

Casey, R. J., & Berman, J. S. (1985). The outcome of psychotherapy with children. *Psychological Bulletin, 98,* 388–400.

Cassell, S. (1965). Effect of brief puppet therapy upon the emotional responses of children undergoing cardiac catheterization. *Journal of Consulting Psychology, 29,* 1–8.

Chethik, M. (1989). *Techniques of child therapy: Psychodynamic strategies.* New York: Guilford Press.

Christiano, B., & Russ, S. (1996). Play as a predictor of coping and distress in children during an invasive dental procedure. *Journal of Clinical Child Psychology, 25,* 130–138.

Chused, J. (1988). The transference neurosis in child analysis. *Psychoanalytic Study of the Child, 43,* 51–81.

Clark, B. E. (1993). Towards an integrated model of time-limited psychodynamic therapy with children. *Dissertation Abstracts International, 54,* 1659-B.

D'Angelo, L. (1995). *Child's play: The relationship between the use of play and adjustment styles.* Unpublished dissertation, Case Western Reserve University, Cleveland, Ohio.

Dansky, I. (1980). Make-believe: A mediator of the relationship between play and associative fluency. *Child Development, 51,* 576–579.

Dansky, J., & Silverman, F. (1973). Effects of play on associative fluency in preschool-aged children. *Developmental Psychology, 9,* 38–43.

Doleys, D. M. (1989). Enuresis and encopresis. In T. H. Ollendick & M. Hersen (Eds.), *Handbook of child psychopathology* (2nd ed., pp. 291–314). New York: Plenum Press.

Dulcan, M., & Piercy, P. (1985). A model for teaching and evaluating brief psychotherapy with children and their families. *Professional Psychology: Research and Practice, 16,* 689–700.

Erikson, E. N. (1963). *Childhood and society.* New York: Norton.

Follick, M., & Turk, D. (1978). *Problem specification by ostomy patients.* Paper presented at the 12th Annual Convention for the Advancement of Behavior Therapy, Chicago.

Fonagy, P., & Moran, G. S. (1990). Studies on the efficacy of child psychoanalysis. *Journal of Consulting and Clinical Psychology, 58,* 684–695.

Freedheim, D. K., & Russ, S. W. (1983). Psychotherapy with children. In C. E. Walker & M. E. Roberts (Eds.), *Handbook of clinical child psychology* (pp. 978–994). New York: Wiley.

Freedheim, D. K., & Russ, S. W. (1992). Psychotherapy with children. In C. E. Walker & M. Roberts (Eds.), *Handbook of clinical child psychology* (2nd ed., pp. 765–780). New York: Wiley.

Freud, A. (1927). Four lectures on child analysis. In *The writings of Anna Freud* (Vol. 1, pp. 3–69). New York: International Universities Press.

Freud, A. (1965). Normality and pathology in childhood: Assessments of development. In *The writings of Anna Freud* (Vol. 6). New York: International Universities Press.

Freud, A. (1966). The ego and the mechanisms of defense. In *The writings of Anna Freud* (Vol. 2). New York: International Universities Press. (Original work published 1936)

Freud, S. (1955). Analysis of phobia in a five-year-old boy. In *Collected papers* (Vol. X). London: Hogarth Press. (Original work published 1909)

Garfield, W. (1980). *Psychotherapy: An eclectic approach.* New York: Wiley.

Gerard, M. W. (1952). Emotional disorders of childhood. In F. Alexander & H. Ross (Eds.), *Dynamic psychiatry* (pp. 165–210). Chicago: University of Chicago Press.

Gil, E. (1991). *The healing power of play.* New York: Guilford Press.

Gilpin, D. (1976). Psychotherapy of borderline psychotic children. *American Journal of Psychotherapy, 30,* 483–496.

Golden, D. (1983). Play therapy for hospitalized children. In C. E. Schaefer & K. J. O'Connor (Eds.), *Handbook of play therapy* (pp. 213–233). New York: Wiley.

Greene, T., & Noice, H. (1988). Influence of positive affect upon creative thinking and problem solving in children. *Psychological Reports, 63,* 895–898.

Grossman-McKee, A. (1990). The relationship between affective expression in fantasy play and pain complaints in first and second grade children. *Dissertation Abstracts International, 50-09B,* 4219.

Guilford, J. P. (1959). *Personality.* New York: McGraw–Hill.

Hug-Hellmuth, H. (1921). On the technique of child-analysis. *International Journal of Psychoanalysis, 2,* 287–305.

Hug-Hellmuth, H. (1924). *New paths to the understanding of youth.* Leipzig-Wien, Germany: Franz Deuticki.

Irwin, E. (1983). The diagnostic and therapeutic use of pretend play. In C. E. Schaefer & K. J. O'Connor (Eds.), *Handbook of play therapy* (pp. 148–173). New York: Wiley.

Isen, A., Daubman, K., & Nowicki, G. (1987). Positive affect facilitates creative problem solving. *Journal of Personality and Social Psychology, 52,* 1122–1131.

Johnson, P. A., & Stockdale, D. E. (1975). Effects of puppet therapy on palmar sweating of hospitalized children. *Johns Hopkins Medical Journal, 137,* 1–5.

Kazdin, A. E. (1990). Psychotherapy for children and adolescents. In M. R. Rosenweig & L. W. Porter (Eds.), *Annual review of psychology* (pp. 21–54). Palo Alto, CA: Annual Review.

Kazdin, A. (1993a, August). Child and adolescent psychotherapy: Models for identifying and developing effective treatments. In S. Eyberg (Chair), *Psychotherapy for children and adolescents.* Symposium conducted at the meeting of the American Psychological Association, Toronto.

Kazdin, A. (1993b). Evaluation in clinical practice: Clinically sensitive and systematic methods of treatment delivery. *Behavior Therapy, 24,* 11–45.

Kenealy, P. (1989). Children's strategies for coping with depression. *Behavior Research Therapy, 27,* 27–34.

Kernberg, P. (1995, October). *Child psychodynamic psychotherapy: Assessing the process.* Paper presented at the meeting of the American Academy of Child and Adolescent Psychiatry, New Orleans.

Kessler, J. (1966). *Psychopathology of childhood.* Englewood Cliffs, NJ: Prentice–Hall.

Kessler, J. (1988). *Psychopathology of childhood* (2nd ed.). Englewood Cliffs, NJ: Prentice–Hall.

Knell, S. (1993). *Cognitive-behavioral play therapy.* Northvale, NJ: Aronson.

Kogan, N. (1983). Stylistic variation in childhood and adolescence: Creativity, metaphor, and cognitive styles. In P. Mussen (Ed.), *Handbook of child psychology* (Vol. 3, pp. 631–706). New York: Wiley.

Kohut, H. (1977). *The restoration of the self.* New York: International Universities Press.

Kohut, H., & Wolfe, ER. (1978). The disorders of the self and their treatment: An outline. *International Journal of Psychoanalysis, 59,* 413–424.

Koocher, G., & D'Angelo, E. J. (1992). Evolution of practice in child psychotherapy. In D. K. Freedheim (Ed.), *History of psychotherapy* (pp. 457–492). Washington, DC: American Psychological Association.

Landreth, G. (1983). Play therapy in elementary school settings. In C. E. Schaefer & K. J. O'Connor (Eds.), *Handbook of play therapy* (pp. 200–212). New York: Wiley.

Lester, E. (1968). Brief psychotherapy in child psychiatry. *Canadian Psychiatric Association Journal, 13,* 301–309.

Lieberman, J. N. (1977). *Playfulness: Its relationship to imagination and creativity.* New York: Academic Press.

Mahler, M. S. (1968). *On human symbiosis and the vicissitudes of individuation.* New York: International Universities Press.

Mahler, M. S. (1975). On human symbiosis and the vicissitudes of individuation. *Journal of the American Psychoanalytic Association, 23,* 740–763.

Mann, E., & McDermott, J. (1983). Play therapy for victims of child abuse and neglect. In C. E. Schaefer & K. J. O'Connor (Eds.), *Handbook of play therapy* (pp. 283–307). New York: Wiley.

Mann, J., & Goldman, R. (1982). *A casebook in time-limited therapy.* New York: McGraw–Hill.

Messer, S. B., & Warren, C. S. (1995). *Models of brief psychodynamic therapy.* New York: Guilford Press.

Milos, M., & Reiss, S. (1982). Effects of three play conditions on separation anxiety in young children. *Journal of Consulting and Clinical Psychology, 50,* 389–395.

Moran, G. S., & Fonagy, P. (1987). Psychoanalysis and diabetic control. A single case study. *British Journal of Medical Psychology, 60,* 352–372.

Moustakas, C. (1953). *Children in play therapy.* New York: McGraw-Hill.

Niec, L., & Russ, S. (1996). Relationships among affect in play, interpersonal themes in fantasy, and children's interpersonal behavior. *Journal of Personality Assessment, 66,* 645–646.

Palmer, J. (1970). *The psychological assessment of children.* New York: Wiley.

Parad, L., & Parad, N. (1968). A study off crisis-oriented planned short-term treatment, Part 1. *Social Casework, 49,* 346–355.

Persons, J. (1991). Psychotherapy outcome studies do not accurately represent current models of psychotherapy: A proposed remedy. *American Psychologist, 46,* 99–106.

Phillips, R. (1985). Whistling in the dark?: A review of play therapy research. *Psychotherapy, 22,* 752–760.

Plank, E. (1962). *Working with children in hospitals.* Cleveland, OH: The Press of Case Western Reserve University.

Proskauer, S. (1969). Some technical issues in time-limited psychotherapy with children. *Journal of the American Academy of Child and Adolescent Psychiatry, 8,* 154–169.

Proskauer, S. (1971). Focused time-limited psychotherapy with children. *Journal of the American Academy of Child and Adolescent Psychiatry, 10,* 619–639.

Rae, W., Worchel, F., Upchurch, J., Sanner, J., & Daniel, C. (1989). The psychosocial impact of play on hospitalized children. *Journal of Pediatric Psychology, 14,* 617–627.

Rosenberg, D. (1984). *The quality and content of preschool fantasy play: Correlates in concurrent social-personality function and early mother–child attachment relationships.* Unpublished dissertation, University of Minnesota, Minneapolis.

Ross, A. O. (1981). On rigor and relevance. *Professional Psychology, 12,* 318–327.

Russ, S. W. (1978). Group consultation: Key variables that effect change. *Professional Psychology, 9,* 145–152.

Russ, S. W. (1987). Assessment of cognitive affective interaction in children: Creativity, fantasy and play research. In J. E. Butcher & C. Spielberger (Eds.), *Advances in personality assessment* (Vol. 6, pp. 141–155). Hillsdale, NJ: Erlbaum.

Russ, S. W. (1991). Child psychopathology: State of the art. (Review of *Handbook of child psychopathology.*) *Contemporary Psychology, 36,* 596–598.

Russ, S. W. (1993). *Affect and creativity: The role of affect and play in the creative process.* Hillsdale, NJ: Erlbaum.

Russ, S. W. (1995). Play psychotherapy research: State of the science. In T. Ollendick & R. Prinz (Eds.), *Advances in clinical child psychology* (Vol. 17, pp. 365–391). New York: Plenum Press.

Russ, S. W., & Grossman-McKee, A. (1990). Affective expression in children's fantasy play, primary process thinking on the Rorschach, and divergent thinking. *Journal of Personality Assessment, 54,* 756–771.

Russ, S. W., & Peterson, N. (1990). *The Affect in Play Scale: Predicting creativity and coping in children.* Unpublished manuscript.

Sandler, J., Kennedy, H., & Tyson, R. L. (1980). *The technique of child psychoanalysis: Discussion with Anna Freud.* Cambridge, MA: Harvard University Press.

Schaefer, C. E., & O'Connor, K. (1983). *Handbook of play therapy.* New York: Wiley.

Shirk, S. R., & Russell, R. (1996). *Change processes in child psychotherapy: Revitalizing treatment and research.* New York: Guilford Press.

Singer, D. (1993). *Playing for their lives.* New York: Free Press.

Singer, D. L., & Rummo, J. (1973). Ideational creativity and behavioral style in kindergarten-age children. *Developmental Psychology, 8,* 154–161.

Singer, D. L., & Singer, J. L. (1990). *The house of make-believe.* Cambridge, MA: Harvard University Press.

Singer, J. L., & Singer, D. (1976). Imaginative play and pretending in early childhood: Some experimental approaches. In A. Davids (Ed.), *Child personality and psychopathology* (Vol. 3, pp. 69–112). New York: Wiley.

Smyrnios, K., & Kirby, R. J. (1993). Long-term comparison of brief versus unlimited psychodynamic treatments with children and their families. *Journal of Counseling and Clinical Psychology, 61,* 1020–1027.

Spielberger, C. D. (1973). *State-Trait Anxiety Inventory for Children.* Palo Alto, CA: Consulting Psychological Press.

Sutton-Smith, B. (1966). Piaget on play—A critique. *Psychological Review, 73,* 104–110.

Tuma, J. M. (1986, August). Current status of traditional therapies with children. In B. Bonner & C. E. Walker (Chairs), *Current status of psychotherapy with children.* Symposium presented at the annual meeting of the American Psychological Association, Washington, DC.

Tuma, J. M. (1989). Traditional therapies with children. In T. H. Ollendick & M. Hersen (Eds.), *Handbook of child psychopathology* (2nd ed., pp. 419–437). New York: Plenum Press.

Tuma, J., & Russ, S. W. (1993). Psychoanalytic psychotherapy with children. In T. Kratochwill & R. Morris (Eds.), *Handbook of psychotherapy with children and adolescents* (pp. 131–161). Boston: Allyn & Bacon.

Tyson, P., & Tyson, R. L. (1990). *Psychoanalytic theories of development: An integration.* New Haven, CT: Yale University Press.

Wachtel, P. (1977). *Psychoanalysis and behavior therapy. Toward an integration.* New York: Basic Books.

Waelder, R. (1933). Psychoanalytic theory of play. *Psychoanalytic Quarterly, 2,* 208–224.

Wallerstein, R. S. (1988). Assessment of structural change in psychoanalytic therapy and research. *Journal of the American Psychoanalytic Association, 36*(Suppl.), 241–261.

Webber, C. (1988). Diagnostic intervention with children at risk. In S. Altschul (Ed.), *Childhood bereavement and its aftermath* (pp. 77–105). New York: International Universities Press.

Weisz, J. (1993, August). Psychotherapy efficacy with children and adolescents? Lab and clinic evidence. In S. Eyberg (Chair) *Psychotherapy for children and adolescents.* Symposium conducted at the meeting of the American Psychological Association, Toronto.

Weisz, J. R., & Weiss, B. (1989). Assessing the effects of clinical-based psychotherapy with children and adolescents. *Journal of Consulting and Clinical Psychology, 57,* 741–746.

Weisz, J., & Weiss, B. (1993). *Effects of psychotherapy with children and adolescents.* Beverly Hills, CA: Sage.

Winnicott, D. W. (1970). *Playing and reality.* London: Tavistock.

23

Family Treatment

MARTIN HERBERT

INTRODUCTION

The title of this chapter highlights a contentious issue in the management of psychological disorders of childhood: the question of whether it is the child referred to a Child and Family Clinic, the parents, or the whole family, to whom the intervention should be directed. The options might include the child (seen alone), the parent(s) (seen alone), the parents and child (seen together), or the members of the family attending as a unit. Proponents of psychodynamic theories are likely to give priority to an exploration of the child's inner life, in the form of individual psychotherapy. Behavior therapists might also opt for focused individual work on, say, a child's phobic fears. Those who still uphold the long-lived aphorism "there are no problem children, only problem parents" (a myth that refuses to die!) would tend to inculpate parents as most in need of remediation by counseling or training. The skills deficit model (which informs some behavioral parent training programs) is sometimes at risk of giving credence to this oversim-

plification. Systems theorists (e.g., family therapists) would look askance at any therapeutic approach that failed to consider, as a priority, the dynamic interactions of the child's family reified as a system that, as a whole, is "larger than the sum of its parts." Then again, several domains might be targeted for change and incorporated into a multimodel/multilevel program of treatment.

Undoubtedly, most psychological therapies require contact with the child's family (notably parents) to some extent or other. The degree of involvement ranges from an initial inquiry about the problem and history-taking (plus occasional review) to an intensive participation in all aspects of the intervention (Herbert, 1991). In a survey of 110 psychologists and psychiatrists, 94% indicated that parents were seen concurrently with children as part of the child's treatment (Koocher & Pedulla, 1977).

Until the 1950s the "child guidance" approach to children's psychological problems was essentially an individual one—the child receiving play therapy or psychotherapy from a therapist while the parent (usually mother) discussed issues with, typically, a social worker (Kaslow, 1980). The conceptual inadequacies of such "lip service" to the role of the child's familial context were clear to see by the early 1950s,

MARTIN HERBERT • Department of Psychology, University of Exeter, Exeter EX4 4QG, England.

Handbook of Child Psychopathology, 3rd edition, edited by Ollendick & Hersen. Plenum Press, New York, 1998.

and professionals from various mental health disciplines began to adopt a truly contextual "whole family" perspective in their assessment and treatment (Haley, 1971). By the 1970s, as Sowder's (1975) survey showed, as many as 34% of children who received outpatient therapy were involved in family therapy (54% received individual therapy).

Today, family therapy, or more accurately the "family therapies," constitute a very fashionable approach to childhood psychological disorder—in the words of Hoffman (1995) "a growth industry in contemporary Child and Family Centres" (p. vii). In the United States, where family therapy has recently been recognized at the federal level as a legitimate profession, there are some 17,000 therapists affiliated with the American Association of Marriage and Family Therapy and well over 300 family therapy training programs. In Britain there are about 1400 members of the Association for Family Therapy. Books and journals have proliferated at a rate that makes it almost impossible for practitioners to keep up with the literature.

There is no one therapeutic entity one can refer to definitively as "family therapy," but rather several schools or paradigms. For example, there is the structural school, which has its roots in the work of Salvador Minuchin and his colleagues in the 1960s, originating in a residential institution for ghetto boys in New York (Minuchin et al., 1975). Strategic family therapy has its origins in the Palo Alto research group led by Gregory Bateson in the early 1950s—working, *inter alia,* on family communication as it affected schizophrenics (e.g., Bateson, Jackson, Haley, & Weakland, 1956). Humanistic, existential therapies of the 1960s, such as Gestalt therapy, psychodrama, client-centered therapy, and the encounter group movement, influenced the theory and methods of various experiential family therapies—challenging the positivistic tenets of the more problem-focused schools of family therapy (e.g., Haley, 1976). Behavioral family therapy found its intellectual roots in Social Learning Theory (Patterson, 1982). Psychoanalytic and object relations perspectives are derived from psychoanalytic theory, but draw on other principles as well. A leading exponent is Nathan Ackerman (1958), who founded the Family Institution, New York. The intergenerational perspective, which looks beyond the immediate family circle and enlists the cooperation of others in resolving the family's distress, is associated with pioneers such as Murray Bowen (1966).

PARADIGMS OF FAMILY THERAPY

There are many variants: the Milan Systemic Approach (Tomm, 1984), the McMaster Family Model (Epstein, Baldwin, & Bishop, 1983), de Shazer's Brief Family Therapy (de Shazer, 1985), problem-solving therapy (Haley, 1976), and Social Network Therapy (Speck & Attneave, 1973), to name but a few.

Not surprisingly, there are significant differences when it comes to defining the activity of treatment covered by the rubric *family therapy* (Dare, 1985). The nearest to a consensus is probably that provided by Gurman and his colleagues:

> Family therapy is: any psychotherapeutic endeavour that explicitly focuses on altering the interactions between or among family members and seeks to improve the functioning of the family as a unit, or its subsystems and/or the functioning of individual members of the family. This is the goal regardless of whether or not an individual is identified as 'the patient.' Family therapy typically involves face to face work with more than one family member . . . although it may involve only a single member for the entire course of treatment. (Gurman, Kniskern, & Pinsolf, 1986, pp. 565–566)

It is impossible to do justice to the different theoretical and practical nuances of the family therapies in this chapter. A helpful summary of their underlying assumptions is provided by Walsh (1982) in Table 1.

When we come to techniques, there are dozens from which to choose. Piercy, Sprenkle, and Associates (1986) described 54 technique skills for the major family therapies. This, perhaps, is

Table 1. Some Basic Assumptions of Various Family Therapies

	Behavioral Family Therapy	Structural Family Therapy	Strategic/Problem Solving	Family System/Intergenerational Therapy	Psychodynamic Family Therapy	Experiential/Humanistic Family Therapy
Focus of therapy and treatment goals	Focus on: behavior, attributions. On the individual and his/her effect on the family. How family members influence (e.g., coerce) each other. Learning adaptive behavior; unlearning dysfunctional interactions. Negotiated goals	Focus on: restructuring/reorganizing family system. Disrupting dysfunctional interactional patterns: e.g., unhealthy coalitions, poor boundaries, excessive enmeshments, inappropriate power relationships	Focus on: resolving presenting problems, setting specific objectives. Symptoms/problems viewed as interpersonal communications. Focus on dyads and triads. Changing dysfunctional sequences between family members	Focus on: entire family and several generations. Also dyadic relationships. Goal: differentiation of self for each family member. Modification of relationships in the family system	Focus on: the individual—his/her effect on family; how members of family feel about/deal with each other. Analysis of projections from past as they affect relationships. Interpretations made to foster insight into projections/other defenses	Focus on: promoting personal growth; expanding awareness/authenticity, enhancing clearer communications. Dyadic relationships—problems within such relationships
Role of the therapist	Mainly collaborative role in imparting child developmental knowledge, behavioral change principles, etc.	An "energetic intruder" in the family system; disrupts dysfunctional patterns by use of various change techniques	Active problem-solver prescriptive paradoxical in style	Directive non-confrontational	Neutral, interpretive, analysis of transference relationships	Facilitates personal growth; provides family with new experiences

(*continued*)

Table 1. (Continued)

	Behavioral Family Therapy	Structural Family Therapy	Strategic/Problem Solving	Family System/Intergenerational Therapy	Psychodynamic Family Therapy	Experiential/Humanistic Family Therapy
View of normal versus dysfunctional family life	Adaptive individual/family; interactions are the norm, encouraged/reinforced. Versus: negative interactions (constant criticism, physical punishment, coercive spirals). Aim to make benefits of family life (parental care/discipline outweigh costs. Attributions discussed when unrealistic etc.	Family has clearly defined boundaries, roles, rules, hierarchies. Flexibility within the system. Versus: weak parental subsystem, poor boundaries and other symptoms of structural imbalance. Inability to change with life circumstances	Flexible; in possession of adequate repertoire of problem-solving strategies. Clear rules and roles within family hierarchy. Versus: limited problem-solving skills. Inability to adjust to life-cycle changes. Malfunctioning hierarchies	Self well differentiated. Intellect and emotions balanced. Versus: family functioning impaired due to role of family of origin. Poor self-differentiation. Anxiety, triangulation	Realistic mature perception of self and relationships. Family tasks and roles based in reality rather than fantasy/projection. Versus: symptoms of unresolved conflict of family origin	Authentic, self-actualization not impeded by family dynamics. Versus: inauthentic style of living. Potential for growth/self-actualization inhibited/impeded by family
Major theoretical rationale	Cognitive-behavioral theory; social learning theory	Structural Family (Systems) Theory	Communication theory. Systems theory. Behavioral theory	Family Systems Theory	Psychoanalysis	Existentialism Phenomenology Humanistic psychology
Main time frame	Mainly current events; here-and-now antecedents and consequences of behavior and beliefs. Reinforcement history taken	Present and past; family's current relationships and its structure (or organization) as it has emerged historically	Current problems maintained by repetitive sequences between family members	Immediate/contemporary experience. Phenomenology of relationships/perceptions	History of client—past experiences/trauma—explored and interpreted	Immediate/contemporary experience. Phenomenology of relationships/perceptions
Major theoretical practitioners	Patterson, Wahler, Webster-Stratton, Liberman, Bandura, Kendall, Alexander	Minuchin, Aponte, Montalvo, Treacher	Haley, Jackson, Selvini-Palazzoli (Milan group), Baseson (Palo Alto group)	Bowen	Ackerman, Lidz, Skynner, Boszormenyl-Nagy	Rogers

Note. Modified from Walsh (1982).

the reason why results of effectiveness in outcome studies of family therapy (where there are so many different levels of therapist expertise and mixed treatment packages) fail, so often, to generate firm conclusions.

What unites most family therapists as they engage in their divergent treatment strategies is a perspective requiring that children's problems be understood as the consequence of the pattern of recursive behavioral sequences that occur in dysfunctional family systems. As Jordan and Franklin (1995) put it in an orchestral metaphor:

> understanding individual family members without understanding the whole family system would be like trying to understand a concert by listening to the instruments one by one. All the instruments synchronized together with their own unique chords, rhythms, and arrangements is what makes the music. Similarly, the way families synchronize together as a group accounts for the functional and dysfunctional behaviour patterns of their members. (p. 199)

This perspective, influenced by a General Systems or Cybernetic paradigm, was originally conceived by Von Bertalanffy in the late 1920s in an attempt to understand living organisms in a holistic way, but it was many years later, in the 1950s (as we have seen), that practitioners such as Jackson (1957) applied it to work with families. The systems approach, as it translates to family work, embraces the concept of reciprocal / circular causation in which each action can be considered as the consequence of the action preceding it and the cause of the action following it. No single element in the sequence controls the operation of the sequence as a whole because it is itself governed by the operation of the other elements in the system. Thus, any individual in a family system is affected by the activities of other members of the family, activities that his or her actions or decisions (in turn) determine. An individual's behavior is both stimulus and response. (It will be appreciated why, with a formulation such as this, it has proved so difficult [or is thought irrelevant] in family therapy, to pin down and measure the traditional in-

dependent and dependent variables of therapy outcome research.)

Family therapists, whatever their methods and theoretical underpinnings, tend to believe that behavior problems in children are symptomatic (or, indeed, artifacts) of dysfunctional family life; the goal of treatment is therefore the improvement of family functioning. Family therapists help families to move from entrenched habits—individual behaviors and interpersonal interactions—that preclude them from finding solutions to the problems of life that confront them. The members are encouraged by a variety of therapeutic strategies and homework tasks, to feel and act differently in order to understand the alliances, conflicts, and attachments that operate within the family unit. Clients are encouraged to look at themselves from a fresh perspective and to seek alternative solutions to their dilemmas.

ASSESSMENT AND INTERVENTION

As we have seen, the family system is viewed as the critical context for an assessment; a typical assessment focuses on the functioning of three subsystems (spouses/partners; parents and children; children alone) all contained within a sometimes ill-defined boundary and, in turn, operating within a multiethnic sociocultural environment. The family, as a small group, can be observed and assessed on a variety of dimensions: patterns of communication, cohesion, processes of decision-making (see Vetere & Gale, 1987). Empirical assessment models have been derived from research on the classification and assessment of family functioning and clinical work with families. Examples are: the Olson Circumplex Family Model (Olson, 1986), the McMaster Family Model (Epstein et al., 1983), and the Beavers Systems Models (Beavers & Hampson, 1990). Jordan and Franklin (1995) provided a useful review of methods and critical issues in this area of assessment. A most important person not to be left out of the assessment is the referrer (Palazzoli, Boscoli, Cecchin, & Piata, 1978), the individual who identified the problem as needing a solution.

The major concepts for an assessment and formulation in family therapy were listed by Dare (1985) as follows:

1. Seeing the family as having an overall structure
2. Understanding the symptom as having a potential function
3. Understanding the location of the family on the life cycle
4. Understanding the intergenerational structure of the family
5. Making an overall formulation linking the preceding four features
6. Linking the formulation to appropriate interventions

There are family therapists who neglect to assess the influence of wider social systems (e.g., school, neighborhood, sociocultural network). Their concentration on therapy with nuclear families within clinical settings tends to impose a form of tunnel vision of family life and difficulties. The family replaces the person/patient as the locus of pathology. The social context is played down as a source of influence. It is an article of faith that outward and visible signs of the families problems, as manifested to a group of observers/commentators behind a one-way screen, represent reliably, what is going wrong. A common criticism of family therapy has to do with the nature of evidence: what it should be; where it should come from; what its status is. How representative of a family's repertoire the samples of interaction (sometimes distorted by observer effects) seen in the clinic, are likely to be, is a crucial issue.

Treacher (1984) questioned whether neglect of the wider social content of families—when they are being assessed—can be justified at a theoretical level. He maintained that it is often best effected by an intervention at another system level. For example, a worker who is attempting to produce change in a family that is experiencing many problems may be better advised to assist in the formation of a housing action group, designed to influence the housing department, than to concentrate on a more limited goal of defining boundaries between the members of a family crowded into a small, damp, and decaying flat.

Family therapy and individual counseling/psychological therapy tend to be polarized by some theorists—unnecessarily, in the author's opinion. The skills of working individually with members of a family are often indispensible to the systems approach—especially when the therapeutic task is to help a child or adolescent learn social skills, overcome a phobia, or cope with an attention deficit. The either/or dichotomy of symptom reduction versus systemic reorganization simply does not apply to some casework, where one or the other or *both* approaches might be called for (see Bennun, 1985; Papp, 1985; Watzlawick, Weakland, & Fisch, 1974).

Assessment

Typically, an assessment by a family therapist (see Lask, 1987) might concern itself with whether there is:

1. Too great a distance between members of the family leading potentially to emotional isolation and physical deprivation
2. Excessive closeness between members of the family leading potentially to overidentification and loss of individuality
3. An inability to work through conflicts, solve problems, or make decisions
4. An inability on the part of parents to form a coalition and to work together, with detrimental effects on the marriage and/or the children
5. An alliance across the generations disrupting family life, as when a grandparent interferes with the mother's childrearing decisions
6. Poor communication between members
7. A failure to respond appropriately to each other's feelings

Some of the ways in which a child may contribute (wittingly or unwittingly) to a family's inability to cope with conflict were described by Lask (1987):

1. *Parent–child coalition,* where one parent attacks the other, using one of the children as an ally
2. *Triangulation,* where both parents attempt to induce a child to take *their* side
3. *Go-between,* where a child is used to transmit messages and feelings
4. *Whipping boy,* where one parent, instead of making a direct attack on the other, uses their child as a whipping boy
5. *Child as weapon,* where one parent attacks the other using the child as a weapon
6. *Sibling transfer,* where the children agree to divert the parents from arguing

The family is thought of as dynamic in the sense that it is subject to continuous change. Children grow into adolescents and bring new interests, ideas, values, and friends into the family system. The peer group gains more influence. The child, becoming an adolescent, learns that friends' families work by different standards and rules. Like individuals, families are believed to pass through developmental life cycle stages. Each life cycle stage is believed to have its own accompanying set of tasks to be accomplished if families are to make successful transitions from one stage to the next (see Carter & McGoldrick, 1988).

Some Conceptual and Theoretical Difficulties

A concept like this of life stages highlights a problem for practitioners assessing families. How do they adopt a standard by which to evaluate functional ("healthy") as opposed to dysfunctional ("unhealthy") patterns of family organization, transitions, boundaries, homeostatic (equilibrium-seeking) strategies, rules, roles, decision-making processes, communications, or any of the other attributes family thera-

pists believe to be significant? Obviously, there are diverse cultural "norms" or values in these matters. The concept of "enmeshment" is a good example of the need for sensitivity to gender, in the pathologizing of family and interpersonal phenomena. Enmeshment of relationships is often referred to perjoratively by structural family therapists. Critics have pointed out that the type of relationship that many women seek (as opposed to men) may involve a greater degree of genuine intimacy, hence "enmeshment" may actually be considered a valued experience of connectedness (Reimers & Treacher, 1995; Walters, Carter, Papp, & Silverstein, 1988). As it happens there was no feminist literature in family therapy until fairly recently. A recurring theme in the feminist critique of family therapy is the isolation of the approach from contemporary theory and research concerning women generated by other disciplines (see Avis, 1986; Goldner, 1985).

There have been disagreements over the years about the appropriate unit of focus in family therapy. Thus, we have exhortations in the 1960s for therapists to win the battle for structure by convening all family members to the first and often ongoing sessions, and some 20 years later, Anderson and Goolishian (1988) challenging the idea of any standard unit of treatment. They questioned the presumption of "individual" or "couple" or "family" as a natural focus for therapy. They chose to work with whichever system can be defined to be relevant to a problem at any one time; its composition may vary over time and should be decided collaboratively by negotiation between the therapist and patient(s).

There are other continuing controversies or gaps in our knowledge: how to assess family patterns that relate functionally to the day-to-day specificities (i.e., changes) and syndrome specificity, of the referred problem; how to bring about change most effectively and how to evaluate such change; how to make a sometimes daunting (to clients) therapy more "user friendly" (Reimers & Treacher, 1995). What hinders assessment in nonbehavioral family therapy is the paucity of adequate microtheo-ries about change processes, a criticism that does not apply to social learning theory-based behavioral family therapy (see Alexander & Par-sons, 1982; Bandura, 1977; Herbert, 1987a, 1991; Patterson & Chamberlain, 1988; Reiss, 1988). The majority of nonbehavioral family therapy processes are formulated at a high level of abstraction. It becomes very difficult to de-fine operationally the key *independent treatment variables* at this level of strategy generality (de Kemp, 1995; Hill, 1982; Marmar, 1990). At the *dependent variable* end of the therapeutic equa-tion, emphasis can be placed on symptom reduction/removal alone (called first-order change), or a more systemic level of family trans-formation (second-order change) adopted. Second-order change is empirically and concep-tually difficult to identify and quantify. Bennun (1986) commented that "if one assumes that sys-tems constantly balance or calibrate themselves to maintain an equilibrium, one may question whether it is possible to obtain first order change without the consequent second order change" (p. 226).

Intervention

The technical elements in family therapy were summarized by Dare (1985) as follows:

1. Making a direct contact with each family member in the meeting or joining
2. Engaging children and adolescents
3. Making the parent(s) feel respected and at ease
4. Eliciting a detailed description of the presenting problem
5. Facilitating direct interaction between family members
6. Helping families develop new strategies to "solve" their problems
7. Drawing up a family tree
8. Devising in-session tasks to facilitate re-alignment of family structure
9. Devising between-session tasks
10. Formulating interpretations

11. Devising and prescribing paradoxes

The primary goals of family therapists, as de-fined by family therapists from several disci-plines, tend to be divergent and are described later.

The following account is a very brief synopsis of what happens in structural approaches to family therapy. It gives something of the flavor of structural family therapy. The focus of atten-tion is very much on the developmental tasks faced by the family and its members, at various stages of its (and their) life span. Day-to-day nu-ances and patterns of relationship—communi-cation and interaction—between members are inferred from highly charged or repetitive se-quences observed and analyzed in the therapy room. The therapist's first step is to "join" with the family, to participate in its transactions and observe members' roles, their communications, and the boundaries within the family and be-tween the family system and other systems. The family "organism," like the individual person, is thought to move between two poles: one repre-senting the security of the known, and the other being the exploration necessary for adaptation to changing conditions. When the family comes to treatment, it may be in difficulty because it is figuratively stuck, trying to maintain old ways that no longer meet the needs of a changed and changing set of circumstances.

Asking clients in the therapy room to move about can intensify an interaction or underline an interpretation being made about a relation-ship. For example, if a husband and wife never confront one another directly, but always use their child as a mediator or channel of commu-nication, the therapist blocks the maneuver (called triangulation) by moving the child from between the parents.

There is a basic sequence through which fam-ily therapy passes. Treacher (1984) described it as follows:

• *The Joining Phase.* Therapists use their skills so that they become absorbed into the family through a process of accommodation. This pro-cess creates a new system—family and therapist.

It may take several sessions to create the new system, but as it is essentially a transitory one, therapists carefully monitor any signs that family members are going to drop out of therapy and thus disrupt the new system.

• *The Middle Therapy Stage*. It is during this phase that the major restructuring "work" occurs. Restructuring interventions are made during sessions, and consolidating homework tasks are set between sessions.

• *The Termination Stage*. This phase involves testing the family's ability to "fire" the therapist and go it alone by getting the family to simulate or rehearse its ability to solve new problems and to deal with old problems if they recur.

• *The Follow-up*. A follow-up session after 3, 6, or 12 months enables the therapist to evaluate the impact of therapy and test whether it has been successful in achieving second-order change, which means the facilitation of changes in family rules and family functions such that the family generates effective solutions to its own problems.

The therapist (according to Minuchin, 1974) acts as an energetic intruder working actively to restructure family organization and channels of communications by modeling, direction, and the use of "action techniques." The techniques for creating crisis or "creative turmoil" might include:

• *Enactments:* the direct illustration by the clients (as opposed to mere description) of the problems that exist between them. Clients are encouraged, where appropriate, to talk directly to one another rather than to (or through) the therapist.

• *Boundary clarification:* the creation or clarification of boundaries between family members is a feature of structural work. A mother who babies her teenager may hear with surprise her daughter's reply to the question "How old to you think your mother treats you as—3 or 13?"

• *Reframing:* involves an alteration in the emotional or conceptual viewpoint within which a situation is experienced. That experience is placed in another "frame" that fits the facts of the situation as well (or more plausibly), thereby transforming its entire meaning. Giving people different "stories" to tell themselves about themselves or about events—stories that are less self-defeating or destructive—is also a feature (under the name of cognitive restructuring) of behavioral family work.

EVALUATIONS OF EFFECTIVENESS

Research on family therapy outcomes with child and adolescent disorders has concentrated mainly on psychosomatic problems, conduct disorders/juvenile delinquency, and mixed emotional/behavioral difficulties. There is very little data from *rigorously controlled* trials or precisely defined problem areas, to provide wholly convincing evidence of whether, how, or where it is effective (Gurman et al., 1986; Kazdin, 1988). However, Piercy et al. (1986) had this to say about behavioral family therapy: "more methodologically sound research has been conducted on behavioral marital and family therapies than on other family therapies, perhaps because of their emphasis on operationalization of treatment components and assessment of change" (p. 80).

Piercy et al. (1986), in their review of the family therapies, commented that most of the articles and books written about structural, strategic, and systemic therapies are nonempirical and anecdotal in nature. They pointed out that the few data-based research studies conducted have used relatively specific presenting problems (e.g., psychosomatic illness, drug addiction) and have not employed alternative family therapy control groups. Evaluations of the Milan method are mainly anecdotal (see Speed, 1984). Likewise, virtually no experimental research has been conducted on the effectiveness of transgenerational family therapies. Experiential family therapists tend to formulate nonspecific goals, such as "self-worth," "self-responsibility," and "growth," which are difficult to operationalize and, in the opinion of practitioners, such attempts (e.g., psychometric techniques) are trivializing. For them, empirical research is incapable of doing justice to the subtleties of lived experience.

Gurman and Kniskern (1981) considered 32 publications on family therapy outcome research. They reported that:

1. About 73% were seen as "improved"; however, as few of the studies used controls, some of the treated families might have improved without any formal intervention.

2. It was impossible to separate the effects of the person of the therapist from the effects of the therapeutic approach.

3. The therapeutic approaches were never "pure" in the sense of being based on one body of theory.

4. The studies never specified what particular aspects of the intervention brought about the improvement.

In a later report, Gurman et al. (1986) drew the following conclusions from several dozen outcome studies of patient populations mixed as to developmental level and/or diagnosis (type and severity):

> little can be gleaned from this aggregate body of research that carried either significant theoretical meaning or clinical implications. Perhaps the most reliable statement that can be made is that, in heterogeneous samples of family therapy with childhood and/or adolescent behavioral problems . . . approximately two-thirds to three-quarters of cases can be expected to improve when treated by any of several well-defined family methods or eclectic methods. (p. 576)

These conclusions would seem to be borne out by the results for children and adolescents adapted from a table published by Gurman et al. (1986) (see Table 2). These findings, collated from 15 models of therapy, suggest that most models are not supported by (or lack) empirical findings. Although Gurman and his colleagues (Gurman et al., 1985) argued that outcome studies generally support the claim that family therapy is effective, only two models (the

behavioral and the psychoeducational) produce convincing results—and these are the models that tend to provide the more precise causal formulations. It is worth noting that all of the methods with at least moderately positive evidence of efficacy for some problems, are directive in nature. Presumably the level of directiveness is moderated, as there is evidence from therapy process research (e.g., Patterson & Forgach, 1985) that too much directiveness leads to patient resistance.

A meta-analysis by Markus, Lange, and Pettigrew (1990) of 19 studies, comparing family therapy with other treatment approaches, found that families treated using a family approach did better than patients receiving alternative treatment, minimal treatment, or no treatment. The effectiveness of components of treatment remains undiscovered or unexplored, and the structure of the families' treatment was not disclosed.

Of course, it is only too easy to criticize the paucity and methodological limitations of family therapy outcome research; it is worth remembering that the formidable problems of operationalizing key concepts are similar to those that hindered outcome research on psychotherapy (see Gurman & Kniskern, 1981). There is the added difficulty of simultaneously measuring change, not only in several people (a family), but also in interactional terms. Furthermore, there is little consensus about which factors constitute evidence of an efficacious outcome. A survey of (*inter alia*) family therapists' primary goals for therapy with a family conducted by the Group for the Advancement of Psychiatry (1970), elicited the following expressed as percentages with regard to *all* families:

Improved communication	86%
Improved autonomy and individuation	56%
Improved empathy	56%
More flexible leadership	34%
Improved role agreement	32%
Reduced conflict	23%
Individual symptomatic improvement	23%
Improved individual task performance	12%

Table 2. *Overall Estimates of the Effectiveness of Various Marital and Family Therapies for Specific Disorders and Problems*

Type of therapy	Adult disorders				Psychosomatic disorders	Child/adolescent disorders			Marital problems	
	Schizophrenia	Substance abuse	Affective disorders	Anxiety disorders		Juvenile delinquency	Conduct disorders	Mixed disorders	Marital discord	Divorce adjustment
Behavioral	2[a]	2[b]	1	3[c]	0	3[d]	3[d]	0	3	1[e]
Bowen FST	0	0	0	0	0	0	0	0	0	0
Contextual[j]	0	0	0	0	0	2	0	0	0	0
Functional[k]	0	0	0	0	0	0	0	0	0	0
Humanistic[f]	0	0	0	0	1	1	1	1	0	0
McMaster PCSTF	0	0	0	0	0	1	1	1	1	0
Milan Systemic	0	0	0	0	0	0	1	1	1	0
MRI Interactional	0	0	0	0	0	0	0	0	1	0
Multigenerational: other[g]	0	0	0	0	0	0	0	0	1	0
Psychoeducational	3	0	1	0	0	0	0	0	0	0
Psychodynamic-Eclectic	0	2[h]	0	0	1	0	1	1	2	1
Strategic	1	2[i]	0	0	1	0	0	0	0	0
Structural	0	2[j]	0	0	2	0	0	0	0	0
Symbolic-Experiential[l]	0	0	0	0	0	0	0	0	0	0
Triadic[m]	0	0	0	0	0	0	0	1	0	0

Note: 3 = effectiveness established; 2 = effectiveness probable; 1 = effectiveness uncertain; 0 = effectiveness untested. Modified from Gurman, Kniskern, and Pinsof (1986) with permission.

[a] Behavioral Family Management
[b] Alcohol abuse
[c] Spouse-assisted exposure therapy
[d] Parent Management Training
[e] Divorce mediation
[f] Satir
[g] Based on Framo and Williamson
[h] Conjoint couples groups for alcoholism
[i] Integrative Structural/Strategic Therapy (Stanton)
[j] Boszormenyi-Nagy
[k] Barton and Alexander
[l] Whitaker
[m] Zuk

Practitioners are not always clear about whether they are concerned with symptom reduction, family restructuring, or both.

Although little is known, in general, about the active therapeutic ingredients in family therapy, there is considerable evidence that the therapist, and how he or she behaves, is a major variable in the outcome of family therapy, regardless of the theoretical approach employed (Gurman & Kniskern, 1981). Todd and Stanton (1983) claimed, on the basis of their review, that the father's participation in family therapy substantially improves treatment outcomes. There seem to be no advantages in short-term/time-limited as opposed to longer-term therapy or between cotherapist participation and solo therapist input.

Dare (1985) concluded on the basis of a review of outcome studies involving children, that approaches employing social learning theory and techniques, as well as a systems approach, were effective in reducing intrafamilial behavior problems (e.g., aggressive behavior in children) and in improving family interactions.

Behavioral Family Therapy

In light of these comments, it is worth looking at the behavioral family therapy perspective. Systems theorists in contemporary behavioral practice—those who work within a behavioral family therapy modality—are like-minded in focusing not only on the individual but also on the system of relationships in which this person acts out his or her life. During the late 1960s and early 1970s, behaviorally orientated clinicians established that families could be taught to use behavioral principles to bring about positive change in the behavior of seriously problematic children. The work of Gerald Patterson in Oregon was part of, and the inspiration for, a rapid proliferation of what might be called "behavioral family therapy" (see Alexander & Parsons, 1982; Griest & Wells, 1983; Herbert, 1991; Kazdin, 1988; Patterson, 1982). This approach is in large part about the assessment and recruitment of naturally occurring environmental in-

fluences, specifically those occurring within the family between parents, siblings, and child, in order to modify deviant behavior and teach new skills and behavior repertoires. Behavioral family therapy, as its name implies, tends to operate much more at a *systemic* level than parent training where the main emphasis is on the parent–child (which usually means the mother–child) dyad rather than the family. Parents, as primary mediators of change, are in situ most of the time, and are in a position to apply contingencies and inductive methods of training, in a variety of situations and over the "long haul" required especially in treating antisocial, aggressive children (Herbert, 1987a).

Behavioral and systems approaches to family therapy are often viewed as being incompatible. Despite their epistemological differences, there are several significant similarities. Both approaches:

1. Focus on interactional rather than intrapsychic causation, i.e., how the problem behavior of one person meshes with the behavior of others

2. Seek to discover regularities or repetitive sequences in interpersonal processes

3. Emphasize observable behavioral events rather than unobservable subjective events

4. View the presenting problem as representative of broader classes of interactional patterns

5. Utilize behavior interventions aimed at changing dysfunctional patterns of interpersonal behavior

Piercy et al. (1986), in their *Family Therapy Sourcebook,* noted that "more methodologically sound research has been conducted on behavioral marital and family therapies than on other therapies, perhaps because of their emphasis on operationalization, treatment components and assessment of change" (p. 80).

PROCESS RESEARCH

Meta-analysts are critical of the reliance in evaluative studies on statistical significance because it misses subtle but meaningful change and does not measure magnitude. This is my cue to examine briefly the trend to more process research. Research into therapeutic process as opposed to therapy outcomes is emerging from its infancy; it is defined as the study (*inter alia*) of the interaction between therapist and family systems. Its goal is to identify change processes in the interaction between these systems (Pinsof, 1989). At present, apart from evidence highlighting the association between treatment outcome and therapist relationship skills, family therapy process research has produced few conclusions about how change (e.g., reducing the antisocial behavior of a child) is linked to therapist–client interactions (de Kemp, 1995; Gurman & Kniskern, 1981).

"User Unfriendliness"

Another important aspect of process in family therapy is the user's experience of therapy. There are aspects of the method, such as the technology (the one-way screen, the video camera) or the ongoing, live supervision that takes place (e.g., the telephone calls, consultations), that are worrying or distasteful to some clients, especially if not explained properly to them. They may be too dissonant with their expectations of what happens, and to whom it happens, in psychological treatment. Such dissonance may arise because patients lack the verbal/reflexive skills for the interaction required of them, a particularly shaming experience when there is known to be an invisible audience.

Howe's (1989) critique of family therapy, carried out by social workers, highlighted this issue. Most families in his sample of 32 clients disliked family therapy, and 23 of them failed to complete treatment.

An overemphasis on formalism—the uncharitable call it "mystique"—is the enemy of *all* therapies. Early in its development, family therapy was unique among therapies in its use of technology—a development that, wittingly or unwittingly, gives it the look of an "expert model" of therapy. The one-way screen, bug-in-the-

ear device, telephones, videos, and associated live supervision of the therapist by a team of colleagues was unusual and provided for the first time the opportunity to observe not only interactional sequences within the family, but also the relationship between therapist and client. What had previously been commonly regarded as an essentially private transaction became now a more public exchange, with the chance for a further team of therapists not only to observe but also to intervene.

Some family therapists insist that such live supervision and its associated technology is a sine qua non of the systems approach (Dallos & Proctor, 1984). It is necessary, in the light of more recent trends in family therapy—away from a rigid methodology to more creative and idiosyncratic approaches to families and their problems—to examine the validity of such a belief. Lask (1987) commented on the paucity of evidence to support live supervision as being more effective than cotherapy or lone therapy with consultation. The settings in which such approaches are applied have had even less research consideration.

Various authors have acknowledged the problems of working in teams (e.g., Roberts, 1982). "Expert teams" are likely to seem threatening to novice family therapists when providing live supervision. They can become very inward looking, a form of collective introspection, that detracts from what should be their main preoccupation—the patients. Conflicts arise; members of teams move on and well-established teams may be difficult to achieve.

Some approaches demand "neutrality" on the part of the therapist. However, effective intervention with a family relies on successful "joining" with them (Treacher, 1984). There is evidence (Speed, 1985) that distancing and maintaining a controlling stance with families leads to a high dropout rate after the first session. Often interpreted as resistance to change, this behavior could reflect the families' perception of the therapist as "cold" and "controlling." Clearly, the line between coldness and neutrality is a fine one, especially for vulnerable clients.

Reimers and Treacher (1995), in their provocative book *Introducing User-friendly Family
Therapy,* reminded us that therapists need to understand that therapy (which to them is an everyday, relatively matter-of-fact way of earning a
living) is a unique, challenging, often threatening experience to their users. It is unfortunate if
the "impedimenta" of cameras and one-way
screen, which are thought of as essential by therapists, should impede the key relationship/
alliance between therapist and patient.

Parenting and the Consultation Method

Interventions referred to as Behavioral Parent Training or the Consultation Model have
been aimed directly (in the main) at parents of
the aggressive/antisocial child; the aim is to
change the child's behavior by changing the
parents' behavior. Kazdin (1987) said of this approach that no other intervention for antisocial
children has been investigated so thoroughly
and has shown as favorable results, a conclusion
with which Gurman et al. (1986) agreed.

Most studies have been concerned with
course content and have neglected process variables (to which we return). With regard to content, a major objective of the varying curricula is
to train parents to alter the reinforcement contingencies that support the antisocial behavior
of their children. The rationale for the approach is that parents of children with conduct
problems tend (in comparison with parents of
non-clinic-attending parents) to exhibit fewer
positive behaviors, to be more aggressive and
critical in their use of discipline, to be more per-
missive, and are more likely to fail to monitor
their children's behaviors. They are also inclined to reinforce inappropriate behaviors and
to ignore or punish prosocial activities (for reviews of the literature see Callias, 1994; Forehand & McMahon, 1981; Herbert, 1987a; Patterson, 1982; Webster-Stratton, 1985, 1992).
Programs also address themselves to the fact
that parents of children with behavior problems
tend to flounder because they issue so many

commands, provide attention following deviant
behavior, are unlikely to perceive deviant behavior as deviant, get frequently embroiled in extended coercive hostile interchanges, give
vague commands, and are generally ineffectual
in bringing their children's deviant behavior to
a halt (Kazdin, 1987; Patterson, 1982). They also
tend to suffer the kinds of socioeconomic disadvantages that have an undermining influence
on parenting and family life.

At a systemic level, Patterson (1982) demonstrated, by means of sequential analyses of family interactions (notably the working of negative
reinforcers) in the home, the pervasiveness of a
family pattern of escalating, coercive interpersonal relationships that have a corrosive influence on family life, in general, and parent–
child relationships, in particular. These prove
antipathetic to the child's normal moral and social development.

One of the child's major acquisitions on the
road to becoming a social being is development
of internal controls over behavior—the "inter-
nalization" of standards of conduct and morali-
ty. Aronfreed (1968), in a series of experiments
on "conduct and conscience" in childhood,
demonstrated the power of cognitive structure
in internalizing inhibition. The role played by
the child's ability to recall behavior in represen-
tational and symbolic form was shown to be of
crucial importance. He found evidence of a subtle interaction between the children's cognitive
structuring of situations, their ability to represent to themselves punishment contingencies,
and the extent of emotional arousal that is associated with their cognitions during the socialization process. Their intellectual level, verbal ability, and ability to make a cognitive structure of
the learning situation are important sources of
control. He also demonstrated that punishment
that is above a certain optimal level of intensity
produces in the child a state of "emotionality"
that appears to interfere with learning. If discrimination of the punished choice is difficult,
intense punishment is actually more likely, subsequently, to lead to transgression. This finding
has clear implications for designers of parent

management programs, particularly with regard to the clear and fair enunciation of rules. A child unable to distinguish what aspect of behavior is being punished (often at high levels of frequency and intensity) will be unable to exercise control over the outcomes of behavior.

The developmental literature provides some useful guidelines to supplement behavioral theory in parent consultation work (e.g., Baumrind, 1971; Wright, 1971). The desiderata for prosocial behavior include the following: a rich supply of positive reinforcement for positive behavior "fueled" by a strong attachment to a caregiver with whom a child can therefore identify; parents' firm moral demands on their offspring; the consistent use of sanctions; techniques of punishment that are psychological rather than physical (i.e., methods that signify or threaten withdrawal of approval); and an intensive use of induction methods (reasoning and explanations).

Despite the documented effectiveness of various types of parent training programs, the literature contains comparatively little discussion of experiential and developmental issues as they affect individuals, or of the actual therapeutic processes utilized by therapists in order to deal with these and other matters, in their intervention programs. Program curricula, and change methods such as Planned Ignoring, Time-Out, Beta Commands, Praise, Differential Attention, Response Cost, and so on, have been carefully detailed (e.g., Dangel & Polster, 1984; Herbert, 1994a). They have an impressive track record for mitigating a wide variety of childhood problems (see Herbert, 1987b). Describing the "technology" alone, however, does not elucidate what happens when therapists try to change or influence parents' behaviors, attitudes, attributions, and practices. How can they encourage regular attendance and persuade parents to keep records or ensure that homework is carried out? How do they help them, when well "defended," to make connections between their own and their child's actions? How do they ensure that training is personally and culturally sensitive? How can therapists promote self-confidence in parents? These are but a few of the questions that require answers.

In that vein, Patterson and Forgatch (1985) reported a microsocial analysis of therapist–client interchanges. They showed that directive therapist behaviors, such as "teach" and "confront," increased the likelihood of parental resistance and lack of cooperation, whereas nondirective therapist behaviors, such as "facilitate" and "support," led to reliable decreases in client noncompliance. Webster-Stratton and Herbert, in the 1994 book *Troubled Families: Problem Children*, analyzed further (by means of detailed qualitative research) such therapist–client interactions, and the transactions of clients (feelings and verbalizations) with the program content. This focus on process is embodied in a collaborative approach to parent consultation work.

A COLLABORATIVE APPROACH

Perceptions of parents with seriously disruptive children have important implications for treatment because their learned helplessness and low self-efficacy beliefs can be reversed by experiences of success. Promotion of effective parenting skills undoubtedly starts such a reversal process giving parents some expectation that they will eventually be able to control outcomes—notably, their children's behavior. The means to this end are a cognitive-behavioral assessment, formulation, and intervention (e.g., Herbert, 1987b, 1992; Kendall & Braswell, 1985). Although the *content* of such programs is widely known and well researched, Webster-Stratton and Herbert (1994) contended that it is not sufficient to bring about success with a substantial proportion of cases (see Schmaling & Jacobson, 1987). They have therefore attempted to categorize operations defining the therapeutic *processes* that arise from adopting a collaborative style with clients. These operations or strategies are classified in terms of knowledge, skills, and values, and are detailed in Table 3.

Table 3. Sources of Increased Self-Empowerment

	Content	Process
Knowledge		
Child development	Developmental norms and tasks	Discussion
Behavior management	Behavioral (learning) principles	Books/pamphlets to read
Individual and temperamental differences	Child management (disciplinary strategies)	Modeling (videotape, live role play, role reversal, rehearsal)
	Relationships (feelings)	Metaphors/analogies
	Self-awareness (self-talk, schema, attributions)	Homework tasks
		Networking
	Interactions (awareness of contingencies, communications)	Developmental counseling
		Videotape viewing and discussion
	Resources (support, sources of assistance)	Self-observation/recording at home
		Discussing records of parents' own data
	Appropriate expectations	
	Parent involvement with children	Teaching, persuading
Skills		
Communication	Self-restraint/anger management	Self-reinforcement
Problem-solving (including problem analysis)	Self-talk (depressive thoughts)	Group and therapist reinforcement
Tactical thinking (use of techniques/methods)	Attend–ignore	Self-observations of interactions at home
	Play–praise–encourage	
Building social relationships	Contracts	Rehearsal
Enhancing children's academic skills	Consistent consequences	Participant modeling
	Sanction effectively (Time Out, loss of privileges, natural consequences)	Homework tasks and practice
		Video modeling and feedback
	Monitoring	Self-disclosure
	Social relationship skills	Therapist use of humor/optimism
	Problem-solving skills	Relaxation training
	Fostering good learning habits	Stress management
	Self-assertion/confidence	Self-instruction
	Empathy for child's perspective	Visual cues at home
	Ways to give and get support	
Values		
Strategic thinking (working out goals, philosophy of child rearing, beliefs)	Treatment/life goals	Discussion/debate
	Objectives (targeted child behaviors)	Sharing
	Ideologies	Listening
	Rules	Respecting/accepting
	Roles	Negotiating
	Relationships	Demystifying
	Emotional barriers	Explaining/interpreting
	Attributions	Reframing
	Prejudices	Resolving conflict
	Past history	Clarifying
		Supporting

Collaboration implies a nonblaming, supportive, reciprocal relationship based on using the therapists' knowledge and the parents' unique strengths and perspectives; it implies respect for each person's contribution. The Rogerian influence here is clear (Rogers, 1951). In a collaborative relationship, the therapist works with parents by actively soliciting their ideas and feelings, understanding their cultural context, involving them in the joint process of setting goals, sharing their experience, discussing and debating ideas, and problem-solving together. The role, as therapeutic partner or collaborator, is to understand the parents' perspectives, to clarify issues, to summarize important ideas and themes raised by the parents, to help them see that their child is trying to solve developmental/life problems just as they are, to teach (coach) and interpret in a way that is culturally sensitive, and finally, to suggest possible alternative approaches or choices when the parents request assistance and when misunderstandings occur.

Webster-Stratton and Herbert (1994) suggested that the collaborative process, which gives parents responsibility for developing solutions (alongside the therapist), is more likely to increase parents' sense of confidence, self-sufficiency, and perceived self-efficacy than are therapy models that do not hold parents responsible for seeking solutions. Support for this approach already comes from the literature on self-efficacy, attribution, helplessness, and locus of control. For example, Bandura (1977) suggested that self-efficacy is the mediating variable between knowledge and behavior. Thus, parents who are self-efficacious will tend to persist at tasks until success is achieved. The literature also indicates that people who "own" outcomes are more likely to persist in the face of difficulties and less likely to show debilitating effects of stress (e.g., Bandura, 1982, 1989). Moreover, evidence (Backeland & Lundwall, 1975; Janis & Mann, 1977; Meichenbaum & Turk, 1987) suggests that the collaborative process of sharing information and thinking has the advantage of reducing attrition rates, increasing motivation and commitment, reducing resistance, increasing temporal and situational generalization, and giving both parents and the therapist a stake in the outcome of the intervention efforts. There are several elements to the collaborative therapist's role.

1. *Developing a supportive relationship.* The collaborative therapist does not present her- or himself as the kind of "expert" who has worked out all of the answers to the parents' problems. She or he attempts to empathize with such difficulties but, at the same time, establish positive expectations for change. There is a deliberate

use of humor to help parents relax and to reduce anger, anxiety, and cynicism. Some videotape vignettes and role-play scenarios are chosen more for their humor value than for their content value.

2. *Empowering parents.* The essential goal of the collaborative approach is to "empower" parents by building on their strengths and experience so that they feel confident about their parenting skills and about their ability to respond to new situations that may arise when the therapist is not there to help them. Bandura (1977) called this strategy strengthening the client's "efficacy expectations," i.e., parents' conviction that they can successfully change their behaviors. There are several strategies to empower parents (see Table 3).

Parents are encouraged to explore different solutions to a problem situation, rather than settling for "quick fixes" or the first solution that comes to mind. The therapist studiously avoids giving any pat answers, keeping the focus of the discussion on the parents' insights. When parents seek professional help for their problems, they usually have experienced or are experiencing thoughts and feelings of powerlessness which is often expressed in terms of feeling victimized by their children—the "Why me?" question. The feeling of helplessness typically is accompanied by intense frustration, anger, and a fear of losing control of themselves when trying to discipline their children. Attention is paid to the "self-talk" of parents and attempts are encouraged to modify cognitions that are negative, distorted, or illogical. Parents are taught actively to formulate positive statements about themselves (e.g., "I was able to stay in control, I stayed calm, I am doing well").

Parents are encouraged to: (1) look at their strengths and think about how effectively they handled a difficult situation, and (2) express positive feelings about their relationship with their child and to remember good times.

3. *Teaching.* Just as the parents have their own expertise concerning their child and have the ultimate responsibility for judging what will be workable in their particular family and com-

munity, the therapist does wear an "expert" hat both when providing information about children's developmental needs, behavior management principles, and communication skills, and when "coaching" parents as they are practicing/rehearsing management strategies. Therapeutic change depends on persuasion, which means demystifying the therapeutic process by giving parents the rationale for each component of the program. It is important for the therapist to voice clear explanations based on valid information and knowledge of the developmental literature. Research has indicated that parents' understanding of the social learning principles underlying the parent-training program leads to enhanced generalization or maintenance of treatment effects (McMahon & Forehand, 1984). However, it is also important that these rationales and theories be presented in such a way that the parent can see the connection with his or her stated goals.

The process of collaborative teaching involves the therapist working with parents to interpret concepts and adapt skills to the particular circumstances of the parents and to the particular temperamental nature of the child. Much use is made of analogies, images, metaphors, charts, cartoons, vignettes, quizzes, playacting, debates, rehearsal, and video feedback to achieve these ends (see Webster-Stratton & Herbert, 1994, for examples). The teacher role involves giving an assignment for every session; at home, parents do some observing and recording of behaviors, thoughts, and feelings. They also experiment with a particular strategy. Assignments and experiments help transfer what is talked about in therapy/training sessions to real life at home and elsewhere.

Role-playing—modeling and rehearsing newly acquired methods—is particularly suited to the dilemma of translating behavioral management principle to public situations such as supermarkets, visiting, and so on. There is evidence that they are effective in producing behavioral changes (Twentyman & McFall, 1975). Self-management skill training for parents and use of telephone contact by therapists facilitate generalization and, indeed, maintenance of change (see Sanders & James, 1983; Sutton, 1995).

Therapeutic change depends on providing explanatory stories and alternative explanations that help clients to reshape their perceptions of, and their beliefs about, the nature of their problems. Reframing by the therapist (cognitive restructuring) is a powerful interpretive tool for helping clients understand experiences by altering their emotional and/or conceptual viewpoint in relation to an experience, or by placing the experience in another "frame" that fits the facts of the situation well, thereby altering its meaning. A common strategy is for the therapist to take a problem a parent is having with a child and reframe it from the child's point of view rather than the parent's perspective. Role reversal is useful for this purpose.

Part of the teacher role is to ensure that each session is evaluated by the parents. This gives the therapist immediate feedback about how each parent is responding to the therapist's style, the quality of the group discussions, and the information presented in the session.

It is often necessary to counter the myths and attributions that get in the way of therapeutic change. Typical examples of some myths and unhelpful attributions are: "It's my child's problem; she's the one who has to change" or "It's me who's to blame" (i.e., sole ownership). "Give him an inch and he takes a mile" (narrow limit-setting). "He won't love me if I insist" or "I feel so guilty if I say no" (broad limit-setting). "There's a demon in her" or "I don't trust him; he has his father in him" (unhelpful attributions). "I'm a complete failure as a parent. I can't forgive myself for the mistakes I've made" (catastrophizing). "Other parents all seem to cope" (unrealistic assumptions).

Another way to interpret the language and culture of the family is to help parents see connections between their own childhood experiences and those of their child. This is a powerful way of promoting empathy and bonding between parent and child.

There are a number of techniques that can be

helpful in facilitating the therapist's teaching role. The Webster-Stratton (1992) group training program relies heavily on videotape modeling as a therapeutic method. This is a series of 16 videotape programs (over 300 vignettes) showing parents and children of different sexes, ages, cultures, socioeconomic backgrounds, and temperamental styles. Parents are shown in natural situations interacting with their children: during mealtimes, getting children dressed in the morning, toilet training, handling child disobedience, playing together, and so forth—some "doing it right" and others "doing it wrong." The intent is to illustrate how parents can learn from their mistakes without feeling "put down." Videotapes are used in a collaborative way—as a catalyst to stimulate group discussion and debate (80% of each session is devoted to just that).

Use of videotape modeling training methods for parents of young conduct-problem children has been shown to be not only more effective in improving parent–child interactions (relative to group discussion approaches and one-to-one therapy with an individual therapist), but also highly cost-effective as prevention (see Webster-Stratton, 1991; Webster-Stratton & Herbert, 1993, 1994). Furthermore, videotape modeling has the potential advantage of being accessible to illiterate parents or to those who simply have difficulties with reading assignments and verbal approaches in general. Videotape modeling has potential for mass dissemination and low individual training cost when used in groups or in self-administered programs (Webster-Stratton, 1992).

SUMMARY

It is clear that the generic term *family therapy* is somewhat misleading. Several divergent schools of family therapy are flourishing in terms of their popularity with practitioners, practice-teachers, and publishers. The growth of the family therapy "industry" since its inception in the 1950s has been prodigious. Development of

evaluative work on the effectiveness of this orientation (i.e., "finely tuned" research that is rigorous in design and execution) has been less impressive. Given the ethical imperative of not foisting invalid or harmful treatments on an unsuspecting and vulnerable section of the public, the output of research testing of these methods, which have been around for some four decades, is disappointing.

Practitioners are faced with a bewildering choice of "brand name" therapy products. They wish to know what works and which method is most effective for which problem area. Confident, i.e., unambiguous or precise answers, are not forthcoming. Admittedly, the methodological difficulties of obtaining definitive answers are daunting. Furthermore, the conventional experimental approach to evaluation is antipathetic to many therapist—to their way of looking at causation, of defining goals or conceptualizing the focus of treatment.

It is on this issue that *behavioral* family therapy, despite some commonalities with other family therapies, parts company with them (see Table 2). Researchers such as Albert Bandura (1977), Robert Wahler (Wahler, House, & Stambaugh, 1976), Gerald Patterson (1982), and Carolyn Webster-Stratton (1991) have reported in great detail the findings of many systematic empirical studies of program content and process, for a variety of childhood disorders (see Herbert, 1987b, 1994a,b, for reviews of this literature).

More is known about program content than therapeutic process variables that contribute to successful treatment. An account of the collaborative model of working was given in order to illustrate the interaction of course content and process in a behaviorally orientated program (Webster-Stratton & Herbert, 1994).

Does Family Therapy Work?

Clearly, this question is too general; we wish to know what works, when and where it works; also why and how. Such attention to detail—the issue of "therapeutic horses for difficult courses"—is somewhat rare. Bennun (1985), who compared specific well-defined forms of family intervention (Milan systemic work and a problem-solving approach) applied to a specific clinical problem (namely, alcoholism), is an exemplar of the kind of research of which we need more. The jury, in the opinion of the present reviewer, is still out, when it comes to the more searching and specific questions about the value of family therapy models (or the nature of their active therapeutic ingredients) when applied to specific problems suffered by children. Only time (and more research) will tell. A particular conceptual difficulty for family therapy work with children is the tendency to polarize the defining of treatment goals into symptom reduction as opposed to systemic reorganization (see Papp, 1985). Such dichotomies are largely inappropriate given the multidimensional, multilevel nature of so many child and family problems (Herbert, 1994a,b).

At a global or undifferentiated level we get a cautious endorsement of family therapy. Thus, Gorell Barnes (1994), concluding a thorough review of the ramifications of family therapy, said that the data "established a crude empirical base for working this way" (p. 948). Gurman et al. (1986) found "a slender empirical basis" for recommending the continued practice and teaching of family therapy as a treatment modality for children. Improvement rates quoted (Gurman & Kniskern, 1981) of 68% for children are close to spontaneous remission rates for many problems, and the success rates of individual psychotherapy (Herbert, 1991).

Gurman (1983) expressed the view that no therapy is superior to another except in specific circumstances and with specific criteria of change. The undoubted superiority of behavioral family therapy to other therapies in the treatment of serious disruptive behavior disorders of childhood might be the circumstances referred to in Gurman's exceptions.

It seems unfortunate that family therapy, which has much in common with, indeed is a more sophisticated elaboration of other psychological therapies, has come to stand so conceptually alone. Is it qualitatively different from the rest; have not other therapies (especially contemporary behavioral work) of necessity become more systemic and less etiologically naive? Process issues were raised in this chapter, notably risks of mystification. Those helpful features, such as the technology, the technical language, and the group supervision, can, if insensitively or self-centeredly applied, create a barrier between therapists and patients, transforming an essentially humane method into an inhumane experience.

The systemic philosophy of family therapy has undoubtedly been a boon to our better understanding of families and children; many of the therapeutic strategies have proved to be powerful agents of change. It was necessary for practitioners to be reminded of the dynamics of family life, of the role of so-called "problem children" as "symptom carriers," and also of the fact that the family as a whole is more than the sum of its parts. The worry is what happens to the "parts." The child as a psychophysiological system may have intrinsic problems that are overlooked or downplayed by systemic workers—especially those without a clinical training.

There is a further issue for clinicians who believe that behaviors ("symptoms") covary to constitute the constellations or syndromes described by factor analysts (Achenbach & Edelbrock, 1983) or classificatory systems such as DSM-IV (APA, 1994). Is there a relationship between dysfunctional patterns of family life and specific childhood disorders? What is their functional relationship with the marked specificity of children's deviant behavior? Answers to these questions are few and far between in the writings of family therapists, perhaps because they are thought to be irrelevant.

To conclude this chapter by saying that more theoretical and process/outcome research is essential sounds trite but is nevertheless a truism. It is not simply a case of more of the same (see Kazdin, 1988). What is required is the discovery and application of more imaginative, sophisticated, microlevel investigatory methods. As Bennun (1986) said: "Until an adequate research methodology is developed, measuring therapeutic outcome will remain an ongoing dilemma" (p. 241).

ACKNOWLEDGMENT

I am indebted to Jenny Wookey, Principal Clinical Psychologist at the Child Development Centre, Plymouth, for critical reading of this chapter and for helpful discussion of the issues raised in it.

REFERENCES

Achenbach, T. M., & Edelbrock, C. S. (1983). Taxonomic issues in child psychology. In T. H. Ollendick & M. Hersen (Eds.), *Handbook of child psychopathology* (pp. 53–73). New York: Plenum Press.

Ackerman, N. (1958). *The psychodynamics of family life.* New York: Basic Books.

Alexander, J. F., & Parsons, B. V. (1982). *Functional family therapy.* Monterey, CA: Brooks/Cole.

American Psychiatric Association. (1994). *Diagnostic and statistical manual of mental disorders* (4th ed.). Washington, DC: Author.

Anderson, H. & Goolishian, H. (1988). Human systems as linguistic systems: Preliminary and evolving ideas about the implications for clinical theory. *Family Process, 27,* 371–393.

Aronfreed, J. (1968). *Conduct and conscience.* New York: Academic Press.

Avis, J. M. (1986). Feminist issues in family therapy. In F. P. Piercy, D. H. Sprenkle, and Associates, *Family therapy sourcebook.* New York: Guilford Press.

Backeland, F., & Lundwall, L. (1975). Dropping out of treatment: A critical review. *Psychological Bulletin, 82,* 738–783.

Bandura, A. (1977). Self-efficacy: Towards a unifying theory of behavioral change. *Psychological Review, 84,* 191–215.

Bandura, A. (1982). Self-efficacy mechanism in human agency. *American Psychologist, 37,* 122–147.

Bandura, A. (1989). Regulation of cognitive processes through perceiver self-efficacy. *Developmental Psychology, 25,* 729–735.

Bateson, G., Jackson, D. D., Haley, J., & Weakland, J. (1956). Toward a theory of schizophrenia. *Behavioral Science, 1,* 251–264.

Baumrind, D. (1971). Current patterns of adult authority. *Developmental Psychology Monograph, 4,* (1, Pt. 2).

Beavers, W. R., & Hampson, R. B. (1990). *Successful families: Assessment and intervention.* New York: Norton.

Bennun, I. (1985). Two approaches to family therapy with alcoholics: Problem-solving and systemic therapy. *Journal of Substance Abuse Treatment, 2,* 19–26.

Bennun, I. (1986). Evaluating family therapy: A comparison of the Milan and problem-solving approaches. *Journal of Family Therapy, 8,* 225–242.

Bowen, M. (1966). Theory in the practice of psychotherapy. In P. J. Guerin (Ed.), *Family therapy: Theory and practice* (pp. 78–92). New York: Gardner.

Callias, M. (1994). Parent training. In M. Rutter, E. Taylor, & L. Hersov (Eds.), *Child and adolescent psychiatry: Modern approaches* (3rd ed., pp. 918–935). London: Blackwell Scientific.

Carter, E. A., & McGoldrick, M. (1988). *The changing family lifecycle: A framework for therapy* (2nd ed.). New York: Gardner.

Dallos, R., & Proctor, H. (1984). *Family processes.* London: Open University Press.

Dangel, R. F., & Polster, R. A. (1984). *Parent training.* New York: Guilford Press.

Dare, C. (1985). Family therapy. In M. Rutter & L. Hersov (Eds.), *Child and adolescent psychiatry* (2nd ed., pp. 204–215). Oxford: Blackwell Scientific.

de Kemp, R. (1995). *Interactions in family therapy: A process research.* Nijmegen: Nederlands.

de Shazer, S. (1985). *Keys to solution in brief therapy.* New York: Newton.

Epstein, N. B., Baldwin, I. M., & Bishop, D. S. (1983). The McMaster Family Assessment Device. *Journal of Marital and Family Therapy, 9,* 171–180.

Forehand, R., & McMahon, R. J. (1981). *Helping the non-compliant child: A clinician's guide to parent training.* New York: Guilford Press.

Goldner, V. (1985). Feminism and family therapy. *Family Process, 24,* 31–47.

Gorell Barnes, G. (1994). Family therapy. In M. Rutter, E. Taylor, & L. Hersov (Eds.), *Child and adolescent psychiatry: Modern approaches* (3rd ed., pp. 946–967). London: Blackwell Scientific.

Griest, D. L., & Wells, K. C. (1983). Behavioral family therapy with conduct disorders in children. *Behavior Therapy, 14,* 37–53.

Group for the Advancement of Psychiatry (GAP). (1970). *The field of family therapy.* New York: Author.

Gurman, H. (1983). Family therapy research and the new epistemology. *Journal of Marital and Family Therapy, 9,* 227–234.

Gurman, A. S., & Kniskern, D. P. (1981). Family therapy outcome research: Knowns and unknowns. In A. S. Gurman & D. P. Kniskern (Eds.), *Handbook of family therapy* (pp. 70–92). New York: Brunner/Mazel.

Gurman, A. S., Kniskern, D. P., & Pinsof, W. M. (1986). Research on the process and outcome of marital and family therapy. In S. L. Garfield & A. E. Bergin (Eds.), *Handbook of psychotherapy and behavior change* (3rd ed., pp. 554–580). New York: Wiley.

Haley, J. (1971). A review of the family therapy field. In J. Haley (Ed.), *Changing families* (pp. 7–24). New York: Grune & Stratton.

Haley, J. (1976). *Problem solving therapy*. San Francisco: Jossey Bass.

Herbert, M. (1987a). *Conduct disorders of childhood and adolescence: A social learning perspective* (2nd ed.). New York: Wiley.

Herbert, M. (1987b). *Behavioral treatment of children with problems*. New York: Academic Press.

Herbert, M. (1991). *Clinical child psychology: Social learning, development and behavior*. New York: Wiley.

Herbert, M. (1992). *Working with children and the children act*. Leicester: British Psychological Society.

Herbert, M. (1994a). Behavioral methods. In M. Rutter, E. Taylor, & L. Hersov (Eds.), *Child and adolescent psychiatry: Modern approaches* (3rd ed., pp. 858–879). Oxford: Blackwell Scientific.

Herbert, M. (1994b). Etiological Issues. In T. Ollendick, N. J. King, & W. Yule (Eds.), *International handbook of phobic and anxiety disorders in children and adolescents* (pp. 3–20). New York: Plenum Press.

Hill, C. E. (1982). Counseling process research: Philosophical and methodological dilemmas. *Counseling Psychologist, 10,* 7–19.

Hoffman, L. (1995). Foreword. In S. Reimers & A. Treacher *Introducing user-friendly family therapy* (pp. vii–xii). London: Routledge.

Howe, D. (1989). *The consumer's view of family therapy*. Aldershot: Gower.

Jackson, D. (1957). The question of family homeostasis. *Psychiatry Quarterly Supplement, 31,* 79–80.

Janis, I. L., & Mann, L. (1977). *Decision making: A psychological analysis of conflict, choice and commitment*. New York: Free Press.

Jordan, C., & Franklin, C. (1995). *Clinical assessment for social workers: Quantitative and qualitative methods*. Chicago: Lyceum.

Kaslow, F. W. (1980). History of family therapy in the United States: A kaleidoscopic overview. *Marriage and Family Review, 3,* 77–111.

Kazdin, A. (1987). Treatment of antisocial behavior in children: Current status and future directions. *Psychological Bulletin, 102,* 187–203.

Kazdin, A. (1988). *Child psychotherapy: Developing and identifying effective treatments*. Elmsford, NY: Pergamon Press.

Kendall, P., & Braswell, L. (1985). *Cognitive-behavioral therapy for impulsive children*. New York: Guilford Press.

Koocher, G. P., & Pedulla, B. M. (1977). Current practices in child psychotherapy. *Professional Psychology,* 275–287.

Lask, B. (1987). Cybernetics—Epistobabble, the emperor's new clothes and other sacred cows. *Journal of Family Therapy, 9,* 207–215.

Markus, E., Lange, A., & Pettigrew, T. (1990). Effectiveness of family therapy: A meta-analysis. *Journal of Family Therapy, 12,* 205–221.

Marmar, C. R. (1990). Psychotherapy process research: Progress, dilemma and future directions. *Journal of Consulting and Clinical Psychology, 58,* 265–272.

McMahon, R., & Forehand, R. (1984). Parent training for the non-compliant child: Treatment outcome, generalization and adjunctive therapy procedures. In R. F. Dangel & R. A. Polster (Eds.), *Parent training: Foundations of research and practice* (pp. 149–176). New York: Guilford Press.

Meichenbaum, D., & Turk, D. (1987). *Facilitating treatment adherence: A practitioner's guidebook*. New York: Plenum Press.

Minuchin, S. (1974). *Families and family therapy*. Cambridge, MA: Harvard University Press.

Minuchin, S., Baker, L., Rosman, B., Liebman, R., Milman, L., & Todd, T. (1975). A conceptual model of psychosomatic illness in children. *Archives of General Psychiatry, 32,* 1031–1038.

Olson, D. H. (1986). Circumplex Model VII: Validation studies and FACES III. *Family Process, 26,* 337–351.

Palazzoli, M., Boscoli, L., Cecchin, G., & Piata, G. (1978). *Paradox and counterparadox*. Northvale, NJ: Aronson.

Papp, P. (1985). *The process of change*. New York: Guilford Press.

Patterson, G. (1982). *Coercive family process*. Eugene, OR: Castalia.

Patterson, G. R., & Chamberlain, P. (1988). Treatment process: A problem at three levels. In L. C. Wynne (Ed.), *The state of the art of family therapy research* (pp. 122–136). New York: Family Process Press.

Patterson, G. R., & Forgatch, M. S. (1985). Therapist behavior as a determinant for client non-compliance: A paradox for the behavior modifier. *Journal of Consulting and Clinical Psychology, 53,* 846–851.

Piercy, F. P., Sprenkle, D., and Associates. (1986). *Family therapy sourcebook*. New York: Guilford Press.

Pinsof, W. M. (1989). A conceptual framework and methodological criteria for family therapy process research. *Journal of Consulting and Clinical Psychology, 57,* 53–59.

Reiss, D. (1988). Theoretical versus tactical inferences: Or how to do family therapy research without dying of boredom. In L. C. Wynne (Ed.), *The state of the art in family therapy research* (pp. 144–158). New York: Family Process Press.

Reimers, S., & Treacher, A. (1995). *Introducing user-friendly family therapy*. London: Routledge.

Roberts, W. (1982). The strengths and weaknesses in cotherapy. In A. Bentovim, G. Gorrell Barnes, & A. Cooklin (Eds.), *Family therapy: Complementary frameworks of theory and practice* (pp. 84–98). New York: Academic Press.

Rogers, C. R. (1951). *Client-centered therapy*. Boston: Houghton–Mifflin.

Sanders, M. R., & James, J. E. (1983). The modification of parent behavior: A review of generalization and maintenance. *Behavior Modification, 7,* 3–27.

Satir, V. (1967). *Conjoint family therapy*. Palo Alto, CA: Science and Behavior Books.

Schmaling, K. B., & Jacobson, N. S. (1987, November). *The clinical significance of treatment resulting from parent training interventions for children with conduct problems: An analysis of outcome data*. Paper presented at the meeting of the Association for the Advancement of Behavior Therapy, Boston.

Sowder, B. J. (1975). *Assessment of child mental health needs* (Vols. I–VIII). McLean, VA: General Research Corp.

Speck, R., & Attneave, C. (1974). *Family networks*. New York: Vintage Books.

Speed, B. (1985). Evaluating the Milan approach. In D. Campbell & R. Draper (Eds.), *Applications of systemic family therapy: The Milan method*. New York: Academic Press.

Sutton, C. (1995). Parent training by telephone: A partial replication. *Behavioral & Cognitive Psychology, 21,* 11–24.

Todd, T. C., & Stanton, M. D. (1983). Research on marital and family therapy: Answers, issues and recommendations for the future. In B. B. Wolman & G. Stricker (Eds.), *Handbook of family and marital therapy* (pp. 196–221). New York: Plenum Press.

Tomm, K. (1984). One perspective of the Milan systemic approach: Part I: Overview of development, theory and practice. *Journal of Marital and Family Therapy, 10,* 253–271.

Treacher, A. (1984). Family therapy with children: The structural approach. In G. Edwards (Ed.), *Current issues in clinical psychology* (Vol. 4, pp. 18–27). New York: Plenum Press.

Twentyman, C. T., & McFall, R. M. (1975). Behavioral training of social skills in shy males. *Journal of Consulting and Clinical Psychology, 43,* 384–395.

Vetere, A., & Gale, A. (1987). *Ecological studies of family life*. New York: Wiley.

Von Bertalanffy, L. (1968). *General systems theory*. Harmondsworth: Penguin.

Wahler, R. G., House, A. E., & Stambaugh, E. E. (1976). *Ecological assessment of child problem behavior*. Elmsford, NY: Pergamon Press.

Walsh, N. (1982). *Normal family process*. New York: Guilford Press.

Walters, M., Carter, B., Papp, P., & Silverstein, O. (1988). *The invisible web: Gender patterns in family relationships*. New York: Guilford Press.

Watzlawick, P., Weakland, J., & Fisch, R. (1974). *Changes: Principles of problem formulation and problem resolution*. New York: Norton.

Webster-Stratton, C. (1988). Parents and children videotape series. Basic and Advanced Programs, 1 to 7. 1411 8th Avenue West, Seattle, WA 98119.

Webster-Stratton, C. (1991). Annotation: Strategies for helping families with conduct disordered children. *Journal of Child Psychology and Psychiatry, 32,* 1047–1062.

Webster-Stratton, C., & Herbert, M. (1993). What really happens in parent training? *Behavior Modification, 17,* 407–456.

Webster-Stratton, C., & Herbert, M. (1994). *Troubled families: Problem children*. Chichester, England: Wiley.

Wright, D. (1971). *The psychology of moral behavior*. Harmondsworth, England: Penguin.

24

Behavioral Treatment

BRIAN P. MARX AND ALAN M. GROSS

INTRODUCTION

The origins of behavior therapy techniques can be found in the work of individuals such as Ivan Pavlov and B. F. Skinner, on which the principles of respondent and operant conditioning are based. Behavioral treatment methods have remained at the forefront of effective intervention for the past 30 years. However, since its inception child behavior therapy has come to include other techniques and strategies for ameliorating child psychopathology. These strategies include observational learning or modeling (Bandura, 1977) and cognitive-behavioral therapies (Meichenbaum & Goodman, 1971).

A defining characteristic of all behavior therapy is its empirical focus. Practitioners systematically examine the sequelae of behavioral difficulties, conduct precise functional analyses, and measure efficacy of specific treatments. Through these empirical methods behavior therapists have made great strides in developing and implementing interventions for various behavior disorders of childhood and adolescence. Although clinicians may disagree as to preferred mode of treatment, most can agree on the importance of empirical demonstrations of treatment effectiveness. Thus, child behavior therapists have shown a strong commitment to treatment outcome research (see Garfield & Bergin, 1986).

As do all behavior therapists, those who treat childhood disorders subscribe to certain tenets (Masters, Burrish, Hollon, & Rimm, 1987). Behavior therapy focuses on observable behavior as opposed to a presumed underlying cause. Symptoms are not seen as manifestations of an underlying process. These maladaptive behaviors are the problem and should be treated accordingly.

Behavior therapists believe that maladaptive behaviors are acquired via the same processes by which adaptive behaviors are acquired. That is, all behavior has similar origins through operant and respondent processes and modeling. A person's learning history holds the key to understanding how his or her behavioral repertoire develops.

Because maladaptive behaviors are believed to be learned, it is posited that techniques based on learning principles may be effective in alter-

BRIAN P. MARX • Department of Psychology, Oklahoma State University, Stillwater, Oklahoma 74047.   ALAN M. GROSS • Department of Psychology, University of Mississippi, University, Mississippi 38677.

Handbook of Child Psychopathology, 3rd edition, edited by Ollendick & Hersen. Plenum Press, New York, 1998.

ing problem responses. Recently, increased recognition of biological influences has led to integration of pharmacological interventions into
some behaviorally based treatment programs
(e.g., attention-deficit hyperactivity disorder
[ADHD]).

Another widely held belief among behavior
therapists is that the focus of therapy should be
on current difficulties. This stands in contrast to
psychodynamically oriented therapists who concentrate their efforts on events that occur early
in life and hold that insight into these events facilitates improved functioning. This point is critical for child behavior therapists, as many children are developmentally incapable of gaining
insight into the relationships between past
events and current behaviors. Although child
behavior therapists believe that a person's learning history is important in the development of
psychopathology, these events cannot be altered. In order to modify current behaviors,
child behavior therapists attempt to affect the
current environmental contingencies that act
to maintain these behaviors. This treatment approach has been viewed by psychodynamic therapists as being limiting in the types of disorders
that it can effectively treat. However, data fail to
support this contention (Mahoney, Kazdin, &
Lesswing, 1974; O'Leary & O'Leary, 1977).

Our chapter will review behavior therapy procedures for behavior problems commonly diagnosed during childhood. Following discussion
of the ethical issues associated with the treatment of children, a review of developmental factors will be presented. Behavioral assessment
will then be discussed. Finally, various behavior
therapy procedures will be considered.

ETHICAL CONSIDERATIONS IN
CHILD BEHAVIOR THERAPY

Behavior therapy with children differs in a
number of ways from such therapy with adults.
Adults usually participate in behavioral treatment programs of their own volition whereas
children do not seek treatment voluntarily.
Rather, they are referred by adults for treatment
(e.g., parents, teachers, public officials). Adults
may also decide when to terminate treatment.
However, children often are denied opportunities to make these choices because referring
adults and therapists may presume that children are developmentally incapable of making
such decisions, or because it may not be in the
child's best interests to allow him or her to decide. This may result in the child becoming confused or responding angrily about coerced
treatment. To avoid the child feeling inconse-
quential in the treatment process, it is suggested
that behavior therapists actively include the
child in deliberations about treatment, and
whenever possible solicit the child's consent to
the goals and procedures of treatment. Child
behavior therapists may also use behavioral contracting procedures to facilitate cooperation
and resolution of differences that remain following mutual discussion (Sulzer-Azaroff &
Mayer, 1977).

Adults are frequently consulted by therapists
when setting specific treatment goals. As noted
above, children often have treatment goals set
for them. At times developmental considerations limit a child's ability to contribute to
treatment planning. No set rules have been established for determining the extent to which
children should be involved in deciding specific
treatment objectives. However, behavior therapists have responded to these concerns regarding a child's competence to make treatment decisions through empirical examination. After
evaluating normal children's responses to several vignettes concerning physical and psychological problems, Weithorn (1980) concluded
that 14-year-olds were comparable to adults in
their understanding of treatment issues. Moreover, 9-year-olds were found basically to agree
with the treatment decisions reached by the older groups, with the qualification that the responses were judged to be more immature.
These findings suggest that often adolescents
are competent to be fully involved in treatment
decision-making. Younger children as well
should contribute to the decision-making process to the extent that they are competent.

Child behavior therapists find themselves committed both to the child as the identified client and to the parents. At times this dual commitment can elicit challenging questions over the issue of confidentiality, especially with preadolescent or adolescent clients. In some cases confidentiality between the therapist and child client may be considered necessary to facilitate effective treatment. However, in most states parents have the right by law to access their child's records (Ehrenreich & Melton, 1983). This problem should be anticipated and the therapist should address issues of confidentiality with children and their parents prior to beginning therapy. It is suggested that an agreement be reached among all three parties about the extent to which communications between the therapist and the child may be restricted from parents.

To help minimize less than optimal sets of conditions, such as those just noted, behavior therapists have adopted a number of ethical standards to guide their work (e.g., see *Behavior Therapy, 8,* 1977). These policies address relevant topics for work with children such as adequate consideration of treatment goals and treatment methods, voluntary participation of children in treatment, interests of subordinated clients, evaluation of adequacy of treatment, and confidentiality of the treatment relationship. It is hoped that by adhering to these guidelines child behavior therapists will ensure that all therapeutic goals are understood by the child, provide the most effectively proven treatment for maladaptive behaviors or provide a range of treatments if the child has been mandated to participate in therapy, make certain that the child and guardian participate in treatment planning as much as the child's abilities permit, and protect the child's therapy records whenever possible.

DEVELOPMENTAL FACTORS

Through both research and clinical work, child behavior therapists have come to realize that developmental factors are essential elements in how children respond to their environments. In addition to the consideration of environmental contingencies, children's behavior should be viewed within the context of their age, social, physical, and cognitive development. For example, it may be considered normal for a 2-year-old to suck his thumb, but it is not considered appropriate for an 11-year-old to engage in this behavior.

The fourth edition of the *Diagnostic and Statistical Manual of Mental Disorders* (DSM-IV) (APA, 1994) separates disorders usually first diagnosed in childhood and adolescence from those diagnosed in adulthood. However, a single criteria set is provided for each disorder that applies to children, adolescents, and adults. Any individual (child or adult) can be diagnosed with a particular disorder, regardless of age, as long as he or she meets the outlined criteria. Variations in presentation of a disorder may be attributable to an individual's developmental stage (e.g., ADHD is more commonly diagnosed in children than adults).

Interventions are also chosen based on age appropriateness, as we can expect children at different stages of development to be capable of different levels of participation in the therapeutic milieu. For example, it may be appropriate to utilize imagery-based fear reduction techniques with an adolescent, but these techniques would be contraindicated for a preschooler (Underwood & Gross, 1989).

Use of normative data is one way in which child behavior therapists may be sensitive to developmental issues. For example, normative data on childhood fears have shown that as children mature, qualitative differences occur with regard to the focus of their fears (Jersild & Holmes, 1935; Kennedy, 1965; Miller, 1983; Ollendick, Matson, & Helsel, 1985; Simon & Ward, 1974). This knowledge allows increased accuracy in targeting appropriate behaviors (Hersen & Van Hasselt, 1987). The contextual matrix of developmental factors is especially important in child behavior therapy because the norms for socially appropriate behavior in children change rapidly as children mature. This is a factor that has considerably less relevance in behavior therapy with adults, where developmental differences over time vary much more slowly. Furthermore, in adhering to a social validation approach in determining the clinical significance of behavior change, norms provide a basis for social comparisons (Kazdin, 1977).

Although age-related norms provide useful information about a child's behavior, child behavior therapists need to be cautious in their interpretation of such data. In some cases data regarding norms may be suspect as a result of methodological flaws. For example, some studies rely on parent and teacher reports (Harris & Ferrari, 1983) rather than independent observers, and are thus subject to bias as parental perception of a child's behavior may be subject to a variety of influences (Graham & Rutter, 1968; Harris & Ferrari, 1983). Another difficulty related to using age-related norms is that the normative database for child psychopathology is still being developed. Adequate norms have not been developed for children of varying ethnic backgrounds, living environments, and levels of socioeconomic status (Underwood & Gross, 1989). To remedy the shortcomings associated with norm-referenced approaches, child behavior therapists should also consider individual or criterion-referenced approaches that emphasize importance of performance in relation to oneself or a predetermined criterion. In this way, behavior therapists can view a child's behavior in the context of both peer performance and individual performance (Nunnally, 1978).

BEHAVIORAL ASSESSMENT

Consistent with behavioral theory, assessment in behavior therapy is directed toward identifying maladaptive behaviors, environmental events that may exacerbate or maintain them, and selective variables that may be used to alter or change current functioning (Ollendick & Cerny, 1981). In behavioral assessment the focus is treatment oriented. For example, through observation and precise recording a behavior therapist attempts to identify which environmental factors are acting to sustain a child's disruptive classroom behavior. Once these factors have been identified, the behavior therapist may elect to treat the child's behavior by interrupting the chain of events that occur in that setting. As a result of behavioral methods being geared more toward treating the individual, the behavior therapist usually assesses continually throughout the treatment period to determine whether or not the elected mode of treatment is effective.

Behavior therapists typically attempt to monitor three response channels. These response channels include cognitive behaviors (subjective/self-report), overt motoric behaviors, and physiological behaviors (Barlow & Hersen, 1984; Lang, 1968, 1971). Research has shown that these three channels of responding are independent of one another.

Because the content focus of assessment may vary widely, a variety of assessment techniques or methods have been developed. These techniques include direct observation, self-reports including self-monitoring, questionnaires, structured interviews, and various types of instrumentation, particularly for the measurement of psychophysiological responding. Though any of these techniques conceivably could be paired with any content domain, current practices favor certain associations between content and method: motor acts with direct observations, cognitive responses with self-report, and physiological responses with instrumentation (Hartmann, Roper, & Bradford, 1979).

Several models of behavioral assessment have been offered as guidelines when conducting a behavioral assessment. These models vary in their complexity and underlying assumptions. For example, Stuart (1970) offered the basic A-B-C (antecedents–behaviors–consequences) model of behavioral assessment, and Kanfer and Saslow (1965) offered the more complex S-O-R-K-C model in which the therapist considers antecedent events (S), the biological condition of the organism (O), observed behaviors

(R), schedules of contingency or other contingency-related conditions (K), and any environmental or organismic consequences of the observed behavior (C). Lazarus (1973) offered the BASIC-ID model in which the therapist considers the behaviors, affect, sensation, imagery, cognition, interpersonal variables, and drugs/biology of the individual. Although these models may differ in complexity and assumptions about which behaviors to target for modification, they all similarly focus on the empirical observation and identification of specific maladaptive behaviors and maintaining factors.

Traditional cognitive assessment has gained increased importance for child behavior therapists. One reason for this is that a growing majority of child referrals may be related to developmental and educational considerations. In these cases traditional cognitive tests can assist in determining whether a behavior problem may be accounted for by a child's maturational and educational level, skill deficits, and learning problems. Another reason for its significance is that standardized tests may be used as outcome measures of treatment effectiveness. Often the measures used by behavior therapists are not standardized and are specifically designed for individual treatment interventions. An evaluation of school achievement, intellectual skill, and/or developmental level through standardized testing can be used to assess more generalized changes that occur, or fail to occur, with specific behavioral programs. Further, these tests are no longer viewed as tests of hypothetical unobservable constructs, but rather as presenting an array of stimulus conditions in which the child can be observed and evaluated in terms of problem-solving skills and in dealing with stressful situations (Ollendick & Cerny, 1981).

BEHAVIORAL TREATMENTS

As noted earlier the techniques of behavior therapy evolved from early work in respondent and operant conditioning. Respondent, or clas-

sical conditioning, therapies are based on the principles of emotional responding derived from the work of Ivan Pavlov (1928). Respondent conditioning principles indicate that individuals develop emotional responses, such as fear and anxiety, through contiguous association or pairing of a neutral stimulus with an aversive stimulus. Following repeated pairings the neutral stimulus evokes an emotional response in the individual that is similar to that evoked by the original aversive stimulus. As such, attempts to eliminate these undesirable emotional responses involve breaking the association.

Operant conditioning therapies are rooted in the work of B. F. Skinner (1953). Skinner demonstrated that much behavior is contingency shaped. That is, an individual's behavior and environment reciprocally affect one another. The basic operant procedure involves identifying environmental factors that support target behaviors. Interventions involve systematically arranging antecedents and consequences of these behaviors in an attempt to alter their probability of occurrence. Below is a description of a number of common child behavior therapy procedures.

Systematic Desensitization

Systematic desensitization, developed by Joseph Wolpe (1958, 1969, 1973, 1982), is a therapeutic procedure that may be used to change, alleviate, or diminish a maladaptive conditioned emotional response to a feared or aversive stimulus. In this technique a state of relaxation in the individual is paired either with the feared stimulus or with an imagined situation in which the individual is confronted with the feared stimulus. According to Wolpe, systematic desensitization reflects the process of counterconditioning or replacing a maladaptive conditioned emotional response with a more adaptive response set. However, experimental data suggest that effectiveness of systematic desensitization may be a result of an extinction process (Gross & Brigham, 1979).

This therapeutic technique involves several components. The first phase of treatment involves teaching the child a progressive relaxation technique in which the patient alternates tensing and relaxing different muscle groups until the body is deeply relaxed. It may prove necessary when training children in relaxation to consider the developmental level of the child. Previous literature notes that relaxation is not indicated for children under 9 years of age, as they may have difficulty maintaining attention to the task. With children it may also be necessary to model the desired relaxation response (Kratochwill & Morris, 1991).

The second phase, construction of a hierarchy of anxiety-provoking stimuli or situations, should only begin after the therapist is sure the child is sufficiently skilled in relaxation. The fear hierarchy is developed by the client with assistance from the therapist and should be arranged in ascending order from the least to the most anxiety-provoking situations. Situations on the hierarchy should relate directly to the child's problem and should reflect past experiences or experiences that he or she anticipates. It has been recommended that the fear hierarchy include enough items so that graduation from one item to the next can be experienced without overwhelming distress. Most fear hierarchies contain 20 to 25 items (Kratochwill & Morris, 1991).

The third step of systematic desensitization involves pairing relaxation with exposure to the anxiety-provoking stimuli on the hierarchy. During the beginning of this phase the child is asked to perform graduated relaxation exercises. The therapist then asks the child to imagine scenes from the hierarchy with scenes presented by the therapist in ascending order. During each presentation the child is asked to imagine the scene until he or she becomes anxious and then is instructed to return to a pleasant image while maintaining the relaxed state. Progression through the fear hierarchy is determined by the speed at which the child learns to imagine the situation with little accompanying anxiety. The process of switching back and forth between relaxing and fear-arousing images continue throughout desensitization sessions until the child can imagine all of the scenes and remain relaxed (Kratochwill & Morris, 1991).

Several variants of systematic desensitization have been developed by clinicians and researchers. A popular variant of this procedure is in vivo desensitization. In this technique, instead of being exposed to imaginal stimuli the child is gradually exposed to real-life anxiety-provoking situations. Child behavior therapists may find this desensitization technique superior to those utilizing imaginal techniques as children may have difficulties imagining aversive situations or may find it difficult to become fearful of mere thoughts of the stimulus (King, Hamilton, & Ollendick, 1988). In vivo desensitization has been used to treat a wide variety of fears and phobias in children including fear of heights (Croghan & Musante, 1975), darkness, separation, and school (Kellerman, 1980; Phillips & Wolpe, 1981), water (Ultee, Griffioen, & Schellekens, 1982), and social situations (Kandel, Ayllon, & Rosenbaum, 1977).

Other variants of systematic desensitization have included using game playing, storytelling, conversation, feeding, and physical contact in place of relaxation. Substitutions for the imaginal component of the procedure have included pictures or toys that represent the feared object (Barrios & O'Dell, 1989).

McGrath, Tsui, Humphries, and Yule (1990) utilized in vivo desensitization to successfully treat a 9-year-old girl's noise phobia. The client was allowed to control timing of the presented noises. Investigators used several anxiety-incompatible responses including conversation, relaxation, and the creation of a playful environment. During the first session, a preliminary hierarchy for presentation of stimuli was drawn up and included doors banging, cap guns popping, balloons bursting, and unexpected explosions of party poppers. It was also during this session that the child was taught progressive relaxation. Fearful stimuli were presented in a progressive fashion over the course of 10 sessions. By the final session the child's fear ratings had significantly declined. At a 3-month follow-up session treatment gains had been maintained. Other fears and phobias in children such as fear of eating (Delgado, Emde, & Pope, 1993), fear of water (Menzies & Clarke, 1993), fear of individuals with mental retardation (Madonna, 1990), fear of social situations (Green & Benjamin, 1990), and fear of dogs (Glasscock & MacLean, 1990) have been successfully treated using in vivo systematic desensitization.

Flooding

Another behavioral technique widely used for treatment of childhood fears and anxiety is flooding. Flooding varies from systematic desensitization in that the subject is exposed in a prolonged fashion to the most intense and fearful aspects of a situation rather than in the graduated manner used in systematic desensitization.

Like systematic desensitization, the flooding procedure has several variations. In imaginal, or in vitro, flooding, the client is asked to imagine scenes from a fear hierarchy much like in systematic desensitization. However, the client is initially exposed to scenes at least halfway up the hierarchy. In an in vivo flooding procedure the subject is presented with the feared object or situation without escape until the fear response diminishes. For example, Saigh (1986) used an in vitro flooding procedure to treat a 6-year-old boy's war-related posttraumatic stress disorder (PTSD). Five anxiety-evoking scenes pertaining to the child's trauma were identified. Prior to treatment the child's psychological sequelae were assessed via several observation inventories, checklists, and several self-report measures. The child was taught deep muscle relaxation exercises involving mental imagery. During the treatment phase each session was initiated by 15 minutes of therapist-directed relaxation exercises. Twenty-four minutes of in vitro flooding was subsequently presented, wherein the child was asked to imagine the exact details of the scene in question. Subjective units of distress probes were conducted at 1-minute intervals

throughout the in vitro flooding process. Ten minutes of relaxation exercises were subsequently presented. Each of the remaining trauma-related scenes was presented for 6 minutes and subjective units of distress (SUDS) assessments were taken at 2-minute intervals. Five minutes of relaxation separated each of the pleasant imagery presentations. Posttreatment and 6-month follow-up results suggested that the flooding intervention decreased the child's symptomatology, as was reflected on behavioral, affective, and cognitive outcome measures. Saigh further demonstrated the efficacy of this procedure in subsequent applications (1987, 1989).

Implosion uses imagined aversive stimuli that are exaggerated versions of the fearful object or situation. In reinforced practice the subject is rewarded for staying in the presence of a feared stimulus for long periods of time (Barrios & O'Dell, 1989). In all of these variations the child is asked to continue until he or she is no longer bothered by the aversive stimulus. Flooding and its variants have been used with a wide variety of child anxiety disorders such as obsessive-compulsive disorder (Harris & Wiebe, 1992), specific phobias (Menzies & Clarke, 1993), and panic attacks with agoraphobia (Kolko, 1984).

Because there are few controlled studies demonstrating efficacy of flooding with children (see Barrios & O'Dell, 1989), many clinicians may have reservations about using it. Additionally, children usually have little input into their treatment regimen, and because flooding may be viewed as an aversive intervention it can be another source of hesitation for child behavior therapists. However, flooding and its variants may prove invaluable in situations that require swift and decisive interventions (e.g., preparation for invasive medical procedures; see Friedman, Campbell, & Evans, 1995).

Graduated Exposure

Another procedure that has become popular with child behavior therapists is graduated exposure. This procedure is similar in some ways to in vivo desensitization and the techniques of flooding and implosion. But graduated exposure also differs from these procedures in several ways. In graduated exposure the child is not provided with a competing response to replace anxiety nor is any care taken to ensure the prevention of avoidance responses (Masters et al., 1987). The subject is provided with a systematic presentation of aversive stimuli gradually moving to more aversive situations. Avoidance behavior is prevented by presenting stimuli that are too weak to elicit the avoidance behavior (Masters et al., 1987). Graduated exposure has been used by clinicians with children suffering from fear of having bowel movements in public toilets (Eisen & Silverman, 1991) and separation anxiety (Hagopian & Slifer, 1993).

Modeling

Modeling procedures are largely based on the work of Albert Bandura. Bandura noted that many behaviors can be learned without direct participation. Fears and phobias may be acquired, inhibited, or eliminated through the observation of models who directly engage in the desired behavior (Bandura, 1969; Barrios & O'Dell, 1989).

Bandura also distinguished between learning and performance of responses. In his seminal study of modeled aggressive responses in children (Bandura, 1965) Bandura discovered that although children may learn modeled responses, the performance of these behaviors was determined by their consequences.

Bandura identified four components of any modeling procedure (Bandura, 1969, 1977): (1) attention to modeled behaviors and situations, (2) retention of what is learned during observation, (3) reproduction of a modeled behavior, and (4) the motivation to reproduce the modeled behavior. Bandura believed that these components were critical to the success of a modeling procedure and that any procedure

not including all components would not be effective.

Modeling techniques are frequently used to teach appropriate use of behaviors currently in the child's repertoire. For example, social skills may be improved by observing a model interact with others in various social situations. Modeling may also lead to disinhibition of behaviors that the client has come to avoid performing. Finally, modeling may also promote the extinction of fear responses associated with an object or situation toward which the behavior was directed. Much of the early research on modeling was centered around decreasing fear and avoidance behaviors (Masters et al., 1987).

All modeling procedures involve exposing the individual to one or more individuals, either in vivo or imaginal, who demonstrate behaviors that the client desires to learn (Masters et al., 1987). Modeling procedures also allow patients to become familiar with antecedents and consequences associated with the desired behavior. In all cases the therapist provides feedback to the client after his or her performance.

Child behavior therapists have developed variations of the basic modeling procedure and have implemented them as therapeutic interventions. In general, most procedures can be reduced to a form of "simple modeling" (observation of a model), "participant modeling" (enactment of the desired behavior during the modeling procedure), or "covert modeling" (imaginal modeling).

"Graduated modeling," "guided modeling," and "guided modeling with reinforcement" are all variants of the simple modeling procedure in which the child first views the model perform a behavior and then practices the behavior while receiving feedback from the model. This approach is typically used to teach new skills or improve existing behaviors.

A frequently used type of modeling procedure is graduated modeling. In this procedure the therapist provides the client with a systematic, graduated presentation of increasingly difficult behaviors and/or situations. Other modeling programs, such as contact desensitization, are well suited to treat individuals with maladaptive fear responses and avoidant behaviors. In contact desensitization, as in other participant modeling procedures, the client's response may be physically guided by the therapist. For example, to treat a child with a dog phobia the therapist may first allow the child to observe a model petting a dog. This is followed by placing the child's hand on the model's hand and gradually moving the child's hand onto the dog. This procedure is commonly used to reduce fear, anxiety, and avoidance behaviors.

In covert modeling the therapist uses a procedure in which the client imagines a model (the client or a contrived model) performing the target behavior. For example, the dog phobic can be asked to imagine that he or she is petting a dog. The therapist instructs the child to imagine performing specific behaviors that are components of adequate coping (Masters et al., 1987). Research shows that this procedure is more effective when the imagined model is close to the child in age, gender, and other physical characteristics (Kazdin, 1974).

Within each modeling procedure a distinction has been made between mastery models and coping models. Coping models depict a model experiencing difficulties with a specific task. The model exhibits a number of coping behaviors and eventually successfully handles the situation. Mastery models display immediate mastery of the situation. There is some evidence that coping model procedures may be more effective than mastery model techniques (e.g., Cunningham, Davis, Bremner, Dunn, & Rzasa, 1993; Kazdin, 1973; Meichenbaum, 1972).

Faust, Olson, and Rodriguez (1991) explored efficacy of a participant modeling procedure in reducing presurgery arousal and distress in pediatric patients. One hour before surgery, participating children were exposed to one of three surgery preparatory conditions: participant modeling, participant modeling accompanied by the presence of the child's mother, and standard hospital presurgery procedures. Partici-

pants exposed to the participant modeling conditions with their mothers either present or absent viewed a 10-minute slide-tape presentation showing a 5-year-old female model undergoing surgery procedures. Both procedural and sensory information were presented through the model. The model also displayed appropriate anxiety accompanied by relevant coping skills (e.g., breathing deeply, imagining floating on a cloud), and encouraged children to practice these skills during the presentation. Children assigned to the control group were exposed to standard presurgery procedures such as surgical information provision and exposure to a mock surgery exhibit. Children also saw and manipulated operating room equipment. Results revealed that relative to children assigned to the control condition and participant modeling with mothers present condition, children exposed to the participant modeling procedures without their mothers had significant reductions in physiological arousal after the presentation. Overall, participant modeling procedures were more effective in relieving distress and arousal than the control procedures. Other participant modeling procedures using videotaped material have demonstrated that this procedure may be especially effective if the child watches her- or himself on video after all maladaptive behaviors are removed via editing (Woltersdorf, 1992).

Child behavior therapists have utilized modeling procedures to treat a wide range of child behavior problems. However, the majority of literature on modeling demonstrates its efficacy in treating children's fears and phobias (see Barrios & O'Dell, 1989; Erfanian & Miltenberger, 1990; Glasscock & MacLean, 1990; Hamilton, 1994; Kearney & Silverman, 1990; Love, Matson, & West, 1990) and social skills training (e.g., Loveland & Tunali, 1991; Matson, Foe, Coe, & Smith, 1991). Recently, modeling procedures have been used to treat childhood behavior problems such as learning and speech disabilities (Holdgrafer, 1994; Lonnecker, Brady, & McPherson, 1994), developmental delays (Biederman, Davey, Ryder, & Franchi, 1994; Summers, Rincover, & Feldman, 1993), anger management (Marion, 1994), aggression (Vidyasagar & Michra, 1993), elective mutism (Holmbeck & Lavigne, 1992), and encopresis (Akande, 1993).

Positive Reinforcement

As previously mentioned, application of behavioral methods in child behavior therapy is a direct result of Skinner's work regarding operant conditioning. Skinner identified those behaviors of an organism that act to modify, shape, or create the surrounding environment as operants. He labeled them as such because he said that they operated on the environment. Operant procedures involve identifying environmental factors that act to sustain target behaviors and then systematically arranging the antecedents and consequences of the behaviors to change the probability of their occurrence.

Reinforcement procedures involve delivering a reinforcing stimulus to the child after he or she exhibits a desired behavior. For this method to be successful the therapist must first identify appropriate reinforcers. Although observing the youngster in the natural environment is the optimum method of identifying potential reinforcers, this procedure is very time consuming. In practice, therapists usually enlist parents or teachers to provide insight into appropriate reinforcers.

Researchers have determined that several variables influence the effectiveness of interventions using positive reinforcement methods. Generally, to maximize its effectiveness a reinforcer should be delivered immediately after the desired response. It has also been noted that with increased amounts of the reinforcer, behaviors are performed with greater frequency. However, this relationship is not linear as the delivery of large amounts of a specified reinforcer may satiate the individual, lessening the reinforcing value of the stimulus. Another factor related to the effectiveness of an operant treatment plan is the schedule of reinforcement. It has been noted (Skinner, 1953) that when initially training an individual a continuous schedule in which an instance of a target behavior results in the delivery of a reinforcing stimulus immediately delivered after each desired response works best. However, after the response has been established it is best maintained by using an intermittent reinforcement schedule. Research has shown that in the most effective treatment regimen therapists provide small reinforcers delivered frequently and immediately after the desired response (Kazdin, 1989).

Child behavior therapists may utilize one or more variants of positive reinforcement methods with their patients. Instead of providing the child with such primary reinforcers as food or treats, the therapist may provide secondary reinforcers such as verbal praise, hugs, smiles, or money.

Use of positive reinforcement techniques with children is easiest when the target response is in the child's response repertoire. When a child must learn a new behavior, shaping is used. In the shaping procedure the child is first observed to determine if he or she can perform any response that is topographically similar to the target response. The next step, through a process called successive approximation, is to reinforce responses that gradually bear more and more resemblance to the desired response. Despite the fact that shaping procedures have been used frequently, there is little research to guide child behavior therapists about the optimal speed at which to progress through a shaping procedure. Researchers have recommended that an 80 to 100% reinforcements-to-attempts ratio be met prior to changing the performance criteria (Ollendick & Cerny, 1981).

Much research has examined the efficacy and utility of positive reinforcement techniques with various child psychopathology populations (see Garfield & Bergin, 1986; Masters et al., 1987). In sum, results of these investigations provide wide support for the application of this technique across time, settings, and behaviors. For example, Hagopian and Slifer (1993) treated a 6-year-old girl with Separation Anxiety Disorder using graduated exposure and positive reinforcement for approximations of independent school attendance. While the mother's proximity and time spent at school increasingly faded out, the child's responses were systematically shaped to increase the duration of school attendance. Shaping occurred by providing a sticker to the child after school each time she remained in her seat while her mother was out of the room. These stickers could be exchanged for prizes at the end of each week. Results showed that the child became increasingly able to tolerate being separated from her mother. Follow-up indicated that the treatment gains were maintained at 2 and 9 months posttreatment.

Aversive Techniques

Behavior therapists typically resist using aversive techniques unless all other possible remedies have been exhausted. Several reasons exist for this hesitance. Aversive procedures may be associated with side effects. Clients may experience emotional reactions such as crying and fear. These reactions may lead the individual to attempt to escape from the aversive situation or even aggress against those implementing the procedure. Another criticism of the use of punishment is that when used alone it does not allow the client to develop new more adaptive responses in place of less adaptive ones. In fact, it has been shown that use of these procedures may increase the very behaviors to be ameliorated (Kazdin, 1989). In addition, it may be argued that through modeling clients will learn, and possibly perform, those aversive procedures used to modify their own behaviors. Fortunately, undesirable side effects can be avoided through implementing a treatment program that combines positive reinforcement and aversive methods.

Behavior therapists have developed several types of punishment procedures based on either the concepts of presenting an aversive stimulus or removing positive consequences after

the performance of an inappropriate behavior. Electric shock, squirts of lemon juice, loud noises, and aversive physical stimulation are all examples of stimuli that have been used as aversive consequences. These aversive events are primarily used in circumstances in which the client engages in behavior that may be dangerous to him- or herself or others. In these situations it is necessary to employ a procedure that offers the possibility of producing dramatically rapid effects.

Numerous child behavior therapists have advocated the use of the Self-Injurious Behavior Inhibiting System (SIBIS). This device emits a controlled small electric shock for the amelioration of severe self-injurious behavior. Attached to the arm or leg, the device emits a well-controlled, completely safe, mild, brief shock equal in intensity to a firm pinch. The shock can be delivered by the use of an automatic blow-detecting helmet or through a remote control device. Research data suggest that this procedure is extremely effective in reducing self-injurious behaviors without producing significant unwanted side effects (Iwata, 1992; Linscheid, Hartel, & Cooley, 1993; Linscheid, Iwata, Ricketts, Williams, & Griffin, 1990; Linscheid, Pejeau, Cohen, & Foote-Lenz, 1994; Ricketts, Gova, & Matese, 1992).

Anderson, Hedden, Justice, and Leslie (1994) reported using the SIBIS to reduce high levels of self-injurious behavior in a child with profound mental retardation. The child, a 10-year-old female, received contingent electric shock via the SIBIS following such undesirable behaviors as punching, slapping, poking her face and ears, biting her hands, scratching herself, head banging, body slamming, and banging extremities against each other or hard surfaces. Instances of self-injurious behavior decreased significantly during the first treatment session and continued to decrease to a near zero level. Results were maintained for 15 months. It was also reported that positive affect increased, negative affect decreased, and adaptive skills improved. No negative side effects were observed.

One widely used form of punishment is overcorrection. In this procedure the youngster is prompted to perform an exaggerated form of the desired behavior following an inappropriate response. Overcorrection is composed of two phases. In the restitution phase the individual makes amends for the exhibited inappropriate behavior. For example, a child who messes up a room during a temper outburst is prompted to clean up the mess. The second component, positive practice, involves the performance of an appropriate alternative response in the target situation. Overcorrection has been used in the treatment of urinary incontinence (Hagopian, Fisher, Piazza, & Wierzbicki, 1993), behavior problems in children with mental retardation (Fisher, Piazza, & Page, 1989; Sisson, Hersen, & Van Hasselt, 1993), and in the elimination of aggressive behavior (Matson, Manikam, & Ladatto, 1990).

Time-out

Time-out involves the removal of all positive reinforcers from a child's environment for a brief time following an instance of undesirable behavior. This is typically accomplished by removing the child from the environment or activity. For example, teachers often place disruptive children in the corner of the classroom for a brief time following a temper outburst. A critical factor in the effectiveness of time-out procedures is the ability to remove all reinforcers from the child's environment. If a child is removed from classroom activities but has access to peer contact, then all reinforcers have not been removed and the undesirable behaviors will not be diminished.

Olson and Roberts (1987) explored treatment alternatives to decrease sibling aggression. In their study 18 pairs of aggressive siblings and their mothers participated in one of three interventions: social skills training, time-out, or a combination of the two treatments. All sibling pairs and their mothers participated in four clinic treatment sessions in which they observed videotaped child models reacting to typical conflict situations, role-played, and obtained parent training. Between treatment sessions all mothers recorded aggressive episodes in the home and consequated such behavior with either discussion, time-out, or a combination of the two. Results showed that time-out training was more effective than social skills training in reducing aggressive behavior. Time-out procedures also have been shown to be an effective intervention for many childhood behavior difficulties, such as stuttering (Ingham, 1993), oppositional child behavior (Roberts, Joe, & Rowe-Halbert, 1992; Roberts & Powers, 1990), sibling aggression in the home (Jones, Sloane, & Roberts, 1992), and conduct disorder (McGuffin, 1991). Therapists agree that the time-out procedure is most easily used with very young children as they can be most easily removed from their environments.

Response Cost

The removal of rewards contingent on occurrence of an undesirable response is called *response cost*. In one form of response cost the children are given rewards that they lose when they perform inappropriate behaviors. Alternatively, on initiation of a treatment program youngsters may be required to deposit a lump sum of money or a few important possessions with a parent and then must forfeit a specified amount for each occurrence of inappropriate behavior. Most frequently, the response cost technique is embedded within a procedure of contingency management in which the individual gains rewards for appropriate behaviors and loses rewards for inappropriate behaviors. Used in this fashion it may assist the youth in making discriminations between appropriate and inappropriate behaviors. Response cost procedures have been demonstrated to be effective in a number of settings and are included in treatment packages covering the whole range of childhood problems, such as inappropriate finger and clothes sucking (Bradley & Houghton, 1992), ADHD (DuPaul, 1991; DuPaul, Guevremont, & Barkley, 1992; Gordon, Thompson, Cooper, & Ivers, 1991), sleep problems (Piazza & Fisher, 1991), chronic nose picking (Pianta & Hudson, 1990), and noncompliance (Little & Kelley, 1989). It has been found particularly useful in decreasing aggressive and disruptive behavior (Ollendick & Cerny, 1981).

Koles and Jenson (1985) designed a multicomponent treatment strategy for a severely behaviorally disordered 10-year-old boy with a 7-year history of fire setting. The treatment sequence included: positive reinforcement for treatment compliance, response cost for noncompliance (withholding of privileges by parents), social skills training, fire safety education, overt sensitization to the dangers of fire (visiting an intensive care burn unit), and overcorrection for fire setting behavior. This treatment was successful in extinguishing fire setting behaviors at the 1-year follow-up.

Extinction

Extinction is also used to reduce the frequency of unwanted behaviors. Instead of removing a reinforcer or presenting an aversive stimulus following undesirable behavior, no consequences are delivered in response to the target behavior. The aim of this procedure is to purposely withhold any reinforcer that is believed to be maintaining the inappropriate response. This technique is usually part of a behavior management program even if it is not explicitly stated, where one desired behavior is selectively reinforced while other behaviors are ignored.

Several factors may influence the effectiveness of extinction procedures used in contingency management programs. It is important that a child behavior therapist properly identify the reinforcers maintaining maladaptive behavior so that they can be withheld when the behavior is performed. Identification of reinforcers is best accomplished through observation of a child's response as consequences for behavior are systematically altered. Failure to correctly identify reinforcers may draw out the extinction process or even result in strengthening behaviors that are deemed inappropriate.

The schedule of reinforcement on which the maladaptive behavior is rewarded also may determine the efficacy of an extinction procedure. Responses that are continually reinforced are more easily extinguished than responses that are intermittently reinforced. Child behavior therapists should take note of behaviors that are maintained on an intermittent schedule of reinforcement as intermittent reinforcement lengthens the extinction process. During this extended extinction process it is possible that the maladaptive response may be inadvertently reinforced, making the behavior even more resistant to extinction.

Identified reinforcers must be withheld consistently so that extinction may occur. This requires careful control over reinforcers, for, as previously mentioned, any accidental reinforcement may strengthen inappropriate behavior, prolonging the extinction process. Thus, it should be cautioned that when a reinforcer is not easily controlled, extinction is not a feasible treatment option.

Application of extinction procedures quite often results in a significant brief increase in frequency and/or severity of the targeted behavior. Such increased responding is referred to as an *extinction burst*. Continued withholding of reinforcement will result in the elimination of this burst of problem behavior.

Withholding of reinforcement may produce negative emotional responses such as crying, frustration, and aggression (e.g., Rekers & Lovaas, 1974). By using positive reinforcement for appropriate behaviors in conjunction with extinction, one can minimize the probability of negative side effects (Kazdin, 1989).

Another characteristic of the extinction process is "spontaneous recovery," a phenomenon in which behaviors eliminated by extinction reoccur. These behaviors quickly will fade away if

they no longer function to yield favorable consequences. However, if reinforcement follows the
behaviors, they will become increasingly resistant to extinction for maladaptive behavior.

Paisey, Fox, Curran, and Hooper (1991)
treated an 11-year-old girl diagnosed with autism who exhibited severe aggression and tantrum behavior. After numerous attempts using
other methods to decrease the problem behavior, control was established when the girl was reinforced for compliance with task demands in
conjunction with extinction for inappropriate
behavior.

Successful application of extinction has been
demonstrated across a wide range of problem
behaviors, including self-injurious behavior
(Howlin, 1993; Pace, Iwata, Cowdery, & Andres,
1993), aggressive behavior (Egan, Zlomke, &
Bush, 1993), ADHD (Douglas & Parry, 1994),
increased food intake (Singer, Nofer, Benson-
Szekely, & Brooks, 1991), sleep disturbances
(France, 1992; Lawton, France, & Blampied,
1991), fears and phobias (Babbitt & Parrish,
1991; Dykeman, 1989), coprolalia (Earles & Myles, 1994), and incontinence (Hagopian et al.,
1993).

Contingency Management

Contingency management involves use of a
combination of reinforcement, extinction, and
punishment procedures. Problem behaviors are
identified and targeted for change by trained
treatment mediators (e.g., parents, teachers,
peers) who may use any of the above-mentioned
strategies. Contingency contracting is one specific contingency management procedure in
which in a written contract the child and the
parents specify behaviors to be performed and
the consequences they will produce. For example, parents and child might agree in a contract
that studying a certain number of hours a day
will allow the child to watch television after the
studying is completed.

Research suggests that five criteria exist for effectively developing a contingency contract
(Williams & Gross, 1994). Contracts should
specify all reinforcers or privileges the child can
obtain. The contrast should also specify any behaviors required to obtain these reinforcers. It is
important that the contract indicate exactly the
required behaviors so that disagreements between parent and child can be avoided. Punishment contingencies included in the contract
should be clearly noted. "Bonus clauses" should
also be included to provide special rewards for
appropriate behaviors that continue over time.
Finally, the contract should include a statement
describing the conditions under which the contract may be either renegotiated or terminated.
Contingency contracts have been successfully
used in treating numerous behavior disorders
such as weight reduction (Epstein, McKenzie,
Valeski, & Klein, 1994), increasing on-task behaviors (Allen, Howard, Sweeney, & McLaughlin, 1993), nocturnal enuresis (Luciano, Molina, Gomez, & Horruzo, 1993), personal
grooming (Allen & Kramer, 1990), and fears
and phobias (Babbitt & Parrish, 1991; Heard,
Dadds, & Conrad, 1992; Singer, Ambuel, Wade,
& Jaffe, 1992).

In a control group design investigation,
Gross, Sanders, Smith, and Samson (1990) evaluated the effectiveness of a behavioral program
designed to increase orthodontic treatment
compliance. Child participants who required
orthodontic treatment (i.e., wearing headgear)
were assigned to either a contingency management or an attention control condition. Children assigned to the contingency management
condition developed a contingency contract
with their families to earn rewards for wearing
headgear. In general, contracts involved specification of the children's daily performance criteria and the daily reward it would earn, as well as
delineation of a weekly performance goal and
reward. Parents in this condition were asked to
monitor their child's headgear wear. During
subsequent treatment sessions, the effectiveness
of the contingency contract was discussed and
adjustments to the contract were made when

necessary. Children assigned to the attention control condition met with investigators and discussed the importance of complying with the prescribed headgear regimen. Results showed that relative to participants assigned to the attention control group, contingency management participants displayed significantly higher levels of treatment compliance. Additionally, these differences were maintained at the 2-month follow-up.

Parent Training Programs

Several parent training programs have been developed to teach parents skills for managing their child's behavior. In general, parents are taught how to issue commands, deliver feedback, and use reinforcement, extinction, and time-out procedures.

An issue in parent training revolves around the extent to which programs emphasize either training in specific behavior management techniques or, in general, principles of child behavior management. The first approach trains parents to target undesirable behaviors and to apply specific behavioral techniques so as to modify these behaviors. The second approach teaches parents general parenting skills based on behavioral principles and encourages parents to use these skills whenever necessary. Research has shown that although training in basic behavioral principles may not significantly increase parents' understanding of behavior modification strategies, it may increase the likelihood that parents apply these new skills to nontrained situations (Glogower & Sloop, 1976; Koegel, Glahn, & Nieminen, 1978; O'Dell, Flynn, & Benlolo, 1977).

Parent training programs have been devised for many child behavior disorders. In particular, investigators have focused on developing parent training programs for noncompliant children and children with disruptive disorders such as ADHD. One such program has been developed by Russell Barkley and his associates (1981, 1987). Their program focuses on the so-

cial processes in the family thought to be responsible for developing or maintaining noncompliance. The goals of the program are to improve parental management skills and competence in dealing with child behavior problems, increase parental knowledge of the causes of childhood misbehavior, and improve child compliance to commands and rules. Parents learn behavioral principles generally important in child management, but particularly relevant to the management of children with ADHD.

The program begins with a thorough evaluation of the child's behavioral strengths and problems. Evaluation methods include clinical interviews with child and parent, review of parent and teacher-completed behavior rating scales, and direct observation of parent–child interactions. Parent training then begins with a discussion with parents concerning typical causes of child misbehavior, including contributions of child characteristics, situational events (e.g., behavioral consequences), and family stressors. Parents are encouraged to make changes in factors over which they have some control. Next, parents learn how to attend to and appropriately interact with their children. They are also shown techniques to increase the effectiveness of their commands for eliciting compliance. Instructors then teach parents to use a shaping procedure to encourage children to play independently. This is accomplished by teaching parents to give periodic positive attention to a child's independent play in order to gradually increase the duration of such play. At this point a reinforcement system is instituted in which the child's privileges are made contingent on compliance with parental instructions. Parents are also instructed to use a time-out procedure to manage noncompliant behavior. The time-out procedure involves isolating the child in a chair in a quiet corner of the home for a specified time immediately after inappropriate behavior. Finally, parents are encouraged to adapt these methods to manage their children's behavior in public places. Throughout the program homework is assigned that consists of activities or procedures that the parents are to complete at home and then review with their therapist. Outcome data show that children with ADHD very typically improve in their compliance following the implementation of these parent-training procedures. This and similar programs designed by Patterson (1976, 1982) and Forehand and McMahon (1981) have been shown to be effective tools in treating noncompliant children.

Cognitive-Behavioral Treatments

Cognitive-behavioral treatments are interventions based on the assumption that maladaptive cognitive processes lead to maladaptive behaviors and that behavior change results from the alteration of these cognitive processes. Cognitive processes, such as perceptions, self-statements, attributions, expectations, beliefs, and images, serve as targets in cognitive-behavior therapy. Whereas treatments described earlier emphasize the relationship between behavior and environmental consequences, cognitive-based treatments emphasize the relationship between internal cognitive events and human responding.

An important concept in cognitive-behavior therapy is reciprocal determinism, which asserts that environmental factors (stimulus–response relationships) interact reciprocally with personal factors (e.g., cognitions) to produce behavior. Thus, changes in cognitions should result in changes and corresponding behaviors and vice versa. Cognitive-behavioral interventions attempt to modify directly both factors (Braswell & Kendall, 1988; Craighead, Meyers, & Craighead, 1985).

Self-Instructional Training was developed by Donald Meichenbaum (e.g., Meichenbaum & Goodman, 1971). It involves teaching children to use "self-talk" to guide themselves through the performance of an overt behavior or a problem situation. Much of the treatment research on self-instruction training has been performed on impulsive children (Masters et al., 1987). Training procedures begin with the therapist modeling appropriate behaviors while overtly producing self-instruction statements. The child then imitates this behavior as the therapist verbalizes self-instructions corresponding to the child's behavior. The youth performs the desired behavior while vocalizing the self-instructional statements that are being whispered by the therapist. This procedure is repeated until the child is performing the desired behavior and producing the self-instructions covertly. Procedures including instructions, modeling, behavioral rehearsal, prompts, feedback, fading, and reinforcement, as well as actual self-instruction, are involved in this approach (Ollendick & Cerny, 1981).

Several case studies and controlled studies have demonstrated the effectiveness of self-instructional training at decreasing impulsive behavior. However, other investigations have demonstrated limited utility using these procedures in naturalistic settings (Kendall & Braswell, 1982; Meichenbaum & Goodman, 1971). Still other investigations have shown that self-instructional training is most effective when it is used as part of a multicomponent behavior therapy program in which operant procedures are employed (Graziano & Mooney, 1980, 1982; Hagopian, Weist, & Ollendick, 1990; Ollendick, Hagopian, & Huntzinger, 1991). Thus, treatments involving a self-instruction component require further exploration to determine clinical utility.

Problem-Solving Skills Training (PSST)

Spivack and Shure (1982) developed a procedure for developing interpersonal problem-solving skills in children. These programs are based on evidence that children and adolescents with adjustment problems have deficits in various cognitive processes that underlie social behavior. Specific problem-solving skills that have been well studied include alternative solution thinking, means–end thinking, sensitivity to interpersonal problems, consequential thinking, and causal thinking (Spivack, Platt, & Shure, 1976).

Problem-solving skills are developed by training children to use problem-solving steps and self-statements via various games, academic tasks, and real-life situations. Training encourages the children to think about the particular task, problem, or situation, the behaviors that need to be performed, and the alternative courses of action that are available, and then to select a particular solution. As in self-instruction training, the children ask specific questions or make specific self-statements to help themselves develop problem-solving skills (e.g., "What am I supposed to do? What is my plan?"). They are trained to answer these questions when confronted with interpersonal situations in which their behavior is problematic, and to identify and carry out socially appropriate solutions to problems. Thus, the focus of training is teaching the youngster how to think and not what to think.

PSST research suggests that children who perform well on PSST tasks tend to show improvements in behavioral adjustment (Spivack et al., 1976) and that these techniques may be effective in treating antisocial youth (Kazdin, 1991). Other research (e.g., Kazdin, Bass, Siegel, & Thomas, 1989) suggests that although these procedures demonstrate promise, they may not decrease maladaptive behaviors to within normal limits. It has been suggested that in order to receive the most gains from these techniques it may be important to individualize PSST procedures such that each child's most problematic domain of functioning is emphasized (e.g., academic functioning, family conflicts) (Kazdin, 1991).

Whereas these and other cognitive techniques have been emphasized by numerous clinicians, there are some who have raised concerns about the efficacy of cognitive-behavior therapy. A meta-analysis of the effectiveness of cognitive-behavior therapy with children found that changes in cognitive processes and behaviors were not significantly related (Durlak, Fuhrman, & Lampman, 1991). They suggested the need for further work delineating the specific mechanisms of therapeutic change. Other reviews of the literature question the effectiveness of cognitive-behavior therapy with children (Powell & Oei, 1991).

SUMMARY

The techniques and procedures of child behavior therapy have enjoyed wide acceptance as effective treatments for childhood behavior problems. These methods, which developed from principles of classical and operant conditioning, have come to include procedures derived from different conceptual models. However, the field of child behavior therapy remains cohesive as a result of sustained emphasis on empirical investigation and validation of treatment procedures.

Systematic desensitization and flooding are therapies derived from principles of classical conditioning. These treatments have been effectively used with childhood anxiety disorders. Modeling therapies evolved from the principles of observational learning. These methods have been successful in treating behavior problems such as fear and anxiety responses, learning disabilities, and social skills deficits.

Therapies based on operant conditioning principles form the basis of behavior change programs. These include positive reinforcement, punishment, and extinction. Such procedures may be used individually or together in a multi-faceted intervention. Existing research provides overwhelming support for the efficacy of these procedures across a wide range of behavior problems.

Cognitive-behavior therapies, based on the assumption that maladaptive cognitive processes lead to maladaptive behaviors, have been applied in the treatment of various childhood behavior problems. However, more empirical investigation is necessary to determine the mechanism by which cognitive-behavior therapy is effective.

REFERENCES

Akande, A. (1993). Improving toilet use (encopresis) in a nine-year-old male through full cleanliness training and token reinforcement. *Early Child Development and Care, 86,* 123–130.

Allen, L. J., Howard, V. F., Sweeney, W. J., & McLaughlin, T. F. (1993). Use of contingency contracting to increase on-task behavior with primary students. *Psychological Reports, 72,* 905–906.

Allen, S. J., & Kramer, J. J. (1990). Modification of personal hygiene and grooming behaviors with contingency contracting: A brief review and case study. *Psychology in the Schools, 27,* 244–251.

American Psychiatric Association. (1994). *Diagnostic and statistical manual of mental disorders* (4th ed.). Washington, DC: Author.

Anderson, J. E., Hedden, C. E., Justice, M. L., & Leslie, L. H. (1994, May). *The self-injurious behavior inhibiting system: Further clinical evaluation with assessment of corresponding affective and adaptive functioning.* Paper presented at the annual meeting of the Association for Applied Behavior Analysis, Chicago.

Babbitt, R. L., & Parrish, J. M. (1991). Phone phobia, phact or phantasy? An operant approach to a child's disruptive behavior induced by telephone usage. *Journal of Behavior Therapy and Experimental Psychiatry, 22,* 123–129.

Bandura, A. (1965). Influence of models' reinforcement contingencies on the acquisition of imitative responses. *Journal of Personality and Social Psychology, 1,* 589–595.

Bandura, A. (1969). *Principles of behavior modification.* New York: Holt, Rinehart & Winston.

Bandura, A. (1977). *Social learning theory.* Englewood Cliffs, NJ: Prentice–Hall.

Barkley, R. B. (1981). *Hyperactive children: A handbook for diagnosis and treatment.* New York: Guilford Press.

Barkley, R. B. (1987). *Defiant children: A clinician's manual for parent training.* New York: Guilford Press.

Barlow, D. H., & Hersen, M. (1984). *Single case experimental designs* (2nd ed.). Elmsford, NY: Pergamon Press.

Barrios, B. A., & O'Dell, S. L. (1989). Fears and anxieties. In E. J. Mash & R. A. Barkley (Eds.), *Treatment of childhood disorders* (pp. 167–221). New York: Guilford Press.

Biederman, G. B., Davey, V. A., Ryder, C., & Franchi, D. (1994). The negative effects of positive reinforcement in teaching children with developmental delay. *Exceptional Children, 60,* 158–165.

Bradley, L., & Houghton, S. (1992). The reduction of inappropriate sucking behavior in a 7-year-old girl through response-cost and social-reinforcement procedures. *Behaviour Change, 9,* 254–257.

Braswell, L., & Kendall, P. C. (1988). Cognitive-behavioral methods with children. In K. S. Dobson (Ed.), *Handbook of cognitive-behavioral therapies* (pp. 167–213). New York: Guilford Press.

Craighead, W. E., Meyers, A. W., & Craighead, L. W. (1985). A conceptual model for cognitive-behavior therapy with children. *Journal of Abnormal Child Psychology, 13,* 331–342.

Croghan, L. M., & Musante, G. J. (1975). The elimination of a boy's high-building phobia by in vivo desensitization and game playing. *Journal of Behavior Therapy and Experimental Psychiatry, 6,* 87–88.

Cunningham, C. E., Davis, J. R., Bremner, R., Dunn, K. W., & Rzasa, T. (1993). Coping modeling problem solving versus mastery modeling: Effects on adherence, in-session process, and skill acquisition in a residential parent-training program. *Journal of Consulting and Clinical Psychology, 61,* 871–877.

Delgado, S. V., Emde, R. N., & Pope, K. K. (1993). An atypical eating disorder in a two-year-old female. *Bulletin of the Menninger Clinic, 57,* 242–251.

Douglas, V. I., & Parry, P. A. (1994). Effects of reward and nonreward on frustration and attention in attention deficit disorder. *Journal of Abnormal Child Psychology, 22,* 281–302.

DuPaul, G. J. (1991). Attention deficit-hyperactivity disorder: Classroom intervention strategies. *School Psychology International, 12,* 85–94.

DuPaul, G. J., Guevrement, D. C., & Barkley, R. A. (1992). Behavioral treatment of attention-deficit hyperactivity disorder in the classroom: The use of the attention training system. *Behavior Modification, 16,* 204–225.

Durlak, J. A., Fuhrman, T., & Lampman, C. (1991). Effectiveness of cognitive behavior therapy for maladapting children: A meta-analysis. *Psychological Bulletin, 110,* 204–214.

Dykeman, B. (1989). A social-learning perspective of treating test anxious students. *College Student Journal, 23,* 123–125.

Earles, T. L., & Myles, B. S. (1994). Using behavioral interventions to decrease coprolalia in a student with Tourette's syndrome and autism: A case study. *Focus on Autistic Behavior, 8,* 1–10.

Erfanian, N., & Miltenberger, R. S. (1990). Contact desensitization in the treatment of dog phobias in persons who have mental retardation. *Behavioral Residential Treatment, 5,* 55–60.

Egan, P. J., Zlomke, L. C., & Bush, B. R. (1993). Utilizing functional assessment, behavioral consultation and videotape review of treatment to reduce aggression: A case study. *Special Services in the Schools, 7,* 27–37.

Ehrenreich, N. S., & Melton, G. B. (1983). Ethical and legal issues in the treatment of children. In E. Walker & M. Roberts (Eds.), *Handbook of clinical child psychology* (pp. 1285–1305). New York: Wiley.

Eisen, A. R., & Silverman, W. K. (1991). Treatment of an adolescent with bowel movement phobia using self-control therapy. *Journal of Behavior Therapy and Experimental Psychiatry, 22,* 45–51.

Epstein, L. H., McKenzie, S. J., Valeski, A., & Klein, K. R. (1994). Effects of mastery criteria and contingent reinforcement for family-based child weight control. *Addictive Behaviors, 19,* 135–145.

Faust, J., Olson, R., & Rodriguez, H. (1991). Same-day surgery preparation: Reduction of pediatric patient arousal and distress through participant. *Journal of Consulting and Clinical Psychology, 59,* 475–478.

Fisher, W., Piazza, C. C., & Page, T. J. (1989). Assessing independent and interactive effects of behavioral and pharmacologic interventions for a client with dual diagnoses. *Journal of Behavior Therapy and Experimental Psychiatry, 20,* 241–250.

Forehand, R. L., & McMahon, R. J. (1981). *Helping the noncompliant child: A clinician's guide to parent training.* New York: Guilford Press.

France, K. G. (1992). Behavior characteristics and security in sleep disturbed infants treated with extinction. *Journal of Pediatric Psychology, 17,* 467–475.

Friedman, A. G., Campbell, T. A., & Evans, I. M. (1993). Multi-dimensional child behavior therapy in the treatment of medically-related anxiety: A practical illustration. *Journal of Behavior Therapy and Experimental Psychiatry, 24,* 241–247.

Garfield, S. L., & Bergin, A. E. (1986). *Handbook of psychotherapy and behavior change* (3rd ed.). New York: Wiley.

Glasscock, S. E., & MacLean, W. E. (1990). Use of contact desensitization and shaping in the treatment of dog phobia and generalized fear of the outdoors. *Journal of Clinical Child Psychology, 19,* 169–172.

Glogower, F., & Sloop, E. W. (1976). Two strategies of group training of parents as effective behavior modifiers. *Behavior Therapy, 7,* 177–184.

Gordon, M., Thompson, D., Cooper, S., & Ivers, C. L. (1991). Nonmedical treatment of ADHD/hyperactivity: The attention training system. *Journal of School Psychology, 29,* 151–159.

Graham, P., & Rutter, M. (1968). The reliability and validity of the psychiatric assessment of the child. *British Journal of Psychiatry, 114,* 581–592.

Graziano, A. M., & Mooney, K. C. (1980). Family self-control instructions for children's nighttime fear reduction. *Journal of Consulting and Clinical Psychology, 48,* 206–213.

Graziano, A. M., & Mooney, K. C. (1982). Behavioral treatment of 'night fears' in children: Maintenance of improvement at 2½ to 3½-year follow-up. *Journal of Clinical and Child Psychology, 50,* 598–599.

Green, J., & Benjamin, C. (1990). Phobic anxiety and clumsiness in a 10-year-old girl. *Developmental Medicine and Child Neurology, 32,* 1089–1092.

Gross, A. M., & Brigham, T. (1979). Self-delivered consequences vs. desensitization in the treatment of fear of rats. *Journal of Clinical Psychology, 35,* 384–390.

Gross, A. M., Sanders, S., Smith, C., & Samson, G. (1990). Increasing compliance with orthodontic treatment. *Child and Family Behavior Therapy, 12,* 13–23.

Hagopian, L. P., Fisher, W., Piazza, C. C., & Wierzbicki, J. J. (1993). A water-prompting procedure for the treatment of urinary incontinence. *Journal of Applied Behavior Analysis, 26,* 473–474.

Hagopian, L. P., & Slifer, K. J. (1993). Treatment of separation anxiety disorder with graduated exposure and reinforcement targeting school attendance: A controlled case study. *Journal of Anxiety Disorders, 7,* 271–280.

Hagopian, L. P., Weist, M. D., & Ollendick, T. H. (1990). Cognitive-behavioral therapy with an 11-year-old girl fearful of AIDS infection, other diseases, and poisoning: A case study. *Journal of Anxiety Disorders, 4,* 257–265.

Hamilton, B. (1994). A systematic approach to a family and school problem: A case study in separation anxiety disorder. *Family Therapy, 21,* 149–152.

Harris, C. V., & Wiebe, D. J. (1992). An analysis of response prevention and flooding procedures in the treatment of adolescent obsessive compulsive disorder. *Journal of Behavior Therapy and Experimental Psychiatry, 23,* 107–115.

Harris, S. L., & Ferrari, M. (1983). Developmental factors in child behavior therapy. *Behavior Therapy, 14,* 54–72.

Hartmann, D. P., Roper, B. L., & Bradford, D. C. (1979). Some relationships between behavioral and traditional assessment. *Journal of Behavioral Assessment, 1,* 3–21.

Heard, P. M., Dadds, M. R., & Conrad, P. (1992). Assessment and treatment of simple phobias in children: Efficacy on family and marital relationships. *Behaviour Change, 9,* 73–82.

Hersen, M., & Van Hasselt, V. B. (1987). Developments and emerging trends. In M. Hersen & V. B. Van Hasselt (Eds.), *Behavior therapy with children and adolescents. A clinical approach* (pp. 3–28). New York: Wiley.

Holdgrafer, G. (1994). Informativeness, imitation, and language play: Factors in word learning. *Perceptual and Motor Skills, 79,* 251–257.

Holmbeck, G. N., & Lavigne, J. V. (1992). Combining self-modeling and stimulus fading in the treatment of an electively mute child. *Psychotherapy, 29,* 661–667.

Howlin, P. (1993). Behavioural techniques to reduce self-injurious behavior in children with autism. *Acta Paedopsychiatrica International-Journal of Child and Adolescent Psychiatry, 56,* 75–84.

Ingham, J. C. (1993). Current status of stuttering and behavior modification: I. Recent trends in the application of behavior modification in children and adults. *Journal of Fluency Disorders, 18,* 27–55.

Iwata, B. (Chair). (1992, May). *Immediate and long-term effects of the Self-Injurious Behavior Inhibiting System (SIBIS) on self-injury and collateral behaviors.* Symposium conducted at the meeting of the Association for Behavior Analysis, San Francisco.

Jersild, A. T., & Holmes, F. B. (Eds.). (1935). *Children's fears*

(Child Development Monograph, No. 20). Chicago: University of Chicago Press.

Jones, R. N., Sloane, H. N., & Roberts, M. W. (1992). Limitations of "don't" instructional control. *Behavior Therapy, 23*, 131–140.

Kandel, H. J., Ayllon, T., & Rosenbaum, M. S. (1977). Flooding or systematic exposure in the treatment of extreme social withdrawal in children. *Journal of Behavior Therapy and Experimental Psychiatry, 8*, 75–81.

Kanfer, F. H., & Saslow, G. (1965). Behavioral analysis: An alternative to diagnostic classification. *Archives of General Psychiatry, 12*, 529–538.

Kazdin, A. E. (1973). The effect of vicarious reinforcement on attentive behavior in the classroom. *Journal of Applied Behavior Analysis, 6*, 71–78.

Kazdin, A. E. (1974). Covert modeling, model similarity, and reduction of avoidance behavior. *Behavior Therapy, 5*, 325–340.

Kazdin, A. E. (1977). Assessing the clinical or implied importance of behavior change through social validation. *Behavior Modification, 1*, 427–452.

Kazdin, A. E. (1989). *Behavior modification in applied settings* (4th ed.). Pacific Grove, CA: Brooks/Cole.

Kazdin, A. E. (1991). Aggressive behavior and conduct disorder. In T. R. Kratochwill & R. J. Morris (Eds.), *The practice of child therapy* (2nd ed., pp. 174–221). Elmsford, NY: Pergamon Press.

Kazdin, A. E., Bass, D., Siegel, T., & Thomas, C. (1989). Cognitive-behavioral therapy and relationship therapy in the treatment of children referred for antisocial behavior. *Journal of Consulting and Clinical Psychology, 57*, 522–535.

Kearney, C. A., & Silverman, W. K. (1990). A preliminary analysis of a functional model of assessment and treatment for school refusal behavior. *Behavior Modification, 14*, 340–366.

Kellerman, J. (1980). Rapid treatment of nocturnal anxiety in children. *Journal of Behavior Therapy and Experimental Psychiatry, 11*, 9–11.

Kendall, P. C., & Braswell, L. (1982). Cognitive-behavioral self-control therapy for children: A components analysis. *Journal of Consulting and Clinical Psychology, 50*, 672–689.

Kennedy, W. A. (1965). School phobia: Rapid treatment of fifty cases. *Journal of Abnormal Psychology, 70*, 285–290.

King, N. J., Hamilton, D. I., & Ollendick, T. H. (1988). *Children's phobias. A behavioural perspective*. New York: Wiley.

Koegel, R. L., Glahn, T. J., & Nieminen, G. S. (1978). Generalization of parent-training results. *Journal of Applied Behavior Analysis, 11*, 95–109.

Koles, M. R., & Jenson, W. R. (1985). Comprehensive treatment of chronic fire setting in a severely disordered boy. *Journal of Behaviour Therapy and Experimental Psychiatry, 16*, 81–85.

Kolko, D. J. (1984). Paradoxical instruction in the elimination of avoidance behavior in an agoraphobic girl. *Journal of Behavior Therapy and Experimental Psychiatry, 15*, 51–58.

Kratochwill, T. R., & Morris, R. J. (Eds.). (1991). *The practice of child therapy* (2nd ed.). Elmsford, NY: Pergamon Press.

Lang, P. J. (1968). Fear reduction and fear behavior: Problems in treating a construct. In J. M. Shlien (Ed.), *Research in psychotherapy* (Vol. 3, pp. 90–103). Washington, DC: American Psychological Association.

Lang, P. J. (1971). The application of psychophysiological methods to the study of psychotherapy and behavior modification. In A. E. Bergin & S. L. Garfield (Eds.), *Handbook of psychotherapy and behavior change* (pp. 75–125). New York: Wiley.

Lawton, C., France, K. G., & Blampied, N. M. (1991). Treatment of infant sleep disturbances by graduated extinction. *Child and Family Behavior Therapy, 13*, 39–56.

Lazarus, A. A. (1973). Multimodal behavior therapy: Treating the "BASIC ID." *Journal of Nervous and Mental Disease, 156*, 404–411.

Linscheid, T. R., Hartel, F., & Cooley, N. (1993). Are aversive procedures durable? A five year follow-up of three individuals treated with contingent electric shock. *Child and Adolescent Mental Health Care, 3*, 67–76.

Linscheid, T. R., Iwata, B. A., Ricketts, R. W., Williams, D. E., & Griffin, J. D. (1990). Clinical evaluation of the Self-Injurious Behavior Inhibiting System (SIBIS). *Journal of Applied Behavior Analysis, 23*, 53–78.

Linscheid, T. R., Pejeau, C., Cohen, S., & Foote-Lenz, M. (1994). Positive side effects in the treatment of SIB using the Self-Injurious Behavior Inhibiting System (SIBIS): Implications for operant and biochemical explanations of SIB. *Research in Developmental Disabilities, 15*, 81–90.

Little, L. M., & Kelley, M. L. (1989). The efficacy of response cost procedures for reducing children's noncompliance to parental instructions. *Behavior Therapy, 20*, 525–534.

Lonnecker, C., Brady, M. P., & McPherson, R. (1994). Video self-modeling and cooperative classroom behavior in children with learning and behavior problems: Training and generalization effects. *Behavioral Disorders, 20*, 24–34.

Love, S. R., Matson, J. L., & West, D. (1990). Mothers as effective therapists for autistic children's phobias. *Journal of Applied Behavior Analysis, 23*, 379–385.

Loveland, K. A., & Tunali, B. (1991). Social scripts for conversational interactions in autism and Down syndrome. *Journal of Autism and Developmental Disorders, 21*, 177–186.

Luciano, M. C., Molina, F. J., Gomez, I., & Horruzo, J. (1993). Response prevention and contingency management in the treatment of nocturnal enuresis: A report of two cases. *Child and Family Behavior Therapy, 15*, 37–51.

McGrath, T., Tsui, E., Humphries, S., & Yule, W. (1990). Successful treatment of a noise phobia in a nine-year-old girl with systematic desensitization in vivo. *Educational Psychology, 10,* 79–83.

McGuffin, P. W. (1991). The effect of timeout duration on frequency of aggression in hospitalized children with conduct disorders. *Behavioral Residential Treatment, 6,* 279–288.

Madonna, J. M. (1990). An integrated approach to the treatment of a specific phobia in a nine-year-old boy. *Phobia Practice and Research Journal, 3,* 95–106.

Mahoney, M. J., Kazdin, A. E., & Lesswing, E. L. (1974). Behavior modification: Delusion or deliverance. In C. M. Franks & G. T. Wilson (Eds.), *Annual review of behavior therapy and practice* (pp. 11–40). New York: Brunner/Mazel.

Marion, M. (1994). Encouraging the development of responsible anger management in young children. *Early Child Development and Care, 97,* 155–163.

Masters, J. C., Burrish, T. G., Hollon, S. D., & Rimm, D. C. (1987). *Behavior therapy: Techniques and empirical findings* (3rd ed.). New York: Harcourt Brace Jovanovich.

Matson, J. L., Foe, V. E., Coe, D. A., & Smith, D. (1991). A social skills program for developmentally delayed preschoolers. *Journal of Clinical Child Psychology, 20,* 429–433.

Matson, J. L., Manikam, R., & Ladatto, J. (1990). A long-term follow-up of a recreate the scene, DRO, overcorrection, and lemon juice therapy program for severe aggressive biting. *Scandinavian Journal of Behavior Therapy, 19,* 33–38.

Meichenbaum, D. (1972). Examination of model characteristics in reducing avoidance behavior. *Journal of Behavior Therapy and Experimental Psychiatry, 3,* 225–227.

Meichenbaum, D., & Goodman, J. (1971). Training impulsive children to talk to themselves: A means of developing self-control. *Journal of Abnormal Psychology, 77,* 115–126.

Menzies, R. G., & Clarke, J. C. (1993). A comparison of in vivo and vicarious exposure in the treatment of childhood water phobia. *Behaviour Research and Therapy, 31,* 9–15.

Miller, L. C. (1983). Fears and anxieties in children. In C. E. Walker & M. C. Roberts (Eds.), *Handbook of clinical child psychology* (pp. 337–380). New York: Wiley.

Nunnally, J. (1978). *Psychometric theory* (2nd ed.). New York: McGraw–Hill.

O'Dell, S. L., Flynn, J., & Benlolo, L. (1977). A comparison of parent training techniques in child behavior modification. *Journal of Behavior Therapy and Experimental Psychiatry, 8,* 261–268.

O'Leary, S. G., & O'Leary, K. D. (1977). Ethical issues of behavior modification research in schools. *Psychology in the Schools, 14,* 299–307.

Ollendick, T. H., & Cerny, J. A. (1981). *Clinical behavior therapy with children.* New York: Plenum Press.

Ollendick, T. H., Hagopian, L. P., & Huntzinger, R. M. (1991). Cognitive-behavior therapy with nighttime fearful children. *Journal of Behavior Therapy and Experimental Psychiatry, 22,* 113–121.

Ollendick, T. H., Matson, J. L., & Helsel, W. J. (1985). Fears in children and adolescents: Normative data. *Behaviour Research and Therapy, 23,* 465–467.

Olson, R. L., & Roberts, M. W. (1987). Alternative treatments for sibling aggression. *Behavior Therapy, 18,* 243–250.

Pace, G. M., Iwata, B. A., Cowdery, G. E., & Andres, P. J. (1993). Stimulus (instructional) fading during extinction of self-injurious escape behavior. *Journal of Applied Behavior Analysis, 26,* 205–212.

Paisey, T. J., Fox, S., Curran, C., & Hooper, K. (1991). Case study: Reinforcement control of severe aggression exhibited by a child with autism in a family home. *Behavioral Residential Treatment, 6,* 289–302.

Patterson, G. R. (1976). *Living with children: New methods for parents and teachers.* Champaign, IL: Research Press.

Patterson, G. R. (1982). *A social learning approach to family intervention: Vol. 3. Coercive family process.* Eugene, OR: Castalia.

Pavlov, I. P. (1928). *Lectures on conditioned reflexes* (W. H. Gantt, Trans.). New York: International Publishers.

Phillips, D., & Wolpe, S. (1981). Multiple behavioral techniques in severe separation anxiety of a twelve-year-old. *Journal of Behavior Therapy and Experimental Psychiatry, 12,* 329–332.

Pianta, M., & Hudson, A. (1990). A simple response cost procedure to reduce nosepicking by a 7-year-old boy. *Behaviour Change, 7,* 58–61.

Piazza, C. C., & Fisher, W. (1991). A faded bedtime with response cost protocol for treatment of multiple sleep problems in children. *Journal of Applied Behavior Analysis, 24,* 129–140.

Powell, M. B., & Oei, T. P. (1991). Cognitive processes underlying the behavior change in cognitive behavior therapy with childhood disorders: A review of experimental evidence. *Behavioural Psychotherapy, 19,* 247–265.

Rekers, G. A., & Lovaas, O. I. (1974). Behavioral treatment of deviant sex role behaviors in a male child. *Journal of Applied Behavioral Analysis, 7,* 173–190.

Ricketts, R. W., Gova, A. B., & Matese, M. (1992). Case study: Effects of naltrexone and SIBIS on self-injury. *Behavioral Residential Treatment, 2,* 315–326.

Roberts, M. W., Joe, V. C., & Rowe-Hallbert, H. A. (1992). Oppositional child behavior and parental locus of control. *Journal of Clinical Child Psychology, 21,* 170–177.

Roberts, M. W., & Powers, S. W. (1990). Adjusting chair timeout enforcement procedures for oppositional children. *Behavior Therapy, 21,* 257–271.

Saigh, P. A. (1986). In vitro flooding in the treatment of a 6-year-old boy's posttraumatic stress disorder. *Behaviour Research and Therapy, 24,* 685–688.

Saigh, P. A. (1987). In vitro flooding of a childhood posttraumatic stress disorder. *School Psychology Review, 16,* 203–211.

Saigh, P. A. (1989). The use of an in vitro flooding package in the treatment of traumatized adolescents. *Journal of Developmental and Behavioral Pediatrics, 10,* 17–21.

Simon, A., & Ward, L. (1974). Variables influencing the sources, frequency, and intensity of worry in secondary school pupils. *British Journal of Social and Clinical Psychology, 13,* 391–396.

Singer, L. T., Ambuel, B., Wade, S., & Jaffe, A. C. (1992). Cognitive-behavioral treatment of health-impairing food phobias in children. *Journal of the American Academy of Child and Adolescent Psychiatry, 31,* 847–852.

Singer, L. T., Nofer, J. A., Benson-Szekely, L. J., & Brooks, L. J. (1991). Behavioral assessment and management of food refusal in children with cystic fibrosis. *Journal of Developmental and Behavioral Pediatrics, 12,* 115–120.

Sisson, L. A., Hersen, M., & Van Hasselt, V. B. (1993). Improving the performance of youth with dual sensory impairment: Analyses and social validation of procedures to reduce maladaptive responding in vocational and leisure settings. *Behavior Therapy, 24,* 553–571.

Skinner, B. F. (1953). *Science and human behavior.* New York: Free Press.

Spivack, G., Platt, J. J., & Shure, M. B. (1976). *The problem-solving approach to adjustment.* San Francisco: Jossey–Bass.

Spivack, G., & Shure, M. B. (1982). The cognition of social adjustment: Interpersonal cognitive problem solving thinking. In B. B. Lahey & A. E. Kazdin (Eds.), *Advances in clinical child psychology* (Vol. 5, pp. 323–372). New York: Plenum Press.

Stuart, R. B. (1970). Situational versus self-control in the treatment of problematic behaviors. In R. D. Rubin (Ed.), *Advances in behavior therapy* (pp. 183–196). New York: Academic Press.

Sulzer-Azaroff, B., & Mayer, J. R. (1977). *Applying behavior*

analysis procedures with children and youth. New York: Holt.

Summers, J. A., Rincover, A., & Feldman, M. A. (1993). Comparison of extra- and within-stimulus prompting to teach propositional discriminations to preschool children with developmental disabilities. *Journal of Behavioral Education, 3,* 287–299.

Ultee, C. A., Griffioen, D., & Schellekens, J. (1982). The reduction of anxiety in children: A comparison of the effects of 'systematic desensitization in vitro' and 'systematic desensitization in vivo.' *Behaviour Research and Therapy, 20,* 61–67.

Underwood, S. L., & Gross, A. M. (1989). Developmental factors in child behavioral assessment. In M. Hersen (Ed.), *Innovations in child behavior therapy* (pp. 57–77). Berlin: Springer.

Vidyasagar, P., & Michra, H. (1993). Effect of modeling on aggression. *Indian Journal of Clinical Psychology, 20,* 50–52.

Weithorn, L. A. (1980). Competency to render informed treatment decisions: A comparison of certain minors and adults. *Dissertation Abstracts International, 42,* 3449B–3450B.

Williams, M. A., & Gross, A. M. (1994). Behavior therapy. In V. B. Van Hasselt & M. Hersen (Eds.), *Advanced abnormal psychology* (pp. 419–439). New York: Plenum Press.

Wolpe, J. (1958). *Psychotherapy by reciprocal inhibition.* Stanford, CA: Stanford University Press.

Wolpe, J. (1969). *The practice of behavior therapy.* Elmsford, NY: Pergamon Press.

Wolpe, J. (1973). *The practice of behavior therapy.* (2nd ed.) Elmsford, NY: Pergamon Press.

Wolpe, J. (1982). *The practice of behavior therapy* (3rd ed.). Elmsford, NY: Pergamon Press.

Woltersdorf, M. A. (1992). Videotape self-modeling in the treatment of attention-deficit hyperactivity disorder. *Child and Family Behavior Therapy, 14,* 53–78.

25

Child and Adolescent Psychopharmacology

Timothy E. Wilens, Thomas J. Spencer, Jean Frazier, and Joseph Biederman

INTRODUCTION

There is a growing awareness of psychiatric disorders in children and adolescents. Many of the children who display psychopathology may benefit from psychopharmacologic treatment. This chapter reviews potential benefits, risks, and treatment guidelines for psychotropic medications used in children and adolescents.

With the increasing recognition of psychopathology in children and adolescents, the field of pediatric psychopharmacology has grown rapidly beyond the use of stimulants for the treatment of minimal brain dysfunction to include many other psychotropics. The interest in using psychotropics in children and adolescents is not surprising given that from 12 to 22% of U.S. children (7.5 to 14 million children) suffer from mental illness and that many of these children might benefit from psychopharmacologic treatment (Anderson, Williams, McGee, & Silva, 1987; Institute of Medicine, 1990). However, there is a paucity of data-based investigations in children, limiting the scope of knowledge on the use of psychotropics in the treatment of childhood psychopathology. In addition, there is an absence of FDA approval for most psychotropics in the pediatric population, further restricting the application of psychopharmacology to potentially treatable conditions in children and adolescents. It is notable that the lack of FDA approval does not preclude the use of any given psychoactive medication in children, but only denotes that the drug was not studied adequately for the particular condition (FDA, 1982). Although in the practice of medicine clinicians frequently use medications for indications not specifically addressed in FDA

TIMOTHY E. WILENS, THOMAS J. SPENCER, AND JEAN FRAZIER • Pediatric Psychopharmacology Unit, Department of Psychiatry, Massachusetts General Hospital, Boston, Massachusetts 02114; and Harvard Medical School, Cambridge, Massachusetts 02138. JOSEPH BIEDERMAN • Joint Program in Pediatric Psychopharmacology, Massachusetts General Hospital and McLean Hospital, Boston, Massachusetts 02114; and Harvard Medical School, Cambridge, Massachusetts 02138.

Handbook of Child Psychopathology, 3rd edition, edited by Ollendick & Hersen. Plenum Press, New York, 1998.

guidelines, risks and potential benefits should be discussed with the family and documented.

Psychotropics can be highly beneficial, as in adults, but their use is not universally successful. A successful pharmacotherapeutic intervention is a process that encompasses the following guidelines:

1. The use of psychotropics should always follow a careful evaluation of the child and the family, including psychiatric, medical, and social evaluations. Prior to commencing pharmacotherapy, a thorough initial diagnostic hypothesis with careful definition of target symptoms should be determined (Biederman, 1991; Gittelman-Klein, 1980).

2. Pharmacotherapy should be integrated into treatment plans as an adjunct to other therapeutic modalities such as individual psychotherapy, family therapy, educational interventions, behavioral interventions, and careful medical management rather than be given as an alternative to these other interventions or only when these other interventions are not as effective or have failed.

3. If the patient has a psychiatric disorder that may respond to psychotropics, the clinician should decide which medication to use, taking into consideration the age of the child and the severity and nature of the symptomatic picture.

4. The family and the child should be familiarized with the risks and benefits of this intervention, the availability of alternative treatments, and the possible adverse effects. Certain adverse effects can be anticipated based on known pharmacologic properties of the drug (e.g., the somnolent effects of clonidine), whereas others, generally rare, are unexpected (idiosyncratic) and difficult to anticipate. Consent should be obtained from the custodial parent or patient's legal guardian. Realistic expectations of treatment need to be reviewed with the child and family.

5. Treatment should be started at the lowest possible dose with frequent contact to determine efficacy, adverse effects, and compliance issues during the initial phase of treatment.

Dose adjustments, medicine changes, and laboratory monitoring need to be periodically addressed during the treatment. Following a sufficient period of clinical stabilization (i.e., 6–12 months), it is prudent to reevaluate the need for continued psychopharmacologic intervention. When a drug is thought to be either ineffective or inappropriate to the current clinical situation, the agent should be tapered and a trial with another medication considered. Appropriate alternative interventions should be reviewed with the family and initiated.

6. Psychologists, social workers, pediatricians, child psychiatrists, and prescribers should work collaboratively in the pharmacologic management of children.

In this chapter we will be presenting the main psychotropic medications used in children and adolescents. Each section is organized by psychiatric disorders accompanied by the major medications used for treatment. Included with the description of the medications are other indications, mechanism of action, clinical efficacy, dosing, and adverse effect profile.

ATTENTION-DEFICIT/ HYPERACTIVITY DISORDER (ADHD)

ADHD may affect from 5 to 9% of school-age children (Anderson et al., 1987; Bird et al., 1988) and persists into adolescence and into adulthood in approximately 50% of childhood cases (Mannuzza, Klein, Bessler, Malloy, & LaPadula, 1993; Weiss, Stein, Trommer, & Refetoff, 1993). A child with ADHD is characterized by a degree of inattentiveness, impulsivity, and often hyperactivity that is inappropriate for the developmental stage of the affected child (Barkley, 1990; see Table 1A). ADHD symptoms vary between children and may adversely influence all areas of function including academic performance, overall behavior, and social/interpersonal relationships with adults and peers (Barkley, 1990). More recent

Table 1. Pharmacotherapy of Common Disorders[a]

Disorder	Main characteristics	Pharmacotherapy
A. Attention-deficit and disruptive behavioral disorders		
Attention-Deficit/Hyperactivity Disorder (ADHD)	Inattentiveness, impulsivity, hyperactivity 50% may continue to manifest the disorder into adulthood Associated with mood, conduct, and anxiety disorders	Stimulants (70% response; for uncomplicated ADHD; careful in patients with tics) TCAs: desipramine, nortriptyline, imipramine (70% response, second line for nonresponders; first line for patients with ADHD + tics) Clonidine (good for preschoolers, severe hyperactivity, aggression, ADHD + tics; nonresponders); guanfacine (Tenex) —generally used if clonidine too sedating Bupropion (second line for nonresponders) Venlafaxine (Effexor) —third line Combined pharmacotherapy for Tx-resistant or comorbid cases

Conduct Disorder (CD)
Oppositional Defiant Disorder (ODD)
	Persistent and pervasive patterns of aggressive and antisocial behaviors
	Often associated with other disorders such as ADHD and depression
		No specific pharmacotherapy available for core disorder
		Behavioral Tx
		For ADHD (see above), complex combinations (clonidine & stimulants)
		For agitation and aggression
		  Clonidine or Tenex
		  Beta blockers (propranolol)
		  Mood stabilizers (lithium, carbamazepine, valproate)
		  Antipsychotics
		Other Axis I Disorders (ADHD, MDD, Psychosis, Anxiety): treat the underlying disorder

B. Mood disorders		
Major Depressive Disorder (MDD)	Sad or irritable mood and associated vegetative symptoms co-occurring for a period of time Similar to the adult disorders with age-specific associated features	SSRIs: Prozac, Zoloft, Luvox, Paxil TCAs: imipramine, amitriptyline, nortriptyline, desipramine Antidepressants + antipsychotics when psychosis develops Adjunct strategies for Tx refractory: antidepressants + low-dose mood stabilizers, + BZDs, + thyroid + stimulants
Bipolar Disorder Depressed	Same as depression	Mood stabilizers (lithium, carbamazepine [Tegretol], valproate [Depakote]) Combine with MDD Tx Use short-acting SSRIs, Serzone

(continued)

Table 1. (Continued)

Disorder	Main characteristics	Pharmacotherapy
Bipolar Disorder Manic	Pervasive and/or severely irritable/angry mood Elevated or expansive mood More frequent psychotic symptoms in juvenile mania	Mood stabilizers Mood stabilizers + antipsychotics if psychosis develops or severe mood lability For Tx refractory: two mood stabilizers (Li + carbamazepine) Mood stabilizers + high-potency BZDs (Klonopin), mood stabilizer + clonidine
Bipolar Disorder Mixed	Mixed depressed and manic symptoms Chronic course Most common presentation of juvenile Bipolar Disorder Usually very severe clinical picture	Mood stabilizers + antipsychotics Mood stabilizers + antidepressants Mood stabilizers + high-potency BZDs (Klonopin, Ativan, Xanax)
C. Anxiety disorders		
Childhood anxiety disorders Overanxious Disorder Separation Anxiety Panic Disorder	Excessive or unrealistic worry about future events Excessive anxiety on separation from caretakers or familial surroundings Recurrent discrete periods of intense fear (panic attacks) Frequent comorbidity with MDD (50%) and ADHD (30%)	BZDs (Valium, Tranxene, and others) Buspirone (Buspar) For panic, use high potency: Ativan, Klonopin, Xanax SSRIs (Zoloft, Luvox, Prozac, Paxil) TCAs (Effexor, imipramine, nortriptyline) Combined pharmacotherapy for refractory or comorbid patients
Obsessive-Compulsive Disorder	Recurrent, severe, and distressing obsessions and/or compulsions Often associated with Tourette's disorder, ADHD, mood, anxiety disorders	Clomipramine SSRIs (Zoloft, Luvox, Prozac, Paxil) Venlafaxine Adjunctive: high-potency BZDs, TCAs, buspirone Combined pharmacotherapy for Tx-refractory or comorbid patients (MDD, ADHD)
D. Other disorders		
Psychotic disorders	Delusions and hallucinations Loose associations Paranoia often present Often associated with mood disorders	Traditional antipsychotics (risk for tardive dyskinesia) High-potency BZDs for agitation Risperdal, olanzapine, sertrindole For Tx-resistant cases: Clozaril Antipsychotics + mood stabilizers Antipsychotics + beta blockers Antipsychotics + BZDs

Tourette's disorder	Multiple motor and one or more vocal tics Frequently associated with OCD and ADHD	Clonidine or Tenex TCAs (desipramine, imipramine, nortriptyline) Beta blockers Antipsychotics (high potency; Haldol, Orap) Combined pharmacotherapy for Tx-resistant or comorbid cases (+ Klonopin)
Enuresis	Bedwetting	DDAVP (vasopressin) TCA (imipramine)
E. Developmental disorders		

Pervasive Developmental Disorders
Autism
	Qualitative impairment in social interactions, acquisition of language, and motor skills
	Stereotypies and self-stimulating behaviors often present
	It can be global, or in specific or multiple areas
		For repetitive behaviors: clomipramine (Anafranil), SSRIs (Zoloft, Luvox, Prozac, Paxil)
		No specific pharmacotherapy for the core disorder
		Pharmacotherapy of complications
		  Aggression and self-abuse
		    Beta blockers (propranolol)
		    Clonidine
		    High-potency BZDs (Xanax, Klonopin)
		    Mood stabilizers (lithium, valproate)
		    Mixed opiate antagonist (Naltraxene)
		  Antipsychosis
		    Antipsychosis
		  Other Axis I Disorders (ADHD, MDD, Psychosis, Anxiety): treat the underlying disorder as in individuals

aAbbreviations: ADHD, Attention-Deficit/Hyperactivity Disorder; BZDs, benzodiazepines; CD, Conduct Disorder; DDAVP, desmopressin; MDD, Major Depressive Disorder; MR, Mental Retardation; OCD, Obsessive-Compulsive Disorder; SSRIs, selective serotonin reuptake inhibitors; TCAs, tricyclic antidepressants; Tx, treatment.

studies indicate that ADHD commonly co-oc-curs with oppositional-defiant, conduct, depres-sive, and anxiety disorders (Biederman, New-corn, & Sprich, 1991). The pharmacologic management of ADHD relies on the stimulants, antidepressants, and antihypertensives.

Stimulants

The most commonly used stimulants are methylphenidate (Ritalin), dextroampheta-mine (Dexedrine), magnesium pemoline (Cy-lert), and amphetamine compounds (Adderall, Desoxyn) (Table 2A). The mechanism of action of this amphetamine class of medication is the potentiation of norepinephrine and dopamine release presynaptically (Elia et al., 1990). De-spite similarities in their chemical structures, there may be differential responses to the chem-ically distinct available stimulants as each may have a different mode of action. For example, methylphenidate and amphetamines affect dif-ferent regions of the presynaptic catecholamine neuron resulting in release of different dopa-minergic neuronal pools (Elia et al., 1990). Stimulants have been shown to be effective in approximately 70% of patients in diminishing symptoms of ADHD including motoric hyperac-tivity, impulsivity, distraction, and inattention (Barkley, 1990; Klein, 1987; Swanson, McBur-nett, Christian, & Wigal, 1995; Wilens & Bieder-man, 1992). In addition, a recent multisite study has shown that at 2-year follow-up when com-pared with intensive multimodal treatment in-cluding psychotherapy, stimulant medications alone are adequate treatment for ADHD (Jen-sen, Vitiello, Leonard, & Laughren, 1994). Stim-ulants have also been shown to function in a dose-dependent manner in improving child–family interactions, peer relationships, aca-demic performance, and classroom behavior (Klein, 1987; Swanson, Granger, & Kliewer, 1987; Wilens & Biederman, 1992). The benefi-cial effects of stimulants are of a similar quality and magnitude in patients of both genders and across different ages, from preschool years to

adulthood (Wilens & Biederman, 1992). Of in-terest, the positive effects of the stimulant medi-cations in reducing ADHD symptoms are not "paradoxical," as they also affect attention and concentration positively in non-ADHD individ-uals (Rapoport et al., 1978).

Methylphenidate and dextroamphetamine are both short-acting compounds with an onset of action within 30 to 60 minutes and a peak clinical effect usually seen between 1 and 4 hours after administration. Given their rela-tively short behavioral half lives, multiple daily administrations may be required for a consis-tent response. Variably absorbed slow-release preparations, with a peak clinical effect between 1 and 6 hours, are available for methylpheni-date (SR) and dextroamphetamine (spansule) and can sometimes allow for a single dose to be administered in the morning that will last dur-ing the school day (Greenhill & Osman, 1991; Wilens & Biederman, 1992). Another stimulant preparation containing the aspartate and sac-charate preparations of amphetamine and dex-troamphetamine (Adderall) may provide more sustained response but remains untested in chil-dren. Magnesium pemoline is a longer-acting compound with a duration of action that also al-lows for a single daily dose. Typically, these com-pounds have similar efficacy and a rapid onset of action so that clinical response will be evident immediately when a therapeutic dose has been obtained (Pelham et al., 1990).

The starting dose of the short-acting stimu-lants is generally 2.5 to 5 mg/day given in the morning with the dose being titrated upward if necessary every few days by 2.5 to 5 mg in a di-vided dose schedule. Suggested daily doses for the short-acting stimulants are: 0.3–1.5 mg/kg for dextroamphetamine and 1.0–2.0 mg/kg for methylphenidate (Greenhill & Osman, 1991; Wilens & Biederman, 1992). Being longer act-ing, magnesium pemoline is typically given as a single daily dose in the morning at a daily dose ranging from 1 to 3 mg/kg per day (ca. 37.5 to 150 mg/day). The typical starting dose of pemoline is 18.75 mg with increments in dose of 18.75 mg every few days thereafter until desired

Table 2. Common Psychotropics Used in Pediatric Psychiatry

Drug (brand name)	Main indications	Daily dose (in mg/kg)	Common adverse effects
A. Stimulants			
Dextroamphetamine (Dexedrine)	ADHD	0.3–1.5	Insomnia, decreased appetite, weight loss Depression
Methylphenidate (Ritalin)	ADHD + comorbidity/Dev disabilities	0.3–2.0	Increase in heart rate and blood pressure (mild)
Amphetamine compound (Adderall)	Adjunct Tx in refractory depression	0.3–1.5	Possible reduction in growth velocity
	ADHD		Rebound phenomena
			Tics (rare)
			Theoretically as above
Magnesium pemoline (Cylert)	As above	1.0–3.0	Same as above
			Abnormal muscle movements
			Liver toxicity
B. Antidepressants			
Tricyclics (TCA) Imipramine (Tofranil) Desipramine (Norpramine, Pertofrane) Nortriptyline (Pamelor)	MDD, enuresis, ADHD, tic disorder + OCD, anxiety disorders	2.0–5.0 (1.0–3.0 for nortriptyline); dose adjusted according to serum levels (therapeutic window for nortriptyline)	Anticholinergic (dry mouth, constipation, blurred vision); weight loss, cardiovascular (mild increase) diastolic blood pressure and ECG conduction parameters with daily doses > 3.5 mg/kg; Treatment requires serum levels and ECG monitoring
Clomipramine (Anafranil)	OCD	2.0–3.0	No known long-term side effects; withdrawal effects can occur (severe gastrointestinal symptoms, malaise), overdoses can be fatal
Monoamine oxidase-A/B inhibitors (MAOIs) Phenelzine (Nardil) Tranylcypromine (Parnate) Selegiline (Deprenyl)	MDD, atypical depression, ADHD, anxiety disorders	0.5–1.0	Severe dietary restrictions (high-tyramine foods); hypertensive crisis with dietetic transgression or with certain drugs; weight gain; drowsiness; changes in blood pressure; insomnia; liver toxicity (remote)
Selective serotonin reuptake inhibitors (SSRIs) Fluoxetine (Prozac) Sertraline (Zoloft) Paroxetine (Paxil) Fluvoxamine (Luvox)	MDD, OCD, anxiety	0.5–1.0 (10–50 mg) 1.5–3.0 (25–200 mg) 0.25–0.70 (10–50 mg) 1.5–4.5 (25–300 mg)	Insomnia, GI symptoms, agitation, headaches Investigational
Venlafaxine (Effexor)	MDD, OCD, anxiety	1–3 (25–150 mg)	Similar to SSRIs, also nausea, dizziness, elevated diastolic blood pressure
Bupropion (Wellbutrin)	ADHD, MDD	1–6 (37.5–225 mg)	Insomnia, irritability, Drug-induced seizures (at doses > 6 mg/kg), contraindicated in bulimics
Trazodone (Desyrel) Serzone (Nefazodone)	MDD, aggression, insomnia	2–5 (25–300 mg)	Priapism, hypotension, sedation, orthostatic

(continued)

Table 2. (Continued)

Drug (brand name)	Main indications	Daily dose (in mg/kg)	Common adverse effects
C. Antipsychotics			
Phenothiazines			
Low potency	Psychosis	3–6	Anticholinergic (dry mouth, constipation, blurred vision—more common with low-potency agents)
Chlorpromazine, thioridiazine (Thorazine, Mellaril)	Mania As last resource for aggressive behavior, severe agitation, severe insomnia, severe self-abuse		Weight gain (lower risk with molindone) Extrapyramidal reactions (dystonia, rigidity, tremor akathisia; higher risk with high potency)
High potency	Tourette's disorder	0.1–0.5	Drowsiness Risk for tardive dyskinesia with chronic administration
Fluphenazine, perphenazine (Prolixin, Trilafon)			Withdrawal dyskinesia
Butyrophenones			
Haloperidol (Haldol)			
Thioxanthenes		1–3	
I.E Thiothixene (Navane)			
Molindone (indole derivative) (Moban)			
Pimozide (Orap)	Tourette's disorder	0.1–1.5 As above Prolonged QTc withdrawal dyskinesia	
Risperidone (Risperdal)	Psychosis, positive and negative symptoms	85 µg/kg	Low incidence of extrapyramidal adverse effects
Olanzapine (Zyprexa)		(1–6 mg)	
Sertrindole (Serlect)		(5–20 mg)	
Clozapine (Clozaril)	Tx-refractory psychosis	(3–5 mg)	Low incidence of extrapyramidal adverse effects, does not induce dystonia; low risk for Tourette's disorder; granulocytopenia/agranulocytosis (treatment requires constant monitoring of blood count); higher risk of seizures (dose related)

D. Antimanic agents

	Dose	Indications	Side effects
Lithium carbonate (Eskalith, LithoBid) Lithium citrate (Cibalith-S)	10–30 (ca. 200–2100 mg) Dose adjusted with serum levels	Bipolar Disorder, Manic Prophylaxis of Bipolar Disorder MDD, hyperaggressive behavior, adjunct Tx in refractory MDD	Polyuria, polydipsia, tremor, nausea, diarrhea, weight gain, drowsiness, skin abnormalities Possible effects on thyroid and renal functioning with chronic administration, therapy requires monitoring of lithium levels, thyroid and renal tests, lithium toxicity (level <2 mEq/liter) can be life threatening
Carbamazepine (Tegretol)	10–20 (ca. 200–1000 mg); dose adjusted with serum levels	Complex partial seizures, bipolar disorder, adjunct Tx in refractory MDD	Bone marrow suppression (requires baseline and close monitoring of blood counts); dizziness, drowsiness, rashes, nausea; toxicity (uncommon)
Valproic acid (Depakote, Depakene, Depakene Sprinkle)	15–50 (ca. 250–1500 mg); dose adjusted with serum levels	Absence seizures, bipolar disorder, adjunct Tx in refractory MDD	Sedation, nausea, liver toxicity (requires baseline and close monitoring); bone marrow suppression

E. Antianxiety drugs

	Dose	Indications	Side effects
High-potency benzodiazepines Long-acting Clonazepam (Klonopin)	0.01–0.04 (ca. 0.5–4 mg)	Anxiety disorders Adjunct Tx in refractory psychosis	Drowsiness, disinhibition, agitation Confusion Depression Withdrawal reactions
Intermediate-acting Diazepam (Valium) Chlorazepate (Tramxene) Oxazepam (Serax)	0.02–1 (10–60 mg)	Adjunct in mania Severe agitation Tourette's disorder Severe insomnia	Potential risk for abuse and dependence Less risk for rebound and withdrawal reactions
Short-acting Alprazolam (Xanax) Lorazepam (Ativan)	0.02–0.08 (0.5–6mg)	MDD + anxiety akathisia	
Atypical Buspirone (Buspar)	0.2–0.6 (10–60 mg)	As above Adjunct treatment	Drowsiness, disinhibition No cross-tolerance to other benzodiazepines

F. Noradrenergic agents

	Dose	Indications	Side effects
Clonidine (Catapres) Guanfacine (Tenex)	3–10 µg/kg (0.05–0.6 mg) (0.5–4 mg)	Tourette's disorder ADHD Aggression/self-abuse Severe agitation Anxiety disorders Adjunct in mania and schizophrenia Withdrawal syndromes	Sedation (very frequent) Hypotension (rare) Dry mouth Confusion (with high dose) Depression Rebound hypertension Localized irritation with transdermal preparation

(continued)

Table 2. (Continued)

Drug (brand name)	Main indications	Daily dose (in mg/kg)	Common adverse effects
Propranolol (Inderal) (β blocker)	Tourette's disorder ADHD Aggression/self-abuse Severe agitation Akathisia	1–8 (20–240 mg)	Similar to clonidine Higher risk for bradycardia and hypotension (dose dependent) and rebound hypertension Bronchospasm (contraindicated in asthmatics) Rebound hypertension on abrupt withdrawal
G. Antihistamine, anticholinergic			
Diphenhydramine (Benadryl)	Sleep disorders, agitation, acute dystonic reactions	1–4 (25–50 mg); divided doses	Sedation, cognitive impairment, anticholinergic (dry mouth, constipation, blurred vision); delirium (rare)
Benztropine (Cogentin)	Sleep disorders, agitation, extrapyramidal reactions (dystonia, rigidity, tremor akathisia)	43–86 μg/kg (0.5–3 mg); divided doses	Same as diphenhydramine
H. Other agents			
Fenfluramine (Pondimin)	PDD (weight loss)	1–2 (18.75–75 mg)	Anorexia, irritability, drowsiness, weight loss, insomnia (when discontinued)
Naltrexone (Trexan, Rivea)	Self-abuse	1–2 (25–75 mg)	Long-acting opioid antagonist minimal adverse effects Hepatotoxicity (rare)
Desmopressin (DDAVP)	Enuresis	3–10 μg/kg (0.1–0.2 ml)	Headache Nausea

effects occur or side effects preclude further increments. Because of the anorexogenic effects of the stimulants it may be beneficial to administer the medicine during or after meals. There appears to be a positive dose–response relationship for both behavioral and cognitive effects of the stimulants in ADHD children, adolescents, and adults (Klein, 1987). Serum stimulant levels are highly variable and are not suggested for routine management (Patrick, Mueller, Gualtieri, & Breese, 1987). The continuous use of methylphenidate and dextroamphetamine on evenings, weekends, and holidays should be determined individually based on the frequency of impairment in the child's social and familial life.

The most commonly reported short-term side effects associated with the stimulants are appetite suppression, sleep disturbances, dysphoria, irritability, and rebound phenomena (Barkley, McMurray, Edelbrock, & Robbins, 1990; Klein & Bessler, 1992). Sleep disturbances may diminish the daytime effectiveness of these medications, requiring alteration of the timing or amount of medicine or the addition of another medication (e.g., clonidine) to aid sleep (Wilens, Biederman, & Spencer, 1994). Whereas irritability or dysphoria occurring 1 to 2 hours after dosing may indicate excessive dosing, the occurrence of these symptoms toward the end of the effective period may indicate withdrawal symptoms. Rebound phenomena can occur in some children between doses creating an uneven, often disturbing clinical course. Usually the overlapping of doses or the change to longer-acting preparations may help reduce both withdrawal symptoms and rebound phenomena (Wilens & Biederman, 1992).

Other infrequent side effects include headaches, stereotypies, dizziness, irritability, abdominal discomfort, choreoathetosis (pemoline), increased lethargy, and fatigue (Wilens & Biederman, 1992). The only studied adverse cardiovascular effects of stimulants are a mild increase in pulse and blood pressure of unclear clinical significance (Barkley et al., 1990; Greenhill & Osman, 1991; Wilens & Biederman,

1992). Stimulant-associated toxic psychosis has rarely been reported and appears in the context of a rapid rise in dose, very high doses, or a preexisting psychotic disorder (Wilens & Biederman, 1992). Administration of magnesium pemoline has been associated with hypersensitivity reactions including serious hepatotoxicity in which elevations in liver function studies (SGOT, AAT) have been noted after several months to years of treatment (Pratt & Dubois, 1990). Thus, educating the family as to the signs of hepatic dysfunction such as change in urine or feces color or jaundice, as well as periodic baseline and repeat liver function tests, are recommended with the administration of this compound.

Areas of previous concern in the use of stimulants have included tic disorders and seizures. The precipitation or exacerbation of a tic disorder following stimulant administration is of clinical concern. A cautious approach to the treatment of patients with ADHD and tics includes an attempt to use nonstimulant treatments such as clonidine or tricyclic antidepressants before stimulants (see below). In refractory cases, stimulants can be used with close observation for stimulant-induced tic exacerbation (Gadow, Sverd, Sprafkin, Nolan, & Ezor, 1995).

Within the PDR, stimulants are reported to be contraindicated in the presence of a seizure disorder secondary to the theoretical concerns of the lowering of the seizure threshold by stimulants. However, scientific investigations of both absolute seizure rates and electroencephalogram recordings in stimulant-treated children do not support this contention (Wilens & Biederman, 1992). Hence, in children with ADHD and seizure disorders, stimulants can be used conjointly with appropriate anticonvulsant agents.

Height and weight growth impairment are other adverse long-term effects of the stimulants (Gittelman & Mannuzza, 1988; Spencer, Biederman, Wright, & Danon, 1992); however, recent data suggest that there may be an ADHD-related growth delay independent of stimulant treatment (Spencer, Biederman, Harding, et al., 1996). Stimulant-associated suppression of growth in height does not appear to be closely associated with weight loss related to appetite suppression. Although stimulant-associated negative effects on growth velocity may be offset by drug holidays (Gittelman, Landa, Mattes, & Klein, 1988), if severe, they may require switching to an alternative treatment. Careful monitoring of growth is indicated during stimulant therapy and should include baseline assessment and at least biyearly height and weight measurements (Spencer, Biederman, Wilens, & Lapey, 1992). If a decrease in growth velocity is sustained, consideration should be given to a drug holiday or other alternative treatments.

Antihypertensives

The antihypertensive clonidine has been used increasingly for the treatment of ADHD particularly in younger children (ages 3 to 10 years), and in children and adolescents with pronounced hyperactivity and/or aggressivity. Clonidine, a nonspecific α-adrenergic agonist (preferably α_2, inhibitory), has achieved increasing prominence in the treatment of ADHD, tics, and aggression (Table 2F).

Clonidine is an imidazoline derivative with α-adrenergic agonist properties that has been primarily used in the treatment of hypertension. At low doses, it appears to stimulate inhibitory, presynaptic autoreceptors in the central nervous system. Clonidine is a relatively short-acting compound with a plasma half-life ranging from approximately 5.5 hours (in children) to 8.5 hours (in adults) (Hunt, Minderaa, & Cohen, 1985). Daily doses should be titrated and individualized. Usual daily dose ranges from 3 to 10 µg/kg (ca. 0.05 to 0.6 mg) given generally in divided doses, up to four times daily. There is also a transdermal preparation, which is associated with high rates of local dermatitis (Hunt, 1987). Therapy is usually initiated at the lowest manufactured dose of a full, half, or even quarter tablet of 0.1 mg depending on the size of the child (ca. 1 to 2 µg/kg) and increased depending on clinical response and adverse effects (Hunt, 1987). Clonidine has been safely used adjunctly with the stimulants and tricyclic antidepressants (TCAs). Initial dosage can more easily be given in the evening hours or before bedtime because of sedation. The most common short-term adverse effect of clonidine is sedation, which tends to subside with continued treatment (Hunt et al., 1985; Steingard, Biederman, Spencer, Wilens, & Gonzalez, 1993). It can also produce, in some cases, hypotension, dry mouth, depression, confusion, and ECG changes (Chandran, 1994; Hunt et al., 1985). Three cases of sudden death in children receiving clonidine and methylphenidate have been reported, although independent review of the extenuating circumstances suggests a lack of association at this time (Popper, 1995). Clonidine is not known to be associated with long-term serious adverse effects. Abrupt withdrawal of clonidine has been associated with rebound hypertension; thus, slow tapering is advised.

Recently, another antihypertensive medication, guanfacine (Tenex), has been used for ADHD (Table 2F). Guanfacine is an α_2 noradrenergic agonist that has been available as an FDA-approved hypotensive agent for more than two decades. An initial open study in 13 ADHD children has indicated improvement in hyperactivity and attention (Hunt, Arnsten, & Asbell, 1995). Although not well delineated, dosing in school-age children should be started at 0.5 mg/day and gradually increased as necessary to a maximum of 4 mg/day in two or three divided doses. Based on preliminary findings, guanfacine may be longer acting, less sedating, and more effective for attentional problems than clonidine (Hunt et al., 1985, 1995). Like clonidine, the occurrence of hypotension in children treated with guanfacine is not problematic. The most common adverse effects included transient somnolence, headaches, stomachaches, early morning sedation, and enuresis (Hunt et al., 1995).

Antidepressants

After the stimulants, the antidepressants have been the most studied pharmacologic treatment for ADHD (Spencer, Biederman, Wilens, et al., 1996; see Table 2B). The tricyclic antidepressants (TCAs) have generally been considered second-line drugs of choice for ADHD (Spencer, Biederman, Wilens, et al., 1996). Possible advantages of TCAs over stimulants include a longer duration of action allowing once-daily dosing without symptom rebound or insomnia, greater flexibility in dosage, and minimal risk of abuse or dependence. In general, TCAs are superior to placebo, although generally not superior to methylphenidate (Rapoport, Quinn, Bradbard, Riddle, & Brooks, 1974; Rapport, Carlson, Kelly, & Pataki, 1993; Spencer, Biederman, Wilens, et al., 1996). Open and controlled studies have reported beneficial effects of TCAs in children and adolescents with ADHD using daily doses ranging from 0.5 to 5 mg/kg (Spencer, Biederman, Wilens, et al., 1996). In these reports, TCAs were tolerated without clinically significant cardiovascular effects despite relatively high doses (Wilens et al., 1996). Recent reports of sudden death in four children on TCAs (Medical Letter, 1990; Riddle, Geller, & Ryan, 1993) have led to increased caution in the use of these compounds (see below).

Besides TCAs, other antidepressants have been evaluated in the treatment of ADHD. The novel dopaminergic antidepressant bupropion has been reported to be superior to placebo and was well tolerated in the treatment of ADHD children (Casat, Pleasants, & Van Wyck Fleet, 1987; Connors et al., 1996; Simeon, Ferguson, & Van Wyck Fleet, 1986). However, bupropion has been reported to be associated with exacerbation of seizures and tic disorders (Spencer, Biederman, Steingard, & Wilens, 1993). Bupropion should be started at 37.5 mg and slowly titrated upward with beneficial effects for ADHD generally noted at less than 150 mg/day in children. One study has reported that mono-amine oxidase inhibitors are helpful in reducing ADHD symptoms (Zametkin, Rapoport, Murphy, Linnoila, & Ismond, 1985); however, treatment is problematic in children because of potential drug–drug and diet interactions and resultant hypertensive crisis.

When ADHD co-occurs with mood or anxiety disorders, treatment of the comorbid disorder with additional nonstimulants or alternative pharmacotherapy (i.e., antidepressants) may result in improved efficacy and clinical stabilization. The large group of children and adolescents with mental retardation and developmental disorders with prominent ADHD symptoms may also benefit from stimulant treatment (Aman, Marks, Turbott, Wilshier, & Merry, 1991), although the treatment of specific developmental disorders (learning disabilities) is largely remedial and supportive.

OPPOSITIONAL AND CONDUCT DISORDERS

Oppositional and conduct disorders are included among the disruptive behavior disorders. The essential features of oppositional defiant disorder are a recurrent pattern of negativistic, defiant, disobedient, and hostile behavior generally directed toward authority figures. These behaviors are characterized by frequent temper outbursts and arguments, deliberately defying, blaming, and annoying other people (Frick et al., 1993; Loeber, Lahey, & Thomas, 1991). Conduct disorder is a repetitive and persistent pattern of behavior that may include threatening physical harm to other people or animals, involvement in property loss or damage, deceitfulness or manipulation, or serious violations of rules (Frick et al., 1993). Although there is no specific pharmacotherapy for oppositional and conduct disorder, the treatment of specific symptoms (e.g., aggressiveness) and comorbid disorders appears helpful in reducing impairment of these disorders (Werry, 1994).

Among the more commonly used agents for these children and adolescents, TCAs, stimulants, antihypertensives, and mood stabilizers appear helpful (Connor, 1993; Klorman et al., 1989; Puig-Antich, 1982; Werry, 1994; Wilens & Biederman, 1992).

MOOD DISORDERS

The suggested pharmacologic approaches for children and adolescents with depressive disorders are based on available data from adults as well as anecdotal, clinical, and research experience. Juvenile mood disorders are commonly classified as bipolar or nonbipolar based on the presence or absence of mania, and as major (i.e., major depression, bipolar depression) or minor (i.e., dysthymia, cyclothymia) based on their severity (see Table 1B). Mood disorders in children tend to be chronic as compared with the more episodic nature typical of adult mood disorders (Geller, 1994; Kovacs, Akiskal, Gatsonis, & Parrone, 1994; Kovacs, Feinberg, Crouse-Novak, Paulauskas, & Finkelstein, 1984; Ryan et al., 1987). Major depression increases in prevalence with age.

Unipolar Depression

Major depression is estimated to affect 0.3% of preschoolers, 1 to 2% of elementary age children, and 5% of adolescents (Anderson et al., 1987; Kashani & Orvaschel, 1988; Kashani & Sherman, 1989). Gender representation is equal until adolescence when the adult pattern emerges with approximately two-thirds of cases affecting females (Kashani & Sherman, 1989). Depressive disorders commonly co-occur with anxiety, conduct, and substance use disorders in older children and adolescents (Kashani & Sherman, 1989).

Major depression in a child may be apparent from a sad or irritable mood or a persistent loss of interest or pleasure in the child's favorite ac-

tivities. Other associated features of depression in children include school difficulties, school refusal, withdrawal, somatic complaints, negativism, aggression, and antisocial behavior (Kashani & Sherman, 1989). Other indicators of depression include physiologic disturbances such as changes in appetite and weight, abnormal sleep patterns, psychomotor abnormalities, fatigue, and diminished ability to think, as well as feelings of worthlessness or guilt and suicidal preoccupation. Additionally, in children the presence of psychotic symptoms is not infrequent. The depressive disorders should be carefully differentiated from temper tantrums or feeling states such as unhappiness or disappointment that commonly occur during childhood. Although these common events are associated with psychosocial stressors and improve spontaneously after the distress is removed, depressive disorders persist.

Juvenile mood disorders appear to be more refractory to pharmacologic intervention than adult disorders (Ambrosini, Bianchi, Rabinovich, & Elia, 1993). Despite promising antidepressant efficacy of TCAs in open studies, control studies have failed to demonstrate significant improvement versus placebo (Geller et al., 1992; Kutcher et al., 1994; Puig-Antich et al., 1987). More recently, attention has been focused on the use of alternative agents including the selective serotonin reuptake inhibitors (SSRIs) for depression (Apter et al., 1994), particularly with a positive controlled investigation demonstrating efficacy of fluoxetine (Prozac) (Emslie, Kowatch, Costello, Travis, & Pierce, 1995). Antidepressant nonresponders may benefit from treatment strategies that include (1) the use of higher doses of the antidepressant in patients without adverse effects and with a relatively low plasma concentration of the drug, (2) the use of a different class of medication, and (3) combined treatment approaches such as use of two antidepressants of a different class, lithium carbonate, stimulants, thyroid hormone (T_3), and antianxiety medications. There are four main families of antidepressant medications: SSRIs, TCAs, atypical antidepressants such as bupropion and venlafaxine, and mono-amine oxidase inhibitors (MAOIs).

SSRIs

The SSRIs include fluoxetine (Prozac), par-oxetine (Paxil), sertraline (Zoloft), and fluvox-amine (Luvox) (see Table 2B). Because of their pharmacologic profile, these medications have less anticholinergic, sedative, and cardiovascu-lar and adverse effects than the TCAs (Baldes-sarini, 1996). The SSRIs as a group are struc-turally dissimilar. Further, these agents vary in their pharmacokinetics and side effect profiles. Whereas Prozac and its active metabolite have a long half-life of approximately 7 to 9 days, par-oxetine and sertraline have half lives of approx-imately 24 hours (Baldessarini, 1996). Because of its long half-life, missed doses of fluoxetine have less effect on overall clinical stabilization than the other SSRIs. In contrast, in children prone to develop mania, the selection of a short-er-acting SSRI may be preferable.

Dosing varies between agents (see Table 2B). For ease in pediatric dosing, fluoxetine is avail-able in both capsule form (10 and 20 mg) and a liquid preparation (20 mg/5cm^3). Although not well established, the suggested daily doses in pediatric subjects approximate those in adults (Riddle et al., 1992; Simeon, Dinicola, Fer-guson, & Copping, 1990). Treatment generally begins with 5–10 mg of Prozac or Paxil, or 25 mg of Zoloft or Luvox and may be titrated upward to full adult doses in some cases (i.e., 20–30 mg of Prozac or Paxil; 150–200 mg of Zoloft or Luvox).

Common adverse effects of SSRIs include ag-itation, gastrointestinal symptoms, irritability, insomnia, and headaches. Fluvoxamine has the unique profile of sedation and is useful in chil-dren with sleep disorders accompanying their psychiatric condition (Apter et al., 1994). All of the SSRIs, in particular fluoxetine and parox-etine, have been found to potently inhibit he-patic (liver) enzymes and thereby increase se-rum levels of TCAs, antibiotics, antihistamines, and similar compounds. In contrast, sertraline

is less likely than the other SSRIs to interact with other drugs (Preskorn et al., 1994).

TCAs

The TCAs include the tertiary amines am-itriptyline, imipramine, doxepin, and trimipra-mine, and the secondary amines desipramine, nortriptyline, and protriptyline (see Table 2B). Although these agents have similar spectra of action, the inhibitory effects on neurotransmit-ter reuptake, anticholinergic effects, and ad-verse effect profiles differ among the various TCAs. Treatment with a TCA should be initiated with a 10- or 25-mg dose and increased slowly ev-ery 4 to 5 days by 20 to 30%. Subjective adverse effects such as dry mouth or dizziness tend to be unrelated to drug serum levels (Biederman et al., 1989). Children and adolescents are more efficient in metabolizing TCAs compared with adults and, despite higher weight-corrected dosing, children often have lower plasma TCA levels than adults (Wilens, Biederman, Bald-essarini, Puopolo, & Flood, 1992). Typical dose ranges for the TCAs are 2.0 to 5.0 mg/kg (1.0– 3.0 mg/kg for nortriptyline).

Common short-term adverse effects of the TCAs include anticholinergic effects, such as dry mouth, blurred vision, and constipation (Bi-ederman et al., 1989; Preskorn, Weller, Weller, & Glotzbach, 1983) as well as rashes, night-mares, and stomachaches. However, there are no known deleterious effects associated with chronic administration of these drugs. Severe headaches, gastrointestinal symptoms, and vomiting may occur when these drugs are dis-continued abruptly; thus, tapering of these medications is recommended. Because the anti-cholinergic effects of TCAs limit salivary flow, they may promote tooth decay.

Evaluations of short- and long-term effects of therapeutic doses of TCAs on the cardiovascular systems of children have found TCAs to be gen-erally well tolerated with minor ECG changes as-sociated with TCA treatment at low and moder-ate doses (Wilens et al., 1996). Several recent case reports of sudden death in children being treated with desipramine (DMI) have raised renewed concern about the potential cardiotoxic risk associated with TCAs in the pediatric population (Medical Letter, 1990; Riddle et al., 1991). Despite uncertainty and imprecise data, a recent epidemiologic evaluation of this issue (Biederman, Thisted, Greenhill, & Ryan, 1994) suggested that the risk of DMI-associated sudden death may be slightly elevated but not much greater than the baseline risk of sudden death in children not on medication.

Other Antidepressants

There are several other chemically unrelated antidepressants that remain unstudied but may also be used for depression. Venlafaxine possesses both serotonergic and noradrenergic properties and is effective in adult depression (Cunningham et al., 1994) and may prove to be useful in the treatment of juvenile mood disorders with ADHD (Adler, Resnick, Kunz, & Devinsky, 1995). When using venlafaxine, unlike the SSRIs, there is a need to monitor for potential cardiac effects including diastolic hypertension. Adverse effects of Effexor are similar to SSRIs with the addition of nausea, which generally improves within the first week of administration.

Bupropion hydrochloride is a novel antidepressant of the aminoketone class pharmacologically distinct from known antidepressants (see Table 2B). Although bupropion seems to have an indirect dopamine agonist effect, its specific site or mechanism of action remains unknown. Bupropion is rapidly absorbed with peak plasma levels usually achieved after 2 hours, with an average elimination half-life of 14 hours (8–24 hours). The usual dose range is 4.0 to 6.0 mg/kg per day in divided doses. The major side effects in children include irritability, anorexia, and insomnia (Casat et al., 1987). It appears to have a somewhat higher (0.4%) rate of drug-induced seizures relative to other antidepressants, particularly in daily doses higher than 6 mg/kg, or in patients with seizures or bulimia. Serzone (nefazadone) has recently been

reported to be helpful for treatment of refractory or bipolar children with depression (Wilens, Spencer, Biederman, & Schleifer, 1997).

The MAOIs include the hydrazine (phenelzine) and nonhydrazine (tranylcypromine) compounds (see Table 2B). MAOIs can be helpful in the treatment of childhood major depression, and atypical depressive disorders with reverse endogenous features and depressive disorders with prominent anxiety features (Ryan, Puig, et al., 1988). Daily doses should be carefully titrated based on response and adverse effects and range from 0.5 to 1.0 mg/kg (Ryan, Puig, et al., 1988). Major general limitations for the use of MAOIs are the dietetic restrictions of tyramine-containing foods (i.e., most cheeses), pressor amines (i.e., sympathomimetic substances), or drug interactions (i.e., most cold medicines, amphetamines), which can induce a hypertensive crisis. Short-term adverse effects include orthostatic hypotension, weight gain, drowsiness, and dizziness. Concurrent use of SSRIs is contraindicated because of reports of potentially fatal hyperserotonism (*Physician's Desk Reference,* 1994). Because of their adverse effect profile, the MAOIs are generally reserved for highly compliant adolescents refractory to other treatments.

Bipolar Disorder

In children, mania is commonly manifested by an extremely irritable or explosive mood with associated poor psychosocial functioning that is often devastating to the child and family (Carlson & Strober, 1978). In milder conditions, additional symptoms include unmodulated high energy such as overtalkativeness, racing thoughts, diminished length and quality of sleep, or increased goal-directed activity (social, work, school, sexual) (Weller, Weller, & Fristad, 1995). In addition, many bipolar children will manifest poor judgment such as thrill-seeking or reckless activities. Although the juvenile symptom complex of mania should be differentiated from ADHD, conduct disorder, depression, and psychotic disorders, these disorders commonly co-occur with childhood mania (Carlson, Fennig, & Bromet, 1994; Carlson & Kashani, 1988; Wozniak & Biederman, 1995). The clinical course of juvenile mania is frequently chronic and commonly mixed with manic and depressive features co-occurring (Geller, Sun, et al., 1995; McElroy, Strakowski, West, Keck, & McConville, 1997; Wozniak et al., 1995).

For juvenile bipolar disorders, treatment with mood stabilizers (lithium, carbamazepine, valproic acid) remains the treatment of choice (Strober et al., 1995). If there is no response to an adequate trial (in dose and time) of a single agent, or the patient cannot tolerate the drug, subsequent trials are recommended. In manic or mixed presentations (those with psychotic symptoms or those with rapid cycling), additional antipsychotic treatment is recommended. In bipolar disorder with prominent symptoms of depression, combined treatment with a mood stabilizer and an antidepressant may be necessary. The management of bipolar disorder with or without comorbid disorders (depression, ADHD) often requires an aggressive treatment approach combining several therapeutic agents targeted for the various disorders (Carlson, 1990; Wozniak & Biederman, 1996).

Lithium Carbonate

Lithium is a simple solid element that has chemical similarities to sodium, potassium, calcium, and magnesium (see Table 2D). Lithium has diverse cellular actions that alter hormonal, metabolic, and neuronal systems. Proposed theories of lithium's mechanism of action include neurotransmission (i.e., interaction with catecholamine, indolamine, cholinergic, and endorphin systems, inhibition of β-adrenoreceptors), endocrine system (i.e., blocking release of thyroid hormone and the synthesis of testosterone), circadian rhythm (i.e., normalization of altered sleep–wake cycles), and cellular processes (i.e., ionic substitution, inhibition of adenylate cyclase) (Alessi, Naylor, Ghaziuddin, & Zubieta, 1994).

In children, the elimination half-life of lithium is approximately 18 hours, and steady state is reached in 5 to 7 days (Alessi et al., 1994; Vitiello et al., 1988). The pharmacokinetics of lithium in children seem to have the same features as in adults, with a shorter elimination half-life and a higher total clearance (Vitiello et al., 1988). The usual lithium starting dosage ranges from 10 to 30 mg/kg or 150 to 300 mg in divided doses once or twice a day. There is no consensus as to therapeutic serum lithium level in pediatric psychiatry. Based on the adult literature, suggested guidelines include serum levels of 0.8 to 1.5 mEq/liter for acute episodes and levels of 0.6 to 0.8 for maintenance or prophylactic therapy (Alessi et al., 1994; Strober, Morrell, Lampert, & Burroughs, 1990; Weller, Weller, & Fristad, 1986). Children with nonspecific mood lability often respond favorably to lower-dose lithium (i.e., 300 mg twice daily) (Campbell, Perry, & Green, 1984). Slow- or controlled-release lithium carbonate preparations are available. Lithium is also available in a liquid form, lithium citrate, which contains 8 mEq of lithium per 5 ml, equivalent to the amount in 300 mg of lithium carbonate.

Common short-term adverse effects in pediatric groups include gastrointestinal symptoms, polyuria and polydipsia, and central nervous symptoms such as tremor, somnolence, and rarely memory impairment (Alessi et al., 1994). The chronic administration of lithium may be associated with metabolic (decreased calcium metabolism, weight gain), endocrine (decreased thyroid functioning), and possible renal impairment. Although systematic data on cumulative nephrotoxicity are not available for children, data collected over the past 10 years for adults suggest that maintenance lithium therapy does not lead to serious nephrotoxicity (Goodwin & Jamison, 1990). Nevertheless, children should be screened for renal function (BUN, creatinine) and thyroid function before lithium treatment is started and every 6 months thereafter. Particular caution should be exercised when lithium is used in patients with neurologic, renal, and cardiovascular disorders (sinus arrhythmias) (Goodwin & Jamison, 1990). In addition, nonsteroidal, anti-inflammatory agents, certain diuretics, and angiotensin-converting enzyme inhibitors may increase lithium levels and monitoring of serum lithium levels is recommended (Vitiello et al., 1988).

Anticonvulsants

Despite the widespread use of lithium in pediatric psychopharmacology, many children do not respond to or cannot tolerate lithium carbonate (Alessi et al., 1994). Alternative mood-stabilizing agents used in children include the anticonvulsants carbamazepine and valproic acid (Mattes, Rosenberg, & Mays, 1984; McElroy, Keck, Pope, & Hudson, 1992) (see Table 2D). Carbamazepine is a heterocyclic compound structurally related to the TCAs. The plasma half-life after chronic administration is between 13 to 17 hours necessitating at least twice-daily dosing that is best tolerated when administered with meals. The suggested therapeutic plasma concentration is between 4 and 12 μg/ml. Because there is substantial variability in the relationship between dose and plasma level, close plasma level monitoring is recommended. Common short-term side effects in children include dizziness, drowsiness, nausea, vomiting, blurred and double vision. Idiosyncratic reactions such as bone marrow suppression, liver toxicity, and skin disorders (including Stevens–Johnson syndrome) have been reported infrequently. However, given the seriousness of these reactions, close contact with the family as well as careful monitoring of complete blood counts and liver function are warranted initially and during treatment.

Valproic acid is another anticonvulsant whose popularity is growing as a second-line treatment for juvenile bipolar disorder (Carlson, 1990). Valproic acid is primarily metabolized by the liver with a plasma half-life of 8–16 hours and a therapeutic plasma concentration of 50–100 μg/ml. Recommended initial daily doses are 15 mg/kg per day gradually titrated to a maximum of 60 mg/kg per day administered three times a day. Valproic acid autoinduces the hepatic enzymes involved in its catabolism, necessitating frequent upward dose adjustments (Wilder, 1992). Common short-term side effects in children include sedation, nausea, vomiting, anorexia, and thinning of hair. Asymptomatic elevation of SGOT may occur but generally resolves spontaneously. Infrequent idiosyncratic reactions such as bone marrow suppression and liver toxicity have been reported (Murphy, Groover, & Hodge, 1993; Wilder, 1992). Hepatic fatalities have been reported in children under 10 with monotherapy, although these deaths have occurred primarily in children under 2 years of age (Murphy et al., 1993). Hence, monitoring of blood counts and liver function is warranted initially and during treatment. Although not yet tested, Neurontin and Lamictal, two new anticonvulsants used in the treatment of partial seizures, may prove to be useful as mood stabilizers.

ANXIETY DISORDERS

The anxiety disorders encompass a wide range of clinical conditions in which anxiety is the predominant feature (Bernstein & Borchardt, 1991) (see Table 1C). These include predominately childhood disorders such as *separation anxiety disorder,* characterized by excessive and persistent anxiety on separation from caretaker or familiar surroundings. Children may also suffer from *social phobia,* a fear of humiliation in social situations. Also considered within the umbrella of anxiety disorders in childhood are *obsessive-compulsive disorder* (see below), and *posttraumatic stress disorder,* in which there is an objective stressor outside the usual human experience along with the recurrent experiencing of the event and accompanying hypervigilance or dissociation. Children may also present with *panic disorder,* characterized by attacks of excessive fear without precipitating events, and *agoraphobia*, a fear of places with limited escape (i.e., school) in which the child restricts travel or requires a companion, similar to separation anxiety. Because of the avoidance pattern that often results from an anxiety disorder, children may develop *school refusal* or *school phobia*. Childhood anxiety disorders are relatively common disorders that bear striking similarities to the adult anxiety disorders and in many cases persist into adult life (Leonard & Rapoport, 1989).

It has been estimated that in 11- to 15-year-olds, 4% have separation anxiety disorder and 5% have simple phobia (Anderson et al., 1987; Kashani & Orvaschel, 1988). Children with anxiety disorders often have other coexisting emotional factors such as depression as well as behavior problems such as ADHD (Anderson et al., 1987; Bernstein, 1991; Jensen, Shervette, Xenakis, & Richters, 1993).

Although there is little information available regarding the efficacy and toxicology of antianxiety agents in pediatric psychiatry (Bernstein, Garfinkel, & Borchardt, 1990), children and adolescents with anxiety disorders appear to respond to the same pharmacologic approaches as adult patients. The benzodiazepines remain some of the most important agents for anxiety (Biederman, 1987; Graae, Milner, Rizzotto, & Klein, 1994). Other available compounds include antidepressants, sedative antihistamines (i.e., diphenhydramine, hydroxycine, and promethazine), and the novel nonbenzodiazepine antianxiety drug, buspirone. Because of their efficacy, safety profiles, and minimal drug interactions, the benzodiazepines and antihistamines are often utilized to treat poorly diagnosed symptoms of agitation and insomnia.

Benzodiazepines

Benzodiazepines are lipophilic and highly bound to plasma proteins with active metabolites that dominate their course of activity (see Table 2E). The primary site of action of ben-

zodiazepines in the central nervous system is the GABA receptor (Shader & Greenblatt, 1993). The fact that benzodiazepines, barbiturates, and ethanol all have related actions on a common receptor type may explain their pharmacologic synergy and cross-tolerance. Most benzodiazepines (e.g., diazepam and lorazepam) are absorbed at an intermediate rate, with peak plasma levels appearing 1 to 3 hours after ingestion. The benzodiazepines are metabolized more rapidly in children, often necessitating relatively higher weight-corrected dosing in children compared with adults (Coffey, Shader, & Greenblatt, 1983; Popper, 1987). Benzodiazepines and related sedative drugs can produce tolerance (and cross-tolerance with most other benzodiazepines). Likewise, in adults the benzodiazepines may cause dependence (physiologic [addiction] and psychologic [habituation]); however, the development of drug dependence does not appear to be clinically significant in pediatric populations (Roy-Byrne & Cowley, 1991).

In recent years, two high-potency benzodiazepines, alprazolam and clonazepam, have received increasing attention as effective and safe treatment for adult panic disorder with and without agoraphobia (Roy-Byrne & Cowley, 1991; Simeon et al., 1992). These agents may not have similar cross-reactive properties with the traditional benzodiazepines. With recent reports suggesting that children manifest adult-like anxiety disorders such as panic disorder and agoraphobia, the high-potency benzodiazepines have been increasingly utilized (Bernstein et al., 1990; Bernstein, Garfinkel, & Borchardt, 1987; Biederman, 1987; Coffey et al., 1983; Graae et al., 1994). Clonazepam, a long-acting, high-potency benzodiazepine, is given one to three times a day with a total daily dose of 3–4 mg. In contrast, the short/intermediate-acting, high-potency benzodiazepines (alprazolam, lorazepam, and oxazepam) must be given three or four times a day because of the higher risk for rebound and withdrawal reactions (Simeon et al., 1992). For children who disinhibit on a benzodiazepine, the use of an intermediate (e.g., clorazepate)- or longer-acting benzodiazepine may ameliorate this difficult clinical problem.

In general, the clinical toxicity of the benzodiazepines is low. Of interest, clonazepam has been utilized in substantially higher doses (e.g., 10–12 mg/day) in the treatment of pediatric seizure disorders (*Physician's Desk Reference,* 1994) than in current pediatric psychiatry for anxiety disorders (e.g., 1–2 mg/day) (Coffey et al., 1993) (see Table 2E). The most commonly encountered short-term adverse effects are sedation, drowsiness, and decreased mental acuity. In adults, benzodiazepines have been reportedly associated with depressogenic adverse effects (Roy-Byrne & Cowley, 1991). Adverse withdrawal effects can occur, and benzodiazepines should be tapered slowly. Lorazepam and oxazepam do not have active metabolites and do not tend to accumulate in tissue, making them preferable for short-term symptomatic use. When long-term use is anticipated, intermediate- or longer-acting benzodiazepines may be preferable.

Other pharmacologic treatments that may be helpful for either uncomplicated or comorbid anxiety disorders include antidepressants such as TCAs, SSRIs, or serzone as single agents (Bernstein et al., 1990; Birmaher et al., 1994), or in combination with the benzodiazepines (Bernstein et al., 1990). In addition, clonidine may be helpful for the acute management of nonspecific symptoms associated with PTSD (e.g., hyperarousal).

Antidepressants

In controlled studies of adults, the antidepressants have been found to be effective in the treatment of anxiety disorders (Rosenbaum, 1982) (see Table 2B). In contrast, controlled studies of TCAs for childhood anxiety have shown mixed results. For instance, early studies with imipramine have reported efficacy superior to placebo in children with school phobia (Gittelman & Klein, 1971) Most of the available evidence suggests that TCAs and MAOIs have antianxiety properties (Bernstein et al., 1990), and the SSRIs appear to share these benefits (Birmaher et al., 1994). Because of their apparent efficacy, reduced monitoring requirements, and adverse effects, the SSRIs are increasingly utilized over the TCAs as first- or second-line drugs of choice.

OBSESSIVE-COMPULSIVE DISORDER (OCD)

OCD is the best-studied juvenile anxiety disorder (March & Leonard, 1996; Rapoport, Swedo, & Leonard, 1992) (see Table 1C). It is characterized by the following symptoms: persistent ideas or impulses (obsessions) that are intrusive and senseless such as thoughts of having caused violence, becoming contaminated, or severe self-doubting. These thoughts may lead to repetitive, purposeful behaviors (compulsions) such as hand washing, counting, checking, or touching in order to neutralize the obsessive worries. This disorder has been estimated to affect 1 to 2% of the population and is thought to commonly begin in childhood or adolescence (Leonard et al., 1989; Swedo, Leonard, & Rapoport, 1992).

Clomipramine

Clomipramine treatment has been reported to be efficacious in children and adolescents with severe OCD and trichotillomania (Leonard et al., 1989). Clomipramine is thought to be effective in OCD because of its blockade of the reuptake of serotonin in the brain (see Table 2B). However, anticholinergic symptoms such as dry mouth, constipation, and blurred vision are common with this medication and limit its usefulness.

SSRIs

There is also an emerging literature on the efficacy of the SSRIs such as fluoxetine for juvenile OCD (Geller, Biederman, Reed, Spencer, & Wilens, 1995; Riddle et al., 1992) (see Table 2B). Preliminary indications suggest that relatively high doses of the SSRIs may be necessary for adequate treatment of the condition (e.g., Prozac does of 40–80 mg daily). The SSRIs are effective in both pre- and postpubertal onset disorder (Geller, Biederman, et al., 1995). Although comparative data of the SSRIs versus clomipramine are lacking, it appears that SSRIs may have a more advantageous side effect profile than clomipramine (Riddle et al., 1992).

TICS AND TOURETTE'S DISORDER

Tourette's disorder is a childhood-onset neuropsychiatric disorder with a long duration that consists of multiform motor and phonic tics and other behavioral and psychological symptoms (Cohen, 1990; Leckman, Riddle, & Cohen, 1988) (see Table 1D). Affected patients commonly have spontaneous waxing, waning, and symptomatic fluctuation. Tourette's disorder is commonly associated with OCD, ADHD, and anxiety disorders (Coffey, Frazier, & Chen, 1992; Cohen, Bruun, & Leckman, 1988; Leckman, Walkup, Riddle, Towbin, & Cohen, 1987). It is noteworthy that in many cases, the comorbid disorders are the major source of distress and disability rather than the tic disorder. There has been much interest in the overlap with ADHD. Some interesting associations include: (1) ADHD appears earlier in life than tics and (2) the use of stimulants may exacerbate tics. The antipsychotic drugs, particularly haloperidol and pimozide, have traditionally been considered the drugs of choice in Tourette's disorder; however, antipsychotics have limited effects on the frequently associated comorbid disorders of ADHD and OCD (Cohen & Leckman, 1994).

Clonidine

Clonidine has been increasingly utilized as a first-line drug of choice for tics and Tourette's disorder (see Table 2F). Recent studies have shown efficacy for clonidine in many children with Tourette's disorder with or without other comorbid psychopathology (Leckman et al., 1991; Steingard et al., 1993) (see below). The mechanism of action of clonidine's effectiveness remains unknown. Dosing for tics or Tourette's disorder appears similar to those employed for the management of ADHD.

Antipsychotics

Pimozide and haloperidol are generally used in doses of up to 0.3 mg/kg in the treatment of Tourette's patients who fail to respond to more conventional treatments (Shapiro, Shapiro, & Fulop, 1987) (see Table 2C). However, antipsychotics have limited effects on the frequently associated comorbid disorders (ADHD and OCD) and carry a risk for the development of tardive dyskinesia when administered chronically (Campbell & Palij, 1985) (see below). Prolongations of QTc of unclear clinical significance have been reported with pimozide treatment.

Antidepressants

More recently, the TCAs have been found to be effective in some children with this disorder (see Table 2B). There have been promising results in multiple case series (desipramine and nortriptyline) and one controlled study of desipramine for ADHD and tic symptoms in juveniles with tic disorder and Tourette's syndrome (Riddle, Hardin, Cho, Woolston, & Leckman, 1988; Singer et al., 1994; Spencer, Biederman, Kerman, Steingard, & Wilens, 1993). Another report indicates that L-deprenyl, a selective, type B, irreversible MAOI, may be a promising new treatment (Jankovic, 1993). Patients with comorbid OCD may need additional pharmacotherapy with serotonergic blocking drugs such as clomipramine, or the SSRIs.

PSYCHOSIS

Psychosis is generally used to refer to abnormal behaviors of children with impaired reality testing. The diagnosis of psychosis is made when children have the presence of delusions (false implausible beliefs), hallucinations (false perceptions that may be visual, auditory, or tactile), or the presence of a thought disorder including looseness of association, or circumferentiality (see Table 1D). Psychotic disorders in children, as in adults, can be "functional" or "organic." Functional psychotic syndromes include schizophrenia and related disorders and the psychotic forms of unipolar or bipolar mood disorders (Frazier et al., 1996; Geller, 1994; Gordon et al., 1994; Werry, McClellan, & Chard, 1991). Organic psychosis can develop secondary to lesions in the central nervous system as a consequence of medical illnesses, trauma, or drug use, both licit and illicit.

Antipsychotics

The major classes of antipsychotic drugs used clinically are: (1) phenothiazines, which include low-potency compounds (requiring high milligram per day dosages) such as chlorpromazine and thioridazine and high-potency compounds such as trifluoperazine and perphenazine, (2) butyrophenones (haloperidol and pimozide), (3) thioxanthenes (thiothixene), (4) indolone derivatives (molindone), and (5) dibenzazepines (loxapine, clozapine, and others) (Baldessarini, 1985) (see Table 2C). These chemically varied drugs are similar pharmacologically and generally yield comparable benefit when given in equivalent doses and induce a similar variety of adverse effects. In addition, those with low potency (e.g., chlorpromazine and thioridazine) are particularly likely to cause autonomic side effects such as hypotension, tachycardia, and sedation.

Both their in vitro receptor binding properties and their in vivo effects confirm that most antipsychotic drugs in current use block the binding of dopamine at the D_2 receptor. Molindone, although structurally distinct, exhibits many similarities to other neuroleptics including dopamine receptor blockade, antipsychotic effects, and anticholinergic adverse effects. Clozapine, an atypical antipsychotic agent, has a relatively strong antagonistic interaction with central α_1-adrenergic, cholinergic, histaminic (H_1), and serotonergic ($5HT_2$) receptors. Although clozapine exerts only weak antagonism of D_2 dopaminergic transmission, it has a high affinity for D_4 receptors with a greater specificity for mesolimbic and mesocortical tracts. Thus, this compound lacks acute extrapyramidal adverse effects, and can be effective in treating both positive and negative symptoms in treatment-resistant cases or in children who develop tardive dyskinesia (Frazier et al., 1994; Kumra, Frazier, & Jacobsen, 1996). Clozapine has a relatively high incidence of dose-related seizures and agranulocytosis, making weekly white blood counts mandatory (Kumra et al., 1996). Risperidone is a novel antipsychotic medication that combines dopaminergic (D_2) and serotonergic ($5HT_2$) antagonist properties and may have fewer extrapyramidal adverse effects than traditional neuroleptics (Mandoki, 1995). Olanzapine, a thienobenzodiazepine similar to clozapine in its mechanism of action, was most recently approved by the FDA. It is effective in treating both positive and negative symptoms of psychotic illness and is free of the concerning side effects associated with clozapine (Tran, Beasley, Tollefson, & Satterlee, 1994).

Antipsychotics are indicated in the treatment of childhood psychotic disorders. The target symptoms that most commonly respond to antipsychotics are so-called positive symptoms. Positive symptoms include hallucinations, delusions, formal thought disorder (incoherency) and/or catatonic symptoms (stupor, negativism, rigidity, excitement, or posturing), or bizarre affect. In contrast, negative symptoms include affective blunting, poverty of speech and thought, apathy, anhedonia, and poor social functioning and are associated with (1) insidious onset, positive premorbid history, chronic deterioration and (2) atrophy on CAT scan, abnormalities on neuropsychological testing, and poor response or worsening on typical antipsychotics.

The atypical antipsychotics, clozapine and risperidone, appear more effective for negative symptoms (Kumra et al., 1996; Remschmidt, Schulz, & Martin, 1994). Systematic data on the efficacy of risperidone in children are lacking; however, case series indicate that it may be a promising treatment (Mandoki, 1995; Simeon, Carrey, Wiggins, Milin, & Hosenbocus, 1995). Other symptoms amenable to typical antipsychotic treatment include excessive motor activity (agitation), aggressiveness, tics, and stereotypies (Campbell, Anderson, & Green, 1983). Antipsychotic agents should not be used as primary agents for the treatment of anxiety or sedation, conditions for which antianxiety medication can be highly effective.

The usual oral dosage of antipsychotic drugs ranges between 3 and 6 mg/kg per day (100–400 mg) for the low-potency phenothiazines and between 0.1 and 0.5 (up to 1.0) mg/kg per day (0.5–20 mg) for the high-potency phenothiazines, butyrophenones, thioxanthenes, and indolederivatives. For major psychopathology, the upper end of the dose range is often required for clinical stabilization, and patients should be given a trial for at least 6 weeks prior to being considered nonresponsive. As with other psychotropics, the neuroleptics are metabolized 30–40% more efficiently in children than adults (Popper, 1987). The dose of clozapine is 3 to 5 mg/kg 100–500 mg); risperidone, up to 85 μg/kg per day (0.5–6 mg). Although systematic data on efficacy, safety, and dose ranges in children are lacking, the current dose range for olanzapine in adults is from 5 to 20 mg and for sertrindole, 12 to 20 mg daily. Antipsychotic medications have a relatively long half-life and, therefore, generally do not have to be administered more than twice daily. Most antipsychotic preparations are available in either tablet or capsule form. In addition, at least one compound from each class of antipsychotics is available in a liquid concentrate form. Several compounds including chlorpromazine, haloperidol, and fluphenazine are available in an injectable form for intramuscular administration.

Common short-term adverse effects of antipsychotic drugs are drowsiness, increase appetite, and significant weight gain. Anticholinergic effects like dry mouth, nasal congestion, and blurred vision are more commonly seen with the low-potency phenothiazines. Extrapyramidal effects are commonly reported in children and may be severe (Campbell & Palij, 1985). These effects, which include acute dystonia, akathisia (motor restlessness), and parkinsonism (bradykinesia, tremor, facial inexpressiveness), are more commonly seen with the high-potency compounds (phenothiazines, butyrophenones, and thioxanthenes).

As in adults, the long-term administration of antipsychotic drugs in children and adolescents may be associated with tardive dyskinesia (Campbell, Adams, Perry, Spencer, & Overall, 1988). Tardive dyskinesia should be distinguished from the more common, generally benign withdrawal dyskinesia associated with the abrupt cessation of antipsychotic drugs that tends to subside after several months of drug discontinuation (Campbell et al., 1988). One approach to minimize withdrawal reactions is to taper antipsychotic drugs *very* slowly over several months. As in adults, early detection with regular monitoring using the abnormal involuntary movement scale (AIMS) is the only available treatment for tardive dyskinesia.

Atypical Antipsychotics

The atypical neuroleptics, clozapine and risperidone, appear to have less extrapyramidal side effects (Frazier et al., 1994; Kumra et al., 1996; Remschmidt et al., 1994) and a reduced risk of tardive dyskinesia (see Table 2C). In the United States as well as Europe there has been a considerable experience with clozapine in adolescents (Frazier et al., 1994; Kumra et al., 1996; Rapoport, 1994; Remschmidt et al., 1994). Although effective in chronic treatment-resistant schizophrenia as well as affective psychosis, there is a dose-related risk of seizures, and an increased risk of leukopenia and agranulocytosis in adolescents which may be slightly more problematic in the younger age group (Kumra et al., 1996).

Another serious idiosyncratic reaction to neuroleptics is the neuroleptic malignant syndrome, which consists of muscle rigidity, delirium, and autonomic instability (instability of blood pressure, pulse, diaphoresis, and hyperpyrexia) often accompanied by high CPK levels, elevated WBC counts, and, less commonly, rhabdomyolysis (Lazarus, Mann, & Caroff, 1989). As in adults, neuroleptic malignant syndrome is potentially lethal in children and requires careful attention. Preliminary evidence indicates that the presentation in juveniles and adults is similar; however, neuroleptic malignant syndrome is often more difficult to distinguish in pediatric groups from the more benign extrapyramidal effects of the neuroleptics (Levenson, 1985). In addition, neuroleptic malignant syndrome needs to be differentiated from primary CNS pathology, concurrent infection, underlying psychosis, and elevated CPK related to injury or intramuscular injections. In children with suspected neuroleptic malignant syndrome, careful behavioral observation of delirium coupled with frequent vital sign checks and laboratory studies (CBC, CPK, BUN/creatine if indicated) should be serially completed. Treatment of neuroleptic malignant syndrome requires intensive medical surveillance and consists of immediate discontinuation of the antipsychotic, symptomatic treatment, and aggressive treatment of concomitant medical conditions, such as acute renal failure from rhabdomyolysis.

Short-term adverse effects of antipsychotics are managed similarly in children and adults. Excessive sedation can be avoided by using less sedating antipsychotics and managed by prescribing most of the daily dose at night. Drowsiness should not be confused with impaired cognition and can usually be corrected by adjusting the dose and timing of administration. In fact, there is little evidence that antipsychotics adversely affect cognition when used in low doses. Anticholinergic adverse effects can be minimized by choosing a medium- or high-potency compound such as haloperidol or perphenazine. Extrapyramidal reactions can be avoided in most cases by slow titration of the antipsychotic dose. If possible, antiparkinsonian agents (e.g., anticholinergic drugs, antihistamines, amantidine) should be avoided because of the added adverse effects that these drugs may produce. Extrapyramidal reactions can be prevented in many cases by avoiding rapid neuroleptization or the use of high-potency antipsychotics such as haloperidol or fluphenazine. When a child or adolescent on antipsychotics develops an acutely agitated clinical picture with associated inability to sit still and aggressive outbursts, the possibility of akathisia should be rapidly considered in the differential diagnosis. If suspected, the dose of the antipsychotic may need to be lowered. Beta blockers (e.g., propranolol) and the high-potency benzodiazepines have been found helpful in relieving symptoms of antipsychotic-induced akathisia in adults and may help relieve similar symptoms in juveniles (Mattes et al., 1984).

In cases where the psychotic process occurs in the context of a mood disorder, the concomitant use of specific treatments for mood disorders is crucial for clinical stabilization. In cases where the clinical picture of psychosis is associated with severe agitation, the adjunct use of high-potency benzodiazepines such as lorazepam and clonazepam can facilitate the management of the patient and may lead to the use of lower doses of antipsychotics. In recent years, the syndrome of postpsychotic depression has received increasing attention (Geller, Fox, & Fletcher, 1993). Initial trials with antidepressant drugs added to the antipsychotic treatment appear to be promising in relieving psychotic patients of associated depression, thus fostering rehabilitation efforts. Postpsychotic depression should be distinguished from akinesia, which is an adverse extrapyramidal effect that can respond to antiparkinsonian agents.

DEVELOPMENTAL DISORDERS

Developmental disorders may include mental retardation, pervasive developmental disorders (autistic, and autistic-like disorders), and the specific developmental disorders (learning disabilities) (see Table 1E). Although pharmacotherapy is generally not effective in correcting the underlying disorder, medications may reduce aggression and self-injurious or other psychiatric symptoms severely impairing the individual. Beta blockers and clonidine have been increasingly reported to be useful in developmentally disordered patients to control aggression to self and others (Connor, 1993; Kemph, DeVane, Levin, Jarecke, & Miller, 1993; Mattes et al., 1984; Williams, Mehl, Yudofsky, Adams, & Roseman, 1982). Considering the relatively low toxicologic profile of these drugs compared with the antipsychotics, they are the preferred first treatment for the management of these complications (Connor, 1993). Finally, although not adequately investigated in children, beta blockers (propranolol) have been reported to be helpful in adults with ADHD and severe impulsive and dyscontrol symptoms (Ratey et al., 1986; Williams et al., 1982).

Propranolol

Of the beta blockers, propranolol is the most commonly used compound (see Table 2F). Propranolol is a nonselective (it affects both β_1 and β_2 receptors) β-adrenergic antagonist. Propranolol effects are mediated through its ability to block β-adrenergic receptors at multiple sites in the body. It also crosses the blood–brain barrier, and this probably accounts for some of its efficacy in psychiatric disorders but also contributes to concerns regarding potential CNS toxicity. As much as a 20-fold variability in interindividual hepatic elimination can occur. The half-life after chronic administration is about 4 hours (Meltzer, 1987). The dose range used in pediatric disorders requiring propranolol is approximately 20–200 mg/day. Short-term ad-

verse effects of propranolol are usually not serious and generally abate on cessation of drug administration. Nausea, vomiting, constipation, and mild diarrhea have been reported. Psychiatric side effects appear to be relatively infrequent but can occur and include vivid dreams, depression, and hallucinations. Allergic reactions manifested by rash, fever, and purpura are infrequent but have been reported and warrant discontinuation of the drug. Propranolol can cause slowed heart rate and hypotension as well as increased airway resistance and is contraindicated in asthmatic and certain cardiac patients. There are no known long-term effects associated with chronic administration of propranolol. Because abrupt cessation of this drug may be associated with rebound hypertension, gradual tapering is recommended. Propranolol has also received considerable attention for its usefulness in drug-induced akathisia, and anxiety disorders, as well as the aggressive and self-abusive behavior disorders.

Clonidine

In addition to beta blockers, clonidine has been increasingly used in aggressive and developmentally disordered patients to control aggression to self and others (Fankhauser, Karumanchi, German, Yates, & Karumanchi, 1992; Kemph et al., 1993) (see Table 2F). Clonidine, a nonspecific α-adrenergic agonist, has achieved an increasing prominence in pediatric psychopharmacology because of the wide range of indications and relative safety. Coadministration of clonidine and beta blockers should be avoided as adverse interactions have been reported with this combination; however, it is commonly used safely with the stimulants.

Antipsychotics

Antipsychotics have also been traditionally used to control symptoms of agitation, aggression, and self-injurious behaviors that occur in children with developmental disorders including mental retardation, and pervasive developmental disorders (autistic, and autistic-like disorders) (Aman et al., 1991; Campbell, Small, et al., 1984) (see Table 2C). Although efficacious, alternate medications should be initially attempted secondary to the long-term adverse effects of the antipsychotics. Whereas a more sedating phenothiazine (e.g., chlorpromazine, thioridazine) may be beneficial for the more agitated patient (Aman et al., 1991), a more potent phenothiazine (e.g., perphenazine, trifluoperazine) or the butyrophenone haloperidol may be helpful in the withdrawn, inactive child (Campbell & Spencer, 1988).

AUTISM

Autism is a pervasive developmental disorder that adversely affects the child's social, speech and language, cognitive, and emotional development (see Table 1E). Motor stereotypies and self-stimulating behavior such as biting and head banging are often associated with this disorder. Although behavioral modification remains the treatment of choice, pharmacotherapy may help in reducing dangerous (self-injurious, aggressive) or dysfunctional symptoms (hyperactivity, obsession).

SSRIs

The SSRIs (Prozac, Zoloft, Luvox, Paxil) are being used increasingly in the treatment of repetitive behaviors commonly seen in autism or pervasive developmental disorders. These agents are also effective for comorbid anxiety and obsessive-compulsive disorders in these children.

Fenfluramine

Fenfluramine has been evaluated as a possible treatment for the autistic syndrome in part because of the finding that 30 to 40% of autistic patients have elevated blood serotonin levels (see Table 2H) (August, Raz, & Baird, 1985; Campbell, 1988; Ritvo et al., 1986). Fenfluramine is a sympathomimetic amine related to the amphetamines and is utilized in adults as an appetite suppressant. Although fenfluramine has been shown to decrease blood and brain serotonin concentrations in animals and reduce hyperactivity scores in autistic children (Ritvo et al., 1986), studies have been unable to document consistent and clinically meaningful long-term efficacy for fenfluramine in autism. In addition, the adverse effects of irritability, restlessness, and weight loss often limit its usefulness (Realmuto et al., 1986).

Naltrexone

Naltrexone is used for the treatment of self-abuse as a result of findings of alterations in the endogenous endorphin system in these patients (see Table 2H). Naltrexone is a potent, long-acting opioid antagonist with fast onset of action that has been used in the treatment of adults with addiction, children with pervasive developmental disorders, and children with severe self-abusive behavior in daily doses of 1 to 2 mg/kg (Campbell, Anderson, Small, Adams, & Gonzalez, 1993; Ratey, 1991). Although the drug is relatively free of serious adverse effects, there have been rare reports of hepatotoxicity.

ENURESIS

Children with functional enuresis usually respond to nonpharmacologic therapies (e.g., behavior modification, psychotherapy) and these treatments should be considered first (see Table 1D). Although the TCAs have been historically used for enuresis, the synthetic antidiuretic hormone desmopressin (DDAVP) has been shown to be effective and is increasingly utilized in clinical practice, particularly given its lack of serious adverse effects (Aladjem et al., 1982; Birkasova, Birkas, Flynn, & Cort, 1978) (see Table 2H). DDAVP therapy should not be continued indefinitely, as enuresis may remit spontaneously. Daily doses are 0.1–0.2 ml by intranasal spray given at bedtime. Although it effectively suppresses urine production for 7 to 10 hours, it lacks the pressor effects of antidiuretic hormone (Aladjem et al., 1982; Birkasova et al., 1978). Its safety has been established in patients requiring long-term therapy. Imipramine and other TCAs have also been shown to be effective (Rapoport, Mikkelsen, & Zavadil, 1978), although in the majority of cases, bedwetting reappeared after the drug was withdrawn. Antidepressant therapy should not be continued indefinitely, as enuresis may remit spontaneously.

COMBINED PHARMACOTHERAPY

Multiple agents have been increasingly utilized both in clinical practice and in research for the treatment of child and adolescent psychiatric disorders (Connor, Ozbayrak, Kusiak, Caponi, & Melloni, 1997). This need has arisen out of an emerging awareness of the high rates of comorbidity described in clinical and epidemiological studies of juvenile psychiatric disorders (Biederman et al., 1991; Bird et al., 1988; Costello, Edelbrock, Costello, Dulcan, & Burns, 1988). In addition, controlled investigations of single agents have often produced inconclusive findings. The law of parsimony previously dictated a single cause for each symptom complex. This led to the use of large doses of individual agents for a given disorder, often resulting in intolerable adverse effects. In contrast, the use of combined pharmacotherapy may permit more targeted treatment and greater efficacy, often achieved with lower doses and fewer adverse effects (Wilens, Spencer, Biederman, Wozniak, & Connor, 1995).

Enhanced response rates have been reported when traditional agents are combined. For instance, controlled studies combining methylphenidate with desipramine have shown an improved ADHD response without untoward adverse effects (Pataki, Carlson, Kelly, Rapport, & Biancaniello, 1993; Rapport et al., 1993). For children with depression refractory to TCAs, lithium augmentation has been shown to be effective (Ryan, Meyer, Dachille, Mazzie, & Puig-Antich, 1988). Children with comorbid depression and ADHD have been reported to benefit from the coadministration of Prozac and methylphenidate (Gammon & Brown, 1993). Tic disorders have been shown to respond more favorably with the use of clonazepam added to antitic agents (Steingard, Goldberg, Lee, & DeMaso, 1994).

General guidelines to assist in determining the appropriateness of using multiple agents include: (1) significant symptoms partially responding to treatment with single agents; (2) potential synergistic effects of combined pharmacotherapeutics; (3) use of lower doses of multiple agents reducing the adverse effect profile associated with higher doses of single agents; (4) when the diagnosis suggests the need for a particular combination, e.g., psychosis with depression; (5) treatment of adverse effects, e.g., extrapyramidal side effects on neuroleptics; and (6) overlapping treatments when changing medications to avoid clinical deterioration (Wilens et al., 1995). Further systematic study of the use of multiple agents in various psychiatric disorders in children is necessary before specific dosing parameters can be established. Until these data are available, clinicians need to be aware of potential drug–drug interactions and toxicity, as well as understanding compliance issues related to combined drug administration.

CONCLUSIONS

The field of pediatric psychopharmacology continues to expand as more agents are used and systematically tested for a broad spectrum of child psychopathological conditions. Using medications for child psychiatric disorders is an ongoing process. An essential feature in treating child psychiatric disorders is to apply a careful differential diagnostic assessment that assesses psychiatric, social, cognitive, educational, and medical / neurological factors that may contribute to the child's clinical presentation. In addition, the use of pharmacotherapy should be integrated as part of a broader treatment plan generally as an adjunct to psychoeducational-behavioral interventions and careful medical management. In defining the role of pharmacotherapy in the treatment plan, realistic expectations of pharmacotherapeutic interventions, careful definition of target symptoms, and careful assessment of the potential risks and benefits of this type of intervention for psychiatrically disturbed children are major ingredients for a successful pharmacologic intervention. In recent years, increasing diagnostic precision has contributed to the recognition of high rates of comorbidity. As in adult psychiatry, the use of combined pharmacotherapy has proven invaluable for resistant and comorbid conditions. Although systematic study of the use of multiple agents is in its early stages, a large clinical experience has led to the adoption of this practice as an acceptable standard of care.

REFERENCES

Adler, L. A., Resnick, S., Kunz, M., & Devinsky, O. (1995). Open label trial of venlafaxine in adults with attention deficit disorder. *Psychopharmacology Bulletin, 31,* 785–788.

Aladjem, M., Wohl, R., Biochis, H., Orda, S., Lotan, D., & Freedman, S. (1982). Desmopressin in nocturnal enuresis. *Archives of Disease in Childhood, 57,* 137–140.

Alessi, N., Naylor, M., Ghaziuddin, M., & Zubieta, J. (1994). Update on lithium carbonate therapy in children and adolescents. *Journal of the American Academy of Child and Adolescent Psychiatry, 33,* 291–304.

Aman, M. G., Marks, R. E., Turbott, S. H., Wilshier, C. P., & Merry, S. N. (1991). Methylphenidate and thioridazine in the treatment of intellectually subaverage children: Effects on cognitive-motor performance. *Journal of the American Academy of Child and Adolescent Psychiatry, 30,* 816–824.

Ambrosini, P., Bianchi, M., Rabinovich, H., & Elia, J. (1993). Antidepressant treatments in children and adolescents: I. Affective disorders. *Journal of the American Academy of Child and Adolescent Psychiatry, 32,* 1–6.

Anderson, J. C., Williams, S., McGee, R., & Silva, P. A. (1987). DSM-III disorders in preadolescent children: Prevalence in a large sample from the general population. *Archives of General Psychiatry, 44,* 69–76.

Apter, A., Ratzoni, G., King, R., Weizman, A., Iancu, I., Binder, M., & Riddle, M. (1994). Fluvoxamine open-label treatment of adolescent inpatients with obsessive-compulsive disorder or depression. *Journal of the American Academy of Child and Adolescent Psychiatry, 33,* 342–348.

August, G. J., Raz, N., & Baird, T. D. (1985). Effects of fenfluramine on behavioral, cognitive, and affective disturbances in autistic children. *Journal of Autism and Developmental Disorders, 15,* 97–107.

Baldessarini, R. J. (1985). *Chemotherapy in psychiatry.* Cambridge, MA: Harvard University Press.

Baldessarini, R. J. (1996). *Chemotherapy in psychiatry* (2nd ed.). Cambridge, MA: Harvard University Press.

Barkley, R. A. (1990). *Attention deficit hyperactivity disorder: A handbook for diagnosis and treatment.* New York: Guilford Press.

Barkley, R. A., McMurray, M. B., Edelbrock, C. S., & Robbins, K. (1990). Side effects of methylphenidate in children with attention deficit hyperactivity disorder: A systematic, placebo-controlled evaluation. *Pediatrics, 86,* 184–192.

Bernstein, G. A. (1991). Comorbidity and severity of anxiety and depressive disorders in a clinic sample. *Journal of the American Academy of Child and Adolescent Psychiatry, 30,* 43–50.

Bernstein, G. A., & Borchardt, C. M. (1991). Anxiety disorders of childhood and adolescence: A critical review. *Journal of the American Academy of Child and Adolescent Psychiatry, 30,* 519–532.

Bernstein, G. A., Garfinkel, B., & Borchardt, C. (1987). *Imipramine versus alprazolam for school phobia.* Paper presented at the annual meeting of the American Academy of Child and Adolescent Psychiatry, Washington, DC.

Bernstein, G. A., Garfinkel, B. D., & Borchardt, C. M. (1990). Comparative studies of pharmacotherapy for school refusal. *Journal of the American Academy of Child and Adolescent Psychiatry, 29,* 773–781.

Biederman, J. (1987). Clonazepam in the treatment of prepubertal children with panic-like symptoms. *Journal of Clinical Psychiatry, 48*(Suppl.), 38–41.

Biederman, J. (1991). Psychopharmacology in children and adolescents. In J. Wiener (Ed.), *Comprehensive textbook of child and adolescent psychiatry* (pp. 545–570). Washington, DC: American Psychiatric Association.

Biederman, J., Baldessarini, R. J., Wright, V., Knee, D., Harmatz, J., & Goldblatt, A. (1989). A double-blind placebo controlled study of desipramine in the treatment of attention deficit disorder II: Serum drug levels and cardiovascular findings. *Journal of the American Academy of Child and Adolescent Psychiatry, 28*, 903–911.

Biederman, J., Newcorn, J., & Sprich, S. (1991). Comorbidity of attention deficit hyperactivity disorder with conduct, depressive, anxiety, and other disorders. *American Journal of Psychiatry, 148*, 564–577.

Biederman, J., Thisted, R., Greenhill, L., & Ryan, N. (1994). Safety of desipramine in children. *Progress Notes of the American Society of Clinical Psychopharmacology, 2–4.*

Bird, H. R., Canino, G., Rubio-Stipec, M., Gould, M. S., Ribera, J., Sesman, M., Woodbury, M., Huertas-Goldman, S., Pagan, A., Sanchez-Lacay, A., & Moscoso, M. (1988). Estimates of the prevalence of childhood maladjustment in a community survey in Puerto Rico. *Archives of General Psychiatry, 45*, 1120–1126.

Birkasova, M., Birkas, O., Flynn, M. J., & Cort, J. H. (1978). Desmopressin in the management of nocturnal enuresis in children: A double-blind study. *Pediatrics, 62*, 970–974.

Birmaher, B., Waterman, S., Ryan, N., Cully, M., Balach, L., & Ingram, J. (1994). Fluoxetine for childhood anxiety disorders. *Journal of the American Academy of Child and Adolescent Psychiatry, 33*, 993–997.

Campbell, M. (1988). Fenfluramine treatment of autism. *Journal of Child Psychology and Psychiatry and Allied Disciplines, 29*, 1–10.

Campbell, M., Adams, P., Perry, R., Spencer, E. K., & Overall, J. E. (1988). Tardive and withdrawal dyskinesia in autistic children: A prospective study. *Psychopharmacology Bulletin, 24*, 251–255.

Campbell, M., Anderson, L. T., & Green, W. H. (1983). Behavior-disordered and aggressive children: New advances in pharmacotherapy. *Journal of Developmental and Behavioral Pediatrics, 4*, 265–271.

Campbell, M., Anderson, L., Small, A., Adams, P., & Gonzalez, N. (1993). Naltrexone in autistic children: Behavioral symptoms and attentional learning. *Journal of the American Academy of Child and Adolescent Psychiatry, 32*, 1283–1291.

Campbell, M., & Palij, M. (1985). Measurement of side effects including tardive dyskinesia. *Psychopharmacology Bulletin, 21*, 1063–1080.

Campbell, M., Perry, R., & Green, W. H. (1984). Use of lithium in children and adolescents. *Psychosomatics, 25*, 95–101.

Campbell, M., Small, A. M., Green, W. H., Jennings, S. J., Perry, R., Bennett, W. G., & Anderson, L. (1984). Behavioral efficacy of haloperidol and lithium carbonate: A comparison in hospitalized aggressive children with conduct disorder. *Archives of General Psychiatry, 41*, 650–656.

Campbell, M., & Spencer, E. K. (1988). Psychopharmacology in child and adolescent psychiatry: A review of the past five years. *Journal of the American Academy of Child and Adolescent Psychiatry, 27*, 269–279.

Carlson, G. A. (1990). Bipolar disorders in children and adolescents. In B. D. Garfinkel, G. A. Carlson, & E. B. Well-

er (Eds.), *Psychiatric disorders in children and adolescents* (pp. 21–36). Philadelphia: Saunders.

Carlson, G., Fennig, S., & Bromet, E. (1994). The confusion between bipolar disorder and schizophrenia in youth: Where does it stand in the 1990's? *Journal of the American Academy of Child and Adolescent Psychiatry, 33*, 453–460.

Carlson, G. A., & Kashani, J. H. (1988). Manic symptoms in a non-referred adolescent population. *Journal of Affective Disorders, 15*, 219–226.

Carlson, G. A., & Strober, M. (1978). Manic-depressive illness in early adolescence: A study of clinical and diagnostic characteristics in six cases. *Journal of the American Academy of Child and Adolescent Psychiatry, 17*, 138–153.

Casat, C. D., Pleasants, D. Z., & Van Wyck Fleet, J. (1987). A double-blind trial of bupropion in children with attention deficit disorder. *Psychopharmacology Bulletin, 23*, 120–122.

Chandran, K. (1994). ECG and clonidine. *Journal of the American Academy of Child and Adolescent Psychiatry, 33*, 1351–1352.

Coffey, B., Frazier, J., & Chen, S. (1992). Comorbidity, Tourette syndrome, and anxiety disorders. In T. N. Chase, A. J. Friedhoff, & D. J. Cohen (Eds.), *Advances in neurology, Tourette syndrome: Genetics, neurobiology, and treatment* (pp. 95–104). New York: Raven Press.

Coffey, B., Shader, R. I., & Greenblatt, D. J. (1983). Pharmacokinetics of benzodiazepines and psychostimulants in children. *Journal of Clinical Psychopharmacology, 3*, 217–225.

Cohen, D. J. (1990). *Tourette's syndrome: Developmental psychopathology of a model neuropsychiatric disorder of childhood.* Lecture presented at the 27th Annual Institute of Pennsylvania Hospital.

Cohen, D. J., Bruun, R. D., & Leckman, J. F. (Eds.). (1988). *Tourette's syndrome and tic disorders: Clinical understanding and treatment.* New York: Wiley.

Cohen, D., & Leckman, J. (1994). Developmental psychopathology and neurobiology of Tourette's syndrome. *Journal of the American Academy of Child and Adolescent Psychiatry, 33*, 2–15.

Conners, C., Casat, C., Gualtieri, C., Weller, E., Reader, M., Reiss, A., Weller, R., Khayrallah, M., & Ascher, J. (1996). Bupropion hydrochloride in attention deficit disorder with hyperactivity. *Journal of the American Academy of Child and Adolescent Psychiatry, 35*, 1314–1321.

Connor, D. (1993). Beta-blockers for aggression: The pediatric experience. *Journal of Child and Adolescent Psychopharmacology, 3*, 99–114.

Connor, D., Ozbayrak, K. R., Kusiak, K., Caponi, A., & Melloni, R. (1997). Combined pharmacotherapy in children and adolescents in a residential treatment center. *Journal of the American Academy of Child and Adolescent Psychiatry, 36*, 248–254.

Costello, E., Edelbrock, C., Costello, A., Dulcan, M., & Burns, B. (1988). Psychopathology in pediatric primary care: The new hidden morbidity. *Journal of Pediatrics, 82*, 415–424.

Cunningham, L., Borison, R., Carmen, J., Chouinard, G., Crowder, J., Diamond, B., Fischer, D., & Hearst, E. (1994). A comparison of venlafaxine, trazodone, and placebo in major depression. *Journal of Clinical Psychopharmacology, 14,* 99–106.

Elia, J., Borcherding, B. G., Potter, W. Z., Mefford, I. N., Rapoport, J. L., & Keysor, C. S. (1990). Stimulant drug treatment of hyperactivity: Biochemical correlates. *Clinical Pharmacology and Therapeutics, 48,* 57–66.

Emslie, G., Kowatch, R., Costello, L., Travis, G., & Pierce, L. (1995). Double-blind study of fluoxetine in depressed children and adolescents. *Proceedings of the American Academy of Child and Adolescent Psychiatry, XI,* 41–42.

Fankhauser, M. P., Karumanchi, V. C., German, M. L., Yates, A., & Karumanchi, S. D. (1992). A double-blind, placebo-controlled study of the efficacy of transdermal clonidine in autism. *Journal of Clinical Psychiatry, 53,* 77–82.

FDA. (1982). Use of approved drugs of unlabeled indications. *Psychopharmacology Bulletin, 18,* 5–20.

Frazier, J., Giedd, J., Hambruger, S., Albus, K., Kaysen, D., Vaituzis, C., Rajapakse, J., Lenane, M., McKenna, K., Jacobsen, L., Gordon, C., Brier, A., & Rapoport, J. (1996). Brain anatomic magnetic resonance imaging in childhood-onset schizophrenia. *Archives of General Psychiatry, 53,* 617–624.

Frazier, J., Giedd, J., McKenna, K., Lenane, M., Jih, D., & Rapoport, J. (1994). An open trial of clozapine in 11 adolescents with childhood onset schizophrenia. *Journal of the American Academy of Child and Adolescent Psychiatry, 33,* 658–663.

Frick, P., Lahey, B., Loeber, R., Tannenbaum, L., Horn, Y., Christ, M., Hart, E., & Hanson, K. (1993). Oppositional defiant disorder and conduct disorder: A meta-analytic review of factor analyses and cross-validation in a clinical sample. *Clinical Psychology Review, 13,* 319–340.

Gadow, K. D., Sverd, J., Sprafkin, J., Nolan, E. E., & Ezor, S. N. (1995). Efficacy of methylphenidate for attention-deficit hyperactivity disorder in children with tic disorder. *Archives of General Psychiatry, 52,* 444–455.

Gammon, G. D., & Brown, T. E. (1993). Fluoxetine and methylphenidate in combination for treatment of attention deficit disorder and comorbid depressive disorder. *Journal of Child and Adolescent Psychopharmacology, 3,* 1–10.

Geller, B. (1994). Phenomenology and course of pediatric bipolar disorders (Grant Application No. 1 R01 MH53063-01). Washington University School of Medicine.

Geller, B., Cooper, T. B., Graham, D. L., Fetner, H. H., Marsteller, F. A., & Wells, J. M. (1992). Pharmacokinetically designed double-blind placebo-controlled study of nortriptyline in 6–12-year-olds with major depressive disorder: Outcome; nortriptyline and hydroxy-nortriptyline plasma levels; EKG, BP and side effects measurements. *Journal of the American Academy of Child and Adolescent Psychiatry, 31,* 34–44.

Geller, B., Fox, L. W., & Fletcher, M. (1993). Effect of tricyclic antidepressants on switching to mania and on the onset of bipolarity in depressed 6- to 12-year-olds. *Journal of the American Academy of Child and Adolescent Psychiatry, 32,* 43–50.

Geller, B., Sun, K., Zimerman, B., Luby, J., Frazier, J., & Williams, M. (1995). Complex and rapid-cycling in bipolar children and adolescents: A preliminary study. *Journal of Affective Disorders, 22,* 1–10.

Geller, D., Biederman, J., Reed, E. D., Spencer, T., & Wilens, T. E. (1995). Similarities in response to fluoxetine in the treatment of children and adolescents with obsessive-compulsive disorder. *Journal of the American Academy of Child and Adolescent Psychiatry, 34,* 36–44.

Gittelman, R., & Klein, D. F. (1971). Controlled imipramine treatment of school phobia. *Archives of General Psychiatry, 25,* 204–207.

Gittelman, R., Landa, B., Mattes, J., & Klein, D. (1988). Methylphenidate and growth in hyperactive children: A controlled withdrawal study. *Archives of General Psychiatry, 45,* 1127–1130.

Gittelman, R., & Mannuzza, S. (1988). Hyperactive boys almost grown up: III. Methylphenidate effects on ultimate height. *Archives of General Psychiatry, 45,* 1131–1134.

Gittelman-Klein, R. (1980). Diagnosis and drug treatment of childhood disorders. In D. F. Klein, R. Gittelman, F. Quitkin, & A. Rifkin (Eds.), *Diagnosis and drug treatment of psychiatric disorders: Adults and children* (pp. 576–775). Baltimore: Williams & Wilkins.

Goodwin, F., & Jamison, K. (1990). *Manic-depressive illness.* London: Oxford University Press.

Gordon, C. T., Frazier, J., McKenna, K., Lenane, M., Jih, D., & Rapoport, J. (1994). Childhood-onset schizophrenia: An NIMH study in progress. *Schizophrenia Bulletin, 20,* 697–712.

Graae, F., Milner, J., Rizzotto, L., & Klein, R. (1994). Clonazepam in childhood anxiety disorders. *Journal of the American Academy of Child and Adolescent Psychiatry, 33,* 372–376.

Greenhill, L. L., & Osman, B. B. (1991). *Ritalin: Theory and patient management.* New York: Mary Ann Liebert.

Hunt, R. D. (1987). Treatment effects of oral and transdermal clonidine in relation to methylphenidate: An open pilot study in ADD-H. *Psychopharmacology Bulletin, 23,* 111–114.

Hunt, R., Arnsten, A., & Asbell, M. (1995). An open trial of guanfacine in the treatment of attention-deficit hyperactivity disorder. *Journal of the American Academy of Child and Adolescent Psychiatry, 34,* 50–54.

Hunt, R. D., Minderaa, R. B., & Cohen, D. J. (1985). Clonidine benefits children with attention deficit disorder and hyperactivity: Report of a double-blind placebo-crossover therapeutic trial. *Journal of the American Academy of Child Psychiatry, 24,* 617–629.

Institute of Medicine. (1990). *Research on children and adolescents with mental, behavioral, and developmental disorders.* Washington, DC: National Institute of Mental Health.

Jankovic, J. (1993). Deprenyl in attention deficit associated with Tourette's syndrome. *Archives of Neurology, 50,* 286–288.

Jensen, P. S., Shervette, R. E., Xenakis, S. N., & Richters, J. (1993). Anxiety and depressive disorders in attention deficit hyperactivity disorder with hyperactivity: New findings. *American Journal of Psychiatry, 150,* 1203–1209.

Jensen, P., Vitiello, B., Leonard, H., & Laughren, T. (1994). Child and adolescent psychopharmacology: Expanding the research base. *Psychopharmacology Bulletin, 30,* 3–8.

Kashani, J. H., & Orvaschel, H. (1988). Anxiety disorders in mid-adolescence: A community sample. *American Journal of Psychiatry, 145,* 960–964.

Kashani, J. H., & Sherman, D. D. (1989). Mood disorders in children and adolescents. In A. Tasman, R. E. Hales, & A. J. Frances (Eds.), *Review of psychiatry* (pp. 197–217). Washington, DC: American Psychiatric Association.

Kemph, J., DeVane, C., Levin, G., Jarecke, R., & Miller, R. (1993). Treatment of aggressive children with clonidine: Results of an open pilot study. *Journal of the American Academy of Child and Adolescent Psychiatry, 32,* 577–581.

Klein, R. G. (1987). Pharmacotherapy of childhood hyperactivity: An update. In H. Y. Meltzer (Ed.), *Psychopharmacology: The third generation of progress* (pp. 1215–1224). New York: Raven Press.

Klein, R. G., & Bessler, A. W. (1992). Stimulant side effects in children. In J. M. Kane & J. A. Lieberman (Eds.), *Adverse effects of psychotropic drugs* (pp. 470–496). New York: Guilford Press.

Klorman, R., Brumaghim, J. T., Salzman, L. F., Strauss, J., Borgstedt, A. D., McBride, M. C., & Loeb, S. (1989). Comparative effects of methylphenidate on attention-deficit hyperactivity disorder with and without aggressive / noncompliant features. *Psychopharmacology Bulletin, 25,* 109–113.

Kovacs, M., Akiskal, H., Gatsonis, C., & Parrone, P. (1994). Childhood-onset dysthymic disorder: Clinical features and prospective naturalistic outcome. *Archives of General Psychiatry, 51,* 365–374.

Kovacs, M., Feinberg, T. L., Crouse-Novak, M., Paulauskas, S. L., & Finkelstein, R. (1984). Depressive disorders in childhood: I. A longitudinal prospective study of characteristics and recovery. *Archives of General Psychiatry, 41,* 229–237.

Kumra, S., Frazier, J. A., & Jacobsen, L. (1996). Childhood onset schizophrenia: A double-blind clozapine trial. *Archives of General Psychiatry, 56,* 1090–1097.

Kutcher, S., Boulos, C., Ward, B., Marton, P., Simeon, J., Ferguson, H. B., Szalai, J., Katic, M., Roberts, N., Dubois, C., & Reed, K. (1994). Response to desipramine treatment in adolescent depression: A fixed-dose, placebo-controlled trial. *Journal of the American Academy of Child and Adolescent Psychiatry, 33,* 686–694.

Lazarus, A., Mann, S. C., & Caroff, S. N. (1989). *The neuroleptic malignant syndrome and related conditions.* Washington, DC: American Psychiatric Association.

Leckman, J. F., Hardin, M. T., Riddle, M. A., Stevenson, J., Ort, S., & Cohen, D. J. (1991). Clonidine treatment of Gilles de la Tourette's syndrome. *Archives of General Psychiatry, 48,* 324–328.

Leckman, J. F., Riddle, M. A., & Cohen, D. J. (1988). Pathobiology of Tourette's syndrome. In D. J. Cohen, R. D. Bruun, & J. F. Leckman (Eds.), *Tourette's syndrome and tic disorders: Clinical understanding and treatment* (pp. 103–118). New York: Wiley.

Leckman, J. F., Walkup, J. T., Riddle, M. A., Towbin, K. E., & Cohen, D. J. (1987). Tic disorders. In H. Y. Meltzer (Ed.), *Psychopharmacology: The third generation of progress* (pp. 1239–1254). New York: Raven Press.

Leonard, H., & Rapoport, J. (1989). Anxiety disorders in childhood and adolescence. In A. Tasman, R. Hales, & A. Frances (Eds.), *Review of psychiatry* (pp. 162–179). Washington, DC: American Psychiatric Association.

Leonard, H. L., Swedo, S. E., Rapoport, J. L., Koby, E. V., Lenane, M. C., Cheslow, D. L., & Hamburger, S. D. (1989). Treatment of obsessive compulsive disorder with clomipramine and desipramine in children and adolescents: A double-blind crossover comparison. *Archives of General Psychiatry, 46,* 1088–1092.

Levenson, J. L. (1985). Neuroleptic malignant syndrome. *American Journal of Psychiatry, 142,* 1137–1145.

Loeber, R., Lahey, B. B., & Thomas, C. (1991). Diagnostic conundrum of oppositional defiant disorder and conduct disorder. *Journal of Abnormal Psychology, 100,* 379–390.

Mandoki, M. (1995). Risperidone treatment of children and adolescents: Increased risk of extrapyramidal side effects? *Journal of Child and Adolescent Psychopharmacology, 5,* 49–67.

Mannuzza, S., Klein, R. G., Bessler, A., Malloy, P., & LaPadula, M. (1993). Adult outcome of hyperactive boys: Educational achievement, occupational rank, and psychiatric status. *Archives of General Psychiatry, 50,* 565–576.

March, J., & Leonard, H. (1996). Obsessive-compulsive disorder in children and adolescents: A review of the past 10 years. *Journal of the American Academy of Child and Adolescent Psychiatry, 35,* 1265–1273.

Mattes, J. A., Rosenberg, J., & Mays, D. (1984). Carbamazepine versus propranolol in patients with uncontrolled rage outbursts: A random assignment study. *Psychopharmacology Bulletin, 20,* 98–100.

McElroy, S. L., Keck, P. E., Pope, H. G., & Hudson, J. I. (1992). Valproate in the treatment of bipolar disorder: Literature review and clinical guidelines. *Journal of Clinical Psychopharmacology, 12,* 42S.

McElroy, S., Strakowski, S., West, S., Keck, P., & McConville, B. (1997). Phenomenology of adolescent and adult mania in hospitalized patients with bipolar disorder. *American Journal of Psychiatry, 154,* 44–49.

Medical Letter. (1990). Sudden death in children treated with a tricyclic antidepressant. *32*(816), 37–40.

Meltzer, H. Y. (Ed.). (1987). *Psychopharmacology: The third generation of progress.* New York: Raven Press.

Murphy, J. V., Groover, R. V., & Hodge, C. (1993). Hepato-toxic effects in a child receiving valproate and carnitine. *Journal of Pediatrics, 123,* 318–320.

Pataki, C., Carlson, G., Kelly, K., Rapport, M., & Biancaniello, T. (1993). Side effects of methylphenidate and desipramine alone and in combination in children. *American Journal of Psychiatry, 32,* 1065–1072.

Patrick, K. S., Mueller, R. A., Gualtieri, C. T., & Breese, G. R. (1987). Pharmacokinetics and actions of methylphenidate. In H. Y. Meltzer (Ed.), *Psychopharmacology: The third generation of progress* (pp. 1387–1395). New York: Raven Press.

Pelham, W., Greenslade, K., Vodde-Hamilton, M., Murphy, D., Greenstein, J., Gnagy, E., Guthrie, K., Hoover, M., & Dahl, R. (1990). Relative efficacy of long-acting stimulants on children with attention deficit-hyperactivity disorder: A comparison of standard methylphenidate, sustained-release methylphenidate, sustained-release dextroamphetamine, and pemoline. *Pediatrics, 86,* 226–237.

Physicians' desk reference (48th ed.). (1994). Montvale, NJ: Medical Economics.

Popper, C. (Ed.). (1987). *Psychiatric pharmacosciences of children and adolescents.* Washington, DC: American Psychiatric Association.

Popper, C. W. (1995). Combining methylphenidate and clonidine: Pharmacologic questions and news reports about sudden death. *Journal of Child and Adolescent Psychopharmacology, 5,* 157–166.

Pratt, D. S., & Dubois, R. S. (1990). Hepatotoxicity due to pemoline (Cylert): A report of two cases. *Journal of Pediatric Gastroenterology, 10,* 239–241.

Preskorn, S., Alderman, J., Chung, M., Harrison, W., Messign, M., & Harris, S. (1994). Pharmacokinetics of desipramine coadministered with sertraline or fluoxetine. *Journal of Clinical Psychopharmacology, 14,* 90–98.

Preskorn, S. H., Weller, E. B., Weller, R. A., & Glotzbach, E. (1983). Plasma levels of imipramine and adverse effects in children. *American Journal of Psychiatry, 140,* 1332–1335.

Puig-Antich, J. (1982). Major depression and conduct disorder in prepuberty. *Journal of the American Academy of Child and Adolescent Psychiatry, 21,* 118–128.

Puig-Antich, J., Perel, J. M., Lupatkin, W., Chambers, W. J., Tabrizi, M. A., King, J., Goetz, R., Davies, M., & Stiller, R. L. (1987). Imipramine in prepubertal major depressive disorders. *Archives of General Psychiatry, 44,* 81–89.

Rapoport, J. (1994). Clozapine and child psychiatry. *Journal of Child and Adolescent Psychopharmacology, 4,* 1–3.

Rapoport, J. L., Buschbaum, M. S., Zahn, T. P., Weingartner, H., Ludlow, C., & Mikkelsen, E. J. (1978). Dextroamphetamine: Cognitive and behavioral effects in prepubertal boys. *Science, 199,* 560–563.

Rapoport, J. L., Mikkelsen, E. J., & Zavadil, A. P. (1978). Plasma imipramine and desmethylimipramine concentration and clinical response in childhood enuresis. *Psychopharmacology Bulletin, 14,* 60–61.

Rapoport, J. L., Quinn, P. Bradbard, G., Riddle, D., & Brooks, E. (1974). Imipramine and methylphenidate treatment of hyperactive boys: A double-blind comparison. *Archives of General Psychiatry, 30,* 789–793.

Rapoport, J., Swedo, S., & Leonard, H. (1992). Childhood obsessive compulsive disorder. *Journal of Clinical Psychiatry, 53,* 11–16.

Rapport, M., Carlson, G., Kelly, K., & Pataki, C. (1993). Methylphenidate and desipramine in hospitalized children: I. Separate and combined effects on cognitive function. *Journal of the American Academy of Child and Adolescent Psychiatry, 32,* 333–342.

Ratey, J. J. (1991). *Mental retardation: Developing pharmacotherapies.* Washington, DC: American Psychiatric Association.

Ratey, J. J., Mikkelsen, E. J., Smith, G. B., Upadhyaya, A., Zuckerman, H. S., Martell, D., Sorgi, P. Polakoff, S., & Bemporad, J. (1986). Beta-blockers in the severely and profoundly mentally retarded. *Journal of Clinical Psychopharmacology, 6,* 103–107.

Realmuto, G. M., Jensen, J., Klykylo, W., Piggott, L., Stubbs, G., Yuwiler, A., Geller, E., Freeman, B. J., & Ritvo, E. (1986). Untoward effects of fenfluramine in autistic children. *Journal of Clinical Psychopharmacology, 6,* 350–355.

Remschmidt, H., Schulz, E., & Martin, P. (1994). An open trial of clozapine in thirty-six adolescents with schizophrenia. *Journal of Child and Adolescent Psychopharmacology, 4,* 31–41.

Riddle, M., Geller, B., & Ryan, N. (1993). Case study: Another sudden death in a child treated with desipramine. *Journal of the American Academy of Child and Adolescent Psychiatry, 32,* 792–797.

Riddle, M. A., Hardin, M. T., Cho, S. C., Woolston, J. L., & Leckman, J. F. (1988). Desipramine treatment of boys with attention-deficit hyperactivity disorder and tics: Preliminary clinical experience. *Journal of the American Academy of Child and Adolescent Psychiatry, 27,* 811–814.

Riddle, M. A., Nelson, J. C., Kleinman, C. S., Rasmussen, A., Leckman, J. F., King, R. A., & Cohen, D. J. (1991). Sudden death in children receiving norpramin: A review of three reported cases and commentary. *Journal of the American Academy of Child and Adolescent Psychiatry, 30,* 104–108.

Riddle, M., Scahill, L., King, R., Hardin, M., Anderson, G., Ort, S., Smith, J., Leckman, J., & Cohen, D. (1992). Double-blind, crossover trial of fluoxetine and placebo in children and adolescents with obsessive-compulsive disorder. *Journal of the American Academy of Child and Adolescent Psychiatry, 31,* 1062–1069.

Ritvo, E. R., Freeman, B. J., Yuwiler, A., Geller, E., Schroth, P., Yokota, A., Mason, B. A., August, G. J., Klykylo, W., & Leventhal, B. (1986). Fenfluramine treatment of autism: UCLA collaborative study of 81 patients at nine medical centers. *Psychopharmacology Bulletin, 22,* 133–140.

Rosenbaum, J. F. (1982). The drug treatment of anxiety. *New England Journal of Medicine, 306,* 401–404.

Roy-Byrne, P. P., & Cowley, D. S. (1991). *Benzodiazepines in clinical practice: Risks and benefits.* Washington, DC: American Psychiatric Association.

Ryan, N. D., Meyer, V., Dachille, S., Mazzie, D., & Puig-Antich, J. (1988). Lithium antidepressant augmentation in TCA-refractory depression in adolescents. *Journal of the American Academy of Child and Adolescent Psychiatry, 27,* 371–376.

Ryan, N. D., Puig, A. J., Rabinovich, H., Fried, J., Ambrosini, P., Meyer, V., Torres, D., Dachille, S., & Mazzie, D. (1988). MAOIs in adolescent major depression unresponsive to tricyclic antidepressants. *Journal of the American Academy of Child and Adolescent Psychiatry, 27,* 755–758.

Ryan, N. D., Puig-Antich, J., Ambrosini, P., Rabinovich, H., Robinson, D., Nelson, B., Iyengar, S., & Twomey, J. (1987). The clinical picture of major depression in children and adolescents. *Archives of General Psychiatry, 44,* 854–861.

Shader, R. I., & Greenblatt, D. J. (1993). Use of benzodiazepines in anxiety disorders. *New England Journal of Medicine, 5,* 1398–1405.

Shapiro, A. K., Shapiro, E., & Fulop, G. (1987). Pimozide treatment of tic and Tourette disorders. *Pediatrics, 79,* 1032–1039.

Simeon, J., Carrey, N., Wiggins, D., Milin, R., & Hosenbocus, S. N. (1995). Risperidone effects in treatment resistant adolescents: Preliminary case reports. *Journal of Child and Adolescent Psychopharmacology, 5,* 69–79.

Simeon, J. G., Dinicola, V. F., Ferguson, H. B., & Copping, W. (1990). Adolescent depression: A placebo-controlled fluoxetine treatment study and follow-up. *Progress in Neuropsychopharmacological and Biological Psychiatry, 14,* 791–795.

Simeon, J. G., Ferguson, H. B., Knott, V., Roberts, N., Gauthier, B., Dubois, C., & Wiggins, D. (1992). Clinical, cognitive, and neurophysiological effects of alprazolam in children and adolescents with over anxious and avoidant disorders. *Journal of the American Academy of Child and Adolescent Psychiatry, 31,* 29–35.

Simeon, J. G., Ferguson, H. B., & Van Wyck Fleet, J. (1986). Bupropion effects in attention deficit and conduct disorders. *Canadian Journal of Psychiatry, 31,* 581–585.

Singer, S., Brown, J., Quaskey, S., Rosenberg, L., Mellits, E., & Denckla, M. (1994). The treatment of attention-deficit hyperactivity disorder in Tourette's syndrome: A double-blind placebo-controlled study with clonidine and desipramine. *Pediatrics, 95,* 74–81.

Spencer, T., Biederman, J., Harding, M., O'Donnell, D., Faraone, S., & Wilens, T. (1996). Growth deficits in ADHD children revisited: Evidence for disorder-associated growth delays? *Journal of the American Academy of Child and Adolescent Psychiatry, 35,* 1460–1469.

Spencer, T., Biederman, J., Kerman, K., Steingard, R., & Wilens, T. (1993). Desipramine in the treatment of children with tic disorder or Tourette's syndrome and attention deficit hyperactivity disorder. *Journal of the American Academy of Child and Adolescent Psychiatry, 32,* 354–360.

Spencer, T. J., Biederman, J., Steingard, R., & Wilens, T. (1993). Bupropion exacerbates tics in children with attention deficit hyperactivity disorder and Tourette's disorder. *Journal of the American Academy of Child and Adolescent Psychiatry, 32,* 211–214.

Spencer, T., Biederman, J., Wilens, T., Harding, M., O'Donnell, D., & Griffin, S. (1996). Pharmacotherapy of attention deficit disorder across the life cycle. *Journal of the American Academy of Child and Adolescent Psychiatry, 35,* 409–432.

Spencer, T., Biederman, J., Wright, V., & Danon, M. (1992). Growth deficits in children treated with desipramine: A controlled study. *Journal of the American Academy of Child and Adolescent Psychiatry, 31,* 235–243.

Spencer, T., Wilens, T., Biederman, J., Fararone, S., Ablon, S., Lapey, K. (1995). A double blind, crossover comparison of methylphenolates and placebo in adults with childhood onset attention deficit hyperactivity disorder. *Archives of General Psychiatry, 52,* 434–443.

Steingard, R., Biederman, J., Spencer, T., Wilens, T., & Gonzalez, A. (1993). Comparison of clonidine response in the treatment of attention deficit hyperactivity disorder with and without comorbid tic disorders. *Journal of the American Academy of Child and Adolescent Psychiatry, 32,* 350–353.

Steingard, R., Goldberg, M., Lee, D., & DeMaso, D. (1994). Adjunctive clonazepam treatment of tic symptoms in children with comorbid tic disorders and ADHD. *Journal of the American Academy of Child and Adolescent Psychiatry, 33,* 394–399.

Strober, M., Morrell, W., Lampert, C., & Burroughs, J. (1990). Relapse following discontinuation of lithium maintenance therapy in adolescents with bipolar I illness: A naturalistic study. *American Journal of Psychiatry, 147,* 457–461.

Strober, M., Schmidt-Lackner, S., Freeman, R., Bower, S., Lampert, C., & DeAntonio, M. (1995). Recovery and relapse in adolescents with bipolar affective illness: A five-year naturalistic, prospective follow-up. *Journal of the American Academy of Child and Adolescent Psychiatry, 34,* 724–731.

Swanson, J. M., Granger, D., & Kliewer, W. (1987). Natural social behaviors in hyperactive children: Dose effects of methylphenidate. *Journal of Consulting and Clinical Psychology, 55,* 187–193.

Swanson, J. M., McBurnett, K., Christian, D. L., & Wigal, T. (1995). Stimulant medications and the treatment of children with ADHD. In T. H. Ollendick & R. Prinz (Eds.), *Advances in clinical child psychology* (Vol. 17, pp. 265–322). New York: Plenum Press.

Swedo, S. E., Leonard, H. L., & Rapoport, J. L. (1992). Childhood-onset obsessive compulsive disorder. *Psychiatric Clinics of North America, 15,* 767–775.

Tran, P., Beasley, C., Tollefson, G. S., & Satterless, W. (1994). *Clinical efficacy and safety of increasing doses of olanzapine: A new atypical antipsychotic agent.* Paper presented at the American College of Neuropharmacology, Puerto Rico.

Vitiello, B., Behar, D., Malone, R., Delaney, M. A., Ryan, P. J., & Simpson, G. M. (1988). Pharmacokinetics of lithium carbonate in children. *Journal of Clinical Psychopharmacology, 8,* 355–359.

Weiss, R., Stein, M., Trommer, B., & Refetoff, S. (1993). Attention-deficit hyperactivity disorder and thyroid function. *Journal of Pediatrics, 123,* 539–545.

Weller, E. B., Weller, R. A., & Fristad, M. A. (1986). Lithium dosage guide for prepubertal children: A preliminary report. *Journal of the American Academy of Child Psychiatry, 25,* 92–95.

Weller, E., Weller, R., & Fristad, M. (1995). Bipolar disorder in children: Misdiagnosis, underdiagnosis, and future directions. *Journal of the American Academy of Child and Adolescent Psychiatry, 34,* 709–714.

Werry, J. (1994). Pharmacotherapy of disruptive behavior disorders. *Child and Adolescent Psychiatric Clinics of North America, 3,* 321–342.

Werry, J. S., McClellan, J. M., & Chard, L. (1991). Childhood and adolescent schizophrenic, bipolar, and schizoaffective disorders: A clinical and outcome study. *Journal of the American Academy of Child and Adolescent Psychiatry, 30,* 457–465.

Wilder, B. J. (1992). Pharmacokinetics of valproate and carbamazepine. *Journal of Clinical Psychopharmacology, 12,* 64S.

Wilens, T., & Biederman, J. (1992). The stimulants. In D. Schaffer (Ed.), *Psychiatric clinics of North America* (pp. 191–222). Philadelphia: Saunders.

Wilens, T., Biederman, J., Baldessarini, J., Geller, B., Schleifer, D., Birmaher, B., & Spencer, T. (1996). The cardiovascular effects of tricyclic antidepressants in children and adolescents. *Journal of the American Academy of Child and Adolescent Psychiatry, 35,* 1491–1501.

Wilens, T. E., Biederman, J., Baldessarini, R. J., Puopolo, P. R., & Flood, J. G. (1992). Developmental changes in serum concentrations of desipramine and 2-hydroxydesipramine during treatment with desipramine. *Journal of the American Academy of Child and Adolescent Psychiatry, 31,* 691–698.

Wilens, T., Biederman, J., & Spencer, T. (1994). Clonidine for sleep disturbances associated with attention-deficit hyperactivity disorder. *Journal of the American Academy of Child and Adolescent Psychiatry, 33,* 424–426.

Wilens, T., Spencer, T., Biederman, J., & Schleifer, D. (1997). Nefazadone for juvenile mood disorders: Case series. *Journal of the American Academy of Child and Adolescent Psychiatry, 36,* 481–485.

Wilens, T., Spencer, T., Biederman, J., Wozniak, J., & Connor, D. (1995). Combined pharmacotherapy: An emerging trend in pediatric psychopharmacology. *Journal of the American Academy of Child and Adolescent Psychiatry, 34,* 110–112.

Williams, D. T., Mehl, R., Yudofsky, S., Adams, D., & Roseman, B. (1982). The effect of propranolol on uncontrolled rage outbursts in children and adolescents with organic brain dysfunction. *Journal of the American Academy of Child and Adolescent Psychiatry, 21,* 129–135.

Wozniak, J., & Biederman, J. (1995). Childhood mania exists (and coexists) with ADHD. *American Society of Clinical Psychopharmacology Progress Notes, 6,* 4–5.

Wozniak, J., & Biederman, J. (1996). A pharmacological approach to the quagmire of comorbidity in juvenile mania. *Journal of the American Academy of Child and Adolescent Psychiatry, 35,* 826–828.

Wozniak, J., Biederman, J., Kiely, K., Ablon, S., Faraone, S. V., Mundy, E., & Mennin, D. (1995). Mania-like symptoms suggestive of childhood-onset bipolar disorder in clinically referred children. *Journal of the American Academy of Child and Adolescent Psychiatry, 34,* 867–876.

Zametkin, A., Rapoport, J. L., Murphy, D. L., Linnoila, M., & Ismond, D. (1985). Treatment of hyperactive children with monoamine oxidase inhibitors: I. Clinical efficacy. *Archives of General Psychiatry, 42,* 962–966.

26

Prevention
A Proactive-Developmental-Ecological Perspective

Richard A. Winett

INTRODUCTION

The Failure of Prevention to Take Hold

Since the late 1960s, there has been a significant amount of discussion about the prevention of health and mental health disorders (U.S. Department of Health and Human Services, 1991). Indeed, there were bold pronouncements of milestones and revolutions in mental health when, with the passage in the United States in 1963 of the Mental Retardation Facilities and Community Mental Health Centers (CMHC) Construction Act, an innovative approach to treatment and prevention was to be undertaken. This legislation emphasized intervention and the training of personnel with new types of skills, community consultation and edu-

cation, and process and outcome research. More than 30 years later, the results of the CMHC movement can be seen as mixed. Its major accomplishments have been to provide more direct services to a wide spectrum of people (particularly the underserved) and to become a pivot point for the development of more effective aftercare for former mental patients. Such care has been facilitated by community follow-up capabilities, and particularly by the advent and widespread use of psychotropic drugs (Hanlon & Pickett, 1984).

The CMHC movement has, however, proved a failure in the conduct of more innovative research, and in the provision of preventive consultation and education activities (Heller, Price, Reinharz, Riger, & Wandersman, 1984). CMHCs have become primarily outpatient therapy clinics. In particular, the CMHC system has not developed its potential as a nationwide system for proactively addressing the mental health needs of children, except for the treatment of already existing problems.

There are several reasons for the failure of prevention efforts to take hold in the 1960s and 1970s and therefore to influence the direction of CMHC in the 1980s and 1990s, including dependence on the medical intervention model

This revised chapter is based on Winett, Riley, King, & Altman, Prevention in Mental Health: A Proactive-Developmental-Ecological Perspective, which appeared in the second edition of this book.

RICHARD A. WINETT • Center for Research in Health Behavior, Virginia Polytechnic Institute and State University, Blacksburg, Virginia 24061.

Handbook of Child Psychopathology, 3rd edition, edited by Ollendick & Hersen. Plenum Press, New York, 1998.

and third-party reimbursement for treatment only. Conceptual issues are involved as well. The public health model that served admirably in the prevention of contagious diseases may be less applicable to the prevention of mental disorders. The model is effective when the relationships between the host characteristics, a disease agent, and a disease outcome can be defined, but may be less helpful when relationships have not been documented clearly, at least at an epidemiological level. This problem has led some researchers to continue the search for specific social, individual, and biological correlates of specific disorders and others are developing more generic interventions to prevent multiple disorders (Coie et al., 1993).

A related problem has been the medical model's orientation to prevention, in which the goal is the prevention of specific disease entities. The continuum of health between ease (total health) and disease is particularly relevant in mental health. Although serious mental illness is clearly disease, there is a range of psychosocial health that falls between the extremes. Continued functioning at the lower end of the continuum is more likely to result in frank disease than is functioning at the higher end. Consequently, support of quality of life is a preventive strategy that is gaining acceptance, although documenting the prevention of specific diseases may be problematic.

A third problem has been reliance on massive programs and federal monies, which are being curtailed sharply. Institutional-level change that entails high-visibility interventions is sometimes required to implement environmental changes that will support a less stressful and more controllable existence, particularly for families. A large-scale perspective in psychology and other mental health professions has not been prominent but has been gaining ground (Edelstein & Michelson, 1986; Weissberg & Elias, 1993). Ironically, the formal training of social services workers, social scientists, and medical personnel that has focused on large-scale interventions may not have a concomitant focus on the importance of efforts by individuals and families and

mediating structures such as schools, clinics, day-care centers, and religious organizations. Thus, the perspective of many professionals who have the ability to influence children each day may be skewed in the direction of only going for "big wins."

Small wins that can provide increased opportunity for children in one community or school are extremely valuable. The literature on many individually focused community interventions, nicely reviewed by Roberts and Peterson (1984), can guide the schoolteacher, the day-care supervisor, and other adults who provide services to children to ensure that those who interact in their setting will do so consistently with the development of social competencies, cognitive ability, and self-worth. Others in the community and workplace who influence policy can play a pivotal role in shaping the environment to support the well-being of families (that they may never meet) by implementing policies responsive to the important needs of families with children at home. Thus, although there is some inevitable tension between an emphasis on system versus more individual change (Rappaport, 1981), this need not be the case. Indeed, a multilevel approach may be more feasible and effective (Weissberg & Elias, 1993).

Behavioral Paradigm

The difficulties in the prevention arena notwithstanding, a conceptual revolution took place during the same period as the CMHC movement. This was the advent of the behavioral paradigm in psychology, that is, behavior analysis, behavior modification, and behavior therapy. By basing therapy and other interventions on laboratory-derived and empirically tested principles, it was believed that within a short time a science of behavior change could have a dramatic impact on virtually all developmental, educational, social, health, and psychiatric problems (Winett, King, & Altman, 1991). Although there has been successes with heretofore untreatable populations and problems

(Kazdin, 1994), as well as intriguing extensions to organizational and community interventions (Greene, Winett, Van Houten, Geller, & Iwata, 1987), there have also been major disappointments, for example, in the maintenance of treatment effects (Brownell, Marlatt, Lichtenstein, & Wilson, 1986). In addition, although earlier efforts emphasized training paraprofessionals and using natural behavior change mediators as well as working in the natural environment (Winett et al., 1995), it is apparent that a good deal of behavior therapy today is conducted by professionals within office settings, that is, within the medical model (Kazdi, 1994). Thus, it can be argued that the behavioral revolution has been a conceptual, procedural innovation but has been sidetracked by events over the last 20 years from making substantial impacts on service delivery modalities or primary prevention.

Community Psychology

Because of dissatisfaction with the direction and the rate of progress, there was a splintering away from the CMHC movement by disappointed but perhaps more zealous psychologists, psychiatrists, and social workers whose orientation was more community- and action-oriented. In psychology, this group called itself community psychologists. Since the late 1960s, this group has searched for a value, conceptual, and research stance consistent with such themes as social justice and welfare, citizen participation, empowerment, and prevention (Heller et al., 1984). Thus, compared with behavior therapy, community psychology is not so much a technical revolution as a call for a different set of rules, a different emphasis, and different values. However, surprisingly, community psychologists have rarely made a close connection with the methods of public health (e.g., Winett et al., 1989).

This chapter has been written within the spirit and the basic tenets of community psychology and public health. The integration of community psychology and public health can form a basis for a true revolution in mental health. This may be particularly the case when the values, perspectives, and strategies of community psychology are enriched by the behavioral and social-cognitive paradigms, with further assistance from the salutogenic, ecological, and developmental perspectives (Winett & Anderson, 1994). In the main, the emphasis throughout this chapter is also on children and families, a focus with a long history in public health (Hanlon & Pickett, 1984). Thus, preventive mental health theory and action is put center stage in psychology and public health.

Areas of Study and Key Questions

However, the history of prior revolutions suggests that before manning the barricades, we need a more guarded pronouncement, a recognition of the advisability of evolutionary steps (e.g., Weick, 1984), more serious questioning and study, and careful investigations. These areas of study form the backbone of this chapter and include the following key questions:

1. Is there a convincing need for the prevention of mental health disorders, with an emphasis on children and families?
2. What are the appropriate targets of preventive interventions?
3. What different approaches to psychological inquiries must be taken when the goal is the prevention, rather than the treatment, of child and family mental health disorders?
4. What conceptualizations and strategies are critical in constructing such preventive interventions?
5. What are particular critical problems in affecting long-term preventive behavior change?
6. What has been learned from the modest successes *and* failures of community health promotion projects targeted toward lifestyle modification?
7. How can interventions be constructed so they are politically feasible in an era of diminishing resources for health and mental health programs?

NEEDS

Selective Review

Since the early 1960s, most significant reports about the incidence and prevalence of mental health disorders have noted that the needs have far outstripped the resources and services at the time of the study (e.g., Gesten & Jason, 1987; Joint Commission on Mental Illness, 1961; USDHHS, 1991). This work over the last two decades is selectively reviewed here.

Munoz, Glish, Soo-Hoo, and Robertson reported in 1982 that whereas the prevalence rate of severe affective disorders was about 6% (a relatively high percentage in itself), mild to moderate depressive symptomatology rates ranged from 9 to 26%. Although it appears that a sizable percentage of mildly to moderately depressed individuals improve without treatment, a reasonable proportion in the mild to moderate range become worse and require extensive intervention or become dysfunctional (O'Leary & Wilson, 1987).

In another domain, a Psychology in the Public Forum series in the *American Psychologist* (Garrison, 1987; Hart & Brassard, 1987; Melton & Davidson, 1987; Rosenberg, 1987) focused on an emerging set of concerns and problems grouped under the term *psychological maltreatment of children*. According to Hart and Brassard (1987), psychological maltreatment appears to be more prevalent and destructive than other forms of child abuse and neglect. In particular, long-term social and emotional dysfunction is associated with early maltreatment. The condition (which is fraught with definitional difficulties) can occur in isolation or as a concomitant of child abuse and neglect. In 1984 (as cited in Hart and Brassard, 1987), there were 1.7 million reported cases of child abuse and neglect. One implication of the series of articles was that even with a stringent definition of psychological maltreatment, it is likely that the prevalence rates of various forms of child abuse, neglect, and maltreatment are much higher than 1.7

million cases. Further, legal, resource, conceptual, and technical limitations (see below) hamper a concerted and effective approach to this problem.

Kiesler (1985) estimated that at any given time, 15–35% of the population needs mental health services. Even at the low end of the estimate, the number of individuals represented far surpasses the capabilities of mental health services as currently constituted and delivered. Gesten and Jason (1987) also cogently noted that although 3.2 million children show evidence of major emotional problems, only 10% of them receive treatment in health care systems. In addition, half of the 7 million children with major learning problems never receive any help (see below).

Using data from Kramer (1982), Gesten and Jason (1987) made some sobering predictions about mental health problems at the turn of the twenty-first century. Unfortunately, these predictions now appear quite accurate:

1. The number of persons with mental health disorders will be about 40 million, up from 33 million in 1980.
2. This estimate may be too modest because of the potential increases in mental health needs as a result of people living longer (with an increase in sick and/or dependent elderly) and an increase in the number of children living in single-parent households.
3. Shifts to high technology, which for some population segments may cause physical relocations and periods of unemployment, may result in increased mental health disorders (Brenner, 1973; Catalono & Dooley, 1983; Dooley & Catalano, 1980; Liem & Ramsay, 1982).

Healthy People 2000

Although *Healthy People 2000* (USDHHS, 1991) is most recognized as the cornerstone for setting priorities, objectives, and specific goals for physical health, it is also the policy setter for mental health and mental disorder. *Healthy*

People 2000 compiled an array of epidemiological and health and social indicators that form the background for each area of focus (e.g., tobacco control, physical activity, unintentional injuries). Obviously, a number of areas dovetail with mental health (e.g., substance abuse, family planning), but an examination of background data for mental health concerns is sufficiently disquieting itself and included these points of reference (USDHHS, 1991, p. 208):

• More than 23 million adults living in communities in the United States are "severely incapacitated" from mental disorders.

• About 45 million adults have experienced at least one diagnosable disorder in their life.

• Mental health disorders cost the nation about $73 billion in 1980, with about half the cost attributable to lost productivity.

• About 30,000 individuals commit suicide each year.

• Schizophrenia affects about 1% of the population.

• Depression and other affective/mood disorders affect about 5% of the population at any given time (see above).

• The number of bed days and other disabilities attributable to depression equals or is greater than bed days and disabilities associated with eight major chronic medical conditions.

• Two-thirds of people with depression are not treated.

• About 10–12% of children and adolescents have diagnosable mental health disorders such as depression, autism, and attention-deficit hyperactivity.

• Developmental delays, skill deficits, and conduct disorders associated with cognitive, emotional, and behavioral dysfunction can determine a child's future and, though these problems are often treatable, only 20–30% of such troubled children receive early identification and treatment programs.

As with all areas of concern, *Healthy People 2000* developed a number of specific priorities, objectives, and goals for reducing the burden of mental health disorders. The overall approach involves using health promotion, health protection, and service provision strategies to reach the goals of increasing the span of healthy life, decreasing the health and disease disparities between different segments of the population, and increasing access to preventive services. Once specific priorities, objectives, and goals are set, tracking systems monitor progress toward meeting predesignated goals, with goals based on past incidence, prevalence, service utilization, and other health indicator rates. With such a monitoring system in place, it is possible to reprioritize resources and make programmatic changes particularly to address recalcitrant problems. For example, progress is apparently being made in reducing suicides and stress-related problems; in contrast, little or no progress has been seen in such areas as reducing teen pregnancies and violent and abusive behavior (McGinnis & Lee, 1995).

Thus, there are some encouraging data showing progress in meeting mental health goals. However, again, what are the most striking points are the large number of people with mental health problems, the enormous individual and societal burden from these problems, and the few individuals who receive treatment. *Healthy People 2000* calls for an amalgamation of health promotion, health protection, and preventive service approaches because the usual restorative interventions are very expensive and often "too little too late." The three approaches from *Healthy People 2000* will be explored later, but it is important here to underscore why more of the same—restorative interventions—is not feasible.

Implications

Even if estimates of current and future incidence and prevalence rates are halved, they suggest an overwhelming number of troubled individuals who do not, or will not, receive mental health services. More to the point, it is almost impossible to estimate the number of mental health service providers needed to deliver effective restorative therapy. This is the case when on the one hand paraprofessionals with limited but focused training are considered integral to treatment programs (Hattie, Sharpley, & Rogers, 1984), particularly within managed care systems, but on the other hand it is realized that chronic problems often require sustained and extensive treatment. Even with high-level intensive intervention, many problems are not reliably responsive to treatment.

It is unwarranted to predict any increases in federal or state funding for mental health services so that service reach and potency can be magnified. In fact, with managed care systems, the emphasis has been on time-limited inpatient or outpatient therapy.

Thus, it appears that millions of people, now and in the future, will be distressed by mental health problems. However, as now constructed, it is difficult to discern how the mental health system of private practitioners in mental health centers can possibly make substantial inroads into this need. Although it cannot be denied that a place will always exit for psychotherapy services, and that some therapy procedures are becoming remarkably effective (especially the behavioral and cognitive-behavioral therapies), the solution (if any) to these problems appears to demand reconceptualizations and reorientations along the lines of prevention. More of the same in mental health is unworkable.

CONCEPTS AND STANCES

The foregoing points and discussion make the case that the so-called CMHC and behavioral revolutions of the 1960s and 1970s were, in actuality, only part of an evolutionary process. There is some agreement that since the early 1960s, significant strides have been made in extending services to wider population segments, for example, poorer people and the developmentally disabled (Heller et al., 1984). However, the product offering has remained essentially the same, the proverbial old wine in a new bottle. Indeed, confusion exists within the field about what constitutes innovation.

Perhaps more important, there has been a basic shortcoming in failing to separate three facets of psychological intervention: timing, conceptualization, and service delivery (Rappaport, 1977). These points will be discussed separately and then brought together in a framework based on *Healthy People 2000.*

Timing

By *timing* it is meant whether an intervention is primary, secondary, or tertiary prevention. Primary prevention is largely a population-focused intervention that occurs before the onset of a disorder. A major example of primary prevention is fluoridation of drinking water to prevent tooth decay. Secondary prevention entails early intervention for those assessed as being at high risk. An example of secondary intervention is providing treatment for teenagers and young adults who are identified at school or at work sites as hypertensive. Tertiary prevention is really the treatment of chronic problems to hasten rehabilitation. Innovative programs that help retarded or autistic children to leave institutions, to live in the community, and to go to regular schools are examples of tertiary prevention. Thus, it is possible to range preventive interventions along a time continuum.

Conceptualization

Historically, considerable effort, energy, and debate in psychology focus on the conceptualization of interventions and not on service delivery modalities or their timing (e.g., Goldfried, 1980; Prochaska, DiClemente, & Norcross, 1992). Often, such debates and new conceptualizations are thought to represent marked innovations. As noted above, this was the case with the ascendance of the behavioral paradigm in the 1960s and 1970s. However, most often, the new behavior therapy treatments were fitted into the prevailing delivery system (i.e., one-to-one psychotherapy). Thus, what innovation existed was mostly in conceptualization. The delivery system and the timing of interventions often remained the same.

Further, debates about the efficacy of different treatments often amount to debates about relatively minor differences in conceptual approach but not structure. For example, cognitive treatment and behavioral treatment for depression demonstrate strong similarities. Either treatment is usually provided by an expert within the confines of weekly or twice-weekly hourly sessions occurring in an office. Both treatments tend to focus on individual deficits, thought patterns, or skills. Both treatments try to provide clients with feedback on present behavioral patterns and to set up corrective experiences or outside sessions for clients to test out new patterns of behavior (Goldfried, 1980). Indeed, recognition of the overlap of different psychotherapy approaches is found in the development of integrative conceptual models (Prochaska et al., 1992).

Service Delivery: Stance and Level

Rarely have sustained debates by mental health professionals examined the service delivery component, which, as we have seen, has been taken as a given. Service delivery can most basically be discussed within the context of two critical aspects: stance and level (Rappaport, 1977).

Stance refers to whether an intervention style can be described as *waiting* or *seeking*. In the waiting mode, professionals remain physically within a service system and, indeed, wait for clients to come to them. This is the most important mode of operation for psychologists and other mental health workers and, not surprisingly, it is the mode supported by third-party payers. The seeking mode is a style in which professionals usually operate physically outside the traditional service system and seek to intervene

in problems before they become chronic. However, in practice, it is acknowledged that waiting and seeking are best thought of as a continuum rather than a dichotomy.

In addition, the waiting mode is usually associated with restorative therapy, whereas seeking is generally associated with prevention. This, however, need not always be the case. For example, a psychoanalytic psychologist may offer advice to many troubled individuals through a newspaper column or television show.

The level of intervention is the other important dimension of service delivery. Suffice it to say that, for the most part, psychological interventions are focused on the individual or group level. Such interventions have the disadvantages of being limited in their reach into a population or community and are expensive, although often reimbursable by third-party payers. Thus, we characterize most mental health services as individual-level, waiting-mode interventions.

Table 1 shows examples of waiting- and seeking-mode interventions at different levels, with the waiting mode emphasizing late tertiary preventive activity and the seeking mode more active, primary prevention. Although it is obvious that the examples in the waiting model are most familiar and acceptable (and it is the waiting-mode individual and group-level interventions that have been reimbursable), it should also be apparent that seeking-mode interventions are relatively untapped, but potentially cost-effective and highly efficacious. Further, it is possible to describe midway interventions, as suggested in our introductory section (e.g., when consultation with schools on student mental health emphasizes individual and organizational change processes). Those interventions in the seeking mode at the organizational, community, and institutional levels are in the most accord with public health interventions. Perhaps, focusing on various seeking-mode interventions can help revitalize clinical psychology at a point where the expense of waiting-mode interventions, delivered by highly trained professionals, serves as a major disincentive to include psychologists in managed care systems.

Table 1. Level and Mode of Mental Health Intervention

Level	Mode	
	Waiting	Seeking
Individual	Therapy for chronic problems	Consultation on mental health with leaders and "gatekeepers" for stressful life events
Group	Therapy for families	Support groups for impending divorces
Organizational/ environmental	Consultation with school administrators and teachers where there is a high prevalence of student mental health problems	Consultation on the organizational structures associated with the mental health problems of students
Institutional	Documentation of the mental health effects on children and families of mass layoffs and unemployment; provision of organized help to those affected	Design and delivery of training on new job skills; testimony on the effects of economic recessions during nonrecession periods

Returning to the overall conceptualization of this chapter, the points concerning timing and level of intervention can also be integrated with the perspective and approaches of *Healthy People 2000*.

Timing and Level of Intervention

Table 2 presents a schema based on Winett (1995) and Winett et al. (1989) that shows how primary, secondary, and tertiary prevention efforts can be enacted at individual, group, organizational, community, and institutional levels of intervention and how such efforts fit within *Healthy People 2000's* provisions of health promotion, health protection, and preventive services. The specific examples are relatively arbitrary and focus particularly on children in school settings. Despite this arbitrariness, Table 2 shows that primary and secondary preventions at individual and group levels are likely to involve health promotion (individual changes) tactics; tertiary prevention is likely to focus on a range of clinical and preventive services (broadly defined); and primary and secondary prevention at organization, community, and institutional levels involves a mix of health promotion and health protection tactics. Note also that the individual- and group-level tertiary prevention ex-

amples are more traditional waiting-mode interventions, whereas all primary and secondary prevention interventions more closely fit the seeking mode. Several other points are also suggested by the schema, including: (1) potentially more effective prevention efforts can synergistically combine programs and strategies from different levels, but that (2) programs at different levels require different implementation skills and resources, and (3) regardless of timing, level, or stance of the intervention, effective programs entail developmentally appropriate content and emphases and an understanding and harnessing of the critical ecology. For example, the individual primary prevention, automated problem-solving intervention must have content that is understandable and fits with particular social, cognitive, and physical abilities but, also, new social skills must be highly functional (reinforced) in particular contexts.

Finally, Table 2 suggests another key point that, quite frankly, makes primary prevention efforts so daunting. Such interventions require *both* stimulus and response generalization and the transposition to potentially different setting modes (Kazdin, 1994). A simple but provocative example is provided by considering developmentally appropriate and ecologically functional skills training at individual and group levels delivered at the third and fourth grades. Preven-

Table 2. Prevention in Mental Health: Level and Timing of Intervention

Level	Timing		
	Primary	Secondary	Tertiary
Individual	Problem-solving training using CD-ROM (A)	Automated skill training program for inappropriately aggressive children (A)	Behavior therapy for conduct-disordered children (C)
Group	Classroom-based problem-solving skill training emphasizing small-group interactions (A)	Classroom-based early skill-building intervention for high-risk children (A)	Family intervention for academically and socially impaired children from dysfunctional families (C)
Organization	Curriculum modifications to emphasize life skills training in K–12 (B)	Mainstreaming system for high-risk children revolving around teacher classroom management skills (B)	Provision for in-school, on-demand counseling for troubled children (C)
Community	Basic parental training featured in newspaper supplements (A)	Expansion of after-school mentoring and other recreational programs for high-risk children (B)	Development of group homes for children unmanageable at school or home (C)
Institutional	State-mandated curriculum change to emphasize life skills training in K–12 (B)	State-mandated screening and early intervention programs for academically or socially impaired children (B)	State-mandated school removal and placement in special program for dangerously aggressive children (C)

A, health promotion; B, health protection; C, clinical services.

tion is *future*-oriented. Skills must *generalize* to new situations and settings in the years to come, and at least somewhat different responses (e.g., assertive behaviors) are required in a new context. Without stimulus and response generalizations, by definition, a behavioral prevention program cannot be effective, let alone long-lasting.

Part of the solution to this problem involves training generic skills that can be transposed over time but also teaching developmentally appropriate, domain-specific skills (Weissberg & Elias, 1993). Such skill training will need to occur at different points in time (e.g., fifth and sixth grades for drug and alcohol experimentation, seventh and eighth grades for sexual experimentation). Thus, an *infrastructure* (or at least supportive context) must be created so that training *does occur* programmatically over time (Weissberg & Elias, 1993), suggesting the need for multilevel prevention programs providing a confluence of personnel, resources,

and mediating structures. This prevention equation emphasizes environmental design and a developmental-ecological perspective to be discussed later.

APPROACHES TO THE INTEGRATION OF PUBLIC HEALTH AND MENTAL HEALTH

To this point, this chapter has argued quite strongly for basing prevention in mental health on community psychology and public health paradigms. In this section, some of the problems in modeling mental health after public health are discussed, leading to different perspectives on how prevention should be mounted for mental health.

Many successful public health efforts have followed a relatively orderly pattern of identifying, through epidemiological research, the specific agents and environmental and host factors that contribute to specific diseases or injuries. After these factors are identified for the populations at risk, specific interventions may focus on host, agent, or environmental factors alone, or in combination. For example, early epidemiological research showed how AIDS was initially spread among homosexual men through sexual contacts, and among intravenous drug users through the sharing of needles (Baltimore & Wolff, 1986). It was also possible to identify high-risk places such as bathhouses and shooting galleries. Note the focus was on specific sexual and drug-related behaviors, and on particular settings whose confluence clearly marked a greatly increased probability of disease for the target populations. Although such analyses do not necessarily ensure that successful programs will be mounted (i.e., given the political, legal, social, and technical constraints and limitations), the emphasis is definitely on the prevention of specific diseases.

Epidemiological methods can identify the populations at risk for mental health problems, but such analyses are not likely to be able to pinpoint the specific agents, environments, and host characteristics leading to specific psychological problems. For example, the same set of conditions (i.e., high stress and social isolation) may result in alcoholism, child abuse, or depression, or in none of these problems (Cassell, 1976).

The picture is further clouded by changes over time in diagnostic categories and continued problems in reliable diagnoses (Albee, 1986). For example, with regard to the first issue, the diagnostic system introduced in 1980 (American Psychiatric Association, 1980) no longer denoted homosexuality as a psychological disorder, and the general category of neurosis was dropped. Thus, a variety of psychological disorders appear to "come and go" as a result of reclassification, as well as changes in political and social fabric.

At least three major perspectives have merged that attempt to deal with these issues

and mesh public health and mental health methods and goals.

An Ecological Perspective

The first perspective, with a decidedly ecological stance, makes the case, as noted above, that the same psychological conditions can result in a variety of psychological problems (Cassell, 1976). It is the conditions—and to some extent the host factors—that are readily identifiable as risk-producing; specific disorders cannot be predicted. From this perspective, it makes sense to mount general intervention programs aimed at common stressors. For example, common stressors for children occur at such milestones, or life transitions, as school transfer (Jason, 1987) or divorce (Bloom, Hodges, Kern, & McFaddin, 1985). During the period of entry into elementary and junior high school, children evidence higher levels of care-seeking for medical and psychological symptoms (Greene & Ollendick, 1994; Schor, 1986).

General programs can be developed to help children negotiate these milestones without the aim of preventing specific pathologies in specific individuals. It is also apparent that large-scale environmental changes such as economic recessions (Liem & Ramsay, 1982) or, indeed, even seemingly moderate economic changes (Catalono & Dooley, 1983) or natural or human-caused disasters (Heller et al., 1984) may set the stage for a range of psychological problems. Proactive efforts that combine individual- and higher-level interventions can lessen the psychological impact of such environmental changes (Felner, Jason, Moritsugu, & Farber, 1983).

Prevention of Specific Disorders

However, in the view of some (e.g., Lorion, 1983), this approach is too amorphous and difficult to justify on scientific grounds. The emphasis of the second perspective is on identifying specific social-psychological and host factors that result in specific disorders (American Psychiatric Association, 1980, 1987, 1994). For example, specific family patterns related to schizophrenia could be identified, and then early intervention programs could be mounted for the families at risk. Presumably, such efforts would eventually lower the incidence and prevalence of schizophrenia (Coie et al., 1993).

The specificity of assessment measures, target populations, and disorders called for by this perspective, as well as its attendant aura of scientific rigor and manageability, has appeal. It is also easier to see this focus (i.e., on pathological family patterns) gaining popular and political support relative to approaches that smack of social engineering (e.g., specifying the criteria that must be met before firms may abandon communities).

Recently, this perspective has been somewhat modified so that the emphasis is on identifiable high-risk populations, that is, populations that are at risk for a *variety* of psychological disorders (Coie et al., 1993). An important example of this approach is an emphasis on helping young, single, female parents to return to school, to receive support from others, and to prevent second pregnancies.

One of the more promising research directions consistent with this perspective is an acquisition-oriented approach to prevention (Chassin, Presson, & Sherman, 1985). Acquisition-oriented means understanding the causal factors involved in a targeted behavior or disorder. It can include both individual-level "host" factors and interventions that seek out higher-level social systems and environmental change. This approach involves determining the functions of the target behavior to be prevented. The research reported by Chassin and her colleagues (Chassin et al., 1985) into the social-psychological factors related to the initiation of adolescent smoking behavior suggested that adolescents who smoke are relatively unconventional and show a relative lack of interest in the goals of

conventional institutions such as school and church. Consequently, the typical program, set in the school and often led by the school leaders, may be missing those adolescents most apt to start smoking. The implications of these data for prevention efforts are far-ranging, and the model has potential for bridging the gap between host and environmental programming. In addition, this model may help to address some of the shortcomings and subsequent modest effects of community health promotion programs, which will be discussed later, and counters the assumption of many psychologists and policymakers that most resources for prevention efforts should be centered in schools (Weissberg & Elias, 1993).

Biological Perspective

A third perspective attempts to more closely follow a medical-biological approach. Increasingly, there is evidence that a number of major mental health disorders and psychological problems have genetic and biochemical bases, for example, manic-depression, schizophrenia, and alcoholism (Lamb & Zusman, 1979; Smith, Schwebel, Dunn, & McIver, 1993). The notion here is that research needs to be focused more clearly on identifying and understanding the biological determinants of mental illness. Once these determinants are marked, appropriate medical interventions (e.g., drugs) may be prescribed. Further, if it is firmly believed that the bases for major mental health disorders are biological, then social-psychological preventive interventions, particularly of the more general kind, are seen at best as being misdirected and futile and at worst as being wasteful. However, even with effective medical treatment for mental health problems, programs would still be needed to help in long-term adjustment and coping.

Quite obviously, strict adherence to this perspective turns back the clock about 100 years to the emergence and then the deification of the medical model of psychopathology. Yet there is enough substance to this approach to give even the staunchest environmentalist pause. It is difficult to deny that genetic-biological factors are associated with the most costly disorders. A major caveat, though, with a long conceptual and research history is that these are "predispositions" that undoubtedly require stressful circumstances to manifest themselves in full-blown disorders. Thus, interventions on one side of the equation (i.e., reducing the stressors in at-risk populations) are one fruitful approach even if it is shown that most major mental health disorders have a biological substrate. Further, our knowledge at this point of the biological bases of mental health disorders is unfortunately quite modest (Coie et al., 1993; Edelstin & Michelson, 1986).

Repeatedly, demands for action, whether in treatment or prevention, have called for a focus—and at times a more optimistic search for cures—for major mental health disorders such as schizophrenia. It is undoubtedly true that these disorders exact an enormous toll on individuals, families, communities, and the mental health and health systems. Thus, the focus appears warranted because enormous savings can be made.

THE DEBATE AND RESOLUTIONS

Concerning these issues, two points need to be made. First, it is not clear if any cures will be forthcoming in the near future because, as noted, our knowledge about the biological bases of mental disorders is still modest. Second, the focus on major mental health disorders and hospitalization obscures the fact that *the vast majority of people are not affected by severe mental illness, and it ignores the personal, community, and societal costs of common pervasive problems in living that have primarily environmental causes.* For example, as noted above, the psychological mistreatment of children appears to be far more pervasive and costly than childhood schizo-

phrenia. The origins of psychological mistreatment are understood to involve the interactions of parents and other caretakers with the child, in the context of a disturbed family system, with inadequate community support and institutional practices that are often unresponsive to the needs of families (Rosenberg, 1987).

Prevention Science

With recognition of these debates and issues, Coie et al. (1993) developed a framework for a new research discipline they call *prevention science.* Coie et al. want efforts of the magnitude of public health directed toward "the systematic study of potential precursors of dysfunction or health called *risk factors* and *protective factors,* respectively" (p. 1013). Risk factors primarily pertain to host characteristics that increase the probability of onset, duration (chronicity), and severity of a disorder. Protective factors include host and environmental factors that decrease the impact of risk factors and subsequent disorders.

The basic biopsychosocial approach of Coie et al. (1993) cannot be faulted and, indeed, there are many consistencies in conceptualization and strategies between that seminal article and this chapter which will be delineated here. However, there are some differences in emphasis which will also be noted.

Coie et al. indicated risk factors are generally not specific to a disorder, and disorders are usually associated with many risk factors. Further, risk factors can differentially affect different functions at different points of development, and exposure to risk factors occurs in many ways in different settings. These points are in contrast to a strictly biologically based approach and other approaches more narrowly following a public health model. Recall that these approaches claim progress in the field of prevention in mental health is dependent on isolating particular risk factors for particular disorders. Presumably, this biological perspective will then mirror the success of prevention of health disorders. However, it is now recognized that a number of diseases (cardiovascular disease, certain cancers) have the same or similar risk factors (e.g., higher fat diet, sedentariness) and, therefore, general lifestyle modification programs can substantially prevent many diseases (USDHHS, 1991). Thus:

> If generic risks can be identified and altered in a population, this can have a positive influence on a range of mental health problems, as well as job productivity, and can reduce the need for many health, social, and correctional services. This strategy has a higher potential payoff for society than does a focused attack on controlling a single major but rarely occurring disorder. (Coie et al., 1993, p. 1014)

Current Emphasis

Points of debate and disagreement between this chapter's emphasis and Coie et al. (1993) concern the potential mix and emphasis of protective factors in prevention programs fostering individual skills and competencies and modifying environments. This chapter emphasizes environmental change more than Coie et al. (1991), at least in terms of developing and sustaining structures to support behavior change. The chapter admittedly, however, does not go far enough in examining and offering remedies for the major environmental determinant of marginalization and ill health, namely, low socioeconomic status (Navarro, 1993).

Other points of agreement with Coie et al. include:

1. Prevention programs should be theoretically based and track risk factors, mediating and moderating variables, and outcomes so that prevention theory may be refined based on research trials.

2. Preventive efforts should be timed so intervention occurs at an appropriate developmental point—the risk factor is contextually relevant but is still amenable to change.

3. Prevention programs can have more impact by focusing on individuals at high risk or targeting social and environmental conditions associated with high or multiple risks and by combining programs focused on high-risk individuals or environments with more universal programs (e.g., skills training programs for youths at high risk for early drug experimentation may work better in schools that have an entire curriculum geared to deterring drug use).

4. Prevention programs need to target multiple levels of intervention so multiple strategies and resources are synergistically brought to bear on ameliorating problems.

As I have noted, it is also possible to have a more environmental focus on prevention in mental health—an ecological stance. For example, only recently have the costs of economic recessions been examined (Catalano & Dooley, 1983). In the past, it has been assumed that the effects of unemployment were relatively benign and short term. However, as unemployment becomes the more permanent lot of particular workers, the psychological and health effects have been studied and have been shown to be substantial, for example, major depression, alcohol abuse, and family disturbance, coupled with loss of medical benefits (Liem & Ramsay, 1982). Likewise, even milder economic downturns appear to have a general negative impact on aggregate and individual indicators of mental health (Catalano & Dooley, 1983). Loss of full-time employment also means for many a loss of health insurance. Interestingly, neither the costs of psychological mistreatment or some rather direct effects of unemployment or economic recessions have typically been included in the costs of mental illness, nor have employment, job training, and economic policies been seen as preventive mental health programs with wide-scale benefits.

It is important at this juncture to clarify what I am and am not proposing. I do not propose the abandonment of medical treatments or of the potential for cures of schizophrenia, autism, and other apparently genetically based disorders. Nor should medical efforts be deemphasized for disorders such as alcoholism, which appear to have a biological (predisposition) component. I also believe that much may be gained by careful assessment and intervention research directed at understanding and reliably preventing specific mental disorders. I am not proposing extreme societal engineering projects that may or may not have preventive mental health outcomes. Further, I am not ignoring the critical role individual deficits play in provoking problems in living. However, I am proposing a balance among perspectives in research and intervention agendas. This balance involves valuing and focusing on investigations of common stressors, modifying the conditions that result in such stressors, and strengthening the competencies of individuals to effectively negotiate common stressors through a variety of individual and collective actions. Thus, our knowledge of the effects of such life transitions as entry into school suggests ways of modifying the stress placed on children and parents as well as ways of developing competencies that will allow them to negotiate these demanding life events.

CONCEPTS AND STRATEGIES

Ecological and Developmental Perspectives

Turning again to the psychological maltreatment of children provides insights into the different conceptualizations and strategies that appear necessary to understand and ameliorate these problems. Two useful approaches to understanding psychological maltreatment are the ecological and the developmental perspectives (Bronfenbrenner, 1979). The ecological perspective emphasizes levels of analysis and the interactions of different levels of analysis. Psychological maltreatment can be examined as it relates to child characteristics and parental beliefs and behaviors, family characteristics and patterns, neighborhood parameters (e.g., degree of stability), subculture and community norms and values, and prevailing cultural con-

ditions. Catalano (1979) showed that the ecological perspective actually has a long history in sociology and, to some extent, in psychology. Besides presenting individual problems within a context, the framework is useful for examining causality at multiple levels, which then suggest multiple avenues for interventions.

The developmental perspective within this chapter means more than, for example, presenting program materials appropriate to children at different ages. Rather, this perspective points to the different issues and problems (and important concomitant systems) that are manifested by the child and the family at different times, and it suggests that maltreatment at different stages of development may have different effects in later life. The combination of the ecological and the developmental perspectives indicates that effectively approaching individual cases and problems in their entirety entails multilevel assessments and congruent interventions aimed at different kinds of families.

Interestingly, in their analyses and recommendations, Melton and Davidson (1987) and Rosenberg (1987) went several steps further than more typical proponents of preventive interventions. Rosenberg cited research on stress resistance and invulnerability (e.g., Garmezy, 1981). Many children exposed to extreme stressors do not manifest present or later difficulties (Cowen, 1994). This intriguing body of research shifts our attention toward examining competencies, resources, and coping abilities. Key questions become "What combination of protective factors at what level(s) are necessary to offset particular vulnerabilities at other level(s)?" and "How would these particular combinations vary according to the developmental stage of the child and family?" (Rosenberg, 1987, p. 169).

Melton and Davidson (1987) detailed the historical aspects and the present legal and psychological issues entailed in family intervention. They noted in conclusion that the usual preventive and intervention strategies (e.g., protective services and foster or institutional care) are not likely to be workable. They recommended as a more fruitful course investigating and promoting positive entitlements (e.g., clean, safe neighborhoods) for children and policies that strengthen families.

Thus, Rosenberg and Melton and Davidson called for a paradigm shift that combines salutogenic, ecological, and developmental perspectives, and that in theory and practice will focus on competencies, strengths, coping, and resources. This perspective is, indeed, far afield from paradigms requiring a specification of particular psychological pathology or genetic deficits resulting in specific mental health disorders. However, the approach is also one step beyond the call for more universal interventions aimed at common stressors (Coie et al., 1993), though it is congruent with other attempts to develop comprehensive salutogenic models (Antonovsky, 1987). At this juncture, it is important to examine work that attempted to follow the strengths, competencies, and resource paradigm, and then to see how such work has been used as a foundation for prevention programs in the 1990s.

The Competencies–Resource Paradigm

Table 3 is (primarily) a distillation of the comprehensive review provided by Gesten and Jason (1987) of preventive work in the 1980s based on the competency, coping, and resource perspective. An attempt is made in Table 3 to place the various studies (noted by reference numbers) within specific categories (e.g., social support) and then to classify them by their focus on agent, host, or environmental factors.

An examination of Table 3 will indicate that except for omnipresent (i.e., poverty) and particular (e.g., specific public school policies) sources of powerlessness, which were treated extensively in Rappaport's classic book (1977), some work still remained to be done. For example, there was still a need for more understanding of the social skills that are important at different developmental levels in specific settings, and that are significant in later adjustment

(Ollendick, 1987). The many analyses of social support and mutual help groups need to provide more than descriptive studies attesting to their role in mental health; in addition, individual, social, and environmental barriers to mutually positive interactions must be discerned (e.g., Fisher, Bell, & Baum, 1984; Humphreys & Rappaport, 1994).

It is apparent from Table 3 that most of these studies and projects attempted to change host factors (i.e., cognitions, behaviors, specific skills, coping strategies, and problem-solving approaches) with less or no focus on environmental change. As most of the work noted in Table 3 has been performed by psychologists, this emphasis is not surprising. Rather than lament this point, I note quite positively that a range of techniques were being developed that were effective in modifying critical host factors and that, most importantly, they appeared to yield preventive outcomes. For example, a special, comprehensive intervention program after separation or divorce resulted in better psychological adjustment 4 years after the intervention (Bloom et al., 1985).

It is also apparent in examining Table 3 that much more needed to be done in designing environmental (setting) changes so that positive behaviors were more likely to occur. Mobilizing community systems for mental health promotion in ways congruent with several well-known community health programs (see Winett et al., 1989) and moving more into the realm of political action in order to promote a more equitable distribution of resources are strategies that have received only scant attention (Humphreys & Rappaport, 1994).

A clear exception is the work by Weissberg and his associates (Weissberg, Caplan, & Harwood, 1991; Weissberg & Elias, 1993) that takes us into the 1990s. Weissberg built on the base of work within the competency, coping, and resource model and defined developmentally appropriate generic and domain-specific skills necessary for children. Yet he went a large step further by delineating the curriculum, school, family, community, and state and federal infra-

Table 3. Categorization of 1980s Preventive Mental Health Efforts[a]

	Competence building	Social support	Mutual help	Behavioral community	Empowerment
Agent	*Assess what are critical skills/behaviors*[b]	*Pinpoint individual, social, and system barriers to social support*	*Identify individual, social, and system barriers to mutual help*	*Ascertain system parameters related to detrimental behaviors*	*Assess multilevel sources of powerlessness* (45)
Host	Increase cognitive and social skills of children at risk (e.g., low SES, disturbed families) (1–8)	Teach skills to gain social support (25, 26)	Provide groups for mutual help with or without professional facilitators (32–35)	Change diverse detrimental behaviors using a variety of behavioral strategies (36–40)	Teach skills to gain access to resources (46–48)
	Teach problem-solving and communication skills early in marriage (9–11) or shortly after divorce with parents and children (12–16)				
	Teach skills to prevent depression (17)				
	Teach skills to prevent child abuse (18, 19)				
	Teach social problem-solving skills (20–23)				
	Teach school transition skills (24)				
Environment	*Modify environments so that competent behaviors are more probable*	Increase access to supportive environments (27–31)	*Modify environments so that mutual help behaviors are more probable*	Provide assessments of environmental change; mobilize community systems (41–44)	*Modify institutionalized disenfranchisement*
		Modify environments so that social support behaviors are more probable			

[a]Table references: 1, Berrata-Clement et al. (1984); 2, Johnson & Breckenridge (1982); 3, Johnson & Walker (1985); 4, Jordon et al. (1985); 5, Pierson et al. (1984); 6, Slaughter (1983); 7, Ruth-Lyons et al. (1984); 8, Goodman (1984); 9, Giblin et al. (1985); 10, Gurney (1986); 11, Markman (1986); 12, Bloom et al. (1985); 13, Warren et al. (1984); 14, Stolberg & Garrison (1985); 15, Pedro-Carroll & Cowen (1985); 16, Pedro-Carroll et al. (1986); 17, Munoz et al. (1982); 18, Olds (1984); 19, Harvey (1985); 20, Shure & Spivack (1982); 21, Feis & Symons (1985); 22, Mannarino et al. (1982); 23, Gesten et al. (1982); 24, Elias et al. (1985); 25, Guerney (1985); 26, Taylor et al. (1984); 27, Henninger & Nelson (1984); 28, Unger & Wanderman (1985); 29, Flener et al. (1983); 30, Wright & Cowen (1987); 31, Roskin (1982); 32, Videka-Sherman (1982); 33, Hinrichsen et al. (1985); 34, George & Gryather (1985); 35, Rappaport et al. (1985); 36, Yokley & Glenwick (1984); 37, Winett et al. (1985); 38, Tartinger et al. (1984); 39, Van Houten et al. (1985); 40, Rudd & Geller (1985); 41, Elder et al. (1985); 42, Jason et al. (1986); 43, Winett & Neale (1981); 44, Seekins et al. (1988); 45, Rappaport (1977); 46, Fawcett et al. (1984); 47, Glidewell (1986); 48, Robers & Thorsherm (1986).

[b]Throughout the table, roman type indicates work that has been done (reference numbers are given in parentheses). Italic type indicates work that has generally not yet been emphasized in this perspective.

structure necessary to support such programs from K to 12. Without such support and continuity, there is little reason to believe that more discrete or categorical programs will succeed. But is this large-scale approach merely a replication of community health programs that have been disappointing in their outcomes? Will these complex interventions fail to reach the most at-risk youths who are alienated from school at young ages or no longer in school at later ages? What has been learned from such efforts that can be applied to prevention in mental health?

LESSONS FROM COMMUNITY HEALTH PROMOTION

Weissberg's multilevel program emphasizing developmentally appropriate generic skills training and domain-specific training with a sustained, supportive infrastructure are akin to community health promotion programs. Such programs were expensive to deliver yet appeared promising for influencing the risk behaviors of large population segments, thus delivering a major public health impact. Unfortunately, although the programs in the United States and other countries report some successful outcomes (see Farquhar et al., 1990; see review in Winett et al., 1989), outcomes of other major trials have been disappointing (Carleton et al., 1995; Luepker et al., 1994). Indeed, it can be said that as these programs represented an amalgamation of the most promising conceptualization and intervention strategies from psychology, public health, and communication and social marketing, their failure is extremely disquieting—indeed, a virtual paradigm crisis (Winett, 1995).

Methodological and strategic arguments have been made by way of explanation of the outcomes and for charting new directions (Carleton et al., 1995; Luepker et al., 1994; Winkelby, 1994). Most large community studies, it appears, at least on the bases of analyses by community level, were "underpowered" (i.e., the unit of analysis was communities). Moreover, comparison communities typically exhibited strong secular trends toward risk reduction (i.e., reduced dietary fat, increased physical activity, decreased smoking prevalence), making differences between treatment and comparison communities more difficult to detect. Although the data from these studies support this interpretation of outcomes, it also can be logically argued that interventions could have been even *more* effective in treatment communities as the interventions were in effect "rowing downstream with the current, not fighting and rowing upstream."

Strategic considerations seem more compelling and have applicability to the large-scale prevention programs discussed in this chapter. These considerations include the following points:

1. Intervention components had shown efficacy in prior smaller-scale studies, i.e., the basic programs were well researched.
2. However, the overall community intervention programs failed to engage enough community residents.
3. People at higher risk, notably people of lower educational and income levels, regardless of ethnic status, need to be especially targeted by these programs if there is to be a significant public health outcome.
4. Supportive policies and structures need more development to maintain behavior change in the face of countervailing forces.

Thus, major concerns for any large-scale prevention efforts include skillful marketing to engage large numbers of people, particularly people at risk because of personal or situation characteristics, and the provision of environmental mechanisms to support change. Without these characteristics, large-scale preventive mental health programs will likely be no more effective than community health promotion programs.

THE PROACTIVE-DEVELOPMENTAL-ECOLOGICAL PREVENTION PARADIGM

In this section, different perspectives noted in this chapter are integrated into one overall paradigm for prevention in mental health. I see this paradigm as appropriate for analyses and intervention directed at children and families at risk, as well as for more general quality-of-life concerns. I first review the earlier points again here:

1.   Mental health interventions should take a proactive approach (i.e., should emphasize the seeking mode), and should not just be reactive or work in the waiting mode (Ollendick & Winett, 1985; Rappaport, 1977).

2.   Mental health interventions should focus on building strength and competencies and not only on treating deficits (Gesten & Jason, 1987). Carrying this idea one step further suggests an emphasis on positive mental health through different empowerment strategies, including more access to resources (Rappaport, 1981).

3.   Preventive interventions need to be planned in terms of targets, scope, resources, and personnel based on the timing and level of intervention. In practice, health promotion and service utilization interventions often need a health-protective element (environmental change) to increase the likelihood of maintenance of change (Winett, 1995).

4.   Effective preventive interventions need to teach both generic and domain-specific skills. However, developmental and response and stimulus generalization considerations suggest such programs require an infrastructure so that training and enactive experiences occur over long time periods and that developmentally appropriate behaviors are more likely to be reinforced (Weissberg & Elias, 1993).

5.   In an era of diminished public resources, there is great added value in considering focusing resources on higher-risk groups, higher-risk settings, or altering behaviors and settings that affect large population segments (Coie et al., 1993).

6.   Programs that attempt to have large-scale impacts will have disappointing outcomes if they do not devise strategies to engage many people, particularly population segments with lower income and education, likely to be at the greatest risk (Luepker et al., 1994; Winkelby, 1994).

7.   A developmental perspective entails understanding how to successfully negotiate life transitions, milestones, and attendant stressors (Felner, Farber, & Primavera, 1983). Particular generic and domain- and time-specific skills need to be taught to make such transitions successful (Weissberg et al., 1991). Examples of life transitions can include seemingly "benign" situations as entering middle or high school or dealing with peer pressure to engage in substance use and other illegal behaviors.

8.   An ecological perspective involves a careful consideration of immediate settings (e.g., interactions at a child-day-care center), organizational structures (e.g., the physical and social environments of day-care settings), the interactions of one setting (e.g., day-care-setting rules) with another setting (e.g., work schedules), and institutional policies (e.g., maternal and paternal leave policies). The basic thrust is an examination of multilevel influence and change in appropriate structures to promote health (Bronfenbrenner, 1979; Winett et al., 1989).

Table 4 is an attempt, although a static one, to illustrate the proactive-developmental-ecological perspective for two different life transitions: the parenting of young children and the adaptation to retirement. For Table 4, we have broadly defined competencies as knowledge or skills of individuals, and resources as both tangible (i.e., time and money) and relatively intangible (i.e., respect and caring from others). The settings include a wide spectrum of places where interactions and care occur and where consideration (i.e., specific policies) of population segments and cultural norms (i.e., mass media) emerge. Rather than focus on the amelioration of spe-

Table 4. Proactive-Developmental-Ecological Prevention Paradigm as Illustrated by Two Different Life Transitions and for Different Levels of Analysis

	Parenting of young children			Adaptation to retirement		
	Competencies	Resources	Settings	Competencies	Resources	Settings
Personal	Appropriate parenting behaviors and development of loving relationships	Enough money for basic home and child care needs	Adequate home setting	Suitable interests and commitments so time and activities are valued; engagement in basic health practices	Enough money for basic home needs and outside interests	Adequate home setting, which may need modification for physical decline
Interpersonal	Family communication skills; mutual support skills; problem-solving abilities; preventive health practices	Relatively stable family existence; supportive social network; access to prevention and medical services	Adequate home setting and proximity to others and their settings; prevention and medical centers	Attachments to social relationships and networks that may or may not be immediate family's; social support and problem-solving skills	Relative family stability; minimally supportive social network	Adequate home setting and proximity to others and their settings
Organizational/ environmental	Child care workers to adequately care for children; general positive regard and value of children in immediate settings; emphasis on preventive health care	Access to child care settings; work schedules to facilitate home and work life without undermining income; preventive health care facilities; general community value	Adequate child care settings; facilitative work environment and general community settings supportive of children; prevention health centers	Regard and value for elderly by various individuals in immediate work, social, and heath settings	Access to settings that provide meaningful interactions with other individuals	Settings that provide access to others, suitable roles and value of the elderly
Institutional	Institutional policies that hold children in highest regard	Specific policies that promote children and families (e.g., parental leaves, subsidized child care at work sites)	Promotion of family and child health and welfare through state and federal legislations, corporate sector, mass media	Institutional policies that promote the continual involvement and wellness of the elderly	Specific policies that enhance quality of life for the elderly (e.g., part-time work, full, comprehensive health care coverage)	Promotion of health for the elderly through state and federal legislations, corporate policies, and depictions in mass media

cific health or mental health problems, the examples in Table 4 more squarely fit with a public health, primary prevention focus attempting to build and support strengths and competencies that can forestall numerous problems and improve the quality of life.

Table 4 does not depict well the sense of interactions and, indeed, the synergistic possibilities between levels or between competencies, resources, and settings that are central to an ecological perspective. For example, parental leave policies and more flexible work schedules may enhance family-support and child-care competencies by allowing more time for family interactions and by reducing the stress engendered by the coordination of work and home life (Winett & Neale, 1981). In turn, a better home life may result in more productive behavior at work, thus further promoting more flexible work hours. An adequate home (setting) and income (resources) set the stage for appropriate parenting behavior. Adequate problem-solving abilities stabilize a family's existence and its access to social and material resources. And, of course, the combination of a more stable and relaxed home life with satisfying and financially rewarding work may have a synergistically positive impact on child development.

Not surprisingly, and as suggested by others (Albee, 1986; Danish, Galambos, & Laquarta, 1983), some of the same competencies (e.g., problem-solving skills), resources (e.g., social support), and settings (e.g., adequate housing) emerge as important at different points in the life cycle. It is the fine points and particulars of the skills, resources, and settings that change over time. If this is indeed the case, it suggests that preventive mental health interventions can be fit into more general finite categories (e.g., those that teach people to increase their social support) and those tailored to particular points in the life cycle (e.g., the birth of a child), i.e., generic skills and domain-specific skills.

Perhaps Table 4 does not suggest the proactive nature of the paradigm. Particular interventions are mounted to ensure target competencies, adequate resources, and supportive settings to promote positive mental health. The range of intervention strategies complements those shown in Tables 1 and 2. For example, mutually supportive parenting and baby-sitting groups may be developed with only very minimal paraprofessional help. Workers can and have banded together to bargain for changes in their work conditions, a collective empowering strategy. Other interventions, however, more clearly call for policy change at the state and federal levels (e.g., personal leave policies). Without such higher-level intervention, substantial barriers will remain to some positive organizational, group, and individual initiatives that all aim to strengthen the family.

WORK AND FAMILY LIFE: AN EXEMPLAR

Background

In the following section, empirical support is developed for approaching one set of problems of many dual-earner families with young children. Not surprisingly, work in this area follows the author's evolving conceptualizations over a 15-year period. That is, the first studies focused almost exclusively on the environmental side of a developmental-ecological perspective. It became apparent that this "one-sided" approach was missing a more developmentally sensitive, individual-level skill-building component. More recently, the author has been concerned with not only integrating the many perspectives, frameworks, and conceptualizations in this chapter, but also how to use such an integration to be sure programs have greater reach and attractiveness particularly for people at higher risk. The last part of the chapter provides one example using the social marketing framework as a point of conceptual integration and program development. At the heart of the intervention described later in this section are the main themes of this chapter: proactive, developmentally appropriate interventions, involving enhancement of skills and competencies, within a supportive ecology. The intervention also is clearly a seeking-mode, multilevel, primary prevention intervention (Table 1) relying on health promotion, health protection, and preventive services tactics (Table 2).

The first area of research on work and family life was not directed toward particular critical incidents (e.g., returning to work after the birth of a child); rather, it was focused on one pervasive problem: When children are young (arbitrarily, under 10 years old), it is difficult to coordinate work and family life, particularly for single parents, or when both parents are working full-time outside the home. In the morning, children need to be given breakfast, to be sent or taken to a child-care situation or school, and later in the day, to be picked up or to be met by a responsible person at home or at the child-care center (i.e., to avoid the latchkey syndrome). In the evening, dinner must be prepared, chores must be done, and children must be cared for, and time is also needed for spouses or partners. Between all of these activities, the person must devote 8–9 hours at the work site and additional time, which may be substantial, for commuting.

This brief overview suggests two problems with the resource of time. Time must be closely regulated so that home, child care, and work responsibilities are coordinated. However, even with good management, there simply may not be enough time for these diverse activities.

In the 1970s there was considerable interest in alternative work schedules, particularly in flexible work hours ("flexitime") (Aldous, 1982; Winett, Neale, & Williams, 1982). The original interest pertained to flexitime as a mechanism for allowing workers greater control over their work life. Under flexitime systems, workers were usually allowed to alter their arrival and departure times within set parameters (e.g., arriving between 7:00 and 9:30 AM) as long as they worked during core hours (e.g., 11:00 AM–3:00 PM) and put in 8 hours per day. In other systems, the hours per day could be altered if a designated number (e.g., 40 hours) were accrued by the end of the week.

Evaluations of such systems suggested that flexitime increased worker morale, decreased absenteeism, and, in some instances, appeared to increase productivity (Nollen, 1982). Another interesting by-product of the system was that in areas where many business establishments worked on flexitime, typical rush-hour traffic was alleviated (Nollen, 1982).

At the same time, a number of experts on family life saw that flexitime could be particularly helpful to families with young children (Bronfenbrenner, 1977). By arriving early at work and then leaving early, parents could be home when their child arrived and could avoid the latchkey syndrome. Overall, flexitime was seen as one simple way of helping a large segment of the population to coordinate work and family life and, hence, also to reduce stress.

Empirical Support for Flexible Work Schedules

This general hypothesis has been tested out in several research studies (Bohen & Viveros-Long, 1981; Winett & Neale, 1981; Winett et al., 1982). The author performed two quasiexperiments with two large federal agencies in Washington, D.C. For these studies, a measure was developed using a time-event log system (Robinson, 1977) in which all study participants monitored their use of time about twice per week for about 2 months before the introduction of flexitime and then for up to 7 months after they were on flexitime. Several different checking methods showed that the time logs were reliable instruments. In this way, it was possible to track the time spent with family members before and during flexitime. Additional measures included evaluations of the quality of time spent and weekly measures that examined the stress involved in typical daily activities (e.g., preparing dinner in the evening).

The flexitime systems were quite limited (i.e., 2-hour leeways in arrival and departure time) but typical of the systems developed in the United States. The studies compared individuals who elected to alter their work schedules and

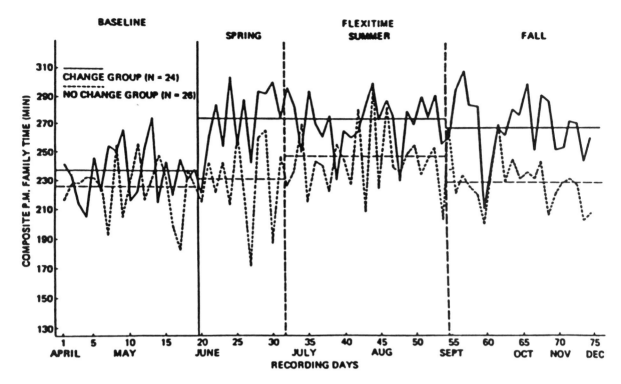

Figure 1. Mean number of minutes spent in composite family time for the change and no-change groups during the phases of the flexitime study. (Adapted from Winett & Neale, 1981.)

similar individuals who decided to remain on their same work schedules. Generally, all participants were from two-parent families where both parents worked full-time and where there was at least one child at home who was under 10 years old. The participants' mean age was about 33, and the average gross family income in 1995 dollars was about $60,000.

The results of the second study are depicted in Figure 1. It is seen that the participants using flexitime were able to increase time with their family by about an hour per day, which was rated as good quality time. In addition, the reported stress involved in daily activities was reduced. The participants sticking to the regular schedule showed no appreciable changes in time use or stress levels.

Although the results of the studies were positive, it was apparent that flexitime was hardly a panacea. There was still much reported diffi-

culty in managing work and family responsibilities. This was made more apparent when all of the time spent at the work site (about 9 hours) and the commuting time (about 2 ½ hours per day) was tallied. There simply was not much time for other activities, and they could only be engaged in at a high personal cost. For example, few people in the study took the time to exercise; the participants' exercise time averaged less than 10 minutes per day. Thus, although flexitime was helpful to parents with young children, it was obviously not a complete solution. The intervention was one-sided and neglected individual skill components.

Individual Level

The prior studies of flexitime evaluated primarily the effects of an environmental (organizational) intervention on individual behavior. In addition to the individual measures, indices focusing on the organization suggested the system was implemented with few problems, and at virtually no cost to the organization (Winett et al., 1982). However, flexitime did not alleviate all problems associated with time management. To some degree, time management problems for parents who have young children and are employed outside the home require other kinds of organizational and institutional changes, which will be discussed later. These same problems also require individual-level change. Individual skills and competencies in personal management and parenting come into play.

King, Winett, and Lovett (1986) undertook another project in family life with a more individual focus. This project was preceded by considerable formative and pilot research (King & Winett, 1986). The formative research included the use of interviews and questionnaires with mostly female clerical staff, as well as female faculty and administrators, who were mothers of younger children and who worked at a large university. The research revealed that the time management problems and stress caused by coordinating home and work life were major difficulties. However, much to our surprise, more flexible work schedules were not highly endorsed by these women as a favored way to alleviate their time and stress problems. Perhaps it was the case that within the conservative climate of this university, flexible hours were not see as a viable alternative; perhaps other problems with flexitime (e.g., not being available for the boss) were envisioned; and perhaps also the short commute of most of the employees obviated some of the need for flexitime. In any case, these female employees strongly endorsed learning about time management skills within a supportive group situation (i.e., with similar women, and with no men included) as their preferred mode of help.

In this study, the major focus became using time management and social support as ways to increase priority time. Priority time was defined individually by each participant as behaviors in her life that were important and on which she wanted to spend more time (e.g., time with the children in the evening; time to be alone and to read; and time to exercise). Such time was reliably tracked by each individual in a way similar to the time logs used in the flexitime studies.

The participants were randomly assigned to four small groups that met twice a week for 4 weeks. The groups differed. In one condition, the participants were directly taught time management skills within a group that was also interactive and emphasized mutual help and support. One group received only time management instruction. One group only followed the precepts of social support. In addition, there was a waiting list control group.

The results of this study, for the priority time measure, are shown in Figure 2. The combination of time management and social support was the most efficacious approach and, indeed, this finding was later replicated with the waiting list control participants. Further, the results appeared to maintain in the follow-up phase. The combination condition also showed some (marginal) reductions in reported stress.

Note also in Figure 2 that time management alone led to increases in priority time, but this was not the case for social support alone. At least within this context and using our priority time measure, even though the social-support-alone condition was reported as highly valued by the participants, it was ineffective. The amorphous concept of social support undoubtedly needs to be unraveled, better defined, and then applied systematically (e.g., Heller, Swindle, & Dusenberg, 1986).

Clearly, this study, in order to better fit our developmental-ecological framework, could have:

1. Worked more exclusively with employees who, for example, were new parents and/or who were just returning to full employment (i.e., a more defined transition point), and

2. Tracked how altered behavior (i.e., priority time), which usually took place in the home, affected other family members and behaviors on the job.

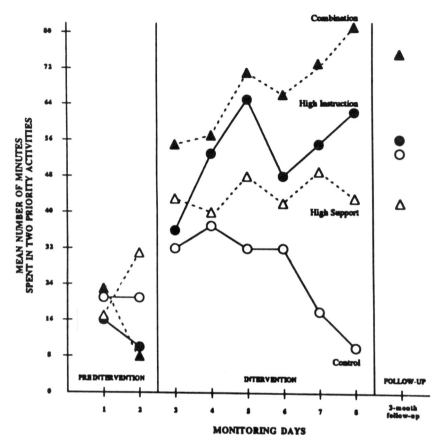

Figure 2. Mean number of minutes spent in two priority activities by the combination, high support, and control groups during phases of the study. (Adapted from King, Winett, & Lovett, 1986.)

Neither the selection-targeting or management-across-settings strategies were followed. However, the study did show that individual interventions that teach specific life skills can be of considerable immediate and enduring value (cf. Danish et al., 1983). Thus, the more usual individual-level conceptual and intervention grounds of psychology may have much significance in preventive efforts, particularly if such efforts are designed to be usable on a large scale.

Conclusions

Not surprisingly, within the general domain of interventions aimed at the problems encoun-

tered in coordinating work and home life, a multilevel approach is favored. For example, the two sets of studies reported in this section certainly suggest that if flexitime, an organizational intervention, could be combined with time management instruction delivered in supportive groups, a particularly effective combination would emerge.

However, the flexitime studies, which were conducted in a large city, showed that when large blocks of time committed to commuting are added to work time, time for other activities may become a very precious resource. Thus, it would appear that one other intervention to help parents with young children entails part-time work (e.g., 66 or 75%) while maintaining status on a job or a career ladder with full accrual of benefits. Also, at certain points, such as the birth of a child, leaves for men and women need to be available that guarantee the same or a similar position on return to work. A recent U.S. Supreme Court case has guaranteed this right. These other kinds of interventions in the work world have required, and will continue to require, changes at the institutional level.

A COMPREHENSIVE APPROACH BASED ON SOCIAL MARKETING

Framework

In these last sections, the prior empirical findings and conclusions are used in conjunction with an overarching social marketing framework to illustrate a more comprehensive approach to the problems of parents working outside the home. Within the context of an overall framework for health promotion and disease prevention, the author (Winett, 1995) has made the case for using social marketing as a conceptual and strategic point of integration for planned interventions. Social marketing essentially adapts the marketing framework (product, price, promotion, place, and positioning) used effectively in the commercial sector to the world of health and mental health interventions.

The framework is a dynamic one where the key variables reciprocally influence each other in the planning and implementation of a program. The *product* is the program or, more specifically, the ideas, beliefs, behaviors, and procedures that are being introduced. New products tend to have a higher probability of adoption if they are triable, show relative advantage through observable, immediate outcomes (feedback), fit into existing lifestyles and systems, are simple to use, and have some capability for adaptation ("reinvention"). *Price* refers to monetary costs

plus effort, social and psychological costs of adopting, and product. In essence, through product design and ready availability, the job of the program implementer is to make use of the product highly reinforcing. *Promotion* refers to various face-to-face and mediated methods to provide information about a product that will increase the rate of adoption. Aspects of the product design, minimal costs for adoption, and tactics of information framing and tailoring to increase the saliency of the product for specific target segments come into play in promotion. *Place* is the distribution point of the product. In essence, the goal is to make the product easily accessible in settings that ensure high-level service and reinforcement of individuals' product procurement efforts.

Place also provides a critical link to the public health model that has advocated more "passive" preventive interventions through structural change. Attention to place and the overall environmental context (including politics; see below) should also increase the probability of behavioral maintenance, a shortcoming in many behavioral interventions and a particular concern in preventive interventions.

Positioning of a product is the special niche of the product and the particular population segment targeted by the product. Thus, product offerings are tailored and matched to specific segments. Such tailoring and matching can be based on demographics, stage of change (for behavioral interventions; Prochaska et al., 1992), developmental point within a life span, and, more likely, all three sets of characteristics. Politics refers to the broad arena of culture, norms, and beliefs. In practice, effective interventions need to be in concert with the current political climate or face considerable reluctance and an early demise.

In practice, through formative and pilot research, the skillful social marketer develops a product offering and intervention while carefully orchestrating the marketing variables so that each variable fits with and supports the other variables, creating a highly synergistic effect within a supportive political context. Winett

(1995) described how current psychological theories can be used to inform and enhance that process, but that discussion is beyond the scope of this chapter. The purpose here is to briefly revisit the problems of families with young children from multilevel and developmental-ecological perspectives, and also to see how a social marketing framework becomes a point of integration for intervention design.

Application

At the individual level, the problem of being a parent with a young child(ren) and also working full-time outside the home is manifested by the challenge of coordinating home and family life activities. More specifically, there is a shortage of time for home and child-care activities, resulting in high levels of stress for a substantial percentage of parents working full-time outside the home. The supposition is that, for a substratum of this population segment, high levels of stress may contribute to a range of problems in mental health (e.g., marital discord) and health (e.g., substance abuse). The word *may* is underscored, as this chain of events is not well documented in the literature. In addition, the goals of the intervention to be described are primarily health enhancement and improved quality of life, rather than the prevention of a specific pathology, although it is certainly possible that decreasing stress may help prevent a range of mental health problems for more at-risk groups.

From a developmental perspective, it is also likely that individual manifestations of the general problem are relatively more intense at certain points. For example, following the birth of a child, returning to work full-time may be particularly stressful, and this represents an important, high-risk point for intervention.

From an ecological perspective, certain environmental impediments and changes may heighten stress. For example, child care using home-based individuals may break down or terminate. Or the transition from day-care center, which extends to 5:30 PM, to public school, which ends at 3:00 PM, may result in considerable problems for parents working outside the home. Thus, life-transition and ecological ("place") considerations are important aspects of defining the problem and of designing programs.

At the interpersonal level, there is also some evidence that because of time constraints and role conflicts, working parents with young children may not have strong social network affiliations or social support (Hopkins & White, 1978), again illustrating the high social and psychological costs faced by single-parent and dual-earner families. If more time were available for social activities, stronger network affiliations might develop. As noted in King et al. (1986), at least some indirect benefits may accrue from regular group interactions with individuals in similar work and family-group situations.

At the organization-environment level, it has been noted (e.g., Kanter, 1977) that work hours have rarely been established with workers' needs as a primary or even secondary consideration. Indeed, within the corporate and labor world, an active effort is made to keep work and family domains separate, with the result that they have infrequently been conjointly studied in the behavioral science (Kanter, 1977). At the level of work organizations, a number of interventions such as flexitime can help working parents. In addition, allowing some individuals (e.g., those with long commutes) to work partly at home (i.e., altering place) may also be helpful. There are, however, trade-offs for individuals working at home (e.g., social isolation, the loss of part of the home to work space, and interruptions and distractions), as well as organizational problems (e.g., supervision) and institutional dilemmas (e.g., tax deductions for home work space).

It has also been noted that other organizations and settings, particularly those involved in child care, may help or hinder the working parent. It is still the case that most of the care of preschool children is done by informal or more formalized means in the parent's home or that of others (i.e., baby-sitters). The advantages of such care are that it may be more personalized and may provide more attention to individual children. Unfortunately, such care may also be haphazard and unsupervised. The effects of center care on child development have been debated through the years. At a minimum, it has been found that high-quality center care is not harmful and may, indeed, have some developmental benefits (Twardosz, 1987). However, in state and federal regulations, quality is generally defined by particular aspects of the child-care setting (e.g., fire safety and the ratio of staff to children at particular ages) and has less to do with the specific interaction styles or environmental parameters that may enhance activities (Twardosz, 1987; Twardosz, Cataldo, & Riskley, 1974). Although it is possible to inform parents what the research literature suggests to be more optimal center care, a center is more likely to be chosen because it is conveniently located and has better hours of operation (e.g., will care for children until 6 PM). Not surprisingly, because there is a limited number of centers, the choice may be the result of fit with immediate needs and scheduling.

A specific problem for families with school-aged children is the latchkey syndrome. The basis of the problem from an ecological perspective is that the school day ends too early and work ends too late. Thus, the child may arrive home from school and be alone for 2–4 hours. As noted above, part of the solution to this problem rests with extending care in the school setting (i.e., again altering place) until the late afternoon and with flexible or part-time work schedules.

Extensions of school-based care and the provision of part-time work, with full job-career-ladder consideration and, perhaps, prorated health benefits, are primarily institutional issues. Although any school district or work organization could develop innovative programs in these domains, such benefits are unlikely to become universally available without state and federal initiative. At a time of fiscal conservatism, innovations that appear to be expensive are most unlikely to garner support unless it can be clearly shown that they result in other positive fiscal outcomes (i.e., less organizational costs, the ability to hire younger workers and phase out older workers). Modification of the school day and part-time work may provide benefits to diverse population segments. For example, after-school programs might be separately paid for by working parents and might thus provide additional jobs for others. Likewise, the option of protected part-time work may provide a predictable pool of hours and work so that additional people may be hired (i.e., new jobs will be created). Such innovations require change at the institutional level.

In a number of cases in which flexitime has been adopted on an experimental basis, labor and management have negotiated so that certain regulations are temporarily suspended. For example, when flexitime systems allow more than 8 hours of work on a particular day, overtime provisions have been dropped (Nollen, 1982). Similarly, small-scale experimentation may be conducted with after-school programs and part-time work.

This overall review and the work described in earlier sections suggest that the problems of time and stress for working parents with young children are the result of combinations of individual, interpersonal, and organizational and institutional factors. The problems may be heightened at difficult transition points and by ecological variables. The discussion has also outlined a number of alternative steps and programs. At this juncture, the conceptual and strategic underpinnings of the proposed interventions are described in the context of the marketing framework.

Intervention Design

As has been noted, parents appear to need both more generic and domain-specific individual skills in managing time, handling critical situations (e.g., the loss of a baby-sitter), negotiating new family arrangements such as the division of labor for child and home care, and giving and receiving social support. These critical skills can be taught starting in high school. In addition, straightforward information on such topics as choosing a mode of child care needs to be imparted. Such diverse skills and specific information fit well into the training curricula developed within social cognitive theory (Bandura, 1986). Behavioral modeling procedures are particularly appropriate. A simple videotape format can be used in which different short scenarios are designed for specific population segments (e.g., single female parent in a large city). Such videotapes may be made generally available through mass market distribution (about 85% of U.S. homes now have a VCR) and through hospitals, pediatricians, libraries, work sites, and rental stores. Other future adaptations of the simple videotape format can include CD-ROM and on-line versions that have much greater potential for individualization, interactivity, mastery learning, and, perhaps, behavioral impacts.

The videotapes (and other formats) may use an interesting storyline and may follow the specific procedures and formats for prosocial action described at length by Winett (1986). Consistent with social cognitive theory, each particular topic (e.g., time management) may be demonstrated; there must be instruction in goal setting, both distal and proximal, and step-by-step individual assignments. The videotapes should be viewed with spouses or partners and friends or acquaintances in small groups and should then be discussed afterward, specifically with regard to carrying out particular steps. This approach follows the notion of a media forum which has been successfully used in the dissemination of innovations (Rogers, 1983). Additional material on later segments of a tape may focus on maintaining skills through varying and trying circumstances, as well as on the developmental hurdles the child will pass and their respective and particular problems. It is also possible to develop a series of such tapes covering different childhood transition periods (e.g., school entry).

Use of the social marketing framework and attendant formative and pilot research strategies can help design the videotapes in these ways: (1) ascertaining which skills, divisions of labor, and means of seeking social support are more acceptable and functional for particular population segments and (2) producing programs that use the same conceptual base but depict particular valued models and relevant settings and skills germane (tailored) to distinct population segments. In this way, the new beliefs and behaviors (the product) are likely to be seen as attractive and adoptable without great costs. The use of a valued model who is shown coping with and mastering difficult behaviors and situations is also a highly effective promotion strategy (Winett, 1995). Thus, through behavioral modeling designed to increase self-efficacy, goal setting, and organization, and through practice and maintenance exercises, the videotapes would be designed in a way that encapsulates what is known about initial and longer-term behavior change (Bandura, 1986; Brownell et al.,1986).

The more didactic information may also be presented in an effective visual manner. For example, actual depictions of optimal and suboptimal child-care situations may be shown. Key points that differentiate such settings and behaviors may be demonstrated, giving the programs more functional value.

Clearly, another notion that underlies the individual-level intervention is personal control. That is, the general goal of teaching time management, parenting, and other family skills is to help individuals gain a measure of control of their behavior and settings. The perception and gaining of control are legitimate goals in their own right, as perceptions of noncontrol have been identified from a variety of perspectives as a key component of ill health (e.g., Antonovsky, 1987). The notion of personal control is also a basis of interventions at organizational and institutional levels, and suggests personal control, choice, and enhancing family values could be a key positioning component of the overall intervention.

Alternative work patterns, such as flexitime,

flexiplace (i.e., work at home), and part-time work, allow individuals more choice in when, where, and how long they will work, and how work will fit in with other responsibilities. Granted that not everyone relishes the idea of such control, but for those who do, alterations in work patterns provide a vehicle for control. Note, however, that alternative work patterns are not being mandated for working parents, an impossibility in this politically conservative era; they are simply one possible choice.

Extensions in school hours also provide an important degree of control by allowing parents to work more routine hours but with the assurance that their child is in a suitably supervised situation. Likewise, extended school days are an option and are not mandated.

As noted above, ecological interventions also fit nicely the public health ideals of creating structural, passive intervention and a core marketing notion that effective interventions need to create a *supportive* "place." Such environmental changes reduce the individual burden of responding to a demanding situation each day. However, the theme (positioning) of personal choice means that such structures and resources should be available, and *not* required, as are some other public health interventions. Thus, by the use of choice, it is anticipated that resistance and, indeed, backlash would be diminished, recognizing the importance of politics.

Targeting and Levels

Consistent with the notion of targeting high-risk groups and situations (Coie et al., 1993), individual-level interventions should be targeted to parents just before and during a transition point. For example, before the birth of a child, some planning and practice should occur, with the most intense part of the intervention (individual instruction) occurring at a critical juncture such as the return to work. A trial period for evaluating the "fit" of different schedules and approaches may also be used to help reduce the

costs of innovation adoption and increase innovation users' "reinvention" of the product. Thus, if an individual can modify the product (e.g., division of labor) to fit his or her circumstances, the product is more likely to be continuously used (behavioral maintenance). A commitment may be made to a particular pattern after the trial period and reinvention, with the commitment to last for at least several months.

An ecological perspective recommends interventions at multiple levels (i.e., individual instruction, plus group support, plus organizational change). Optimistically, it is expected that this strategy will result in interactive and synergistic benefits. For example, more skilled and less stressed parents should be more productive workers, and more optimal work conditions should enhance family life and should contribute to a reduction in the potential for childhood psychopathology. Thus, in today's political climate, such programs are seen as pro-family values and business.

Goals and Measures

The general goal of the interventions is to provide parents working outside the home with skills and environmental mechanisms to better coordinate their home and work life at particular transition points and during highly demanding periods. This general goal should be manifested by a self-reported increase in feelings of control over scheduling and responsibilities and by less reported stress, more quality time spent with children and one's spouse or partner, better child-adjustment development, and more satisfaction and productivity at work. Measurement must consider a person's cognitions, affect, and behavior in multiple situations and in the face of particular critical incidents; the effects of the person's interactions on others (spouse, child, and co-workers); and the effect of individual, group, and setting processes and changes on each other. It is also possible this intervention could reduce health care utilization and costs, a critical area to document.

In addition, it appears important to assess the costs and benefits for work and school settings. For example, all employees' satisfaction and productivity may be measured after the introduction of alternative work patterns that may be used by only a minority of employees. The effects of flexitime and part-time work on supervisory efficiency and additions to the work force, along with the attendant costs (e.g., for training), need to be determined. In short, evaluation needs to be pinpointed, yet comprehensive, to verify the utility of this multifaceted intervention. If utility to different sectors is demonstrated, the effect should be to diffuse this intervention to more individuals and settings.

Product Fit and Redesign

In some respects, the design of this overall program, the product, appears to be exceedingly complex because it involves multiple strategies in multiple settings plus the tailoring of the individual intervention. Although by no means dismissing the difficulty in implementing such an effort, I note that, in the spirit of public health, parts of the overall intervention are relatively passive. For example, once the rules and supervisory systems for alternative work patterns are in place (by no means a simple task, as part-time work, flexitime, and flexiplace require institutional actions), they should not require constant prompting and surveillance for behavior change, but should involve only periodic review and revision. Likewise, once an after-school program is established, it may continue with only routine supervision and administration. Further, such programs may be used by successive waves of parents and children. Thus, these interventions also fit Cowen's notion (1980) of prevention through structural change.

The individual-level intervention, although made relatively permanent by the use of videotape (and other formats), does require diverse and considerable staffing (Winett, 1987, 1995).

For example, an array of production professionals (from scriptwriters to camerapeople, tape editors, and computer scientists for newer formats) is needed. Marketing professionals, using formative research strategies, are needed to capture the nuances of critical behaviors and situations for different people (e.g., a middle-income single parent living in a large city) at different transition points (e.g., pubescence) so there is a basis for tailoring programs. Subtle yet important differences between target audiences may be studied, and important points may be communicated by behavioral scientists working in concert with scriptwriters and other production personnel. Relevant scenarios need to be created for the videotapes, and these scenarios should adhere to the structures of social cognitive theory in storyline, modeling, and format (Winett, 1986). It was noted above that the videotapes would be "relatively permanent." In order to continue to be effective, it is likely that the videotapes would have to be periodically updated and altered to reflect changing conditions and mores (politics). In fact, the ease of individualizing and updating programs is a major advantage of computer-based formats. Thus, it is clear the individual part of the intervention would require considerable resources and personnel to design, produce, and promote the videotapes.

The group part of the intervention is seen as informal, although the videotapes may include pointers for mutual help and feedback in practice assignments, topics for discussion, and so on. Except for opportunity costs, this part of the overall program should be neither cumbersome nor expensive.

Pilot Tests and Program Implementation

An important caveat is that all large-scale efforts should be preceded by a series of small-scale pilot studies (Winett, 1995). For example, several cooperative firms could test the feasibility of alternative work schedules with parents returning to the work force after the birth of a child. The individual and group components emphasizing information dissemination, skill development, and mutual help and support would also be enacted. And a detailed and comprehensive measurement system (discussed above) would examine the multiple impacts and program areas in need of change.

Additional pilot studies would help to refine the overall program and marketing plan. However, it is likely a series of pilot studies would need to be undertaken for programs aimed at different target groups at different points in the life cycle. At the end of a series of pilot studies, not only will refined programs emerge, but there will be a good estimation of the relative costs and benefits to individuals, organizations, and communities of alterations in family patterns, child-care settings, and work sites. Such a research enterprise needs to adhere to the basic tenets of the developmental-ecological and marketing frameworks so that the studies are a test of these frameworks and the overall orientation.

SUMMARY

The multifaceted intervention described in the last sections of this chapter is certainly more extensive than the more individual-based "strength and competency" programs described in Table 3. The intervention is also quite far removed from programs designed to prevent a particular mental disorder, and seemingly from a different world from a medical-model orientation seeking to cure major mental health disorders by finding their biological substrates. The interventions proposed in this chapter will not cure major mental health illnesses, although it is likely that, if effectively implemented, such interventions could reduce the incidence and prevalence rates of child psychopathology. These interventions are, therefore, in no way seen as panaceas (i.e., eliminating all individual pathology and problems in living).

It is also important to underscore that not every effort and intervention needs to be as comprehensive and encompassing as the example outlined in the last sections of this chapter. Prevention activity requires many smaller and successful efforts, much in the spirit of Cowen's call (1980) for "baby steps" to prevention and Weick's notion (1984) of "small wins." In the final analysis, the willingness to try one facsimile of a developmental-ecological program is probably the most important step to be taken and a sure small win.

REFERENCES

Albee, G. W. (1986). Toward a just society: Lessons from observations on the primary prevention of psychopathology. *American Psychologist, 41,* 891–898.

Aldous, J. (1982). *Two paychecks: Life in dual-earner families.* Beverly Hills, CA: Sage.

American Psychiatric Association. (1980). *Diagnostic and statistical manual of mental disorders* (3rd ed.). Washington, DC: Author.

American Psychiatric Association. (1987). *Diagnostic and statistical manual of mental disorders* (3rd ed. rev.). Washington, DC: Author.

American Psychiatric Association. (1994). *Diagnostic and statistical manual of mental disorders* (4th ed.). Washington, DC: Author.

Antonovsky, A. (1987). *Unraveling the mystery of health.* San Francisco: Jossey–Bass.

Baltimore, D., & Wolff, S. M. (1986). *Confronting AIDS: Directions for public health, health care, and research.* Washington, DC: Institute of Medicine, National Academy of Sciences.

Bandura, A. (1986). *Social foundations of thought and action: A social cognitive theory.* Englewood Cliffs, NJ: Prentice–Hall.

Berrata-Clement, J. R., Schweinhart, L. J., Barnett, M. W., Epstein, A. S., & Weikart, D. P. (1984). *Changed lives: The effects of the Perry Preschool Program on youths through age 19.* Ypsilanti, MI: High/Scope Educational Research Foundation.

Bloom, B. L., Hodges, W. F., Kern, M. B., & McFaddin, S. C. (1985). A prevention program for the newly separated: Final evaluations. *American Journal of Orthopsychiatry, 55,* 9–26.

Bohen, H., & Viveros-Long, A. (1981). *Balancing job and family life: Do flexible work schedules help?* Philadelphia: Temple University Press.

Brenner, M. H. (1973). *Mental illness and the economy.* Cambridge, MA: Harvard University Press.

Bronfenbrenner, U. (1977). Toward an experimental ecology of human development. *American Psychologist, 32,* 513–531.

Bronfenbrenner, U. (1979). *The ecology of human development: Experiments by nature and design.* Cambridge, MA: Harvard University Press.

Brownell, K. D., Marlatt, A., Lichtenstein, E., & Wilson, G. T. (1986). Understanding and preventing relapse. *American Psychologist, 41,* 765–782.

Carleton, R. A., Lasater, T. M., Assaf, A. R., Feldman, H. A., McKinlay, S., & Pawtucket Heart Health Program Writing Group. (1995). The Pawtucket Heart Health Program: Community changes in cardiovascular risk factors and projected disease risk. *American Journal of Public Health, 85,* 777–785.

Cassell, J. (1976). The contribution of the social environment to host resistance. *American Journal of Epidemiology, 104,* 107–123.

Catalano, R. A. (1979). *Health, behavior, and community.* Elmsford, NY: Pergamon Press.

Catalano, R. A., & Dooley, D. (1983). The health effects of economics instability: A test of the economic stress hypothesis. *Journal of Health and Social Behavior, 23,* 133–147.

Chassin, L. A., Presson, C. C., & Sherman, S. J. (1985). Stepping backward in order to step forward: An acquisition-oriented approach to primary prevention. *Journal of Consulting and Clinical Psychology, 53,* 612–622.

Coie, J. D., Watt, N. F., West, S. G., Hawkins, J. D., Asarnow, J. R., Markman, H. J., Ramey, S. L., Shure, M. B., & Long, B. (1993). The science of prevention: A conceptual framework and some directions for a national research program. *American Psychologist, 48,* 1013–1022.

Cowen, E. L. (1980). The wooing of primary prevention. *American Journal of Community Psychology, 8,* 258–284.

Cowen, E. L. (1994). The enhancement of psychological wellness: Challenges and opportunities. *American Journal of Community Psychology, 22,* 149–179.

Danish, S. J., Galambos, N. L., & Laquarta, I. (1983). Life development intervention: Skill training for personal competence. In R. D. Feiner, L. A. Jason, J. N. Moritsugu, & S. S. Farber (Eds.), *Preventive psychology: Theory, research, and practice* (pp. 127–151). Elmsford, NY: Pergamon Press.

Dooley, D., & Catalano, R. (1980). Economic change as a cause of behavior disorder. *Psychological Bulletin, 87,* 450–468.

Edelstein, B. A., & Michelson, L. (Eds.). (1986). *Handbook of prevention.* New York: Plenum Press.

Elder, J. P., Howell, M. F., Lasater, T. M., Wells, B. L., & Carleton, R. A. (1985). Applications of behavior modification to community health education: The case of heart disease prevention. *Health Education Quarterly, 12,* 151–168.

Elias, M., Bruene, L., Clabby, J., Barbiere, M., & Heckelman, S. (1985). A multidisciplinary social problem-solving intervention for middle school students with behavior and learning disorders. *Advances in Learning and Behavioral Disabilities, 4,* 49–75. Fairfield, CT: JAI Press.

Farquhar, J. W., Fortmann, S. P., Flora, J. A., Taylor, C. B., Haskell, W. L., Williams, P. T., Maccoby, N., & Wood, P. D. (1990). Effects of community-wide education on cardiovascular risk factors. *Journal of the American Medical Association, 264,* 359–365.

Fawcett, S. B., Seekins, T., Whang, P. L., & Muiu, S. (1984). Creating and using social technologies for community empowerment. *Prevention in Human Services, 3,* 145–172.

Feis, C. L., & Symons, C. (1985). Training preschool children in interpersonal cognitive problem-solving skills: A replication. *Prevention in Human Services, 4,* 59–70.

Felner, R. D., Farber, S. S., & Primavera, J. (1983). Transitions and stressful life events: A model for primary prevention. In R. D. Felner, L. A. Jason, J. N. Moritsugu, & S. S. Farber (Eds.), *Preventive psychology: Theory, research, and practice* (pp. 216–257). Elmsford, NY: Pergamon Press.

Felner, R. D., Jason, L. A., Moritsugu, J. N., & Farber, S. S. (Eds.). (1983). *Preventive psychology: Theory, research, and practice.* Elmsford, NY: Pergamon Press.

Fisher, J. D., Bell, P. A., & Baum, A. (1984). *Environmental psychology* (2nd ed.). New York: Holt, Rinehart & Winston.

Garmezy, N. (1981). Children under stress: Perspectives on antecedents and correlates of vulnerability and resistance to psychopathology. In A. I. Rubin, J. Aronoff, A. M. Barclay, & R. A. Zucker (Eds.), *Further explorations in personality* (pp. 98–117). New York: Wiley.

Garrison, E. G. (1987). Psychological maltreatment of children: An emerging focus for inquiry and concern. *American Psychologist, 42,* 157–159.

George, L. K., & Gryather, L. P. (1985). *Support groups for caregivers of memory-impaired elderly: Easing caregiver burden.* Paper presented at the Annual Vermont Conference on Primary Prevention, Burlington.

Gesten, E. L., & Jason, L. A. (1987). Social and community interventions. *Annual Review of Psychology* (Vol. 38). Palo Alto, CA: Annual Reviews.

Gesten, E. L., Rains, M. H., Rapkin, B. D., Weissberg, R. P., Flores do Apodaca, R., Cowen, E. L., & Bowen, R. (1982). Training children in social problem-solving competencies: A first and second look. *American Journal of Community Psychology, 10,* 95–115.

Giblin, P., Sprenkle, D. H., & Sheehan, R. (1985). Enrichment outcome research: A meta-analysis of premarital, marital, and family intervention. *Journal of Marital Family Therapy, 11,* 257–271.

Glidewell, J. C. (1986). *Psychosocial empowerment in community action.* Unpublished manuscript, Vanderbilt University.

Goldfried, M. R. (1980). Toward the delineation of therapeutic change principles. *American Psychologist, 35,* 991–996.

Goldston, S. E. (1986). Primary prevention: Historical perspectives and blueprint for action. *American Psychologist, 41,* 453–468.

Goodman, S. H. (1984). Children of disturbed parents: The

interface between research and intervention. *American Journal of Community Psychology, 12,* 663–687.

Greene, B. F., Winett, R. A., Van Houten, R., Geller, E. S., & Iwata, B. A. (1987). *Behavior analysis in the community.* Lawrence, KS: Society for the Experimental Analyses of Behavior.

Greene, R. W., & Ollendick, T. H. (1994). Evaluation of a multidimensional program for sixth graders in transition from elementary to middle school. *Journal of Community Psychology, 21,* 162–176.

Guerney, B. G. (1985). *Phone Friend Child Helpline: A community primary prevention service.* Paper presented at the Annual Vermont Conference on Primary Prevention, Burlington.

Guerney, B. G. (1986). Family relationship enhancement: A skill training approach. In L. Bond (Ed.), *Families in transition: Primary prevention programs that work* (pp.72–87). Beverly Hills, CA: Sage.

Hanlon, J. J., & Pickett, G. E. (1984). *Public health: Administration and practice* (8th ed.). St. Louis, MO: Times Mirror/Mosby.

Hart, S. N., & Brassard, M. R. (1987). A major threat to children's mental health: Psychological maltreatment. *American Psychologist, 42,* 160–165.

Harvey, M. R. (1985). *Exemplary rape crisis programs: A cross-site analysis and case studies* (DHHS Publication ADM 85-1423). Washington, DC: U.S. Government Printing Office.

Hattie, J. A., Sharpley, C. F., & Rogers, H. J. (1984). Comparative effectiveness of professionals and paraprofessional helpers. *Psychological Bulletin, 95,* 534–541.

Heller, K., Price, R. H., Reinharz, S., Riger, S., & Wandersman, A. (1984). *Psychology and community change.* Homewood, IL: Dorsey Press.

Heller, K., Swindle, R. W., & Dusenberg, L. (1986). Component social support processes: Comments and integration. *Journal of Consulting and Clinical Psychology, 54,* 466–470.

Henninger, D. G., & Nelson, G. (1984). Evaluation of a social support program for young unwed mothers. *Journal of Primary Prevention, 5,* 3–16.

Hinrichsen, G. A., Revenson, T. A., & Shinn, M. (1985). Does self-help help? An empirical investigation of scoliosis peer support groups. *Journal of Social Issues, 41,* 65–87.

Hopkins, J., & White, P. (1978). The dual-earner couple: Constraints and supports. *The Family Coordinator, July,* 253–259.

Humphreys, K., & Rappaport, J. (1994). Researching self-help/mutual aid groups and organizations: Many roads, one journey. *Applied and Preventive Psychology, 3,* 217–231.

Jason, L. A. (1987). *Ongoing NIMH project on social transitions.* Department of Psychology, DePaul University.

Johnson, D. L., & Breckenridge, J. N. (1982). The Houston Parent-Child Development Center and the primary prevention of behavior problems in young children. *American Journal of Community Psychology, 10,* 305–316.

Johnson, D. L., & Walker, T. (1985). *The primary prevention of behavior problems in Mexican-American children.* Paper presented at the Social Research and Child Development Convention, Toronto.

Joint Commission on Mental Illness. (1961). *Action for mental health.* New York: Basic Books.

Jordon, T. J., Grallo, R., Deutsch, M., & Deutsch, C. P. (1985). Long-term effects of early enrichment: A 20-year perspective on persistence and change. *American Journal of Community Psychology, 13,* 393–416.

Kanter, R. M. (1977). *Work and family in the United States: A critical review and agenda for research and policy.* Beverly Hills, CA: Sage.

Kazdin, A. E. (1994). *Behavior modification in applied settings* (5th ed.). Homewood, IL: Dorsey Press.

Kiesler, C. A. (1985). Prevention and public policy. In J. C. Posey & L. J. Soloman (Eds.), *Prevention in health psychology* (pp. 237–252). Hanover, VT: University Press of New England.

King, A. C., & Winett, R. A. (1986). Stress reduction for individuals at risk: Comparisons of women from dual-earner and dual-career families. *Family and Community Health, 9,* 42–50.

King, A. C., Winett, R. A., & Lovett, S. B. (1986). Enhancing coping behaviors in at-risk populations: The effects of time management instruction and social support in women from dual-career families. *Behavior Therapy, 17,* 57–66.

Kramer, M. (1982). The continuing challenge: The rising prevalence of mental disorders, associated chronic diseases, and disabling conditions. In M. O. Wagenfield, P. V. Lemkau, & B. Justice (Eds.), *Public mental health* (pp. 58–84). Beverly Hills, CA: Sage.

Lamb, H. R., & Zusman, J. (1979). Primary prevention in perspective. *American Journal of Psychiatry, 136,* 12–17.

Liem, R., & Ramsay, P. (1982). Health and social costs of unemployment: Research and policy considerations. *American Psychologist, 37,* 1116–1123.

Lorion, R. P. (1983). Evaluating preventive interventions: Guidelines for the serious social change agent. In R. D. Felner, L. A. Jason, J. N. Moritsugu, & S. S. Farber (Eds.), *Preventive psychology: Theory, research, and practice.* Elmsford, NY: Pergamon Press.

Luepker, R. V., Murray, D. M., Jacobs, D. R., Jr., Mittelmark, M. B., Bracht, N., Carlaw, R., Crow, R., Elmer, P., Finnegan, J., Folsom, A. R., Grimm, R., Hannan, P. J., Jeffrey, R., Lando, H., McGovern, P., Mullis, R., Perry, C. L., Pechacek, T., Pirie, P., Sprafka, J. M., Weisbrod, R., & Blackburn, H. (1994). Community education for cardiovascular disease prevention: Risk factor changes in the Minnesota Heart Health Program. *American Journal of Public Health, 84,* 1383–1393.

Mannarino, A. P., Christy, M., Durlak, J. A., & Magnussen, M. G. (1982). Evaluation of social competence training in the schools. *Journal of School Psychology, 20*, 11–19.

McGinnis, J. M., & Lee, P. R. (1995). Healthy People 2000 at mid-decade. *Journal of the American Medical Association, 273*, 1123–1129.

Melton, G. B., & Davidson, H. A. (1987). Child protection and society: When should the state intervene? *American Psychologist, 42*, 172–175.

Munoz, R. F., Glish, M., Soo-Hoo, T., & Robertson, J. (1982). The San Francisco mood survey project: Preliminary work toward the prevention of depression. *American Journal of Community Psychology, 10*, 317–329.

Murkman, H. J., Jamieson, K., & Floyd, F. (1983). The assessment and modification of premarital relationships: Preliminary findings on the etiology and prevention of marital and family distress. In J. Vincent (Ed.), *Advances in family interventions, assessment and therapy.* (Vol. 3, pp. 41–90). Greenwich, CT: JAI.

Navarro, V. (1993). *Dangerous to your health: Capitalism in health care.* New York: Monthly Review Press.

Nollen, S. D. (1982). *New work schedules in practice: Managing time in a changing society.* Princeton, NJ: Van Nostrand–Reinhold.

Olds, D. L. (1984). *Final report: Prenatal/early infancy project.* Washington, DC: Maternal and Child Health Research, NIMH.

O'Leary, K. D., & Wilson, G. T. (1987). *Principles of behavior therapy* (2nd ed.). New York: Holt, Rinehart & Winston.

Ollendick, T. H. (1986). Children and adolescent behavior therapy. In S. L. Garfield & A. E. Bergin (Eds.), *Handbook of psychotherapy and behavior change* (3rd ed., pp. 272–298). New York: Wiley.

Ollendick, T. H., & Winett, R. A. (1985). Behavioral-preventive interventions with children. In P. H. Bornstein & A. E. Kazdin (Eds.), *Handbook of clinical behavior therapy with children* (pp. 805–832). Homewood, IL: Dorsey Press.

Pedro-Carroll, J. L., & Cowen, E. L. (1985). The children of divorce intervention program: An investigation of the efficacy of a school-based prevention program. *Journal of Consulting and Clinical Psychology, 53*, 603–611.

Pedro-Carroll, J. L., Cowen, E. L., Hightower, A. D., & Guare, J. C. (1986). Preventive intervention with latency-aged children of divorce: A replication study. *American Journal of Community Psychology, 13*, 117–126.

Pierson, D. E., Walker, D. E., & Tivnan, T. (1984). A school-based program from infancy to kindergarten for children and their parents. *Personal Guidance Journal, 62*, 448–454.

Prochaska, J. O., DiClemente, C. C., & Norcross, J. C. (1992). In search of how people change: Applications to addictive behaviors. *American Psychologist, 47*, 1102–1114.

Rappaport, J. (1977). *Community psychology: Values, research, and action.* New York: Holt, Rinehart & Winston.

Rappaport, J. (1981). In praise of paradox: A social policy of empowerment over prevention. *American Journal of Community Psychology, 9*, 1–25.

Rappaport, J. (1987). Terms of empowerment/exemplars of prevention: Toward a theory for community psychology. *American Journal of Community Psychology, 15*, 121–148.

Roberts, B. B., & Thorsheim, H. I. (1986). A partnership approach to consultation: The process and results of a major primary prevention field experiment. In J. Kelly (Ed.), *Ecological theory: Guidelines for doing consultation as a preventive services: Prevention in Human Services* (Vol. 10, pp. 122–139). New York: Haworth Press.

Roberts, M. C., & Peterson, L. (Eds.). (1984). *Prevention of problems in childhood: Psychological research and applications.* New York: Wiley–Interscience.

Robinson, J. P. (1977). *How Americans use time.* New York: Praeger.

Rogers, E. M. (1983). *Diffusion of innovation* (3rd ed.). New York: Free Press.

Rosenberg, M. S. (1987). New directions for research in psychological maltreatment of children. *American Psychologist, 42*, 166–171.

Roskin, M. (1982). Coping with life changes: A preventive social work approach. *American Journal of Community Psychology, 10*, 331–340.

Rudd, J. R., & Geller, E. S. (1985). A university-based incentive program to increase safety belt use: Toward cost-effective institutionalization. *Journal of Applied Behavior Analysis, 18*, 215–226.

Ruth-Lyons, K., Botein, S., & Grunebaum, H. U. (1984). Reaching the hard-to-reach: Serving isolated and depressed mothers with infants in the community. In B. Cohen & J. Musick (Eds.), *Parents and their young children* (pp. 297–312). San Francisco: Jossey–Bass.

Schor, E. L. (1986). Use of health care services by children and diagnoses received during presumably stressful life transitions. *Pediatrics, 77*, 834–841.

Seekins, T., Fawcett, S. B., Elder, J. P., Jason, L. A., Schnelle, J., & Winett, R. A. (1988). Interstate evaluation of child restraint laws. *Journal of Applied Behavioral Analyses, 21*, 233–244.

Shure, M. B., & Spivack, G. (1982). Interpersonal problem-solving in young children: A cognitive approach to prevention. *American Journal of Community Psychology, 10*, 341–356.

Slaughter, D. T. (1983). Early intervention and its effect on maternal and child development. *Monograph of Social Research and Child Development, 48*(4, No. 202), 99.

Smith, G. B., Schwebel, A. I., Dunn, R. L., & McIver, S. D. (1993). The role of psychologists in the treatment, management, and prevention of chronic mental illness. *American Psychologist, 48*, 966–971.

Stolberg, J. C., & Garrison, R. S. (1985). Preventive intervention with children of divorced couples. *Journal of Marriage and Family Counseling, 14*, 28–42.

Tartinger, D. A., Greene, B. R., & Lutzker, J. R. (1984).

Home safety: Development and validation of one component of an eco-behavioral treatment for abused and neglected children. *Journal of Applied Behavior Analysis, 7,* 159–174.

Taylor, R. M., Lam, D. J., Roppel, C. E., & Barter, J. J. (1984). Friends can be good medicine: An excursion into mental health promotion. *Community Mental Health Journal, 20,* 294–303.

Twardosz, S. (1987). The importance of day-care ecology. *The Community Psychologist, 20,* 18.

Twardosz, S., Cataldo, M. F., & Riskley, T. R. (1974). Open environment for infant toddler day care. *Journal of Applied Behavior Analysis, 7,* 529–546.

Unger, D. G., & Wandersman, A. (1985). The importance of neighbors: The social, cognitive, and affective components of neighboring. *American Journal of Community Psychology, 13,* 139–169.

U.S. Department of Health and Human Services. (1991). *Healthy People 2000: National health promotion and disease prevention objectives* (Publication No. PHS 91-50212). Washington, DC: Author.

Van Houten, R., & Nau, P. A. (1983). Feedback interventions and driving speed: A parametric and comparative analysis. *Journal of Applied Behavior Analysis, 16,* 253–281.

Videka-Sherman, L. (1982). Effects of participation in a self-help group for bereaved parents: Compassionate Friends. *Prevention in Human Services, 1,* 69–78.

Warren, N. J., Grew, R. S., Ilgen, E. R., et al. (1984). *Parenting after divorce: Preventive measures for divorcing families.* Synopsis of research prepared for NIMH conference, "Children and Divorce," Washington, DC.

Weick, K. (1984). Small wins: Redefining the scale of social problems. *American Psychologist, 39,* 40–49.

Weissberg, R. P., Caplan, M., & Harwood, R. L. (1991). Promoting competent young people in competence-enhancing environments: A systems-based perspective on primary prevention. *Journal of Consulting and Clinical Psychology, 59,* 830–841.

Weissberg, R. P., & Elias, M. J. (1993). Enhancing young people's social competence and health behavior: An important challenge for educators, scientists, policy makers, and funders. *Applied and Preventive Psychology, 2,* 179–190.

Winett, R. A. (1986). *Information and behavior: Systems of influence.* Hillsdale, NJ: Erlbaum.

Winett, R. A. (1987). Prosocial television for solving community problems. In L. Jason, R. D. Feiner, R. Hoss, & J. D. Moritsugu (Eds.), *Communities: Contributions from allied professions* (pp. 117–160). New York: Haworth Press.

Winett, R. A. (1995). A framework for health promotion and disease prevention. *American Psychologist, 50,* 341–350.

Winett, R. A., & Anderson, E. S. (1994). Preventing HIV in youths: A framework for research and action. In T. H. Ollendick & R. J. Prinz (Eds.), *Advances in clinical child psychology* (Vol. 16, pp. 1–43). New York: Plenum Press.

Winett, R. A., Desiderato, L. L., Anderson, E. S., Solomon, L. J., Perry, M., Kelly, J. A., Sikkema, K. J., Roffman, R. A., Norman, A. D., Lombard, D. N., & Lombard, T. N. (1995). Enhancing social diffusion theory as a basis for prevention intervention: A conceptual and strategic framework. *Applied and Preventive Psychology, 4,* 233–245.

Winett, R. A., King, A. C., & Altman, D. G. (1989). *Health psychology and public health: An integrative approach.* Elmsford, NY: Pergamon Press.

Winett, R. A., King, A. C., & Altman, D. G. (1991). Extending applications of behavior therapy to large-scale interventions. In P. R. Martin (Ed.), *Handbook of behavior therapy and psychological science: An integrative approach* (pp. 454–486). Elmsford, NY: Pergamon Press.

Winett, R. A., Leckliter, I. N., Chinn, D. E., Stahl, B., & Love, S. Q. (1985). Effects of television modeling on residential energy conservation. *Journal of Applied Behavior Analysis, 18,* 33–34.

Winett, R. A., & Neale, M. S. (1981). Flexitime and family time allocation: Use of a self-report log to assess the effects of a system change on individual behavior. *Journal of Applied Behavior Analysis, 14,* 39–46.

Winett, R. A., Neale, M. S., & Williams, K. R. (1982). The effects of flexible work schedules on urban families with young children: Quasi-experimental, ecological studies. *American Journal of Community Psychology, 10,* 49–54.

Winkelby, M. A. (1994). The future of community-based cardiovascular disease intervention studies. *American Journal of Public Health, 84,* 1369–1371.

Wright, S., & Cowen, E. L. (1987). The effects of peer teaching on students' perceptions of class environment, adjustment, and academic performance. *American Journal of Community Psychology, 13,* 417–431.

Yokley, J. M., & Glenwick, D. S. (1984). Increasing the immunization of preschool children: An evaluation of applied community interventions. *Journal of Applied Behavior Analysis, 17,* 313–325.

Index

ISBN 0-306-45321-5

90000